Surgery of the Knee

Surgery of the Knee

Edited by
John N. Insall, M.D.

Professor of Orthopedic Surgery
Cornell University Medical Center
Attending Orthopedic Surgeon
The Hospital for Special Surgery and
The New York Hospital
Chief of the Knee Service
The Hospital for Special Surgery
New York, New York
Honorary Consultant Surgeon
The London Hospital
London, England

With 23 Contributors

Churchill Livingstone
New York, Edinburgh, London, and Melbourne
1984

Copy Editor: Michael Kelley
Production Editor: Charlie Lebeda
Production Supervisor: Kerry A. O'Rourke
Compositor: Waldman Graphics, Inc.
Printer: The Murray Printing Co.
Binder: The Murray Printing Company

© **Churchill Livingstone Inc. 1984**

Distributed in the United Kingdom by Churchill Livingstone, Robert Stevenson House, 1-3 Baxter's Place, Leith Walk, Edinburgh EH1 3AF and by associated companies, branches and representatives throughout the world.

First published 1984

Printed in USA

ISBN 0-443-08087-9

7 6 5 4 3 2

Library of Congress Cataloging in Publication Data

Main entry under title:

Surgery of the knee.

  Bibliography: p.
  Includes index.
  1. Knee—Surgery.   I. Insall, John N.
[DNLM: 1. Knee—Surgery. WE 870 S961]
RD561.S87   1983   617'.582   83-15075
ISBN 0-443-08087-9

Contributors

Paul Aichroth, M.S., F.R.C.S.
Consultant Orthopedic Surgeon, Westminster Hospital, London, S.W.1, England; Westminster Children's Hospital and Queen Mary's Hospital, Roehampton, England

Paolo Aglietti, M.D.
Associate Professor of Orthopedic Surgery and Traumatology, University of Florence, Florence, Italy

Steven Paul Arnoczky, D.V.M., Diplomate, A.C.V.S.
Director, Laboratory of Comparative Orthopédics, Associate Research Scientist, The Hospital for Special Surgery; Associate Professor of Comparative Orthopedics in Surgery, Cornell University Medical College, New York, New York

Peter G. Bullough, M.D.
Chief of Orthopedic Pathology, The Hospital for Special Surgery; Professor of Pathology, Cornell University Medical College, New York, New York

Albert H. Burstein, Ph.D.
Director, Department of Biomechanics, Senior Scientist, Department of Research, The Hospital for Special Surgery; Professor of Applied Biomechanics in Surgery, Cornell University Medical College, New York, New York

John E. Carvell, M.B., Ch.B., M.M.Sc., F.R.C.S.
Consultant Orthopedic Surgeon, Odstock Hospital and Salisbury General Infirmary, Salisbury, England

Pierre Chambat, M.D.
Chef de Clinique dans le service de Chirurgie Orthopédique et Traumatologique du Centre Hospitalier, Lyon-Sud, Lyon, France

Charles L. Christian, M.D.
Physician-in-Chief, The Hospital for Special Surgery; Professor of Medicine, Cornell University Medical College, New York, New York

Henri DeJour, M.D.
Professeur de Clinique de Chirurgie Orthopédique et Traumatologique à l'Université Lyon I; Chef du Service d'Orthopédie et Traumatologie, Centre Hospitalier, Lyon-Sud, Lyon, France

Robert B. Duthie, M.A. (Oxon.), Ch.M. (Edinburgh), F.R.C.S. (Edinburgh and England) Hon. D.Sc. (U. of Rochester)
Nuffield Professor of Orthopedic Surgery, University of Oxford; Honorary Consultant, Nuffield Orthopedic Center, and Accident Department, John Radcliffe Hospital, Oxford, England

Robert L. Fisher, M.D.
Chief of Orthopedics, Hartford Hospital, Hartford, Connecticut; Attending Orthopedic Surgeon, Newington Children's Hospital, Newington, Connecticut; Assistant Clinical Professor, University of Connecticut Health Center, Farmington, Connecticut; Clinical Associate in Orthopedic Surgery, Yale Medical School, New Haven, Connecticut

M. A. R. Freeman, B.A., M.B., B.Ch., M.D., F.R.C.S.
Honorary Consultant Orthopedic Surgeon, The London Hospital, London, England

Robert H. Freiberger, M.D.
Director, Department of Radiology, The Hospital for Special Surgery, Professor of Radiology, Cornell University Medical Center; Attending Radiologist, The New York Hospital, New York, New York

Brian J. Hurson, M.Ch., F.R.C.S.(I)
Clinical Fellow in Orthopedic Oncology, Memorial Sloan-Kettering Cancer Center; Research Fellow, The Hospital for Special Surgery, New York, New York

John N. Insall, M.D.
Attending Orthopedic Surgeon, The Hospital for Special Surgery and The New York Hospital; Chief of The Knee Service, The Hospital for Special Surgery; Professor of Orthopedic Surgery, Cornell University Medical Center, New York, New York

Joseph M. Lane, M.D.
Chief, Metabolic Bone Disease Service, The Hospital for Special Surgery; Chief, Orthopedic Division, Memorial Sloan-Kettering Cancer Center; Professor of Orthopedic Surgery, Cornell University Medical Center; Attending Orthopedic Surgeon, The Hospital for Special Surgery and The New York Hospital, New York, New York

I. Martin Levy, M.D.
Assistant Attending Orthopedic Surgeon, Montefiore Medical Center and Albert Einstein College of Medicine; Instructor in Orthopedic Surgery, Albert Einstein College of Medicine, Bronx, New York

John B. McGinty, M.D.
Clinical Professor of Orthopedic Surgery, Tufts University School of Medicine, Boston, Massachusetts; Chief, Orthopedic Service, Newton Wellesley Hospital, Newton, Massachusetts

Jo Miller, M.D., F.R.C.S. (C)
Orthopedic Surgeon-in-Chief, The Montreal General Hospital; Professor and Chairman, Division of Orthopedic Surgery, McGill University, Montreal, Canada

Helene Pavlov, M.D.
Attending Radiologist, The Hospital for Special Surgery; Associate Attending Radiologist, The New York Hospital and Cornell University Medical College; Assistant Professor of Radiology, Cornell University Medical College, New York, New York

Clement B. Sledge, M.D.
Chairman, Department of Orthopedic Surgery, Brigham and Women's Hospital; John B. and Buckminster Brown Professor of Orthopedic Surgery, Harvard Medical School, Boston, Massachusetts

Frederick Vosburgh, M.D.
Senior Staff Fellow, Mineralized Tissue Research Branch, The National Institute of Dental Research, Bethesda, Maryland

Peter S. Walker, Ph.D.
Director, Orthopedic Biomechanics Laboratory, Brigham and Women's Hospital, Boston, Massachusetts; Director, Orthopedic Biomechanics Laboratory, VA Medical Center, West Roxbury, Massachusetts; Associate Professor of Orthopedic Surgery, Harvard Medical School, Boston, Massachusetts

Russell F. Warren, M.D.
Associate Attending Orthopedic Surgeon and Director of Sports Medicine Service, The Hospital for Special Surgery; Associate Professor of Orthopedic Surgery, Cornell University Medical Center, New York, New York

Foreword

This comprehensive work encompasses the advances that have been made over the past 15 years in the knowledge of knee joint biomechanics, the understanding of common pathologic processes affecting the knee whether due to injury or to other causes, surveys of newer diagnostic measures and methods, refinements of traditional treatment modalities, and the development of newer surgical methods such as total knee arthroplasty and arthroscopic surgery.

It brings together the expertise of many authorities in the field, but the main core of the material has been provided by scientists and physicians from The Hospital for Special Surgery. Balance, however, has been provided through the eight chapters written by authorities from other institutions, including four Europeans, one Canadian, and three Americans. Readers will find the chapters comprehensive and authoritative, yet not lacking in controversy where practice is not yet fully scientifically founded and differences of opinion still exist.

The work should become a must on the shelves of all orthopedic surgeons, and particularly for surgeons whose primary interest is surgery of the knee.

Dr. Insall, who is singularly suited by experience and research to have undertaken this task, is to be complimented for bringing together so much useful information in a field where there has been, and continues to be, such an explosion of scientific knowledge, technology, and technique.

Philip D. Wilson, Jr. M.D.
Surgeon-in-Chief
The Hospital for Special Surgery &
Professor of Surgery (Orthopedics)
Cornell University Medical College

Preface

If the 1960s saw a revolution in hip surgery, the knee had its turn during the 1970s. Much has changed and is still changing. Arthroscopic surgery has emerged as a new discipline; knee arthroplasty has become a reliable treatment for gonarthrosis; and concepts in the treatment of ligament injuries have altered radically in the last 10 years. Also, surgeons interested in the knee have separated into three groups, their major involvement being either in arthroscopy, sports medicine, or knee replacement. As one who has dabbled in all of these areas, it is my hope that this book will have some unifying benefit.

However, there is still no unanimity of opinion about how to treat all disorders of the knee joint, and for one who has the temerity to edit a textbook on the subject, there is the certain knowledge that he cannot please everyone. On the other hand, a textbook must have cohesion so that one chapter does not contradict the next. My solution to this dilemma is to present the current opinion and practice at The Hospital for Special Surgery, and, therefore, most of the contributors are past or present members of the staff. Where there are significant areas of controversy, I have also sought other viewpoints, notably on ligament surgery, the place of the cruciate ligaments in knee arthroplasty, and the fixation of prosthetic components to bone. I have also reached beyond the walls of my own hospital for additional expertise, and well-known authorities have written chapters on osteochondritis dissecans, hemophilia, surgical pathology of arthritis, and arthroscopy.

With regard to the chapter on arthroscopy, I foresee that this chapter may be considered too short in an era when arthroscopic surgery and knee surgery are becoming synonymous in the minds of many surgeons. This decision to keep this chapter short was made deliberately and for two reasons: (1) Excellent textbooks devoted specifically to the techniques of arthroscopic surgery already exist, and (2) both Doctor McGinty and I feel that, because arthroscopic surgery has not yet been placed in full perspective, some currently popular arthroscopic techniques may become discredited with time.

I also decided not to include specific details of AO surgical techniques in the fracture chapter as these are also very well described elsewhere.

It would not have been possible to complete this book without the invaluable assistance of my secretary, Mrs. Martha Moore, who has put in as much effort as I and must now know every word and every reference by heart. I also wish to thank Ms. Joelle Pacht for her endless retyping of the manuscript, Miss Dottie Page and the Photographic Department at The Hospital for Special Surgery for their assistance in preparing the photographic material, and Mr. William Thackeray who has done most of the book's illustrations and drawings.

John N. Insall, M.D.

Contents

Surgery of the Knee

1 Anatomy of the Knee

John N. Insall

The knee joint possesses very little inherent stability by virtue of its shape. It is also one of the most flexible joints in the body. For both reasons, proper function is unusually dependent on ligament integrity.

The description that follows is partly taken from standard anatomic texts.[2,3,14,21] The joint may be considered as having three distinct and partially separated compartments (Fig. 1.1). In the anterior or patellofemoral compartment, the patella articulates with the femoral groove or sulcus until about 90 degrees, after which the medial and lateral facets articulate separately with the corresponding femoral condyles. In extreme flexion, patellofemoral contact passes from the medial facet onto the odd facet of the patella.

The patella is described as possessing seven facets. Both medial and lateral facets are divided vertically into approximately equal thirds, while the seventh or odd facet lies along the extreme medial border of the patella. Overall, the medial facet is smaller and slightly convex and the lateral, which consists of roughly two-thirds of the bone, has a sagittal convexity and coronal concavity. The patella fits the patellar surface of the femur imperfectly. The femoral sulcus has medial and lateral lips of which the lateral is wider and higher and both of which have a sagittal convexity. The femoral groove is separated from the medial and lateral femoral condyles by an indistinct ridge more prominent laterally. The contact patch between the patella and femur varies with position as the patella sweeps across the femoral surface. The contact patch has been investigated by dye[8] and casting techniques.[1] Both methods give very similar results and indicate that the area of contact never exceeds about one-third the total patellar surface available, the most extensive contact being made at 45 degrees in which position it shows as an ellipse occupying the central medial, and lateral facets. In full extension, the lower medial and lateral patellar facets rest against the upper portion of the femoral groove. At 90 degrees the contact area has shifted to the upper medial and lateral patellar facets and with further flexion the contact patch separates into distinct medial and lateral areas. Because the odd facet only makes contact with the femur in extreme flexion (as in the act of squatting), this facet is habitually a noncontact zone in Western man, a fact that is thought to have some pathologic significance.

In shape and dimensions, the femoral condyles are asymmetric, with the larger medial condyle having a more symmetric curvature. The lateral condyle viewed from the side has a sharply increasing curvature posteriorly. The femoral condyles viewed from the surface articulating with the tibia show that the lateral

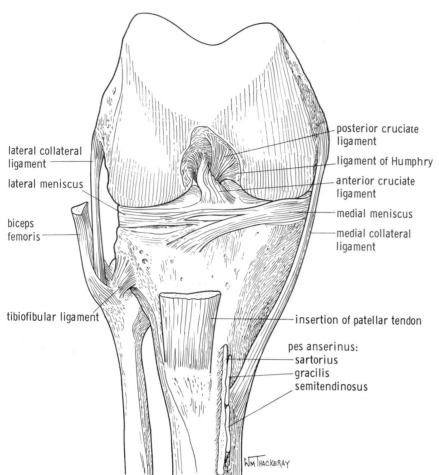

lateral collateral
ligament

lateral meniscus

biceps
femoris

tibiofibular ligament

posterior cruciate
ligament

ligament of Humphry

anterior cruciate
ligament

medial meniscus

medial collateral
ligament

insertion of patellar tendon

pes anserinus:
sartorius
gracilis
semitendinosus

WM THACKERAY

Fig. 1.1. Anterior view of a
partially dissected knee joint.

condyle is slightly shorter than the medial. The long
axis of the lateral condyle is slightly longer than the
long axis of the medial condyle and is placed in a more
sagittal plane, while the medial is placed at an angle
of about 22 degrees on average and opened posteriorly. The width of the lateral condyle is slightly
greater than that of the medial condyle at the center
of the intercondylar notch.

In the macerated skeletons, inspection of the tibial
plateaus would suggest that femoral and tibial surfaces do not conform at all. The larger medial tibial
plateau is nearly flat, whereas the lateral plateau is
actually concave. Both have a posterior inclination
with respect to the shaft of the tibia of approximately
10 degrees. This lack of conformity between the joint
surfaces is more apparent than real, however, because in the intact knee the menisci enlarge the contact area considerably and provide a degree of con-

formity between the joint surfaces that is not present
in their absence.

The median portion of the tibia between the plateau is occupied by an elevation—the spine of the
tibia. Anteriorly there is a depression, the anterior
intercondyloid fossa, to which from anterior to posterior are attached the anterior horn of the medial
meniscus, the anterior cruciate ligament, and the anterior horn of the lateral meniscus. Behind this region
are two elevations, the medial and lateral tubercles.
They are divided by a gutterlike depression, the in-
tertubercular sulcus. The ligaments and menisci are
not attached to the tubercles, which act by projecting
toward the inner sides of the femoral condyles as side-
to-side stabilizers. Taken with the menisci the tibial
spine enhances the impression of cupping seen in intact specimens. In the posterior intercondyloid fossa
behind the tubercles are attached first the medial and

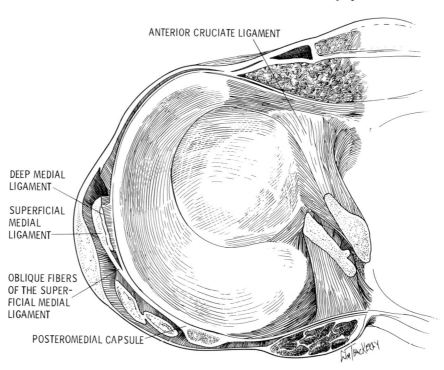

ANTERIOR CRUCIATE LIGAMENT

DEEP MEDIAL
LIGAMENT

SUPERFICIAL
MEDIAL
LIGAMENT

OBLIQUE FIBERS
OF THE SUPER-
FICIAL MEDIAL
LIGAMENT

POSTEROMEDIAL CAPSULE

Fig. 1.2. Superior view of the medial meniscus showing the order of attachments in the intercondylar notch. Also shown is the attachment of the medial meniscus to the medial collateral ligament and the arrangement of the three fascial layers on the medial aspect of the knee. (From Warren, L.F., and Marshall, J.L.: The supporting structures and layers on the medial side of the knee. An anatomical analysis. J. Bone Joint Surg. [Am.], *61*: 56, 1979, with permission.)

then the lateral menisci and behind them on the margin of the tibia between the condyles, the posterior cruciate ligament.

The menisci are two crescentic lamellae that serve to deepen the surfaces of the articular fossae of the head of the tibia for reception of the condyles of the femur. Each meniscus covers approximately the peripheral two-thirds of the corresponding articular surface of the tibia. The peripheral border of each meniscus is thick, convex, and attached to the capsule of the joint; the opposite border tapers to a thin, free edge. The proximal surfaces of the menisci are concave and in contact with the condyles of the femur; their distal surfaces are flat and rest on the head of the tibia.

The medial meniscus is nearly semicircular in form and about 3.5 cm in length. It has a triangular cross-section and is considerably wider posteriorly than it is anteriorly. It is firmly attached to the posterior intercondylar fossa of the tibia (Fig. 1.2). The anterior attachment is more variable; it is usually firmly attached to the anterior intercondylar fossa, but this attachment can be quite flimsy, within the realm of normal variation. There is also a fibrous band of variable thickness and identity that connects the anterior horn of the medial meniscus with the lateral meniscus

(the transverse ligament). Peripherally, the medial meniscus is attached to the capsule of the knee to both tibia and femur. The tibial attachment is sometimes known as the coronary ligament. At its midpoint it is more firmly attached to the femur and the tibia via a condensation in the capsule known as the deep medial ligament.

The coronary ligament attaches to the tibial margin a few millimeters distal to the articular surface, giving rise to a synovial recess. Posteromedially, according to Kaplan,[10] the meniscus receives a portion of the insertion of the semimembranosus via the capsule.

The lateral meniscus is nearly circular and covers a larger portion of the articular surface than the medial meniscus. Its anterior horn is attached to the intercondylar fossa, lateral and posterior to the anterior cruciate ligament. The posterior horn is attached to the intercondylar fossa anterior to the posterior end of the medial meniscus. Its posterior attachment, consisting of somewhat variable fibrous bands, connect the posterior arc of the lateral meniscus to the medial condyle of the femur in the intercondylar fossa, embracing the posterior cruciate ligament. These are known as the ligaments of Humphry and Wrisberg (Fig. 1.3). Posterolaterally, the meniscus is grooved by the tendon of popliteus, some fibers

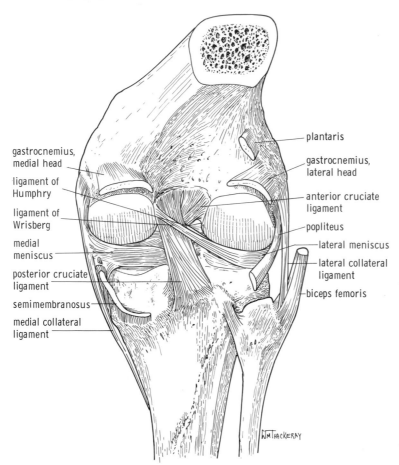

gastrocnemius,
medial head

ligament of
Humphry

ligament of
Wrisberg

medial
meniscus

posterior cruciate
ligament

semimembranosus

medial collateral
ligament

plantaris

gastrocnemius,
lateral head

anterior cruciate
ligament

popliteus

lateral meniscus

lateral collateral
ligament

biceps femoris

Fig. 1.3. Drawing of partially dissected specimen showing the posterior aspect of the knee. The ligaments of Humphry and Wrisberg attach the posterior horn of the lateral meniscus to the medial femoral condyle embracing the posterior cruciate ligament. The popliteus tendon partially inserts into the posterolateral aspect of the lateral meniscus. Similarly there is a partial insertion of the semimembranosus into the posteromedial aspect of the medial meniscus.

of which are inserted into the periphery and superior border of the meniscus.[12]

The patellar ligament is the central portion of the common tendon of the quadriceps femoris, which is continued from the patella to the tuberosity of the tibia. It is a strong, flat, ligamentous band about 6 cm in length attached proximally to the apex and adjoining margins of the patella and the rough depression on its posterior surface, and distally to the tuberosity of the tibia; superficial fibers are continuous over the front of the patella with those of the tendon of the quadriceps femoris. Medial and lateral portions of the quadriceps tendon pass down on either side of the patella to be inserted into the proximal extremity of the tibia on either side of the tuberosity. These portions merge into the capsule forming the medial and lateral patellar retinacula. The posterior surface of the ligamentum patellae is separated from the synovial membrane of the joint by a large infrapatellar pad of fat and from the tibia by a bursa.

LIGAMENTS OF THE KNEE

The articular capsule is a fibrous membrane of variable thickness containing areas of thickening that may be referred to as discrete ligaments. Anteriorly the capsule is replaced by the patellar ligament. Posteriorly the capsule consists of vertical fibers that arise from the condyles and from the sides of the intercondylar fossa of the femur. It is augmented by fibers derived from the tendon of the semimembranosus, forming the oblique popliteal ligament, a broad, flat band attached proximally to the margin of the intercondylar fossa and posterior surface of the femur, close to the articular margins of the condyles, and distally to the posterior margin of the head of the tibia. The fibers pass mainly downward and medially, and the fasciculae are separated by apertures for the passage of vessels and nerves. The oblique popliteal ligament forms part of the floor of the popliteal fossa and the popliteal artery rests on it.

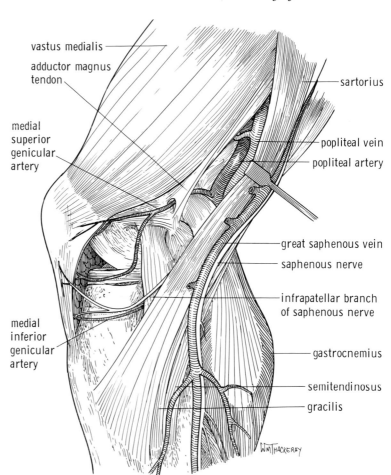

vastus medialis

adductor magnus tendon

medial superior genicular artery

sartorius

popliteal vein

popliteal artery

great saphenous vein

saphenous nerve

infrapatellar branch of saphenous nerve

medial inferior genicular artery

gastrocnemius

semitendinosus

gracilis

WM THACKERAY

Fig. 1.4. Layer 1 of the fascial layers on the medial side of the knee is defined by the sartorius tendon. In this specimen the fascia anterior to the tendon has been partially excised. The saphenous nerve and its infrapatellar branch and the saphenous vein lie superficial to this layer.

On the medial side of the knee the supporting structures can be divided into three layers, according to Warren and Marshall.[19] Layer 1 (Fig. 1.4) is the most superficial, being the first fascial plane encountered after a skin incision is made on the medial side of the knee. This layer is the deep fascia, and its plane is defined by the fascia that invests the sartorius muscle. The sartorius inserts into this network of fascial fibers and does not have a distinct tendon of insertion as do the underlying gracilis and semitendinosus muscles. Proceeding posteriorly, layer 1 is a sheet that overlies the two heads of the gastrocnemius and the structures of the popliteal fossa. This layer serves as a support for the muscle bellies and the neurovascular structures in the popliteal region. Layer 1 can always be separated from the underlying parallel and oblique portions of the superficial medial ligament, and if a vertical incision is made posterior to the parallel fibers of the ligament, the anterior portion of layer 1 can be reflected forward, exposing the entire superficial medial ligament. Further anteriorly, layer 1 blends with the anterior part of layer 2 and the medial patellar retinaculum derived from vastus medialis. Posteriorly there is a layer of fatty tissue that lies between layer 1 and the deeper structures. The tendons of gracilis and semitendinosus lie in this region. Anteriorly and distally layer 1 joins the periosteum of the tibia.

Layer 2 is the plane of the superficial medial ligament (Fig. 1.5). The superficial medial ligament, as described by Brantigan and Voshell,[5] consists of parallel and oblique portions. The anterior or parallel fibers arise from the medial epicondyle of the femur and consist of heavy and vertically oriented fibers running distally to an insertion on the medial surface of the tibia on an average of 4.6 cm inferior to the tibial articular surface, immediately posterior to the insertion of the pes anserinus. The posterior oblique

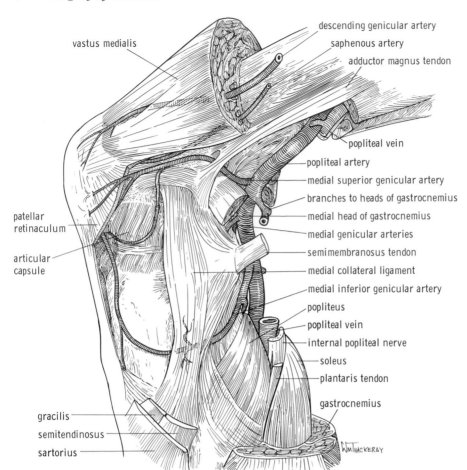

vastus medialis

descending genicular artery

saphenous artery

adductor magnus tendon

popliteal vein

popliteal artery

medial superior genicular artery

branches to heads of gastrocnemius

medial head of gastrocnemius

medial genicular arteries

semimembranosus tendon

medial collateral ligament

medial inferior genicular artery

popliteus

popliteal vein

internal popliteal nerve

soleus

plantaris tendon

gastrocnemius

patellar retinaculum

articular capsule

gracilis

semitendinosus

sartorius

W.M. THACKERAY

Fig. 1.5 Layer 2 is the superficial medial ligament consisting of parallel and oblique portions. Posteriorly this layer blends with layer 3.

fibers run from the femoral epicondyle and blend with the underlying layer 3 (capsule), and are thus attached immediately inferior to the posterior tibial articular surface and to the medial meniscus. The fibers are augmented by contributions from the semimembranosus tendon sheath.

Anteriorly, according to Warren and Marshall,[19] layer 2 splits vertically. The fibers anterior to the split proceed cephalad to the vastus medialis and join the plane of layer 1 forming the parapatellar retinaculum fibers. The fibers posterior to the split run cephalad to the femoral condyle from which transverse fibers run forward in the plane of layer 2 to the patella forming the patellofemoral ligament. The patellofemoral ligament, which is a continuation of layer 2, thus lies deep to the plane of layer 1.

Layer 3, the capsule of the knee joint, (Fig. 1.6) can be separated from layer 2, except toward the margin of the patella; anteriorly the capsule is very thin.

Beneath the superficial medial ligament, layer 3 becomes thicker and forms a vertically oriented band of short fibers known as the deep medial ligament. The deep ligament extends from the femur to the midportion of the peripheral margin of the meniscus and tibia. Anteriorly the deep ligament is clearly separated from the superficial ligament, with a bursa interposed, but posteriorly the layers blend as the meniscal-femoral portion of the deep ligament tends to merge with the overlying superficial ligament near its cephalad attachment. The meniscotibial portion, however, is readily separated from the overlying superficial ligament. Further posteriorly, layer 3 merges with layer 2 to form a conjoined posteromedial capsule that envelopes the medial condyle of the femur.

Thus the three layers are most obviously separated in the region of the superficial medial ligament. Posteriorly the deep and middle layers blend and the superficial layer becomes the deep fascia. Anteriorly,

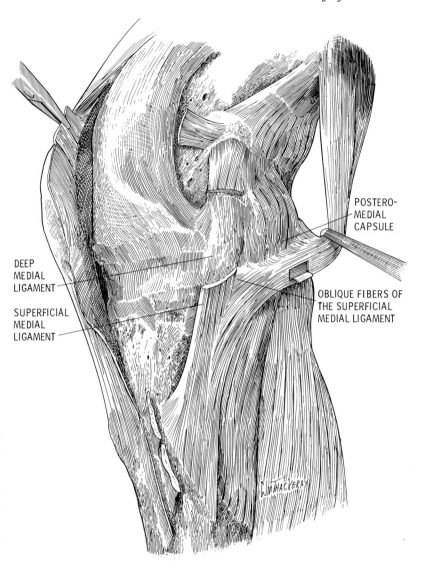

DEEP
MEDIAL
LIGAMENT

SUPERFICIAL
MEDIAL
LIGAMENT

POSTERO-
MEDIAL
CAPSULE

OBLIQUE FIBERS OF
THE SUPERFICIAL
MEDIAL LIGAMENT

Fig. 1.6. Layer 3 is the capsule of the knee joint very thin anteriorly but posteriorly blending with layer 2 to form the posteromedial capsule. There is partial blending of the layers 2 and 3 beneath the superficial medial ligament that still remains distinct anteriorly (see also Fig. 1.2). (From Warren, L.F., and Marshall, J.L.: The supporting structures and layers on the medial side of the knee. An anatomical analysis. J. Bone Joint Surg [Am.], *61:* 56, 1979, with permission.)

the superficial and middle layers blend and merge with the overlying retinacular expansion from the quadriceps. The deep layer, although it remains separate, becomes extremely thin. The middle layer splits anterior to the superficial medial ligament, so that the cephalad portion persists as a separate layer forming the patellofemoral ligament.

The supporting structures on the lateral side of the knee may also be described as consisting of three layers. Most superficial is the lateral knee retinaculum, the middle layer is made up of the lateral collateral ligament, the fabellofibular ligament and the arcuate ligament, and the deep layer is the lateral capsule.

The lateral knee retinaculum (Fig. 1.7) has been described by Fulkerson and Gossling.[6] Starting at the lateral border of the patella, the fibrous expansion of the vastus lateralis is oriented longitudinally along the lateral patellar border proceeding distally to become part of the patellar tendon. Interdigitating with these fibers is the superficial oblique retinaculum, originating in the iliotibial band. Most of these fibers merge into the anterior part of the patellar tendon. Posteriorly lie the fascia lata and iliotibial band, running longitudinally along the lateral side of the knee and inserting into Gerdy's tubercle on the tibia. Some of the fibers proceed across Gerdy's tubercle to the tibial tuberosity. Proximally the fascia lata is adherent to the lateral intramuscular septum, whereby it is at-

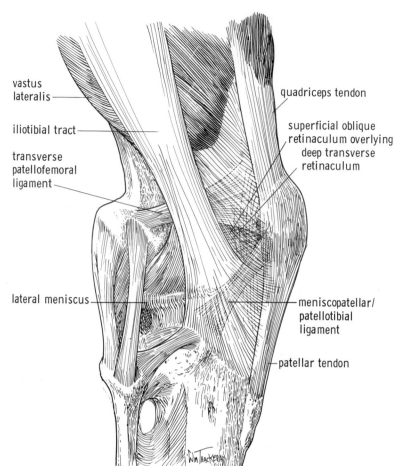

vastus
lateralis

iliotibial tract

transverse
patellofemoral
ligament

lateral meniscus

quadriceps tendon

superficial oblique
retinaculum overlying
deep transverse
retinaculum

meniscopatellar/
patellotibial
ligament

patellar tendon

Fig. 1.7. Structures of the lateral retinaculum (see text).

tached to the femur. Posteriorly the fascia lata merges into the biceps fascia. There is a distinct deeper portion to this layer running more or less transversely from the fascia lata to the lateral patella and caudally running more obliquely to connect the patella with the upper tibia. Cephalad a band of fibers can be found running from the lateral intramuscular septum and lateral epicondyle to the lateral patella (the epicondylopatellar ligament described by Kaplan).[11]

The lateral collateral ligament originates in the lateral epicondyle of the femur anterior to the origin of gastrocnemius, forming a cordlike structure that runs beneath the lateral retinaculum to insert into the head of the fibula, blending with the tendon of insertion of biceps femoris. The fabellofibular ligament[9] is a condensation of fibers lying between the lateral and arcuate ligaments, running from the lateral head of gastrocnemius to the fibular styloid. In most knees both

the fabellofibular and arcuate ligaments are present, but in the case of a large fabella, there may be no arcuate ligament, and in the absence of a fabella, the fabellofibular ligament is absent as well.[18]

The arcuate ligament has been variously described; according to Last, "In truth there is at this part of the capsule such a complexity of fibers running in many directions that by artful dissection almost any pattern desired by the dissector could be made."[13] Some fibers extend from the lateral condyle of the femur to the posterior part of the capsule. The strongest and most consistent fibers of the arcuate ligament, however, form a triangular sheet that diverges upward from the fibular styloid. The lateral limb of this mass is dense and strong and is attached to the femur and the popliteus tendon; while the weaker medial limb curves over the popliteus muscle, is attached to the posterior arc of the lateral meniscus, and from that point, passes upward, to be lost on the posterior part of the capsule. The free edge of this medial limb is crescentic; beneath it, the lateral or femoral part of the popliteus emerges to approach its tibial attachment. The lateral capsule is a thin, weak layer that blends posteriorly with the arcuate ligament and posterior capsule; anteriorly it forms the weak, lax coronary ligament aligned with the synovial membrane, attaching the inferior border of the lateral meniscus to the edge of the articular surface of the tibia.

The popliteus muscle arises by a strong tendon about 2.5 cm long from a depression at the anterior part of the groove on the lateral condyle of the femur. The tendon, which is invested in synovial membrane, passes beneath the medial limb of the arcuate ligament and forms a thin, flat, triangular muscle that inserts into the medial two-thirds of the triangular surface proximal to the popliteal line on the posterior surface of the tibia. The tendon is attached to the arcuate ligament; according to Last, up to one-half its fibers are attached to the lateral meniscus.[13] The synovial membrane below the meniscus herniates deep to the muscle as the popliteus bursa.

CRUCIATE LIGAMENTS

The anatomy of the cruciate ligaments has been studied by Girgis et al (Figs. 1.8 and 1.9).[7]

The anterior cruciate ligament is attached to the femur at the posterior part of the medial surface of the lateral femoral condyle in the form of a segment of a circle. The anterior side is almost straight and the posterior side convex. The attachment is in an oblique direction. The average length of the ligament is 38 mm and the average width 11 mm. About 10 mm below the femoral attachment the ligament stands out as it proceeds distally to the tibial attachment, which is to a wide depressed area in front of and lateral to the anterior tibial spine. There is a well-marked slip to the anterior horn of the lateral meniscus.

The posterior cruciate ligament is attached to the posterior part of the lateral surface of the medial condyle of the femur and, like the anterior cruciate, this attachment is in the form of a segment of a circle. It is horizontal in its general direction. The upper boundary of the attachment is straight and the lower boundary convex. The posterior cruciate has an average length of 38 mm and an average width of 13 mm and is narrowest in its middle portion, fanning out to a greater extent superiorly than it does inferiorly. The fibers are attached to the tibia in a lateromedial direction, while in the femur they are in an anteroposterior direction. The tibial attachment is to a depression behind the intraarticular upper surface of the tibia. The attachment extends for a few millimeters onto the adjoining posterior surface of the tibia; shortly above its tibial attachment, the posterior cruciate sends a slip to blend with the posterior horn of the lateral meniscus. The ligaments of Humphry and Wrisberg have never been observed together and are sometimes absent.

The nature of the superior attachment of the cruciate ligaments results in the bands being twisted around their longitudinal axes upon flexion. They are twisted in opposite directions, since they are attached to opposing surfaces. From the front, the direction of the torsion will appear to be toward the center of the joint.

MOTION OF THE NORMAL KNEE JOINT AND FUNCTION OF THE LIGAMENTS

The motion of the joint is controlled both by the bony architecture and by the ligamentous attachments.[4] In a completely extended knee joint, both collateral and cruciate ligaments are taut and the anterior aspects of both menisci are snugly held between the condyles of the tibia and the femur. At the beginning of flexion the knee "unlocks," and there is a medial rotation of the tibia on the femur which, according to Last, is brought about by contraction of the popliteus muscle.[13] The articular surface of the medial femoral condyle is larger than that of the lateral femoral condyle; when the direction of motion is reversed, the lateral compartment reaches a position of full extension first and before the medial compartment is fully extended. Terminal extension is achieved and the knee is "locked" by the tibia rotating externally until the medial compartment also reaches the limits of extension.

As the knee is flexed, there is initially during the first 30 degrees a rollback of the femur on the tibia that is more pronounced laterally than medially. After 30 degrees the femoral condyles spin at one point on

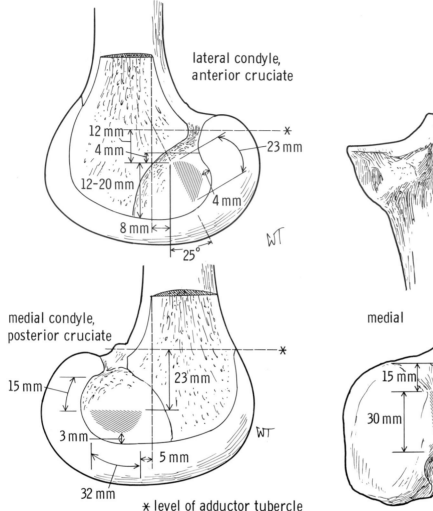

Fig. 1.8. Attachments of the anterior and posterior cruciate ligaments to the femur. (From Girgis, F.G., Marshall, J.L., and Al Monajem, A.R.S.: The cruciate ligaments of the knee joint. Clin. Orthop., *106*: 216, 1975, with permission.)

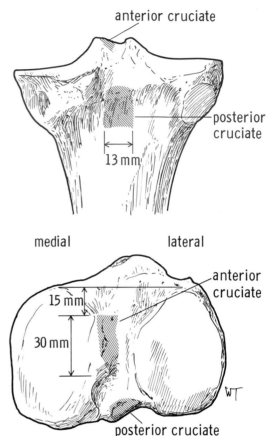

Fig. 1.9 The attachments of the anterior and posterior cruciate ligaments to the tibia. (From Girgis, F.G., Marshall, J.L. and Al Monajem, A.R.S.: The cruciate ligaments of the knee joint. Clin. Orthop., *106*: 216, 1975, with permission.)

the tibial condyles.[16] The menisci, which are squeezed between the joint surfaces in extension, move backward with the femur in flexion—the lateral more so than the medial.

The tibia rotates on the femur more in the lateral than in the medial direction, and the center of rotation is through the medial femoral condyle. Some portion of the superficial medial ligament remains taut throughout flexion, whereas the lateral collateral ligament is taut only in extension and relaxes as soon as the knee is flexed, thereby permitting a greater excursion of the lateral tibial condyle.

The superficial medial collateral ligament is the most important medial stabilizer.[20] The parallel fibers move in a posterior direction as the knee is flexed. The attachments to the femoral condyle are such that with the knee in extension the posterior fibers are taut and the anterior fibers relax and are drawn in under the posterior part of the ligament (Fig. 1.10). With flexion of the knee the anterior fibers move proximally and become tight and are subjected to increasing tension as the joint is flexed (Fig. 1.11). This action, according to Palmer,[16] is attributable to the oval shape of the femoral origin, which changes its orientation in flex-

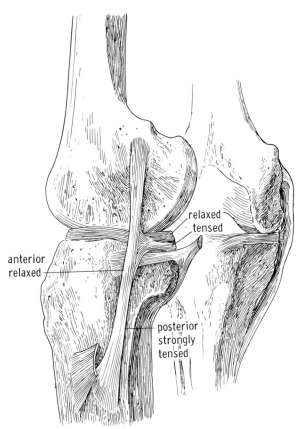

Fig. 1.10. In extension, the posterior margin of the medial collateral ligament is tense and the anterior border relatively relaxed. Proximal anterior fibers are drawn underneath the posterior fibers.

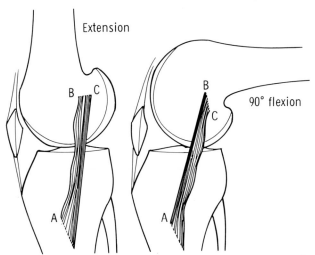

Fig. 1.11. Diagram of the superficial medial ligament with flexion and extension of the knee. Because point B moves superiorly, the anterior border is tightened in flexion. Conversely, in extension point C moves proximally, tightening the posterior margin of the ligament. (From Warren, L.F., Marshall, J.L., and Girgis, F.G.: The prime static stabilizer of the medial side of the knee. J. Bone Joint Surg. [Am.], 56: 665, 1974, with permission.)

ion such that the attachments of the most anterior fibers are elevated. As the anterior border becomes tight, the posterior fibers slacken as the knee flexes and remain relaxed throughout flexion. The posterior oblique fibers are relaxed in extension and lie partially beneath the parallel fibers. In flexion the fibers are drawn out (Fig. 1.12); according to Palmer, because of their attachment to the capsule and periphery of the medial meniscus, they check the backward sliding of the meniscus that occurs in flexion.

In the presence of intact parallel fibers, there is approximately 1 mm of medial opening to valgus stress. The joint is slightly tighter in full extension; the greatest degree of medial opening occurs at 45 degrees. The long fibers of the superficial medial ligament also control rotation and sectioning the capsule, deep medial ligament, and the oblique fibers of the superficial medial ligament cause little or no increase in rotation.

Sectioning the long fibers, on the other hand, not only increases the amount of medial opening to valgus stress, but causes a significant increase in external rotation as well.[20]

Lateral stability is provided by several structures. In extension the fibers of the iliotibial band are probably the most important and, because these fibers attach proximally to the femur, they may be regarded as a true ligament. It is probable that contraction of tensor fascia lata and gluteus maximus is not transmitted to the tibia. Kaplan[11] states that this is proved by electrical stimulation of the tensor fascia lata and by traction on the iliotibial tract in experiments on cadavers. As the knee flexes, the iliotibial tract moves posteriorly and becomes somewhat relaxed; in this position the tendon of biceps femoris may become an important stabilizer.[15]

The lateral ligament is also taut in extension but is

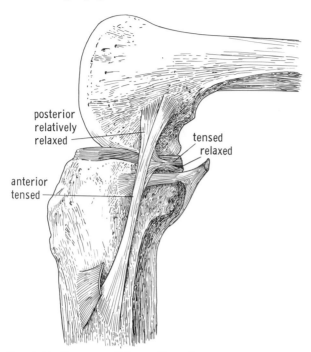

posterior
relatively
relaxed

tensed
relaxed

anterior
tensed

Fig. 1.12. Posterior oblique fibers become more tense in flexion. (From Palmer, I.: On the injuries to the ligaments of the knee joint. A clinical study. Acta Chir. Scand. Suppl., 53: 1938, with permission.)

relaxed throughout flexion. This is also true of the arcuate ligament. Thus in flexion a much greater degree of rotation is possible laterally than medially. This rotation is permitted by the attachments of the lateral meniscus and by relaxation of the supporting ligaments in flexion. There is also a greater degree of rolling of the femur on the tibia, whereas medially this motion is only slight. The attachment of the popliteus tendon to the lateral meniscus, according to Last,[13] draws the meniscus posteriorly and prevents entrapment as the knee is flexed.

The anterior cruciate ligament consists of two parts—an anteromedial band and a stronger, thicker posterolateral part. In extension the ligament appears as a flat band and the posterolateral bulk of the ligament is taut (Fig. 1.13). Almost immediately after flexion begins, the smaller anteromedial band becomes tight and the bulk of the ligament slackens. In flexion it is the anteromedial band that provides the primary restraint against anterior displacement of the tibia.

The posterior cruciate ligament consists of two in-

separable parts. An anterior portion forms the bulk of the ligament and a smaller posterior part runs obliquely to the back of the tibia. In extension the bulk of the ligament is relaxed and only the posterior band is tight. In flexion the major portion of the ligament becomes tight and the small posterior band is loose (Fig. 1.14).

The anterior cruciate ligament is a check against both hyperextension and internal and external rotation. The posterior cruciate ligament is a check against posterior instability in the flexed knee, but not against hyperextension, provided that the anterior cruciate is intact.

According to Palmer,[16] the tightening of the anterior cruciate in extension fixes the lateral femoral condyle anteriorly; thus a continuation of the movement into hyperextension is only possible where there is a simultaneous inward rotation of the femur, that is, a supination movement in the joint. This so-called *compulsory final rotation* is caused by the tensing of the anterior band.

Rotation takes place around an axis through the center of the medial femoral condyle, arising from the tighter anchorage of this condyle by the superficial medial ligament. If this ligament is ruptured, the axis shifts laterally.

According to Palmer,[16] because of the medially shifted axis of rotation, external rotation of the tibia relaxes the anterior cruciate ligament through the traveling forward of the lateral femoral condyle, at the same time stretching the posterior cruciate. Internal rotation reverses this sequence, tensing the anterior cruciate and relaxing the posterior cruciate.

A fibrous band connects the posterior cruciate with the posterior margin of the lateral meniscus (the tibiomeniscal ligament of Kaplan). This probably restricts the forward sliding motion of the lateral meniscus in internal rotation.

According to Girgis and associates,[7] rotary movements of the tibia on the femur occur in all ranges of motion. Their studies indicate that the anterior cruciate is a check against external rotation in flexion but does not significantly limit internal rotation. In extension the anterior cruciate ligament is a check against external rotation and to a lesser degree against internal rotation. There is therefore some disagreement as to the precise function of the cruciate ligaments in regard to rotation.

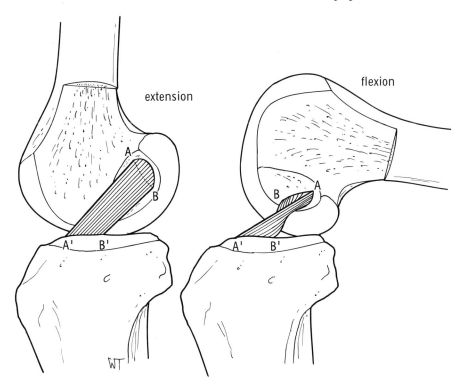

Fig. 1.13. Diagram of the anterior cruciate ligament in extension and flexion. Note that in extension the posterolateral bulk is taut, whereas in flexion the anteromedial band is tight and the posterolateral bulk relatively relaxed. (From Girgis, F.G., Marshall, J.L., and Al Monajem, A.R.S.: The cruciate ligaments of the knee joint. Clin. Orthop., *106*: 216, 1975, with permission.)

SYNOVIAL CAVITY

The synovium invests the knee and extends superiorly into the suprapatellar pouch for three fingerbreadths above the patella. The suprapatellar pouch is separated from the anterior femur by a layer of fat, and the upper most limit of the pouch has attached to it a small muscle, the articularis genus, which originates from the anterior surface of the femoral shaft. The articularis genus serves to prevent invagination of the suprapatellar pouch beneath the patella.

The synovium invests the cruciate ligaments and the popliteus tendon. A synovial recess or sleeve extends around the popliteus tendon for a variable distance beyond the posterolateral capsule. The synovium also lines the coronal recesses beneath the menisci and anteriorly invests the fat pad. The ligamentum mucosum forms an incomplete septum between the anterior intercondylar notch of the femur and the fat pad. It is more developed in some animals. Reduplication or synovial folds occur quite frequently, particularly in the suprapatellar pouch.

The posterior synovial cavity communicates in about 50 percent of persons with a popliteal bursa lying between the semimembranosus tendon and the medial head of gastrocnemius.[22] Thus, the popliteal bursa often becomes filled when dye is injected into the knee; the bursa can become enlarged causing a popliteal cyst when there is a chronic synovitis. With this exception, the synovial cavity does not normally communicate with any other of the numerous bursae around the knee. Of these bursae, three have clinical significance. The prepatellar bursa is large and lies subcutaneously anterior to the patella. The infrapatellar bursa lies beneath the patellar ligament, separating the ligament from the tibia and lower portion of the fat pad. The pes anserinus bursa lies between the tendons of sartorius, gracilis, and semitendinosus and the tibia. Another bursa separates the superficial medial ligament from the same tendons.

The fat pad lies beneath the patellar ligament, filling the space between the femoral condyles and the ligamentum patellae and adjusting its shape as the size of this potential cavity varies with movement. It is covered within by synovium and is pierced by nu-

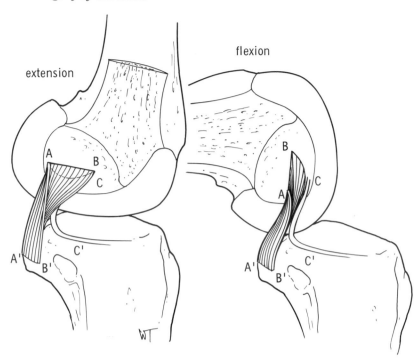

extension

flexion

Fig. 1.14. Posterior cruciate ligament: in flexion the bulk of the ligament becomes tight whereas in extension it is relaxed. (From Girgis, F.G., Marshall, J.L., and Al Mona-jem, A.R.S.: The cruciate ligaments of the knee joint. Clin. Orthop., *106*: 216, 1975, with permission.)

merous blood vessels derived from the genicular arteries.

ARTERIES AND VEINS

The popliteal artery (Fig. 1.15) leaves Hunter's canal and enters the popliteal fossa at the junction of the middle and lower thirds of the femur, passing through an aperture in adductor magnus. Before leaving the subsartorial canal, the descending genicular artery is given off. This vessel in turn gives off the superficial branch that accompanies the saphenous nerve and an articular branch. The femoral artery enters the popliteal fossa and runs vertically downward, separated above from the femur by a thick pad of fat, but at the back of the knee in direct contact with the oblique posterior ligament. Distally, the artery runs superficial to the popliteus fascia and ends at the lower border of the popliteus by dividing into the anterior and posterior tibial arteries. The artery gives off numerous muscular branches and five articular branches. The middle genicular artery arises from the anterior aspect and pierces the posterior oblique ligament to supply the intracapsular structures and cruciate ligaments. Medial and lateral superior genicular arteries

wind around the lower end of the femur immediately proximal to the condyles. The lateral inferior genicular artery lies immediately adjacent to the lateral joint line and is thus frequently injured in the course of open lateral meniscectomy. The inferior medial genicular artery passes two fingerbreadths distal to the medial joint line.

The anastomosis around the knee is formed by the five genicular arteries, the articular branch of the descending genicular artery, descending branch of the lateral circumflex femoral artery, and recurrent branches of the anterior tibial artery, which form an arterial network. The anastomosis thus connects the femoral artery at the origin of its profundus branch with the popliteal and anterior tibial arteries (Fig. 1.16). Anteriorly, an anastomosis forms a vascular circle around the patella from which, according to Scapinelli (Fig. 1.17), nine to 12 nutrient arteries arise at the lower pole of the patella, running upward on the anterior surface of the bone in a series of furrows.[17] The popliteal vein enters the popliteal fossa on the lateral side of the artery; it crosses superficial to the artery and lies on the medial side in the lower part of the space. Throughout it is interposed between the artery and the medial popliteal nerve.

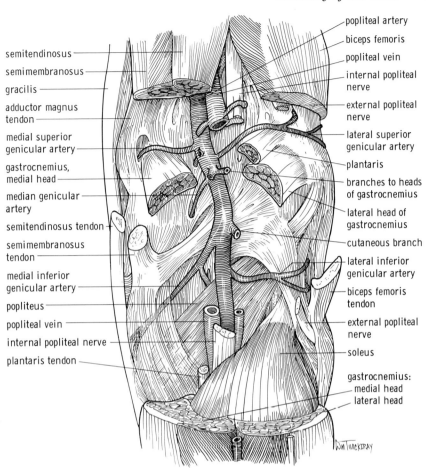

semitendinosus

semimembranosus

gracilis

adductor magnus tendon

medial superior genicular artery

gastrocnemius, medial head

median genicular artery

semitendinosus tendon

semimembranosus tendon

medial inferior genicular artery

popliteus

popliteal vein

internal popliteal nerve

plantaris tendon

popliteal artery

biceps femoris

popliteal vein

internal popliteal nerve

external popliteal nerve

lateral superior genicular artery

plantaris

branches to heads of gastrocnemius

lateral head of gastrocnemius

cutaneous branch

lateral inferior genicular artery

biceps femoris tendon

external popliteal nerve

soleus

gastrocnemius: medial head lateral head

Fig. 1.15. Branches of the popliteal artery in the popliteal space. The artery lies on the oblique posterior ligament at the back of the knee, although superiorly it is separated by a layer of fat. The femoral vein is interposed between the artery and the medial popliteal nerve throughout.

NERVES

The medial popliteal nerve arises from the sciatic nerve halfway down the thigh (Fig. 1.18). It runs downward through the popliteal fossa, lying at first in the fat beneath the deep fascia. Distally, it is placed more deeply in the interval between the two heads of the gastrocnemius. The artery crosses the popliteal vessels from lateral to medial, with the popliteal vein intervening between the nerve and the artery. A cutaneous branch, the sural nerve, descends on the surface of gastrocnemius. Muscular branches are given to both heads of gastrocnemius, plantaris, soleus, and popliteus muscles. There are several articular branches. The lateral popliteal nerve enters the popliteal fossa on the lateral side of the medial popliteal nerve and runs distally at the medial side of the biceps tendon. The lateral popliteal nerve passes between the tendon and the lateral head of the gastrocnemius, running downward behind the head of the fibula and winding around the lateral aspect of the neck of the fibula, piercing the peroneus longus through a fibrous tunnel and dividing into the musculocutaneous and anterior tibial nerves. Cutaneous branches are the sural communicating nerve, which joins the sural nerve and gives a small branch to the skin over the upper anterolateral aspect of the leg. There are also three articular branches. The patellar plexus lies in front of the patella and ligamentum patellae. It is formed by the numerous communications between the terminal branches of the lateral, intermediate, and medial cutaneous nerves of the thigh and the infrapatellar branch of the saphenous nerve. The saphenous nerve arises from the posterior division of the femoral nerve. At the lower end of the subsartorial canal, the nerve pierces deep fascia on the medial side of the knee between the sartorius and gracilis tendons. The infrapatellar branch pierces the sartorius muscle and joins the patellar plexus. The saphenous nerve is joined

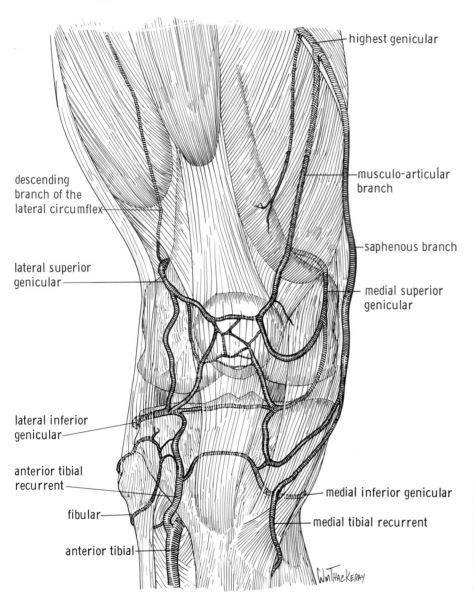

highest genicular

musculo-articular branch

descending branch of the lateral circumflex

saphenous branch

lateral superior genicular

medial superior genicular

lateral inferior genicular

anterior tibial recurrent

fibular

anterior tibial

medial inferior genicular

medial tibial recurrent

WmThackeray

Fig. 1.16 Anastomosis at the front of the knee formed by genicular branches from the popliteal artery and descending branches, which connect the femoral artery proximally with the popliteal and anterior tibial arteries distally.

by the long saphenous vein and runs distally to the medial aspect of the leg.

MUSCULAR ATTACHMENTS

The quadriceps muscle consists of four distinct parts that share a common tendon of insertion (Fig. 1.19). The rectus femoris arises from two heads on the ilium that unite and form a muscular belly that runs down the front of the thigh. Vastus lateralis arises from a broad linear strip, beginning at the upper end of the trochanteric line and extending halfway down the linea aspera. It also arises from the lateral intermuscular septum. From the lower margin of the vastus lateralis, a fibrous expansion is given to the lateral patellar retinaculum through which there is a direct attachment to the tibia. The vastus medialis originates in the lower part of the trochanteric line and follows the spiral line to the medial lip of the linea aspera. The lowest fibers of the muscle arise from the tendon of the adductor magnus and pass almost horizontally forward to the insertion into the common tendon and the medial border of the patella. This part of the mus-

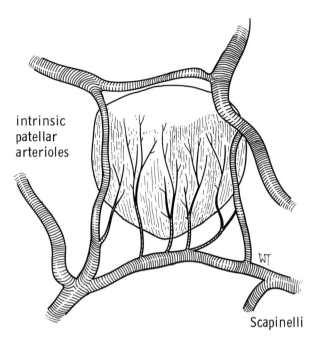

intrinsic
patellar
arterioles

Scapinelli

Fig. 1.17. Vascular circle around the patella, which according to Scapinelli supplies the patella by nutrient arteries that enter predominantly at the inferior pole. The genicular arteries and their branches lie in the most superficial layer of the deep fascia.

cle is sometimes described as the vastus medialis obliquus. Like the vastus lateralis, the vastus medialis gives a fibrous expansion to the medial patellar retinaculum. The vastus intermedius arises from the anterior and lateral aspects of the shaft of the femur; medially it partly blends with the vastus medialis. The quadriceps tendon is trilaminar, the anterior layer being formed by the rectus femoris, the intermediate layer by the vastus medialis and lateralis, and the deep layer by the tendon of vastus intermedius. The tendon inserts into the patella with an expansion that passes longitudinally anterior to the patella. In addition, extensions from the medial and lateral vasti insert directly into the tibia via the patellar retinaculum. The ligamentum patellae runs from the lower border of the patella to the tubercle of the tibia. Because there is an inclination to the shaft of the femur, the quadriceps muscle does not pull in a direct line with the ligamentum patellae. The angle formed is always valgus, and the average is 12 degrees in males and 15 degrees in females. The quadriceps (Q) angle is accentuated by internal rotation of the femur. The resulting tendency toward lateral patellar displace-

ment is resisted by the lateral lip of the femoral sulcus and the horizontal fibers of vastus medialis obliquus, together with the medial patellar retinaculum. The four segments of the quadriceps femoris are supplied by the femoral nerve.

The popliteal fossa is bounded laterally by the biceps femoris and medially by the semimembranosus and semitendinosus tendons. In its lower part, the space is closed by the two heads of the gastrocnemius. The roof of the fossa is formed by the deep fascia; the floor consists of the popliteal surface of the femur, posterior ligament of the knee joint, and the popliteus muscle with its fascial covering.

The biceps femoris arises as a long head in common with the semitendinosus and as a short head from the lateral lip of the linea aspera, the lateral supracondylar line, and the lateral intramuscular septum. The two heads unite above the knee joint in a common tendon that inserts into the head of the fibula in front of the styloid process folding around the lateral ligament. An expansion crosses to the adjoining part of the tibia. The nerve supply is derived from the sciatic nerve (the long head medial and short head lateral popliteal nerve).

The semitendinosus arises from the ischial tuberosity and runs downward medially on the surface of semimembranosus. The semimembranosus arises from the upper and lateral impression on the ischial tuberosity by a long tendon. It passes downward and medially deep to the origin of biceps and semitendinosus and more distally is overlapped by semitendinosus. Its tendon forms the upper and medial boundary of the popliteal fossa and inserts into a groove on the posteromedial aspect of the medial condyle of the tibia. From the tendon a strong expansion passes upward and laterally, forming the oblique posterior ligament of the knee. The nerve supply to the hamstring muscles is derived from the sciatic nerve. The gracilis muscle arises from the pubic arch and adjoining parts of the body of the pubis and runs distally along the medial side of the thigh. In the lower third of the thigh, the fibers end in a long tendon that lies medial to the tendon of semitendinosus. It is supplied by the obturator nerve. The sartorius muscle arises from the anterior superior iliac spine and runs downward and medially across the front of the thigh. It forms the roof of the subsartorial canal. Its nerve supply is derived from the femoral nerve. The sartorius tendon is shorter and wider than those of gracilis and semi-

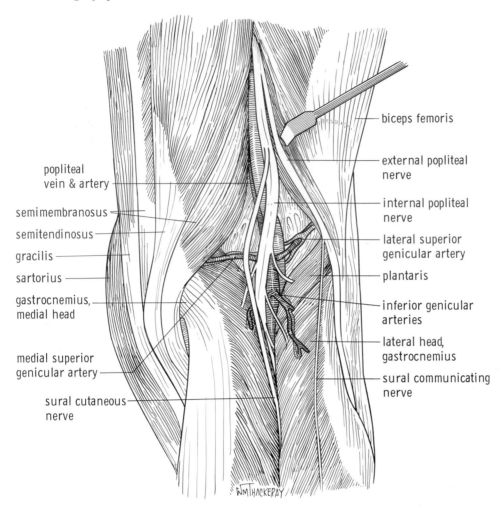

popliteal
vein & artery

semimembranosus

semitendinosus

gracilis

sartorius

gastrocnemius,
medial head

medial superior
genicular artery

sural cutaneous
nerve

biceps femoris

external popliteal
nerve

internal popliteal
nerve

lateral superior
genicular artery

plantaris

inferior genicular
arteries

lateral head,
gastrocnemius

sural communicating
nerve

WM THACKERAY

tendinosus. The muscle fibers do not diminish in width until they end in the tendon just above the knee. Together the tendons of sartorius, gracilis, and semitendinosus form the pes anserinus. The sartorius tendon has an expanded insertion into the medial upper tibia, which covers the insertions of gracilis and semitendinosus. The semitendinosus is inserted just below the gracilis.

When the knee is flexed, the biceps tendon can be felt subcutaneously on the lateral side. Medially, two tendons are prominent, the gracilis lying medial to the semitendinosus.

The ischial fibers of adductor magnus are a derivative of the hamstring group. The fibers run vertically downward and end in a short tendon, which inserts into the adductor tubercle on the medial condyle of the femur. Through a gap in the insertion of this mus-

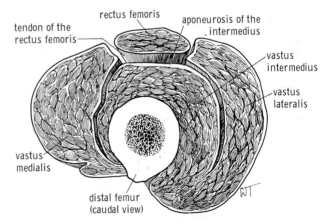

rectus femoris

tendon of the
rectus femoris

aponeurosis of the
intermedius

vastus
intermedius

vastus
lateralis

vastus
medialis

distal femur
(caudal view)

WT

Fig. 1.19. Four components of the quadriceps muscle shown through a cross section at the junction of middle and distal thirds of the femur. The four components then fuse to form the trilaminar tendon of the quadriceps muscle.

cle, the femoral vessels enter the popliteal fossa. Like the hamstrings, this portion of the adductor magnus is supplied by the sciatic nerve.

The gastrocnemius muscle arises as a lateral head from the lateral aspect of the lateral femoral condyle, and as a medial head from the popliteal surface of the femur and the medial aspect of the medial femoral condyle. The lateral head has a largely fleshy origin, but the portion of the medial head that arises from the medial condyle, adjoining the attachment of the medial collateral ligament, is tendinous. The two heads insert into the posterior aspect of a common tendon, which narrows below into the tendocalcaneous. The plantaris has a small, fleshy belly that arises from the lateral supracondylar line of the femur under cover of the lateral head of the gastrocnemius. It gives rise to a very long, narrow tendon that runs deep to the medial head of the gastrocnemius. The soleus arises (1) from the upper fourth of the posterior surface of the shaft of the fibula, extending upward onto the head of the bone, (2) from the tendinous arch crossing the posterior tibial vessels and nerve, and (3) from the soleal line on the posterior surface of the tibia. Its tendon joins the deep surface of the tendoachilles. The gastrocnemius, plantaris and soleus are supplied by the medial popliteal nerve. The popliteus has an intra-articular origin by a tendon from the lateral surface of the lateral condyle of the femur. The most medial fibers of the muscle take origin from the posterior aspect of the capsular ligament of the knee joint and the lateral semilunar cartilage. The tendon passes distally and backward separating the lateral meniscus from the lateral ligament of the knee. The fibers run in a distal and medial direction to be inserted into the posterior surface of the tibia above the soleal line. The muscle is covered distally by a thick fascia. The nerve to the popliteus arises from the medial popliteal nerve and runs downward across the popliteal vessels, to reach the lower border of the muscle, where it enters its deep surface.

ACTION OF THE MUSCLES

The movements of the knee are flexion, extension, and rotation. Flexion is performed by the hamstrings and biceps femoris and to a lesser extent by gastrocnemius and popliteus; it is limited by the soft tissues at the back of the knee. Extension is performed by

the quadriceps and, because of the shape of the articulation and the ligament attachments, the femur rotates medially on the tibia in terminal extension— the "screw home" mechanism that locks the joint. This movement is purely passive, as are other rotary movements occurring during activity; the exception is the lateral rotation of the femur that precedes flexion by unlocking the joint. This movement is performed by popliteus. Sartorius, gracilis, and the hamstrings are weak rotators of the knee, but probably do not act as such. Sartorius, gracilis, and semitendinosus medially and the iliotibial tract laterally mostly act as "guy ropes" to stabilize the pelvis.

FIBULA

The superior tibiofibular joint is lined with synovial membrane and possesses a capsular ligament that is strengthened by anterior and posterior ligaments. In contrast, the inferior tibiofibular joint is a syndesmosis and the bones are joined by a strong intraosseous ligament. The intraosseous membrane stretches from the intraosseous border of the fibula, the fibers running distal and medial to be attached to the intraosseous border of the tibia. A large opening is present in its uppermost part for the passage of the anterior tibial vessels.

The articular surface of the head of the fibula is directed upward and slightly forward and medially to articulate with the posterior part of the lateral condyle of the tibia. The styloid process projects upward from the posterolateral aspect and to it is attached the lateral ligament of the knee joint and the bifurcated insertion of the biceps femoris. The anterior aspect of the superior tibiofibular joint and adjoining portions of the tibia and fibula give rise to the origins of tibialis anterior, extensor digitorum longus, and peroneus longus muscles. The posterior aspect of the same region gives rise to a portion of the soleus muscle. The anterior tibial artery, the terminal branch of the popliteal artery enters the anterior compartment of the leg through an aperture in the intraosseous membrane, two fingerbreadths below the superior tibiofibular joint. In this situation, it lies on the intraosseous membrane between the tibialis anterior and extensor digitorum longus. A recurrent branch takes part in the anastomosis around the knee. The anterior tibial nerve and a terminal branch of the lateral popliteal nerve pierce the anterior intramuscular septum between the extensor digitorum longus and the fibula and come to lie at the lateral side of the artery. The musculocutaneous nerve arises from the lateral popliteal nerve on the lateral side of the neck of the fibula and runs distally and forward in the substance of the peroneus longus muscle.

REFERENCES

1. Aglietti, P., Insall, J.N., Walker, P.S., et al: A new patella prosthesis. Design and application. Clin. Orthop., *107:* 175, 1975.
2. Anderson, J.E., ed.: Grant's Atlas of Anatomy, 7th Ed. Baltimore, Williams & Wilkins, 1978.
3. Basmajian, J.V., ed.: Grant's Method of Anatomy, 10th Ed. Baltimore, Williams & Wilkins, 1980.
4. Brantigan, O.C., and Voshell, A.F.: The mechanics of the ligaments and menisci of the knee joint. J. Bone Joint Surg. *23:* 44, 1941.
5. Brantigan, O.C., and Voshell, A.F.: The tibial collateral ligament: Its function, its bursae, and its relation to the medial meniscus. J Bone Joint Surg., *25:* 121, 1943.
6. Fulkerson, J.P., and Gossling, H.R.: Anatomy of the knee joint lateral retinaculum. Clin. Orthop., *153:* 183, 1980.
7. Girgis, F.G., Marshall, J.L., and Al Monajem, A.R.S.: The cruciate ligaments of the knee joint. Clin. Orthop., *106:* 216, 1975.
8. Goodfellow, J., Hungerford, D.S., and Zindel, M.: Patello-femoral mechanics and pathology. I. Functional anatomy of the patello-femoral joint. J. Bone Joint Surg. [Br.], *58:* 287, 1976.
9. Kaplan, E.B.: The fabellofibular and short lateral ligaments of the knee joint. J. Bone Joint Surg. [Am.], *43:* 169, 1961.
10. Kaplan, E.B.: Some aspects of functional anatomy of the human knee joint. Clin. Orthop., *23:* 18, 1962.
11. Kaplan, E.B.: The iliotibial tract. Clinical and morphological significance. J. Bone Joint Surg. [Am.], *40:* 817, 1958.
12. Last, R.J.: Some anatomical details of the knee joint. J. Bone Joint Surg. [Br.], *30:* 683, 1948.
13. Last, R.J.: The popliteus muscle and the lateral meniscus. J. Bone Joint Surg. [Br.], *32:* 93, 1950.
14. Last, R.J.: Anatomy. Regional and Applied, 6th Ed. Edinburgh, Churchill Livingstone, 1978.
15. Marshall, J.L., Girgis, F.G., and Zelko, R.R.: The biceps femoris tendon and its functional significance. J Bone Joint Surg. [Am.], *54:* 1444, 1972.
16. Palmer, I.: On the injuries to the ligaments of the knee joint. A clinical study. Acta Chir. Scand. Suppl. *53:* 1938.
17. Scapinelli, R.: Blood supply of the human patella. Its relation to ischaemic necrosis after fracture. J. Bone Joint Surg. [Br.], *49:* 563, 1967.
18. Seebacher, J.R., Inglis, A.E., Marshall, J.L., et al: The structure of the posterolateral aspect of the knee. J. Bone Joint Surg. [Am.], *64:* 536, 1982.
19. Warren, L.F., and Marshall, J.L.: The supporting structures and layers on the medial side of the knee. An anatomical analysis. J. Bone Joint Surg. [Am.], *61:* 56, 1979.
20. Warren, L.F., Marshall, J.L., and Girgis, F.G.: The prime static stabilizer of the medial side of the knee. J. Bone Joint Surg. [Am.], *56:* 665, 1974.
21. Williams, P.L., and Warwick, R., eds.: Gray's Anatomy, 36th British Ed. Philadelphia, W.B. Saunders, 1980.
22. Wilson, P.D., Eyre-Brook, A.L., and Francis, J.D.: A clinical and anatomical study of the semimembranosus bursa in relation to popliteal cyst. J. Bone Joint Surg. *20:* 963, 1938.

2 Biomechanics of the Knee

Albert H. Burstein

FUNCTION OF NORMAL JOINT

The mechanical function of any of the joints of the skeleton is to permit motion of the bone segments while these segments are carrying functional loads. For the knee joint, the desired motions are usually associated with ambulatory processes, including running, walking, and ascending and descending stairs and ramps. The functional loads during these activities are either the ground reaction force applied to the foot during the stance phase of the activity or the inertial load of the leg during the swing phase of the activity. Except for static postural activities, such as standing, the knee must carry varying loads; at the same time, it must permit motion between its three bony components. The major voluntarily controlled component of knee motion is flexion/extension. It is well recognized that the knee can and does undergo other motions (e.g., varus/valgus angulation). Nevertheless, it is the flexion/extension component motion that is directly controlled voluntarily and that must be present if normal function of the knee is to be achieved.

The concepts of load carrying and kinematic function are often treated as if they are separate entities in gross studies of knee function. Such a treatment may be acceptable. The purpose of this chapter, however, is to elucidate the fundamental issues of the biomechanics of the knee joint so that the complexity of its mechanical interactions may be more fully understood. If these fundamental aspects are to be understood, the simplistic notion of distinguishing between load transfer and motion must be avoided. The process of load carrying influences the motion of the knee joint as alterations of the kinematics of the knee joint can alter the loads borne by that joint. This chapter describes the basic mechanical function of the knee joint necessary to understand the function of the joint in its natural, diseased, and mechanically altered states.

FUNCTIONAL LOADING

The knee joint is required to resist the loads imposed on the foot during its contact with the ground for all ambulatory processes as well as to provide the necessary forces and moments to overcome the inertial effects of the leg during the swing phase of gait. The ground contact forces during various ambulatory activities have been measured by several investigators.[2,3,7,9] These forces vary during the gait cycle from a maximum of about 1.3 times body weight for normal walking to more than twice body weight for running activities. The direction of this foot/floor contact force is also variable during the gait cycle. During the heel-

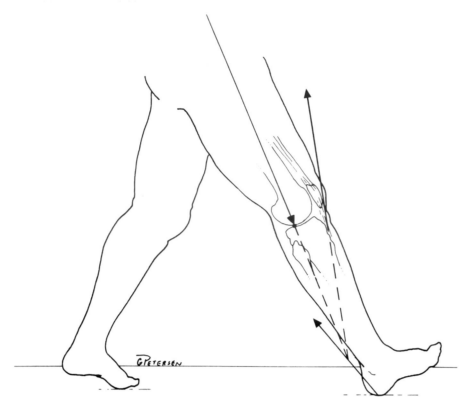

Fig. 2.1. During the early part of stance phase of gait, the ground/foot reaction force is directed upward and posteriorly. This force tends to flex the knee and is resisted by the quadriceps mechanism. The contact force at the heel, taken together with the force induced by the patellar tendon, creates a net upward force on the tibia which is, in turn, resisted by a downwardly directed force acting on the tibia at the knee joint. In this case, the point of application of the joint load is on the posterior aspects of the tibial plateau.

strike portion of the stance phase, the force is directed upward and posteriorly. During the midstance portion of the stance phase, the force is directed upward and slightly anteriorly. In each case the functional load induces a moment about the knee joint, and this moment must be resisted by the agonist muscle or muscle group. The magnitude of the moment produced by the functional load is dependent on the actual center of rotation or, as will be shown later, the point of contact of the knee joint. The amount of force required for the agonist muscle group to balance this externally applied moment is also dependent on the center of rotation of the joint. In the two examples shown, the center of joint rotation has shifted from its posterior position in Figure 2.1 to a more anterior position in Figure 2.2. The location of these points of contact is not based on any clinical observation, but rather on the assumption that the leg is in equilibrium and that the three dominant forces—the functional load, the muscle force, and the joint reaction—must provide this equilibrium. The equilibrium condition results in a particular line of application of the joint contact force. That is to say, the direction and magnitude of the functional load, taken together with the

direction of the applied muscle force, induce a particular direction and magnitude of joint reaction. This joint reaction can be achieved in both illustrated cases without the necessity of evoking tensile forces in the cruciate or collateral ligaments, since at the point of application of the joint contact force, the line of application of the joint force is perpendicular to the joint surfaces. Because the force is perpendicular to the surfaces, no additional force is required from the ligaments to provide an equilibrium situation. If the joint reaction force and joint surface are not perpendicular, additional forces will be required across the knee joint. These will be provided by stretching the cruciate or collateral ligaments, or both. These simple examples illustrate the interaction between the nature of the applied functional loads and the resulting contact surfaces of the knee joint.

The concept of instant center of relative motion has been applied to studies of the knee joint.[4] The mechanics of normal joint motion require that the instant center be located along the line that is perpendicular to the joint surfaces at the point of contact of the joint surfaces (Fig. 2.3). This is, in effect, another form of the statement that joint surfaces slide when they are

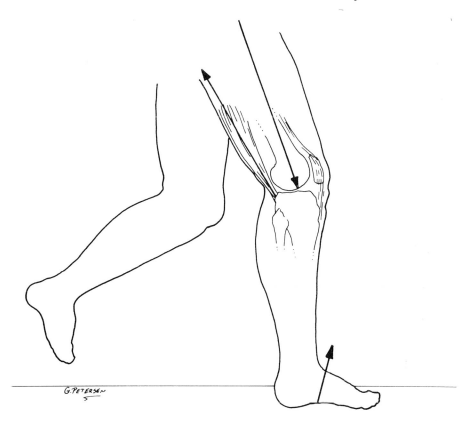

Fig. 2.2. When the foot is in mid stance, the foot/floor reaction lies anterior to the knee joint. This force tends to extend the knee and is resisted by muscle forces which tend to flex the knee. These forces in combination require a joint reaction force on the tibial plateau which is located in the anterior region of the plateau.

functioning normally. If the surfaces are sliding one over the other, then the instant center must lie along the line perpendicular to the joint surface. If the joint surfaces are not sliding, but rather tending to separate (Fig. 2.4) or penetrate one another, then the instant center will lie off this perpendicular line. This condition may occur when either the surface or ligamentous structures, or both, are not in their normal anatomical positions or when a brace or other orthotic device is superimposed over the knee, forcing motion in an unnatural way. If the point of contact of the knee is forced to shift from the posterior position to the anterior position as a result of the normal forces applied to the knee, then the instant center of motion of the knee would likewise shift from a location along the perpendicular line from the posterior point of contact to the location along the perpendicular line above the anterior point of contact. The example shown in Figure 2.5A illustrates why studies of kinematics of the knee on the basis of a fixed anatomic location of the instant center are difficult to repeat. For any given angle of flexion or extension, the instant center of the knee is not determined by the kinematic constraints of the ligaments and the joint surfaces alone, but by the position of the point of contact as well. The range of these positions will vary, especially with absent or stretched cruciate ligaments. The cruciate ligaments can therefore be thought of as those structures that limit the position of the instant center of the knee joint. In doing so it must be realized that the cruciates themselves are elastic structures. With minimal force imposed on these structures, they can allow alteration of the relative position of the tibia and femur by 1 or 2 mm.[5,8] This alteration is sufficient to cause significant changes in the location of the contact point, which will result, of course, in altered kinematic function of the knee joint. The more congruent the surfaces within the knee joint, the more dramatic the change in the point of contact between the two surfaces may be for small shifts in their relative positions. Figure 2.5A shows that with more congruent surfaces, a shift of 2 mm of the tibia may result in movement of the contact point by as much as 8 to 10 mm, while those surfaces that are less congruent (Fig. 2.5B) will require larger shifts of the tibia to produce the same shift of the contact point.

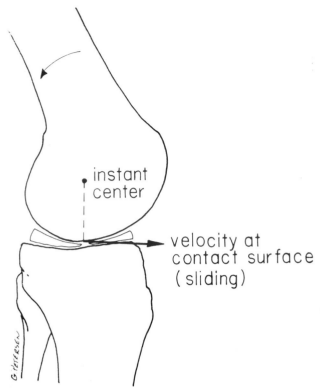

hence the center of rotation, results in an increase in the moment arm of the extensor mechanism and a decrease in the moment arm of the functional load. When the load is moved anteriorly, the instant center shifts posteriorly as a result of a shift of the point of contact. In this case, the flexors enjoy a greater moment arm while the moment arm of the functional load is concomitantly decreased. If the joint is restricted in its motion, and therefore in the allowable shift of the instant center, the muscles will not enjoy the effect of the shift in the moment arms. Muscle forces will be increased, ultimately resulting in increased joint loads.

In both examples (Figs. 2.1 and 2.2), we have seen that the magnitude of the muscle force required to overcome the externally applied functional load is

Fig. 2.3. During knee joint motion we can appreciate the relative surface velocity by considering the tibia to be stationary and the femur to be rotating. Furthermore, the femur may be thought of as rotating about a particular point on the stationary tibia called the 'instant center'. The velocity of the femur at its contact point with the tibia must be perpendicular to a line connecting the contact point with the instant center. For normal knee motion the velocity of this contact point is parallel to the surface of the tibia.

These examples illustrate one effect of the meniscus in that it permits greater shifts in the contact point with smaller relative motions of the two bony surfaces. The menisci accomplish this in two ways. First, they increase the stiffness of the joint by permitting less overall joint deflection under the application of compressive loads. This means other joint surfaces, together with the menisci, can retain their inherent congruency. Second, they increase the congruency of the joint as witnessed by their efficiency in increasing joint contact area and decreasing joint contact stress.[6]

The mobility of the point of contact between joint surfaces obviously has beneficial results in terms of joint mechanics. As shown in Figure 2.1, the relatively posterior placement of the contact point, and

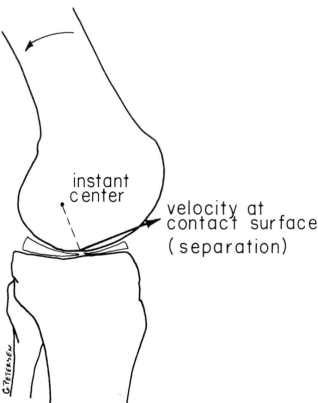

Fig. 2.4. If the location of the instant center relative to the contact surface of the joint is such that the velocity of the contact point is not parallel to the joint surface, then a condition of joint separation or joint distraction will occur. In this case, the velocity of the contact point is diverging from the tibial surface and therefore we consider this as separation.

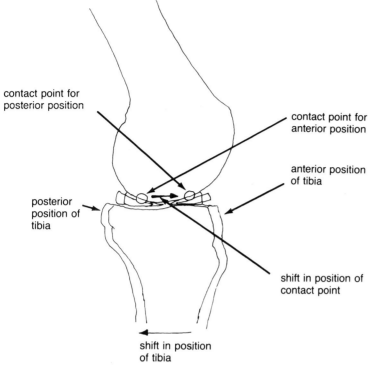

contact point for
posterior position

contact point for
anterior position

anterior position
of tibia

posterior
position of
tibia

shift in position of
contact point

shift in position
of tibia

A

Fig. 2.5. (A) In the normal knee, anterior and posterior shifts of the tibia with respect to the femur produce different contact points on the joint surfaces. When the tibia is in the anterior position, the contact point between the femur and the tibia moves to a relatively posterior position on both joint surfaces. A small shift in the position of the tibia posteriorly will result in a large shift in the position of the contact point in the anterior direction. (B) In the less congruent joint, for example one with absent menisci, larger anterior and posterior shifts in the tibia are required to produce equivalent shifts in the point of contact of the joint surfaces.

considerably greater than the functional load. In both cases, muscle force was approximately three times the magnitude of the applied load. Such large muscle forces may be appreciated intuitively, on the basis of observation of the relative lengths of the moment arms of the two forces. In general, the moment arm enjoyed by the functional load can vary widely and, for the lower limb, may be as large as the length of the leg itself. Straight leg raising while wearing weighted boots is an example of a function load having a very large moment arm. Conversely, the moment arms of the muscle forces are relatively fixed by the anatomic positions of the muscles. The only means of altering

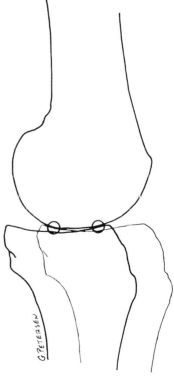

Less Congruent Surfaces

B

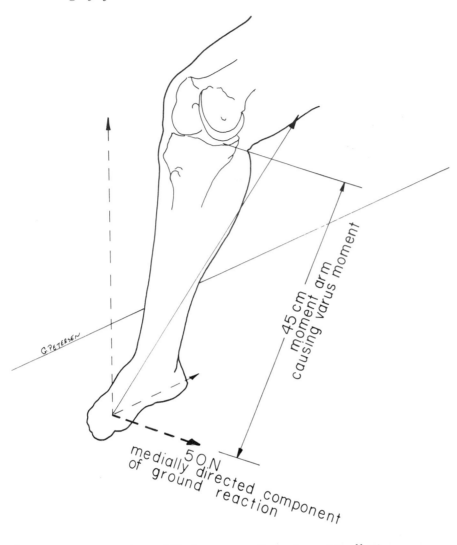

G. PETERSEN

45 cm moment arm
causing varus moment

50 N
medially directed component
of ground reaction

Fig. 2.6. When the foot/ground contact force is examined in three-dimensions, the component which can produce valgus, or in this case, varus knee joint moments must be considered if the forces about the knee joint are to be determined. In this example the ground reaction force has a 50N component which is responsible for the production of the varus moment.

these moment arms is to shift the center of rotation of the joint itself. Generally, the ratio of moment arm advantage enjoyed by the external load is somewhere between 1:1 and 6:1. As a result, numerous investigators,[10,11] when calculating forces about the knee joint, find that very large forces exist. If we examine the simplest possible equilibrium configuration in which only three forces are considered (Figs. 2.1 and 2.2), it is seen that the magnitude of the joint reaction force is approximately equal to that of the muscle force. Since it is the muscle force that is responsible for most of the joint reaction, it is no surprise that these same investigators have shown theoretical joint reaction loads that range from two to five times body weight for normal ambulatory activities and considerably higher, up to 24 times body weight, for more vigorous activ-

ities.[11] Thus, a person with a body weight of 700 N would generate joint contact forces that might vary anywhere from 1,400 to 3,500 N.

The ground reaction force imposed on the foot during ambulatory activities was previously described as having vertical and horizontal components. The horizontal component of this contact force may be further considered as having effects both in the anterior–posterior and in the lateral directions. Under conditions of loads that tend to produce varus–valgus moments about the knee joint, three mechanisms can occur within the joint that will resist these applied moments. Since the forces producing varus–valgus moments are applied concomitantly with the forces that tend to produce flexion and extension moments, we may consider that either the extensor or flexor

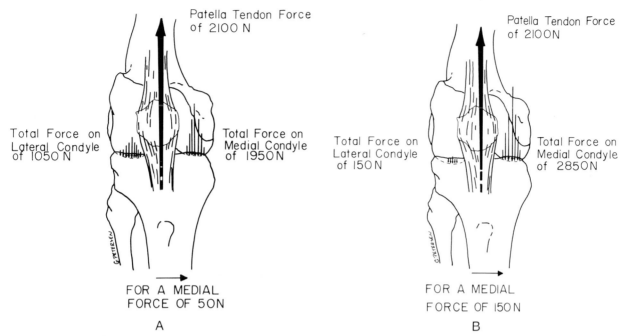

Fig. 2.7. (A) In order for equilibrium to exist a total joint contact force of 3000N must be applied. Because of the medial force of 50N applied at the foot, unequal contact force distribution will result in the medial-lateral direction. The medial condyle will have the larger contact force while the lateral condyle will enjoy lower loads. The results of this load distribution will be the production of a valgus moment in the knee joint to counteract the externally applied varus moment. (B) The medial force acting on the foot has been increased to 150N. Stability is still maintained without the imposition of any additional constraints by virtue of the fact that the force on the medial condyle has increased to 2850N, while the force on the lateral condyle has decreased to 150N. This results in a sufficient valgus moment at the knee to counterbalance the varus moment induced by the medial foot load.

muscle groups would be active. With the force passing posterior to the joint, as in Figure 2.6, the quadriceps would be active.

We will now examine the mechanics of the knee joint that enable it to resist that component of the ground reaction force that is producing a varus moment about the knee joint. The three methods that the knee joint has available to overcome this moment are (1) redistribution of joint contact force, (2) redistribution of augmented joint contact force, and (3) production of ligamentous loads by large varus–valgus displacement.

The first method is illustrated in Fig. 2.7A,B. In this example, the varus–valgus moment is approximately 2,250 N-cm (obtained by multiplying the 50 N medially directed contact force component by the 45-cm moment arm between the force and the center of contact of the knee joint). As we have previously seen in this example, the quadriceps force is 2,100 N. This force, in concert with the ground reaction

force as applied to the tibia, produces a total joint reaction of 3,000 N. This total 3,000-N joint contact force is divided between the medial and lateral condyles in such a way that the joint must be in equilibrium not only in the flexion–extension mode, but in the varus–valgus mode as well (Fig. 2.7A). Therefore, the total force acting on the medial condyle is going to be larger than that acting on the lateral condyle. In this case, 1,950 N of the 3,000-N contact force is transferred by the medial condyle. The force on the lateral condyle has been reduced to 1,050 N. If we consider the moments produced by medial and lateral condylar forces about the center of the joint, we will observe that the force on the medial condyle produces 2,250 N-cm of moment in excess of that produced by the lateral condyle, that is

$$(1950 \text{ N} \times 2.5 \text{ cm}) - (1050 \text{ N} \times 2.5 \text{ cm}) = 2250 = \text{N} - \text{cm}$$

Because we have chosen the center of the joint as our

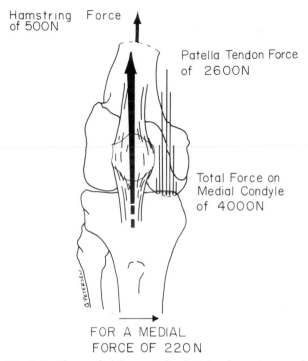

Hamstring Force
of 500N

Patella Tendon Force
of 2600N

Total Force on
Medial Condyle
of 4000N

FOR A MEDIAL
FORCE OF 220N

Fig. 2.8. The medial force at the foot has been increased to 220N and the knee joint contact forces are no longer able to supply a sufficient balancing valgus moment. Therefore, a force on the hamstrings and additional patellar tendon force are required to increase joint contact forces. In this case, a 500N of additional force for each muscle group produce 4000N of compression on the medial condyle. This is sufficient to balance the medial force at the foot.

arbitrary center of rotation in order to examine the moments, the quadriceps force has no moment effect. The quadriceps force passes through this point, hence its moment arm is zero. This is, in fact, the reason why this arbitrary point was chosen, a choice that simplifies the calculation. In this example, the 50-N medial load was a realistic choice in terms of ordinary ambulatory activities. It can be seen that balancing a varus moment can be accomplished by a moderate shift in the joint reaction load between the condyles. If a more severe loading situation were studied (e.g., Fig. 2.7B), in which the 50-N medial ground contact force were increased to 150 N, then a varus moment of 6,750 N-cm would be produced. To resist such a moment, the load on the medial condyle would increase to 2,850 N, while the load on the lateral condyle would drop off to 150 N. Thus, a medial force of slightly over 150 N can be tolerated by this mechanism of equilibrium.

Changes in contact load distribution across the joint surfaces must be accomplished by a slight varus angulation of the knee joint. This angulation would result from the increased compressive strain on the medial condyle and the decreased compressive strain on the lateral condyle. Since the resulting total displacement of the surfaces of the cartilaginous coverings of the joint is of the order of magnitude of a fraction of a millimeter, the amount of varus–valgus angulation produced by the increase in medial compressive load and the decrease in lateral compressive load is quite small, actually on the order of 1 or 2 degrees.

If medial forces greater than 167 N are applied to the foot (Fig. 2.8), the lateral side of the joint will begin to separate, losing contact and reducing the lateral contact force to zero. Once this happens, there can no longer be any increase in the load felt by the medial compartment, leaving the knee joint incapable of providing any additional valgus moment to overcome the externally applied varus load. Additional medial force at the foot will simply result in a greater opening of the joint and stretching of the ligaments.

At this point, the second method of varus–valgus moment production may go into effect to alleviate imposed varus deformity on the knee: the voluntary contraction of both the quadriceps and the hamstrings. If both quadriceps and hamstrings are contracted in proportional amounts, the net effect of a flexion–extension moment may be negated. The equilibrium would not be altered in the flexion–extension direction, but clearly if both muscle groups increased their force, the joint compressive load would increase. This is illustrated in Figure 2.8, in which voluntary action has raised the joint compressive load from its previous level of 3,000 to 4,000 N. This may be accomplished by an increase of muscle force of roughly 500 N in each of the two muscle groups. By increasing the muscle force, and hence the joint compression load, contact pressure on the medial side of the joint will be increased. The net valgus moment that can be produced by such a load will also be increased. Thus, at the time that the lateral side of the joint is tending to separate, voluntary muscle contraction can increase joint load, which would lead to increased medial compartment pressure, in turn producing a stabilizing moment to resist the externally applied load. In this case, an externally applied load of approximately 220 N may be resisted without the joint angulating more than a few degrees.

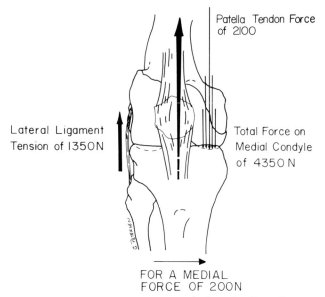

Patella Tendon Force of 2100

Lateral Ligament Tension of 1350N

Total Force on Medial Condyle of 4350 N

FOR A MEDIAL FORCE OF 200N

Fig. 2.9. With a medial force applied at the foot of 200N and no contraction of the hamstrings or additional contraction of the quadriceps, the lateral ligaments will be elongated and forced to produce tension. In this case, with a patellar tendon force remaining constant at 2100N a lateral ligament tension of 1350N will be required and this will result in a total medial condyle contact force of 4350N.

The third method of joint stabilization would come into effect if either the internal valgus moment required were to exceed the capacity of the equilibrating moment provided by voluntary muscle contraction or if the external load were applied in a rapid, unexpected manner such that the muscles would not have a chance to contract voluntarily. The ligaments would then have to be stretched to produce tensile forces that would contribute toward the production of an equilibrating valgus moment. Consider the contributions of the cruciates and the lateral–collateral ligaments separately. Studies have shown that the collateral ligaments develop their maximum loads at elongations of approximately 5 percent. In order to develop significant loads, these ligaments would have to be stretched approximately 1 or 2 percent of their length. This would amount to changes in length on the order of 1 to 2 mm. We may then envision the mechanism of stabilization as occurring when the lateral side of the knee joint has opened (angulated) sufficiently to stretch the collateral ligaments to the extent that their loads become significant factors in providing moment equilibrium.

As an example, we can determine the amount of varus angulation required to in turn produce the required ligamentous force when the applied medial load is 200 N (Fig. 2.9). In this diagram, the dimension from the lateral side of the knee, where the collateral ligaments are located, to the center of pressure of the medial condyle, where all the joint force may be considered to be concentrated, is about 6.7 cm. The first mechanism of joint stabilization has been overpowered, and we assume that the second mechanism is not operable. Therefore, there is an excessive varus moment (applied varus–valgus moment caused by eccentric loading) of 9,000 N-cm, which must be overcome by the resistance of the collateral ligaments. For a lever arm of 6.7 cm, the amount of lateral–collateral tension that must be developed would be equal to 1,350 N. This is the amount of force that must be applied with the 6.7-cm moment arm to produce 9,000 N-cm of valgus moment in order to balance the excessive varus moment.

We can generalize the discussion just presented by examining Figure 2.10. For each increment of rotation (labeled θ), the collateral ligaments will stretch an amount equal to θ times W The stiffness of the ligament, that is, the amount of load required to induce a unit of elongation, may be called *k;* hence the amount of force produced in the ligament will be

$$\text{Lateral ligament force} = \theta W k$$

The amount of valgus moment that this ligament force will produce (considering moment equilibrium about the contact point on the medial condyle) will be equal to the ligamentous force multiplied by its moment arm to the point of joint contact. In this case, that amount would be

$$\text{Force} \times \text{moment arm} = \text{valgus moment}$$
$$(\theta W k)W = \text{valgus moment}$$

or

$$\theta k W^2 = \text{valgus moment}$$

Thus, the amount of correctional valgus moment that would be produced is proportional to the opening of the knee joint, the stiffness of the collateral ligament and the square of the characteristic joint dimension *W*. Note that in order for this third joint stabilization mechanism to exist, the amount of angulation at the joint would be on the order of several degrees, while the first two stabilization mechanisms

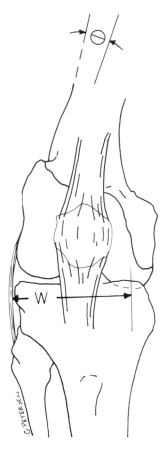

Fig. 2.10. The amount of stretch in the lateral ligament that is produced by each increment of varus angulation is related to the dimension W, the distance between the contact point in the medial condyle and the lateral-collateral ligament.

discussed would require angulation only on the order of 1 or 2 degrees.

When the collateral ligament produces tension in response to the excess varus–valgus moment, a new equilibrium condition is created for the leg. The upward pull of the collateral ligament on the tibia requires an additional downward push on the tibia at the medial condyle. This increases the total joint reaction by an amount equal to the tensile force in the collateral ligament. The original joint reaction of 3,000 N is then increased by the amount of ligament tension, or 1,350 N, for a total joint reaction force of 4,350 N (Fig. 2.9). This entire force would be applied to the medial condyle.

The cruciate ligaments may also contribute to the varus–valgus stability of the knee joint. The previous method of analysis could be applied to the cruciate ligaments, except that because of the oblique direction of the cruciate ligaments, forces produced in the cruciates would tend to be higher for equal contributions to varus–valgus stability. However, a more

important factor moderating contributions of the cruciate ligaments to the varus–valgus stability is their distance from the contact point on the joint surfaces. In Figure 2.11, it can be seen that the distance W' at which the cruciate ligaments act is considerably closer than the distance W for the collateral ligaments. In this case, the analysis of the force in the cruciate ligaments for each unit of varus angulation would still hold. Since the distance of W' is less than half of W, the contribution of the cruciate ligaments, even for equal amounts of angulation, can be expected to be one-quarter that of the collateral ligaments. This is not inconsistent with experimental studies that have described the cruciate ligaments as "secondary" stabilizers; furthermore, it is clinically recognized that an absent cruciate ligament is difficult to appreciate when applying varus–valgus moments to the relaxed knee.

In all the foregoing analyses, the knee had to develop an internal moment in order to be able to resist the moment attributable to the external functional load. In each case, the moment was resisted by two forces acting on the tibia and located in close proximity to the joint. In the case of the functional load being applied in a plane of flexion–extension, the two forces were the muscle force applied through the pa-

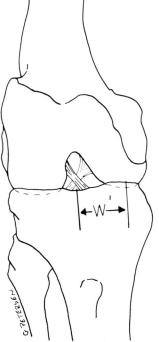

Fig. 2.11. The cruciate ligaments can also provide a valgus righting moment to balance a varus load at the foot. In this case, however, the functional lever arm is W' which is the distance between the contact point on the medial condyle and the center of effort of the collateral ligaments.

tellar tendon and the joint reaction on the tibial condyles. The combined effect of these two forces produces the moment that equilibrated the externally applied functional load. When varus–valgus moments were applied, again, for each of the three methods of maintaining equilibrium, two forces were generated to resist the external moment. In the first method, the force pair consisted of the quadriceps force as transmitted through the patellar tendon and the joint reaction force of the medial femoral condyle as applied to the medial tibial condyle. For the second method, the force pair again consisted of a patellar tendon force and a joint reaction force. In the third method of moment production, the previous force pair was augmented by a force pair consisting of a collateral ligament force and the additional joint reaction force caused by the collateral ligament force.

As a general condition, therefore, moments are created in joints by the application of force pairs. These force pairs usually consist of a joint reaction force and a muscle or ligament force. However, if the functional external load that is being resisted is an axial torque (a force that causes torque about the axis of the tibia), it is possible that the force pair will consist of ligamentous forces alone. Consider, for example, the case in which a torque is applied to the foot during the stance phase in gait. Such torques have been measured in amounts of approximately 10 N-m during ambulatory activities. In the absence of muscle forces, such torques must be resisted by the development of tension in a pair of ligaments. For example, virtually all the ligamentous structures surrounding the knee joint are capable of exerting force in oblique directions. Any pair, such as the medial collateral and lateral collateral ligaments, can exert such forces and counterbalance the applied external torque. One of the pairs of forces counterbalancing the torque may also be a muscle-induced force, since there are muscles that cross the knee joint obliquely. It is important to note that these torques must be generated by pairs of forces. Therefore, when considering the functions of ligaments in resisting torsional loads, it is important to think of these functions in terms of pairs of ligaments. One ligament may be absent, necessitating the substitution of an additional ligament, but if more than one ligament is absent, the substitution patterns become more complex, making the function less predictable.

The mechanics of the patellofemoral joint differ considerably from those of the femorotibial joint. The patellofemoral joint forces do not result from equilibrium requirements of functional load. Rather, they result from the necessity to change the direction of the load of the quadriceps as it passes about the knee joint before it is applied to the tibia through the patellar tendon. The mechanical function of the patella, then, is to provide a means for a mechanically compatible change of force direction. The patella responds to a set of three forces: the pull of the quadriceps, the pull of the patellar tendon, and the compressive force at the patellofemoral surface. If these three forces must be essentially coplanar, we can think of the force acting on the patellofemoral surface as an integrated effect in which a single force replaces the distribution of forces on the surface. Again, conceptually, we may consider the pull of the quadriceps and the patellar tendon as pure forces not having any components of moment.

The questions most often asked when considering clinical problems of the patella involve the magnitude and direction of the forces acting on the patella. The net reaction force of the quadriceps against the patella, accepting the assumption stated above, have been shown to be quite large for various types of activities, reaching four to five times body weight.

There are several factors concerning the biomechanical analyses that are quite important. First, the patellofemoral joint, like the femorotibial joint, does not have a fixed relationship between the kinematic function of the joint and the relative position of its bony elements. For any given angle of knee flexion, or for that matter any given position of patellofemoral contact, the actual region of contact may vary depending on the particular set of loads applied. Thus, any experiment that employs only one set of loading conditions can only be interpreted in terms of that particular condition. Other loading conditions (e.g., walking as compared with stair climbing), even though they may involve similar angles of flexion, will produce different loading conditions on the joint surface. It is not difficult to appreciate the fact that different activities will produce different loads in the patellofemoral joint at the same degree of flexion. For example, it is well understood that when doing straight leg raises the functional load induced by gravity varies if the patient is supine and extends the leg from 90 degrees to 0 degrees of flexion. In the 90-degree position, the functional load is essentially zero, since the

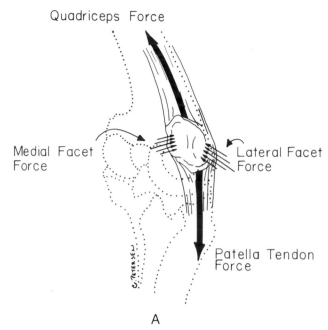

Quadriceps Force

Medial Facet
Force

Lateral Facet
Force

Patella Tendon
Force

A

Fig. 2.12. (A) The patella is acted upon by four major forces: the force of the quadriceps muscle, the tension in the patellar tendon, the contact force on the lateral facet, and the contact force on the medial facet. (B) The forces on the lateral and medial facets may be thought of as combining to produce a resultant joint contact force which must lie in the plane of the quadriceps and patellar tendon forces.

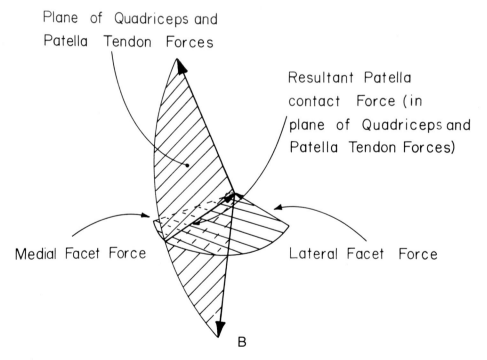

Plane of Quadriceps and
Patella Tendon Forces

Resultant Patella
contact Force (in
plane of Quadriceps and
Patella Tendon Forces)

Medial Facet Force

Lateral Facet Force

B

gravitational attraction force on the leg passes through the center of the joint. When the leg is brought into full extension, the functional load is maximum. When climbing stairs, however, in the region of 90 degrees of flexion, the functional load may be very severe, hence the amount of force required in the quadriceps to maintain equilibrium may be very large. Conversely, when standing in a position of full extension, the muscle load on the patella may be very low, since the functional load applied to the leg passes very close to the center of rotation of the knee joint. In any given case, once the required quadriceps force is determined and the particular geometric configuration of the joint is known, the question arises as to the load distribution over the femoral condyles. Again, the biomechanical principle that applies is that the forces are essentially coplanar. Therefore, the distribution of forces on the load-bearing portion of the patella must resolve into a resultant force that is coplanar with the applied muscle force and the induced patellar tendon load.

Clinical measurement parameters, such as the quadriceps (Q) angle, are important in understanding the influence of anatomy on the forces so as to allow the forces to be coplanar. However, care must be taken to observe the three-dimensional nature of the joint. Thus, in a position of 20 degrees of flexion, the Q angle may be thought of as describing the plane of the patellar force system (Fig. 2.12), but at 90 degrees of flexion the concept does not apply.

In the above illustration, the relative magnitude of the medial and lateral patellar joint contact forces are created in such proportions that the resulting patellar force is in the plane of the quadriceps force and the patellar tendon force. In visualizing the angle of intersection of this plane with the femoral condyles, the relative magnitudes of the two joint contact forces can be determined. Remember that the direction of these two contact forces is controlled by the orientation of the contact surfaces of the joint (i.e., perpendicular to these surfaces). Therefore, to alter the direction of the resulting total force, the relative magnitudes of the components of the force will have to vary.

APPLICATIONS OF BIOMECHANICS TO PRINCIPLES OF TOTAL KNEE REPLACEMENT

At the beginning of this chapter, we examined the interaction between kinematic function and load transmission in the natural joint. We shall now examine the same relationship in the knee joint that has been a recipient of a total knee replacement prosthesis. We shall focus mainly on the condylar types of prostheses, since this is the design class that has met with the greatest clinical success and represents the vast majority of prostheses currently in use.

The mechanics of loading in the limb with a total knee prosthesis do not differ substantially from those of the natural limb. If we were to examine Figures 2.1 and 2.2 and assume that the joint surface is replaced by artificial components, we would see that the loading system produces much the same result. There is no reason for either the magnitudes of the forces or the lines of force application to change. The concept of the point of application of the load deserves closer scrutiny. Condylar style prostheses are available with a wide range of tibial condyle curvatures. They vary all the way from the relatively flat geometry, used most frequently in cruciate-retaining prostheses, to the more curved geometry commonly associated with cruciate-sacrificing prostheses. In any case, the principles of mechanics do not change and, if the joint reaction force is to be composed solely of transmitted compressive load between the femur and tibia, the load line must lie perpendicular to the surface of the joint at its point of contact. For the natural joint, with its remarkably low coefficient of friction, deviation from the perpendicularity condition of approximately one part per thousand was required if no cruciate force was to be applied. For total joint prostheses with somewhat higher coefficients of friction, deviation from perpendicularity can be of the order of several parts per hundred. While this deviation is considerably more than that of the natural joint, for practical purposes we may still consider the requirement that the load be perpendicular to the contact surface as a valid condition.

Consider those prostheses that require sacrifice of the cruciate ligaments. The loads usually borne by the surface of the natural joint, without incurring cruciate force, can only vary over a relative narrow angle. In Figure 2.13, the angular variation of an allowable normal force is only about 8 degrees. Required angular deviations greater than 8 degrees would result in load application by the cruciate ligaments. To get a general idea of what the required angular deviation would be for a normal set of forces, we might consider, as a rough guideline, the ratio of normal to cruciate force reported in the literature. In these studies, cruciate loads did not exceed one-quarter of the normal loads. This would limit the angular deviation to approximately 22 degrees. That is, the combination of the normal force and the cruciate force can be replaced by a single force inclined at an angle of 22 degrees to the tibial axis. The implication for total knee replacement is that if the curvature of the tibial component can have an included angle of 22 degrees, then it should be possible to replace cruciate

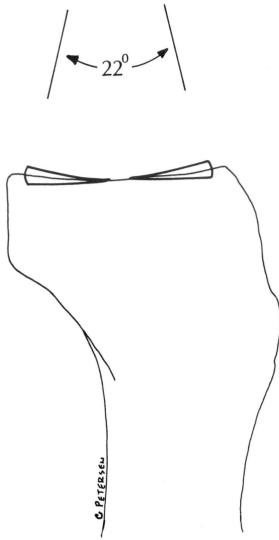

Fig. 2.13. While the surface contours of the medial and lateral condyles are not the same, in the natural knee joint the range of position through which normal force can traverse is relatively small.

such a large included angle in the tibial plateau, or if it is inappropriate to allow the contact point to shift to the extreme anterior position, then supplementary mechanisms can be used to provide the necessary cruciate equivalent force. An example of this is the posterior stabilized condylar prosthesis (Fig. 2.14). Although the included angle of the tibial plateau is 42 degrees, during activities involving flexion, it is desirable to maintain contact in the posterior region of the plateau. Therefore, the posterior motion of the tibia is controlled and limited by the contacting cam surfaces on both tibial and femoral components, and the contact between the femur and tibia is maintained in the posterior region of the prosthesis. For positions of flexion greater than about 40 degrees, the instant center is also maintained in the posterior region because of the contact between both the cam surfaces and the condylar surfaces.

In examining the mechanisms involved in producing varus–valgus stability with total knee replacements, the previously derived three mechanisms for joint stabilization are still applicable for most prostheses. Figure 2.15A shows such a set of artificial surfaces, and the analogy with the previous argu-

function with the simple mechanical substitution of varying the line of application of contact force. For those prostheses that do not have this much of an included angle, large joint displacements would be expected, requiring the secondary anteroposterior constraints, namely the collateral ligaments, to provide the restraining force. If it is not desirable to have

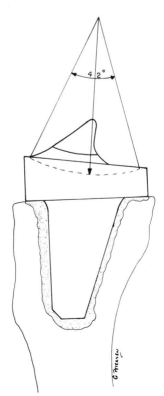

Fig. 2.14. The included angle of the tibia in many prosthetic designs is rather large. This allows correspondingly large variations in the angular positions in the normal contact force.

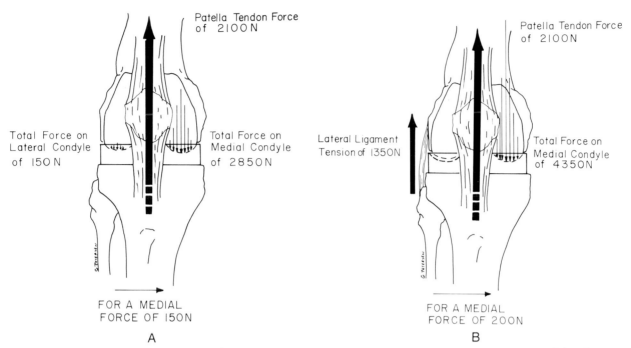

Fig. 2.15. (A) In the artificial knee as with the natural knee, varus/valgus equilibrium can be maintained by changing the distribution of the joint contact forces. In this case, a medial force at the foot of 150N can be resisted in a manner similar to that of the natural knee. The lateral contact force is greatly reduced while medial contact force increases. The patellar tendon force remains constant. (B) The mechanism of resisting excessive medial forces applied at the foot is similar in an artificial joint if the joint retains the characteristic behavior of being able to separate the contact surfaces on one condyle. In this case the lateral condyle is separating and lateral ligament tension is induced. This ligament tension, even in the presence of constant patellar tendon force, increases the total force on the medial condyle.

ments is demonstrated. In this case, because the knee consists of two condyles, varus–valgus equilibrium can be obtained by shifting load from the lateral condyle to the medial condyle. Because the artificial materials are considerably stiffer than the natural cartilage, the amount of angulation required to relieve the load in the lateral surface is greatly reduced. In this case, it might be considered to be a major fraction of 1 degree. Because the surfaces are bicondylar, the second stabilization mechanism (i.e., the supplementing of the valgus moment by the addition of agonist and antagonist muscle activity) will operate as well. Likewise, the third mechanism (the production of a moment by the collateral ligaments) would also be valid (Fig. 2.15B). Note that the surgeon can influence dimension W (refer to Fig. 2.9) by the choice of prosthesis. In the natural knee joint, this dimension is obviously fixed. However, in artificial joints, the dimension W may be varied by choice. Because the production of the lateral moment is proportional to

W^2, the value of W is very important. As an illustration, consider a choice between prostheses for which dimension W may be either 50 or 55 mm. In identical situations wherein equal varus moments must be resisted, the choice of the prosthesis with the 55 mm dimension would result in a reduction of approximately 20 percent in the amount of ligamentous force required to produce a given moment. This 20 percent reduction in ligament force would result in a corresponding decrease in the contribution of the ligament force to the total joint reaction. Thus, not only would the ligamentous force be lower, but the compressive force acting on the artificial joint would receive direct benefit as well.

Although these same equilibrium mechanisms are present in the natural knee joint, there are some important distinctions in the total knee replacement joint. In the natural knee joint, the stiffness of the cartilage is considerably less than the stiffness of the polyethylene found in most total knee replacements. Because of this difference in stiffness, less angulation will be .required in the total knee replacement to produce dramatic shifts in the load distribution between medial and lateral condyles. This may be thought of as an increased sensitivity in the total knee replacement to changes in pressure distribution as a result of small angulations of the tibia. Thus, although the mechanism is the same, the sensitivity of load with respect to deflection is considerably greater. There do not appear to be any immediately discernible disadvantages to this heightened response, but it should be noted that if a patient with a total knee prosthesis is examined for varus–valgus stability in the presence of voluntary contraction of the quadriceps, the clinical feel of the knee will be different from that of a natural knee, even though the mechanisms and quality of the varus–valgus stability may be virtually identical.

Knees that have varus moments applied beyond the capability of resistance by the first mechanism (the shifting of load) or the second mechanism (supplemental muscle force) require the lifting off of one condyle and the stretching of the collateral ligaments to obtain equilibrium. In some total knee designs, this may result in a very inappropriate contact geometry. For example, consider those prostheses that are essentially flat in the anteroposterior view. Lateral tipping would result in point contact, or line contact, at the extreme edge of the prosthesis. This is inappropriate from the point of view of function and longevity of the polyethylene and also from the point of view of load distribution in the tibial plateau (see next section). Those prostheses having curved surfaces, either convex or concave, which allow for a gradual change in the region of contact or which maintain the region of contact in the central region of the plateau are more desirable. For the prosthesis shown in Figure 2.15B, the same force distribution exists as was found in the example illustrated in Figure 2.9. The prosthesis geometry matches the natural joint geometry and, because it has the appropriate surface geometry, the force distribution across the contact surface is similar to that of the natural joint. If a prosthesis does not have the capability of lifting off and separating on one condyle, this last mechanism of stability is unavailable. This mechanism is totally unavailable, for example, to any prosthesis that is rigidly hinged between the femoral and tibial components.

For the total knee replacement, the interaction between joint motion and load transmission has another important effect: the stress distribution within the tibial plateau. It is commonly recognized that within the joint, the more severe loading environment is the tibial plateau, since this is the component that is most often involved in clinical complications. The clinical problem of tibial loosening has been associated with the mechanism of load transmission in that one probable cause of tibial loosening is thought to be either inappropriately high stresses in the interface region between the tibia and the prosthesis or inappropriately high stresses within the cancellous bone immediately below the interface region. In either case, concern is expressed as to the nature of the transmitted forces and the distribution throughout the natural and artificial structure.

In order to describe this load distribution, three questions may be asked. The first question concerns the overall design concept of using a peg on the tibial tray. The nominal purpose of the peg is to provide a backup fixation mode in the event of degradation of the interface between the plateau and the tibia. The question arises as to what sort of load distribution function exists between peg and plateau and whether this distribution results in alterations of bone density because of undesirable paths of load transfer. The second question concerns the choice of materials for the tibial plateau. Specifically, the question of the comparative effect between a polyethylene tibial plateau with a metal layer (metal backing) and a plain polyethylene tibial plateau on the distribution of forces and stresses is pertinent. The third question is related to the influence of load position on the stress distribution within the tibial plateau. In particular, we have previously seen that asymmetric loads are quite feasible, and the effect of such loads on the stress distribution should be determined.

The conventionally accepted method for answering such questions is the use of a finite element model. By use of such techniques,[1] these questions have been examined; the following discussion summarizes the common opinions. Figure 2.16 shows three models used to answer the previous questions: the upper model represents a polyethylene tibial component without a peg; the middle model, a polyethylene tibial component with a polyethylene peg; and the lower model, a polyethylene tibial component encased in a metal tray on which there is a metal peg. Dimensionally, all models are similar, with the exception of the omitted peg from the upper model. The tibial components were incorporated into the bone–cement–prosthesis

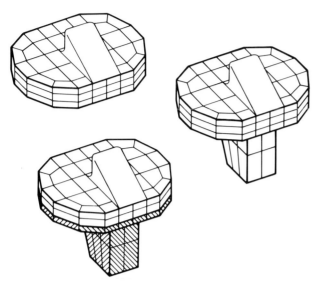

metal peg plays only a moderate role in the proximal region and would not be expected to have a major influence on the remodeling of the bone in the region of the peg.

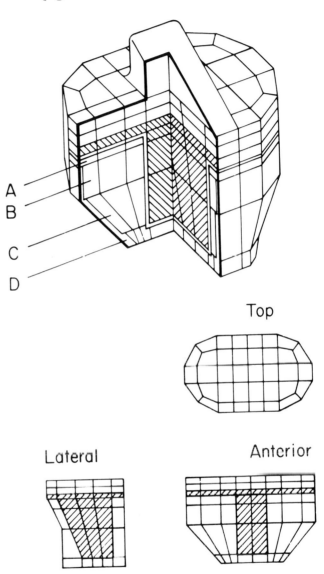

Fig. 2.16. Finite element models approximate the geometry of the real structures. In this case, a polyethylene tibial component without a peg is represented in the upper model. The middle model represents the same component with a polyethylene peg, while the lower model represents a similar geometry which contains a polyethylene articulating surface encased in a metal tray which itself is attached to a metal peg. (From Bartel, A.H., Burstein, E.A., Santavicca, E.A., et al: Performance of the tibial component in total knee replacement: conventional and revision designs. J. Bone Joint Surg. *64A* (No. 7). 1026, 1982, with permission.)

Fig. 2.17. The components shown in the previous Figure are now shown encased in the model of the proximal tibia. Again, the finite element model is a replica of the natural geometry and the model contains elements which represent cortical bone, cancellous bone, and PMMA. In addition, the model has a representation of the anterior/posterior asymmetry of the tibia. (From Bartel, A.H., Burstein, E.A., Santavicca, E.A., et al: Performance of the tibial component in total knee replacement: conventional and revision designs. J. Bone Joint Surg. *64A* (No. 7): 1026, 1982, with permission.)

model shown in Figure 2.17. To permit determination of the effects of the peg as well as the effects of the metal tray, a severe loading condition was examined. The load was placed entirely on one side of the joint in a position representing slight posterior subluxation (Fig. 2.18, case 4).

As can be seen in Table 2.1, the amount of load transferred at the various sections A, B, and C are only slightly different when comparing a plastic plateau having no peg with one that does have a peg. Throughout its length, the peg does not appear to transfer more than about 8 percent of the total load and, more importantly, the load distribution reaching the cortical bone is virtually the same with and without a peg. The metal tray and the metal peg do affect the load distribution in that the metal peg may carry as much as 25 percent of the load in the most proximal section. This still leaves more than 70 percent of the load to be borne by the tibial plateau. Thus, the conclusion can be reached that the plastic peg plays a minimal structural role in transferring load, while the

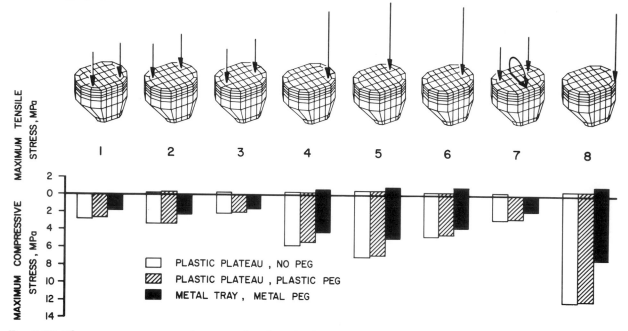

Fig. 2.18. The maximum stresses that are induced in the bone material underneath the tibial plateau is displayed for each loading case. The bars below the line represent compressive stresses while those above the line represent tensile stresses. Results are shown for the three classes of trays previously described. The magnitude of the single joint loads is equal to the sum of the symmetrical loads. This is consistent with the previous examples which show the shifting of load from one condyle to the other in response to an application of a varus moment. (From Bartel, A.H., Burstein, E.A., Santavicca, E.A., et al: Performance of the tibial component in total knee replacement: conventional and revision designs. J. Bone Joint Surg. *64A* (No. 7): 1026, 1982, with permission.)

To examine the effect of load placement on the tibial plateau, eight load cases were investigated. In Figure 2.18, cases 1–3 represent the anterior, posterior, and centrally loaded conditions in which the load is placed symmetrically on the tibial plateau. In these cases, no varus–valgus moment would be pro-

Table 2.1. Percentages of an Anteromedial Load Borne by the Different Components of the Three Models Within Each of the Three Layers Just Beneath the Plateau[a]

Model	Layer[b]	Cancellous Bone	Peg	Cement	Cortical Bone
Plastic plateau, no peg	A	100.0	—	—	—
	B	43.9	—	—	56.1
	C	15.0	—	—	85.0
Plastic plateau, with peg	A	85.5	6.5	8.0	—
	B	33.6	7.9	6.8	51.7
	C	9.7	3.1	2.7	84.5
Metal tray and peg	A	72.5	26.8	0.7	—
	B	27.3	23.0	0.2	49.5
	C	9.3	7.2	0.7	82.8

[a]Case 4, Figure 2.18.
[b]See Figure 2.17.

duced. In cases 4–6 there is, again, an anterior, posterior, and centrally placed load, but here the load is concentrated entirely on one plateau. These cases represent the maximum condition for the attainment of varus–valgus equilibrium for this particular component. The magnitude of load in cases 4–6 is the same as the sum of the two magnitudes of the individual loads in cases 1–3. In other words, this is a realistic condition, in which the total equilibrium force is kept constant but the load is shifted entirely to one plateau. Again, the load in cases 4–6 maintains the load in the central region of the single plateau. This represents a condition consistent with the geometry of total condylar prostheses, in which the load will remain essentially in the center of the concavity. In case 8, the load application point is allowed to shift to the extreme edge of the prosthesis. This represents the case in which the maximum varus–valgus moment is supported by a prosthesis which has either a flat profile in the anteroposterior view, or a condylar-type prosthesis that is displaced so as to make contact at the extreme outer edge. Finally, case 7 is included to show the load condition comparable to case 2, in which a posterior stabilizing feature is added to the prosthesis. The purpose of this case is simply to compare prostheses containing posterior stabilizing features with those that omit it.

The graphic results in Figure 2.18 depict the maximum stress in the cancellous bone. For those bars appearing beneath the line, the representation is the maximum compressive stress in the cancellous bone. This always occurred in the region of the cancellous bone directly beneath the points of application of the load. Those bars that appear above the line represent the maximum tensile stresses. For the tensile stresses, the maximum stress always occurred in the opposite condyle from the point of application of the joint load.

Examining Figure 2.18, we can readily see that the highest stresses are produced in those cases in which a single load is applied to the condyle. In that case in which the load is applied most eccentrically (case 8), the magnitude of the stresses in the cancellous bone is greatest. Note that in all cases the metal tray with the metal peg produced lower maximum cancellous bone stresses than did either of the other two configurations. Also note that the metal tray induced some tension stress at the interface.

CONCLUSIONS

Several conclusions can be drawn:
1. The most severe, but nevertheless, expected loading configuration occurs when load is concentrated in one condyle. A more severe, but unexpected, load condition occurs when a concentrated load is placed at the extreme edge of the prosthesis.
2. Metal trays reduce the magnitude of the maximum compressive stress in the cancellous bone for all loading conditions.

3. The tibial peg does not play a major role in the primary load transmission mechanism of the tibial plateau.

REFERENCES

1. Bartel, D.L., Burstein, A.H., Santavicca, E.A., et al.: Performance of the tibial component in total knee replacement. Conventional and revision designs. J. Bone Joint Surg. [Am.], *64*:1026, 1982.
2. Cavanagh, P.R., and Lafortune, M.A.: Ground reaction forces in distance running. J. Biomech., *13*:397, 1980.
3. Elftman, H.: The forces exerted by the ground in walking. Arb. Physiol., *10*:485, 1939.
4. Frankel, V.H., Burstein, A.H., and Brooks, D.B.: Biomechanics of internal derangement of the knee. J. Bone Joint Surg. [Am.], *53*:945, 1971.
5. Grood, E.S., and Noyes, F.R.: Cruciate ligament prosthesis: Strength, creep and fatigue properties. J. Bone Joint Surg. [Am.], *58*:1083, 1976.
6. Kurosawa, H., Fukubayashi, T., and Nakajima, H.: Load bearing mode of the knee joint: Physical behavior of the knee joint with or without menisci. Clin. Orthop., *149*:283, 1980.
7. Morrison, J.B.: The Forces Transmitted to the Human Knee Joint During Activity. Doctoral thesis, University of Strathclyde, 1967.
8. Noyes, F.R., Grood, E.S., Butler, D.L., et al.: Clinical laxity tests and functional stability of the knee: Biomechanical concepts. Clin. Orthop., *146*:84, 1980.
9. Paul, J.P.: Forces at the Human Hip Joint. Doctoral thesis, University of Strathclyde, 1967.
10. Seedhom, B.B., and Terayama, K.: Knee forces during the activity of getting out of a chair with and without the aid of arms. Biomed. Eng., *2*:278, 1976.
11. Smith, A.J.: A Study of the Forces on the Body in Athletic Activities with Particular Reference to Jumping. Doctoral thesis, Leeds University, 1972.

3 Surgical Approaches to the Knee

John N. Insall

It is not the purpose of this chapter to provide an exhaustive survey of all the described approaches to the knee,[1,5] but rather to discuss the exposures I have personally found useful. Through them all aspects of the knee can be reached and any type of knee surgery performed. Some of the approaches are extensile, and often only a portion of the approach is required to achieve the desired objective.

In regard to skin incisions, I would make a plea for one long incision rather than two short ones, provided that the amount of skin undermining is not excessive. For example, through a gently curved lateral parapatellar skin incision, both anteromedial and posterolateral capsular incisions can be made. If the skin incision is curved to the medial side, both anteromedial and posteromedial incisions in the capsule can be done easily. However, when it is necessary to approach the anterior, posteromedial, and posterolateral compartments, it may be necessary to reach the posterolateral compartment through a separate skin incision.

Skin necrosis after knee surgery is an ever-present hazard in young and old alike. Necrosis is particularly likely when there are previous scars on the knee. A skin incision that too closely parallels a former incision may result in necrosis of the skin bridge between them, even when the time between operations is long. For example, it was at one time the practice in our hospital to perform synovectomy of the knee through two incisions, one internal and one external. Some of these knees later required an arthroplasty, and it was then found that neither of the previous incisions was suitable, one being too medial and the other too lateral: Hobson's choice decreed that a single midline skin incision be made to do the arthroplasty. Extensive skin necrosis occurred in some cases. On the other hand, transverse skin incisions, such as are used for tibial osteotomy, can be crossed at right angles with impunity. We have never seen a case of skin necrosis occurring in such circumstances.

It is therefore the responsibility of the surgeon to remember that the currently planned operation may not be the last on that knee and to plan incisions accordingly. Henry's dictum[7] that a straight incision is generally preferable to a curved one seems sound, and most extensive knee surgery can be done very well through a single straight anterior midline incision of appropriate length. By extension proximally or distally, the lower femur and upper tibia can be beautifully exposed. Thus, quadricepsplasty or supracondylar osteotomy of the femur can be done very well through proximal extension of the midline incision and tibial osteotomy through distal extension. A straight anterior skin incision heals well and, in spite of its exposed position, causes neither tenderness nor discomfort when kneeling. There is some tendency for the superior part of the incision to stretch with

41

motion, but certainly no more than occurs with medial parapatellar skin incisions. Cosmetically, however, a slightly curved lateral parapatellar skin incision is preferable and can be used for this reason in
young women. Because the lymphatic drainage of the
knee is from lateral to medial, the traditionally curved
medial parapatellar skin incisions are the least desirable and should be avoided unless a simultaneous approach to the posteromedial compartment is intended
(Fig. 3.1).

A straight anterior incision can be reopened as many
times as necessary and can provide access to both
sides of the knee when this is necessary without making further skin incisions. Posteromedial and posterolateral skin incisions should also be straight. Lazy S
incisions at the side of the joint have no virtue.

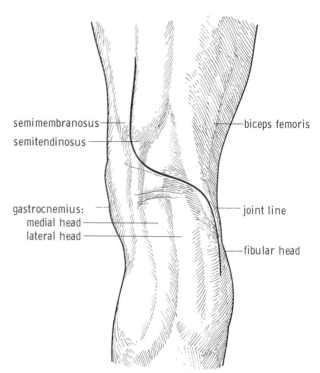

Fig. 3.2. The skin incision for posterior exposure of the
knee. This S-shaped incision is an exception to the rule of
straight skin incisions about the knee.

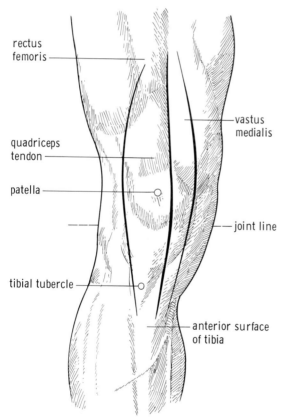

Fig. 3.1. Anterior skin incisions should be extensile to permit further proximal or distal exposure. The incision may
be straight anterior or gently curved in a lateral or medial
direction, particularly if a simultaneous posterolateral or
posteromedial capsular incision is required.

Skin incisions for open meniscal operations can be
made transverse. On the lateral side this is the preferred approach.[2] On the medial side an oblique skin
incision, provided that it is short, has never posed
difficulty with future surgery and need not be avoided.
Transverse incisions are not extensile, constituting the
major disadvantage of this approach.

The posterior skin creases do not correspond with
Langer's lines.[7] However, transverse skin incisions in
this region seem to heal well, and when there is the
infrequent need to expose the popliteal fossa widely,
one exception to the "straight" rule is made by using
a curved incision (Fig. 3.2).

Whether it is necessary to preserve branches of
cutaneous nerves is open to debate. Naturally, when
wide exposure is required, this is not possible, and
an area of numbness will result. Preservation of the
infrapatellar branch of the saphenous nerve during
meniscectomy is feasible and can be done if this is
the surgeon's preference. For many years I have ignored this branch and have not had cause to regret

the policy. The resulting numbness is trivial and usually disappears. Neuroma formation seems more related to the patient's temperament than to any actual pathologic process.

ANTERIOR APPROACHES

The skin incision can be straight anterior or C-shaped lateral parapatella, the latter giving a slightly better cosmetic appearance. The patella and extensor mechanism are then exposed. The straight skin incision has the advantage of requiring minimal mobilization of skin flaps to view the entire extensor apparatus.

The capsular incisions may be made in a variety of ways.

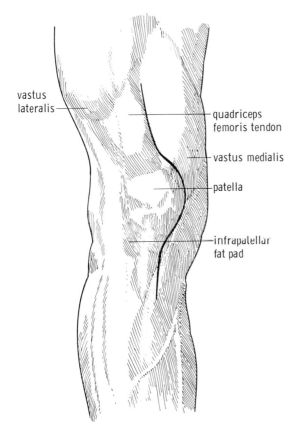

vastus lateralis

quadriceps femoris tendon

vastus medialis

patella

infrapatellar fat pad

Fig. 3.3. von Langenbeck approach. This incision divides transversely the lower fibers of vastus medialis that insert to the quadriceps tendon and adjoining part of the upper pole of the patella. The incision is susceptible to rupture at this point with early motion of the knee and should be discarded in favor of a straight capsular incision.

ANTEROMEDIAL APPROACH

In the anteromedial approach of von Langenbeck (Fig. 3.3),[10] the vastus medialis is dissected free from the quadriceps expansion, and the incision is extended medially through the patellar retinaculum in a curved manner, extending back to the margin of the patellar ligament beyond the patella and then distally along the line of the patellar ligament. The synovium is entered and a portion of the fat pad divided to permit a lateral dislocation of the patella.

This "standard" utility incision into the knee is mentioned only to condemn its use. Incisions that divide the insertion of the vastus medialis into the patella and further divide the medial retinaculum are akin to hip joint approaches that divide the abductor musculature. Repair of the quadriceps muscle and medial retinaculum is never as sound as it was before, unless prolonged immobilization is given, a condition that is seldom desirable or necessary. The following incision provides all the advantages of the medial parapatellar approach without these disadvantages.

MIDLINE INCISION

The midline incision (Fig. 3.4)[8] has been used for many years for all types of knee surgery requiring full exposure. I find it the exposure of choice for total knee arthroplasty, cruciate ligament repair, patellar realignment procedures, synovectomy (combined with a short posterolateral incision), and debridement of the knee. In concept, this approach is a modification of the split patellar approach of Jones[5] and that of Timbrell Fisher.[6] When the extensor mechanism is exposed, a straight incision is made beginning at the apex of the quadriceps tendon. The incision proceeds distally in the substance of the quadriceps tendon immediately adjacent to the vastus medialis insertion and is extended distally over the medial quarter of the patella and then through the anterior capsule and onto the subcutaneous surface of the tibia. The quadriceps expansion is peeled from the anterior surface of the patella by sharp dissection until the medial border of the patella is reached. The synovium is incised and the fat pad split in the midline to avoid injury to the medial meniscus. The transverse ligament can be divided. The patella is everted and dislocated laterally.

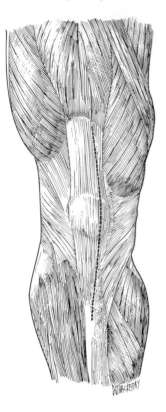

Fig. 3.4. The midline approach crosses the medial border of the patella and the quadriceps expansion can be peeled from the patella without directly dividing the insertion of vastus medialis. For this reason, closure of the incision has inherent stability. (From Insall, J.: A midline approach to the knee. J. Bone Joint Surg. 53A: 1584, 1971, with permission.)

When this incision is used for total knee arthroplasty, the distal extension onto the tibia is continued for several inches through the periosteum, at least 1 cm medial to the tibial tubercle. This allows a cuff of thick periosteum reinforced by the insertion of the pes anserinus insertion to be elevated from the tibia in continuity with the ligamentum patellae.

The advantage of this placement is that in a tight or stiff knee, accidental avulsion of the tibial tubercle is much less likely, and even if it does happen, the ligamentum patellae remains in continuity with a sleeve of the periosteum covering the tibia, which effectively anchors the ligament to the tibial tubercle. A second advantage of making the distal extension of the incision in this manner is that the periosteum thickened by the fibrous expansion of the pes anserinus holds sutures more effectively.

Proximal extension, if required, is made through the muscle medial to, but adjoining, the rectus femoris tendon. Full exposure of the lower third of the femur can be obtained; I have found this the best exposure for supracondylar osteotomy, as it allows circumferential exposure of the lower femur as the two

halves of the divided muscle fall backward when the knee is flexed.

The midline incision is usually closed by suturing the divided expansion side to side; because the incision is straight, an intact portion of the quadriceps expansion remains crossing the patella. The closure is inherently stable as can be demonstrated by flexing the knee as soon as the suturing is completed. Separation and retraction of the vastus medialis are not expected and the knee can be mobilized early without fear of capsular separation. The security of this closure has been demonstrated when early reexploration of the knee was required. On one occasion, as early as 2 weeks, the previous capsular incision was barely visible, and a new arthrotomy was made in the same manner. However extensive the midline incision, the

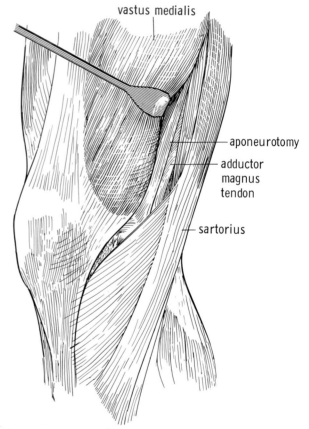

Fig. 3.5. Anteromedial incision preserving vastus medialis. The oblique portion of vastus medialis is separated from the adductor magnus tendon and mobilized proximally until the patella can be dislocated laterally.

aftercare requires no special precautions, although to prevent wound drainage, a few days in a compression dressing is recommended. Early weight-bearing is permitted.

ANTEROMEDIAL INCISION PRESERVING VASTUS MEDIALIS

In this approach (Fig. 3.5), the distal part of the incision is a slightly modified version of the midline approach. Proximally, instead of extending the incision in the manner described above, the deep fascia over vastus medialis is incised to expose the vastus medialis obliquus. The distal border of the muscle is mobilized by a combination of sharp and blunt dissection, until the origin from the adductor magnus tendon and aponeurosis is reached. The fleshy muscle fibers are separated from the aponeurosis as far proximally as the aperture for the femoral artery and vein. The synovium is entered and the patella dislocated laterally. In most patients the exposure obtained is only slightly less than by the midline route, and postoperative recovery is rapid. A minor disadvantage is that the vastus medialis is stretched by retraction. Also, vastus medialis tension cannot be adjusted during closure; with the midline approach, this is accomplished by overlapping the medial "flap" containing the muscle.

ANTEROLATERAL APPROACH

In the anterolateral approach described by Kocher (Fig. 3.6),[9] the capsular incision is made lateral to the quadriceps tendon in the substance of vastus lateralis and is continued distally along the lateral margin of the patella (it is in fact an extended "lateral release"). The approach permits imperfect visualization of the knee because the patella does not displace medially with ease, and only partial eversion is possible. The incision can be extended distally through the fat pad and gives a satisfactory view of the lateral compartment. Lateral meniscectomy can be done by this approach.

Otherwise, the anterolateral approach is mainly useful for three purposes:

1. *Quadricepsplasty*, allowing as it does good visualization of the vastus lateralis and vastus inter-

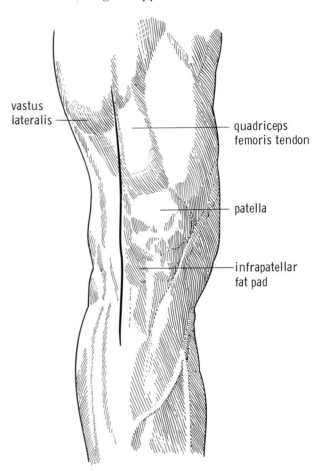

Fig. 3.6. Kocher anterolateral approach.

medius as well as sufficient intra-articular access to divide peripatellar adhesions.
2. *Lateral release*, in which a short longitudinal skin incision is sufficient, the release can be done by undermining the skin above and below the incision.
3. *Removal of loose bodies from the suprapatellar pouch*, where again, only the short central part of the incision is used.

MODIFIED INVERTED V APPROACH

Coonse and Adams[4] described an incision whereby a Y or V incision was made into the quadriceps tendon extending distally at the sides of the patella and patellar ligament to the tibia (Fig. 3.7A,B). The patella and patellar tendon were then reflected distally to expose the knee. Because of the need for a broad-based distal attachment to preserve a reasonable blood

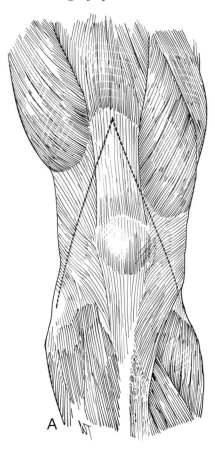

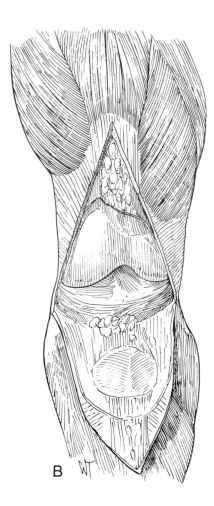

Fig. 3.7. Coonse and Adams inverted-**V** approach, showing (A) the markings of the capsular incisions, and (B) quadriceps tendon and patella turned distally on a broad-based flap based on the tibia.

supply, the decision to use this approach must be made in advance. I have modified this patellar turndown approach so that it can be adopted at any stage of the operation if there is difficulty in exposure or if quadriceps tightness imposes excessive tension on the patellar ligament insertion into the tibia. It is perhaps appropriate to stress that inadvertent avulsion of the patellar ligament from the tibia can be a disaster and adequate reattachment may not be obtained. A weak fibrous bond may occur, causing a permanent extension lag to result. Avulsion is most likely during an arthroplasty, when additional soft-tissue stripping of the upper tibia may devascularize the bone. In addition, prosthetic pegs or stems hamper the use of staples or screws for fixation of the avulsed tendon. Avulsion of the tibial tubercle should be prevented. The following approach provides a means of doing so.

PATELLAR TURNDOWN APPROACH

In the patellar turndown approach (Fig. 3.8A, B), the skin incision is straight midline, and the capsular incision crosses the medial quarter of the patella in exactly the same manner as described for the standard midline approach. In a knee that is stiff or in which the quadriceps is tight, further attempts to expose the joint may cause soft-tissue tearing or peeling from the tibia even though a periosteal "cuff" was developed. Before this occurs, a second incision is made inclined at 45 degrees from the apex of the quadriceps tendon extending laterally through the vastus lateralis and upper portion of the iliotibial tract. The second incision stops short of the vessels arising from the inferior lateral genicular artery to preserve the blood supply.

The exposure is comparable to that obtained by the

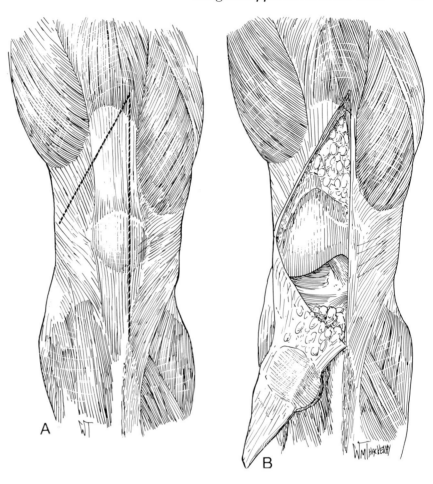

Fig. 3.8. (A) Patellar turndown approach. (B) This modification of the Coonse and Adams incision allows a conventional midline capsular approach to be converted into a patellar turndown.

Coonse and Adams approach and, in addition to increased versatility, it holds other advantages. The vastus medialis attachment to the tibia through the medial "flap" remains undisturbed and thus a more secure closure is obtained. The vertical incision and the apex of the quadriceps tendon are always repaired, but the oblique lateral incision into the vastus lateralis needs only partial repair or may indeed be left open if patellar tracking suggests that this is desirable. Flexion should be delayed for 2 weeks. Initially there will be an extension lag, but 6 months after surgery the lag will have almost invariably disappeared, and recovery of quadriceps strength to near normal has been the rule.

In addition to exposing stiff or ankylosed knees, the patellar turndown approach is being used with increasing frequency for arthroplasty revision operations.

INCISIONS FOR LATERAL MENISCECTOMY

ANTEROLATERAL APPROACH

The lateral meniscus can be excised through the lower portion of the anterolateral Kocher incision. This approach has the advantage of permitting proximal extension. However, if the lower portion alone is used, the approach is cramped and the posterior horn of the lateral meniscus may be difficult to mobilize.

TRANSVERSE APPROACH

The transverse approach of Bruser (Fig. 3.9)[2] takes advantage of the orientation of the iliotibial tract when the knee is flexed and the fibers more or less parallel

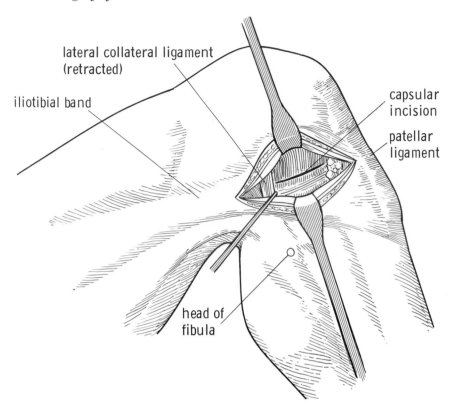

lateral collateral ligament
(retracted)

iliotibial band

capsular
incision

patellar
ligament

head of
fibula

Fig. 3.9. Bruser transverse approach for lateral meniscectomy.

the lateral joint line. With the knee fully flexed, a transverse skin incision is made beginning at the lateral border of the patellar tendon. The iliotibial band is split in the direction of its fibers and in the posterior part of the incision the lateral collateral ligament is identified and protected. The capsule and synovium are opened transversely superior to the lateral meniscus and the fat pad retracted anteriorly. This exposure provides limited access for the purposes of exploration, but is particularly suitable for the removal of discoid lateral menisci and cysts of the lateral meniscus.

INCISIONS FOR MEDIAL MENISCECTOMY

OBLIQUE ANTEROMEDIAL APPROACH

A short oblique anteromedial incision (Fig. 3.10) is made through skin, capsule, and synovium. The incision is aligned in a direction passing from the tibial tubercle to the midpoint between the patellar margin and medial epicondyle exposing the periphery of the

meniscus. It cannot, however, be extended without dividing the medial retinaculum and vastus medialis insertion. The infrapatellar branch of the saphenous nerve passes across the line of the incision and can be preserved if desired.

TRANSVERSE INCISIONS

A transverse incision at the level of the joint line provides access to the medial capsule in front and behind the medial collateral ligament. With suitable undermining of the skin, an oblique incision can be made through the anterior capsule and, through the posterior part of the incision, a vertical capsular incision provides access to the posterior compartment. The Cave approach (Fig. 3.11)[10] converts the transverse skin incision to the shape of a hockey stick, with an upward curve posteriorly.

POSTERIOR APPROACHES

Henry[3] describes posterior, posteromedial, and posterolateral approaches to the back of the lower femur and knee.

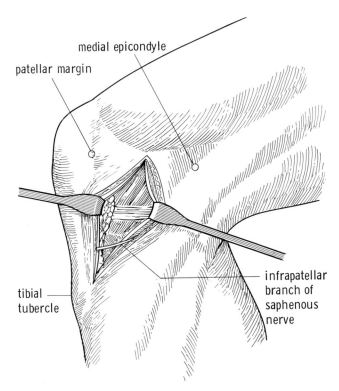

Fig. 3.10. Oblique anteromedial incision for medial meniscectomy.

nosus. Semimembranosus passing to the tibia is found in the posterior part of the incision. The saphenous nerve is found in front of the tendon of adductor magnus and, during the exposure, may be found in the wound or lying on the deep aspect of sartorius. In distal extension of the incision, the nerve is particularly likely to be encountered. The saphenous vein, on the other hand, lying on the surface of sartorius, is usually not seen.

Proximal extension of the incision exposes the popliteal fossa and the popliteal vessels, which lie one fingerbreadth from the bone. To reach the popliteal surface of the femur, some vessels must be divided, and to reach the back of the knee, it is usually necessary to ligate the medial superior genicular and the middle genicular arteries. Extended further proximally and displacing sartorius, the roof of Hunter's canal can be divided after ligating some large vessels that pass into the vastus medialis; the femoral and popliteal trunks can be mobilized and displaced. The medial half of the femur is then exposed by displacing

POSTEROMEDIAL APPROACH

The leg is positioned with the hip externally rotated and the knee partially flexed in the posteromedial approach (Fig. 3.12A–C). The adductor tubercle is identified and indicates the position of the skin incision, which is made vertically. Alternatively, when it is necessary to expose the anterior part of the knee simultaneously, an anteromedial skin incision is used and the posterior skin flap reflected. The incision is deepened in the interval between vastus medialis and sartorius to expose the upper aspect of the posteromedial capsule. The medial head of gastrocnemius attaches here with a fibrous origin adjoining the femoral insertion of the medial collateral ligament, the fibers becoming fleshy as the origin moves onto the popliteal face of the femur. An incision can be made into the knee behind the tibial collateral ligament and medial to gastrocnemius. Distal extension demonstrates the length of the tibial collateral ligament and the insertion of sartorius, gracilis, and semitendi-

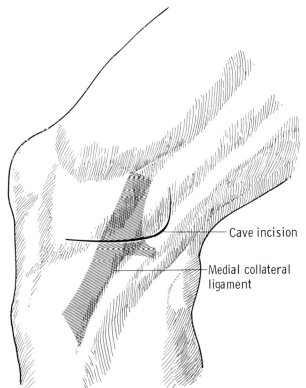

Fig. 3.11. Cave hockey-stick skin incision permits anterior and posterior capsular incisions.

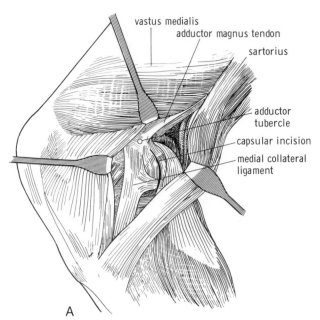

vastus medialis
adductor magnus tendon
sartorius
adductor tubercle
capsular incision
medial collateral ligament

A

Fig. 3.12. Posteromedial approach. (A) A vertical capsular incision posterior to the medial collateral ligament permits exposure of the posterior compartment and posterior horn of the medial meniscus. (B) Access to the posterior compartment. (C) Wider exposure is obtained by proximal extension separating the proximal capsule with the adjoining origin of medial head of gastrocnemius from the femur.

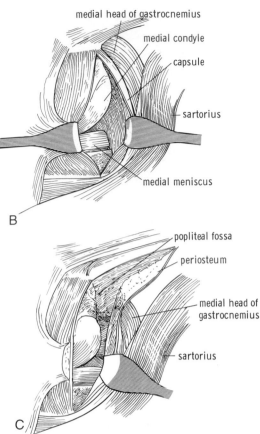

medial head of gastrocnemius
medial condyle
capsule
sartorius
medial meniscus

B

popliteal fossa
periosteum
medial head of gastrocnemius
sartorius

C

Fig. 3.13. A posterolateral approach between the lateral collateral ligament and arcuate ligament. The popliteus tendon crosses this space and cramps access. The tendon can, to some degree, be mobilized and retracted distally and because of its attachment to the lateral meniscus to a lesser degree proximally.

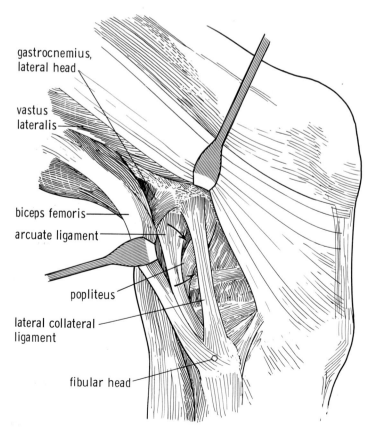

gastrocnemius, lateral head
vastus lateralis
biceps femoris
arcuate ligament
popliteus
lateral collateral ligament
fibular head

vastus medialis forwards and dividing the origin of the muscle from the adductor tendon and medial lip of the linea aspera.

POSTEROLATERAL APPROACH

The incision is placed vertically at the posterior margin of the iliotibial tract to develop the interval between this and the biceps, in the posterolateral approach. The knee is flexed slightly, and a skin incision is made vertically at this point, extending distally to the head of the fibula. Separating the interval between iliotibial tract and biceps tendon by dividing the deep fascia just above the lateral femoral condyle leads to the popliteal fossa. The posterolateral aspect of the knee capsule can be entered by identifying the tendon of popliteus, which is mobilized to retract distally. The lateral head of gastrocnemius and plantaris muscles can be mobilized and retracted medially and posteriorly (Fig. 3.13).

Alternatively, the lateral superior genicular artery

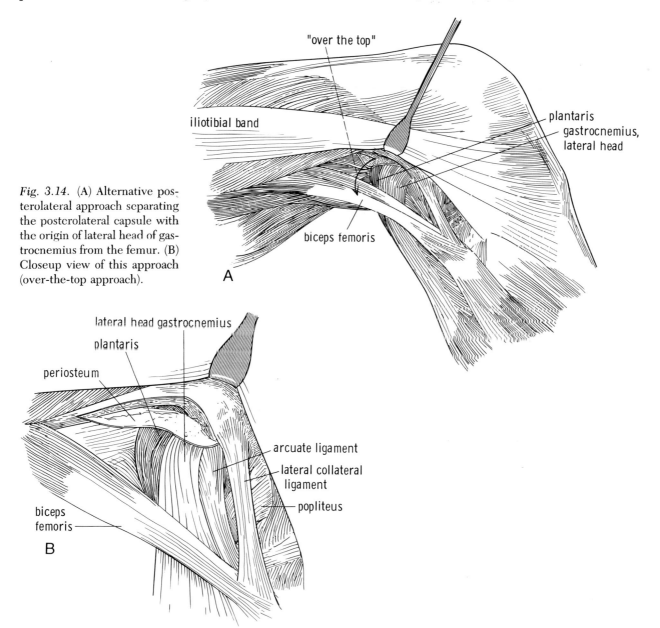

Fig. 3.14. (A) Alternative posterolateral approach separating the posterolateral capsule with the origin of lateral head of gastrocnemius from the femur. (B) Closeup view of this approach (over-the-top approach).

is ligated and the femoral shaft approached two fingerbreadths above the femoral condyle. The periosteum is incised and stripped from the posterior aspect of the femur until the condyle is reached. The posterior capsule is incised along its attachment to the condyle to enter the posterolateral compartment medial to the lateral head of gastrocnemius, which is retracted (or reflected) laterally (Fig 3.14A,B). When approaching the lateral compartment from above in this manner, it is sometimes easier to split the iliotibial tract, passing behind vastus lateralis to approach the lower femoral shaft directly. This route is also used to place a fascial graft for anterior cruciate substitution in the "over-the-top" manner. Proximal extension exposes the lateral femoral shaft by stripping vastus lateralis and dividing the lower perforating vessels from the profunda femoris. Distal extension of the incision exposes the fibular head and the peroneal nerve as it passes around the neck of the fibula.

POSTERIOR APPROACH

This approach provides access to the popliteal surface of the femur, the posterior capsule, and, extended distally, the posterior aspect of the tibia. The skin incision as it is generally made begins on the medial side along the tendon of semitendinosus, curving across the back of the knee before turning distally again. Alternatively, a straight skin incision crossing the flexor crease may be used (and in fact may be better, as this follows Langers' lines). The short saphenous vein lying on the deep fascia and the sural nerve lying beneath the fascia are the guides to the dissection (Fig. 3.15). The fascia is incised and the sural nerve is traced proximally until the medial popliteal nerve is reached. The fascia is incised proximally along the trunk of the medial popliteal nerve and the lateral popliteal nerve is identified. Dissecting the lateral popliteal nerve distally shows the lateral cutaneous nerve of the calf and the sural communicating nerve.

After the medial popliteal nerve is exposed distally, the twin heads of the gastrocnemius that join together in a shallow V are seen. Separating the two heads permits further distal exposure and identification of the muscular branches from the medial popliteal nerve to gastrocnemius, plantaris, soleus, and popliteus (Fig. 3.16). Beneath the medial popliteal nerve lie the popliteal vessels, approaching the nerve from the medial

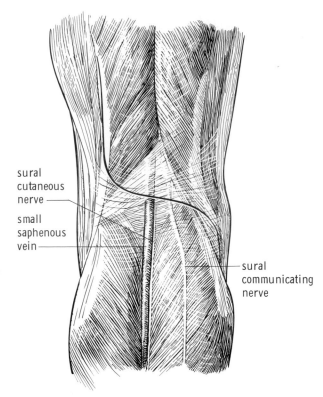

Fig. 3.15. The posterior approach to the knee is marked by the short saphenous vein and the sural cutaneous nerve.

side above and crossing anterior to the nerve to lie laterally below. One or more of the genicular vessels can be ligated for greater exposure. The posteromedial compartment is approached by freeing the medial head of gastrocnemius and retracting the muscle laterally to protect the popliteal vessels and nerves (Fig. 3.17). The posterolateral aspect of the knee is exposed by elevating the lateral head of gastrocnemius. The vessels and nerve may be retracted together; alternatively, the vessels may be retracted medially and the nerve laterally, in which case only the muscular branch to medial head of gastrocnemius will cross.

Distal extension below the knee is done by transecting popliteus, cutting along its medial aspect as indicated by the vertical fibers that pass distally from the semimembranosus expansion. The inferior medial genicular artery can be divided and the muscle belly mobilized laterally. The nerve to popliteus curves around the distal border of the muscle to enter its deep surface. Retracting the popliteus toward the fibula exposes the upper proximal tibia.

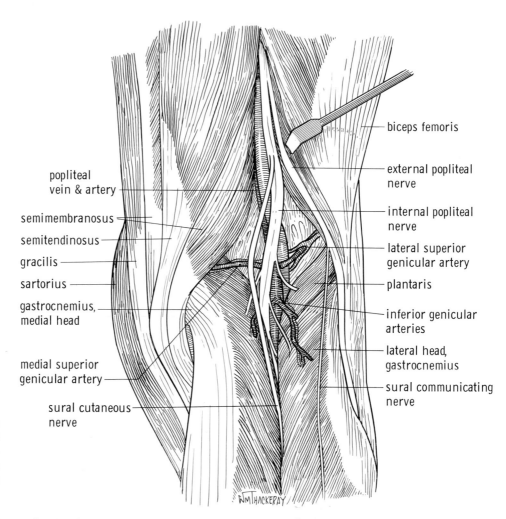

popliteal
vein & artery

semimembranosus

semitendinosus

gracilis

sartorius

gastrocnemius,
medial head

medial superior
genicular artery

sural cutaneous
nerve

biceps femoris

external popliteal
nerve

internal popliteal
nerve

lateral superior
genicular artery

plantaris

inferior genicular
arteries

lateral head,
gastrocnemius

sural communicating
nerve

WMTHACKERAY

Fig. 3.16. After the deep fascia are incised, the gastrocnemii are separated to expose the popliteal neurovascular structures.

Fig. 3.17. Division of the medial head of gastrocnemius allows lateral retraction together with the nerves, arteries, and veins and provides access to the posterior capsule of the knee.

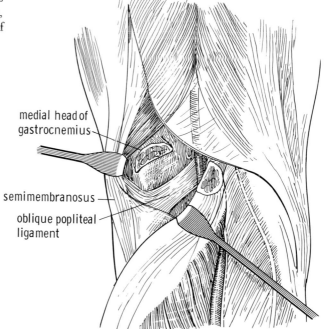

medial head of
gastrocnemius

semimembranosus

oblique popliteal
ligament

53

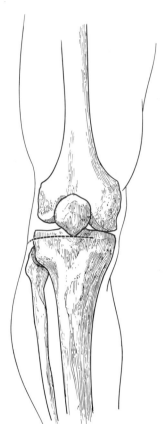

Fig. 3.18. The transverse lateral approach to the upper tibia.

TRANSVERSE LATERAL APPROACH TO THE UPPER TIBIA

A transverse skin incision is made one fingersbreadth proximal to the tibial tubercle extending laterally to the fibular head (Fig. 3.18). A vertical fascial incision is made along the lateral margin of the patellar ligament from which a horizontal incision is made

at the upper margin of the anterolateral musculature to the superior tibiofibular joint. The muscles are stripped from the anterolateral tibia, and the superior tibiofibular joint is divided with a periosteal elevator. Popliteus muscle is then separated from the posterior aspect of the tibia and a retractor inserted. With retraction of the patellar ligament forward, the upper tibia lies exposed.

REFERENCES

1. Abbott, L.C., and Carpenter, W.F.: Surgical approaches to the knee joint. J. Bone Joint Surg., 27: 277, 1945.
2. Bruser, D.M.: A direct lateral approach to the lateral compartment of the knee joint. J. Bone Joint Surg. [Br.], 42: 348, 1960.
3. Cave, E.F.: Combined anterior-posterior approach to the knee joint. J. Bone Joint Surg., 17: 427, 1935.
4. Coonse, K., and Adams, J.D.: A new operative approach to the knee joint. Surg. Gynecol. Obstet., 77: 344, 1943.
5. Edmonson, A.S., and Crenshaw, A.H., eds.: Campbell's Operative Orthopaedics, 6th Ed., Vol. 1. St. Louis, C.V. Mosby, 1980.
6. Fisher, A.G. Timbrell: The treatment of internal derangements of the knee-joint. A new method of operative exposure. Lancet, 1: 945, 1923.
7. Henry, A.K.: Extensile Exposure, 2nd Ed. Baltimore, Williams & Wilkins, 1970.
8. Insall, J.: A midline approach to the knee. J. Bone Joint Surg. [Am.], 53: 1584, 1971.
9. Kocher, T.: Text-book of Operative Surgery, 2nd Ed. (translated from 4th German Ed.). London, Adam and Charles Black, 1903.
10. von Langenbeck, B.: Zur Resection des Kniegelenks. Verh. Dtsch. Ges. Chir., 7: 34, 1878.

4 Examination of the Knee

John N. Insall

A good history and clinical examination will, in many cases, reveal the source of the complaints that bring a patient to the physician. Given the opportunity, the patient will often tell you the problem: "My knee cap went out," or "I felt something rip inside my knee." Similarly, a systematic and thorough clinical examination is invaluable. Watching how a patient stands and walks, for example, is sometimes omitted. However, a subtle varus deformity will not be appreciated with the patient supine, and the concomitant laxity of the medial ligament, which is actually secondary to bone erosion, may be mistakenly diagnosed as a primary ligament injury.

It is equally important that the surgeon know which conditions are most likely to be encountered in a given patient. This information, which will clearly differ for a 16-year-old athletic young man and a frail 70-year-old woman, will affect the thrust of the questioning, the interpretation of the answers, and the focus of the examination. Thus, for example, subtle tests for meniscal tears or ligamentous instability are inappropriate in a patient who has gross and obvious osteoarthritis.

It becomes apparent that a problem-oriented approach to examination, taking into strict account the variability in the types of disorders encountered among different age groups, can be extremely valuable and time saving. This chapter therefore begins by consid-

ering the examination of the knee in two different patient populations—those under age 45, and those over 45 years of age. The choice of this approach is not meant to imply that there are no uniformly applicable principles or that there is no overlap between these groups, but rather to emphasize the value of identifying a hierarchy of probable causes and directing one's examination along a pathway that is most likely to yield a diagnosis in the shortest time, minimizing both the expense and discomfort to the patient.

GENERAL CONSIDERATION OF DIAGNOSIS

PATIENTS UNDER 45 YEARS OF AGE

The most frequent conditions encountered in this patient population are meniscal lesions, ligament injuries, and patellar syndromes (pain and instability). In children, osteochondritis, monarticular arthritis, and tumors must be considered as well. The presenting complaint is nearly always either pain or instability with lesser complaints of swelling and locking.

Meniscal and Ligament Injuries

Such injuries are produced by trauma and are unilateral. A twisting or pivoting injury with the foot planted on the ground is most likely to injure a meniscus and sometimes the anterior cruciate ligament (ACL) as well; thus it is important to have the patient give as precise a description of the event as possible (Fig. 4.1). The sensation of a "pop" is very characteristic of a tear of the anterior cruciate ligament. This type of injury often occurs in sports such as tennis and skiing. Sometimes these injuries may seem relatively trivial and occur in the course of everyday activity, for example, while squatting in an awkward

position. Nevertheless, the precise moment of injury is usually fixed in the patient's mind. More severe injury occurring in contact sports suggests additional injury to the collateral ligament and the posterior cruciate ligament. Again, the patient's description of the event, if it can be elicited, is important, particularly in the assessment of the acute injury.

Patellar Dislocation

Similar types of injury can produce patellar dislocation. More typically, however, patellar instability—as well as other patellar pain syndromes—begins more

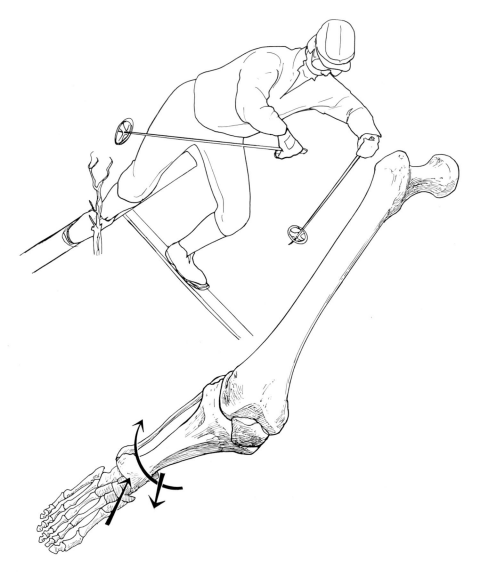

Fig. 4.1. A precise description of the mechanism of injury is important. Shown is the most common mechanism causing damage to the anterior cruciate ligament and the medial collateral ligament. (From Palmer, I.: On the injuries to the ligaments of the knee joint. A clinical study. Acta Chir. Scand. Suppl. 53: 1938, with permission.)

insidiously and is often bilateral. Bilaterality suggests an anatomic etiology, and a patellar problem should be suspected until proved otherwise. Patellar syndromes give rise to symptoms that are usually fairly constant (although varying in degree from time to time), whereas symptoms caused by a meniscal or ligament injury occur in episodes between which the knee is relatively symptom free. Inquiry must also be made into the severity of symptoms: Are they disabling or merely an inconvenience? Do they occur only in sports or in the course of everyday activities such as walking, climbing stairs, or sitting in a confined space (movie sign)? Are the symptoms of recent onset, or have they been present for years?

Site of Pain

Whereas the site of pain may be helpful in making the diagnosis, it is also often misleading. For example, tears of the medial meniscus produce pain and tenderness along the medial joint margin and are often strictly localized. However, patients with patellar disorders will often localize their pain to the same place. Similarly (although less frequently), lateral symptoms may arise from both lateral meniscus disorders and patellar derangements.

Details of Instability

The patient is often aware of what is happening and will describe how "my knee cap goes out." A statement such as "my knee comes apart" or a description of "sliding" sensations are given by patients with ligamentous instabilities. Instability may occur on a daily basis, but more often it is episodic, occurring during certain activities, particularly sports. In episodic cases, one needs to know the answers to the following questions: How often and how severe is the reaction? Is there much pain afterward? Can weight be borne on the leg, or are crutches required? A severe reaction after giving way suggests ligament instability. On the other hand, if buckling is very frequent and not followed by much pain or swelling, the cause is probably patellar. It is worthwhile trying to distinguish between forward buckling or giving way, which is patellar in origin, and buckling caused by abnormal motion from ligament insufficiency. A description that the knee goes backward or that it hyperextends on walking is usually a sensation produced by patellar

derangements (unless hyperextension is actually confirmed on physical examination).

Swelling

Often swelling of the knee is only a subjective sensation that cannot be objectively confirmed. True swelling is most noticeable above the patella, whereas subjective swelling is usually described as being in the infrapatellar region. Swelling after injury occurs immediately after ligament injuries and fractures, and the effusion is bloody when aspirated. Swelling that occurs several hours after injury is more likely to be caused by tears of the meniscus or patellar subluxation (although a traumatic patellar dislocation in a knee without a predisposing anatomic weakness is a severe injury and will present as one).

Locking

Mechanical causes, such as an interposed meniscal fragment, can cause locking of the knee and may be marked by characteristic diagnostic features. For example, transient locking in which the patient is aware of a loose body and may even be able to palpate the fragment is unlikely to be mistaken for anything else. Likewise, locking associated with a palpable meniscal tag cannot be misinterpreted. Locking can be caused by any abnormality that interferes with the complex gliding and rotational movements of the joint. Any disturbance of the instant center of rotation causes "jamming" of the joint surfaces and the appearance of a locked knee.[4] Thus, the interpretation of locking must be made with caution. I have seen a knee that remained locked in 15 degrees of flexion for 2 months after a patellar subluxation.

Inquiry into Athletic Activities

It can be informative to inquire into athletic activities. Patients adjust to their limitations and avoid motions that will cause them difficulty. Meniscal tears, cruciate injuries, and patellar subluxation all cause difficulty in "cutting," as well as a sensation of instability and apprehension. In regard to jumping, pain on takeoff has a patellar origin, whereas instability on landing suggests cruciate insufficiency.

Above all, look for patterns; common things occur

commonly, and the same history is given by different people with only minor variations over and over again. Familiarity with the usual patterns will also bring awareness when something does not fit. A discordant note, be it symptom or sign that is out of the ordinary, should alert the examiner, suggest care in evaluation, and necessitate a search for unusual causes.

PATIENTS OVER 45 YEARS OF AGE

Among older patients, degenerative conditions and osteonecrosis predominate. Acute meniscal tears do occur, but meniscal lesions are more commonly degenerative in origin. Patellar symptoms result from patellofemoral arthritis rather than malalignment. Pain and inability to walk are the usual presenting complaints. Buckling is described less frequently.

Description

A precise description of the onset of symptoms is helpful, particularly in relationship to injury. Degenerative disorders are often bilateral and usually of insidious onset. Osteonecrosis presents with dramatic suddenness,[13,18] and the patient recalls the very instant of the onset of symptoms ("I was crossing the street when. . . ." "I got out of bed and had this terrible pain. . . .").

Site of Pain

As in younger patients, the site of pain is not always helpful. For example, patellofemoral arthritis often causes popliteal pain; if there is, in addition, an associated popliteal cyst, the pain and the cyst may be erroneously connected. The phenomenon of hip arthritis presenting as knee pain is well known. Similar referral of pain takes place within the knee itself, and the site of pain sensation is not a good indication of its source. This seems particularly true of the patella, perhaps because of the wide derivation of its nerve supply. Examples, already cited, include localized medial pain and popliteal pain.

Giving Way and Locking

Less common symptoms in this age group are giving way and locking. When they do occur, these symptoms are usually caused by a loose body. The patient is typically aware of a loose body and can feel it moving around in the knee. Loose bodies are frequently seen in arthritic knees and are usually not significant in and of themselves. They should be ignored unless the patient has a specific complaint and is aware that the fragment is loose. The assumption that loose bodies cause pain without the patient sensing the presence of the fragment is wrong.

Assessment of Disability

In arthritic joints, an assessment of disability must be made, taking into account walking distance, standing ability, stair climbing, transferring from a chair, shopping, and the use of walking aids. The severity of pain is assessed during activity and rest. The knee rating form of the Hospital for Special Surgery (HSS) (Fig. 20.119) is an example of this type of assessment.

Among this patient population, other joint abnormalities must be considered. Lumbar radicular pain and the pain of hip arthritis may both refer to the knee. In rheumatoid arthritis, foot and ankle pain limit activity, which will be reflected in the knee rating. Stiffness and swelling in the fingers may signify a rheumatic origin of synovitis of the knee.

Current emphasis on physical fitness and activity has created a generation of older athletes who jog, ski, and enthusiastically play tennis and squash. More and more of these people end up in the orthopedic surgeon's office with knee complaints. The source of their symptoms is most frequently early degenerative arthritis of the patellofemoral joint, which is not readily apparent from routine radiographs.

SPECIFIC TESTS

ALIGNMENT

Alignment is best judged with the patient standing and walking; in this way, varus and valgus alignments and asymmetry between the two legs are more apparent than with the patient lying down. Torsional abnormalities such as femoral anteversion, external torsion of the tibia, and infacing of the patellae are most apparent when the patient stands with his feet together.

A thrust is a medial or lateral movement of the knee in the stance phase of walking (Fig. 4.2). It is usually present in arthritic knees that have developed an an-

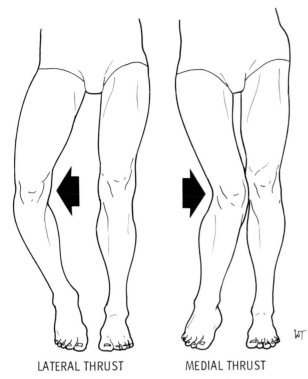

LATERAL THRUST   MEDIAL THRUST

Fig. 4.2. A "thrust" is a sideways movement of the knee in the stance phase of gait indicative of osteoarthritic erosion and secondary ligamentous instability.

gular deformity secondary to bone and cartilage erosion with secondary stretching of the opposite collateral ligament. The thrust is therefore lateral in medial osteoarthritis and medial in lateral osteoarthritis, and is caused by collapse of the joint into the position of deformity until it is limited by the tautness in the opposite ligament.

Both malalignment and thrust can be masked to some extent. For example, in varus malalignment the deformity is partially under voluntary control, and muscular patients are able to straighten the leg and disguise a thrust by muscular contraction acting through the iliotibial band. The thrust may therefore be most apparent after the patient has walked sufficiently to fatigue the muscles. Similarly, the full extent of valgus deformity is often lost because the knees come in contact with one another, preventing further angulation. Having the patient stand on one leg at a time will therefore be more informative.

A thrust backward into recurvatum is occasionally seen and may actually indicate a posterior capsular laxity. More often it is merely a symptom of an in-

ternal derangement, usually of the patella. Probably because the patient fears anterior buckling, the knee is thrust into hyperextension during the stance phase suggesting recurvatum, but careful inspection will demonstrate that the actual degree of extension is the same in both knees.

EFFUSION

An effusion is often visible as a fullness and swelling in the suprapatellar pouch. It is confirmed by palpation by ballotting the patella onto the femoral groove when a tap is felt. Lesser degrees of fluid in the knee may fail to actually separate the patella from the femur, and the presence of free fluid is then demonstrated by placing one hand on the suprapatellar pouch and the other hand more distally at the sides of the patella. Squeezing with one hand displaces fluid toward the other and a fluid thrill can be felt (Fig. 4.3). Very small effusions are best demonstrated by milking the fluid upward into the suprapatellar pouch and then milking it down again and observing the medial side of the joint where the capsule is thinnest. A fluid "wave" is seen.

Synovitis may be difficult to separate from an effusion. Synovial thickening and hypertrophy may occasionally be palpated, indicated by a lumpy enlargement, unlike the uniformly smooth swelling caused by fluid.

Crepitus can be felt and sometimes heard on joint motion and usually indicates articular degeneration, although this can sometimes be mimicked by para patellar synovial hypertrophy with synovial fringes becoming interposed between patella and femur. Crepitus may be quite normal in older patients and is not necessarily significant unless it is also painful. Patellar crepitus is best demonstrated by active extension of the knee from a flexed position with the examiner's hand placed over the patella.

Muscle strength is assessed by testing active extension against resistance and palpating quadriceps muscle bulk (Fig. 4.4).

MENISCUS TESTS

Numerous rotation tests for meniscus pathology have been described. Their purpose is to trap abnormally mobile or torn fragments of the menisci between the

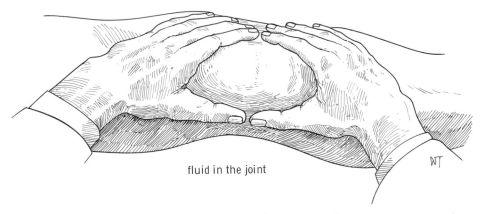

fluid in the joint

Fig. 4.3. Synovitis and effusion are detected by palpating the synovium. When the swelling is primarily caused by fluid, a fluid thrill can be transmitted by alternately compressing with the thumb and fingers of one hand and then the other. When the swelling is caused by synovial thickening, such a fluid thrill will not be appreciated, and the synovium has a lumpy feeling to palpation.

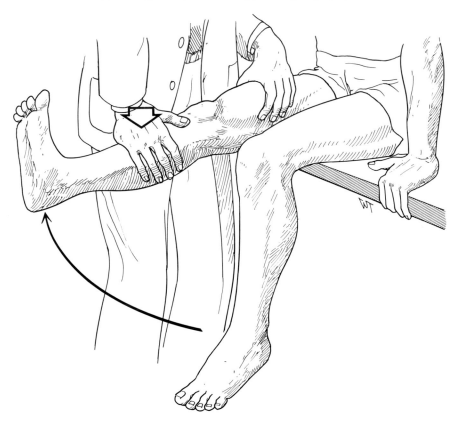

Fig. 4.4. Active extension of the knee against resistance elicits patellar crepitus and pain and gives an indication of quadriceps bulk and strength.

joint surfaces, thereby causing either pain or clicking. The three tests most widely used are the McMurray test, the Apley test, and the Steinmann test.

The McMurray test[15] is intended to diagnose lesions of the posterior horn of the meniscus. As described by its originator, it is done with the patient supine, the hip flexed 90 degrees and the knee flexed more than 90 degrees (Fig. 4.5). For examining the right knee, the examiner stands to the right of the patient with the left hand on the knee and the right hand holding the foot. The foot is taken from a position of abduction and external rotation to one of adduction and internal rotation. The maneuver is repeated for various angles between full flexion and 90 degrees. Entrapment of a damaged meniscus is demonstrated by a cartilage "jump" that can be felt by the fingers of the left hand appropriately placed on the medial or lateral joint line. The McMurray test has been frequently modified and is often done in another manner. The knee is placed in a position of flexion and external rotation and is then straightened to a position of full extension. It is not clear who originated this modification. Although the test may be useful in diagnosing bucket handle or other extensive tears of the meniscus, it is not specifically designed for lesions of the posterior horn and should not be called a McMurray test.

The Apley test[1] is a modification of the McMurray performed with the patient prone. The hip is extended and the knee is flexed more than 90 degrees. Downward pressure is applied on the foot, and the joint surfaces are thereby rotated and compressed slightly, changing the flexion angle (Fig. 4.6A). The maneuver is then repeated, but this time the joint is distracted rather than compressed (Fig. 4.6B). Meniscal lesions will be shown by clicking or pain in the compression part of the test, whereas ligamentous injuries will be apparent when the joint is distracted. This test is nullified when there is synovitis or a painful patellar disorder because of the pressure exerted on the knee by the examining table.

The third rotation test is the Steinmann,[17] and it is perhaps the best and most reliable. The Steinmann test is done with the patient seated and with the knee hanging loose over the edge of the examining table. With a flexion angle of at least 90 degrees, the foot is grasped and the tibia sharply rotated, first in an internal and then in an external direction (Fig. 4.7). A meniscal lesion is demonstrated by sharp pain at the appropriate joint line.

All these tibial rotation tests have diagnostic limitations that should be realized. All produce a painful response in patients with collateral ligament injuries, and the response may differ in the same knee from time to time.

Squatting and duck walking are also useful meniscal tests. Both usually cause difficulty in the presence of a damaged meniscus, but can be done easily by patients with other conditions that may mimic and be

confused with a torn meniscus. On the other hand, the half squat position is most difficult for patients with painful patellar disorders.

PATELLAR TESTS

A painful and tender patellar articular surface can be examined in three ways.

Direct palpation with the fingers is possible by alternate medial and lateral displacement; however, the soft tissues, particularly the synovium and capsule, are interposed, and if they are inflamed can give misleading results.

The same objection applies to compressing the patella against the femur in full extension, particularly if the maneuver is accompanied by quadriceps contraction on the part of the patient. Entrapment of the synovium from the suprapatellar pouch is common in these circumstances, and exquisite pain can be produced even in the normal knee by this test (Fig. 4.8).

Patellar pain is most reliably elicited with the knee in sufficient flexion to draw the patella into the femoral groove. This can be conveniently achieved by simply crossing one knee over the other (Fig. 4.9) or by placing a pillow beneath the knee. Patellar pain is then sought by compressing the patella with the thumb, first medially then laterally (Fig. 4.10). The lateral displacement test causes apprehension and guarding in cases of patellar instability, and the patient becomes fearful of a dislocation as the patella approaches the lateral lip of the femoral groove. With the thumbs placed on the lateral patellar border, compressing in a medial direction, pain is elicited in chondromalacia and osteoarthritis. The test is highly reliable and specific, and pain is seldom produced in a normal knee.

LIGAMENT TESTS

Laxity of the knee can vary from one person to another, so that the patient's opposite and presumably normal knee must be used as a control. The clinical examination of laxity is highly subjective, and the terms mild, moderate, and severe, or 1+, 2+, 3+, and 4+ can have different meanings. It is better to describe laxity in terms of estimated abnormal displacement (in millimeters). While the estimate may not be entirely accurate, there is at least a chance

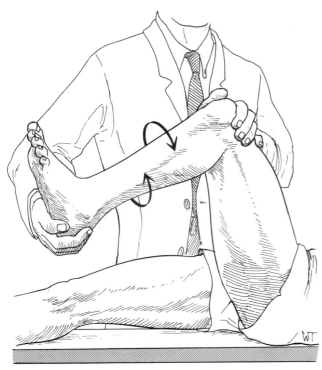

Fig. 4.5. The McMurray test is performed with the knee in flexion alternately internally and externally rotating the foot. A cartilage snap or jump is appreciated by the fingers of the other hand placed on the joint line.

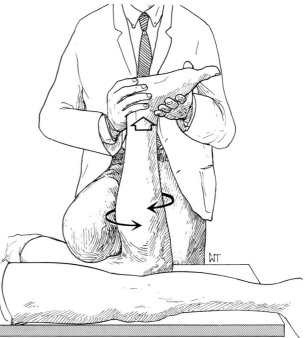

Fig. 4.6. The Apley test is a variation of the McMurray test. (A) The tibia is rotated on the femur applying axial compression. This part of the test is positive when there is a meniscal tear. (B) The maneuver is repeated but this time distracting the knee joint. The maneuver is supposed to differentiate between meniscal and ligamentous injuries.

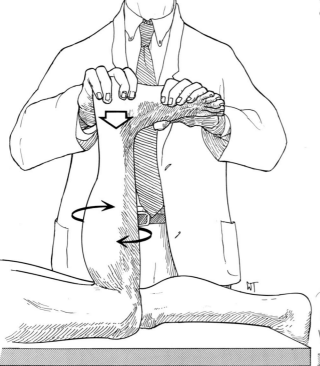

A

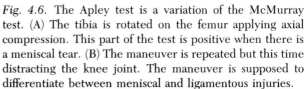

B

difficult of all. The interpretation of abnormal knee instability is open to controversy and debate, and the examiner will do well to assess first and foremost knee laxity in the four primary directions: medial, lateral, anterior, and posterior.

Although assessing straight medial or lateral instability is generally uncomplicated, there are some pitfalls that must be avoided. Convention has it that medial and lateral instability should be sought with the knee positioned at 30 degrees flexion on the assumption that in this position the posterior capsule and cruciate ligaments are relaxed. However, with the knee in this much flexion, rotary movements of the femur can easily occur unless the knee is precisely stabilized, and these motions may accentuate or be mistaken for medial and lateral laxity (Fig. 4.11). It is therefore recommended that this assessment be made in varying degrees of flexion from full extension (i.e., extension but not hyperextension) to 30 degrees. Only the very slightest degree of flexion is required to relax the posterior capsule, and with the knee flexed this almost imperceptible amount, it is much easier to stabilize the femur and prevent rotation. The test should be done with the hands, one holding the foot and the other placed at the side of

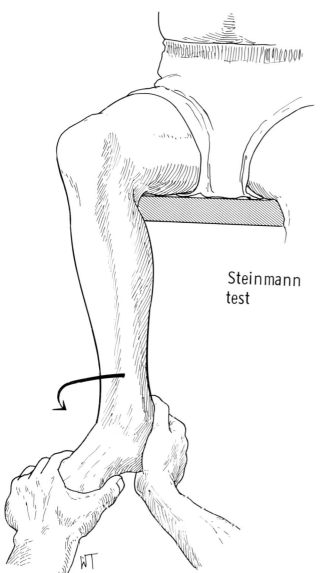

Steinmann test

Fig. 4.7. The Steinmann test is performed with the knee hanging loose over the edge of the table. The examiner sharply rotates the foot in both internal and external directions. When done as shown, the test is positive when pain is felt medially.

that this method may be reproducible by others who may later examine the knee on subsequent occasions. Stress radiographs may in some circumstances be used to confirm the clinical impression. Most examiners have little difficulty in assessing medial and lateral instability; anteroposterior instability is more difficult, and combined or rotary instabilities are the most

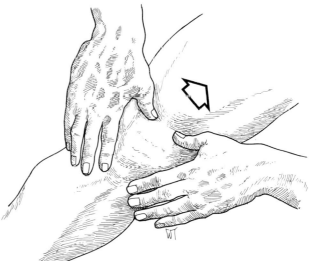

Fig. 4.8. The patellofemoral joint is frequently tested by holding the patella distally and asking the patient to tighten the quadriceps muscle. Unfortunately the synovium of the suprapatellar pouch is often trapped in this maneuver, giving a false-positive result.

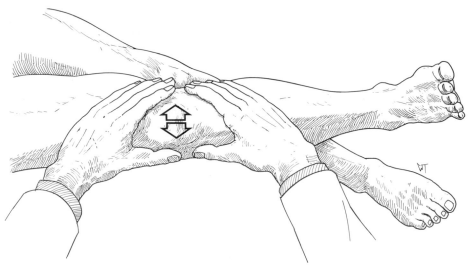

Fig. 4.9. Patellar testing should be done with the knee in sufficient flexion to draw the patella into the femoral groove thus avoiding the possibility of synovial entrapment. This can be done either by crossing one knee over the other or by placing a bolster beneath the knee.

the knee joint (Fig. 4.12A,B). Forcible stress will often be painful, and the motion should be most gentle.

Anteroposterior instability can also be assessed with the knee in the same position of almost full extension (the Lachman test) (Fig. 4.13).[20] This testing is diffi-

cult for examiners who have small hands, particularly when the patient is muscular and the thigh is large. Again the sensation of instability transmitted through the hands and fingers is as important as the amount of visible displacement, which in any case is often

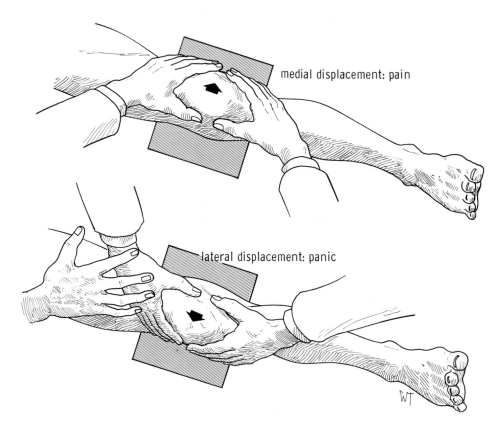

medial displacement: pain

lateral displacement: panic

Fig. 4.10. (Top) Medial compression displacement in the slightly flexed knee reproduces pain. (Bottom) Lateral displacement can cause great apprehension when the patella is unstable.

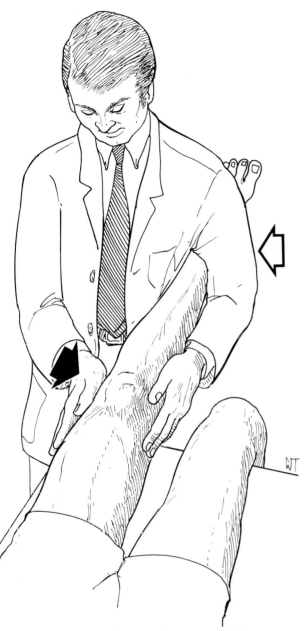

Fig. 4.11. Lateral instability is often tested in this manner, the foot held beneath the examiner's arm. Unfortunately it is difficult to prevent femoral rotation which, if accompanied by slight flexion of the knee, can mimic or accentuate collateral ligament instability.

more apparent to an observer than it is to the examiner. (For this reason, the experience of the examiner is all important.) There are other difficulties with the Lachman test. It is seldom possible to estimate with any precision the actual amount of dis-

placement in millimeters, nor is it possible to say precisely whether the laxity is anterior, posterior, or both. However, this test has the advantage that it does not require patient cooperation, and the laxity is not masked by lack of muscular relaxation. The drawer test[14] done at 90 degrees of flexion, on the other hand, permits a more precise description of laxity and—from a comparison of the appearance of the two knees—permits an estimate of whether the displacement is anterior or posterior. In the case of posterior laxity, a dropback of the tibia in the resting position can be seen when the contour of the knee is compared with that of the opposite side. Tibial dropback can also be assessed with hips and knees flexed 90 degrees and the feet supported. When the neutral position appears visually the same on the two sides, abnormal anterior laxity can be attributed solely to the anterior cruciate ligament (Fig. 4.14) and posterior laxity to a lesion of the posterior cruciate ligament. With the knee in flexion, a quantitative assessment of laxity is also easier and should be described. Unfortunately, the anterior drawer test is quite dependent on patient cooperation, as tension in the hamstring muscles can negate the test.

The anterior and posterior drawer tests are usually done with the patient supine, the knee flexed 90 degrees, and the feet stabilized by the examiner seating himself upon them (Fig. 4.15). The upper tibia is grasped between fingers and thumb with the fingers palpating the hamstring and biceps tendons to ensure relaxation. A firm discrete pull forward gives evidence of laxity by vision and touch, and the tactile sensation can be enhanced if the thumbs are extended upward to press on the femoral condyles. The "end point" at the limit of the anterior excursion denotes continuity in the anterior cruciate ligament. The end point, however, is extremely subjective and may not be reproducible. The feeling is that motion is sharply limited, a sensation similar to tugging on the end of a rope. When the ligament is absent, the end point is spongy and not firm.

Posterior cruciate lesions are indicated by tibial dropback, and the extent of further posterior laxity to the "end point" is assessed by anterior pressure on the upper tibia (Fig. 4.16). To some extent the posterior drawer is influenced by the pull of the ligamentum patellae; therefore, the quadriceps muscle should be relaxed. In a tense patient, the drawer test can be done with the patient seated and the knees

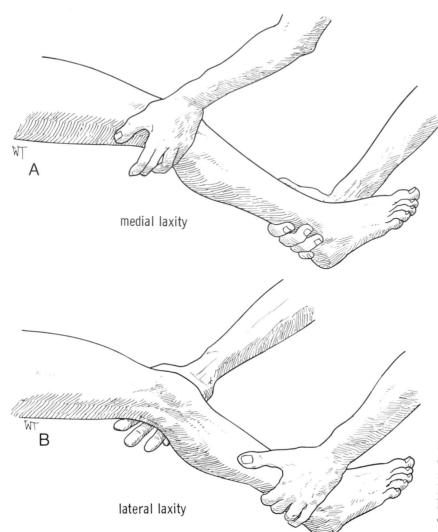

medial laxity

lateral laxity

Fig. 4.12. (A, B) To avoid femoral rotation, it is recommended that medial and lateral laxity be tested, thus using the hands alone. Tests should be done extremely gently to avoid causing pain.

flexed over the table. The foot can be stabilized between the examiner's knees. Muscle relaxation is often better in this position, but the measurement of laxity is less precise, and the neutral point not so clearly defined.

Definition of the neutral point is critical to any assessment of anteroposterior instability. Without it, posterior laxity may be erroneously diagnosed as anterior, and combined cruciate injuries will not be appreciated. Most errors in diagnosis are therefore made in the anteroposterior plane. Combined instability is present when there is two-plane laxity (medial and anterior are the most common). This subject is discussed further in Chapter 12. It will suffice here

to describe an extremely useful test known variously as the lateral pivot shift test,[5] the jerk test,[7] the Losee test,[12] and the anterolateral rotary instability test.[19] The manner of performing the test and its interpretation depend on the particular originator. I am most familiar with the pivot shift (Fig. 4.17), which is performed as follows. The patient lies supine with the knee extended. The foot is grasped in one hand while the other hand is placed fingers forward with the palm behind the fibular head. The foot is slightly internally rotated and, with the patient relaxed, the knee is flexed by pressure applied posterolaterally, at the same time exerting a mild valgus stress. The normal knee, without laxity, tested in this manner, moves in a smooth

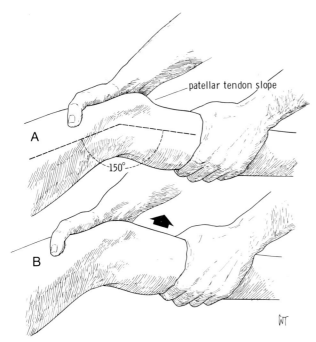

Fig. 4.13. The Lachman test performed with the knee in slight flexion. Although the test is sensitive for anteroposterior instability, because the effect of muscle contraction is eliminated, it is difficult to assess the *direction* of the instability with accuracy.

METHOD OF EXAMINATION

It is strongly recommended that examination of the knee proceed in a stepwise manner in order to avoid omission. The examination is modified, however, according to age and probable diagnosis. For example, one does not normally look for thrust in teenage patients, nor is it appropriate to ask an elderly woman who has obvious osteoarthritis to squat or duck walk. Similarly, a detailed ligament examination is not necessary in severe osteoarthritis. That is not to say that ligament instability in the arthritic knee is unimportant, but rather that the parameters are different. In patients with arthritis, one is more concerned with collateral ligament balance than with anteroposterior instability to the extent that alterations in ligament length contribute to fixed angular deformity.

Taking it for granted that common sense dictates these modifications, the examination should proceed as follows. There should be sufficient space to view the patient standing and walking, and the patient should be undressed or in shorts to view the whole length of the limb. Beginning with the patient standing with the feet together, angulation, flexion deformity, hyperextension, and patellar "squinting" can be seen. Walking may display a limp or a thrust. Sometimes the character of the limp may suggest a hip disorder presenting as referred pain to the knee. Asymmetry in the limbs can be noted.

Younger patients should be asked to assume a half knee bend, progressing to a squatting position, followed by an attempt at duck walking. Loss of flexion and the location of pain, when present, are noted. Running in place, hopping on one leg, and a standing broad jump are performed.[2] The broad jump should be done barefooted, jumping off and landing on one foot at a time. Patients with ligament insufficiency or patellar subluxation usually have difficulty with this test, and the difference between performance on the two legs should be measured.

Older patients should be asked to sit in and rise from a straightbacked chair, and the need for hand assisted pushoff should be noted. The ease with which the examining table is mounted is observed. A stool permits assessment of stair-climbing ability, particularly in older patients, and the need for the use of hands is again noted.

The next series of observations are made with the patient sitting with the knee flexed over the exam-

arc, whereas when the test is positive, at or about 30 degrees of flexion, a sudden, posterior shift of tibia on femur will be seen or felt, sometimes appreciated as a clunk. The shift is caused by reduction of anterior subluxation of the tibia and is accentuated by compressing the knee by axial pressure on the foot as the knee is flexed. The interpretation of the pivot shift phenomenon is open to debate. It is my personal observation that the pivot shift is diagnostic of anteroposterior laxity. The most common cause is anterior cruciate insufficiency.[3] A true pivot shift is not obtained in posterior cruciate laxity, but something similar to it can occur if the tibia subluxes backward in flexion.[10] Usually the motion is more gentle and can be prevented when the tibia is held forward as the knee is flexed.[12] The phenomenon is never produced by collateral laxity alone; it can occur when collateral stability is normal, but is more pronounced when there is combined anteroposterior and mediolateral laxity. In addition to its diagnostic value, the pivot shift seems of more functional significance than the other static tests, correlating better with complaints of instability.

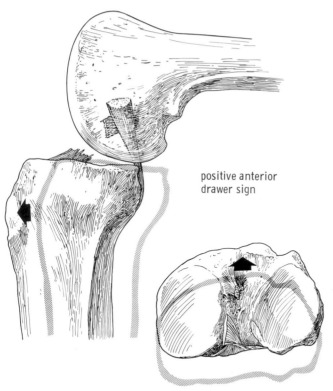

positive anterior
drawer sign

Fig. 4.14. When the neutral position of the two knees in flexion is the same, anterior instability can be confidently attributed to incompetence of the anterior cruciate ligament.

ining table. From the flexed position, the knee is actively extended and the motion repeated against resistance. Crepitus, muscle weakness, extension lag, and patellar tracking are assessed. Pain, when present, is noted. The Steinmann rotation test is next performed, followed by the anterior drawer test.

The patient now lies down; swelling around the knee, both generalized and local, is sought. Skin changes (e.g., the bluish-red discoloration of sympathetic dystrophy) and previous scars are recorded. The quadriceps bulk is assessed visually and by measurement and the muscle tone palpated when contracted. The knee is then palpated for swelling, effusion, synovitis, cysts located around the joint line and in the popliteal fossa, and enlargement of bursae. Tenderness is sought over the joint line, the bony landmarks of the femur and tibia, and tendon insertions. The knee is flexed across the other and the patellar compression test performed. The precise range of motion compared with the opposite side is recorded, noting any loss in extension when the legs are lifted by the heels, and a heel-to-buttock measurement is

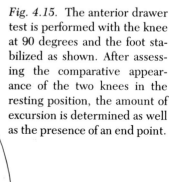

Fig. 4.15. The anterior drawer test is performed with the knee at 90 degrees and the foot stabilized as shown. After assessing the comparative appearance of the two knees in the resting position, the amount of excursion is determined as well as the presence of an end point.

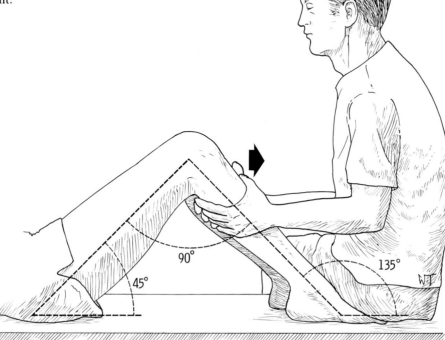

90°

45°

135°

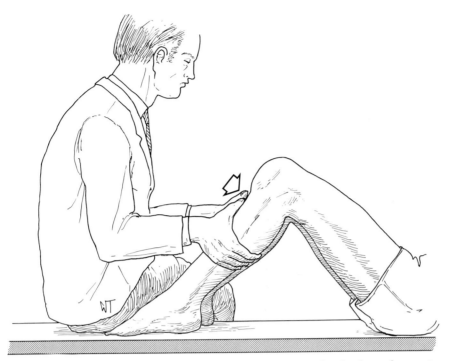

Fig. 4.16. Usually with posterior cruciate laxity there is a dropback in the resting position, so that there is a concavity beneath the patella on the affected side. Further backward pressure by the examiner demonstrates the extent of the laxity.

Fig. 4.17. The pivot shift test for anterior cruciate insufficiency. As the knee is brought from flexion into extension, a jump is noticed at 30 degrees of flexion caused by anterior tibial subluxation.

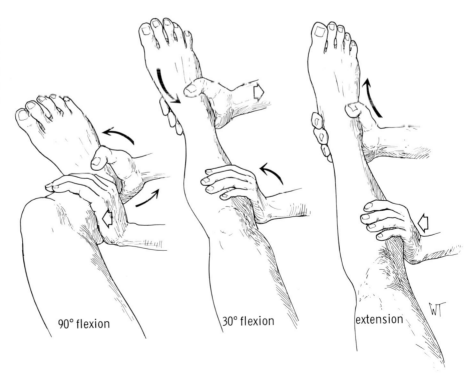

90° flexion   30° flexion   extension

made on both sides. Abnormal motion is recorded next, concentrating on detailed ligament assessment or ligament balance as seems appropriate. The McMurray test is done and the patient then turned prone for the Apley test. In this position, the back of the knee and popliteal fossa are examined.

Local examination of the knee should always include the hips, ankles, and feet, as well as palpation of the peripheral pulses; a more detailed general examination is done at this stage as needed.

ADDITIONAL INVESTIGATIONS

RADIOLOGIC EVALUATION

Radiographs of both knees should always be made for comparative purposes. Standard views should include a standing anteroposterior view of sufficient length to permit measurement of alignment, a true lateral view with the knee in partial flexion, and a patellofemoral skyline view. Oblique and tunnel views are not generally helpful and should not be done as a routine, but only as indicated in specific cases.

The standing anteroposterior view is often omitted, with the result that joint space narrowing diagnostic of arthritis may not be seen on supine views. Moreover, even when the diagnosis of arthritis is obvious, the full extent of deformity and instability will not be apparent unless a weight-bearing view is made. The standing film is the single most important observation to be made in a patient over 40 years of age, and to omit it is to deprive oneself of often critical information, regarding both diagnosis and alignment.

The lateral view is primarily of interest in regard to patellar position. Partial flexion ensures that the patellar ligament is taut. The diagonal length of the patella and the distance from lower pole to tibial tubercle should be measured.[8] Normally these are equal; if the patellar ligament is longer, the patella is high riding (suggesting that perhaps the patient's complaints are patellar in origin). The skyline view[11,16] is also a patellar view, and patellar osteoarthritis and patellofemoral incongruence can be assessed.

The radiographs also provide helpful information in cases of osteochondritis, loose bodies, trauma, and, more rarely, tumors.

ARTHROGRAPHY

To be useful, the arthrogram must be of the highest quality; an examination that does not show clear tangential views of the meniscus is not only useless, but misleading. Erroneous interpretation of a poor-quality arthrogram has probably led to many unnecessary meniscectomies, and unless good quality arthrography is available, the test should be omitted. However, a double-contrast arthrogram performed by an expert radiologist is arguably the most accurate method of diagnosing meniscal lesions and, with the proper technique, provides useful information about the integrity of the anterior cruciate ligament. The arthrogram may also provide information about osteochondritic lesions, outline loose bodies, and show soft-tissue synovial tumors (e.g., in patients with pigmented villonodular synovitis). Thinning and irregularity of articular cartilage (particularly femorotibial) can sometimes be seen, but the arthrogram is not very useful for the assessment of the patellofemoral joint.

ARTHROSCOPY

I do not recommend routine diagnostic arthroscopy, except when good-quality arthrography is unavailable. Patellar disorders and ligament insufficiency are best diagnosed by clinical examination, so that unless the state of the meniscus is in doubt, there seems little reason to arthroscope the knee except for learning purposes. However, it is recognized that arthrographic skills vary greatly; for many surgeons, the arthroscope is therefore essential. The danger of routine arthroscopy is that its limitations may not be realized, or that a too mechanistic approach to the knee will be made. It is now well accepted that asymptomatic meniscal tears and patchy erosions of the articular cartilage are common and age dependent. An arthroscopic confirmation of their presence does not necessarily provide a diagnosis.[6] On the other hand, one of the commonest causes of knee pain is patellofemoral incongruence, in which there may be no articular damage at all. In this condition, the arthroscope is useless and the diagnosis must be made from a combination of clinical examination and the patellofemoral skyline view.

STRESS RADIOGRAPHS

Varus and valgus stress films provide objective and quantitative measurement of collateral ligament instability. They are particularly useful in the assessment of acute ligament injuries and may be done under anesthesia when pain prevents an adequate examination. Anteroposterior stress radiographs done by the method of Jacobsen[9] can sometimes provide information that is not available by any other means. For example, in doubtful cases the direction of instability (anterior, posterior, or both) can only be determined by radiographically assessing the neutral point in comparison with the normal side.[21] However, the measurement required is somewhat complicated and sensitive to any out-of-plane motion that may occur during the course of the test. For example, femoral or tibial rotation can produce measurement errors of such a degree as to render the result invalid; conclusions can only be drawn when the position is comparable on all the views. Stress films usually require the development of some kind of jig or testing machine and are not really applicable for general use.

SCINTIMETRY

Scintimetric examination by technetium-99m scan is diagnostic in cases of osteonecrosis when routine radiographs are normal. Scintimetry may indicate early degenerative arthritis as well, also not apparent on routine radiographs; this finding may be significant and relevant in making the decision to remove a degenerative meniscus diagnosed by arthrography or arthroscopy. Scintimetry may also indicate an unsuspected tumor.

REFERENCES

1. Apley, A. G.: The diagnosis of meniscus injuries. Some new clinical methods. J. Bone Joint Surg., 29: 78, 1947.
2. Daniel, D., Malcom, L., Stone, M.L., et al.: Quantification of knee stability and function. Contemp. Orthop., 5: 83, 1982.
3. Fetto, J.F., and Marshall, J.L.: Injury to the anterior cruciate ligament producing the pivot-shift sign. J. Bone Joint Surg. [Am.], 61: 710, 1979.
4. Frankel, V.H., Burstein, A.H., and Brooks, D.B.: Biomechanics of internal derangement of the knee. Pathomechanics as determined by analysis of the instant centers of motion. J. Bone Joint Surg. [Am.], 53: 945, 1971.
5. Galway, R.D., Beaupré, A., and MacIntosh, D.L.: Pivot shift: A clinical sign of symptomatic anterior cruciate insufficiency. J. Bone Joint Surg. [Br.], 54: 763, 1972.
6. Goodfellow, J.: He who hesitates is saved (Editorial). J. Bone Joint Surg. [Br.], 62: 1, 1980.
7. Hughston, J.C., Andrews, J.R., Cross, M.J., et al.: Classification of knee ligament instabilities. Part II. The lateral compartment. J. Bone Joint Surg. [Am.], 58: 173, 1976.
8. Insall, J., and Salvati, E.: Patella position in the normal knee joint. Radiology, 101: 101, 1971.
9. Jacobsen, K.: Stress radiographical measurement of the anteroposterior, medial and lateral stability of the knee joint. Acta Orthop. Scand., 47: 335, 1976.
10. Jakob, P., and Staubli, H.U.: The reversed pivot shift sign—A new diagnostic aid for posterolateral rotatory instability of the knee. Its distinction from the true pivot shift sign. Orthop. Trans., 5: 487, 1981.
11. Laurin, C.A., Dussault, R., and Levesque, H.P.: The tangential x-ray investigation of the patellofemoral joint: X-ray technique, diagnostic criteria and their interpretation. Clin. Orthop., 144: 16, 1979.
12. Losee, R.E., Johnson, T.R., and Southwick, W.O.: Anterior subluxation of the lateral tibial plateau. A diagnostic test and operative repair. J. Bone Joint Surg. [Am.], 60: 1015, 1978.
13. Lotke, P.A., Ecker, M.L., and Alavi, A.: Painful knees in older patients. Radionuclide diagnosis of possible osteonecrosis with spontaneous resolution. J. Bone Joint Surg. [Am.], 59: 617, 1977.
14. Marshall, J.L., Wang, J.B., Furman, W., et al.: The anterior drawer sign: What is it? J. Sports Med., 3: 152, 1975.
15. McMurray, T.P.: The semilunar cartilages. Br. J. Surg., 29: 407, 1941.
16. Merchant, A.C., Mercer, R.L., Jacobsen, R.H., et al.: Roentgenographic analysis of patellofemoral congruence. J. Bone Joint Surg. [Am.], 56: 1391, 1974.
17. Ricklin, P., Ruttiman, A., and del Buono, M.S.: Meniscal Lesions. Practical Problems of Clinical Diagnosis, Arthrography, and Therapy. New York, Grune & Stratton, 1971.
18. Rozing, P.M., Insall, J., and Bohne, W.H.: Spontaneous osteonecrosis of the knee. J. Bone Joint Surg. [Am.], 62: 2, 1980.

19. Slocum, D.B., James, S.L., Larson, R.L., et al.: Clinical test for anterolateral rotary instability of the knee. Clin. Orthop., *118*: 63, 1976.

20. Torg, J.S., Conrad, W., and Kalen, V.: Clinical diagnosis of anterior cruciate ligament instability in the athlete. Am. J. Sports Med., *4*: 84, 1976.

21. Torzilli, P.A., Greenberg, R.L., and Insall, J.: An in vivo biomechanical evaluation of anterior-posterior motion of the knee. Roentgenographic measurement technique, stress machine, and stable population. J. Bone Joint Surg. [Am.], *63*: 960, 1981.

5 Radiographic Examination of the Knee

Helene Pavlov

A routine radiographic examination of the knee must include a minimum of two views: anteroposterior (AP) and lateral. In addition to the AP and lateral views, two other projections are usually included in the routine knee examination: a tunnel and a patellofemoral view.

The AP view is obtained with the knee extended, the cassette placed posterior to the knee, and the central ray perpendicular to the cassette. The patient should be standing, but if the affected knee is unable to bear weight, a supine AP view is acceptable. An abnormality, particularly if related to alignment, is enhanced on a standing weight-bearing projection. Demonstrated on the AP view are the medial and lateral soft tissues, the weight-bearing aspects of the medial and lateral femoral condyles, the proximal tibia and fibula, the patella, the medial and lateral joint compartments, and the femoral–tibial alignment (Fig. 5.1A).

The lateral view of the knee is obtained with the knee in 30 degrees of flexion and the patient lying on the affected limb. The cassette is placed posterior to the knee and the central ray is perpendicular to the cassette. If the clinical concern is the femoral–tibial alignment, the lateral view should be obtained with the patient standing with a straight knee. Demonstrated on the lateral view are the suprapatellar pouch, the quadriceps tendon, the patellar tendon, the distal femur, the proximal tibia and fibula, the patella, and the patellofemoral alignment (Fig. 5.1B).

A tunnel view is a frontal view obtained with the knee in 60 degrees of flexion. It can be an AP view performed with the patient supine, the cassette posterior to the knee, and the central ray perpendicular to the tibia, or it can be a posteroanterior (PA) view obtained with the patient kneeling on the cassette, the tibia parallel to the cassette, and the central ray perpendicular to the tibia. Demonstrated on the tunnel view are the posterior aspect of the medial and lateral femoral condyles, the intercondylar notch, the tibial spines, and the tibial plateau (Fig. 5.1C).

A patellofemoral view can be obtained in numerous ways, but the Merchant or mountain view is preferred to the skyline.[4,5,20] The Merchant view is obtained with the patient supine, the knees flexed 45 degrees, the cassette distal to the patella and the central ray inclined inferiorly 30 degrees from the horizontal (Fig. 5.1D). Both knees are usually examined together but lateral divergence of the x-ray beam is minimized if each knee is examined separately. The patellofemoral joint is demonstrated on the Merchant or mountain view (Fig. 5.1E). The skyline view, obtained with the knee in maximum flexion, also demonstrates the posterior surface of the patella and the anterior surface of the femur but the femoral surface is distal to the patellofemoral joint.[4] Patellofemoral

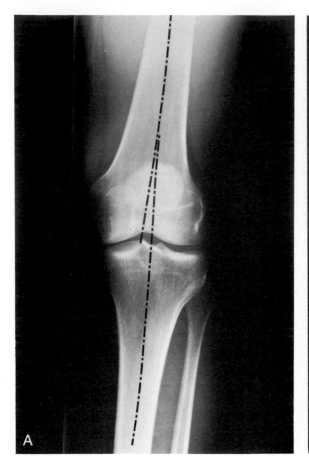

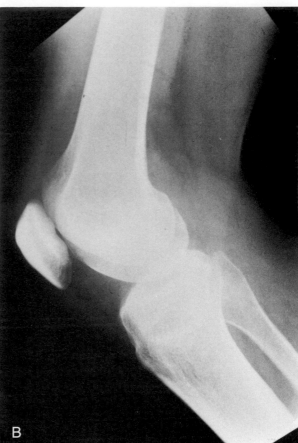

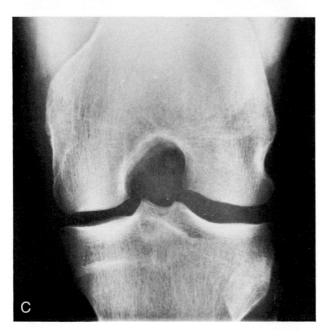

Fig. 5.1 (A) Standing AP view of the knee. The osseous structures are normally mineralized and the articular cortices are smooth. The femoral tibial alignment is in 7° of genu valgus. The lateral joint compartment is slightly wider than the medial joint compartment. (B) Lateral view of the knee obtained with the patient lying on the affected side. The osseous structures are normally mineralized and the articular cortices are smooth although detail is less than optimal because the film is under penetrated to demonstrate the soft tissues. The posterior surface of the quadriceps tendon and patellar tendon are demarcated against the suprapatellar pouch and Hoffa's fat pad respectively. The patellar length: patellar tendon length is 1:1.2. (C) Tunnel view demonstrating the posterior aspect of the femoral condyles, the tibial spines, the articular cortices of the tibial plateau, and the intercondylar notch.

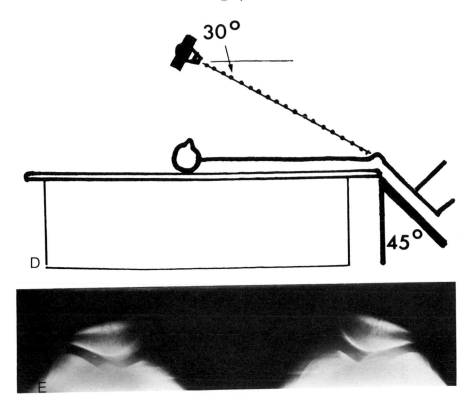

(D) Diagrammatic representation of the positioning for the Merchant view. (E) Merchant view demonstrating the patellae in tangent. The patellofemoral joints are normal bilaterally.

alignment can be analyzed on the Merchant or mountain view, but not on the skyline view.

Oblique views of the knee are not a necessary part of the routine knee examination except to evaluate further a radiographic finding identified on the routine views. For the two oblique views, one at 45 degrees of external rotation and the other at 45 degrees of internal rotation, the patient is supine, lying on the cassette with the knee extended. Demonstrated on the oblique views are the posterior articular surface of the medial and lateral femoral condyles and the patella.

NORMAL RADIOGRAPHIC FINDINGS

SOFT TISSUES

The soft tissues of the knee are optimally demonstrated with low kilovoltage (kV) (Fig. 5.1B). The soft tissues examined on the lateral view are the suprapatellar pouch, the quadriceps tendon, and the patellar tendon. The suprapatellar pouch is the lucent triangular area between the distal femur and the quadriceps tendon. The quadriceps tendon inserts on the superior aspect of the patella, and its posterior surface is demarcated by the suprapatellar pouch. The patellar tendon originates on the inferior surface of the patella and inserts on the tibial tubercle; its posterior surface is adjacent to Hoffa's fat pad. The normal tendons are straight, clearly demarcated posteriorly and uniform in thickness.

The soft tissues demonstrated on the AP view are the medial and lateral supporting ligaments; however, they have no distinguishing radiographic characteristics unless they are calcified.

OSSEOUS STRUCTURES

The osseous structures of the knee include the bones and their articulations. Radiographically, the mineralization, alignment and the integrity of the bones, as well as their articulation, are examined. The bones of the knee are the distal femur, proximal tibia and fibula, patella, and on occasion a fabella or cyamella, or both. A fabella is a sesamoid bone in the lateral head of the gastrocnemius and is identified on the lateral view

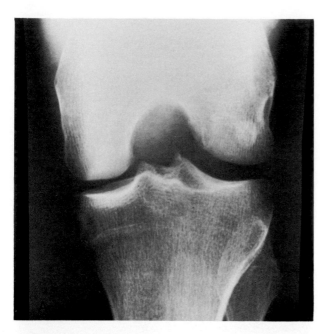

Fig. 5.2. A fabella is a circular osseous density, a sesamoid, in the lateral head of the gastrocnemius. (A) On the AP view, the fabella is superimposed on the lateral femoral condyle. (B) On the lateral view, the fabella is posterior to the femoral condyles. (C) A cyamella is a circular osseous density, a sesamoid, in the popliteus tendon. On the AP view, a cyamella is present within the notch in the lateral aspect of the lateral femoral condyle.

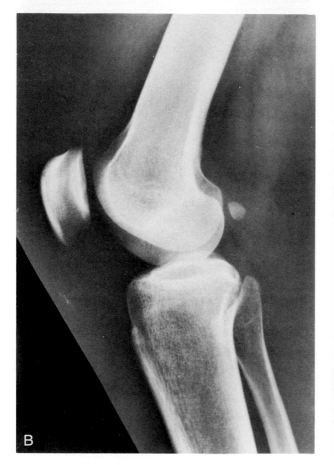

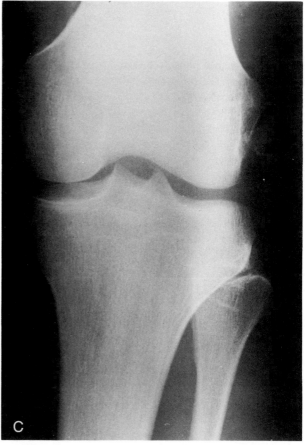

posterior to the distal femur and on the AP view, superimposed on the lateral femoral condyle (Fig. 5.2A,B). A cyamella is a sesamoid bone in the popliteus tendon and is identified on the AP and oblique views in the groove in the lateral aspect of the lateral femoral condyle (Fig. 5.2C).

There are three articular compartments within the knee: the medial and lateral femoral tibial compartments and the patellofemoral compartment.

MINERALIZATION

An accurate determination of bone density cannot be made on the basis of routine radiographs, but a subjective evaluation can be established. A bone of normal mineralization has a uniform cortex, a sharp cortex medullary interface, and compact trabeculae.

ALIGNMENT

Femoral-tibial alignment is measured on the AP view. Alignment is measured by the intersection of a line through the vertical axis of the femur and through the vertical axis of the tibia. On the standing AP view, the tibia is normally directed 7 degrees laterally from the femoral axis (Fig. 5.1A).[15]

Patellofemoral alignment is demonstrated both on the lateral view and the Merchant view. On the lateral view, patellar position is measured relative to the patellar tendon, that is, the maximum vertical dimension of the patella to the length of the patellar tendon. The normal patellar length:patellar tendon ratio is 1:1.2 (Fig. 5.1B).[14]

On the Merchant view, patellar position is determined relative to the femoral component of the patellofemoral joint, which forms the congruence angle (Fig. 5.3). The mean normal congruence angle is −6 degrees (SD 11 degrees).[20]

INTEGRITY

Osseous integrity is determined by continuity of the cortex, except in the immature and adolescent skeleton at the site of the open epiphyses, and by uniformity of the medullary cavity trabeculae and the cortical medullary interface. Normal developmental

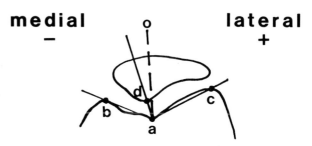

congruence angle

Fig. 5.3. The congruence angle measures the patellofemoral alignment. The femoral component of the patellofemoral joint is the sulcus angle (bac), constructed by determining the highest points of the medial femoral condyle (b) and the lateral femoral condyle (c), with the lowest point of the intercondylar sulcus (a). The sulcus angle is bisected; reference line (ao). The congruence angle (dao) is formed by connecting the lowest point of the intercondylar sulcus (a) with the lowest point of the articular edge of the patella (d). A congruence angle medial to the reference line is minus (−) and an angle lateral to the reference line is plus (+). A congruence angle of > +16° is abnormal.

variations in the immature skeleton can be confused with an abnormality. These skeletal variants are usually incidental findings and asymptomatic. The most common sites for these variations are: (1) the posterior articular cortical surface of the medial or lateral femoral condyles, or both; (2) the distal metaphysis of the medial femoral condyle; (3) the tibial tubercle; and (4) the patella.

The irregularity on the posterior aspect of the femoral condyles is best visualized on the tunnel or the oblique views (Fig. 5.4A,B). The cartilage covering the osseous area of irregularity is thick and intact.

The metaphyseal defect of the distal medial femoral condyle is at the insertion site of the adductor muscles and is best visualized on the oblique view (Fig. 5.4C,D). It may represent a benign cortical defect or a reaction to microtrauma. It must be recognized in order to avoid an unnecessary biopsy.[2,7,36]

Tibial tubercle and patellar irregularities result from variations in the number of ossification centers and in their pattern of fusion. The size and shape of the tibial tubercle are varied, it may be either fragmented or ununited to the tibia, or both. A bipartite or tripartite patella has separate osseous centers at the superior-lateral pole. The individual osseous fragments are usually corticated (Fig. 5.4E,F).

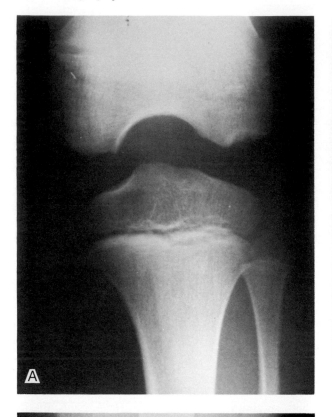

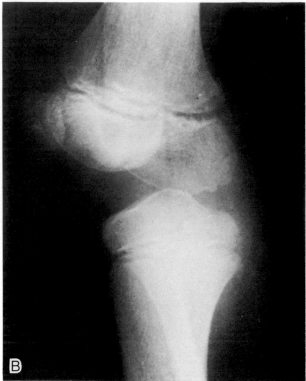

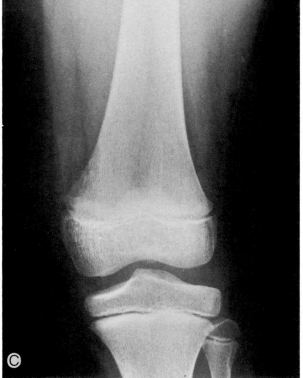

Fig. 5.4. (A,B) AP and oblique views of a child's knee demonstrate irregularity and fragmentation of the posterior articular surface of the lateral femoral condyle. This is a normal variation, and the articular cartilage over this defect is intact. (C,D) AP and oblique views of the distal femur in a youngster demonstrates a cortical irregularity in the distal medial metaphysis. The cortical defect is an asymptomatic incidental finding that should not be biopsied.

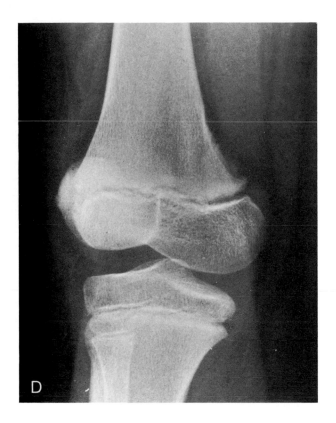

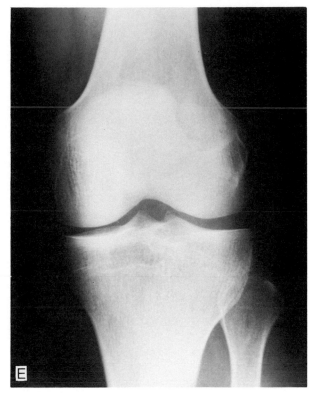

(E,F) AP and Merchant views demonstrate a bipartite patella. A corticated separate osseous fragment forms the supralateral pole of the patella.

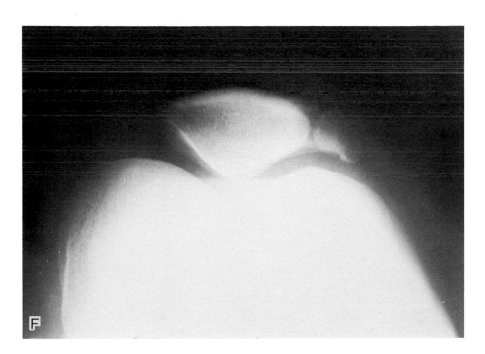

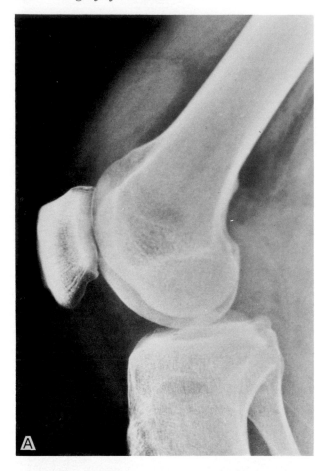

ARTICULATION

The joint articulations are examined indirectly on routine radiographs by the distance between the bones. Direct radiographic demonstration requires arthrography. There are three joint compartments: the medial, the lateral tibial-femoral articulation, and the patellar femoral articulation. On the AP view, the lateral compartment is slightly wider than the medial compartment (Fig. 5.1A). On the lateral and patellofemoral views, the width of the patellofemoral joint compartment approximates the width of the other two compartments (Fig. 5.1B,D). The articular cortices are smooth, thin, and continuous.

ABNORMAL RADIOGRAPHIC FINDINGS

SOFT TISSUES

Radiographically, the most common soft tissue abnormality in the knee is an oval soft tissue density posterior to the quadriceps tendon (Fig. 5.5A). It indicates an abnormal distention of the suprapatellar pouch by either a joint effusion or by synovial hypertrophic tissue. A joint effusion may be synovial fluid, blood, or pus. Synovial hypertrophic tissue may rep-

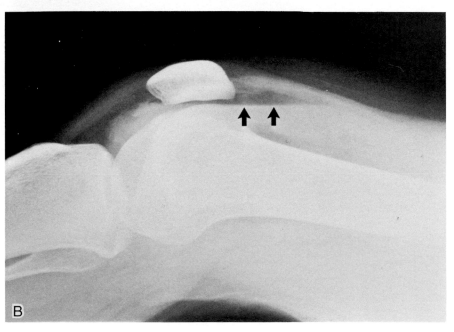

Fig. 5.5. (A) Lateral view demonstrates an oval soft tissue density within the suprapatellar pouch posterior to the quadriceps tendon, representing a joint effusion or synovial hypertrophic tissue. (B) A cross-table lateral view demonstrates a fat–fluid level (arrows). The lucent intra-articular bone marrow fat layers on hemarthrosis and is diagnostic of an intra-articular fracture. (Part B from Torg, J.S., Pavlov, H., Morris, V.B.: Salter Harris Type III fracture of the medial femoral condyle occurring in the adolescent athlete. J. Bone Joint Surg., *63A*: 586–591, 1981, with permission.)

resent a nonspecific synovitis or pigmented villonodular synovitis.

When a joint effusion is present in a patient with a clinically suspected fracture that is not seen radiographically, a cross-table lateral view is mandatory. A cross-table lateral view is obtained with the patient supine, the cassette perpendicular to the tabletop, and the central ray perpendicular to the cassette. A fracture that involves an articular surface bleeds into the joint; the blood contains bone marrow fat. Fat has a lower specific gravity than that of blood; thus the fat separates from the blood and floats on it much as oil floats on vinegar; the difference in specific gravity can be distinguished radiographically (Fig. 5.5B). The presence of a fat fluid level confirms an intra-articular fracture.

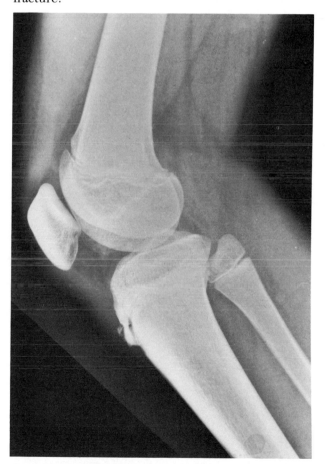

Fig. 5.6. Lateral view, using soft tissue technique, demonstrates the roentgen findings of Osgood Schlatter's disease: (1) a thick patellar tendon with an ill-defined posterior surface, (2) fragmentation of the tibial tubercle, and (3) a soft tissue swelling anterior to the tibial tubercle.

Tendon injuries can also be radiographically diagnosed on the routine lateral view. A rupture of the quadriceps or patellar tendon, or both, is diagnosed when the tendon is thick and wavy instead of straight, or when the posterior surface of the tendon interface is lost. In adolescents, one cause of patellar tendon thickening is Osgood Schlatter's disease. Osgood Schlatter's disease is diagnosed radiographically by such findings as thickening of the patellar tendon, loss of the posterior definition of the tendon, a soft tissue bulge anterior to the tibial tubercle, and fragmentation of the tibial tubercle (Fig. 5.6). These findings must be correlated with appropriate clinical signs and symptoms.[24,26,35]

Other soft tissue abnormalities around the knee are radiographically apparent if they calcify. Calcification within the soft tissues of the knee results from previous trauma or degeneration and in association with systemic conditions such as hyperparathyroidism and scleroderma. Calcifications may be linear, speckled, dense, clumped, or fragmented.

Linear calcification within the medial collateral or lateral capsular ligaments observed on the AP and tunnel views, is usually post-traumatic. Pellegrini Stieda's disease (calcification in the medial collateral ligament) can range from minimal calcification to extensive myositis ossification (Fig. 5.7A,B).[22,23] A chronic intra-articular ligament injury may also calcify (Fig. 5.7C). Quadriceps tendon calcification is usually the result of a direct traumatic insult (Fig. 5.7D), although it can be associated with hyperparathyroidism.[10]

Cartilage calcification (chondrocalcinosis) within the articular or meniscal cartilage may be identified on routine radiographs. This calcification can be thin and linear, speckled, or dense and follows the contour of the cartilaginous structure (Fig. 5.8A,B).[13,17,18,27] Chondrocalcinosis is a nonspecific finding that occurs with pseudogout, degenerative arthritis, hyperparathyroidism, gout, or ochronosis.

Circular calcifications resembling popcorn indicate intra-articular osteocartilaginous bodies. Intra-articular loose bodies result from cartilaginous fragments that grow, nourished by synovial fluid. Loose bodies commonly rest within the intercondylar notch, the suprapatellar pouch, a popliteal cyst, or the popliteal bursa. They can be a result or a source of degenerative changes. Posterior loose bodies can be overlooked or misinterpreted as a normal cyamella or fabella

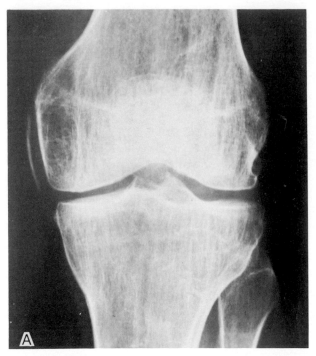

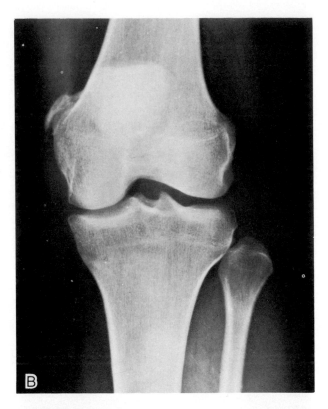

Fig. 5.7. Pelligrini Stieda's disease involves calcification in the medial collateral ligament and can be in the body of the ligament (A), or at its proximal attachment site (B). (C) Coned lateral view of the posterior lateral joint compartment demonstrates an ossified popliteus tendon. (D) A lateral view of the femur demonstrates myositis ossificans anterior to the femur; characteristically, the ossification is denser peripherally than centrally. (From Pavlov, H.: Radiology for the orthopaedic surgeon. Contemporary Orthopaedics, 6: 85–88, 1983, with permission.)

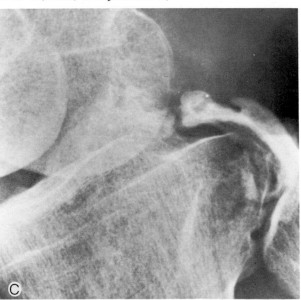

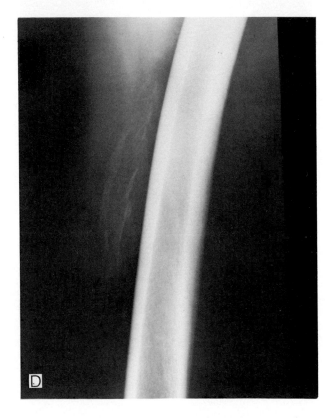

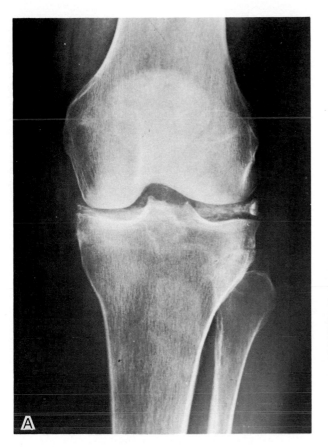

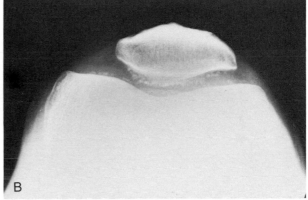

Fig. 5.8. (A) AP view demonstrates chondrocalcinosis in the lateral meniscal cartilage and the articular cartilage of the medial tibial plateau. (B) Tangent view of the patella demonstrates chondrocalcinosis of the posterior articular cartilage of the patella and the anterior articular cartilage of the distal femur.

(Fig. 5.9A,B). Multiple and extensive osteochondral bodies may be loose within the joint or part of the synovium, as with secondary synovial chondromatosis (Fig. 5.10A,B).

Small, irregular, calcific flecks or dense, calcific clumps represent different entities depending on their locations, inferior to the patella, it is Hoffa's disease or necrosis of the infrapatellar fat pad (Fig. 5.11A), whereas anterior to the patella, it is calcific prepatellar bursitis or housemaid's knee (Fig. 5.11B). The presence of thin flecks of calcification throughout the synovium indicates primary synovial chondromatosis; if located distant from the joint, it can signify a synovial sarcoma.

OSSEOUS STRUCTURES

MINERALIZATION

Osteopenia involves diminished bone density; this disorder is suggested if the cortex is thin, the cortical medullary interface is poorly defined, and/or the tra-

beculae are loosely packed. Osteopenia may indicate osteoporosis or osteomalacia, but in the knee it is usually secondary to postmenopausal or disuse osteoporosis. Localized osteoporosis can be symptomatic representing transient migratory or regional osteoporosis.

Osteosclerosis is suggested if the cortex is thick and the cortex medullary demarcation is poorly defined and continuous with the densely packed trabeculae. Osteosclerosis occurs with myelo-fibrosis, fluorosis, and various systemic illnesses. Mixed density patterns may be generalized or localized and are associated with infection, Paget's disease, primary and secondary neoplasms, and other disorders.

ALIGNMENT

Femoral tibial malalignment is described in terms of genu varus, genu valgus, or genu recurvatum. The genu varus or valgus deformities are best measured on the standing AP view. A genu varus deformity describes a knee in which the tibia is directed toward

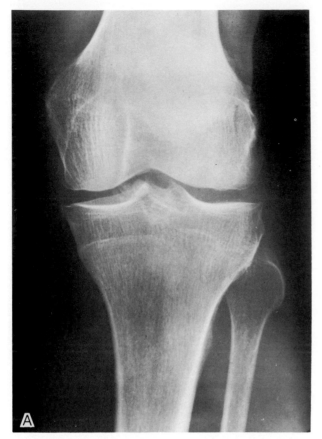
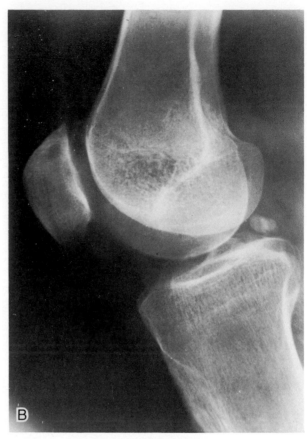

Fig. 5.9. (A,B) AP and lateral views demonstrate two osseous densities posterior to the medial joint compartment (arrows). These densities represent intra-articular loose bodies and should not be confused with a fabella or a cyamella, both of which are laterally located and are more proximal (see Fig. 2A–C).

the midline (Fig. 5.12A); a patient with bilateral genu varus deformities has bowlegs. A genu valgus deformity describes a knee in which the tibia is directed over 7 degrees laterally from the femoral axis; a patient with bilateral genu valgus deformities has knock-knees (Fig. 5.12B). A hyperextended knee represents genu recurvatum and is best diagnosed on a standing lateral view (Fig. 5.12C).

In the immature and adolescent skeleton, the malalignment may be within the tibia and represents a tibia vara or Blount's disease. Blount's disease is diagnosed by an acute angulation between the tibial metaphyses and the tibial shaft, fragmentation and irregularity of the medial posterior aspect of the metaphyses and the epiphyses, flattening of the medial tibial epiphyses, and posterior beaking of the tibial metaphyses (Fig. 5.13). Blount's disease can be symmetric or asymmetric and can be initially diagnosed in a patient over 2 years old or during adolescence.[3]

Patellar femoral malalignment usually refers to one of two conditions: either a patella that is too high, known as patella alta, or a patella that is laterally subluxed. Patella alta is diagnosed when the patellar length:patellar tendon ratio on the lateral view is > 1:1.2 (Fig. 5.14A).[15] The most common causes of patella alta are cerebral palsy and patellar tendon ruptures. Patellar subluxation is determined on the Merchant or mountain view by a congruence angle of > +16 degrees (Fig. 5.14B).[20]

INTEGRITY

Osseous integrity is interrupted by a fracture or a neoplasm. Fractures may be complete or partial, impacted, epiphyseal, avulsion, or osteochondral. Neoplasms can be benign or malignant.

A complete fracture involves both cortices and is

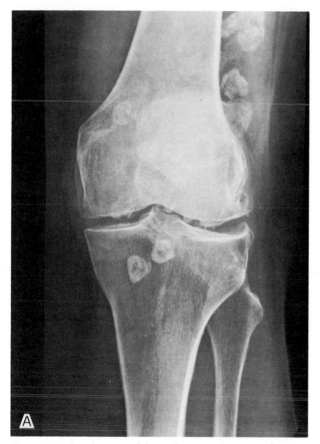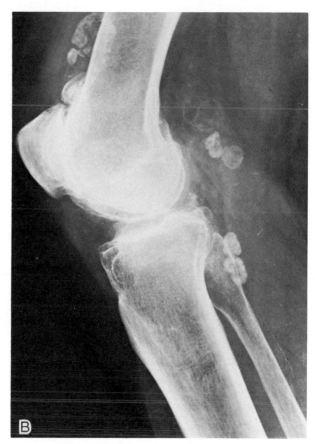

Fig. 5.10. (A,B) AP and lateral views demonstrate multiple intra-articular osteochondral densities representing loose bodies or synovial chondromatosis. There are degenerative changes of the patellofemoral and lateral joint compartments.

either simple or comminuted. It can be horizontal, oblique, spiral, or vertical. A fracture is radiographically described according to the displacement and angulation of the distal fracture fragment relative to the proximal fragment.

Partial fractures that do not involve both cortices are stress fractures. The location of a stress fracture is predictable. Such fractures can be cortical or cancellous.[32,34,38] In the femur, stress fractures are supracondylar and involve the anterior or posterior cortex. In the proximal tibia, cortical stress fractures occur in the posterior cortex at the junction of the proximal and middle thirds; cancellous fractures occur inferior to the medial or lateral plateau (Fig. 5.15A,B). Cortical stress fractures are lucent and linear and are usually within an area of localized cortical thickening or hyperostosis. Cancellous stress fractures are dense because of impaction of the fractured trabeculae and osteoblastic activity. Cortical and cancellous stress

fractures may be difficult to identify radiographically; a radionuclide bone scan is suggested whenever a fracture is clinically suspected (Fig. 5.15C).[19]

Impacted fractures occur most commonly at the articular surface of the tibia (Fig. 5.16A) or at the medial facet of the patella (Fig 5.16B). The tibial fracture is best diagnosed on the AP view. A small fracture adjacent to a flattened medial facet of the patella indicates a prior patellar dislocation and is best diagnosed on the Merchant view.[9,19]

Epiphyseal and avulsion fractures occur in children. They are the result of severe stress on a joint. In the immature skeleton, the ligaments are elastic and more resistant to injury than the epiphyseal plate or the ligamentous attachment site. Epiphyseal fractures are described according to the Salter–Harris classification (Fig. 5.17).[31] There are five types of Salter fractures. Types I, III, and V, when occurring in the femur can be radiographically subtle. A Salter I

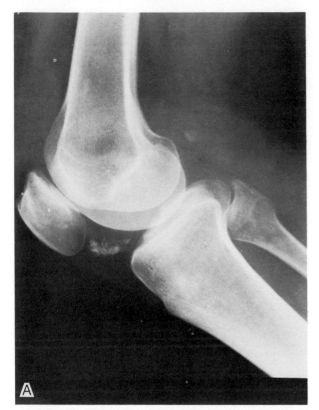
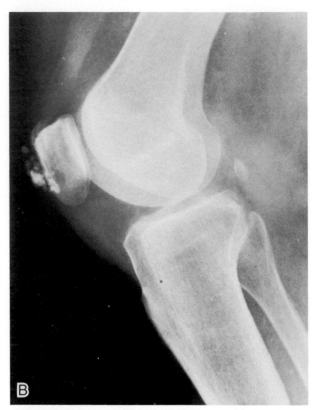

Fig. 5.11. (A) Calcific flecks are present inferior to the patella in Hoffa's fat pad, representing Hoffa's disease or necrosis of the fat pad. (B) Calcific flecks are present anterior to the patella in the prepatellar bursa, representing calcific bursitis or housemaid's knee.

or III fracture should be suspected when the epiphysis is wider than usual, and a type V if the epiphysis appears narrower than usual, especially if only part of the epiphysis is affected.[28,37] A joint effusion in any patient, (especially a child), with a possible fracture should be checked with a cross-table lateral view to determine the presence of fat fluid level.

Two avulsion fractures that occur near the knee are associated with specific ligament injuries. The first is an osseous fragment anterior and superior to the tibial spines that results from an avulsion of the bony insertion of the anterior cruciate ligament, with the ligament remaining intact. This injury is best demonstrated on the AP and lateral views (Fig. 5.18A,B). The second avulsion fracture is characterized by a small, linear fracture fragment adjacent to the lateral aspect of the lateral tibial plateau, a capsular sign, produced by the avulsion of the bony insertion of the meniscal capsular component of the lateral capsular ligament. This injury is usually associated with a torn

anterior cruciate ligament and is identified on the AP or tunnel views (Fig. 5.19).[39]

The cartilaginous articular surfaces of the femur are occasionally injured, especially in adolescents. When the injury is acute and confined completely to the cartilage, it cannot be diagnosed on routine films, but if the abnormality extends into the bone, radiographic changes are apparent. Chondral and osteochondral fractures occur primarily in one of the following locations: the posterior aspect of the medial or the lateral femoral condyle and the superior anterior aspect to the lateral femoral condyle.[1,6,11,16,21,25,29,30,33] Osteochondritis dissecans is commonly seen on the intercondylar aspect of the medial femoral condyle. An osteochondral fracture or osteochondritis dissecans can have several roentgenographic presentations: (1) a lucent osseous defect (Fig. 5.20A,B), (2) a fragmented osseous density within a lucent defect (Fig. 5.20C), or (3) a corticated osseous density within a lucent defect (Fig. 5.20D,E). Arthrography is helpful in deter-

(Text continues on p. 93.)

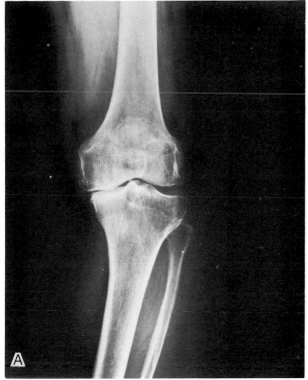

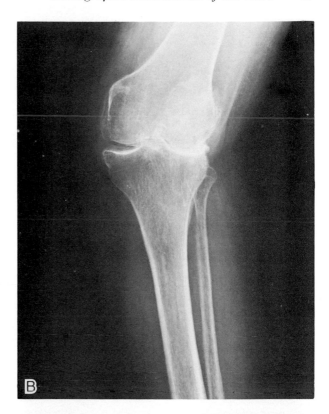

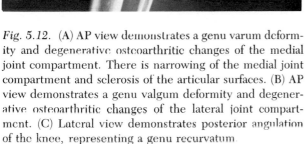

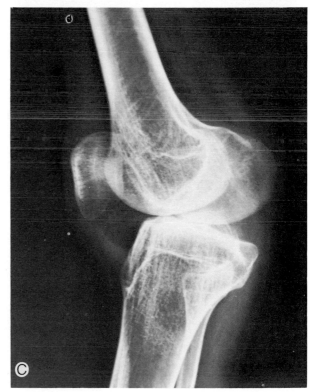

Fig. 5.12. (A) AP view demonstrates a genu varum deformity and degenerative osteoarthritic changes of the medial joint compartment. There is narrowing of the medial joint compartment and sclerosis of the articular surfaces. (B) AP view demonstrates a genu valgum deformity and degenerative osteoarthritic changes of the lateral joint compartment. (C) Lateral view demonstrates posterior angulation of the knee, representing a genu recurvatum.

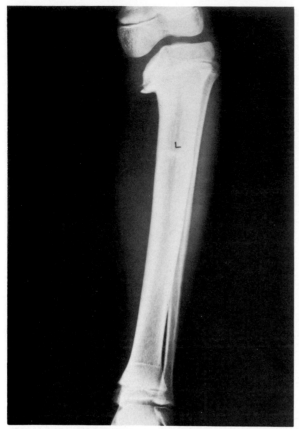

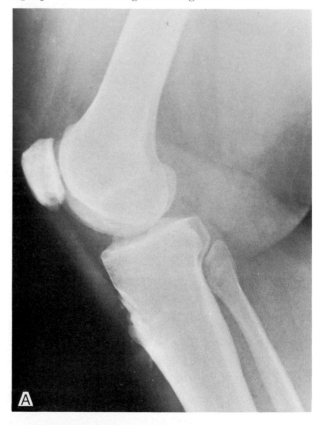

Fig. 5.14. (A) Lateral view demonstrates patella alta. The patellar length: patellar tendon length ratio exceeds 1:1.2. (B) Merchant view demonstrates lateral subluxation of the right patella with a congruence angle of > +16°.

Fig. 5.13. AP view of the tibia demonstrates tibia vara or Blount's disease. Shortening of the entire medial aspect of the proximal tibia, flattening and fragmentation of the medial metaphysis and epiphysis, and increased angulation between the metaphysis and the tibial shaft are seen. Such findings are physiologic in a child under 2 years of age but are abnormal in the older child.

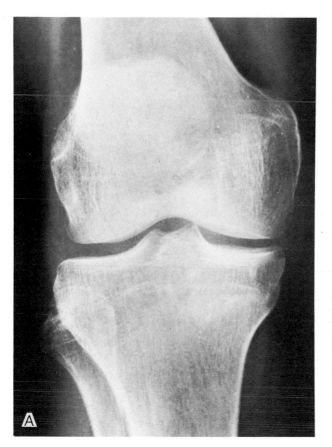

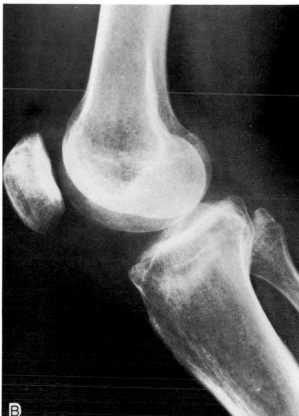

Fig. 5.15. (A,B) AP and lateral views demonstrate a cancellous stress fracture in the medial tibial plateau represented as a horizontal linear density. Generalized osteopenia is seen. (C) A radionuclide bone scan of the cancellous stress fracture in the left medial tibial plateau (A,B) is represented by intense augmented isotope uptake. The small area of augmented uptake located on the right may represent a subclinical fracture or early degenerative arthritis.

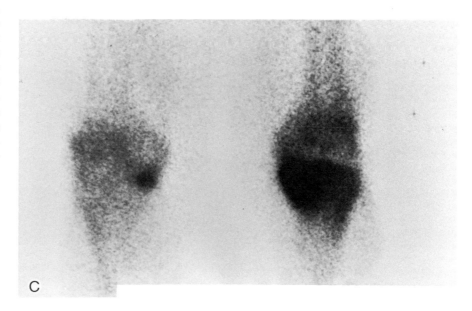

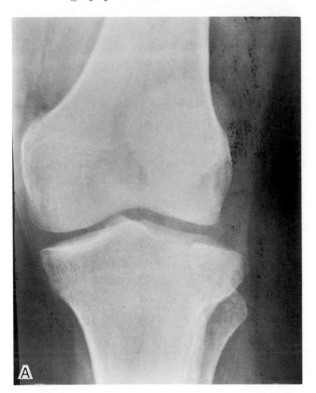

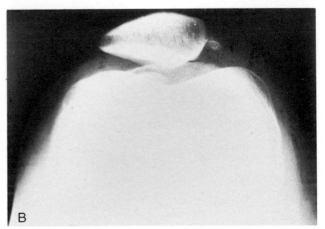

Fig. 5.16. (A) AP view demonstrates an impacted fracture of the lateral tibial plateau. The articular cortical border of the tibial plateau is interrupted and the lateral fragment is depressed. (B) A tangential view of the patella demonstrates flattening of the medial facet of the patella and an adjacent osseous fragment to the patella. These findings are consistent with a prior fracture/dislocation of the patella.

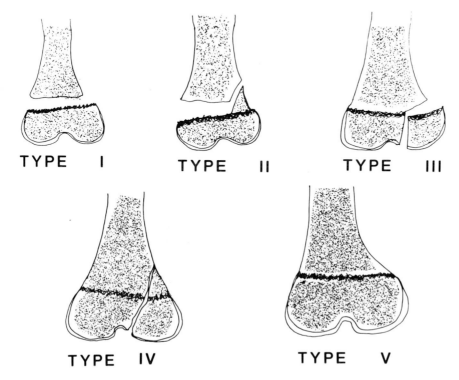

Fig. 5.17. Diagrammatic representation of the Salter–Harris classification of epiphyseal fractures. (From Pavlov, H.: Radiology for the orthopaedic surgeon. Contemporary Orthopaedics, *4:* 515–519, 1982, with permission.)

TYPE I TYPE II TYPE III

TYPE IV TYPE V

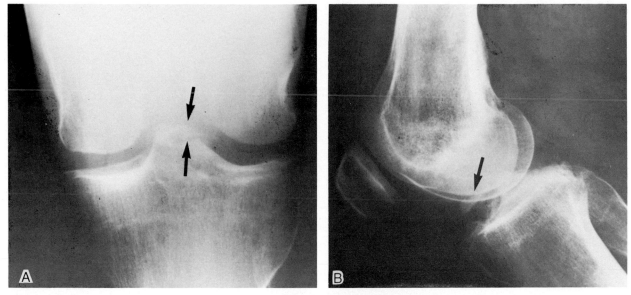

Fig. 5.18. (A,B) AP and lateral views demonstrate a corticated osseous density anterior and superior to the tibial spines (arrow), representing the avulsed bony attachment of the anterior cruciate ligament.

Fig. 5.19. A small osseous fragment lateral to the lateral tibial plateau (arrow) is a capsular sign. The fragment represents the avulsed attachment of the meniscal capsular portion of the lateral capsular ligament. This injury is usually associated with an anterior cruciate ligament injury.

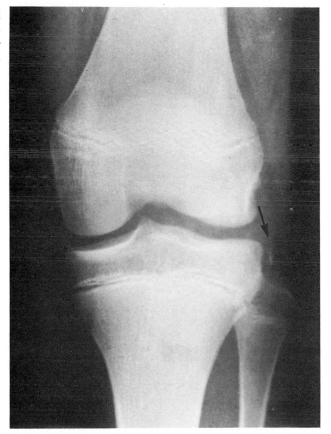

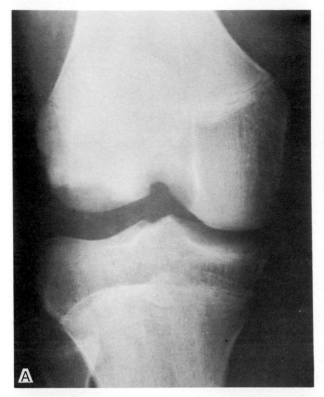

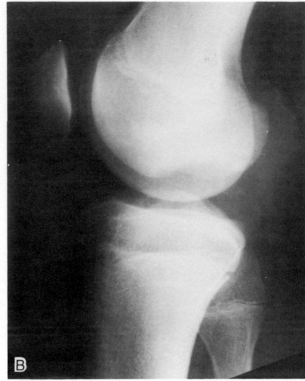

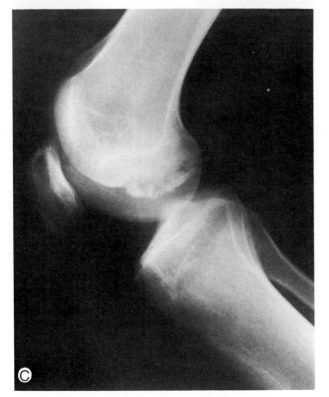

Fig. 5.20. Radiographic manifestations of an osteochondral fracture and/or osteochondritis dissecans. (A,B) AP and lateral views demonstrating a lucent saucer-shaped defect on the posterior aspect of the lateral femoral condyle. (C) Lateral view demonstrating fragmented osseous density within a lucent defect on the posterior aspect of the lateral femoral condyle. (D,E) Lateral and tunnel views demonstrate a corticated osseous density within a lucent defect in the intercondylar aspect of the medial femoral condyle.

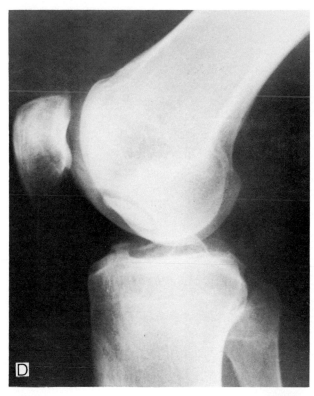

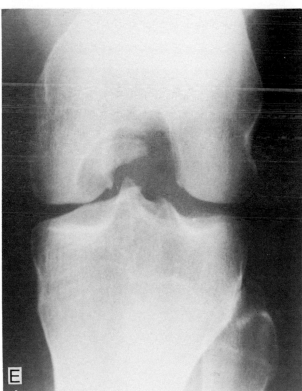

mining whether the cartilage overlying the osseous defect is intact or whether there is a loose cartilaginous or osseous fragment within the defect.[11,33]

A neoplasm, either benign or malignant, can destroy the normal architecture or bony integrity, or both. A neoplasm is evident by a localized alteration in density, expansion, or a destruction of the cortex and/or medullary cavity. A benign tumor usually has a sharp line of demarcation, that is, a narrow zone of transition. A malignant tumor usually has an ill-defined line of demarcation, that is, a wide zone of transition. Radiologic diagnosis of a tumor as benign or malignant, is made on the basis of the type of matrix, the periosteal reaction, as well as the age of the patient and location, solitary or multiple surrounding soft tissue involvement, and other factors. Osseous tumors are usually categorized by their matrix, which may be cystic, fibrous, cartilaginous, or osseous.

ARTICULAR PATHOLOGY

Signs of intra-articular pathology are a joint effusion or synovial tissue hypertrophy (Fig. 5.5A), joint compartment narrowing, sclerosis along the articular border, hypertrophic osteophytic spurring, subchondral cysts, cortical erosions, malalignment, and/or periarticular osteoporosis.

Degenerative osteoarthritis is diagnosed by joint space narrowing, articular sclerosis, subchondral cysts, and hypertrophic osteophytic spurring involving one, two, or all three joint compartments, but usually not to the same degree (Fig. 5.21A). A severe medial or lateral joint involvement is usually associated with degeneration of the corresponding meniscus and a genu varus or a genu valgus deformity. Osteoarthritic changes confined to the patellar femoral joint is associated with pseudogout or chronic abnormal patellofemoral tracking.

Flattening of the weight-bearing surface of the femoral condyle, sclerosis, and large subchondral cysts may represent osteonecrosis (Fig. 5.21B) or severe osteoarthritis. Osteonecrosis most commonly occurs in the medial femoral condyle of elderly patients. Osteonecrosis is not associated with joint space narrowing unless degenerative changes are superimposed.

An inflammatory arthritis, such as a rheumatoid, rheumatoid variant, or sepsis, is usually associated

(Text continues on p. 97.)

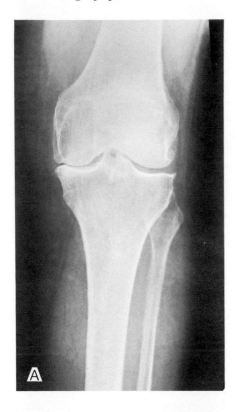

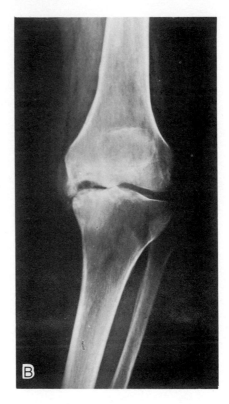

Fig. 5.21. (A) AP view demonstrates degenerative osteoarthritis of the medial and lateral joint compartments. There is joint compartment narrowing more severe medially, marginal hypertrophic spurs and sclerosis of the articular borders of the medial and lateral tibial plateaus. (B) Medial osteonecrosis with superimposed degenerative arthritis. The articular surface of the medial femoral condyle is concave and bordered by sclerosis. There are large hypertrophic spurs along the medial joint compartment and a genu varus deformity.

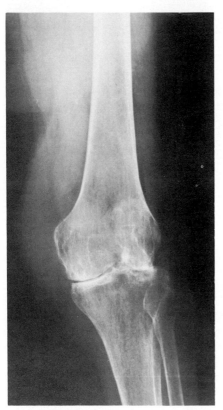

Fig. 5.22. Standing AP view demonstrates changes consistent with an inflammatory arthritides such as rheumatoid arthritis. Uniform narrowing of the medial and lateral joint compartments, subchondral cysts on both the femoral and tibial joint surfaces, periarticular osteopenia, and a genu valgus deformity are shown.

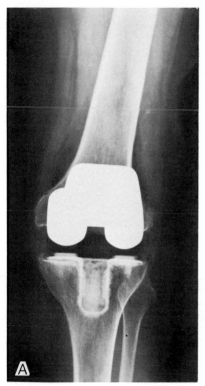 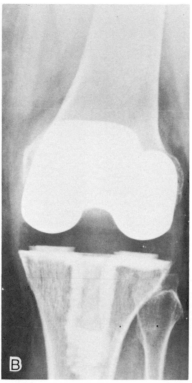 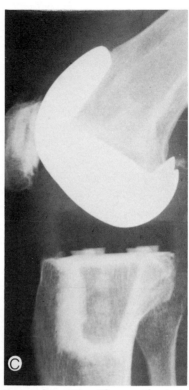

Fig. 5.23. (A–C) Two AP views and a lateral view of various total knee prosthesis in normal position. The prosthesis is embedded in radiopaque cement with contact between the metal and cement and the cement and bone interface. The radiolucent plastic tibial component cannot be evaluated radiographically. The femoral tibial alignment is anatomic.

Fig. 5.24. A lateral view of a total knee prosthesis obtained through an encircling cast demonstrates posterior dislocation of the tibial component with respect to the femoral component.

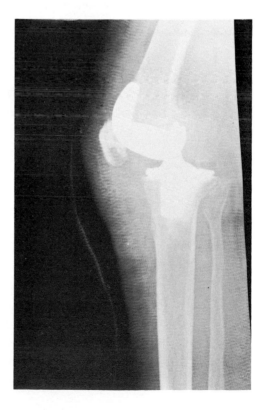

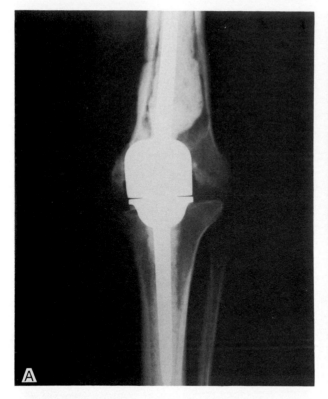

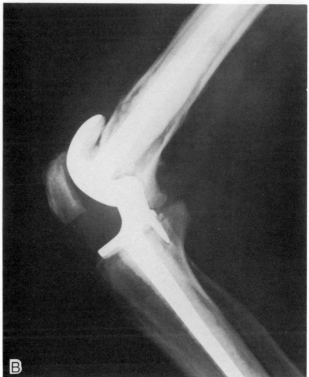

Fig. 5.25. (A,B) AP and lateral view of a total knee prosthesis demonstrates a wide lucent zone between the cement–bone interface surrounding the femoral component. This lucency is obviously over 2 mm and represents an infected or loose femoral component.

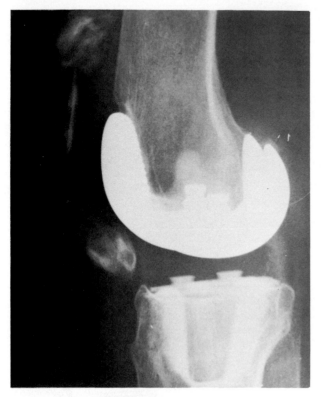

Fig. 5.26. Lateral view demonstrates a fractured patella. The superior and inferior patellar poles are avulsed from the prosthetic button.

with periarticular osteoporosis, uniform joint compartment narrowing, subarticular cortical erosions and a lack of signs of repair, that is, sclerosis and/or hypertrophic spurring (Fig. 5.22). Rheumatoid arthritis is usually polyarticular, whereas septic arthritis is generally monarticular.

POSTSURGICAL KNEE

Normal

The roentgenographic evaluation of a knee after surgery requires AP and lateral views.

Immediately after surgery, air is usually seen in the joint or surrounding soft tissues. After immobilization, subcortical disuse osteoporosis is usually present.

Metal staples, pins, screws, wires, or an osteotomy confirm a surgical procedure. After ligamentous surgery, a bone block, in which the ligament has been attached, or a track line, where the ligament has been pulled through the bone may be observed.

Prosthetic knee replacements vary in design. A total knee prosthesis replaces the distal femur, proximal tibia, and posterior patella. Most prostheses are embedded in radiopaque cement and have metal and plastic components. The metal components of a total knee prostheses are examined for alignment, metal–cement and cement–bone interfaces, and the integrity of the metal and the cement. The plastic portion of the total knee prosthesis cannot be fully evaluated radiographically.

On the AP view, the alignment of the tibial and femoral prosthetic components is determined by drawing two lines, one tangent to the prosthetic femoral condyles and the other line tangent to the tibial plateau; normally these two lines are approximately parallel to each other and perpendicular to the weight-bearing line (Fig. 5.23A,B). On the lateral view, the tibial and femoral prosthetic components should be in anatomic position (Fig. 5.23C). On the Merchant view and the lateral view, the prosthetic patellofemoral components are in anatomic alignment.

The interface between the metal and cement is nil and between the cement and bone is normally a uniform linear lucency < 2 mm.[8] The borders of the metallic components are smooth and intact, and the surrounding cement is uniform and homogeneous.

Abnormal

Signs of abnormality related to the various surgical procedures include a joint effusion, infection and/or extensive osteoporosis, displaced metallic implants and/or lucency around the screws and/or staples.

Abnormality of prosthetic components includes malalignment, subluxation and/or dislocation, loosening and/or infection, or fracture. Malalignment is diagnosed as genu varus, genu valgus, tibial subluxation, dislocation (Fig. 5.24), or patellar subluxation. Loosening and/or infection is suggested when the lucency between the cement and bone is > 2 mm, especially if this lucent interface widens on serial films (Fig. 5.25A,B).[8] Differentiating loosening from infection is not usually possible on routine films unless there are signs of osteomyelitis. Any lucency between the cement and the prosthetic component is abnormal.

The metallic components and/or the surrounding cement can fracture from direct trauma or from stress. The tibial plateau and the patella may fracture. The tibial plateau fracture is usually depressed. The fracture of the patella is usually at the superior or inferior pole, with the fragments avulsed from the prosthetic resurfacing (Fig. 5.26).

ACKNOWLEDGMENTS

This manuscript could not have been prepared without the editorial assistance of Jill Spiller, the typing skills, patience, and endurance of Patricia Boggia, and the support of Dr. Robert H. Freiberger.

REFERENCES

1. Ahuja, S.C., and Bullough, P.G.: Osteonecrosis of the knee. A clinicopathological study in twenty-eight patients. J. Bone Joint Surg [Am.], *60*: 191, 1978.
2. Barnes, G.R. Jr., and Gwinn, J.L.: Distal irregularities of the femur simulating malignancy. Am. J. Roentgenol., *122*: 180, 1974.
3. Blount, W.P.: Tibia vara. Osteochondrosis deformans tibiae. J. Bone Joint Surg., *19*: 1, 1937.
4. Bradley, W.G., and Ominsky, S.H.: Mountain view of the patella. Am. J. Roentgenol., *136*, 53, 1981.
5. Brattström, H.: Shape of the intercondylar groove normally and in recurrent dislocation of patella. Acta Orthop. Scand., *68*: (suppl.), 1, 1964.

6. Coventry, M.B.: Osteochondral fracture of the femoral condyles. Surg. Gynecol. Obstet., *100*: 591, 1955.
7. Dunham, W.K., Marcus, N.W., Enneking, W.F., et al.: Developmental defects of the distal femoral metaphysis. J. Bone Joint Surg [Am.], *62*: 801, 1980.
8. Dussault, R.G., Goldman, A.B., and Ghelman, B.G.: Radiologic diagnosis of loosening and infection in hip prostheses. J. Can. Assoc. Radiol., *28*: 119, 1977.
9. Freiberger, R.H., and Kotzen, L.M.: Fracture of the medial margin of the patella, a finding diagnostic of lateral dislocation. Radiology, *88*: 902, 1967.
10. Gayler, B.W., and Brogdon, B.G.: Soft tissue calcification in the extremities in systemic diseases. Am. J. Med. Sci., *249*: 590, 1965.
11. Gilley, J.S., Gelman, M.I., Edson, D.M., et al.: Chondral fractures of the knee, arthrographic, arthroscopic, and clinical manifestations. Radiology, *138*: 51, 1981.
12. Geslien, G.E., Thrall, J.H., Espinosa, J.L., et al.: Early detection of stress fractures using 99mTc polyphosphate. Radiology, *121*: 683, 1976.
13. Hosking, G.E., and Clennar, G.: Calcification in articular cartilage. J. Bone Joint Surg. [Br.], *42*: 530, 1960.
14. Insall, J., and Salvati, E.: Patella position in the normal knee joint. Radiology, *101*: 101, 1971.
15. Insall, J.: Personal communication.
16. Kennedy, J.C., Grainger, R.W., and McGraw, R.W.: Osteochondral fractures of the femoral condyles. J. Bone Joint Surg. [Br.], *48*: 436, 1966.
17. McCarty, D.J., Jr., Kohn, N.N., and Faires, J.S.: Significance of calcium phosphate crystals in synovial fluid of arthritic patients: The "pseudogout syndrome" I. clinical aspects. Ann. Intern. Med., *56*: 711, 1962.
18. McCarty, D.J., Jr., and Haskin, M.E.: The roentgenographic aspects of pseudogout (articular chondrocalcinosis). An analysis of 20 cases. Am. J. Roentgenol., *90*: 1248, 1963.
19. McNab, I.: Recurrent dislocation of the patella. J. Bone Joint Surg [Am.], *34*: 957, 1952.
20. Merchant, A.C., Mercer, R.L., Jacobsen, R.H., et al.: Roentgenographic analysis of patellofemoral congruence. J. Bone Joint Surg. [Am.], *56*: 1391, 1974.
21. Milgram, J.W., Rodgers, L.F., Miller, J.W.: Osteochondral fractures; mechanism of injury and fate of fragments. Am. J. Roentgenol., *130*: 651, 1978.
22. Nachlas, I.W., and Olpp, J.L.: Para-articular calcification (Pellegrini-Stieda) in affections of the knee. Surg. Gynecol. Obstet., *81*: 206, 1945.
23. Norman, A., and Dorfman, H.D.: Juxtacortical circumscribed myositis ossificans; evolution and radiographic features. Radiology, *96*: 301, 1970.
24. Ogden, J.A., and Southwick, W.O.: Osgood-Schlatter's disease and tibial tuberosity development. Clin. Orthop., *116*: 180, 1976.
25. O'Donoghue, D.H.: Chondral and osteochondral fractures. J. Trauma, *6*: 469, 1966.
26. Osgood, R.B.: Lesions of the tibial tubercle occurring during adolescence. Boston Med. Surg. J., *148*: 114, 1903.
27. Resnick, D., Niwayama, G., Goergen, T.G., et al.: Clinical, radiographic and pathologic abnormalities in calcium pyrophosphate dihydrate deposition disease (CPPD): Pseudogout. Radiology, *122*: 1, 1977.
28. Rogers, L.F., Jones, S., Davis, A.R., et al.: "Clipping injury" fracture of the epiphysis in the adolescent football player: an occult lesion of the knee. Am. J. Roentgenol., *121*: 69, 1974.
29. Rosenberg, N.J.: Osteochondral fractures of the lateral femoral condyle. J. Bone Joint Surg. [Am.], *46*: 1013, 1964.
30. Rozing, P.M., Insall, J., and Bohne, W.H.: Spontaneous osteonecrosis of the knee. J. Bone Joint Surg. [Am.], *62*: 2, 1980.
31. Salter, R.B., and Harris, W.R.: Injuries involving the epiphyseal plate. J. Bone Joint Surg [Am.], *45*: 587, 1963.
32. Savoca, C.J.: Stress fractures: A classification of the earliest radiographic signs. Radiology, *100*: 519, 1971.
33. Schneider, R.: Extra-meniscal abnormalities. In Freiberger, R.H., and Kaye, J.J. eds.: Arthrography. New York, Appleton-Century-Crofts, p. 109, 1979.
34. Schneider, R., and Kaye, J.J.: Insufficiency and stress fractures of long bones occurring in patients with rheumatoid arthritis. Radiology *116*: 595, 1975.
35. Scotti, D.M., Sadhu, V.K., Heimberg, F., et al.: Osgood Schlatter's disease, an emphasis on soft tissue changes in roentgen diagnosis. Skeletal Radiol., *4*: 21, 1979.
36. Sontag, L.W., and Pyle, S.I.: The appearance and nature of cyst-like areas in the distal femoral metaphyses of children. Am. J. Roentgenol., *46*: 185, 1941.
37. Torg, J.S., Pavlov, H., and Morris, V.B.: Salter-Harris Type III fracture of the medial femoral condyle occurring in the adolescent athlete. J. Bone Joint Surg. [Am.], *63*: 586, 1981.
38. Wilson, E.S., and Katz, F.N.: Stress fractures: An analysis of 250 consecutive cases. Radiology, *92*: 481, 1969.
39. Woods, G.W., Stanley, R.F., Jr., and Tullos, H.S.: Lateral capsular sign: x-ray clue to a significant knee instability. Am. J. Sports Med., *7*: 27, 1979.

6 Arthrography of the Knee

Robert H. Freiberger

Arthrography of the knee is an accurate means of diagnosing tears of the medial and lateral menisci and the cruciate ligaments. Acute capsular tears and tears of the medial collateral ligament, osteochondral fractures, osteochondritis dissecans, chondromalacia, and synovial lesions can be diagnosed, but not with the same high accuracy possible with meniscal and cruciate ligament tears.

Arthrography of the knee is by no means a new diagnostic procedure. The first report of knee arthrography by Werndorff and Robinson[6] was published in 1905, less than 10 years after Roentgen's announcement of the discovery of the x-ray. At first, either air or oxygen was used as a contrast medium, because positive-contrast agents were toxic. Later, when nontoxic positive-contrast agents had been developed primarily for use in intravenous pyelography, they were also used for arthrography and found to be more satisfactory than gases. One of the most comprehensive early studies on positive-contrast knee arthrography showing its high degree of accuracy was published by Lindblom[5] in 1948. Our studies of double-contrast arthrography[2,3,4] using air and a positive-contrast agent suggest that this method has a slight superiority over single positive-contrast arthrography. Approximately 30,000 arthrograms, using a double-contrast method with air and a meglumine salt positive-contrast agent, have been performed at the Hospital for Special Surgery and form the basis for this chapter. At present a fluoroscopic spot film method is used[2] that is more accurate than the previously used horizontal beam method described by Andrén.[1] Serious complications of arthrography are extremely rare, a single infection occurring in the 17-year period covered by this series. Rarely, only about once per 1,000 arthrograms, does a patient experience acute painful swelling of the knee because of rapid fluid accumulation. This appears to be caused by synovitis produced by the injected contrast agent. When this occurs, the knee joint is aspirated and fluid sent to the laboratory for culture. The aspiration cures the patient's symptoms. A less important and equally rare complication is urticaria, which has been controlled by oral administration of an antihistamine agent. The more serious allergic complications associated with the intravenous injection of positive-contrast agents have not occurred with arthrography.

High-quality modern radiographic and fluoroscopic equipment, as well as meticulous attention to detail of examination are required to produce optimal arthrographic radiographs. Evaluation of the arthrographic radiographs requires both knowledge of the technique of arthrography in order to ascertain that a complete and optimal study has been performed, as well as a detailed knowledge of the intracapsular anatomy of the knee joint. For this reason, the highlights of technique and the important features of normal anatomy of the knee are reviewed.

TECHNIQUE OF ARTHROGRAPHY

EQUIPMENT

An image-amplified fluoroscope with an x-ray tube that has a focal spot of smaller than 0.6 mm diameter for spot filming is essential. A 0.3-mm focal spot is optimal at the present time; in the future, smaller focal spot tubes may become available. At focal spot sizes of greater than 0.6 mm, radiographs become hazy and, while major meniscal tears can be seen, other abnormalities will be missed. A spot film device that places six to nine exposures on one film is normally used. A device that will stabilize the distal thigh to permit distraction of the knee joint during filming must be available. This can be a sling fastened to the edge of the table or a more sophisticated holding device. A small, firm pillow placed under the distal thigh is used at times to elevate the knee from the table in order to permit optimal tangential views.

INJECTION EQUIPMENT

Equipment consisting of swabs to scrub the knee joint, as well as drapes, syringes, and needles is available in commercially prepared sterile trays or can be assembled and autoclaved.

INJECTION TECHNIQUE

After povidone-iodine skin preparation, a 20-gauge, 1½-inch disposable needle is placed into the sulcus between the patella and the femoral condyle, on either the medial or the lateral side. Local lidocaine anesthesia is optional. When fluid is present, be it blood or clear synovial fluid, it must be aspirated as completely as possible. Any appreciable quantity of fluid remaining in the knee joint interferes with obtaining an optimal arthrogram. Complete aspiration, although time consuming, is necessary; even massive hemarthroses can be aspirated to the point at which excellent arthrograms can be obtained. When no excessive fluid is present or excess fluid has been adequately aspirated, 20 cc of room air is injected into the knee joint followed by 5 cc of a mixture of 60 percent meglumine contrast agent (RenoM60) mixed with three-tenths of a 1-cc 1/1,000 solution of epi-

nephrine. Epinephrine can be used to slow the absorption of the positive-contrast medium, providing more time in which to obtain optimal radiographs. If there are medical contraindications to the use of epinephrine, it is omitted. After a positive-contrast agent has been injected, another 20 cc of air is injected and the needle withdrawn. Since some of the air leaks through the needle when the syringes are changed, the amount of air in the knee varies between 30 and 40 cc, which is adequate for performing the arthrogram and does not cause painful overdistention of the knee joint.

Extracapsular injections of air or positive-contrast medium should be avoided, since either no arthrogram can be obtained or the partially extra-articular contrast agent interferes with interpretation. Extra-articular injection of meglumine positive-contrast agent may cause minor discomfort to the patient, but in our experience it has not caused permanent harm. Sodium salt contrast agents should not be used because their extra-articular injection causes severe pain. Immediately after the injection, the patient is placed prone and the knee flexed gently in order to distribute the contrast agent and thereby obtain good positive-contrast coating of the anterior cruciate ligament. The cruciate ligaments are examined next.

CRUCIATE LIGAMENT EXAMINATION

The patient sits at the edge of the x-ray table. A hard bolster is placed behind the calf and the foot, and the ankle is forced backward and held in this position either by a weighted chair or by a sling attached to the table. The bolster acts as a fulcrum to force the proximal tibia forward at the knee joint and keep the anterior cruciate ligament taut. A grid cassette is placed between the patient's knees, and a sharply collimated, overpenetrated radiograph of the knee is made with a horizontal x-ray beam (Fig. 6.1).

The patient then lies on the x-ray table with the knee in lateral position. A sling is placed around the calf and fastened to the side of the table. Using the sling as a fulcrum, the foot and ankle are pushed backward and downward to keep the cruciate ligaments, particularly the anterior cruciate ligament, taut. One or more spot films are taken with the knee in lateral position. A true lateral position can be confirmed by

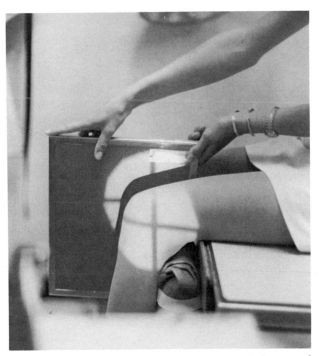

Fig. 6.1. Cruciate ligament examination with horizontal x-ray beam. The leg is forcibly flexed over a hard bolster that pushes the tibia forward to tense the anterior cruciate ligament. The patient holds a grid cassette. (From Freiberger, R.H., Kaye, J.J.: Arthrography. Appleton-Century-Crofts, New York, 1979, p. 97, with permission.)

seeing the femoral condyles superimposed. Other exposures are made with the sling around the distal thigh and pulling the foot and ankle downward and backward. This tightens the anterior and posterior cruciate ligaments. The menisci are then examined.

EXAMINATION OF THE MENISCI

The patient is placed prone, a sling or other restraining device is placed around the distal thigh and a determination made whether the medial or lateral side should be examined first. In children the lateral side is usually examined first because of the likelihood of a discoid or torn discoid lateral meniscus. In adults one is guided by the patient's symptoms; most often the medial side is examined first (Fig. 6.2). Initially the knee should be placed in a completely lateral position with the condyles overlapping. The knee is then turned slightly until the meniscus being examined is seen clear of the opposite condyle. A series of expo-

sures is made as the knee is turned, until the femoral condyles are again almost, but not completely, overlapping. Spot films should be large enough so that the degree of overlapping of the condyles in the most anterior and posterior portions of the menisci can be seen. Twelve to 18 spot film exposures of each meniscus are usually made for a complete examination.

If clinically indicated, the articular surfaces of the patella can be examined.

EXAMINATION OF THE PATELLA

The knee is fully extended; an elastic bandage may be applied to compress the suprapatellar bursa compressing it. By taking fluoroscopic spot films in the lateral and slightly off-lateral projections, the cartilaginous articular surfaces of the patella can be demonstrated.

POPLITEAL CYSTS

A large film to show the complete size and location of a popliteal cyst can be made at the end of the examination either with the spot film device or with an overhead x-ray tube. The popliteal cyst is usually seen partially on the spot films taken while the menisci are being examined.

The arthrographic films are reviewed immediately after the examination so that further exposures can be made if deemed necessary.

TECHNICAL POINTS

It is important that the interpreter of the arthrogram check the degree of overlapping of femoral condyles in the most anterior and posterior projections of the menisci. It is not unusual to see arthrograms in which only the midportions of the menisci have been adequately examined and which can be recognized by the lack of adequate overlapping of the condyles. Haziness of the contrast-coated cartilaginous contours or of the trabecular pattern of the condyles is an indication of either a large focal spot or of motion during the exposures. Both are detrimental to adequate evaluation. Haziness of contours may also be caused by absorption of the positive-contrast medium that results from a delay in filming. This effect can be minimized by the addition of epinephrine.

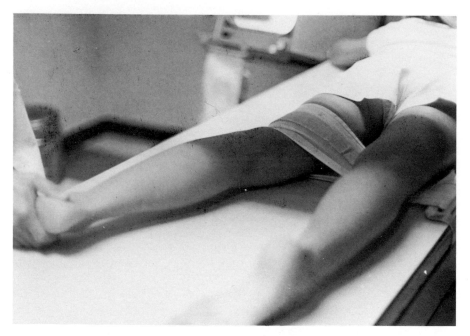

Fig. 6.2. The leg is positioned for spot filming the posterior segment of the medial meniscus. A sling around the distal thigh and fastened to the table permits distraction of the articular surfaces. (From Frieberger, R.H., Kay, J.J: Arthrography. Appleton-Century-Crofts, New York, 1979, p. 14, with permission.)

Fig. 6.3. Normal cruciate ligaments. The synovial surfaces of the cruciate ligaments (arrows) are coated with radiopaque contrast substance. The anterior surface of the anterior cruciate ligament is perfectly straight and inserts posterior to the anterior margin of the tibia.

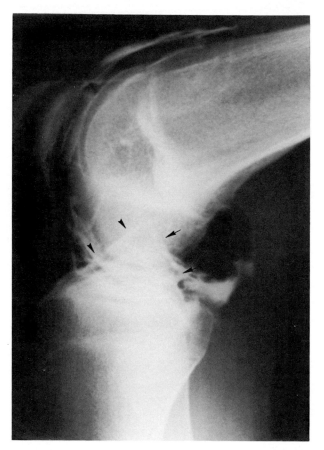

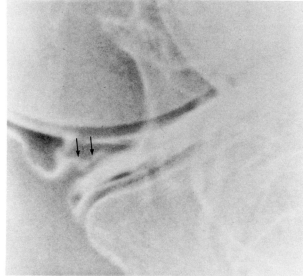

Fig. 6.4. The wavy horizontal line (arrowheads), representing contrast agent at the bottom of the synovial meniscal recess, is not a tear. (From Freiberger, R.H., Kaye, J.J.: Arthrography. Appleton-Century-Crofts, New York, 1979, p. 39, with permission.)

ANATOMY

CRUCIATE LIGAMENTS

The cruciate ligaments are intra-articular extra-synovial structures that are coated by contrast agent only at their synovial surfaces and that are therefore not completely surrounded by contrast agent. Essentially only the anterior surface of the anterior cruciate ligament and posterior surface of the posterior cruciate ligament can be seen on the arthrogram. The anterior cruciate ligament inserts into the tibia approximately 8 mm posterior from its anterior margin. When normal and properly tensed during the examination, it is seen as a sharp, straight line on both the horizontal beam film and on the fluoroscopic spot films (Fig. 6.3). The posterior cruciate ligament extends over the posterior margin of the tibia and is also depicted by a straight or slightly posteriorly bowed line of contrast depicting its posterior synovial surface. While the cruciate ligaments can be seen on a tunnel view of the knee taken after the injection of contrast media, this view is not usable for the evaluation of tears.

MEDIAL MENISCUS

The medial meniscus is a crescent-shaped fibrocartilaginous structure, triangular in vertical section, and having a complete peripheral capsular attachment. It is wider posteriorly than it is anteriorly. The synovial attachments of the meniscus are slightly lax, forming small recesses at the meniscal–synovial junction. Because of its complete capsular attachment, no contrast agent normally penetrates between the meniscus and the capsule or within the meniscus. Positive-contrast agent in the meniscal synovial recesses can be projected through the meniscus and has been mistaken for a horizontal tear (Fig. 6.4). The opacified capsular recesses projected through the meniscus can, however, be easily differentiated from tears because the horizontal lines of opaque contrast agent always end exactly at the apex of the meniscal synovial recess seen in profile.

LATERAL MENISCUS

The lateral meniscus is also a fibrocartilaginous structure which is more circular than the medial meniscus and which has approximately the same width from front to back. Its cross section is triangular. The lateral meniscus is not completely attached to the capsule. In its posterior portion it is partially separated from the capsule by the popliteus hiatus that communicates with the knee joint and fills with contrast agent. Therefore, normally, contrast agent can be seen peripheral to the posterior portion of the lateral meniscus. At the superior end of the popliteus hiatus the superior margin of the lateral meniscus lacks a capsular attachment. The capsular attachment starts again immediately posterior to the superior orifice of the hiatus and forms the roof of the hiatus. A second inferior capsular attachment that forms the floor of the hiatus becomes progressively thinner as it proceeds posteriorly (Fig. 6.5). Commonly there is a defect in the inferior attachment of the lateral meniscus where it crosses the tibial plateau (Fig. 6.6). At this point there is a thick superior meniscal attachment so that the meniscus is not loose or detached. The defect in the inferior attachment of the lateral meniscus can be seen on arthrograms and on anatomic dissection and should not be mistaken for a clinically significant lesion. The popliteus hiatus therefore communicates with the intracapsular space of the knee not only superiorly but usually also inferiorly, and it is normally possible during an arthrotomy or arthroscopy to place a probe under the lateral meniscus and into the popliteus hiatus.

Because the lateral meniscus is more circular than the medial meniscus its most anterior and posterior portions cannot be completely examined by arthrography. Fortunately it is uncommon to have tears totally confined to the small areas that cannot be seen on the arthrogram. Although the contrast containing popliteus hiatus causes some problems in interpretation of the arthrogram, its normal appearance is recognizable by knowing its anatomy. Distortions of the contours of the popliteus hiatus serve as an arthrographic clue to abnormalities of the posterior segment of the lateral meniscus.

MENISCAL ABNORMALITIES

Meniscal tears, which can be perceived as fractures of the meniscus, are identified arthrographically by seeing contrast medium within the meniscus coating the surfaces of the tear. If meniscal fragments are in close apposition, only a thin line of positive contrast agent between the fragments may be evident (Fig.

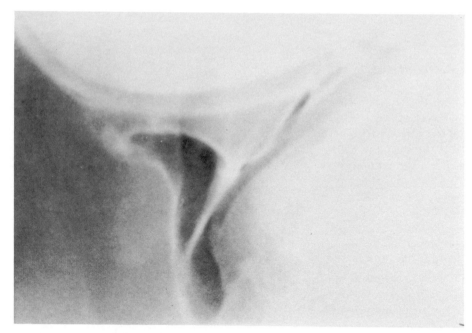

Fig. 6.5. Normal posterior horn of the lateral meniscus. The popliteus tendon forms the lateral border of the hiatus, the superior capsular attachment the roof, and the inferior capsular attachment the floor of the hiatus. (From Freiberger, R.H., Kaye, J.J.: Arthrography. Appleton-Century-Crofts, New York, 1979, p. 46, with permission.)

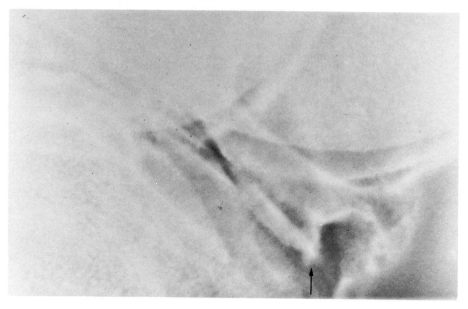

Fig. 6.6. A defect in the inferior capsular attachment of the lateral meniscus far posteriorly (arrow) is normal. (From Freiberger, R.H., Kaye, J.J.: Arthrography. Appleton-Century-Crofts, New York, 1979, p. 48, with permission.)

6.7). When the fragments are separated the surfaces of the tear are coated by positive contrast agent and air fills the space between the separated fragments (Fig. 6.8). If there is wide separation of the fragments as in a bucket-handle tear in which the inner fragment has displaced into the intercondylar notch, arthrographic evidence is a deformed narrow outer fragment and absence of the normal wedge-shaped inner fragment (Fig. 6.9). The tear may be completely vertical in orientation or it may be horizontal extending into the meniscus from either its superior or inferior articular surface (Fig. 6.10). A combination of vertical and horizontal components forming a complex tear is common. Occasionally particularly in older people, the inner normally sharp margin of the meniscus is rounded or somewhat irregular in appearance with

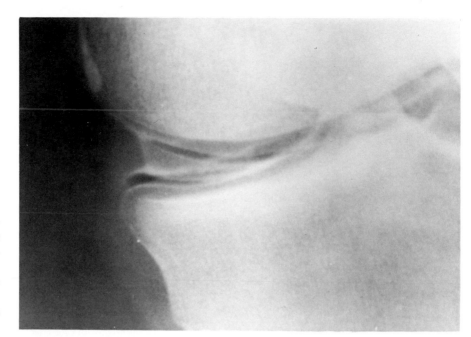

Fig. 6.7. A vertical longitudinal tear of the medial meniscus with the fragments in close apposition. (From Freiberger, R.H., Kaye, J.J.: Arthrography. Appleton-Century-Crofts, New York, 1979, p. 61, with permission.)

Fig. 6.8. A tear of the medial meniscus with considerable separation of fragments.

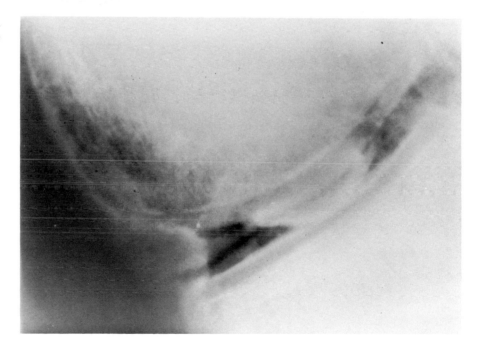

opacification of the inner apex of the meniscus. This is an indication of one or more small inner marginal tears representing degenerative changes rather than an acute traumatic tear.

Cysts of the menisci are seen more commonly in the lateral meniscus, where they tend to be in the anterior portion rather than in the medial meniscus where they tend to be posterior. The arthrographic diagnosis of meniscal cyst is made when a horizontal or oblique tear opacified by contrast agent extends beyond the periphery of the meniscus with contrast agent opacifying a portion of the cyst (Fig. 6.11). The

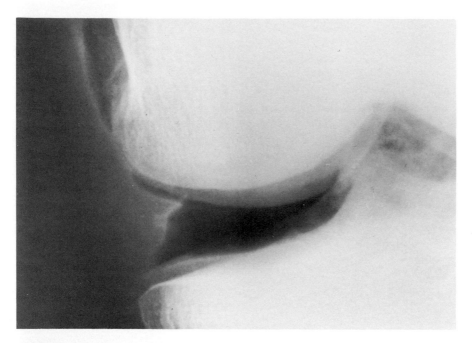

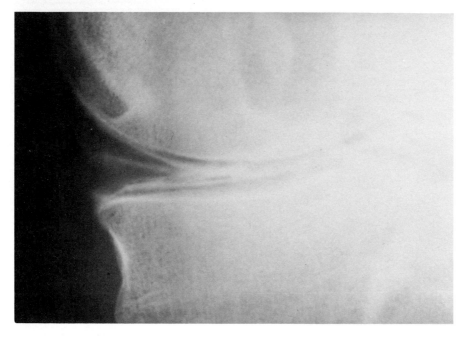

Fig. 6.9. The inner fragment of the medial meniscus has displaced into the intercondylar notch. Only the deformed outer fragment remains visible. (From Freiberger, R.H., Kaye, J.J.: Arthrography. Appleton-Century-Crofts, New York, 1979, p. 65, with permission.)

Fig. 6.10. A horizontal meniscal tear. (From Freiberger, R.H., Kaye, J.J.: Arthrography. Appleton-Century-Crofts, New York, 1979, p. 71, with permission.)

complete opacification of the peripheral portion of the tear and of the cyst may not be evident on the exposures made in the early part of the examination and therefore, when a horizontal tear is seen and the presence of a cyst suspected, delayed exposures should be made after the patient has walked for a few minutes to permit contrast filling of the peripheral portion of the tear and of the cyst.

Discoid menisci are much more common in the lateral than in the medial meniscus and are likely to be the cause of the symptoms of internal derangement of the knee in the child. A discoid meniscus is recognized by its abnormal width and thickness and by loss of the inner apex and wedge shape of the meniscus. Discoid menisci are commonly torn. If the inner fragment is displaced, it is not difficult to make

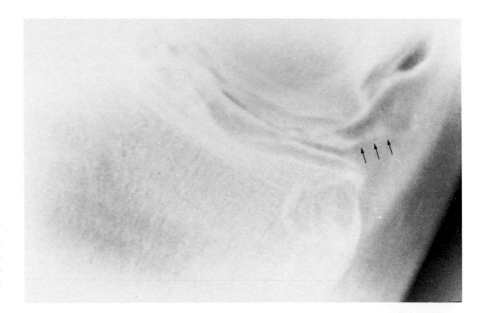

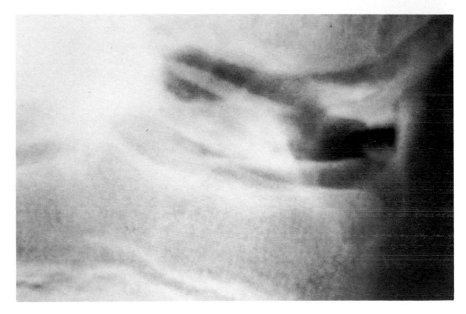

Fig. 6.11. A horizontal tear extends peripherally into a small collection of peripherally placed contrast agent (arrows), indicating a torn cystic lateral meniscus.

Fig. 6.12. A torn discoid lateral meniscus in a child. The inner fragment is abnormally wide, indicating that the tear is in a discoid meniscus. (From Freiberger, R.H., Kaye, J.J.: Arthrography. Appleton-Century-Crofts, New York, 1979, p. 81, with permission.)

the diagnosis of a tear, however, it may not be evident that the tear has occurred in a discoid meniscus (Fig. 6.12). Conversely the discoid shape of the meniscus may be recognized but a tear might not be evident. In either case the arthrogram has visualized the abnormality of the knee joint and permits the surgeon a course of action that depends on the patient's symptoms and disability.

CRUCIATE LIGAMENT TEARS

When the arthrogram has been technically properly performed and the exposures made with the cruciate ligaments taut, absence of visualization of a straight anterior margin of the anterior cruciate ligament or laxity with posterior bowing of the anterior cruciate ligament's contour is a sign of either a com-

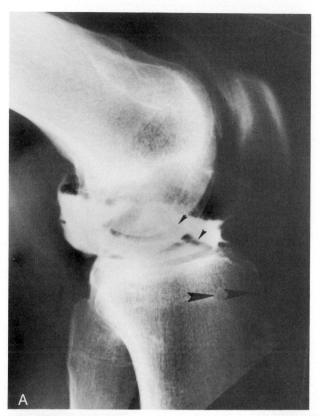

plete or subsynovial cruciate ligament tear (Fig. 6.13A, B). Absence of the contour of the posterior cruciate ligament indicates a tear. A slight posterior bowing of the cruciate ligament contour is normal.

CAPSULAR TEARS

Leakage of contrast agent medially is evidence of a tear of the capsule and medial collateral ligament. Lateral leakage is indicative of a capsular tear. Leakage from the capsule indicates a tear; however, the absence of contrast leakage more than 3 days after an injury does not rule out the possibility of a capsular or medial collateral ligament tear, since the synovial lining can heal water-tight by this period, whereas a structural defect in the capsule or ligament is still present. Leakage of contrast occasionally occurs posteriorly from a popliteal cyst. This is usually not of clinical significance and can be the result of overdistention of the knee joint. Care must be taken not to mistake extra-articularly injected contrast medium for leakage from the joint.

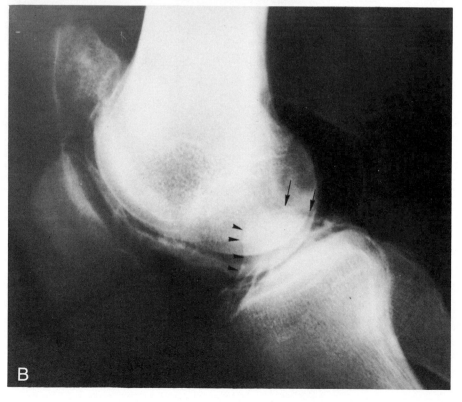

Fig. 6.13. A posteriorly bowed irregular anterior cruciate ligament surface (arrows) indicates a subsynovial tear. (*A*) Horizontal beam examination. (*B*) Vertical beam spot film examination. (Part A from Freiberger, R.H., Kaye, J.J.: Arthrography. Appleton-Century-Crofts, New York, 1979, p. 104, with permission.)

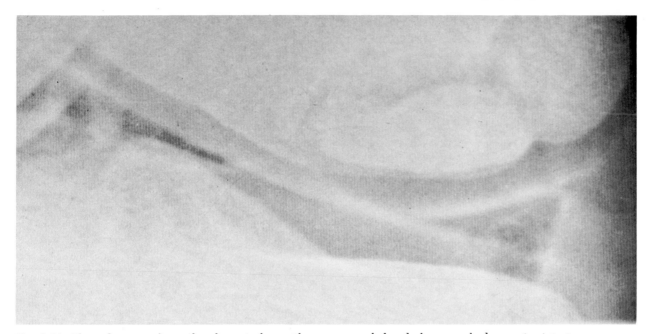

Fig. 6.14. The arthrogram shows that the articular cartilage over a subchondral osseous body remains intact.

MISCELLANEOUS INTRA-ARTICULAR ABNORMALITIES

Chondral fractures not involving underlying bone can be demonstrated if they are located tangential to the x-ray beam. Osteochondral fractures and osteochondritis dissecans can similarly be identified and it is possible to determine whether the overlying articular cartilage remains intact or whether contrast agent extends between the fragments indicating a fracture of the overlying cartilage (Fig. 6.14), and loosening of the fragment. Loose cartilaginous or osseous bodies can be identified as being intra-articular, however, the contrast-coated bubbles of a double-contrast arthrogram may interfere with the identification of these bodies. Single-contrast arthrograms either with diluted positive-contrast agent or with air are preferable for finding loose cartilaginous bodies and the combination of positive-contrast arthrography and tomography is useful. Synovial masses, as seen in pigmented villonodular synovitis, can be identified (Fig. 6.15).

CONCLUSION

Knee arthrography is a simple, accurate diagnostic examination which does not require hospitalization of the patient and has practically no complications or post-examination morbidity. Arthrograms must be performed with meticulous attention to detail of pro-

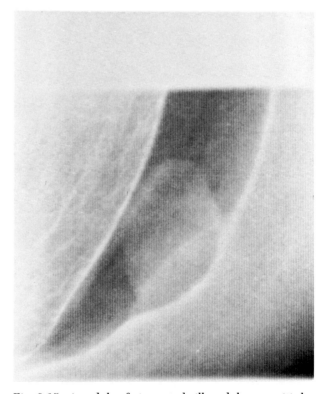

Fig. 6.15. A nodule of pigmented villonodular synovitis located in the suprapatellar bursa becomes visible on a double-contrast arthrogram. (From Freiberger, R.H., Kaye, J.J.: Arthrography. Appleton-Century-Crofts, New York, 1979, p. 115, with permission.)

cedure and with modern x-ray equipment having image-amplified fluoroscopy and small focal spot filming. Properly performed arthrograms can be interpreted by any physician familiar with the intra-articular anatomy of the knee joint and sufficiently familiar with the arthrographic procedure to determine whether a technically adequate arthrogram has been submitted.

REFERENCES

1. Andrén, L., and Wehlin, L.: Double-contrast arthrography of the knee with horizontal roentgen ray beam. Acta Orthop Scand 29: 307, 1960.
2. Freiberger, R.H., and Kaye, J.J.: Arthrography. New York, Appleton-Century-Crofts, 1979.
3. Freiberger, R.H., Killoran, P.J., and Cardona, G.: Arthrography of the knee by double contrast method. Am J Roentgenol Radium Ther Nucl Med 97: 736, 1966.
4. Furuya, M., Harrison-Stubbs, M.O., and Freiberger, R.H.: Arthrography of the knee: analysis of 2101 arthrograms and 623 surgical findings. Rev Hosp Spec Surg 2: 11, 1972.
5. Lindblom, K.: Arthrography of the knee: roengenographic and anatomic study. Acta Radiol (Suppl) 74: 1, 1948.
6. Werndorff, K. R., and Robinson, H.: Verhandlung d. deutsch. Gesellsch. f. orthop. Chir., 4th Congress, 1905.

7 Arthroscopy of the Knee

John B. McGinty

During the past decade, arthroscopy has grown from an innovative curiosity into an accepted diagnostic procedure in the armamentarium of orthopedic surgeons. It is becoming commonplace in North America to see arthrotomy of the knee preceded by an endoscopic examination to confirm the diagnosis, establish the specific details of the pathology, and formulate the plan for the subsequent surgical management. In the past 5 years arthroscopic techniques have been adapted to surgery of the knee as a treatment modality, thereby reducing the morbidity associated with the more traditional approaches to intraarticular pathology. Although these surgical approaches are still controversial in some situations, they are gradually coming into perspective in relationship to the overall management of musculoskeletal pathology.

HISTORY

The first arthroscopic examinations were performed in Tokyo in 1918 by Takagi using a cystoscope to examine cadaver knees in a gas medium.[38] Two years later, he developed the No. 1 arthroscope, the precursor to modern instruments. The techniques were introduced to North America in 1931 by Michael Burman, when he examined multiple joints in a cadaver and subsequently reviewed a series of his patients with rheumatoid arthritis.[1,2] Interest dropped in the United States, and further development returned to Japan, where Watanabe developed the No. 21 arthroscope[41] and published his classic atlas.[42] The No. 21 arthroscope became the instrument with which many of the leaders of the 1970s learned their techniques. This instrument, however, used a tungsten bulb in a light carrier for illumination, a situation which resulted in relatively easy loss of illumination and breakage in the knee. Today virtually all arthroscopic examinations are performed with a rigid telescope and fiberoptic illumination.

The decade beginning in 1970 brought the most rapid advances in the use of arthroscopy with both diagnostic and therapeutic techniques. Casscells[4] published his own series with an accuracy of 80 percent. McGinty and Freedman[22] reviewed 225 cases with an accuracy of 90 percent. However, it was Dandy and Jackson's review of 800 consecutive cases, with an accuracy of more than 98 percent, that firmly established arthroscopy in the diagnostic repertoire of orthopedic surgeons.[6] DeHaven and Collins[7] published a prospective study of 100 cases comparing physical examination, arthrography, and arthroscopy and showed that arthroscopy was of definite value in increasing diagnostic accuracy.

On the basis of O'Connor's pioneering efforts in the mid-1970s and the development of the operating arthroscope, arthroscopic surgery was initiated.[33] Johnson[18] initiated the use of power instrumentation in the knee to trim menisci, excise synovium, shave articular cartilage, and abrade articular surfaces. Investigative work is now under way using carbon dioxide and nitrogen as a medium for arthroscopy, trying different sources of energy, such as laser energy for arthroscopic surgery, attempting to repair and reconstruct the anterior cruciate ligament, attempting to repair peripheral detachments of posterior tears of the menisci, and using the arthroscope for various purposes in other joints including the spine.

ANESTHESIA

Diagnostic arthroscopy can be performed satisfactorily with local anesthesia. In comparing consecutive arthroscopic examinations under general or spinal anesthesia and examinations under local anesthesia, McGinty and Matza[26] attained a diagnostic accuracy of 91 percent and 95 percent respectively. Assessment of accuracy was done on the basis of subsequent arthrotomy in 104 knees examined under local anesthesia and 124 knees examined with general or spinal anesthesia. A loss in diagnostic accuracy did not accompany the use of local anesthesia.

In 228 knees examined with general or spinal anesthesia, one pulmonary embolus, two significant hemarthroses, and two infections in procedures immediately followed by arthrotomy occurred. In 297 knees examined with local anesthesia no complications were seen.

The use of local anesthesia eliminates the morbidity of general anesthesia including potential airway problems and central nervous system depression. The cost of a recovery room and an anesthesiologist is also eliminated. The patient is awake and aware and can leave the hospital immediately at the conclusion of the procedure.

The technique involves the use of 0.5 percent lidocaine (Xylocaine) without epinephrine for entry into skin, subcutaneous tissue, capsule, and synovium. It is imperative to wait at least 3 minutes from the instillation of anesthesia until starting the procedure. After entry into the joint, 10 cm^3 of 0.5 percent bupivacaine hydrochloride (Marcaine) is injected directly into the knee. This technique has allowed anesthesia for up to 1 hour without additional anesthesia.

Johnson[17] has shown the successful use of local anesthesia with the small-diameter arthroscope and multiple-puncture techniques. In our experience there have been no adverse reactions to local anesthetic agents.

The use of local anesthesia in arthroscopic surgical procedures is somewhat more difficult. The required maneuvering of changing portals of viewing and operating instruments and the patient relaxation required make the use of general or spinal anesthesia more desirable. On the other hand, Stone[37] recently performed more than 100 consecutive surgical procedures satisfactorily under local anesthesia.

INSTRUMENTS AND OPERATING ROOM SETUP

Arthroscopic examinations are performed with rigid instruments and illumination through fiberoptic cables (Fig. 7.1). These instruments vary in diameter from 1.7 to 6.0 mm. Instruments with outside sheath diameters of 4.0 to 6.0 mm are satisfactory for examination of the knee. The entire knee, including the posterior compartments, can be examined satisfactorily with large-diameter arthroscopes. The larger-diameter arthroscopes provide a larger field of vision, better illumination for both visualization and photography, a more efficient irrigation system, and adequate illumination if television is to be used. A tungsten light source with a 150-watt bulb is adequate for direct visualization through the arthroscope. However, for photography, a strobe unit or a high-intensity light source, although not necessary, is desirable. To use television satisfactorily, a high-intensity or xenon light source is also desirable (Fig. 7.2). It should be emphasized that direct viewing through the arthroscope with a xenon light source has some attendant danger. Retinal burns have been reported by surgeons who have repeatedly examined directly with a xenon light source.[36]

A good source of irrigation is essential for adequate visualization of the inside of the knee. This source should be normal saline at room temperature connected from a sterile reservoir 1 meter above the operating table in a gravity feed (Fig. 7.3A). Using pressure greater than gravity may result in soft tissue extravasation, which can produce a compartment syndrome. The irrigation system can be connected to the

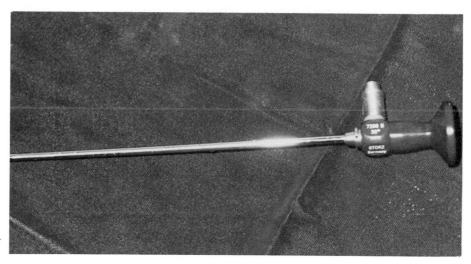

Fig. 7.1. Standard 4.5-mm fiberoptic arthroscope.

sheath of the arthroscope and used intermittently or can enter through a suprapatellar portal as a continuous irrigation system. The outflow of the system may be connected to suction in an intermittent system: The inflow valve is open during the procedure and closed while the outflow valve is opened to evacuate the joint, or is connected to gravity drainage in a continuous system (Fig. 7.3B).

Accessory instruments for diagnostic arthroscopy should include a probe and a biopsy forceps. A probe should be used in every diagnostic examination (Fig. 7.4). It provides a sense of touch as well as sight. By palpating the meniscus, tears may be detected that might otherwise go unrecognized. The examiner can palpate the anterior cruciate ligament and detect subsynovial tears. The probe also gives the examiner a

Fig. 7.2. Standard tungsten (150-watt) light course on top of xenon light source.

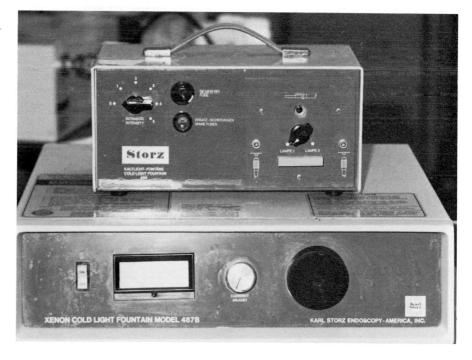

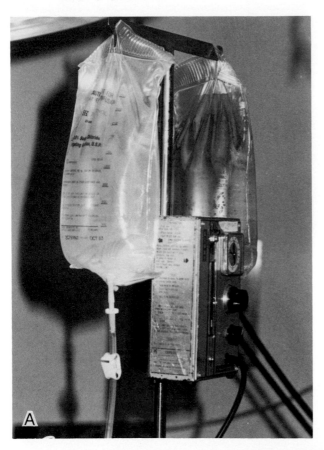

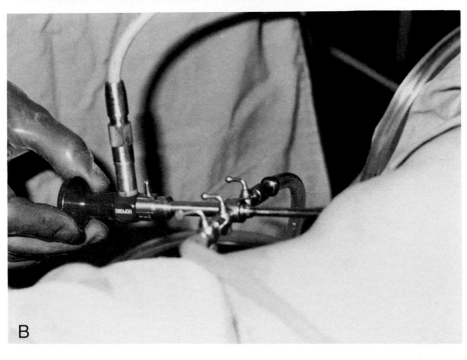

Fig. 7.3 (A) Irrigation reservoir on pole with tourniquet box. Two bags of sterile saline are connected by a Y tube to arthroscopy sheath. (B) Inflow tube in foreground connected to saline reservoir proximally. Second valve is connected to vacuum system for outflow.

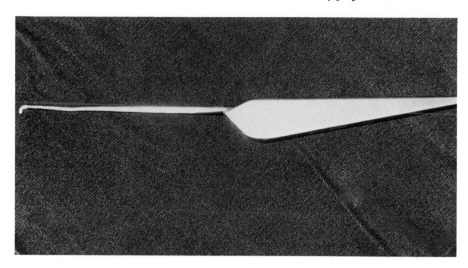

Fig. 7.4. Probe may be calibrated in shaft for reference. Tip is 4 mm long.

sense of firmness or softness of articular cartilage. Finally, the probe enables the arthroscopist to develop and practice triangulation, a skill essential to bringing two points together inside the knee, a skill without which arthroscopic surgery is impossible (Fig. 7.5).

The best method of synovial biopsy is the use of techniques of arthroscopic surgery. Therefore, biopsy forceps of different sizes are essential, both for blind synovial biopsy and for biopsy under direct vision.

Arthroscopic surgery has provided a milieu for a proliferation of instruments (Fig. 7.6). There are a plethora of knives (Fig. 7.7), scissors, grasping forceps, and retractors (Fig. 7.8). There are several systems of power instruments, including shavers, cut-

Fig. 7.5. Arthroscope in anterolateral portal and probe in anteromedial portal in position for triangulation.

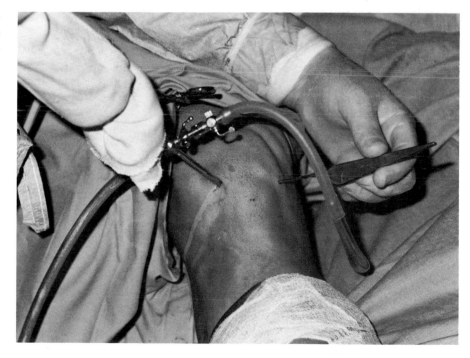

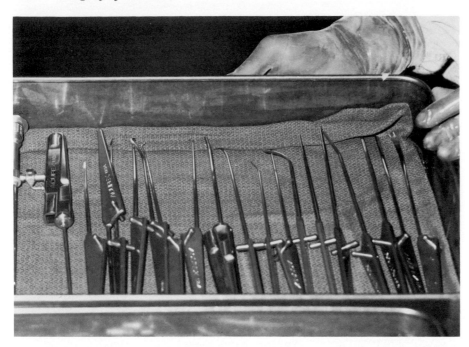

Fib. 7.6. Tray with assortment of knives and scissors.

ters, drills, and abraders (Fig. 7.9). These are systems driven by electric motors, air systems, and mechanical linkages, run directly from house current, and some from rechargeable batteries.

Various types of legholders are marketed to fix the thigh of the involved extremity so that varus and valgus stress can be applied to open up the lateral and medial compartments (Fig. 7.10). A leg holder is very helpful, particularly for meniscal surgery. Providing a fixation point proximal to the knee stabilizes the

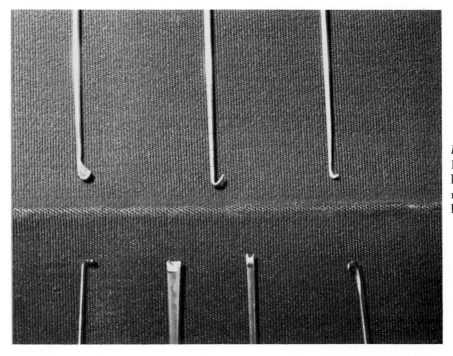

Fig. 7.7. Variety of knives (Top) Hockey stick knife, curved probe, hooked knife. (Bottom) Probe, large meniscotome, small meniscotome, back cutting knife.

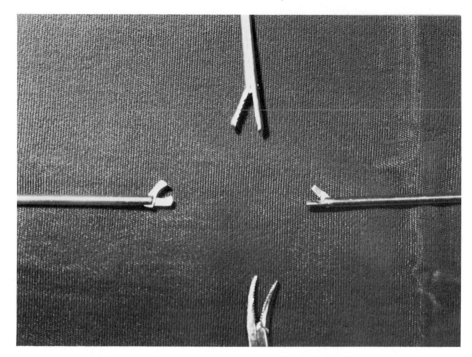

Fig. 7.8. Clockwise from top: loose body forceps, basket forceps, grasping forceps, scissors.

operative field when stress is applied, thereby making instrumentation in the knee much easier. If the leg holder is applied with the hip in 30 degrees of flexion, the knee can be moved from full extension to 90 degrees of flexion without breaking the foot of the table.

The operating team is extremely important in the performance of arthroscopic surgery. An assistant familiar with the instruments, manipulations, and techniques is invaluable to the procedure.[16] Arthroscopic instruments are fragile and sophisticated. They must

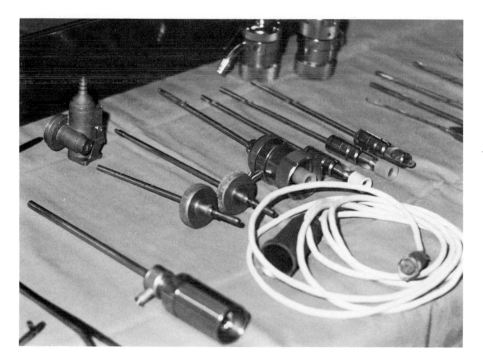

Fig. 7.9. Three types of power instruments.

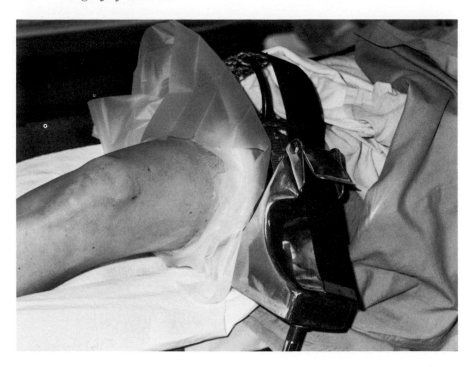

Fig. 7.10. Leg holder to fix thigh and act as fulcrum for varus and valgus stress.

be handled with care to maintain sharp edges. Most operating room personnel, without special interest and training, do not understand the care of these instruments and therefore end up using inadequate instrumentation to perform the task at hand.

The use of television in arthroscopic surgery, although not necessary, is extremely helpful in several ways (Fig. 7.11). First television gets the team involved in the procedure so that the assistant can really help if he can see what he is doing; if the assistant can hold the camera, you now have two hands with which to work. By learning to examine and work with a television monitor, you are in a more comfortable position and can therefore concentrate better and work more efficiently. Also with a cassette recorder the surgeon can record any sequence of the procedure desired. Television also has great educational value in arthroscopy and probably represents the best method of learning these skills, first by observing someone either live or on tape, and later doing the examination (one-to-one) while the instructor gives instruction, watching the monitor.

Arthroscopy must be done in the operating room with the same aseptic technique one would use for an arthrotomy. Two infections occurred several years ago when I followed an arthroscopy with an arthrot-

omy without a second skin preparation. If the arthroscopy is to be followed directly by arthrotomy, complete reprepping, regowning, and redraping must be carried out by the entire team.

The use of a tourniquet is not necessary for diagnostic arthroscopy. A tourniquet is helpful in most arthroscopic surgical procedures in order to completely eliminate bleeding as a distraction. However, bleeding can be handled by irrigation in most instances, with the exception of lateral retinacular release and synovectomy, two procedures for which the use of a tourniquet is essential.

INDICATIONS

Not every painful knee requires an arthroscopic examination. Arthroscopy is an ancillary diagnostic procedure; like arthrography, it should never replace a good clinical routine. Before considering arthroscopy, a good history, a thorough physical examination, and appropriate radiographic studies must be performed. If indicated, laboratory studies should next be done. The use of an arthrogram has become somewhat more controversial and probably should be done if the local talent is more proficient in arthrography rather than

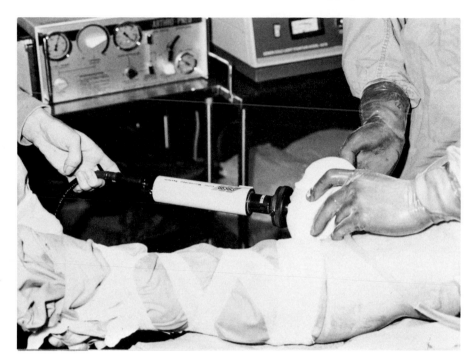

Fig. 7.11. Six-ounce video-camera attached to eyepiece of arthroscope at beginning of procedure before being wrapped with sterile stockinette.

arthroscopy.[31] However, there is no area of the knee that a good arthroscopist cannot visualize.

Arthroscopy is indicated, like a myelogram in spine surgery, when surgery is contemplated in the knee, particularly meniscal surgery. This allows specific definition of the lesion and planning of arthrotomy. It is also indicated in diagnostic problems of the knee, particularly with synovial lesions. It is not indicated when extensive operative procedures, such as ligament reconstructions or total knee replacements, are planned. Arthroscopy is indicated before proximal tibial osteotomy for unicompartmental osteoarthritis to confirm the status of the articular cartilage in the more normal compartment.

Arthroscopy is indicated in the acutely injured stable knee with a hemarthrosis to define the status of the anterior cruciate ligament.[32] Arthroscopy is not indicated in the unstable knee with acute injury. In this situation arthroscopy may result in extravasation of fluid into the extracellular compartment, making ligament repair more difficult.

Arthroscopy may be indicated in the patient with a worker's compensation injury or a legal liability injury who has failed to respond to treatment and has a paucity of physical or radiographic findings.

Pain per se is not an indication for arthroscopy. The procedure should only be performed for pain in the presence of objective physical or radiographic findings, a clinical pattern suggesting a specific diagnosis, or a failure to respond to established treatment.

TECHNIQUE

There are several different techniques for performing arthroscopic examinations. The technique I use to perform routine examinations is presented here.[24]

The examination should always be performed in a routine fashion, following the same course each time. The examiner can return to any area or make special approaches after the routine look through the knee. It is recommended to start in the suprapatellar pouch, to look at the patellofemoral joint, move into the anteromedial compartment, then to the intercondylar notch, and conclude with the anterolateral compartment. After this routine, a look in the posterior compartments or probing can be done if it is considered necessary.

The examination must be performed in the operating room under the same aseptic precautions taken for an arthrotomy. These precautions must not be compromised. The patient is in the supine position

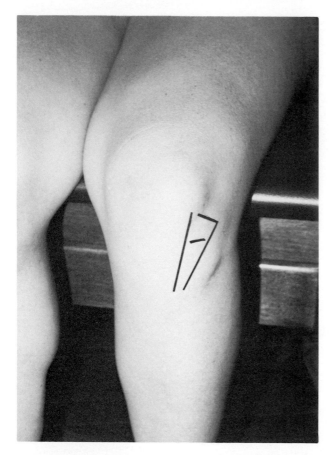

Fig. 7.12. Routine anteolateral incision in triangle bounded by lateral border of patellar tendon, anterior border of iliotibial band, and transverse band of lateral retinaculum.

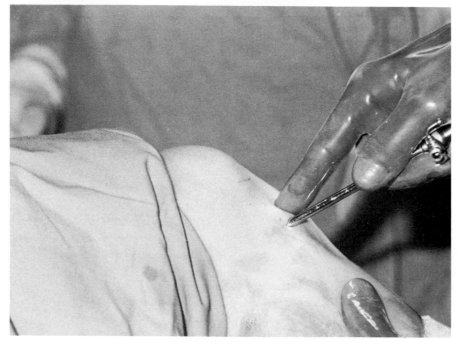

Fig. 7.13. Note position of examiner's index finger to prevent overpenetration of the sharp trochar and damage to articular cartilage.

on the operating table. The table is not broken. A tourniquet and leg holder are not necessary for arthroscopic examination without surgery. The anterolateral portal is used for routine examination.

After the induction of appropriate anesthesia, preparation of the skin of the lower extremity, and draping, an incision is made in the anterior knee in a triangle bounded anteriorly by the lateral border of the patellar tendon, posteriorly by the anterior border of the iliotibial band, and superiorly by the patelloepicondylar fibers of the lateral retinaculum (Fig. 7.12). The sheath with the sharp trochar is then inserted through the capsule (Fig. 7.13). The sharp trochar is replaced with a blunt trochar to prevent damage to articular cartilage; the sheath is inserted through the synovium into the intercondylar notch and up under the patella into the suprapatellar pouch. The trochar is removed, and a fiberoptic arthroscope is placed in the sheath. The surgeon must be certain that the tip of the telescope does not extend beyond the end of the sheath more than 2 or 3 mm; otherwise, damage to the telescope may occur.

The knee is extended and the suprapatellar pouch is scanned and the lateral suprapatellar recess explored to the joint line (Fig. 7.14). The quality of the synovium is noted in this location and can subsequently be biopsied. The undersurface of the patella is examined from superior to inferior pole and scanned from medial to lateral border, both by moving the telescope and manipulating the patella with the opposite hand. The instrument is then guided into the anteromedial compartment by flexing the knee to 45 degrees and using the horizon of the medial condyle as a reference (Fig. 7.15). The medial condylar surface and anterior two-thirds of the medial meniscus are inspected with the foot off the side of the table. The surgeon can apply a valgus force, leaning against the lateral side of the knee and thereby visualize about 40 percent of the posterior horn of the medial meniscus. The telescope is then moved into the intercondylar notch and the anterior cruciate ligament visualized (Fig. 7.16). Care must be taken not to confuse the ligamentum mucosum with the anterior cruciate ligament. If the anterior cruciate ligament is intact, the posterior cruciate ligament cannot be visualized. The knee is then flexed to 90 degrees and the hip externally rotated, allowing the lateral malleolus of the involved side to rest on the proximal tibia of the uninvolved side in the so-called 4 position (Fig. 7.17).

Gravity then allows the knee to drop into varus opening the lateral compartment. The telescope is then dropped off the anterior cruciate into the posterolateral compartment. The entire posterior horn of the lateral meniscus can be seen from the ligament of Humphry to the popliteus sheath. By slowly extending the knee, the middle and anterior thirds of the lateral meniscus can be visualized. The surgeon can then return to areas of particular concern for a more detailed examination or photographic documentation.[25] The surgeon may also use alternate approaches and tactile examination with a probe.

APPROACHES

There are six basic approaches to examination of the knee.

1. Anterolateral. This approach represents the best portal for the most comprehensive examination of the knee (see above for detailed description). Other approaches should be supplemental to it in exploring areas of the knee that cannot be reached through the anterolateral approach.

2. Anteromedial. This approach is valuable in examining the anterolateral compartment and in getting an overview of the anterior half of the lateral meniscus, particularly if using instrumentation on the lateral meniscus through the anterolateral portal. It is made through an incision just medial to the patellar tendon and about 1 cm above the medial tibial plateau. The arthroscope is then brought across the joint to the anterolateral compartment in the mirror image of the anterolateral approach. The suprapatellar medial recess can be visualized through this approach (Fig. 7.18A,B).

3. Central. This approach has three variations. It is useful for examining the posteromedial and posterolateral compartments. The central approach was described by Gillquist and co-workers[9–11] and involves passing the sheath and sharp trochar through a midline incision 1 cm below the inferior pole of the patella either medial or lateral to the anterior cruciate ligament in the intracondylar notch and on into the posteromedial or posterolateral compartment. The 70-degree telescope is then placed into the sheath and, by rotating the arthroscope, the entire posterior compartment and posterior cruciate ligament can be ex-

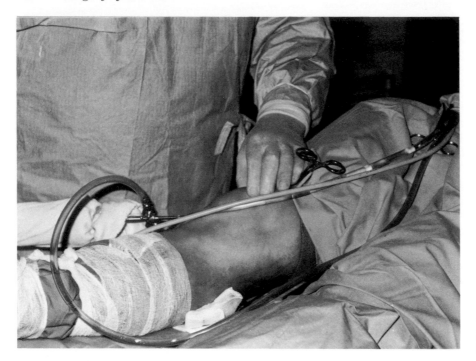

Fig. 7.14. Examination of suprapateller pouch and patellofemoral joint.

Fig. 7.15. Examination of the anteromedial compartment.

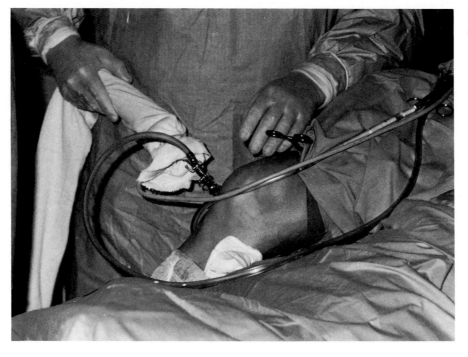

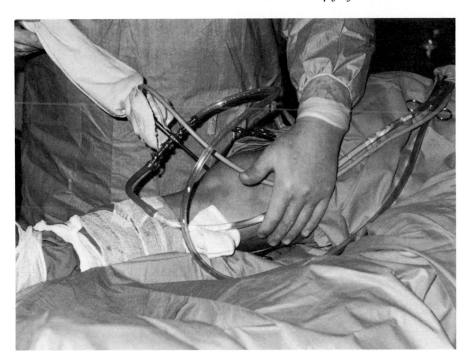

Fig. 7.16. Examination of the intercondylar notch.

Fig. 7.17. Examination of the anterolateral compartment.

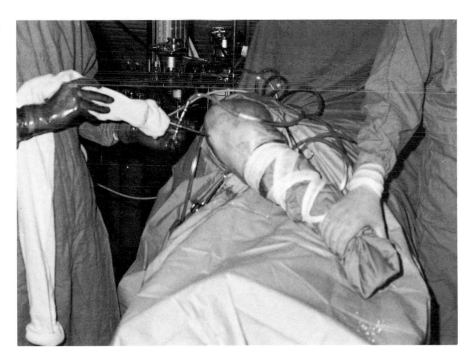

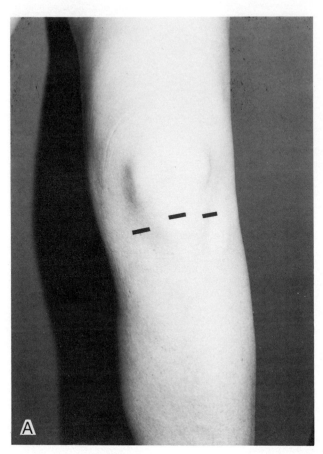

amined. Visualization of the posterior attachments of the meniscus is readily attained. A probe can be inserted behind the respective collateral ligament and tactile examination completed.

A variation of this central approach is possible using the anterolateral and anteromedial portals, thereby avoiding puncture of the patellar tendon. After routine examination through an anterolateral portal, the telescope is removed and a blunt trochar is inserted into the sheath. The medial condyle is palpated with the tip of the trochar until the interval between the lateral surface of the medial condyle and the anterior cruciate ligament is entered (Fig. 7.19A). The soft tissue around the sheath where it enters the skin is pushed toward the midline with the knee in 30 degrees of flexion; slight pressure is applied to the sheath, and the tip will drop into the posteromedial compartment (Fig. 7.19B). The 70-degree telescope can then replace the trochar and the posteromedial compartment can be examined (Fig. 7.19C). Similarly, by using an anteromedial portal and the interval between the medial surface of the lateral femoral condyle and the anterior cruciate ligament, the posterolateral compartment can be explored. To explore the posterior compartments adequately, the knee must be in 90 degrees of flexion to allow the posterior capsule and soft tissue structures to fall away.

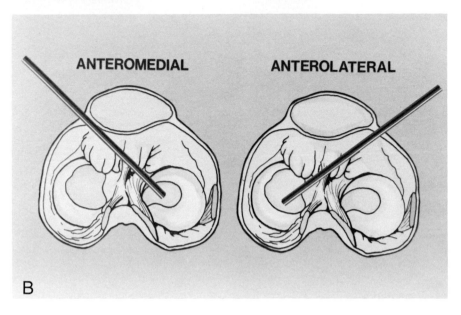

ANTEROMEDIAL   ANTEROLATERAL

Fig. 7.18. (A) Incisions for anterolateral (right), anteromedial (left), and central approaches. (B) Diagrammatic position of arthroscope for anterolateral and anteromedial approaches.

4. Supra- or Midpatellar. This approach, described by Patel,[35] is useful for thoroughly exploring the most anterior aspects of the anteromedial and anterolateral compartments and the anterior horns of the menisci (Fig. 7.20A). The lateral approach is used to visualize the anteromedial compartment and the medial suprapatellar approach to see the anterolateral compartment. A point is taken at the desired location in the anterior compartment and a second point at the midpoint of the sulcus in the anterior distal femur (Fig. 7.20B). These two points are connected by an imaginary line extended proximally to the point of incision, usually between the superior pole and midpoint of the patella. The sharp trochar is inserted into the suprapatellar pouch and replaced with a blunt trochar. The sheath is placed under the patella, through the femoral sulcus into the appropriate anterior compartment. The knee must be in a position between full extension and 30 degrees of flexion.

5. Posteromedial. This approach can be used for arthroscopic visualization or for instrumentation when examining through the central approach. The point of entry is just behind the medial collateral ligament and just above the posteromedial joint line (Fig. 7.21A). The joint must be distended to enter safely at this point. The sheath and sharp trochar are inserted through the posterior oblique ligament and distended synovial cavity (Fig. 7.21B). If saline returns, the trochar is replaced with a telescope and the examiner sees the posterior condylar surface, posterior attachment of the medial meniscus, and the posterior cruciate ligament. Metcalf[30] has described a variation of this approach wherein the sheath with a sharp trochar is inserted through the same incision and held against the posterior capsule and synovium. A large bolus of saline is rapidly blown into the knee through a syringe with a large-bore needle, thereby pushing the synovium and capsule against the sharp trochar and gaining entry (Fig. 7.21C).

6. Posterolateral. This approach is very similar to the posteromedial. An incision is made just behind the fibular collateral ligament and just above the joint line (Fig. 7.22). It must be superior to the insertion of the biceps femoris to avoid the peroneal nerve. The sheath and sharp trochar are inserted through the distended arcuate ligament and synovium into the posterolateral compartment for visualization or instrumentation.

TECHNICAL PROBLEMS

Proliferative synovium or the fat pad may interfere with visualization inside the knee. This problem can usually be avoided by keeping the synovial cavity well distended and working from deep to superficial. Difficulties in interpretation of lesions can occur unless the examiner is familiar with the results of optical magnification. Disorientation can be a problem, particularly with angled arthroscopes, and can only be remedied by practice. I recommend the 30-degree four-oblique arthroscope for most routine work. This telescope is not so angled as to cause disorientation, yet the angle permits about a 50 percent increase in field size simply by rotating the instrument.

Instrument breakage is a serious problem. Instruments are small and fragile and must be used with care. The tip of an arthroscope must not be left unprotected. Scissors and knife blades break in the joint. I have even seen the end of a probe break. If an instrument breaks during a procedure, the surgeon, upon recognizing the problem, should stop all motion and freeze for about 30 seconds. The surgeon should not move before formulating a plan of action and should then retrieve the broken part with great deliberation trying not to let it get out of the field of view.

PATHOLOGIC LESIONS: DIAGNOSIS AND TREATMENT

SYNOVIUM

Lesions of the synovium are particularly amenable to inspection and biopsy by arthroscopic techniques. Chronic proliferative synovitis, nonspecific or rheumatoid, can certainly be inspected and biopsied. If villous formation and proliferation are extensive (Plate 7.1) visualization can be difficult. Adequate distention of the synovial cavity is essential for proper inspection. Pigmented villonodular synovitis (Plate 7.2) presents similar problems but can frequently be recognized by the brownish pigmentation.

In the hands of an experienced arthroscopic surgeon, synovectomy can be performed fairly completely, using multiple portals. Synovectomy requires the use of larger-diameter-powered intraarticular shavers, a good system of irrigation through large-

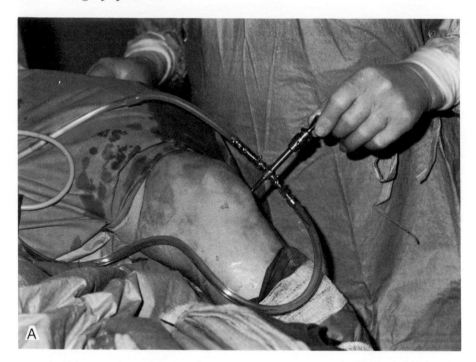

Fig. 7.19. (A) Blunt trochar in sheath and tip of trochar palpating medial condyle until interval between medial condyle and anterior cruciate is identified. (B) Note thumb of left hand pushing sheath toward midline before pushing it into posterior compartment. (C) Diagrammatic representation of looking at posteromedial compartment through intercondylar notch.

bore cannulae, and adequate vacuum suction with a trap to collect pathologic material. Although synovectomy with this technique is tedious, as material is removed, visualization becomes easier. The great advantage is less morbidity and stiffness. After endoscopic synovectomy, it is not unusual to see a patient achieve a straight-leg raise in full extension and flex to 90 degrees in the recovery room immediately after surgery. This eliminates the need for postoperative manipulation under anesthesia frequently required after traditional synovectomy.

The crystal synovitis of gout and the chondrocalcinosis of pseudogout are readily identified arthroscopically. The crystals have a characteristic appearance and can be seen adherent to the synovium and menisci (Plate 7.3).

Arthroscopic technique is the method of choice in the diagnosis and treatment of acute pyogenic arthritis. The arthroscopic sheath gives ready access to the joint to obtain material for culture. The degree of damage to internal structures can be readily arrested. Copious irrigation can be attained and closed systems of irrigation can be left in place if desired. The joint can be readily debrided of fibrinous debris either by irrigation or powered shavers. Finally, if necessary, repeat examinations or irrigation of the knee can be performed with minimal morbidity (Plate 7.4).

Synovial plicae can be identified and treated arthroscopically (Plate 7.5). Hughston et al.[14] described the medial plica and recommended resection by arthrotomy. Patel[34] defined arthroscopic management. About 35 percent of persons will demonstrate a medial plica, only a small percentage of which are symptomatic. These few will present with medial pain, snapping, and occasionally buckling. The plica may be palpated under the medial retinaculum. Resection can most easily be accomplished after visualization through a lateral midpatellar portal by basket forceps through an anterolateral portal. Our results in more than 60 patients have showed an 85 percent improvement rate with a minimum 2-year follow-up.

PATELLOFEMORAL JOINT

Patellofemoral malalignment of the knee can be evaluated and treated by arthroscopic techniques. In patients with patellofemoral malalignment, lateral overhang of the patella can be visualized with the knee in 40 to 60 degrees of flexion. Lateral overhang (Plate 7.6) is seen with the arthroscope in an anterolateral portal looking upward at the lateral facet of the patella and its relationship to the lateral femoral condyle. Normally less than 5 percent of the patella can

Figure 7.19. (Continued.)

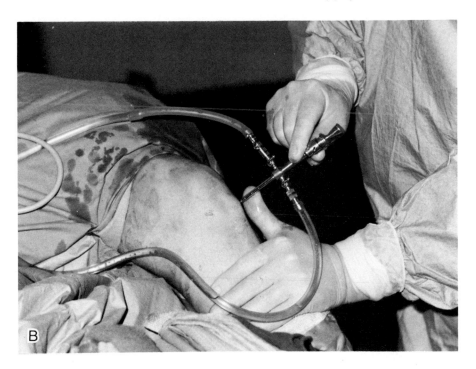

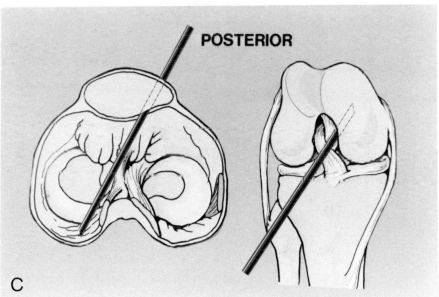

be seen. With patellofemoral malalignment, 20 to 50 percent of the patella will hang over the lateral femoral condyle. Since with the knee in extension and distended a false-positive appearance may occur, it is essential that this determination be made with the knee in flexion. Also, while visualizing the articulation of the patella with the femur, lateral tilt of the

patella may be seen with patellofemoral malalignment.

In patellofemoral malalignment with objective findings, such as internal femoral torsion, medial facet tenderness, patella alta, increased Q angle, lateral position in flexion or extension, and abnormal patellar tilt in tangential x-rays, and in a patient who has not

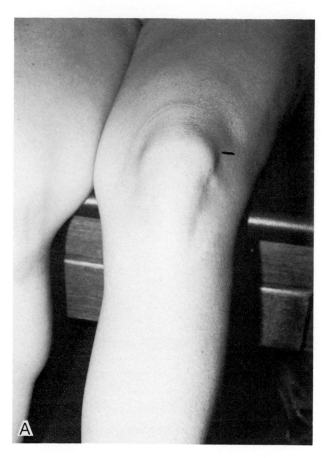

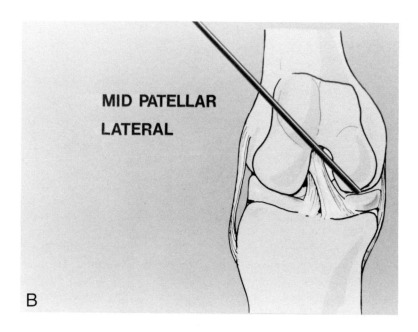

Fig. 7.20. (A) Incision for midpatellar approach. (B) Diagrammatic representation of midpatellar approach to examine anteromedial compartment.

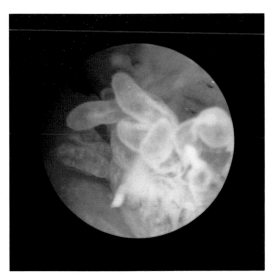

Plate 7.1. Chronic proliferative synovitis—rheumatoid.

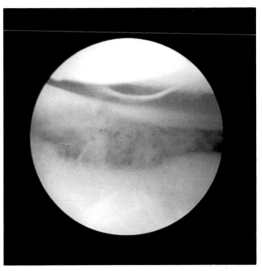

Plate 7.2. Pigmented villonodular synovitis from posterior compartment visualized under lateral meniscus.

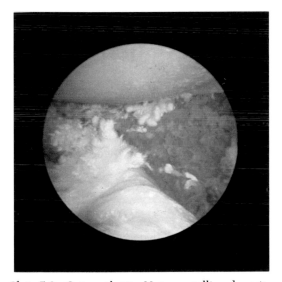

Plate 7.3. Osteoarthritis. Note crystalline deposits.

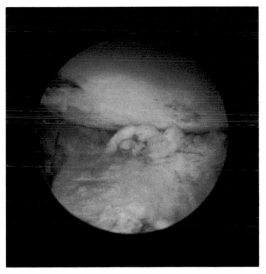

Plate 7.4. Pyogenic arthritis. Note fibrinous debris in meniscus and loss of articular cartilage.

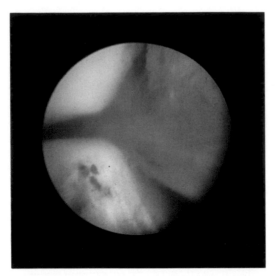

Plate 7.5. Hypertrophic medial plica viewed from pateral suprapatellar portal. Patella above, medial femoral condyle below.

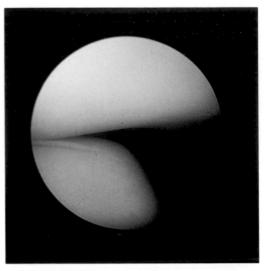

Plate 7.6. Patellofemoral malalignment with lateral overhang. Patella above, lateral femoral condyle below.

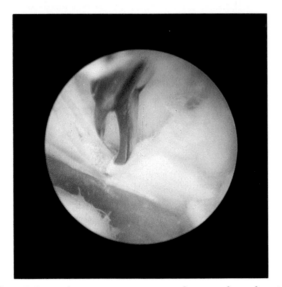

Plate 7.7. Encloscopic scissors completing a lateral retinacular release.

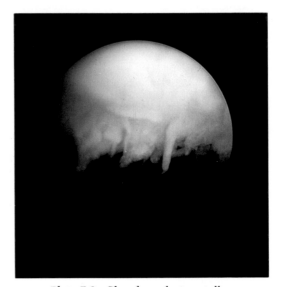

Plate 7.8. Chondromalacia patellae.

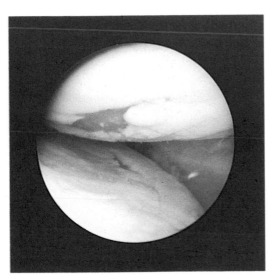

Plate 7.9. Chondromalacia of medial femoral condyle 8 years after total meniscectomy.

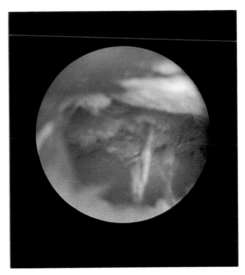

Plate 7.10. Osteoarthritis, medial compartment. Note loss of articular cartilage and degenerative meniscus.

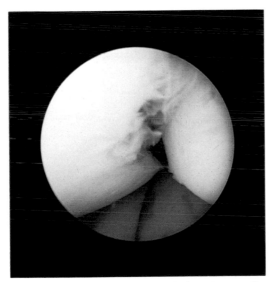

Plate 7.11. Large separated fragment from lesion of osteochondritis dissecans in 23-year-old man. Femoral condyle is on left with loose fragment on right. Note medial meniscus.

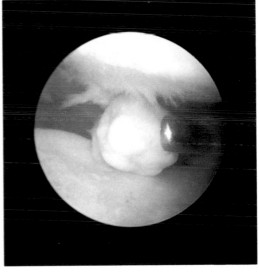

Plate 7.12. Loose body being removed with grasping forceps under patella.

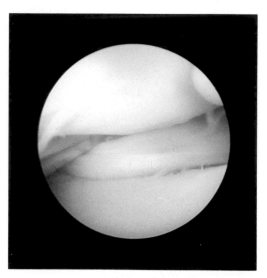 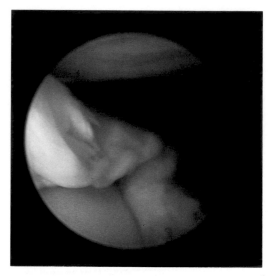

Plate 7.13. Fragment from longitudinal tear of posterior horn of medial meniscus being delivered with a probe.

Plate 7.14. Bucket handle tear of medial meniscus.

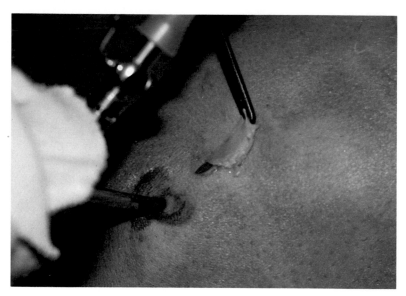

Plate 7.15. Meniscal fragment being removed.

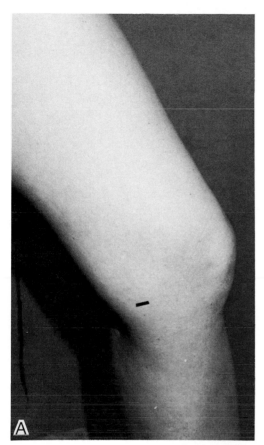

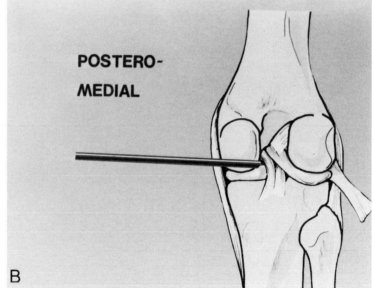

Fig. 7.21. (A) Incision for posteromedial approach. (B) Diagrammatic representation of posteromedial approach. (C) Instruments placed in posteromedial approach while visualizing posteromedial compartment through intercondylar notch. Note spinal needle used to identify direction of insertion of instrument.

POSTERO-
MEDIAL

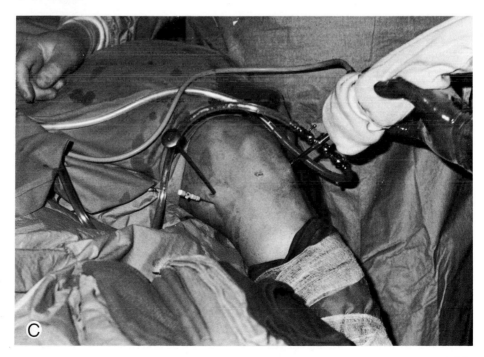

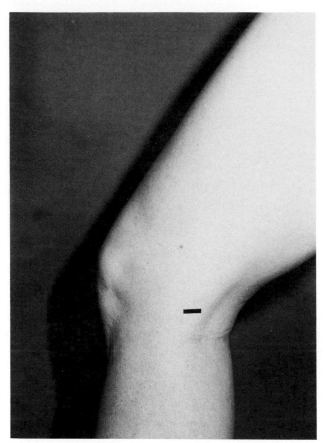

Fig. 7.22. Incision for posterolateral incision.

responded to conservative therapy, lateral retinacular release by endoscopic methods may be the initial surgical treatment of choice. This procedure can be accomplished with minimal morbidity and minimal cosmetic scarring, using two 1-cm endoscopic incisions. After completion of the arthroscopic examination, a partial release up to the midpatella is performed blindly with a Mayo scissors. The cut retinaculum is then identified with the arthroscope and the release completed up to the interval of the vastus lateralis and rectus femoris with endoscopic scissors under arthroscopic control through a second incision 1 cm proximal to the anterolateral portal (Plate 7.7). The dissection must be proximal enough to release the vastus lateralis completely. By means of this technique, a review of 39 consecutive cases with an average follow-up of 16 months showed 85 percent improvement, a rate consistent with that published for open lateral re-

lease.[21,27,29] However a subsequent review of the same series showed that the results deteriorated to 65 percent satisfactory after an average follow-up of 40 months.

Chondromalacia of the patella can be readily seen and evaluated with an arthroscope (Plate 7.8). There has been in the past several years a tendency to shave the articular surface of the patella with powered intra-articular shavers for chondromalacia. The efficacy of this procedure requires some long-term follow-up studies to document the value. Early results suggest improvement of pain. However, patients with knee pain with negative arthroscopic examinations show 86 percent improvement in our review of 225 consecutive knee arthroscopies.[22]

ARTICULAR CARTILAGE

Lesions of articular cartilage can be divided into chondromalacia, osteoarthritis, osteochondritis dissecans, and loose bodies.

CHONDROMALACIA

Chondromalacia of the femoral condyles can be assessed and diagnosed arthroscopically (Plate 7.9). This is frequently associated with degenerative lesions of the meniscus. It has been established that the menisci have a load-bearing and cartilage-sparing effect on articular cartilage.[20,40] Therefore, degenerative menisci should be preserved whenever possible in the presence of chondromalacia or osteoarthritis. We debride these joints arthroscopically in an effort to preserve as much meniscal tissue as possible, removing only those portions that are unstable. Associated with this, the joint is debrided with a powered intraarticular shaver and loose tissue is removed.

OSTEOARTHRITIS

In the presence of osteoarthritis with exposed and sclerotic bone, there is no established arthroscopic solution (Plate 7.10). Some arthroscopic surgeons are attempting abrasive chondroplasty; that is, abrading articular surface down to subchondral bone in an attempt to attain healing by a fibrocartilage surface. Follow-up results are of insufficient length and detail to give credence to the value of this procedure.

OSTEOCHONDRITIS DISSECANS

Osteochondritis dissecans is a lesion of subchondral bone with localized necrosis and secondary changes in the overlying articular cartilage (Plate 7.11). When the diagnosis is made by x-ray, arthroscopic examination of the overlying cartilage is mandatory. Guhl[12] has classified these lesions for appropriate arthroscopic management. If, in a patient over the age of 12 years, there is no loosening of the intraarticular lesion, the treatment is drilling with a small-diameter Kirschner wire to stimulate vascularity and healing. If the lesion is loose and not displaced, it should be drilled and pinned arthroscopically with one or two Kirschner wires which are removed in 6 weeks. If the lesion is loose and attached with a hinge, it should be elevated, the base curetted, replaced, and pinned. The pins are again removed in 6 weeks. In a patient over 20 years of age, if the lesion is completely free, the loose body should be removed and the base drilled. Guhl recommended grafting the lesions arthroscopically with grafts inserted arthroscopically in a tract made with a cannulated reamer over a guide pin. Regardless of what methods are used to treat the lesion of osteochondritis dissecans, arthroscopy provides an excellent method of examining the lesion under local anesthesia.

LOOSE BODIES

Loose bodies usually originate from articular cartilage lesions. They are quite easily discovered in a systematic arthroscopic examination. It is surprising how often nonradiopaque loose bodies are unexpectedly found during arthroscopic examinations. Loose bodies are easy to remove through a second portal after they are located (Plate 7.12). The most common location is in the lateral suprapatellar recess, followed by the posteromedial compartment. Occasionally they will be found in the popliteus sheath and can be delivered by milking the sheath from outside the knee.

The largest loose body I have removed without en-

larging the incision is 2.5 cm. When the loose body is firmly grasped, the incision can be enlarged with a No. 11 blade if necessary. A large loose body can be delivered to the suprapatellar pouch and pushed up, tenting the soft tissues. An incision can then be made over it, and it can be delivered from inside out. Extremely large loose bodies can be broken up and removed in pieces.

LESIONS OF THE MENISCUS

Meniscal lesions present the greatest challenge to the arthroscopist. These lesions can be very specifically defined with the arthroscope, particularly when supplemented with examination with the probe (Plate 7.13). However, to communicate information in meniscal lesions, a system of classification is helpful.[28] Basic tears can be defined in terms of one of the three planes of the meniscus: longitudinal (perpendicular to the surface of the meniscus and parallel to its arc), radial (perpendicular to the surface and parallel to its radius), and cleavage (parallel to the surface, thereby splitting the meniscus). Most tears can be defined as combinations of these three types. Also, there are discoid menisci, complex tears, and degenerative tears.

Having made a diagnosis of a torn meniscus, it is feasible to remove the torn portions with arthroscopic techniques by means of multiple portals. Traditional teaching states that total meniscectomy results in the best replica of the original.[36A] However, this hypothesis has not been confirmed by the observations of most arthroscopists. Fairbank[8] has shown degenerative changes in the knee by x-ray after meniscectomy. Johnson et al[19] and Walker and Erkman[40] have shown a definite load-bearing effect of the meniscus. Several investigators have demonstrated degenerative changes in the knee after total meniscectomy.[5,8,13,15,20,39] Cargill and Jackson[3] demonstrated better results after partial meniscectomy for bucket-handle tears. In our own series of 89 total and 39 partial meniscectomies with an average of 6 years follow-up,[23] the patients with partial meniscectomy showed better functional results, less objective findings, fewer complications, and 50 percent fewer x-ray changes on follow-up. The trend is therefore to remove only the damaged portion of a meniscus and to retain as much of a stable rim as possible.

It becomes feasible to perform most partial meniscectomies using endoscopic techniques. The lesion must first be defined (Plate 7.14), then converted into a flap of tissue that can be grasped through a second portal, the base of the flap divided by a knife or scissors through a third portal, and the torn fragment removed. The rim must then be carefully inspected for a secondary tear, then smoothed with either a basket forceps or a meniscal cutter so that the remaining rim will be stable and can take at least part of the original load-bearing function of the meniscus (Plate 7.15).

GENERAL COMMENTS

A surgeon starting arthroscopy should precede every arthrotomy with an arthroscopic examination for no more than 30 minutes. The next step is to reprep, regown, redrape, and proceed with the arthrotomy. With increasing experience, the surgeon will become facile until the day comes when he or she finds nothing and does not proceed with the arthrotomy.

Before making the step from diagnostic to surgical arthroscopy, the surgeon should meet three prerequisites:

1. Approach the diagnostic accuracy of 98 percent published by Dandy and Jackson[6]
2. Be completely familiar and comfortable with all approaches and feel no hesitation about using any of them
3. Be thoroughly skilled in triangulation, the skill of bringing an instrument and a telescope together in a defined area in the knee (The surgeon will rapidly acquire this skill by using a probe in every diagnostic arthroscopy.)

A surgeon learning operative arthroscopy should set a definite time for the procedure (1 hour). If the goal has not been accomplished arthroscopically at the end of this time, the surgeon should reprep, regown, redrape, and proceed with an arthrotomy. It is far better to treat a knee lesion with a good arthrotomy than a poor arthroscopy. Arthrotomy is a viable and accepted method of treating all surgical intra-articular pathology of the knee.

Arthroscopy is rapidly assuming its place in orthopedic surgery. The decade of the 1980s will see this procedure fall into proper perspective. It is a discipline that has grown mostly through the efforts of surgeons in private practice. This procedure awaits good laboratory research in animals in order to develop instruments and techniques and good long-range follow-up studies. With these efforts, arthroscopy can look forward to a bright future.

REFERENCES

1. Burman, M.S.: Arthroscopy or direct visualization of joints: An experimental cadaver study. J. Bone Joint Surg. [Am.], *13*: 669, 1931.
2. Burman, M.S., Finkelstein, H., and Mayer, L.: Arthroscopy of the knee joint. J. Bone Joint Surg., *16*: 255, 1934.
3. Cargill, A.O., and Jackson, J.P.: Bucket-handle tear of the medial meniscus. J. Bone Joint Surg. [Am.], *58*: 248, 1976.
4. Casscells S.W.: Arthroscopy of the knee joint. J. Bone Joint Surg. [Am.], *53*: 287, 1971.
5. Cox, J.S., Nye, C.E., and Schaefer, W.W.: The degenerative effects of partial and total resection of the medial meniscus in dogs' knees. Clin. Orthop., *109*: 178, 1975.
6. Dandy, D.J., and Jackson, R.W.: The impact of arthroscopy in the management of disorders of the knee. J. Bone Joint Surg. [Br.], *57*: 346, 1975.
7. DeHaven, K.E., and Collins, H.R.: Diagnosis of internal derangements of the knee. The role of arthroscopy. J. Bone Joint Surg. [Am.], *57*: 802, 1975.
8. Fairbank, T.J.: Knee joint changes after meniscectomy. J. Bone Joint Surg. [Br.], *30*: 664, 1948.
9. Gillquist, J., and Hagberg, G.: A new modification of the technique of arthroscopy of the knee joint. Acta Chir. Scand., *142*: 123, 1976.
10. Gillquist, J., and Liljedahl, S.: Arthroscopy. In Berci, G., ed.: *Endoscopy.* New York, Appleton-Century-Crofts, 1976, p. 677.
11. Gillquist, J., Hagberg, G., and Oretrop, N.: Arthroscopic visualization of the posteromedial compartment of the knee joint. Orthop. Clin. North Am., *10*(3): 545, 1979.
12. Guhl, J.F.: Arthroscopic treatment of osteochondritis dissecans: Preliminary report. Orthop. Clin. North Am., *10*(3): 671, 1979.
13. Huckell, J.R.: Is meniscectomy a benign procedure? A long term follow-up study. Can. J. Surg., *8*: 254, 1965.
14. Hughston, J.C., Andrews, J.R., and Waddell, D.D.: The suprapatellar plica: Its role in internal derangement of the knee. Orthop. Trans., *2*: 199, 1978.
15. Jackson, J.P.: Degenerative changes in the knee after meniscectomy. Br. Med. J., *2*: 525, 1968.
16. Johnson, L.L., and Becker, R.L.: Arthroscopy: tech-

nique and the role of the assistant. Orthop. Rev., 5(9): 31, 1976.

17. Johnson, L.L.: Comprehensive Arthroscopic Examination of the Knee. St Louis, C.V. Mosby, 1977.
18. Johnson, L.L.: Diagnostic and Surgical Arthroscopy. St Louis, C.V. Mosby, 1981.
19. Johnson, R.J., Kettelkamp, D.B., Clark, W., et al: Factors affecting late results after meniscectomy. J Bone Joint Surg. [Am.], 56: 719, 1974.
20. Kettelkamp, D.B., and Jacobs, A.W.: Tibiofemoral contract area—determination and implications. J. Bone Joint Surg. [Am.], 54: 349, 1972.
21. Larson, R.L., Caubaud, H.E., Slocum, D.B., et al: The patellar compression syndrome. Clin. Orthop., 134: 158, 1978.
22. McGinty, J.B., and Freedman, P.A.: Arthroscopy of the knee. Clin. Orthop., 121: 173, 1976.
23. McGinty, J.B., Geuss, L.F., and Marvin, R.A.: Partial or total meniscectomy: a comparative analysis. J. Bone Joint Surg. [Am.], 59: 763, 1977.
24. McGinty, J.B.: Technique of arthroscopy. AAOS Symposium on Arthroscopy and Arthrography of the Knee. St. Louis, C.V. Mosby, 1978, p. 61.
25. McGinty, J.B.: Photography in arthroscopy. AAOS Symposium on Arthroscopy and Arthrography of the Knee. St. Louis, C.V. Mosby, 1978, p. 282.
26. McGinty, J.B., and Matza, R.A.: Arthroscopy of the Knee. Evaluation of an out-patient procedure under local anesthesia. J. Bone Joint Surg. [Am.], 60: 787, 1978.
27. McGinty, J.B., and McCarthy, J.C.: Endoscopic lateral retinacular release. A preliminary report. Clin. Orthop., 158: 120, 1981.
28. McGinty, J.B.: Arthroscopy of the knee: Update and review. Orthop. Digest, 7: 17, 1979.
29. Merchant, A.C., Mercer, R.L.: Lateral release of the patella: a preliminary report. Clin. Orthop., 103: 40, 1974.
30. Metcalf, R.W.: Personal communication.
31. Nicholas, J.A., Freiberger, R.H., and Killoran, P.J.: Double contrast arthrography of the knee. J. Bone Joint Surg. [Am.], 52: 203, 1970.
32. Noyes, F.R., Bassett, R.W., Grood, E.S., et al: Arthroscopy in acute traumatic hemarthrosis of the knee. Incidence of anterior cruciate tears and other injuries. J. Bone Joint Surg. [Am.], 62: 687, 1980.
33. O'Connor, R.: Arthroscopy. Philadelphia, J.B. Lippincott, 1977.
34. Patel, D.: Arthroscopy of the plicae-synovial folds and their significance. Am. J. Sports Med., 6: 217, 1978.
35. Patel, D.: Personal communication.
36. Rosenberg, T.: Personal communication, 1972.
36A. Smillie, I.S.: Injuries of the Knee Joint, 4th Ed. Edinburgh, Churchill Livingstone, 1970.
37. Stone, R.: Personal communication.
38. Takagi, K.: Practical experience using Takagi's arthroscope. J. Jpn. Orthop. Assoc., 8: 132, 1933.
39. Tapper, E.M., and Hoover, N.W.: Late results after meniscectomy. J. Bone Joint Surg. [Am.], 51: 517, 1969.
40. Walker, P.S., and Erkman, M.J.: The role of the menisci in force transmission across the knee. Clin. Orthop., 109: 184, 1975.
41. Watanabe, M.: The development and present status of the arthroscope. J. Jpn. Med Inst., 25: 11, 1954.
42. Watanabe, M., Takeda, S., and Ikeuchi, H.: Atlas of Arthroscopy. Tokyo, Igaku Shoin Ltd., 1969.

8 The Menisci of the Knee

Peter G. Bullough
Frederick Vosburgh
Steven Paul Arnoczky
and
I. Martin Levy

EVOLUTION

As animals began millions of years ago to walk on land, the structure of their knees changed to suit these new mechanical demands. Part of this adaptation was the evolution of menisci, which are functional extensions of the tibial condyles that mate the tibia to the femur.[18]

The first creatures with meniscus-like structures were the amphibians. In some primitive, tailed amphibians the space between the femur and tibia is entirely filled with a pliant fibrovascular tissue. In the salamander, which possesses a true joint cavity, this tissue is limited to the medial portion of the joint and has been referred to as a medial meniscus. In the knee joint of the bullfrog there exist two distinct elliptical structures interposed between the tibial and femoral condyles.

In the knee joint of the crocodile, the only living relation to the dinosaur, the menisci appear as two large, nonperforate masses of fibrocartilage. The lizard possesses comparatively smaller menisci with the lateral being discoid in shape and the medial circular, with a central perforation through which intra-articular ligaments pass.

Birds, which arose from a reptilian ancestor, possess somewhat similar meniscal structures. The medial meniscus has become C shaped, however, while the lateral meniscus remains discoid in appearance. The tetra- and bipedal mammals have the most developed fibrocartilaginous menisci. While the attachments of the menisci to the tibia vary among different orders, the crescent-like shape of the menisci prevails in most cases, the horse being an exception with discoid menisci. Discoid lateral menisci do occur at times in dogs and humans. However, these appear to be only anomalies within an expected range of morphologic variation as an end product of development.

MENISCAL DEVELOPMENT

The menisci exist first in the embryo as a condensation of intermediate layer mesenchymal tissue and by the eighth week are clearly defined. At this stage,

135

the meniscus consists largely of fibroblasts without much extracellular matrix, and vascular channels permeate the entire structure. As the fetus develops, the matrix of the meniscus becomes more collagenous with a gradual orientation of the collagen bundles into a circumferential arrangement. The increases in collagen content and fibrous organization continues into the postnatal period. Vessels are present through much of the meniscus at birth; however, by mid to late adolescence the internal and intermediate regions of the menisci appear avascular.

GROSS ANATOMY

The menisci or semilunar cartilages of the human knee joint, although sometimes referred to as intra-articular structures (structures that are shared equally by the femoral condyles and the tibial plateaus), are properly regarded as functional extensions of the tibial articulation of the knee. With the menisci in place, the tibial articulation displays a biconcavity providing a surface more or less congruent with the femoral condyles. Without the menisci, the tibial plateaus are almost flat, and indeed the lateral portion of the tibial articulation has a convex profile in the sagittal plane.

The medial meniscus is crescentic in form, but its limbs lie wider apart than do those in the lateral meniscus. In addition, the medial meniscus is broader behind than in front. The anterior end of the medial meniscus is attached slightly below the front edge of the articular surface of the tibia in front of the anterior cruciate ligament. The posterior fibers of the anterior horn merge with the transverse ligament. The posterior end of the meniscus is fixed to the posterior intercondylar area between the attachments of the lateral meniscus and the posterior cruciate ligament. The peripheral border of the medial meniscus adheres firmly to the deep surface of the medial collateral ligament.

The lateral meniscus forms approximately four-fifths of a complete ring and is approximately the same width from front to back. It covers a larger area of the articular surface on the tibia than does the medial meniscus. Its anterior end is attached in front of the intercondylar eminence of the tibia and behind the attachment of the anterior cruciate ligament, with which it partly blends. The posterior end of the me-

niscus is attached behind the intercondylar eminence of the tibia in front of the posterior end of the medial meniscus. There is no attachment of the lateral meniscus to the lateral collateral ligament. However, the midportion of the capsular ligament attaches to the meniscus as far posteriorly as the recess for the popliteus tendon. In addition, the popliteus tendon sends a slip into the posterior horn of the lateral meniscus. The anterior horns of both menisci attach to the patella by fibrous bands in such a fashion that extending the knee draws the menisci forward. Finally, several ligaments run from the posterior horn of the lateral meniscus into the medial femoral condyle, either just in front of or behind the origin of the posterior cruciate ligament. These ligaments are the ligaments of Humphry (the anterior meniscal–femoral ligament), and Wrisberg (the posterior meniscal–femoral ligament).

Opinion as to the function of the menisci has varied considerably. These structures were long regarded as merely vestigial remnants, but today it is generally accepted that they provide for various functions, including an aid to lubrication, provision of shock absorption, increasing congruity, limiting the extremes of flexion and extension, and most importantly, providing for stability and the transmission of load across the joint (see below).

STRUCTURE OF THE MENISCI

The menisci are constructed principally of collagen, although some proteoglycan is also present. As a result of examining carefully oriented sections, it has been shown that the principal orientation of the collagen fibers in both menisci is circumferential. The few, small, radially disposed fibers that do occur exist primarily on the tibial surface, but also to some extent on the femoral surface and in the midzone. Some of these radially disposed fibers curl and change direction, becoming perpendicular to the surface. The circumferential orientation of most of the collagen fibers appears designed to withstand the circumferential tension that develops in the meniscus during normal loading.[3] The radially disposed fibers probably act as ties to resist any longitudinal splitting of the menisci that may result from undue compression (Fig. 8.1).

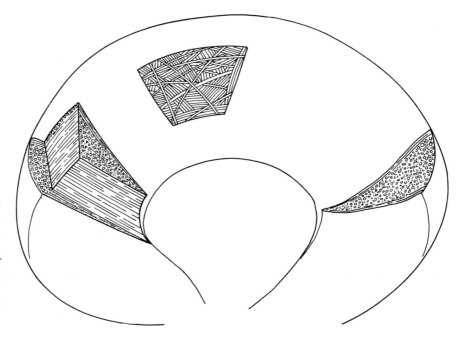

Fig. 8.1. Organization of the collagen fibers in the meniscus. (Adapted from Bullough, P.G., Murphy, J., and Weinstein, A.: The strength of the meniscus of the knee as it relates to the knee structure. J. Bone Joint Surg., *52B*: 564, 1970, with permission.)

VASCULAR ANATOMY OF THE MENISCUS

The vascular supply to the menisci of the human knee originates predominantly in the lateral and medial genicular arteries (both inferior and superior). Branches from these vessels give rise to a plexus of perimeniscal capillaries that lies within the synovial and capsular tissues.[2] These perimeniscal capillaries lie in a predominantly circumferential pattern, with radial projections into the meniscus, toward the center of the joint (Fig. 8.2).

The degree of vascular penetration from the periphery in the medial meniscus ranges from 10 to 30 percent of the width. The degree of vascular penetration in the lateral meniscus ranges from 10 to 25 percent.

The middle genicular artery and a few terminal branches of the medial and lateral genicular arteries also supply vessels to the menisci by way of the vascularized synovium that covers the anterior and posterior horns. Both the anterior and posterior horns of the lateral meniscus are covered with such a layer of vascularized synovial tissue, which appears to be continuous with that of the synovial sheath surrounding the cruciate ligaments (Fig. 8.3).

BIOCHEMICAL CONSIDERATIONS

In the extracellular matrix in the meniscus, the proteoglycans are the principal macromolecules other than collagen. Proteoglycans (PG) consist of glycosaminoglycans (GAG) and protein. The size and composition of the PGs trapped between the collagen fibers lend the tissue its ability to carry load by deforming viscoelastically. The proteoglycans and GAG in the fibrocartilaginous menisci seem to resemble in many ways those in hyaline cartilage.[1,13] We shall present, therefore, what is known about the proteoglycans in hyaline tissue and point out the differences for those in the meniscus.

The GAGs, which comprise as much as 93 percent of the weight of the PG in the articular cartilage in young adults, are long chains of repeating disaccharide units attached at one end to a protein core that comprises the remainder of the PG molecule. The presence of many GAG chains radiating from the core of protein yields a structure that resembles a bottle brush. Hyaline cartilage contains two GAGs, chondroitin sulfate (CS) and keratin sulfate (KS), each of which has a strongly negative charge owing to the presence of sulfate and carboxyl groups on the aminosugar in each disaccharide. The affinity of the PG

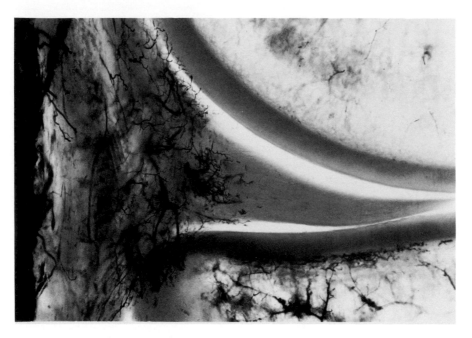

Fig. 8.2. Frontal section of the medial compartment of the knee demonstrating vessels from the perimeniscal capillary plexus penetrating the peripheral border of the medial meniscus. (From Arnoczky, S.P., and Warren, R.F.: Micro-vasculature of the human meniscus. Am. J. Sports Med., *10:* 90, 1982, with permission, © 1982, Am. Orthopaedic Soc. for Sports Medicine.)

for water depends in large part on this charge. Also lending an attraction for water is the size of the PG. A single molecule, also termed a proteoglycan subunit (PGS), has a molecular weight of approximately 2.5 million. In articular cartilage, hyaluronic acid (HA), an unsulfated GAG, links PGS molecules reversibly together in an aggregate that typically has a molecular weight greater than 20 million, aggregate size being limited only by the length of the HA chain. The size of either the PGS or the aggregate is large enough that neither will flow out of intact tissue with the water expressed during loading. This retention of pro-

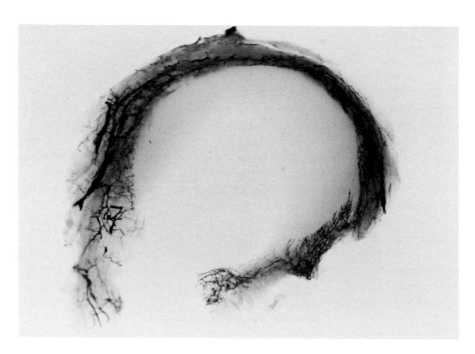

Fig. 8.3. Superior aspect of the medial meniscus, illustrating the peripheral vasculature as well as the vascular synovial tissues that cover the anterior and posterior horns. (From Arnoczky, S.P., and Warren, R.F.: Microvasculature of the human meniscus. Am. J. Sports Med., *10:* 90, 1982, with permission, © 1982, Am. Orthopaedic Soc. for Sports Medicine.)

teoglycans is thought to be crucial for the maintenance of a healthy, functional joint. For without the proteoglycans to induce swelling, the tissue is flaccid and quickly fibrillated.

The most obvious contrasts between the proteoglycans in the meniscus and hyaline cartilage are in concentration and composition. The meniscus contains only about one-eighth the concentration of PG in hyaline cartilage. In the dog, less occurs in the medial than in the lateral meniscus. The PGs in the meniscus, whether in humans or dogs, appear to form aggregates under appropriate conditions and yield profiles on gel chromatography that closely resemble those for the PG in articular cartilage under the same conditions. Aggregation by proteoglycans from the meniscus appears, however, to be effected by disulfide bonds rather than by accretion along a molecule of HA. Proteolytic digestion of the PG releases sulfated GAGs that on gel chromatography are indistinguishable in size from those in articular cartilage.

While the structural characteristics of PGs are quite similar between the meniscus and hyaline tissue, the GAG compositions differ. The most conspicuous difference is the presence in the meniscus of dermatan sulfate (DS). The balance of the population of GAG in the meniscus consists of the CS and KS found as well in hyaline cartilage. The DS, which accounts for about 20 percent of the GAG, occurs primarily in the low-density, protein-rich PGs. CS occurs, by contrast, in the high-density PGs, which are rich in GAG and poor in protein. KS accounts for about one-third of the GAG pool in the adult meniscus, as it does in adult articular cartilage.

Age-related changes in the PGs in the meniscus are several. The PG can be more completely extracted from the menisci of older people. This trend is opposite that of decreasing extraction from hyaline cartilage. The protein content decreases and the GAG content increases with age. That the ratio of galactosamine (in CS and DS) to glucosamine (in KS) increases with aging indicates that KS accumulates more than does either CS or DS. The apparent size on gel chromatography of the PG from the meniscus also increases, although neither the cause nor function of this change is yet clear. While the changes in structure and composition that occur with aging produce a larger, more carbohydrate-rich PG in the meniscus, the apparent viscosity of the molecule does not change detectably with aging. We note, however, that PGs in situ do not flow in bulk, being immobilized by the collagen fibers in the tissue. As a result, the usefulness of a viscosity test in monitoring functional change in the tissue is unclear.

MECHANICAL CONSIDERATIONS

The forces of weight and muscle action in physical activity of the knee cause a load to act between the tibia and the femur.[14] The knee as a structure must deal with two consequences of this loading: (1) it must prevent dislocation, and (2) it must sustain the mechanical stresses that develop in the various tissues. As functional extensions of the load-bearing condyles of the tibia, the fibrocartilaginous menisci act as shims that mate the femur to the tibia. Thus the menisci help stabilize the knee[7,9,10] and modify the stress in the articular cartilage on the condyles. This modification of stress and, apparently, the maintenance of a healthy joint depends on the architecture and the composition of the menisci.

Without the menisci, the parts of the knee do not fit together well. Lacking the ball-and-socket fit of the hip, the knee depends solely on the menisci and the surrounding ligaments for stability and fit. The menisci on the tibial condyles present the femur with a double concavity whose shape is compliant in service of this fit, as well as transmitting loads equitably between the tibia and femur.

For small loads, all of the force passing from the femur to the tibia passes through the menisci.[20] As a result, for small forces, stress is induced only in the tibial cartilage beneath the menisci. As the magnitude of the force increases, the portions of the tibial condyles not covered by the menisci also bear load. Axial loading by the femur on the triagonal section of each meniscus causes a radial displacement (Fig. 8.4) that is opposed by the tethering of the horns to the plateau.[17] By opposing radial displacement, this tethering force creates a circumferential, tensile stress that accompanies the axial, compressive stress in the tissue. The work required for these deformations of the menisci and the adjacent hyaline tissue determines the structural stiffness of the knee in compression until the two sets of condyles come into contact. Removal or sectioning of one or both menisci reduces the resistance of the knee to axial compression.[17] Removal of the menisci creates a gap between the bones and decreases the structural compliance of the knee. Sectioning the menisci precludes the development of circumferential stress in the menisci to oppose their compression (Fig. 8.4).

The fibrous morphology of the meniscus suits it well for the tensile stresses that normally develop in the circumferential direction.[3,10] Collagen fibers, the strongest tension-resisting fibers in the body, trace circumferential trajectories in all but the most superficial layers of these semilunar cartilages. Tensile tests of specimens cut from the menisci along or across the circumferentially arrayed fibers clearly demonstrate that the tensile strength of the menisci is greater in the direction of the fibers than any other. This design for circumferential stress, however, may predispose the meniscus to splitting (see below).

The distribution of stress in the cartilage covering the tibial condyles depends in part on the match in shape of the femoral condyles with the menisci and the tibial condyles, which together function as the tibial side of the joint. The better the match, the smoother the distribution of stress. Each of the menisci, being a compliant structure, deforms somewhat as the knee flexes and thereby maintains the congruency of the two sets of complexly shaped condyles. The shape, manner of attachment, and the mechanical properties of the tissue all contribute to the mechanical compliance of the meniscus. Semilunar structures that each taper to thin interior margins, the menisci are loosely but strongly moored by the horns and capsular attachments. This less than rigid mooring permits the menisci to slide and rotate some-

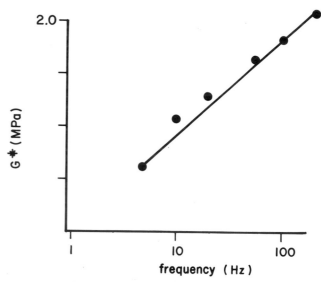

Fig. 8.5. Relationship of the dynamic shear modulus to the frequency of shear. Data represent response of a single slice. The modulus varies linearly with the frequency of shear over the range of 5 to 250 Hz.

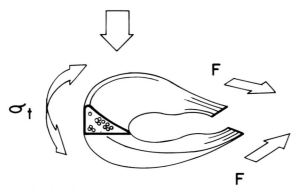

Fig. 8.4. Schematic of the loaded meniscus. The femoral condyle compresses the meniscus. The tethering force from the horns prevents its lateral extrusion and induces a circumferential stress (σ_τ) that is carried by the collagen fibers.

what on the tibial condyles while cupping the femoral condyles, which present a changing curvature with flexion of the knee. The taper toward the inner margin of the meniscus also contributes to the compliance in service of congruency in the joint.

The mechanical properties of the tissue in the meniscus, properties that are divorced from the size, shape or manner of attachment of the meniscus, also contribute to the mechanical response of the meniscus to loading in the intact knee. Our studies to date show in preliminary fashion that the menisci in healthy, adult dogs deform viscoelastically in shear with a stiffness characterized by a dynamic modulus similar to that for articular cartilage.

The dynamic shear modulus is a rate-specific measure of the resistance to distortion in the tissue. We find that this modulus varies with the rate of distortion and the concentration of PG in the tissue, although less closely than for hyaline cartilage.[6] For each meniscus, the modulus increases linearly with the log of the rate of distortion (Fig. 8.5.). At higher rates of distortion, the tissue can be said to resist more forcefully. It is possible to calculate a mean value of the modulus at any rate of distortion for comparison among specimens. Done at 50 Hz, in the midrange of the rates used in these tests, this calculation yields a value similar to that reported for the articular cartilage on the femoral condyles in the cow (Table 8.1). This similarity in modulus is worthy of note in light of the marked differences in fibrous architecture and proteoglycan content between the two types of tissue. Preliminary data also suggest that there may also be a difference in stiffness between the medial and lateral menisci (Table 8.1).

At any frequency, the modulus varies among specimens cut from a single meniscus in linear proportion to the water content (Fig. 8.6), which reflects the hydrophilic characteristics of the extracellular matrix. This correlation obtains for an individual meniscus but lacks statistical significance for data pooled among menisci. Several factors may contribute variation that is not accounted for by a universal regression. Stiffness in the menisci may be less sensitive to PG content, as there is substantially less present. Instead, fibrous architecture may have a detectable influence. The stiffness also may differ between medial and lateral menisci for reasons other than PG content. Differences among animals and variation that arises in experimentation also may mask some of the correlation.

A dynamic modulus has components that reflect the work done in elastic or viscous deformation. The work of elastic deformation drives the recoil of the tissue when load is removed. The work of viscous deformation is lost, being dissipated ultimately as heat. The ratio of the viscous and elastic components equals the experimentally derived value for tan Δ, explained clearly in Ferry[5] and discussed in a biomechanical context by Wainwright et al.[19] In the meniscus, the value for tan Δ is approximately 0.3, indicating that the tissue elastically stores approximately two-thirds of the work of deformation. The variation in tan Δ over the range of frequencies tested so far is small.

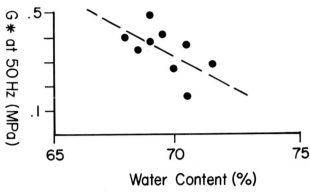

Fig. 8.6. Relationship between the dynamic shear modulus and the water content in the meniscus. Data represent coronal slices from a single lateral meniscus. The modulus is inversely related to the water content. A linear regression of the data has a coefficient of correlation of -0.59, demonstrating that the relationship is statistically significant at $p < 0.05$.

As such it provides little information on the molecular mechanism of deformation. Study of the tissue over a wide range of rates of distortion should lend insight into the supramolecular basis of mechanical behavior in the extracellular matrix.

In summary, the tissue in the menisci in the knee of the dog has a shear stiffness similar to that of articular cartilage. Each meniscus contains substantially less proteoglycan than does hyaline tissue. Yet, the difference in stiffness between the fibrocartilage and the hyaline cartilage is small. These two facts together may suggest a larger role for fibrous architecture in the determination of the tissue properties than considered likely to date. Differences among animals, as well as residual technical variation, may mask significant correlation in the data thereby accounting for the weaker correlations between stiffness and the proteoglycan content of the tissue. The accumulation of data on similar specimens as well as specimens cut in the two perpendicular planes in the meniscus will make clearer the mechanical design in the meniscus and cartilaginous tissues in general.

FUNCTION

Clinical observers of knee motion have suggested that knee stability may be intimately related to the presence of normal menisci. Huckell[8] suggested that

Table 8.1. Dynamic Shear Modulus of Meniscus[a]

Dog	Lateral		Medial
1	0.54 ± 0.062 (N = 17)	b	0.12 ± 0.028 (N = 8)
2	0.47 ± 0.018 (N = 8)	b	0.33 ± 0.028 (N = 8)
3	0.43 ± 0.036 (N = 8)	NS	0.38 ± 0.039 (N = 8)

Abbreviation: N, number of specimens.
[a]Values are reported in megapascals ± SE.
[b]Significant differences between the medial and lateral menisci.

the loss of meniscal mass after meniscectomy may contribute to the relative looseness of the knee. Johnson et al.,[9] evaluated a group of 99 patients, an average of 17.5 years after meniscectomy, and found more knees with ligamentous laxity postoperatively than noted preoperatively. Factors other than undiagnosed injury were implicated, including the fact that the meniscus had a stabilizing function. Mechanical studies have supported these clinical findings.

Wang and Walker[21] examined single-axis rotational motion of the tibia on the femur at 25 degrees of knee flexion. A cyclic internal and external rotational torque was applied to the tibia, and resulting internal and external tibial rotations were recorded. After dual medial–lateral meniscectomy, three of the six specimens had increases in rotation of 14 percent at a torque of 5 kg-cm. These workers concluded that the menisci resisted rotation and therefore aided the control of internal–external rotational motion of the tibia on the femur. In another mechanical test, Hsieh and Walker[7] evaluated the effect of dual meniscectomy on total anterior–posterior motion of one cadaveric knee at 0 and 30 degrees of knee flexion, with and without compressive load. Medial–lateral meniscectomy had little effect on induced anterior–posterior knee displacement. However, in another knee, when excision of both menisci followed cutting of both cruciates, total anterior–posterior tibial displacement was found to be greater than that obtained by section of the cruciates alone. These findings were true for the loaded or unloaded joint.

Seale et al.,[16] used an in vitro test apparatus to measure varus–valgus and tibial rotation of cadaveric knees. Measurements were made while an axial load of 50 lbs compressed the joint. These workers found that removal of the medial meniscus from a loaded joint had an effect on internal rotation, allowing greater rotation with increasingly applied torque. Lateral meniscectomy allowed for increases in both internal and external rotation. Valgus rotation resulting from an applied bending moment increased after medial meniscectomy. Valgus rotations were even greater after lateral meniscectomy. Dual meniscectomy was accompanied by internal and external tibial rotations and varus–valgus tibial rotation that were greater than those observed after isolated cuts.

Markolf et al.,[12] using a three-component knee-testing apparatus, evaluated rotational, anterior–posterior, and valgus–varus stability of the knee joint

at 0 and 20 degrees of knee flexion in the loaded and unloaded joint. They found that axial load served as an important stabilizer of the knee joint and that medial–lateral meniscectomy caused a decrease in anterior–posterior neutral stiffness and varus–valgus neutral stiffness in the fully extended, unloaded knee. When no compressive load was applied across the knee joint lacking both menisci, anterior–posterior neutral stiffness decreased by one-third.

Levy et al.,[11] evaluated the effect of medial meniscectomy on induced anteroposterior knee motion, before and after section of the anterior cruciate ligament in the unloaded knee. A cyclic 100-newton anterior–posterior force was applied to the tibia by the actuator ram of a hydraulic testing machine. Resulting anterior–posterior motion of the tibia on the femur was recorded for flexion angles 0, 30, 60, and 90 degrees (Fig. 8.7). Induced anterior–posterior motion of the knee was unaffected by medial meniscectomy at all flexion angles. In eight knees with combined medial meniscectomy and section of the anterior cruciate ligament, the anterior tibial displacements were greater for flexion angles 30, 60, and 90 degrees than the displacements seen in knees with isolated anterior cruciate cuts. Although the greatest anterior displacement occurred at 30 degrees of flexion, the greatest increase, 58 percent, occurred at 90 degrees.

These results suggest that the meniscus may not restrict anterior–posterior displacement in the intact knee, but anterior cruciate rupture may permit sufficient excursion of the tibia on the femur for the posterior horn of the medial meniscus to limit further excursion of the tibia (Fig. 8.8). As the tibia slides forward in the anterior cruciate-insufficient knee, the other supportive ligaments act to compress the joint, increasing the effect of the posterior wedge.

Both mechanical tests and clinical observation implicate the menisci as contributors to knee joint stability. It seems likely that the effect of this contribution is greatest in the unloaded joint. In addition, their importance may increase in the face of ligament disruption.

That a significant proportion of the load transferred across the knee joint may be carried through the menisci may be inferred from the classic work of Fairbank, published in 1948.[4] Fairbank reported on radiologic changes after meniscectomy in 107 cases. The changes he reported on were of three types: formation of an anteroposterior ridge projecting down from

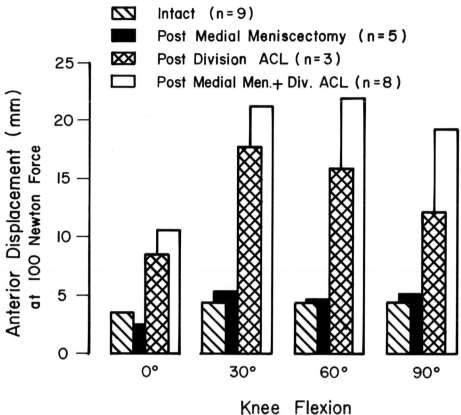

Fig. 8.7. Anterior displacement of the tibia on the femur resulting from a 100-newton anterior force plotted as a function of the four-tested flexion angle.

Fig. 8.8. (A) In the intact knee an anterior force applied to the tibia is restrained primarily by the anterior cruciate ligament (dotted outline). (B) In the absence of an anterior cruciate ligament, the medial meniscus is wedged between the medial femoral condyle and tibial plateau and contributes to the restraint of anterior tibial displacement.

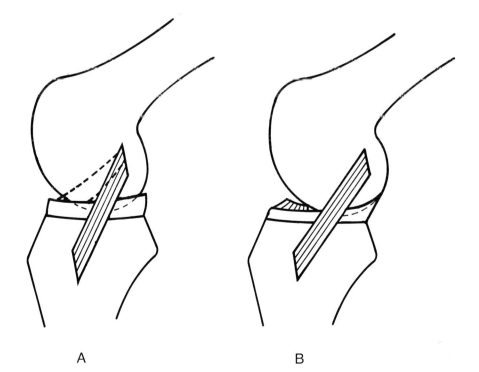

A   B

the margin of the femoral condyle over the site of the meniscus; generalized flattening of the marginal half of the femoral articular surface; and narrowing of the joint space on the side of the operation. One or all of these changes were seen in a significant number of patients. In the study of the late results after meniscectomy, Johnson et al.[9] have reported that 74 of 99 knees examined after removal of the meniscus had at least one of the changes described by Fairbank.[4] However, only 6 percent of the opposite unoperated knees showed these sort of changes. Fairbank attributed the changes to loss of the weight-bearing function of the meniscus.

The anatomy, microscopic and chemical structure, and mechanical properties of the meniscus which have been described above, all support the contention that the menisci transmit load between the femur and the tibia.

AGING IN THE MENISCUS

The menisci of young persons are generally white, have a translucent quality, and are supple on palpation. The menisci in older persons lose their translucency and become more opaque and yellow in color. In addition, they feel less supple. Mechanical testing of meniscal tissue shows that the tissue becomes stronger but less extensible with age, probably because of increased cross-linking in the collagen. The resulting tendency toward failure of the collagen fibers probably contributes significantly to the splitting and fraying of the menisci that is common in older persons.

MORBID ANATOMY

The most common congenital abnormality of the meniscus is the so-called discoid meniscus. It is almost exclusively seen in the lateral side of the knee and in a recent review of 200 cases at autopsy showed an incidence of discoid meniscus in 7 percent. In 4.5 percent of cases, the malformation was present in both knees. A familial pattern has been reported. Other abnormalities of the meniscus, such as circular formation, partial absence, and reduplication, have also been reported, although their incidence is difficult to establish.

TRAUMA

Lacerations of the meniscus lead to symptoms that require surgical treatment in two groups of patients: young active patients in whom injury is frequently related to some sport, and older patients in whom degeneration leads to laceration. Most lacerations occur in the posterior horn of the menisci and more commonly in the medial meniscus. They usually occur as clefts that run along the circumferentially directed collagen fibers. Such a cleft may extend in time to the medial margin of the meniscus and create a tag, which eventually may become quite smooth. Extension of the tear may lead to the bucket-handle deformity. On occasion, the meniscus shows peripheral detachment, again usually posteriorly.

The advent of arthroscopy and arthrography have assisted in the clinical diagnosis of tears in the menisci. They help localize tears and, where injury is limited in scope, have facilitated partial meniscectomies.

In histologic sections, evidence of both injury and repair may be seen, and the findings are likely to be time dependent. It is difficult to determine whether histological changes seen at the time of meniscectomy are the result of or contribute to the tear. In older patients, the presence of a horizontal cleavage in the posterior horn of the meniscus is commonly found at autopsy. In a report of 100 necropsy examinations, Noble and Hamblen[15] reported that 60 percent of the subjects had at least one such tear, the incidence being 29 percent of the 400 menisci examined. The lesions were commoner in the medial menisci and in males, and the coincidence of such lesions with osteoarthritis was frequent.

Calcification within the meniscus is commonly seen. At autopsy in the series of Noble and Hamblen, 34 percent of the menisci were calcified. The calcium salt is generally calcium pyrophosphate dihydrate (CPPD). On microscopic examination, typical crystals can frequently be identified, although this is not always the case. Sometimes the calcium appears quite amorphous in character; however, x-ray defraction studies have demonstrated that this noncrystalline form is also usually CPPD.

It is easy to miss small calcium deposits in the meniscus by naked eye examination or on clinical x-ray films. However, calcium deposition may be clearly demonstrated by the use of fine-grain-specimen

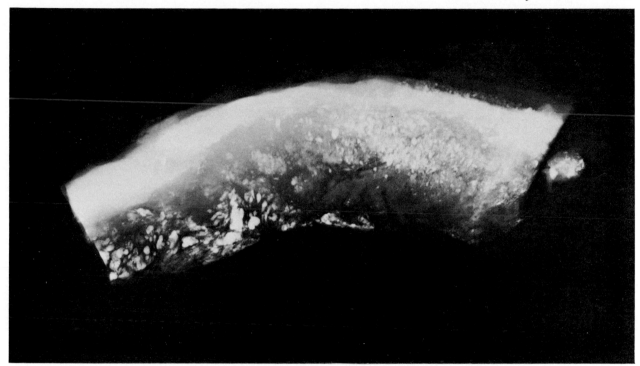

Fig. 8.9. Roentgenogram of a piece of meniscus to illustrate the distribution of mineral salt in a patient with calcium pyrophosphate crystal deposition disease (chondrocalcinosis).

radiographs using a high-resolution x-ray machine (Fig. 8.9). Such calcium deposits within the menisci of older persons must affect the mechanical properties of the meniscal tissue and contribute to accelerated break down of the structure with subsequent effects on the joint as a whole.

SUMMARY

The gross anatomy, the microscopic arrangement of the collagen fibers, and the biochemical composition in the meniscus all taken together lead us to conclude that the meniscus is important for load transfer in the knee joint. The mechanical properties of the isolated tissue and of the entire knee joint after various manipulations of the menisci support this view as well. Disturbances in joint function resulting from morbid changes in the menisci may be expected to affect the function of the joint as a whole and lead eventually to arthritis.

ACKNOWLEDGMENTS

We are indebted to Dr. W. C. Hayes, director of the biomechanics laboratory at the Beth-Israel Hospital, Boston, for his generous assistance in providing facilities to us for mechanical testing

REFERENCES

1. Adams, M.E., and Muir, H.: The glycosaminoglycans of canine menisci. Biochem. J. *197:* 385, 1981.
2. Arnoczky, S.P., and Warren, R.F.: Micro-vasculature of the human meniscus. Am. J. Sports Med. *10:* 90, 1982.
3. Bullough, P.G., Munuera, L., Murphy, J., et al.: The strength of the menisci of the knee as it relates to their fine structure. J. Bone Joint Surg. [Br.], *52:* 564, 1970.
4. Fairbank, T.J.: Knee joint changes after meniscectomy. J Bone Joint Surg. [Br.], *30:* 664, 1948.
5. Ferry, J.D.: Viscoelastic Behavior of Polymers, 2nd Ed. New York, Wiley, 1970.

6. Hayes, W.C., and Bodine, A.J.: Flow-independent viscoelastic properties of articular cartilage matrix. J. Biomech., *11:* 407, 1978.

7. Hsieh, H.H., and Walker, P.S.: Stabilizing mechanisms of the loaded and unloaded knee joint. J. Bone Joint Surg. [Am.], *58:* 87, 1976.

8. Huckell, J.R.: Is meniscectomy a benign procedure? Can. J. Surg. *8:* 254, 1965.

9. Johnson, R.J., Kettelkamp, D.B., Clark, W., et al.: Factors affecting late results after meniscectomy. J. Bone Joint Surg. [Am.], *56:* 719, 1974.

10. Krause, W.R., Pope, M.H., Johnson, R.J., et al.: Mechanical changes in the knee after meniscectomy. J Bone Joint Surg. [Am.], *58:* 599, 1976.

11. Levy, I.M., Torzilli, P.A., and Warren, R.F.: The effect of medial meniscectomy on anterior-posterior motion of the knee. J. Bone Joint Surg. [Am.], *64:* 883, 1982.

12. Markolf, K.L., Bargar, W.L., Shoemaker, S.C., et al.: The role of joint load in knee stability. J. Bone Joint Surg. [Am.], *63:* 570, 1981.

13. McNicol, D., and Roughley, P.J.: Extraction and characterization of proteoglycan from human meniscus. Biochem. J., *185:* 705, 1980.

14. Minns, R.J.: Forces at the knee joint: Anatomical considerations. J. Biomech., *14:* 633, 1981.

15. Noble, J., and Hamblen, D.L.: The pathology of the degenerate meniscus lesion. J. Bone Joint Surg. [Br.], *57:* 180, 1975.

16. Seale, K.S., Haynes, D.W., Nelson, C.L., et al.: The effect of meniscectomy on knee stability. Transactions of the 27th Annual Meeting of the Orthopaedic Research Society, Feb. 24–26, 1981, p. 236.

17. Shrive, N.: The weight-bearing role of the menisci of the knee. In proceedings J. Bone Joint Surg. [Br.], *56:* 381, 1974.

18. Van Sickle, D.C., and Kincaid, S.A.: Comparative arthrology. In Sokoloff, L. (ed.): The Joints and Synovial Fluid. New York, Academic Press, 1978, p. 1.

19. Wainwright, S.A., Biggs, W.D., Currey, J.D., et al.: Mechanical Design in Organisms. London, Edward Arnold, 1976.

20. Walker, P.S., and Erkman, M.J.: The role of the menisci in force transmission across the knee. Clin. Orthop., *109:* 184, 1975.

21. Wang, C.J., and Walker, P.S.: Rotatory laxity of the human knee joint. J. Bone Joint Surg. [Am.], *56:* 161, 1974.

9 Meniscectomy

John N. Insall

For many years meniscectomy has been one of the most frequently performed orthopedic operations, indeed, it had become the orthopedic appendectomy. It was also generally assumed that the results of a properly performed meniscectomy were uniformly good provided that there was no associated articular or ligament damage. Perey[55] found that most patients returned to heavy manual labor after meniscectomy; Wynn-Parry et al.,[67] in a review of 1,723 meniscectomies, found that patients returned to athletic competition without difficulty.

It was generally advised that once the diagnosis of a torn meniscus was made prompt operation was advisable to prevent articular damage.[24] This view received support from an arthroscopic study by Dandy and Jackson,[14] who found that severity of chondromalacia on the femoral condyles correlated directly with the time interval from injury until the arthroscopic examination. On this basis, these workers concluded that prompt identification and early removal of meniscal tears would preserve the joint surfaces. They did not, however, offer any direct evidence that this is so.

After Watson-Jones'[65] teaching, total meniscectomy has generally been preferred to partial excision. Smillie[61] recommends total meniscectomy for several reasons:

1. Multiple tears are not uncommon, they are difficult to identify, hence partial meniscectomy may leave a meniscal fragment with a tear in it.
2. The hardest tears to see are of the horizontal cleavage type, and these are usually found in the posterior horn. Smillie therefore considers excision of the anterior horn alone an inadequate operation.
3. Partial removal of the meniscus, for example, in a bucket-handle tear does not permit meniscal regeneration. In his experience, a regenerated meniscus often resembles the original structure, although it is composed of fibrous tissue, rather than cartilage.

These assumptions, although widely accepted for many years, have undergone recent reappraisals.[3,6,27,42]

FUNCTION OF THE MENISCI

The preceding opinions were held in the belief that the meniscus functions mainly as a space filler and a means whereby lubrication of the joint is enhanced. However, Fairbank[20] had suggested that the meniscus probably had a weight-bearing function as well. He based this opinion on a radiographic study of patients who had undergone meniscectomy (Fig. 9.1) and some subsequent cadaver experiments in which he showed that upon compression the meniscus was

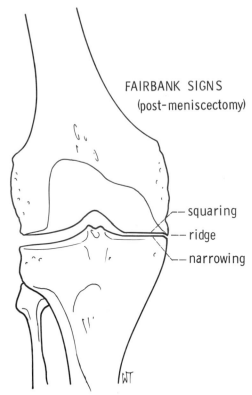

FAIRBANK SIGNS
(post-meniscectomy)

-- squaring
-- ridge
-- narrowing

Fig. 9.1. Joint changes after meniscectomy showing (1) a medial ridge of the femoral condyle, (2) squaring of the contour of the femoral condyle, and (3) narrowing of the joint space. (From Fairbank, T.J.: Knee joint changes after meniscectomy. J. Bone Joint Surg. [Br.], *30:* 664, 1948, with permission.)

extruded from between the joint surfaces in the same manner as a pip is squeezed from between the fingers. However, extrusion was prevented by the fibrous peripheral attachment of the meniscus, which under load became firm and tense. These observations provided strong circumstantial evidence that the menisci transmitted load.

Walker and Erkman[64] studied the role of menisci in force transmission across the knee. Two methods were employed: (1) a measurement of the areas of contact under varying loads using a self-curing methylmethacrylate casting technique, and (2) direct measurements of contact pressure using a miniature pressure transducer. These workers concluded, "The cartilage beneath the menisci will be under load most of the time, whereas the exposed cartilage will carry load only when the joint is highly loaded."

Removal of the menisci will increase the stress on the cartilage on the underlying bone and will also change the locations of the contact areas. This is particularly significant to the future viability of the exposed cartilage because in this area it is usually soft and fibrillated.

Krause et al.,[41] using a compression testing machine, showed that the menisci performed a load-transmitting and energy-absorbing function in the knee joint.

Using essentially the same experimental models, Shrive[60] calculated that the menisci carried 40 to 60 percent of the total load transmitted across the joint. Seedhom and associates[59] found that in full extension the menisci carried 50 percent or more of the load.

RELATIONSHIP OF MENISCAL TEARS AND OSTEOARTHRITIS

On the basis of the evidence, there can be no question but that the menisci substantially increase the area of contact (and conformity) between femur and tibia, and in addition, transmit at least one-half the load across the joint. The menisci are then far from being vestigial or dispensable structures.[37] The removal of a normal meniscus profoundly alters load transmission across the knee, and removal of an intact but so-called "hypermobile" meniscus must be regarded as a questionable practice. Furthermore, it may be asked whether old damaged menisci require removal, particularly when the symptoms they cause are intermittent and infrequent. On this last point there are no definitive data. Dandy and Jackson[14] could correlate severity of chondromalacia with the duration of symptoms from a meniscal tear, but their study raises several questions: First, their patients were arthroscoped before arthrotomy and meniscectomy and presumably had persistently severe symptoms that mandated operation. Does the same degree of chondromalacia occur with asymptomatic meniscal tears? Second, the most severe chondromalacia occurred in older patients, suggesting that the meniscal tear might itself be degenerative in nature. Third, they were unable to show that chondromalacia would have been prevented by early meniscectomy.

Tapper and Hoover,[63] on the other hand, found that the duration of symptoms seemed to have no bearing on the long-term effects of meniscectomy. These investigators found fewer excellent results when operation was delayed more than 2 years, but the proportion of overall satisfactory results (excellent plus good) was substantially the same, and the proportion of poor results was no higher than among those operated on sooner after their injury. They stated, "We may conclude that delay of meniscectomy is not prejudicial to satisfactory recovery, and therefore adequate time can be allowed for recovery from the initial injury to ensure accuracy of diagnosis, as long as no major ligamentous injury is present. In other words, the longer one waits, the more episodes of locking the patient has, the more specific the diagnosis, the more confident the surgeon, and the more precise the operation. Therefore, good results occurring after delay in treatment may possibly be explained by better diagnosis."

Northmore-Ball and Dandy[52] in an arthroscopic study concluded, "The development of chondromalacia is an age related process largely independent of meniscal pathology."

From a study of 115 cadaveric knees, Fahmy et al.[19] found little evidence that tears of the meniscus caused osteoarthritis or vice versa.

On the basis of this evidence, I believe that the demonstration of a meniscal tear is not in itself a reason for meniscectomy (Fig. 9.2).[10]

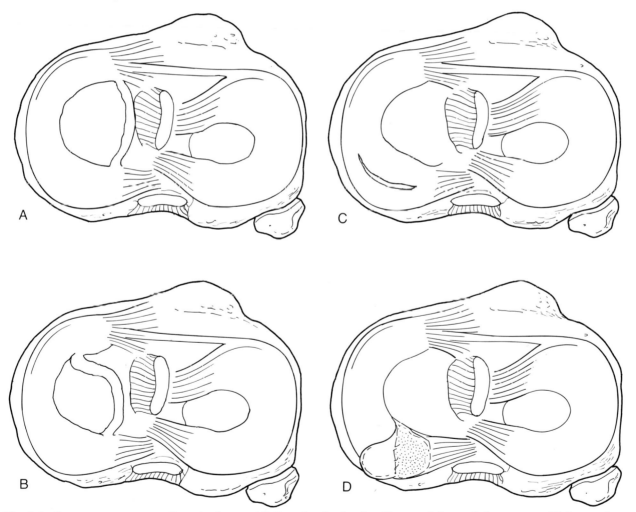

Fig. 9.2. Some common types of meniscal tears. (A) Complete bucket-handle tear of the medial meniscus. (B) Incomplete bucket-handle tear of medial meniscus. (C) Concealed incomplete bucket-handle tear of posterior horn of the medial meniscus. (D) Superior flap tear of posterior horn of the medial meniscus (Figure continues).

DIAGNOSIS

Good clinicians claim an accuracy of diagnosis approaching 90 percent by examination alone.

The characteristic injury that produces a meniscal tear is a twisting motion with the foot fixed to the ground. Sudden pain over the joint line is experienced, followed in an hour or so by swelling. Sometimes the injury may be caused by squatting or such everyday activities as climbing into a car. Although it is true that particularly in older people the menisci may tear in the absence of injury, a specific *occurrence*, however trivial, is the rule and insidious onset of symptoms should raise serious suspicion that the cause of symptoms lies elsewhere. For example, bilaterality of symptoms is much more likely to be patella in origin than the result of meniscal injury.

Meniscal tears tend to cause trouble intermittently. Characteristically a bout of pain, locking, or swelling is produced by a pivoting or cutting movement. Symptoms typically settle down within 1 or 2 weeks,

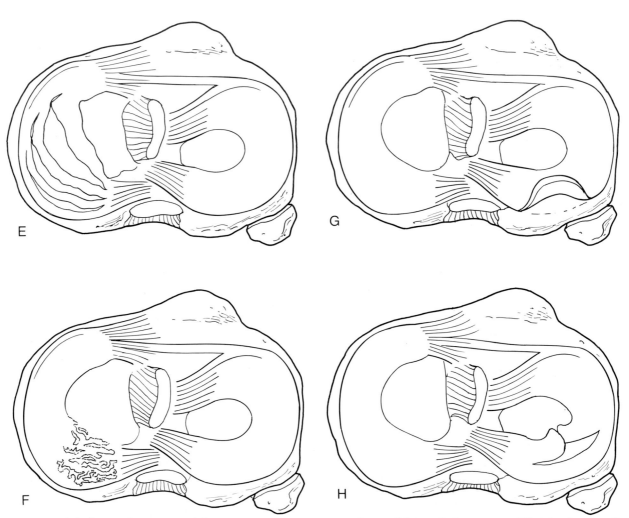

Figure 9.2 (E) Shattered meniscus. (F) Degenerative tear posterior horn of the medial meniscus. (G) A bucket-handle tear of the lateral meniscus involving the whole thickness of the posterior half. (H) A bucket-handle fragment of the lateral meniscus ruptured in its center (Figure continues).

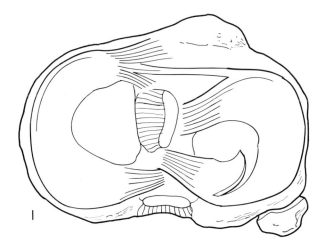

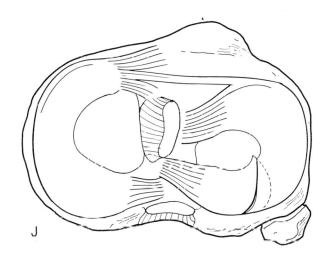

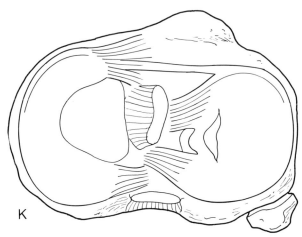

Fig. 9.2 (I) Posterior flap tear of the lateral meniscus. (J) A parrot-beak tear of the posterior third of the lateral meniscus in the region of popliteus tunnel. (K) A discoid lateral meniscus with a small central tear. (From Dandy, D.J.: Arthroscopic Surgery of the Knee. Edinburgh, Churchill Livingstone, 1981, with permission.)

be sought with particular care when the symptom of giving way is present.

Even if a trial of function is intended confirmation of the diagnosis is desirable although not mandatory. However, with recurrent or persistent symptoms requiring surgery, arthrography[39] or arthroscopy[7,12,16,32] is needed. Because of access to expert arthrography the arthrogram is the author's personal first preference, but this choice will vary according to circumstance.[32]

Arthrography is most useful in diagnosing peripheral posteromedial tears of the medial meniscus, least useful for lateral meniscal tears. Daniel et al.[15] recommend both arthrography and arthroscopy except for suspected lateral meniscal tears and meniscal extension blocks; in these circumstances arthroscopy is done without a prior arthrogram. These workers found that most of the medial compartment arthrogram errors were false-positives owing to overinterpretation of anterior horn anatomy. Many proficient arthroscopists consider arthroscopy superior to arthrography (Table 9.1) even for posteromedial tears of the meniscus provided that (1) the meniscus is probed, and (2) a posteromedial puncture is used.

Only when convinced of both the need for surgery and the accuracy of diagnosis should meniscectomy be performed.

after which the knee feels relatively normal. The physical signs also vary and in an asymptomatic phase examination of the knee may show little or no abnormalities. However, some degree of quadriceps atrophy is nearly always present. In the symptomatic phase there is loss of motion in either extension or flexion, and squatting causes pain. The tibial rotation tests (Apley,[2] McMurray,[46] Steinmann[57]) are positive and refer pain to the affected compartment. There is usually an effusion. Joint line tenderness is nearly always present, but as this can also be found in ligamentous or patellar disorders, it must be interpreted with caution. Joint line tenderness when it is the only finding is probably not meniscal in origin.

Associated ligament injury, particularly of the anterior cruciate ligament (ACL), is common and must

Table 9.1 Accuracy of Diagnosis

Investigators	Clinical	Arthrogram	Arthroscopy
Nicholas et al.[49]		97%	
Casscells[7]			80%
Jackson and Abe[34]	68.5%	68.2%	95%
McGinty and Metza[45]			91% G.A.
			95% L.A.
DeHaven and Collins[16]	72%	78% (84% medial 72% lateral)	94%
Gillies and Seligson[25]	85%	83%	68%

MANAGEMENT OF MENISCAL TEARS AND INDICATIONS FOR MENISCAL EXCISION

In a retrospective study of patients undergoing meniscectomy at the Hospital for Special Surgery between 1935 and 1955, 121 patients were seen and examined by me (unpublished observations). In this study, the conclusions were very similar to those of Tapper and Hoover.[63] Clearly, meniscectomy was not a benign procedure, and the proportion of about 70 percent satisfactory results left something to be desired. Associated ligament instability, usually of the ACL, was found in about 30 percent but did not contribute greatly to the unsatisfactory results. The two main causes for a poor result were degenerative arthritis in the affected compartment and patellar pain. Patellar crepitus and tenderness were found in one-quarter of patients. How often this was present before surgery is impossible to say, but in some of these cases the meniscus was described as hypermobile, suggesting the possibility of mistaken diagnosis. In other cases the arthrotomy incision (medial parapatellar) may have precipitated a patellar tracking problem that did not exist before surgery.

Radiographically, 11 patients had grade III degenerative arthritis, and almost all the remainder showed the characteristic changes described by Fairbank.

Partly because of this study and partly because reliable arthrography became available, a conservative policy toward meniscectomy was adopted. The logistics of obtaining an arthrogram inevitably imposed delay between injury and the confirmation of the diagnosis. Often this delay amounted to several weeks, and by that time the patient's acute symptoms had often subsided making a trial of function desirable. Patients were told of their diagnosis and given the arguments in favor of meniscectomy. They were also informed that degenerative arthritis often occurred after meniscectomy so that no guarantee could be made of its prevention. Armed with this information, most patients elected to "wait and see." Subsequently fewer than one-quarter have required surgery because of sufficiently annoying or disabling symptoms. It is as yet too soon to know how many will later develop clinically evident osteoarthritis, but in those who have been re-examined radiographically, the typical Fairbank changes were seen, which we believe indicate loss of normal meniscal function.

It is our belief that once the meniscus is torn degenerative arthritis becomes more likely with[33] or without meniscectomy, and thus procrastination and trial of function are justified: once the diagnosis has been established, the choice regarding surgery can be left to the patient, who will then ask for it or not depending on the severity of the symptoms. Obviously repeated episodes of locking followed by painful effusions are a clear indication for surgery, but when the knee remains virtually asymptomatic, it is difficult to believe that the meniscal tear, simply by its presence, can cause rapid articular deterioration.[50]

MANAGEMENT OF THE LOCKED KNEE

It is widely believed that a locked knee (defined as inability to fully extend the joint) is a semi-emergency that should be corrected immediately by manipulation (under anesthesia if necessary), traction, or even immediate meniscectomy. It is questionable that any of these approaches is justified. Sometimes the patient can unlock the knee by making certain movements, but passive manipulation is seldom useful, and forcible pressure applied under anesthesia is likely to do damage. According to Frankel et al.,[23] locking is seldom caused by actual interposition of a meniscal fragment, but rather by a disturbance of the instant center of motion that inhibits the normal spinning and gliding motions, causing the joint surfaces to jam into each other. Almost invariably, unlocking occurs spontaneously within a few days if the patient is begun on a series of straight-leg-raising exercises. Traction which usually means hospitalization therefore seems unnecessary. Initially weight-bearing is painful and, for this reason, crutches are prescribed, but weight-bearing is then permitted according to the patient's tolerance.

Immediate open surgery is not advisable for a number of reasons, not least because by no means is all locking caused by the meniscus. Errors in diagnosis should be avoidable by the use of arthrography and of arthroscopy, so that a normal meniscus is not removed inadvertently.

REPAIR OF PERIPHERAL MENISCAL TEARS

Annandale[1] repaired a torn meniscus by suturing as early as 1889. The operation was an apparent clinical success in that the patient returned to work 6 months later. King[40] showed experimentally that peripheral lesions of the meniscus can heal. He demonstrated that while tears in the substance of the meniscus probably never heal, cuts in the meniscus which extend peripherally into the synovium may heal by the invasion of synovial cells into the cut. However, until recently, there has been little interest in attempting meniscal repair. Heatley[29] performed a number of experiments in rabbits that showed the

meniscus to possess a considerable potential for healing and that an essential prelude is invasion by synovial cells. Healing occurred more quickly and with less scarring when sutures were used to provide stability and reduce the size of the gap. Similar results were reported by Cabaud et al.[5] in experiments on canine and rhesus knee joints. A simulated parrot-beak laceration of the anterior horn of the meniscus was produced contiguous with the synovium and coronary ligament. The laceration was then repaired with a single dexon suture. Four months postoperatively only two of 32 repaired menisci had failed to heal.

Cassidy and Shaffer[8] reported on surgical repair of tears in the peripheral one-third of the meniscus in 29 cases. The knee was first examined under anesthesia and arthroscoped to confirm that there were no other injuries. A posteromedial incision was made behind the tibial collateral ligament. The meniscus and the tear were exposed and identified. Incomplete tears were converted to complete ones and the edges of the tear were debrided or excised. The periphery of the meniscus was then sutured to the posterior capsule by a series of sutures placed 3 to 4 mm apart (Fig. 9.3A, B). Four of their cases had a postoperative

Fig. 9.3. Repair of a peripherally detached meniscus. (A) Type of peripheral tear amenable to repair. (B) When the tear is old, the edges should be freshened and any peripheral rim of meniscus excised. The body of the meniscus is reattached to the capsule with interrupted sutures.

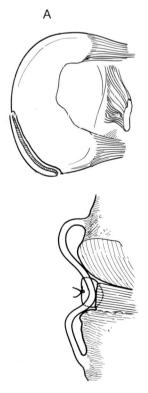

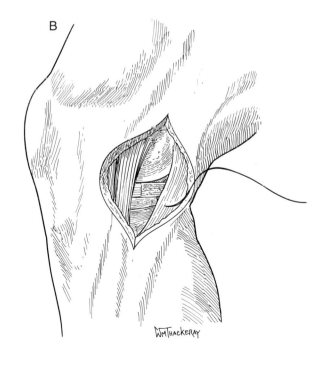

arthrogram, all of which indicated that the tears had completely healed. Two patients reinjured the knee, permitting an inspection of the repair. Both were found to be intact. These workers recommend that this technique be restricted to peripheral vertical tears in the outer one-third of the meniscus and emphasize that it is important to debride the edges of the meniscus before suturing particularly when the tear is an old one. DeHaven[17] has used a similar technique since 1976, immobilizing the knee in flexion for approximately 6 weeks. He reports four confirmed retears in 75 cases.

Repair of a peripheral tear of the meniscus would seem to be feasible treatment on the basis of this evidence.

ARTHROTOMY OR ARTHROSCOPY?

Experts in arthroscopic surgery have predicted that arthrotomy for meniscectomy will soon be obsolete. Public awareness of arthroscopic techniques has made patients request them and certainly the reduced morbidity makes arthroscopic surgery very attractive. Nonetheless, perspective is needed and a recognition that arthroscopic surgery is difficult, requires special training, and may indeed be beyond the capabilities of all. The key issue is avoidance of articular damage, and if severe scuffing results from an arthroscopic meniscectomy that patient would have been better treated by arthrotomy. The factors that influence this decision are individual skill and the type of meniscal tear. There will always be some indications for open meniscectomy, and a good arthrotomy is better than a bad arthroscopy.

Bucket-handle tears, flap tears of the anterior and middle thirds, and degenerative tears are the easiest to treat arthroscopically, particularly when slight ligament laxity allows the joint to open. Complex tears requiring total meniscectomy and tight joints make for difficulty and increase the chance of articular scuffing. When an arthroscopic meniscectomy is not going well and nothing has been accomplished in an hour of operating time, it is sensible to abort the procedure, redrape the knee and open the joint. This can happen even in skilled hands. Gillquist and Oretorp[26] report that in 12 percent of their cases endoscopic meniscectomy failed and arthrotomy was required.

This figure is perhaps higher than would be expected and probably represents a learning phase in their experience.

PARTIAL OR TOTAL MENISCECTOMY?

Tapper and Hoover[63] found that the highest proportion of satisfactory results was obtained when, for bucket-handle tears, removal of the detached fragment only was done, leaving the peripheral rim intact. This procedure yielded the highest percentage of excellent knees (67 percent). Partial meniscectomy of another type in which the posterior horn was left intact gave results significantly worse than total meniscectomy. These investigators recommended that when it was possible to remove the bucket-handle portion of the tear leaving an intact peripheral rim, this should be done, but leaving an intact posterior horn was not advisable. They believed that in these circumstances a second incision should be made to remove the posterior horn.

McGinty and associates[44] studied a total of 128 cases of meniscectomy of which 89 were total and 39 partial. The type of tear was classified as anterior third, middle third, posterior third, bucket handle, or discoid. The patients selected for partial meniscectomy were those in which the torn fragment could be easily removed (bucket handle or flap tear). The tears were classified as anterior third in 12 and bucket handle in 27.

The patients undergoing partial meniscectomy had fewer postoperative complications, a shorter hospital course, and a shorter period on crutches.

Sixty-eight of these patients were examined in a follow-up study. Only three of 20 partial meniscectomy patients had any subjective symptoms: one had some pain and two had difficulty squatting. All 20 scored over 90 points on Larson's scale and 19 scored 99 or 100 points.

In the total meniscectomy group of 48 patients, the symptoms were recorded as follows: pain, 17; difficulty walking, 10; difficulty climbing stairs, 13; difficulty running, 19; difficulty jumping, 9; and difficulty squatting, 14. Nine patients in this group scored below 80, and the largest point loss was attributable to pain.

The criteria of Fairbank were used to examine the radiographs. In general the patients with partial meniscectomy had less narrowing of the joint interval than the patients with total meniscectomy. Condylar flattening was present in 20 percent of the instances of partial meniscectomy and in 38 percent of those of total meniscectomy.

They concluded that they could find no evidence, subjective or objective, to favor total meniscectomy over partial excision in the management of bucket-handle tears and anterior horn tears of the menisci. In the functional rating, patients scored 95 points or better after partial meniscectomy compared with 73 percent of the patients in this category after total meniscectomy. On the basis of the review of the literature and the findings in their series, they recommended that partial meniscectomy be done in lesions of the meniscus where a relatively normal rim of fibrocartilage can be retained.

Clearly, in the era of endoscopic surgery these findings have a special significance. Bucket-handle and flap tears can be removed relatively easily under endoscopic control, whereas total meniscectomy is not only more difficult but carries with it a significant risk of articular damage.

Jackson and Dandy[35] have suggested the following criteria for partial meniscectomy. (1) a bucket-handle tear should be vertical and not obliquely sliced, (2) the peripheral rim must be intact, (3) supporting ligaments and capsule should be intact, and (4) a flap tear should be less than one-third of the total area of the meniscus, and its removal should not create an "unbalanced" knee.

Today those experienced in endoscopic surgery treat most meniscal tears by closed partial meniscectomy even lesions of the posterior horn (Table 9.2).

By the conventional open-technique removal of bucket-handle,[6] flap, and parrot-beak tears should be done whenever a sound peripheral rim can be left.

Table 9.2 Meniscal Lesions

	Medial	*Lateral*
Bucket handle	29	12
Anterior third	1	7
Middle third	1	1
Posterior third	15	3
	46	23

From Northmore-Ball, M.D., and Dandy, D.J.: Long-term results of arthroscopic partial meniscectomy. Clin. Orthop., *167*: 34, 1982.

MENISCECTOMY AND LIGAMENT INJURIES

Tears of the menisci are frequently associated with ligament injuries most often of the anterior cruciate ligament.[11] While the precise incidence of co-occurrence is uncertain, it is known that about two-thirds of acute ruptures of the anterior cruciate ligament are accompanied by meniscal tears,[53] and further attritional tears may follow in cruciate insufficient knees. The immediate repair of acute anterior cruciate ruptures is controversial; in a patient with chronic symptoms after injury, it may be difficult to decide whether meniscectomy alone will be sufficient or whether a cruciate reconstruction should also be done. In favor of early repair of anterior cruciate rupture is the opportunity to return the knee to a near-normal state; against is the knowledge that many primary repairs fail with time. McDaniel and Dameron show (see Chapter 13) roughly two-thirds of patients are able to return to strenuous sports without repair of a ruptured anterior criciate ligament. Thus, for acute injuries it seems reasonable to recommend conservative management for older patients and those not particularly interested in energetic sports, reserving arthroscopy, aspiration of the hemarthrosis, and endoscopic meniscectomy when necessary for athletic persons. Perhaps it will soon be possible to predict which patients with a ruptured anterior cruciate ligament will not do well without repair or reconstruction; until then, it is my view that primary repair can only be justified in very high level of professional athletes.

When symptoms are chronic, the pattern is usually (1) primarily mechanical with episodes of catching, locking, and swelling, or (2) associated with anterior cruciate insufficiency. In the former case, meniscectomy alone seems preferable, recognizing that some of these patients may later need a reconstruction.

On the other hand, when the characteristic syndrome of anterior cruciate insufficiency is present (and the meniscal tear seems largely incidental), a cruciate reconstruction is indicated. These patients are usually, although not always, those with the most pronounced physical signs of instability, most often with a pronounced pivot shift test. Also, the athletic pretensions of the patient as well as age and sex must be considered. Obviously, not all cases are clear cut and may be difficult to categorize satisfactorily. Naturally, the patient must fully understand these issues and have a part in the decision making; most are very willing to accept the lesser procedure.

DEGENERATED MENISCI AND DEBRIDEMENT OF THE KNEE

Osteonecrosis of the medial femoral condyle is sometimes misdiagnosed as a tear of the medial meniscus, but this error can be prevented by obtaining a bone scan, which in the case of osteonecrosis will reveal the characteristically high uptake in the medial femoral condyle.

Noble and Hamblen[51] have reported that about one-half the population over 50 years of age have asymptomatic degenerative tears of the meniscus on the basis of autopsy studies. This fact clearly raises a difficulty when dealing with older patients complaining of pain in the knee. First and foremost, any such patient must first be assessed with weight-bearing radiographs as any significant narrowing of the joint space is a contraindication to meniscectomy; these cases are better treated by osteotomy.

The true dilemma arises in a patient with a near normal joint space in the weight-bearing radiograph (Fig. 9.4) and a knee scan that shows a mildly increased uptake suggesting early osteoarthritis. The meniscal tear is usually of the horizontal cleavage variety; Smillie[61] has recommended that these menisci be removed to prevent progression of gonarthrosis. It is my impression that many do not fare well after meniscectomy. The pain attributed to the meniscal tear is often not relieved, in fact, some patients may actually be worse. The findings of Lotke et al.[43] confirm this view. In a study of 101 patients who were over age 45 at meniscectomy, the end result correlated with the preoperative severity of arthritis. Whereas 90 percent of those with normal radiographs did well after meniscectomy, when there was moderate to severe arthritis beforehand, meniscectomy had a low chance of success. They recommend arthroscopic evaluation deferring meniscectomy in those with a considerable degree of articular damage.

Lotke's patients with minimal detectable arthritis also had unpredictable results after meniscectomy especially when symptoms were chronic and the onset not related to a specific episode of trauma.

An opposing opinion is expressed by Sprague,[62] who cites his experience with arthroscopic debridement for gonarthrosis. Most of his patients had a tear of at least one meniscus and, with an admittedly short follow-up, 84 percent were found to be satisfactory after the procedure. Sprague argues that arthroscopic meniscectomy involves minor morbidity and risk and does not preclude more major surgery at a later date.

The evaluation of older patients for meniscectomy requires much care and judgment, and most should be treated conservatively for a lengthy period before considering surgery. Clearly, degenerative tears occur with great frequency, and it has not been shown that the presence of a damaged meniscus increases clinically significant gonarthrosis. In the natural his-

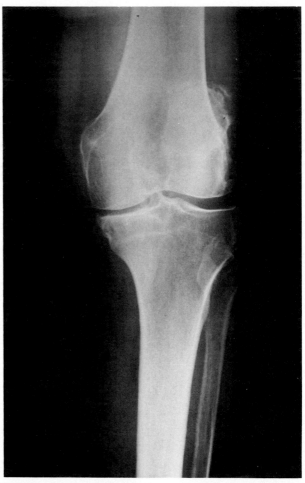

Fig. 9.4. Osteotomy or meniscectomy? The correct choice of procedure may be difficult to make. See text for discussion.

tory of gonarthrosis, there is a painful phase during which there is little degeneration of the articular cartilage, although the bone scan is abnormal. This painful phase is often self-limiting, and curiously the symptoms may subside with the appearance of radiographic evidence of osteoarthritis. There is a parallel in the development of Heberden's nodes. It seems well recognized that a finger joint becomes painful before the characteristic enlargement, whereas in later stages the joint ceases to hurt even when considerable deformity is present.

This point is made to emphasize a belief that in older patients a meniscal tear, unless clearly traumatic, is merely part of a more generalized degenerative process, which may even be accelerated by meniscectomy.

Interest in debridement of the knee has been renewed by arthroscopic surgery. As an open operation it had some popularity two and three decades ago. Magnuson[47] considered that roughened surfaces within a joint acted as a source of irritation perpetuating degenerative changes and giving rise to the symptoms of osteoarthritis. He suggested that the removal of all mechanical irritants would relieve the symptoms and perhaps arrest future progression of the disease. Haggart[28] described an operation in which all intra-articular abnormalities were removed as far as was feasible. He pointed out that degenerative changes were most advanced in the patellofemoral region and that the patella was often enlarged by osteophyte formation. He recommended that the patella should be either reduced in size so that it might move easily in the femoral groove or excised completely. Magnuson used the term debridement for this type of operation. He emphasized that surgery must be thorough and that "no half-way procedure will give satisfactory results; the success of the procedure depends on complete removal of all mechanical irritants." Haggart reported the results in 30 patients with osteoarthritis of the knee. The follow-up was from 18 months to 7 years. Twelve patients had no symptoms, eight had aching pain, seven had periodic mild discomfort, and three were unrelieved. Both Haggart and Magnuson stated that the procedure was suitable for only a few patients and should not be done on knees that are too severely disorganized.

A similar type of operation was done by Pridie.[56] Hypertrophic or inflamed synovium was excised from the anterior compartment and the fat pad. Osteo-phytes were trimmed from around the patella and femoral condyles. All softened, fissured, or fibrillated cartilage was shaved, and torn or degenerated menisci and any loose osteocartilaginous bodies were removed. Pridie introduced the modification of drilling exposed subchondral bone. These drill holes breeched the dense eburnated bone and permitted vascular cancellous bone beneath to bring regenerative tissue to the surface, so that the drill holes later become filled with fibrocartilage[58] (Fig. 9.5 A–D). Tibial osteotomy was done to correct significant malalignment. Pridie's approach was more empirical than the standardized operation advocated by Magnuson and Haggart. Although agreeing that the aim of the operation was to remove mechanical irritants, Pridie believed it desirable to do no more than necessary.

Insall[31] reviewed 62 knees that had been operated on by Pridie. Results in 48 knees (77 percent) were pleasing to the patient. However, only 40 knees (64 percent) were objectively rated as good at review. The operation seemed most suitable for relatively active healthy people and most of the bad results were associated with removal of the patella.

Joint debridement of the magnitude advocated by Pridie fell into disrepute because it was an extensive and painful procedure that gave somewhat unpredictable results. Also, better alternatives became available. As a closed procedure these objections seem less important. Done in this manner, patients can begin walking the day after surgery and begin range of motion and muscle-strengthening exercises at 2 to 3 days. In general, the endoscopic procedure follows the same general principles used in the open operation. A limited synovectomy, excision of osteophytes and trimming of degenerated minisci are done. Flaking and fibrillated cartilage is removed with a power tool. Johnson[36] has introduced a mechanical burr to abrade exposed bone to bleeding tissue (abrasion arthroplasty). Good results are reported with these techniques, and Johnson has shown by repeat arthroscopy that some fibrocartilaginous healing can occur. Sprague[62] has reported a short follow-up on 63 patients of whom 51 (74 percent) had a good result. Abrasion arthroplasty was not a part of his procedure. Complaints were few and mild in nature and there was little morbidity.

These new techniques justify a second look at debridement, but more follow-up information is needed before a final judgment on its merits can be made.

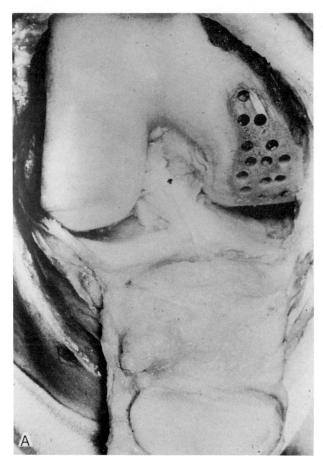

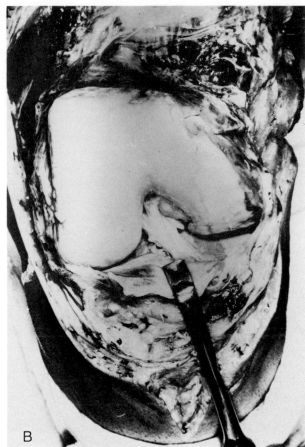

LATE RESULTS OF MENISCECTOMY

Tapper and Hoover[63] reviewed the records of patients who had undergone meniscectomy at the Mayo Clinic between 1936 and 1956. Patients who had evidence of osteochondritis dissecans, loose bodies, degenerative arthritis, chondromalacia, and torn ligaments at operation were excluded. Questionnaires were sent to 494 patients, and 255 were completed and returned; 126 of these patients returned to the Clinic for examination. Their series was composed of two groups: group I, 113 patients who had a single meniscectomy and returned for examination, and group II, 100 patients who had a single meniscectomy and responded by questionnaire.

The following grading system was used: excellent, the patient had no symptoms and no disability; good, the patient had minimum symptoms but there was essentially no disability; fair, the patient had symptoms that interfered with everyday activities and the patient thought he had some disability; poor, the symptoms were severe and the patient was clearly disabled and his activities, including walking, were definitely limited.

Overall, the results were 38 percent excellent, 30 percent good, 19 percent fair, and 13 percent poor. In discussing these results, the authors point out an inherent problem in clinical studies:

> The excellent and poor results are easily identified but represent only about half the patients. Thus, after meniscectomy about 40 percent of patients will have a normally functioning knee and 10 percent will have a bad outcome. This leaves about 50 percent who have varying degrees of symptoms and disability following their meniscus tear and surgical removal of the meniscus. Depending on the examiner's judgment of this group, one can therefore report anywhere from 40 to 90 percent of good or satisfactory results.

There was no difference in results that could be

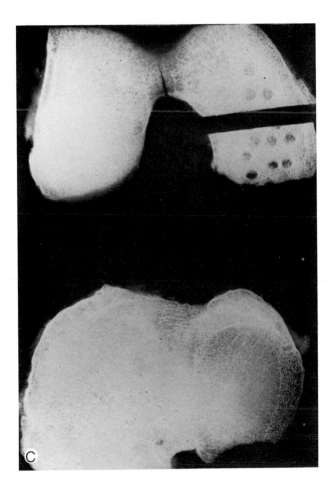

related to the length of follow-up, but patients who were 20 years old or less at operation had significantly fewer excellent or good results than did those aged 21 or over. The most common surgical lesion encountered was the longitudinal bucket-handle tear, which occurred in 50 percent of patients. Thirty-two patients had no tear but a meniscus that was judged to be loose or hypermobile. One-half these patients were women (compared with a 4:1 ratio of men to women in the entire group). Of these 32 patients, only 12 had excellent or good results, suggesting that the correct diagnosis was either not made preoperatively or not apparent at operation.

Roentgenographic changes as described by Fairbank were present in 85 percent of patients. In the remaining 16 patients there were no changes at all in six patients, and minimum changes in three others. More advanced degenerative changes were present in the remaining seven knees.

In general, the severity of radiographic changes correlated with the clinical results: "It is possible to have a good clinical result with a poor appearance on the roentgenogram and vice-versa, but this was unusual."

There is no comparable follow-up for endoscopic meniscectomy, but the short-term results are encouraging. Northmore-Ball and Dandy[52] report 90 percent excellent or good results after arthroscopic

Fig. 9-5. A case of osteoarthritis treated by the Pridie technique. (A) At the debridement operation, the medial condyle was extensively drilled. (B) The knee was reoperated because of persistent pain, affording a second look at the joint. The previously drilled area was covered with fibrocartilage. (C) A section was taken through this region of the medial femoral condyle. (D) Photomicrograph through one of the drill holes showing the rather cellular fibrocartilage that had filled the defect. (From Insall, J.N.: Intra-articular surgery for degenerative arthritis of the knee. J. Bone Joint Surg. [Br.], *49*: 211, 1967, with permission.)

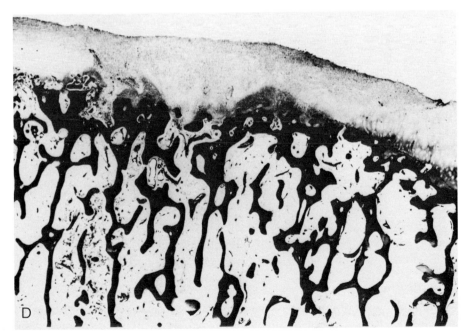

partial meniscectomy with a minimum 2-year follow-up. The results were better in group I cases (no ligament instability or marked articular damage) than in group II (knees with anterior cruciate lesions, osteoarthritis, or previous meniscal surgery). The results were also better after treatment of bucket-handle tears than following excision of flap tears; the presence of chondromalacia at the time of surgery also affected the outcome. Contrary to the findings of Tapper and Hoover younger patients in their series were more likely to have a satisfactory result than the older ones.

DISCOID LATERAL MENISCUS

It has been suggested that the so-called congenital discoid meniscus[9,18,21,48] represents the arrested development of an embryonic stage when the menisci form a solid plate or disc which entirely separates femur and tibia. However, according to Kaplan,[38] there is no stage in human development in which the meniscus is present as a disc in this manner. Rather, Kaplan believes the discoid shape is acquired and attributable to abnormal attachments of the ligaments of Wrisberg and Humphry. These ligaments being unduly shortened prevent the lateral meniscus from moving backwards with the femur on flexion of the knee. The result is that the femur rides over the posterior margin of the meniscus, which in time is pushed forward into the joint, so that the central concavity is lost and the meniscus assumes the shape of a disc.

A discoid meniscus may present in childhood as a clicking[48] knee caused by the lateral femoral condyle jumping over the posterior margin of the meniscus. The click at times can be quite violent so that the jump is audible and visible.

The discoid meniscus is unusually vulnerable to injury because of its relative lack of mobility and therefore is apt to tear rather easily. An alternative presentation can be that of a torn lateral meniscus, the onset occurring either spontaneously or following trivial trauma.

The diagnosis may sometimes be suspected from routine anteroposterior radiographs because of widening of the lateral joint space, and the abnormal meniscus shape can be readily recognized by arthrography (Fig. 9.6 A,B).

The decision to remove a discoid lateral meniscus in childhood can often be a difficult one, for even

when clicking is pronounced there is usually no pain. The reason for removing the meniscus is the presumption that disturbance of joint mechanics will eventually cause articular cartilage damage. There is no definitive evidence that this is true and each case can be judged on its merits. A period of observation after the onset of symptoms is justified in the hope that the clicking will diminish in time.

Technically a discoid meniscus is harder to remove than one with normal anatomy. The posterior part of the meniscus is quite rigidly fixed and will neither pull forward nor displace into the intercondylar notch with the same ease as a normal meniscus. Therefore the posterior attachments have to be surgically divided so that the Bruser approach,[4] which gives better access to the posterior compartment, is helpful.

Arthroscopic removal of a discoid lateral meniscus[30] can be very difficult; the meniscus usually must be removed in sections or piecemeal.

CYSTS OF THE MENISCUS

Cystic degeneration of the meniscus[66] sometimes occurs and presents as a swelling on/or adjoining the joint line and often there is a chronic aching pain in the knee. Cysts occur much more frequently associated with the lateral meniscus (the ratio according to Smillie is 4:1) and characteristically vary in size. While usually quite small, they can at times measure 2 or 3 cm in diameter. Meniscal cysts must be distinguished from the rare ganglion, which is not connected to the meniscus, and from even more unusual solid para-articular swellings (e.g., fibroma or synovioma). In the latter case if there is serious doubt, a cyst can be identified by aspiration with a wide bore needle.

Lateral cysts are usually more prominent with the knee flexed than they are in extension because in the latter position the bulk of the iliotibial band is taut and overlies the cyst (Fig. 9.7).

TREATMENT

Small cysts that cause little trouble do not need excision and can be observed. In more troublesome cases, there is the choice between excision of the cyst alone or excision of the cyst and meniscus. If the meniscus is itself intact (as seen by arthrography or arthroscopy) simple excision of the cyst may be enough.

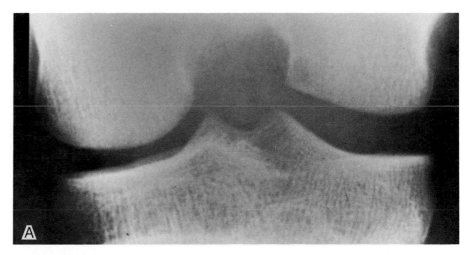

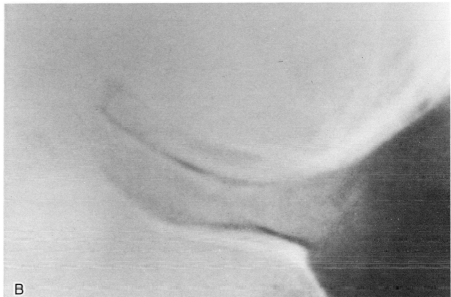

Fig. 9.6. (A) Radiograph of a discoid lateral meniscus. Widening of the lateral joint space is obvious. (B) Arthrogram in the same patient showing a discoid lateral meniscus.

Satisfactory results with this method have been accomplished.[22] When the meniscus is torn, or if the cyst recurs after simple excision, meniscectomy should be done.

TECHNIQUE OF OPEN MENISCECTOMY

MEDIAL MENISCECTOMY

The best incision is a short oblique one that provides a compromise between access to the peripheral rim of the meniscus and the intercondylar notch. There are two tricks to a clean and neat meniscectomy. The first is to place the peripheral incision in the correct plane, that is to say, at the exact rim of the meniscus, separating this from the capsular attachment. If the separation is made within the substance of meniscus leaving a small peripheral rim of meniscus behind, it is much more difficult to mobilize the posterior horn. On the other hand, if the plane is initially in the synovium, there is risk of injuring the medial ligament. Provided that the anterior horn is mobilized and the line of separation identified anteriorly, it is relatively simple to remain in the same plane in a posterior direction. The second is to separate fully the meniscus from the deep medial ligament before

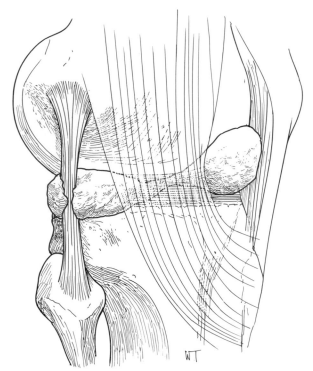

Fig. 9.7. Cysts of the lateral meniscus often envelop the lateral collateral ligament but usually lie beneath the iliotibial tract.

attempting to mobilize the posterior horn (Fig. 9.8). The capsular attachments of the meniscus are much firmer in this region than they are anteriorly and posteriorly, and the scalpel should be directed posteriorly into the posteromedial corner of the capsule. There are no vital structures that may be injured in this region, so the scalpel blade can be passed backward without concern. Once the separation from the medial ligament is complete the posterior horn can be easily separated with a curved Smillie knife and the entire meniscus displaced into the intercondylar notch. With regard to instruments, solid knives are best but disposable blades are satisfactory provided that very small sizes are not used (there is too great a risk of breakage).

LATERAL MENISCECTOMY

There are two acceptable incisions: the vertical anterolateral and the transverse (Bruser). The Bruser incision is preferred for removal of cystic menisci and discoid menisci because it provides better posterior exposure and allows the dissection of cystic proliferations around the lateral ligament. On the other hand, the exposure is very limited: the joint and meniscus are poorly seen until the anterior horn is mobilized. The anterolateral vertical incision provides a much better view of the entire lateral compartment. The trick of lateral meniscectomy is to accurately divide the popliteus attachment to the meniscus (Fig. 9.9), for when this is done, the meniscus is easily displaced into the notch. The lateral genicular artery is nearly always damaged during the course of lateral meniscectomy so that it is advisable to deflate the tourniquet to allow ligation of the artery. Reinflation can be done before closure.

RETAINED POSTERIOR HORN

Even though partial meniscectomy is now in favor, it is generally believed that leaving a sizable posterior fragment, particularly of the medial meniscus, is inadvisable. Tapper and Hoover found that the worst results were with partial meniscectomy leaving the posterior horn. However, symptoms caused by a retained posterior horn do not occur as frequently as opinions expressed in the literature would suggest, and seldom are symptoms unequivocally the result of a residual meniscal fragment.[13] This is not very surprising, as unless the posterior horn of the meniscus is grossly torn there seems little difference between leaving a part of it behind and removing the detached portion of a bucket-handle tear. Moreover, as the semimembranosus has an insertion into the posterior part of the medial meniscus as the popliteus does into the corresponding part of the lateral meniscus, one would expect this portion to be drawn out of harm's way when the knee is flexed. While it may be that in occasional cases persistent symptoms are caused by the remaining fragment, often they may be attributable to other causes. The posterior horn is most likely to be left in degenerative tears where the midsection is attenuated, so that the meniscus is likely to break at this point. These cases tend not to do well with any kind of meniscectomy (see above). Other causes of persistent symptoms may be rupture of the anterior cruciate ligament or unrecognized patellar disorders which refer pain to the back of the knee. Therefore, if total meniscectomy is indicated, a reasonable at-

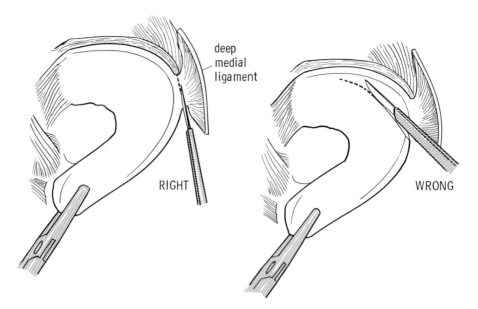

Fig. 9.8. The periphery of the medial meniscus must be sharply divided from its attachment to the deep medial ligament.

tempt should be made to remove the whole meniscus, and if a large fragment is left that may well contain a tear, removal through a separate posterior incision is indicated.[65] However, there should be no hesitation about leaving small fragments behind. Above all, attempts to perform a complete meniscectomy should never result in articular damage.

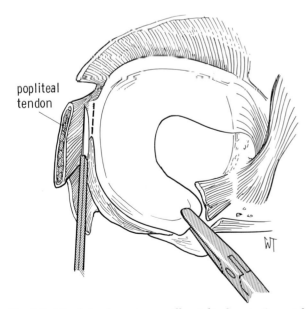

Fig. 9.9. The lateral meniscus will not displace to the notch until the popliteus attachment is divided.

COMPLICATIONS OF MENISCECTOMY

DAMAGE TO OTHER TISSUES

The most frequent occurrence is inadvertent laceration or scuffing of the articular surfaces. It is unlikely that these lesions will ever heal, and there is experimental animal data which indicates that they may predispose to degenerative arthritis. It is impossible to gauge the true incidence, but every surgeon must know from his own experience that it does occur, particularly when the meniscectomy is "difficult." One must assume that abrasions are more likely with arthroscopic techniques because the subject has received more attention than it ever did before in the era of open meniscectomy. Clearly this may be an unrecognized factor affecting the long-term results. The means whereby articular abrasions may be avoided have already been discussed, namely surgical care, selection of the type of meniscectomy—open or arthroscopic—and willingness to leave small fragments behind.

Other structures should not be damaged but lacerations of both collateral ligaments and of the popliteal artery have occurred. Laceration of the medial ligament is caused by failure to keep the scalpel blade parallel to the long fibers of the ligament. The lateral ligament can be more easily injured particularly with the Bruser incision unless the ligament is properly identified. Fortunately the injury is of less serious consequence. Arterial lacerations are almost always due to the use of meniscal knives to free the posterior horn. Again, the desire to perform a complete meniscectomy may be a contributing factor. Meniscal knives should be used with extreme gentleness; in fact, there is no cause for forcible maneuvers of any kind in meniscectomy. An arterial laceration usually causes blood to well up in the joint even when a tourniquet is used. However, there have been reports of unrecognized laceration leading to arteriovenous aneurysm.[54]

Postoperative hemarthrosis is caused either by unrecognized arterial bleeding (most often from the lateral genicular artery) or as a result of too vigorous postoperative physical therapy. Occasionally reoperation is required for the former type.

Chronic synovitis may be found in patients who resume their occupation or too vigorous activity before healing has taken place and the muscles have been redeveloped. The treatment is rest (with perhaps partial immobilization) until the synovitis has subsided, followed by a graduated program of quadriceps rebuilding. The possibility that chronic synovitis may represent a low grade infection should be considered and a diagnostic aspiration performed. Established sepsis should generally be treated by incision and drainage followed by intravenous antibiotic therapy. A so-called synovial fistula is usually a manifestation of low-grade sepsis.

Finally, there are the general complications associated with any surgery. In particular, thromboembolism does occur even in young patients, and I personally know of a case of fatal pulmonary embolism after uncomplicated meniscectomy in a healthy young adult male.

AFTERCARE FOLLOWING MENISCECTOMY

A heavily padded pressure dressing of the Robert Jones type is preferred for the partial immobilization and compression that it provides. The tourniquet should be released to identify bleeding points with subsequent reinflation before closure. This method plus the compression dressing practically eliminate postoperative hemarthrosis. My own approach to

physical therapy is considered somewhat unorthodox. Weight-bearing is allowed early, on the first or second postoperative day as tolerated and without restriction. On the other hand, contrary to the usual advice quadriceps exercises and motion are deferred until about 2 weeks after surgery, at which time the sutures are removed. Early and vigorous physical therapy may encourage postoperative swelling, hemarthrosis and the development of chronic synovitis. By delaying exercises there is no particular difficulty in regaining quadriceps strength, and the avoidance of early straight leg raising certainly spares the patient pain and frustration. At 2 weeks straight leg raising can be done by most people without difficulty, and the initial exercises are done without weights several hundred times a day. About 4 weeks postsurgery, progressive weight lifting is begun using sets of ten repetitions with an increasing weight. The exercises are done with the knee in extension and, in those without evidence of patellar problems, from a flexed position.

Regaining motion should seldom be a problem, but it is a mistake to resume normal activity too early. At least 3 weeks of convalescence is advisable after open meniscectomy to avoid chronic synovitis. Running can begin at 2 months and sports at 3 months.

Endoscopic meniscectomy can be done as a day case or with at most 1 to 2 days' hospitalization. One of its most attractive features is the rapid postoperative recovery. Morbidity is much less than with the open type of operation, so that rehabilitation can begin almost at once.

REFERENCES

1. Annandale, T.: Excision of the internal semilunar cartilage resulting in perfect restoration of the joint movement. Br. Med. J., *1:* 291, 1889.
2. Apley, A.G.: The diagnosis of meniscus injuries. Some new clinical methods. J. Bone Joint Surg. *29:* 78, 1947.
3. Appel, H.: Late results after meniscectomy in the knee joint. Acta Orthop. Scand., *133:* suppl. 1, 1970.
4. Bruser, D.M.: A direct lateral approach to the lateral compartment of the knee joint. J. Bone Joint Surg. [Br.], *42:* 348, 1960.
5. Cabaud, H.E., Rodkey, W.G., and Fitzwater, J.E.: Medial meniscus repair. Am. J. Sports Med., *9:* 129, 1981.

6. Cargill, A.O., and Jackson, J.P.: Bucket-handle tear of the medial meniscus. A case for conservative surgery. J. Bone Joint Surg. [Am.], *58:* 248, 1976.

7. Casscells, S.W.: Arthroscopy of the knee joint: A review of 150 cases. J. Bone Joint Surg. [Am.], *53:* 287, 1971.

8. Cassidy, R.E., and Shaffer, A.J.: Repair of peripheral meniscus tears. Am. J. Sports Med., *9:* 209, 1981.

9. Cave, E.F., and Staples, O.S.: Congenital discoid meniscus: A cause of internal derangement of the knee. Am. J. Surg., *54:* 371, 1941.

10. Dandy, D.J.: Arthroscopic Surgery of the Knee. Edinburgh, Churchill Livingstone, 1981.

11. Dandy D.J., Flanagan, J.P., and Steenmeyer, V.: Arthroscopy and the management of the ruptured anterior cruciate ligament. Clin. Orthop., *167:* 43, 1982.

12. Dandy, D.J., and Jackson, R.W.: The impact of arthroscopy on the management of disorders of the knee. J. Bone Joint Surg. [Br.], *57:* 346, 1975.

13. Dandy, D.J., and Jackson, R.W.: The diagnosis of problems after meniscectomy. J. Bone Joint Surg. [Br.], *57:* 349, 1975.

14. Dandy, D.J., and Jackson R.W.: Meniscectomy and chondromalacia of the femoral condyle. J. Bone Joint Surg. [Am.], *57:* 1116, 1975.

15. Daniel, D., Daniels, E., and Aronson, D.: The diagnosis of meniscus pathology. Clin. Orthop., *163:* 218, 1982.

16. DeHaven, K.E., and Collins, H.R.: Diagnosis of internal derangements of the knee. The role of arthroscopy. J. Bone Joint Surg. [Am.], *57:* 802, 1975.

17. DeHaven, K.E.: Commentary. Repair of peripheral meniscus tears. A preliminary report. Am. J. Sports Med., *9:* 213, 1981.

18. Dwyer, F.C., and Taylor, C.: Congenital discoid internal cartilage. Br. Med. J., *2:* 287, 1945.

19. Fahmy, N.R.M., Noble, J., and Williams, E.A.: Relationship between meniscal tears and osteoarthritis of the knee. In proceedings J. Bone Joint Surg. [Br.], *63:* 629, 1981.

20. Fairbank, T.J.: Knee joint changes after meniscectomy. J. Bone Joint Surg. [Br.], *30:* 664, 1948.

21. Finder, J.G.: Discoid external semilunar cartilage. A cause of internal derangement of the knee joint. J. Bone Joint Surg., *16:* 804, 1934.

22. Flynn, M., and Kelly, J.P.: Local excision of cyst of lateral meniscus of knee without recurrence. J. Bone Joint Surg. [Br.], *58:* 88, 1976.

23. Frankel, V.H., Burstein, A.H., and Brooks, D.B.: Biomechanics of internal derangement of the knee. Pathomechanics as determined by analysis of the instant centers of motion. J. Bone Joint Surg. [Am.] *53:* 945, 1971.

24. Gear, M.W.: The late results of meniscectomy. Br. J. Surg., *54:* 270, 1967.

25. Gillies, H., and Seligson, D.: Precision in the diagnosis of meniscal lesions. A comparison of clinical evaluation, arthrography, and arthroscopy. J. Bone Joint Surg. [Am.], *61:* 343, 1979.

26. Gillquist, J., and Oretorp, N.: Arthroscopic partial meniscectomy. Technique and long-term results. Clin. Orthop., *167:* 29, 1982.

27. Goodfellow, J.: He who hesitates is saved. Editorials and annotations. J. Bone Joint Surg. [Br.], *62:* 1, 1980.

28. Haggart, G.E.: Surgical treatment of degenerative arthritis of the knee joint. N. Engl. J. Med., *236:* 971, 1947.

29. Heatley, F.W.: The meniscus—Can it be repaired? An experimental investigation in rabbits. J. Bone Joint Surg. [Br.] *62:* 397, 1980.

30. Ikeuchi, H.: Arthroscopic treatment of the discoid lateral meniscus. Clin. Orthop., *167:* 19, 1982.

31. Insall, J.N.: Intra-articular surgery for degenerative arthritis of the knee. J. Bone Joint Surg. [Br.], *49:* 211, 1967.

32. Ireland, J., Trickey, E.L., and Stoker, D.J.: Arthroscopy and arthrography of the knee. J. Bone Joint Surg. [Br.], *62:* 3, 1980.

33. Jackson, J.P.: Degenerative changes in the knee after meniscectomy. Br. Med. J., *2:* 525, 1968.

34. Jackson, R.W., and Abe, I.: The role of arthroscopy in the management of disorders of the knee. An analysis of 200 consecutive examinations. J. Bone Joint Surg. [Br.], *54:* 310, 1972.

35. Jackson, R.W., and Dandy, D.J.: Partial meniscectomy. J. Bone Joint Surg. [Br.], *58:* 142, 1976.

36. Johnson, L.L.: Diagnostic and Surgical Arthroscopy: The Knee and Other Joints, 2nd Ed. St. Louis, C.V. Mosby, 1981.

37. Johnson, R.J., Kettelkamp, D.B., Clark, W., et al.: Factors affecting late results after meniscectomy. J. Bone Joint Surg. [Am.] *56:* 719, 1974.

38. Kaplan, E.B.: Discoid lateral meniscus of the knee joint. Nature, mechanism and operative treatment. J. Bone Joint Surg. [Am.], *39:* 77, 1957.

39. Kaye, J.J., and Freiberger, R.H.: Arthrography of the knee. Clin. Orthop., *107:* 73, 1975.

40. King, D.: The healing of the semilunar cartilages. J. Bone Joint Surg. *18:* 333, 1936.

41. Krause, W.R., Pope, M.H., Johnson, R.J., et al.: Mechanical changes in the knee after meniscectomy. J. Bone Joint Surg. [Am.], *58:* 599, 1976.

42. Editorial: Unnecessary meniscectomy. Lancet, *1:* 235, 1976.

43. Lotke, P.A., Lefkoe, R.T., and Ecker, M.L.: Late re-

sults following medial meniscectomy in an older population. J. Bone Joint Surg. [Am.], *63:* 115, 1981.

44. McGinty, J.B., Geuss, L.F., and Marvin, R.A.: Partial or total meniscectomy. A comparative analysis. J. Bone Joint Surg. [Am.], *59:* 763, 1977.

45. McGinty, J.B., and Matza, R.A.: Arthroscopy of the knee. Evaluation of an out-patient procedure under local anesthesia. J. Bone Joint Surg. [Am.], *60:* 787, 1978.

46. McMurray, T.P.: The semilunar cartilages. Br. J. Surg., *29:* 407, 1941.

47. Magnuson, P.B.: Joint debridement. Surgical treatment of degenerative arthritis. Surg. Gynec. Obstet., *73:* 1, 1941.

48. Middleton, D.S.: Congenital disc-shaped lateral meniscus with snapping knee. Br. J. Surg., *24:* 246, 1936.

49. Nicholas, J.A., Freiberger, R.H., and Killoran, P.J.: Double-contrast arthrography of the knee. J. Bone Joint Surg. [Am.], *52:* 203, 1970.

50. Noble, J., and Erat, K.: In defence of the meniscus. A prospective study of 200 meniscectomy patients. J. Bone Joint Surg. [Br.], *62:* 7, 1980.

51. Noble, J., and Hamblen, D.L.: The pathology of the degenerate meniscus lesion. J. Bone Joint Surg. [Br.], *57:* 180, 1975.

52. Northmore-Ball, M.D., and Dandy, D.J.: Long-term results of arthroscopic partial meniscectomy. Clin. Orthop., *167:* 34, 1982.

53. Noyes, F.R., Bassett, R.W., Grood, E.S., et al.: Arthroscopy in acute traumatic hemarthrosis of the knee. J. Bone Joint Surg. [Am.], *62:* 687, 1980.

54. Patrick, J.: Aneurysm of the popliteal vessels after meniscectomy. J. Bone Joint Surg. [Br.], *45:* 570, 1963.

55. Perey, O.: Follow-up results of meniscectomy with regard to the working capacity. Acta Orthop. Scand., *32:* 457, 1962.

56. Pridie, K.H.: A method of resurfacing osteoarthritic knee joints. In proceedings J. Bone Joint Surg. [Br.], *41:* 618, 1959.

57. Ricklin, P., Ruttiman, A., and del Buono, M.S.: Meniscal lesions. Practical problems of clinical diagnosis, arthrography, and therapy. New York, Grune & Stratton, 1971.

58. Salter, R.B., Simmonds, D.F., and Malcolm, B.W.: The biological effect of continuous passive motion on the healing of full-thickness defects in articular cartilage. An experimental investigation in the rabbit. J. Bone Joint Surg. [Am.], *62:* 1232, 1980.

59. Seedhom, B.B., Dowson, D., and Wright, V.: The functions of the menisci—A preliminary study. In proceedings J. Bone Joint Surg. [Br.], *56:* 381, 1974.

60. Shrive, N.: The weight-bearing role of the menisci of the knee. In proceedings J. Bone Joint Surg. [Br.], *56:* 381, 1974.

61. Smillie, I.S.: Injuries of the Knee Joint, 5th Ed. Edinburgh, Churchill Livingstone, 1978.

62. Sprague, N.F.: Arthroscopic debridement for degenerative knee joint disease. Clin. Orthop., *160:* 118, 1981.

63. Tapper, E.M., and Hoover, N.W.: Late results after meniscectomy. J. Bone Joint Surg. [Am.], *51:* 517, 1969.

64. Walker, P.S., and Erkman, M.J.: The role of the menisci in force transmission across the knee. Clin. Orthop., *109:* 184, 1975.

65. Watson-Jones, R.: Fractures and Other Bone and Joint Injuries, Baltimore, William Wilkins Co., 1940.

66. Wroblewski, B.M.: Trauma and the cystic meniscus: Review of 500 cases. Injury, *4:* 319, 1973.

67. Wynn-Parry, C.B., Nichols, P.J., and Lewis, N.R.: Meniscectomy: A review of 1723 cases. Ann. Phys. Med., *4:* 201, 1958.

10 Osteochondritis Dissecans of the Knee

Paul Aichroth

Osteochondritis dissecans is the process whereby a segment of cartilage together with subchondral bone separates from an articular surface. It may be found in many joints but is most common in the knee. The lesion is usually unilateral, but bilateral and symmetric lesions are not unusual.

Osteochondritis dissecans is the most common cause of a loose body in the knee joint in the young person. The fragment may stay in its crater, remaining silent or alternatively producing symptoms of pain, giving way, swelling, and occasionally locking. The cause of the separation of the fragment has been the subject of much discussion and many theories over the past century. There have been two main schools, one supporting injury[11,16,25] and the other supporting vascular insufficiency leading to bone infarction.[6,27,31]

HISTORIC REVIEW

Loose bodies in joints were first recognized by Ambroise Paré[26] in the sixth century, who must be credited not only with the first recognition of the disease, but also with the first reported case of the surgical removal of a loose body from the knee joint. Monro Primus was the first of three Munros to hold the chair of anatomy in Edinburgh. In the early 1700s he advocated the theory that loose bodies in the knee were of a traumatic origin (Fig. 10.1). Paget's classic description of the disease in 1870 mentioned in the first case a girl who had the habit of breaking thick pieces of wood across her thigh. The second case was of an athletic schoolboy from Harrow who had sustained many blows and strains of the knee (Fig. 10.2). König in 1887[16] was the first to name the disease osteochondritis dissecans; and he believed the cause of this dissection to be traumatic (Fig. 10.3).

Fairbank[11] endorsed the suggestion that osteochondritis dissecans might be caused by an un-united subchondral fracture; he envisaged such a lesion as being frequently sustained in sports in the heat of a game. Koch in 1879[15] performed a series of experiments on bone necrosis and stated that he had proved conclusively that articular bone infarction with loose body formation was the result of obstruction of the whole capillary bed of the area concerned. Many experiments since have advocated an embolic theory; as late as 1952, Watson-Jones[31] suggested that osteochondritis dissecans in multiple sites in the adolescent was caused by clumping of red blood cells leading to bone infarction. A large number of systemic diseases in which areas of avascular necrosis of bone develop include the postrenal transplant arthropathies, decompression syndrome, haemoglobinopathies, alcoholism, and steroid therapy. The lesions produced in these conditions are strikingly similar and often symmetric.

167

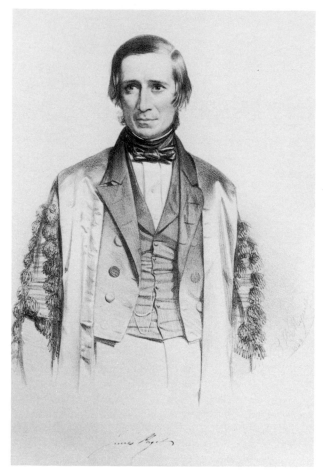

Fig. 10.1. Sir James Paget (1870).

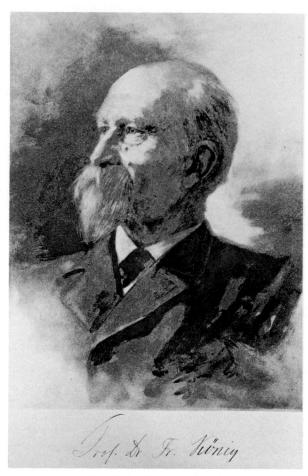

Fig. 10.2. F. König (1887).

There is, however, one essential difference from osteochondritis dissecans, for in this disease the crater from which the fragments separate is normally vascularized bone, whereas in the hemoglobinopathies and so forth a vast area of the femoral condyle is avascular and the peripheral separation of the segment is a small portion of the infarct. It is this peripheral separation of a fragment from an avascular bed that should be called osteonecrosis (Fig. 10.3); it should be differentiated from the condition seen so frequently in the athletic young man in whom the segment separates from vascularized normal bone and is traditionally called an osteochondritis dissecans (Fig. 10.4).

Smillie[30] believed that in many patients there was a relationship to abnormalities of endocrine function and that hormonal imbalance was responsible for abnormalities of epiphyseal growth. This is illustrated by the association of the Fröhlich-like syndrome and slipped femoral epiphysis.

Smillie believed that there were four types of osteochondritis dissecans and that all were interrelated in the etiology of the disease:

1. The lesion seen at age 10 was an anomaly of ossification.
2. The lesion seen at age 15 was described as a juvenile type.
3. The lesion appearing initially in the adult was termed adult osteochondritis dissecans.
4. Certain other lesions were tangential osteochondral fractures.

He stressed that the basic pathology of the disease

CLINICAL FEATURES

The clinical features of this condition are taken from a survey of 200 patients with osteochondritis dissecans of the knee.[3,4] The lesion was seen most commonly on the femoral condyle; the positions of the fragments are shown in Fig. 10.5. The patella is infrequently affected, and very rarely has osteochondritis dissecans of the upper tibial plateau been seen. Unilateral lesions were present in 74 percent and bilateral lesions in 26 percent of cases. Males were affected twice as frequently as females (males 68 percent, females 32 percent), and in 46 percent of patients the whole fragment or part of it had separated to form a loose body (Fig. 10.6).

Osteochondritis dissecans is a condition of young people with an average age of onset of symptoms at 18 years. The age range was from 6 to 53 years, but the large majority of patients seen were between 10 and 20 years of age (Fig. 10.7).

TRAUMA

A significant injury to the knee joint was sustained in 46 percent of cases, and in each case the patient was taken to a doctor or to a hospital for treatment. Anything less definite was not counted. A direct blow occurred in 35 percent and a severe rotational injury in 11 percent.

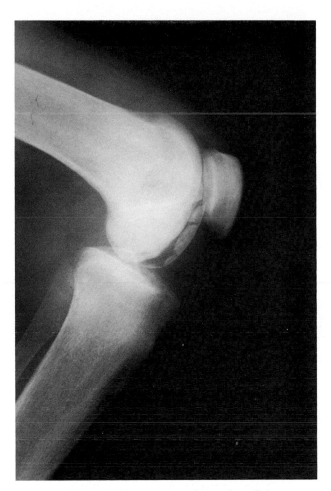

Fig. 10.3. Osteonecrosis femoral condyle.

was local ischemia, relative or absolute. In the first group the transition from an anomaly of ossification to a pathologic process was attributable to interruption of the blood supply; in the second group trauma was superimposed on an ischemic bone to produce the lesion; in the third adult type trauma produced the ischemia and when it continued produced the lesion; and in the fourth type there was a single traumatic incident producing a fracture that may or may not separate immediately. The end result was a loose body and a condylar crater not materially different from that encountered in true osteochondritis dissecans.

The following experimental and clinical features, however, seem to indicate that this last concept of Smillie is the most important.

ATHLETIC ABILITY

The athletic pursuits and abilities of each patient in this series were investigated. They were graded as follows:

Excellent: International or county
standard ..... 14 percent
Good: Participation in a league or
school first team ..... 47 percent
Moderate: Regular participation ..... 17 percent
Poor: Nil ..... 22 percent

More than 60 percent were therefore classified excellent or good at their sports and were nearly all concerned with field games and athletics. This is a remarkably high figure in any group of young people and was considered a significant etiologic factor.

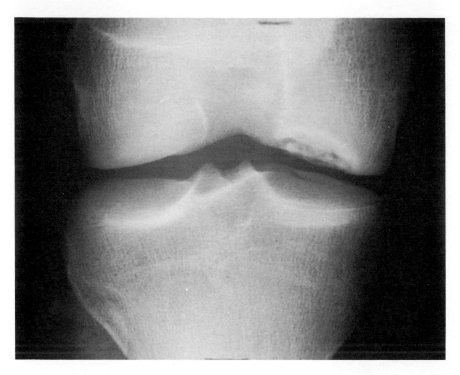

Fig. 10.4. Osteochondritis dissecans.

ASSOCIATED MECHANICAL ABNORMALITIES AND INTERNAL DERANGEMENTS

A significant genu valgum of more than 10 degrees was present in 5 percent and genu varum in 9 percent. Of those patients with a deformed knee it was interesting to note that one-half had bilateral osteochondritic lesions of a symmetric type. Easily demonstrable ligament laxity was found in 15 percent. In 4 percent of patients there was medial and anterior cruciate laxity with anterolateral rotary instability. In 7 percent the anterior cruciate alone appeared unstable, and in 4 percent there was anteromedial instability.

The patella dislocated in 7 percent, but in a further 9 percent patellar subluxation was possible. Most of the femoral condylar lesions in those patients with patellar instability were on the lateral side and those seen on the anterior aspect of this condyle were only present in the patients in whom there had been a full patellar dislocation with gross violence (Fig. 10.8).

Only three patients in this series had a meniscal tear, but it has recently been recognized from a survey of patients with discoid menisci that a lateral femoral condyle osteochondral defect is present in 20 percent.[5]

EPIPHYSEAL ABNORMALITIES AND JOINT SURFACE DEFORMITIES

Patients with epiphysealis dysplasia multiplex congenita and other similar conditions in which the joint surfaces are very irregular do present osteochondritis dissecans at the knee. The patient shown in Figure 10.9 has gross bone abnormality labeled a boomerang bone disease. At his knees the patient presented bilateral symmetric osteochondritis dissecans lesions; it was postulated that with such irregularity of joint surfaces, high-stress raising at abnormal anatomic points was a possible etiologic explanation.

ASSOCIATED OSTEOCHONDRITIC LESIONS IN OTHER JOINTS

After routine x-ray films of the knees, elbows, and ankles, additional lesions were discovered in asymptomatic joints in seven patients. In three, the other

Fig. 10.5. Sites of osteochondritis dissecans. (From Aichroth, P.: Osteochondritis dissecans of the knee. J. Bone Joint Surg. [Br.], 53:440–447, 1971, with permission.

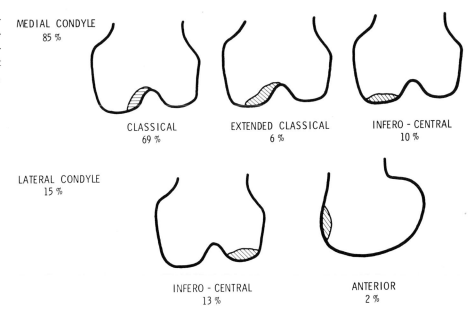

MEDIAL CONDYLE
85 %

CLASSICAL
69 %

EXTENDED CLASSICAL
6 %

INFERO - CENTRAL
10 %

LATERAL CONDYLE
15 %

INFERO - CENTRAL
13 %

ANTERIOR
2 %

knee presented symmetric medial femoral condylar lesions, in two patients the capitellum was involved, and in two patients the upper lateral aspect of the talus presented an osteochondritis dissecans.

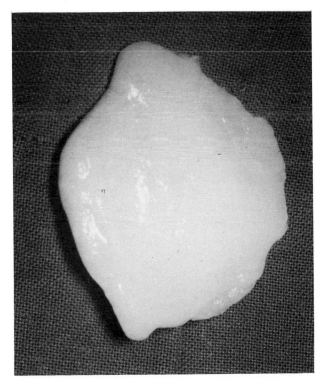

Fig. 10.6. Separated loose body.

OSTEOCHONDRAL FRACTURES AT THE KNEE

Osteochondral fractures of any part of the articular surface of the knee may occur in a variety of traumatic incidents. Direct blows, ligament ruptures, and patellar dislocations are frequently responsible. Matthewson and Dandy[21] have pointed out that indirect violence and especially pivoting on an extending knee produces shearing forces severe enough to avulse segments of articular cartilage and subchondral bone. The lateral femoral condyle is especially involved with an osteochondral fracture after this type of sports injury. Osteochondral fractures of the patella have been recognized since the beginning of this century; Milgram[22] was the first to describe the tangential osteochondral fracture so characteristic of a patellar dislocation.

Kennedy et al.[14] classified two groups: (1) exogenous fractures resulting from direct injury, and (2) endogenous fractures resulting from combined rotary and compression forces. These workers found clinical examples where fractures of most areas of both condyles were present with separation of a fragment. They further studied these endogenous fractures setting up experiments in the cadaver knee in which strong axial compression and rotary forces were applied. They found that certain osteochondral fractures of the weight-bearing surface could be produced by this method.

In clinical practice, osteochondral fractures of the

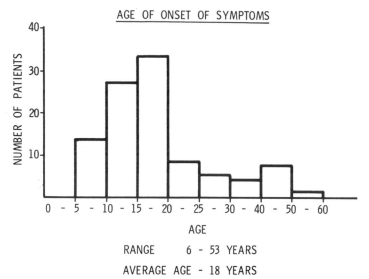

Fig. 10.7. Osteochondritis dissecans. Age of onset of symptoms. (From Aichroth, P.: Osteochondritis dissecans of the knee. J. Bone Joint Surg. [Br.], 53:440–447, 1971, with permission.)

medial and lateral condylar weight-bearing surfaces may be sustained by rotary forces on the flexed knee as in football and skiing injuries. A direct shearing force on the anterior surface of the medial condyle may occur in a fall on the flexed knee, and a direct shearing force on the lateral condyle may be sustained by a kick on the outside of the knee.

It has been pointed out by Landells[17] and Rosenberg[28] that adult articular cartilage tears at the junction between the calcified and uncalcified zones. The immature adolescent cartilage does not have this calcified zone, hence shearing forces are transmitted to the subchondral bone; it is here that osteochondral fractures occur. Clinically, the osteochondral fracture is nearly always confined to the adolescent. O'Donoghue[24] believes there is no real difference between an osteochondral fracture and osteochondritis dissecans. This idea is further explored in this chapter.

ETIOLOGY OF OSTEOCHONDRITIS DISSECANS AT THE KNEE

The clinical survey showed that joint trauma was the principal etiologic factor. Sixty percent showed remarkable prowess at athletics. Many had associated internal derangements, knee deformities, or patellar instability. In this survey 10 percent of the lesions

were considered acute osteochondral fractures, but it is probable that more patients were affected by this injury; the lesion was later called an osteochondritis dissecans.[4]

Kennedy et al.[14] demonstrated ways in which osteochondral fractures were sustained clinically. They also showed experimentally that osteochondral fractures of most parts of the weight bearing surfaces of the femoral condyles could be produced in the cadaver joint using a variably loaded stress machine, applying strong axial compression and rotary forces. It was therefore believed necessary to investigate the natural history of experimental osteochondral fractures of various types in an attempt to relate these osteochondral fractures to the clinical disease.

EXPERIMENTAL OSTEOCHONDRAL FRACTURES IN ANIMALS

Sixty adult New Zealand white rabbits were used. A knee arthrotomy was undertaken under general anaesthetic and various osteochondral cuts were made into the medial femoral condyle (Fig. 10.10).

In 31 animals fragments were fully separated from the joint surface. In group I the fragments were cut in such a way that they remained unstable and would shift on joint movement. In group II the fragments were cut in such a way that when they were replaced

Fig. 10.8. Dissecans of the anterior aspect of the lateral femoral condyle after patellar dislocation.

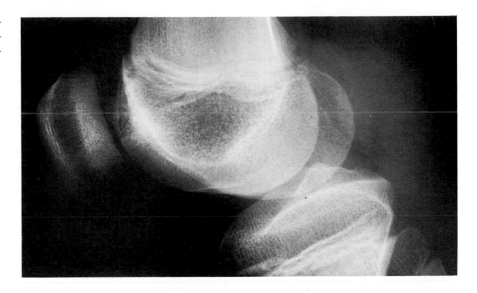

in their crater they remained in situ, well embedded and fairly stable. In group III the fragments were returned to their crater and internally fixed with fine stainless steel pins. In 29 animals fractures were made through the femoral condyle. In group IV a substantial intercondylar bridge of bone was left. In group V a minimal intercondylar bridge of bone remained, leaving a bridge that was unstable and that usually broke when the animals were exercised.

The union and nonunion rates in each group were noted. In group I, in which the fragment was shifting, most fragments remained un-united. In group II, in which there was a more stable fragment in situ, eight of the 13 animals' fragments united. Those in which internal fixation pins stabilized the fragments, all united rapidly. In group IV the osteochondral cut was made in such a way that it was totally stabilized, and all fractures united rapidly. In group V the medial femoral condylar cut was made leaving only a minimal bridge of intercondylar bone. This bridge proved unstable and eight of the 17 united with nine of the 17 remaining un-united.

To summarize these results, osteochondral fractures, which were cut in such a way that shift occurred, progressed to a nonunion state. Those adequately fixed united. Nonunion of an osteochondral fragment was characterized by a necrotic osseous portion with viable cartilage. The junctional zone between the crater and the fragment contained much fibrous tissue and fibrocartilaginous material. The ap-

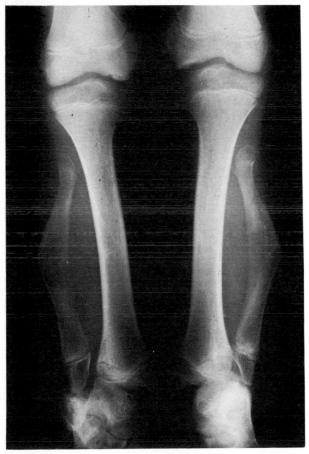

Fig. 10.9. Boomerang bone disease and osteochondritis dissecans.

60 ANIMALS

	31 FRAGMENTS			29 FRACTURES	
Group 1	Group 2	Group 3	Group 4	Group 5
SHIFTING	STABLE	PINNED	BRIDGED	UNSTABLE BRIDGE
ANIMALS 8	13	10	12	17
UNITED 1	8	10	12	8
NOT UNITED 7	5	0	0	9

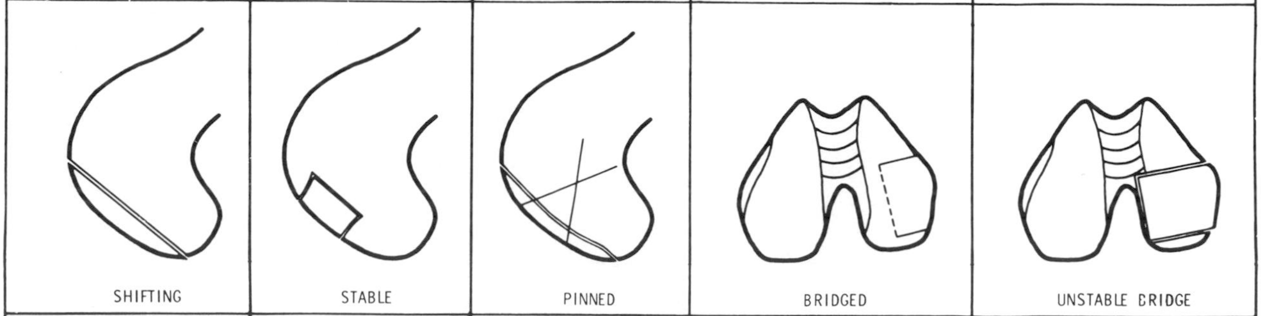

Fig. 10.10. The experimental plan. Osteochondral fractures in animals. (From Aichroth, P.: Osteochondral fractures and their relationship to osteochondritis dissecans of the knee. J. Bone Joint Surg. [Br.], 53:448–454, with permission.)

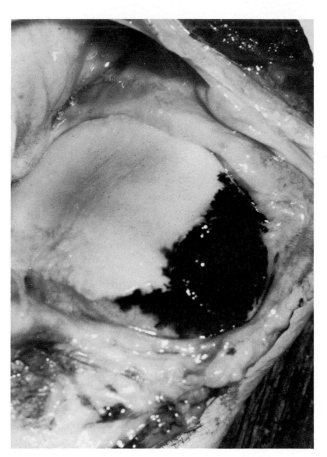

Fig. 10.11. Dye on medial patellar facet.

pearance of the un-united osteochondral fragment was similar to that in osteochondritis dissecans in the human.

CADAVER STUDIES

Osteochondritis dissecans at the knee joint occurs most commonly (69 percent) at the classic site on the intercondylar aspect of the medial femoral condyle. At first glance, this site appears protected and placed away from areas that could be affected by osteochondral fractures, but this is not so. Cadaver dissection demonstrated that this classical site could be injured. Bonney's blue dye was placed on the medial articular facet of the patella (Fig. 10.11), and with normal patellar articulation the knee joint was flexed. Increasing flexion of the joint demonstrated the areas of contact between the patella and the medial femoral condyle (Fig. 10.12). In full flexion the classic site was colored.

With an anterior blow on the flexed knee, osteochondral fractures could be anticipated by the impact of the patella on the medial condyle. Kennedy et al.[14] have shown that osteochondral fractures of the rest of the weight-bearing surfaces of the condyles do occur both clinically and in an experiment using a cadaver joint. Osteochondral fractures may therefore be sustained in any area of the joint affected by osteochondritis dissecans. Direct blows to the flexed knee may

Fig. 10.12. Dyed area of the medial femoral condyle.

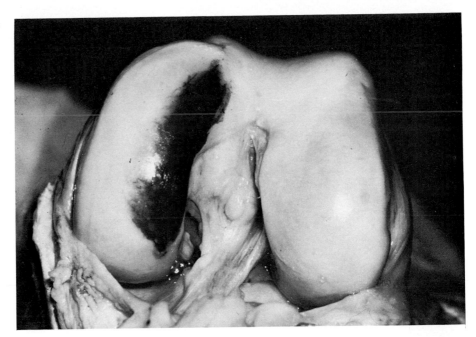

injure the femoral condyles and, in full flexion, forces may be transmitted via the patella to the classic site.

Twisting injuries of the knee may avulse areas of the weight-bearing surface, and here particularly the lateral femoral condyle is involved.

OSTEONECROSIS

Loose bodies in joints may develop from lesions resembling osteochondritis dissecans in multiple systemic disease processes. In the hemoglobinopathies, bone infarcts are common and loose bodies may be shed from the joint surfaces with their histologic appearance closely resembling the lesion in osteochondritis dissecans. In the painful crises of a hemoglobinopathy, the abnormal red cells clump together and peripheral emboli of this intravascular mass infarct many tissues, including bone. In caisson's disease, painful episodes called the bends develop and occur in divers or workers in pressurized tunnels who have been inadequately depressurized when returning to the surface. Intravascular nitrogen bubbles develop; these embolize peripherally, and again many tissues including bone become infarcted. The arthropathy is characterized by loose bodies detaching from a joint surface. There are many other systemic abnormalities in which identical changes occur. Gaucher's disease,

hyperuricemias, alcoholism, and posttransplantation arthropathy are all examples. It is probable that a similar embolic pathogenic mechanism occurs in these diseases, and there is increasing evidence that fat emboli are responsible for the alcoholic and posttransplantation arthropathies (Fig. 10.13).

The appearance of a knee joint at postmortem in a patient who suffered from a postrenal transplant arthropathy is shown in Figure 10.14. Multiple loose bodies were present as well as attached osteochondral fragments which remained in their crater. Slabs of the femoral condyle were prepared; the slab radiographs indicated large zones of infarcted necrotic bone and loose osteoarticular fragments were found to be peripheral portions of this avascular area. The fragments therefore separate from necrotic bone, and the actual line of demarcation is through an avascular area. In osteochondritis dissecans the loose bodies separate from underlying normal vascularized bone. The crater in osteochondritis dissecans of the femoral condyle is covered with a layer of fibrous tissue and fibrocartilage. If this fibrous layer is removed at operation, normal bleeding bone is revealed (Fig. 10.15).

Avascular necrosis of the femoral head with segmental separation has been well recognized for many years. Corticosteroid-induced necrosis and postrenal transplantation necrosis have been studied in detail.[9,12] It has been found that the risk of avascular

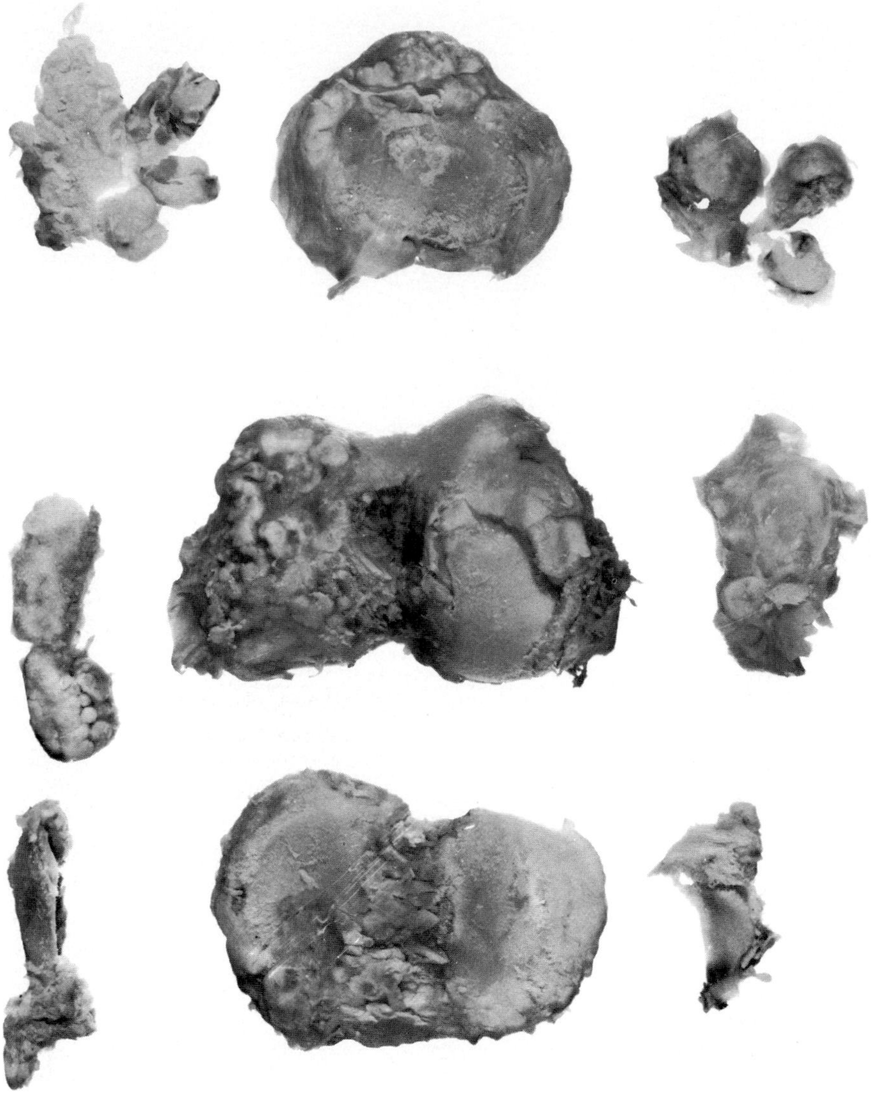

Fig. 10.13. Knee joint surfaces in postrenal transplant arthropathy.

necrosis is correlated with the total steroid dose, but the precise amount of cortisone required to cause the lesion is unknown. Steroid administration produces a fatty liver,[23] and it is postulated that fat embolism to the subchondral region of bone is responsible for the avascular collapse.

SPONTANEOUS OSTEONECROSIS AT THE KNEE

Subchondral idiopathic avascular necrosis in the femoral condyle was initially described by Ahlbäch et al.[1] They initially described radiolucent lesions in the medial femoral condyles in whom core biopsies were performed revealing necrotic bone and bone marrow. The classic syndrome is one of sudden onset of knee pain in the elderly patient.[20] They initially described 12 patients in whom there was a clinical picture identical to that of osteonecrosis, in which the radiographs were not characteristic but there were positive bone scans. Eventually they became asymptomatic and their bone scans returned to normal within a few months.

A careful pathologic study of 28 patients was undertaken by Ahuja and Bullough.[2] Tissues were removed from 29 knees during total knee replacements, and there were some other biopsy specimens. Their cases were grouped into three types:

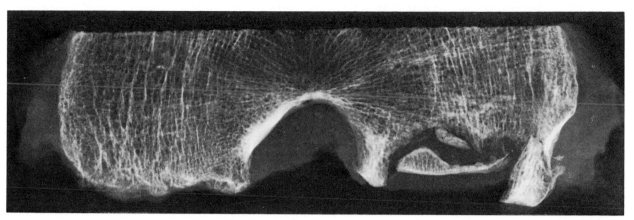

Fig. 10.14. Slab radiograph of osteonecrosis femoral condyle.

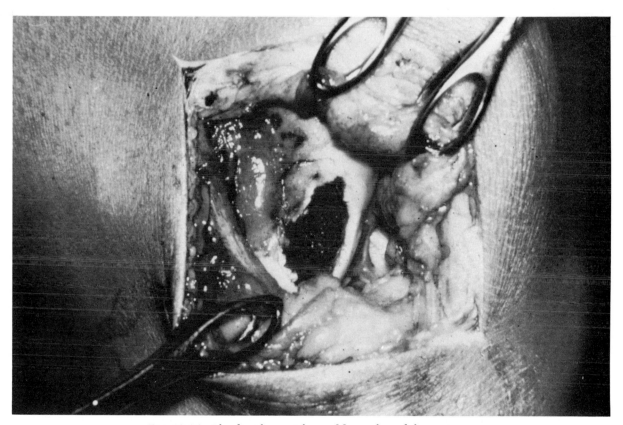

Fig. 10.15. Bleeding bone at base of femoral condylar crater.

Group I: Idiopathic primary osteonecrosis

Group II: Osteoarthrosis with associated osteone-crosis

Group III: Rheumatoid disease and osteonecrosis

These workers pointed out that in patients with osteonecrosis, the lesion may be demonstrated by iso-topic studies before x-ray changes become evident.

Marked deformities of the joint developed with fracture of necrotic bone and fragmentation and col-lapse of the articular cartilage. Secondary osteoar-thritis also occurred. Those patients with rheumatoid arthritis had a long history of steroid therapy. They pointed out, however, that from their observation of many patients with untreated rheumatoid arthritis, osteonecrosis was extremely uncommon. Spontaneous osteonecrosis in 90 knees was carefully assessed by Rozing et al.[29] In their cases a radiologic lesion developed within 6 months, characterized by a high uptake on scintimetric studies. They found that the prognosis depended on the size of the radiologic lesion and in those with an area affected of > 2.3 cm², osteoarthritis was likely to develop. Rozing et al. advocated conservative treatment with weight restriction and anti-inflammatory drugs together with some physiotherapy exercises once the diagnosis had been established. In two-thirds of their patients, the symptoms resolved within 6 months, but one-third continued to have persistent, disabling symptoms. Simple drilling of the lesion at arthrotomy proved ineffective, and osteotomy was preferred for the younger patient. Total knee replacements were more suitable for the older and less active.

In summary, idiopathic osteonecrosis differs in several ways from true osteochondritis dissecans. The latter is present in the younger person who is athletic and a history of trauma precedes the lesion in 50 percent. The area affected in osteochondritis dissecans is at the classic site on the intercondylar region of the medial femoral condyle in contrast to the weight-bearing surface of the medial femoral condyle in patients with idiopathic osteonecrosis. Loose bodies occur much more frequently in osteochondritis than in osteonecrosis; in the latter, they separate from a bed of avascular bone. In osteochondritis dissecans the crater consists of fibrous tissue and of fibrocartilaginous material that shows bleeding bone upon removal.

OSTEOCHONDRITIS DISSECANS IN THE YOUNG CHILD

Most patients with osteochondritis dissecans are between 10 and 20 years of age; the vigorous sports-orientated teenager is the most affected. Osteochondritis dissecans does occur in the young child and, although most fragments heal, loose bodies may be shed from the joint surface.

The arthroscope has permitted clear differentiation of osteochondritis dissecans from ossification defects seen so frequently and considered by Smillie[30] to be an etiologic factor. The young child's femoral condyle normally presents radiographic epiphyseal irregular-

ity beneath the articular cartilage. The appearance is that of an irregular mosaic (Fig. 10.16) and naturally develops into the smooth epiphyseal bone surface of the teenager. In the young child the appearance of osteochondritis dissecans is that of a fragment in a definite crater in two projections. The arthroscopic appearance is that shown in Figure 10.17, with a definite break in the articular cartilage.

The child's osteochondritis dissecans confirmed arthroscopically readily heals and particularly so on the more posterior surfaces of the condyles (Fig. 10.18). The classic site is not so common in the young child but the inferocentral area of the weight-bearing surface is seen more frequently. If there is doubt as to whether a symptomatic knee is affected by osteochondritis dissecans, or that the radiologic lesion is an ossification defect, arthroscopy is an important means of providing a definite answer and a firm prognosis. It is so easy for the clinician when first faced with a child with a symptomatic knee to decide that the whole painful syndrome is caused by a defect in the articular surface. Nevertheless, the defect may in fact be an ossification defect. The true dissecans lesion does persist as a fragment in a crater and, although it is sometimes possible for this to be confirmed on an arthrogram,[32] it is usually necessary to arthroscope the joint if the worrying symptoms persist.

NATURAL HISTORY OF OSTEOCHONDRITIS DISSECANS

The osteochondritis dissecans lesion in a young child will frequently heal, especially if the femoral condylar fragment is posterior. During this phase, pain may be experienced with intermittent swelling of the joint. Pain tends to be a little worse if the lesion is in the classic site; this may be caused by some associated synovial irritation over the cruciate ligament area. The child may also externally rotate the tibia on the femur and the gait may be affected by this external rotary sign described by Wilson.[33]

The knee joint may now start to feel unstable; the patient describes definite episodes of giving way. This is caused by a movement of the fragment in its crater and, for the first time the patient's activities are affected; causing him to seek medical help at this stage. A click or pop may now be experienced, caused by

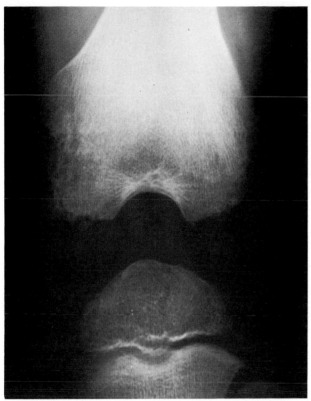

Fig. 10.16. Irregular epiphyseal appearance of child's femoral condyle.

movement of the fragment and sometimes early hinging of the fragment in its crater. A major movement of the fragment that still retains attachment by a hinge may lock the joint, which either remains locked or unlocks as the main fragment returns to the crater. The joint is now painful, irritable, and swollen. On arthroscopy, the hinged fragment is seen with surrounding erythema of the synovium in the intercondylar region. When the fragment fully separates, a loose body is formed displaying all the specific symptoms of this internal derangement.

Osteochondritis dissecans of the lateral femoral condyle occurs in 15 percent of cases. The lesions on the anterior aspect of the condyle are most closely associated with patients who have a dislocating patella. Osteochondritis dissecans in the young child that affects the weight-bearing surface of the lateral femoral condyle may be associated with a discoid meniscus.

OSTEOCHONDRITIS DISSECANS PATELLAE

This uncommon condition (Fig. 10.19) has been well reviewed by Edwards and Bentley.[10] Most patients affected have associated patellar subluxation and, al-

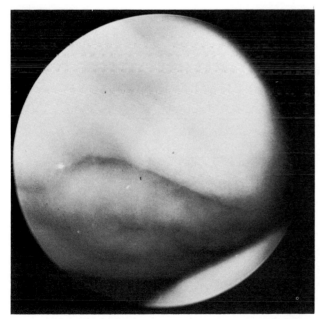

Fig. 10.17. Articular cartilage fracture. Arthroscopic appearance.

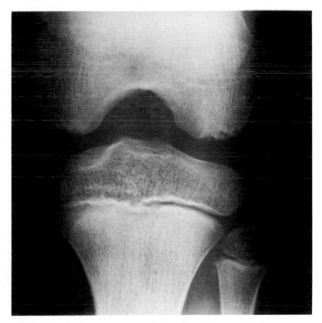

Fig. 10.18. Posterior condylar dissecans. Child's knee.

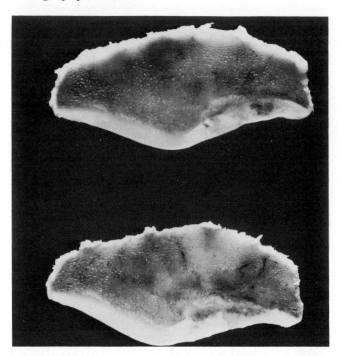

Fig. 10.19. Osteochondritis dissecans patellae. Cut section and slab radiograph.

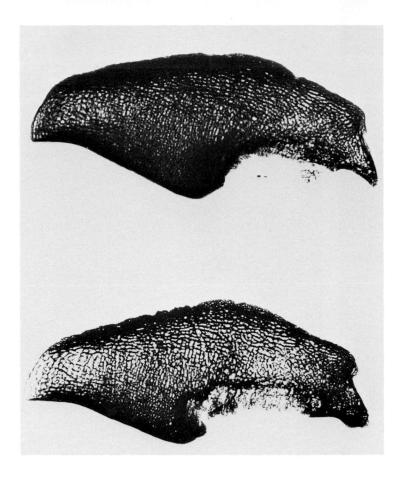

though a loose body may develop, the fragment usually remains in situ, producing retropatellar crepitus and pain. The indication for operation closely resembles that seen in osteochondritis dissecans of the femoral condyles, for a loose fragment or a fragment partly detached from the articular surface of the patella is most easily treated by excision of the affected area with drilling of the underlying bone.

LOOSE BODY AT THE KNEE

A loose body at the knee may be produced by an acute osteochondral fracture or osteochondritis dissecans. In the older patient, osteonecrosis or osteoarthritis produces the loose body and rarely synovial osteochondromatosis may be present. In this disease metaplasia of the synovial membrane produces a multitude of cartilaginous plaques that may then loosen as showers of cartilaginous or osteocartilaginous loose fragments within the knee joint cavity and sometimes within a posterior synovial pouch. Cartilaginous loose bodies may break from the hyaline articular surface in a chondral fracture and may sometimes become totally detached from the menisci as a fibrocartilaginous loose body, both of the fragments being radiolucent.

The loose body acts like a joint mouse, moving and sometimes darting around the knee joint cavity, appearing at one site and then on flexion or palpation moving to another. The joint mouse may initially be a source of amusement to the patient, but this soon disappears as the loose body produces severe symptoms of locking, pain, and swelling. Repeated locking and unlocking will produce such a functional disability that the patient demands removal of the joint mouse. More frequently, the patient presents with the above symptoms of an internal derangement and the loose body is then found by the examiner's fingers or by radiography. Loose bodies from chondral fractures are often first detected on arthroscopic examination, for without an osseous center they are undetected on x-ray examination and rarely picked up on arthrography. Full views of the knee are required in an attempt to confirm a loose body and anteroposterior, lateral, tunnel, and skyline views are mandatory. Oblique views may also be helpful.

The patient with an osteoarthritic knee frequently possesses loose totally asymptomatic bodies seen radiographically. The fragments usually loosen from the peripheral osteophytes and may become attached to the synovium or to the synovium in the suprapatellar pouch. However, they may break loose and produce all the symptoms and signs of a joint mouse.

REMOVAL OF LOOSE BODIES

The loose fragment must be removed if the internal derangement symptoms of pain, locking, and swelling are present. If such locking continues repeatedly, secondary degenerative changes in the knee joint are certain.

REMOVAL OF LOOSE BODY BY OPEN OPERATION

The initial position of the loose body must be determined by palpation and by x-ray examination in the position in which the knee will be opened. If the loose body is in the suprapatellar pouch, it is best removed with the knee extended, but if the fragment is in the posteromedial or posterolateral compartment, the knee should be flexed over the edge of the table to permit appropriate access. It is important to follow these preoperative precautions carefully to avoid opening the joint in the wrong position, for the fragment frequently and easily moves to another area.

LOOSE BODY REMOVAL FROM THE SUPRAPATELLAR POUCH AND ANTERIOR CAVITY

A vertical parapatellar incision is recommended. This incision may be extended to permit inspection of the condylar crater from which the loose body came. After incision of the synovium, the loose fragment frequently pops through the opening with a rush of synovial fluid. More commonly, it is obscured by a synovial fold. As soon as it is seen, a large curette should be positioned behind it and the fragment may then be grasped by a rongeur or a toothed forceps. A Kocher forceps may also be helpful in grasping this very slippery fragment. If the loose body is seen to move to another part of the joint, it may be retrieved by milking it into view with the fingers; flexing and extending the joint may also be helpful. If this fails, syringing the cavity with normal saline may also be helpful. A second glove may be donned and joint cavity exploration with a finger may also be necessary.

REMOVAL OF THE LOOSE BODY FROM THE POSTERIOR COMPARTMENTS

The posterior cruciate ligament and its synovial reflection separate the posterior aspect of the knee into two compartments. It is therefore important to identify the particular compartment containing the loose body. The posteromedial approach is undertaken with the knee flexed; a vertical incision is made centered on the joint line posteriorly behind the medial collateral ligament. Through the capsular and synovial incision, the posterior horn of the medial meniscus and the posterior compartment are exposed. The posterolateral approach is also undertaken with the knee flexed; a curved incision is made anterior to the fibular head and the biceps femoris tendon. The popliteus tendon is positioned between the biceps and the lateral collateral ligament. The synovium is incised in the same vertical line, and the posterior compartment is opened and explored.

ARTHROSCOPIC REMOVAL OF LOOSE BODIES

Removal of a loose body by an arthroscopic technique can be either the easiest procedure or the most difficult. It should be undertaken only by someone fully conversant with diagnostic arthroscopy, for all arthroscopic approaches may be necessary to identify, localize, and withdraw the loose fragment.

IDENTIFICATION

It is still a wise precaution to x-ray the knee before beginning an arthroscopic search. The loose fragment, however, may alter its position as soon as the knee is distended with saline, and one can never be certain that it will remain in the same position once irrigation commences. Nevertheless, it will give some idea of where the loose body is located. If it is present in the posteromedial or posterolateral compartment, all but experienced arthroscopists should probably consider removal of the loose body by open arthrotomy into these posterior areas.

The usual anterolateral arthroscopic approach is preferred, and a systematic search of the whole synovial cavity must be undertaken. The suprapatellar pouch is carefully inspected, and the irrigation needle, which ideally is already in the suprapatellar pouch, can be used to help in this exploration by pushing back synovial folds and identifying any loose fragment that may be hiding behind and beneath the suprapatellar plica. The retropatellar surface must now be carefully inspected for, although a loose fragment is rarely seen at this site, an osteochondral defect may be present that corresponds in size and shape to the loose body. It is now very important to inspect the medial and lateral synovial gutters carefully, for the loose fragments frequently fall from the suprapatellar pouch into these gutters. If a fragment is in the gutter and the knee is flexed, it is likely to pass inferiorly and posteriorly into one of the two posterior compartments. It is therefore important to resist flexion of the knee at this point before the gutters are fully inspected. It is a good idea to milk the gutters by digital pressure from behind forward; sometimes the loose fragment will pop into view. When the surgeon is convinced that there is no loose fragment in the two gutters, the knee may be flexed and the medial and lateral anterior compartments inspected. The loose body is sometimes nicely placed in the anterior compartments or in the intercondylar region. The latter site is sometimes difficult to see because the fat pad obscures the view; it is wise to insert a hook through an anteromedial portal to search the intercondylar region and also to look under remnants of the ligamentum mucosum and beneath the menisci, because rarely a loose fragment can hide in such a recess. If the fragment has still not been found, it is important to attempt to enter the posteromedial and posterolateral compartments through the intercondylar notch; using a 70-degree angle telescope, the loose fragment may be found tucked away in these recesses above the posterior horns of the menisci.

LOCALIZATION

Once the loose body has been identified, it is important to fix the position of the fragment to permit grasping and removal of the body. It may be possible to fix it with a needle, but this may be difficult to achieve because of the very hard nature of some loose bodies. Finger pressure may hold its position, particularly in the gutters. I have found it possible to hold the fragment in these recesses by inserting a barrier of two or three needles behind the lesion. A hook may be used in the anterior compartment to maneuver the fragment into a position from which it is easier to remove.

HOLDING THE FRAGMENT

Once the fragment is localized and to some extent fixed, a pituitary rongeur, Kocher forceps, or some other similar meniscus holder must be inserted by a portal that easily trangresses the synovial cavity, permitting one to grab the fragment under arthroscopic vision. Blind grabbing at the fragment with an appropriate forceps is a fool's game; only rarely will this succeed, and usually the fragment skids off to another part of the joint making another portal of entry necessary. Taking time to plan the portal of entry is considered to be a very important and worthwhile exercise and some arthroscopists use a long needle to make sure that their planned track is realistic.

REMOVAL

Once the fragment is grasped firmly with the pituitary rongeur or some other forceps, it must be brought through the synovium and capsule. If the fragment is soft, the pituitary rongeur may take a bite out of the fragment and leave the main body of it in the joint. Caution is therefore necessary in using this instrument. A large fragment will not be easily withdrawn through the initial capsular incision; extension of the capsular incision is therefore made with a No. 15 blade, and the fragment is gradually worked through this opening rather like bringing a baby's head through an episiotomy incision. The fragment may come off the forceps at this point, in which case it may fall back into the joint cavity or remain stuck in the synovium. Sometimes it is possible to grab the fragment again and continue the exercise. More frequently, the fragment floats free again and should be grasped in the usual way.

The most difficult removal is from the posteromedial and posterolateral recesses. It is sometimes possible to identify the fragment through the intercondylar region and grasp it with a fine pituitary rongeur, but more frequently it is tucked away behind the femoral condyle, making a formal posteromedial or posterolateral arthroscopic approach necessary. Once the fragment is identified in this site, it is sometimes possible to insert a forceps above the arthroscope and to achieve adequate triangulation of the two instruments to grasp the loose body. However, there may not be enough room for this maneuver, in which case a fine forceps or rongeur may be inserted through the arthroscope cannula, so that the fragment can be grabbed in a blind fashion. This is a doubtful technique, however, and a formal posterolateral or posteromedial arthrotomy may be required.

REPLACEMENT AND FIXATION OF A LOOSE FRAGMENT

An acute osteochondral fracture with a substantial portion of bone that fits accurately into the crater from which it was detached may be replaced and internally fixed with success. It must be emphasized that it is the acute osteochondral fracture that may be treated in this way. There is no place for reattachment of a chronic osteochondritis dissecans loose body, for the osseous fragment is always covered by fibrous tissue or by hyperplastic hyaline cartilage. When this tissue is removed, bone apposition is usually totally inadequate, and the fragment poorly fits into its crater. If such a fragment is internally fixed, the chances of success are very slim. The method of internal fixation recommended is by means of wires that transfix the fragment into the crater and then emerge medially or laterally through the sides of the femoral condyle. It is sometimes possible to undertake this procedure arthroscopically, but as the knee joint must be immobilized for approximately 6 weeks to allow the fragment to unite, there is no particular advantage to an arthroscopic technique. Arthroscopic advantages are only those of immediate mobilization of the joint postoperation. The wires may be removed from the medial or lateral femoral condylar sites at a later stage with great ease if the wire ends are left in a subcutaneous position.

TREATMENT OF THE UNSTABLE HINGED OSTEOCHONDRITIS DISSECANS FRAGMENT

Avulsion of an osteochondral fragment from its crater may be incomplete, and the lesion remains hinged, frequently producing a feeling of instability or of intermittent locking of the joint. Arthroscopic examination is recommended, for again it is only rarely possible to fix such a fragment internally. If the osteochondral fracture has only recently been produced, the fragment may fit accurately; it is possible to internally fix it using wires as described above. This osteochondritis dissecans lesion, however, may have been unstable in its crater for a very long time, in which case there is much fibrous tissue and fibrocartilaginous material in the crater and on the surface of the fragment. It is recommended in this situation that the fragment be removed and that the crater be curetted down to bleeding bone. This is undertaken either by arthrotomy or readily by arthroscopy. Scissors or a knife inserted arthroscopically will satisfactorily divide the cartilaginous hinge; the loose body is then removed by the technique described above. Curved pituitary rongeurs or a curette inserted through an appropriate portal will readily remove the fibrocartilaginous material from the crater surface, leaving bleeding bone.

Satisfactory resurfacing of the crater can then occur with fibrocartilaginous material. When inspected at a later stage arthroscopically, it is frequently found to be of satisfactory quality for weight bearing.

Internal fixation of the fragment has been undertaken with a multitude of different methods over the years, and screws, ivory bone pegs, and Smillie's pins have all been advocated. The replacement and fixation with readily removed pins as described before has been readvocated recently by Lipscomb et al.[19a] Transplants of cortical bone pegs have been found successful to fix fragments in both the knee joint and the hip.[18,19]

TREATMENT OF THE UNSTABLE OSTEOCHONDRITIS DISSECANS FRAGMENT IN SITU

Arthroscopic examination is important in determining the stability of the fragment seen radiographically in situ. The stable fragment in the child particularly will heal in most cases. However, the unstable fragment in the child, and especially the adult, is unlikely to heal in the future and a decision must be made as to whether the fragment should be removed or internally fixed. If there is evidence that it is a very recent lesion, internal fixation with easily removable

pins may be indicated, but this is only rarely the case. A chronic osteochondritis dissecans with much fibrous tissue and fibrocartilaginous material in the pseudarthrosis will rarely heal even if internal fixation is stable and satisfactory. It is therefore recommended that the fragment is removed and the crater from which it came is carefully curetted to bleeding bone. This may be undertaken by means of the arthroscopic instruments or by open arthrotomy. The advantage of the arthroscopic method is the very rapid rehabilitation postoperatively. Once the unstable fragment has been fixed internally, it must be carefully reviewed radiographically at regular intervals. Ideally there should be a period of immobilization after the internal fixation, in order to give the pseudarthrosis a chance to unite. If the internal fixation is unsatisfactory, a further procedure will be necessary to remove the fragment and to remove the wire.

TREATMENT OF THE STABLE OSTEOCHONDRITIS DISSECANS FRAGMENT IN SITU

Arthroscopic examination of this fragment is recommended, for it is impossible to determine stability or instability of the lesion by radiographic methods. The stable fragment in situ may not be readily identified at inspection, as the lesion is sometimes totally subchondral without a breach in the hyaline articular cartilaginous surface. There may be a roughness and irregularity of the articular cartilage overlying the fragment, but particularly in the child the articular surface may appear totally intact with a definite proven radiographic osteochondritis dissecans beneath. It is always recommended that a hook is inserted through a separate portal so that the arthroscopic assessment may be undertaken both visually and also by feel. The articular cartilage surface may be soft or may indent. The stable fragment may also present with a breach in the articular cartilage; when a hook is placed into this cartilage defect, the bony fragment beneath is found to be fixed. A decision must now be made as to whether the pseudarthrosis should be drilled. This is best undertaken using a drill from above entering through the femoral condyle and approaching the articular surface from the condylar side. With the arthroscope in place, the drill should be seen to come up to, but not through, the hyaline surface.

Some surgeons advocate the insertion of a drill through the articular surface; multiple drill holes are then made through the pseudarthrosis, disturbing the articular cartilage as little as possible. Although this is a very attractive method of treating such a fragment stable in situ there is little evidence that it is effective.[3] It is probably better to leave the fragment alone and to review the situation regularly both clinically and radiographically. If the fragment heals or becomes totally asymptomatic, it should be left alone. If it loosens or becomes more symptomatic, it should be removed.

THE CONDYLAR DEFECT

Most knees affected by osteochondritis dissecans in which a loose body has been shed demonstrate an obvious defect on the condylar surface from which the fragment came. However, in some knees examined radiologically or by arthroscopy or arthrotomy, the site of separation cannot be detected and the weight-bearing surfaces, the classic site, and the retropatellar region all appear pristine. The quality of resurfacing of the osteochondritis dissecans defect has been so good in these cases that the examiner cannot determine the original site of origin. The defect fills with fibrous tissue and with fibrocartilaginous material that appears smooth and may be of good weight-bearing quality. The quality and quantity of repair in fibrocartilage depend on the depth of the crater and its size.[8] The patient in whom a cartilage fragment without bone is avulsed from the weight-bearing surface of the femoral condyle (usually lateral) develops only a minimal covering of the defect. The deep crater that was curetted down to bleeding bone developed a good surface at 3 months at arthroscopic inspection, and the fibrocartilaginous material had developed to a normal height. The surface quality appeared fairly smooth even at this very early stage of repair (Fig. 10.20).

Experiments in large animals confirm that articular cartilage has very limited capacity for repair if of partial thickness. Full-thickness defects are replaced by a major ingrowth of vascularized connective tissue, with the primitive stem cells from which it arises being the mesenchymal cells of the exposed bone.[8] The completeness of repair, however, seems to depend on the size of the osteochondral defect. Poor quality

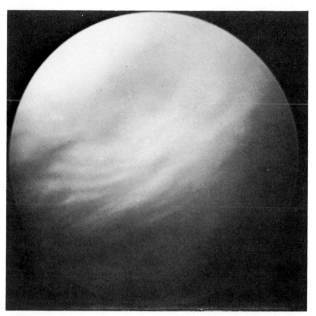

Fig. 10.20. Arthroscopic appearance of a crater filled with repair cartilage.

and quantity of repair material in the defect will have an increasingly deleterious effect on the articular cartilage on the opposite side of the joint.

The incomplete repair of large defects has stimulated much research into the possibility of replacement with auto- and allografts. Bentley[7] has shown that grafts of chondrocytes isolated from epiphyseal growth plates will allow rapid resurfacing of small defects with good quality hyaline cartilage. This research continues.

Much work in both small animals and sheep has shown that shell allografts of articular hyaline cartilage and subchondral bone will produce satisfactory resurfacing and union of the graft if fixation is perfect. The combined thickness must be satisfactory to permit early weight-bearing; the ideal shape of the graft was found to be a shell allograft with dowels that fit appropriate holes on the host condylar surface, as shown in Figure 10.21. Allografts of this type do show cartilage erosion and destruction in the long term, owing to immunologic attack, although the short-term results are excellent.[3] Gross and Langer[13] have extended this line of research to the human and are now regularly replacing the knee hemi-joint with cadaver allografts with good early results.

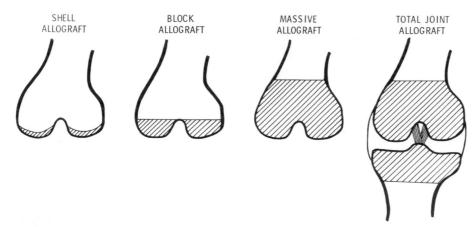

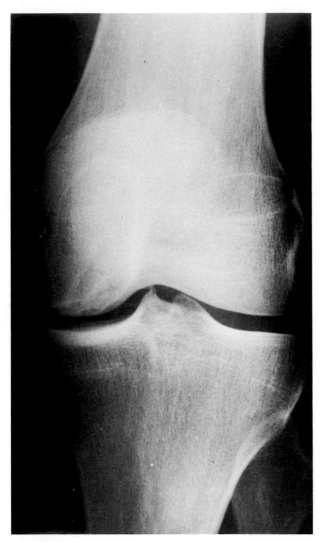

Fig. 10.22. Osteoarthritis after medial femoral condyle dissecans.

OSTEOARTHRITIS AFTER OSTEOCHONDRITIS DISSECANS

A radiograph of a patient in whom an osteochondritis dissecans of the medial femoral condyle had been removed 17 years previously is shown in Figure 10.22. A large, hinged fragment that had separated from the weight-bearing surface was removed at arthrotomy, and the base was curetted. The fragment measured 4 × 2 cm; after a short period of restricted weight-bearing, the patient returned to all sports with the knee remaining asymptomatic. After 15 years, however, pain and recurrent effusions occurred and a very slight deformity became evident. Degenerative changes undoubtedly occur in a substantial number of patients following large osteochondral defects of this type. The surprising feature of osteochondritis dissecans at the knee is the large number of patients who, when followed up, present no degenerative change whatsoever. It is assumed that the good-quality resurfacing that occurs in most cases produces little effect on the long-term health of the joint.

OSTEOCHONDRITIS DISSECANS AT THE KNEE: A TREATMENT PLAN

THE LOOSE BODY

OSTEOCHONDRITIS DISSECANS

1. Remove the loose body by arthroscopic or arthrotomy technique.
2. Inspect crater and curette to bleeding bone.

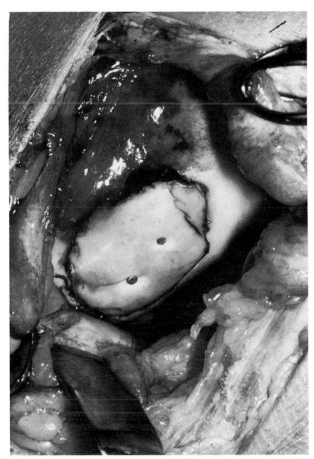

Fig. 10.23. Acute osteochondral fracture. Fragment pinned.

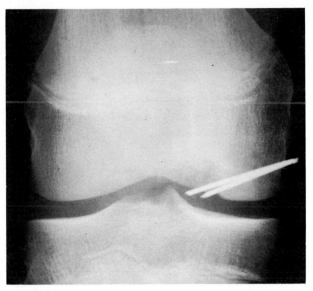

Fig. 10.24. Pinned acute osteochondral fracture.

THE HINGED FRAGMENT

1. If of recent origin and the fragment reduces accurately with good stability, consider internal fixation with pins or wires (arthroscopic or arthrotomy technique).
2. If well established, cut through the hinge, remove the fragment, and curette the crater (arthroscopic or arthrotomy technique).

THE FRAGMENT IN SITU

Arthroscopic examination of the joint is recommended in order to establish the stability of the fragment in situ. A hook probe will be useful to help assess this stability. All areas of the joint should be inspected.

IF UNSTABLE

1. Pin the fragment only if the lesion is considered a recent traumatic osteochondral fracture.
2. If the lesion is well established, remove the fragment and curette the base (arthroscopic or arthrotomy technique).

FRESH OSTEOCHONDRAL FRACTURE

1. Pin back if the fragment fits the crater exactly with good stability (Fig. 10.23, 10.24). Easily removable pins and wires are advocated (arthroscopic or arthrotomy technique).
2. If the fragment is broken or replaces poorly, remove it and curette the crater (arthroscopic or arthrotomy technique).

It is always necessary to inspect the knee joint fully (preferably by arthroscopic technique) to look for other loose bodies and for other lesions affecting the internal structures.

IF STABLE

In the Child

The child's lesion will almost certainly heal and should be left alone if it is found stable on arthroscopy or if the lesion is essentially subchondral without breach of the hyaline cartilage. The child should be followed up clinically, radiographically, and sometimes arthroscopically.

In the Late Teenager or Adult

Leave alone and await events if the fragment is tightly in situ with full stability and there is little disturbance of the articular surface. Alternatively, the fragment may be drilled from the condylar surface or through the articular cartilage by arthroscopic technique (one drill entry only through the cartilage surface).

It should be noted, however, that there is no definite evidence either of revascularization of the fragment or of healing of the pseudarthrosis after drilling.

OSTEOCHONDRITIS DISSECANS? OSSIFICATION DEFECT?

In the child with a symptomatic knee, there may be some confusion as to whether the lesion is truly an osteochondritis dissecans or an ossification defect of the femoral condyle. If there is still doubt after full and careful radiographic examination, arthroscopy is advisable. The lesion, if present, should be treated as above.

OSTEOCHONDRITIS DISSECANS ASSOCIATED WITH OTHER KNEE DERANGEMENTS

Osteochondritis dissecans of the anterior aspect of the lateral femoral condyle or of the patellar surface is usually associated with recurrent patellar dislocation. The dissecans lesion should be treated as above, and patellar stability should be achieved by surgical operation.

The child's lateral discoid meniscus may be associated with a dissecans lesion on the weight-bearing surface of the lateral femoral condyle. The discoid meniscus should be removed or trimmed and the osteochondritis treated as above.

REFERENCES

1. Ahlbäch, S., Bauer, G.C.H., and Bohne W.H.: Spontaneous osteonecrosis of the knee. Arthritis Rheum., *11:* 705, 1968.
2. Ahuja, S.C., and Bullough, P.G.: Osteonecrosis of the knee. J. Bone Joint Surg. [Am.], *60:* 191, 1978.
3. Aichroth, P.: Osteochondritis dissecans of the knee. J. Bone Joint Surg. [Br.], *53:* 440, 1971.
4. Aichroth, P.M.: Osteochondral fracture and osteochondritis dissecans in sportsmen's knee injuries. In proceedings J. Bone Joint Surg. [Br.], *59:* 108, 1977.
5. Aichroth, P.M., Baird, P.R.E., and Glasgow, M.: The discord lateral meniscus: a clinical review. J. Bone Joint Surg. [Br.], *64:* 245, 1982.
6. Axhausen, G.: Zur Histologie und Pathogenese der Gelenkmaus Bildung im Kniegelenk. Beitr. Klin. Chir., *133:* 89, 1925.
7. Bentley, G.: Transplantation of isolated chondrocytes into joint surfaces. In proceedings J. Bone Joint Surg. [Br.], *55:* 209, 1973.
8. Convery, F.R., Akeson, W.H., and Keown, G.H.: The repair of large osteochondral defects. Clin. Orthop., *82:* 253, 1972.
9. Creuss, R.L.: Cortisone-induced avascular necrosis of the femoral head. J. Bone Joint Surg. [Br.], *59:* 308, 1977.
10. Edwards, D.H., and Bentley, G.: Osteochondritis dissecans patellae. J. Bone Joint Surg. [Br.], *59:* 58, 1977.
11. Fairbank, H.A.T.: Osteochondritis dissecans. Br. J. Surg., *21:* 67, 1933.
12. Fisher, D.E., and Bickel, W.H.: Corticosteroid-induced avascular necrosis. J. Bone Joint Surg. [Am.], *53:* 859, 1971.
13. Gross, A., and Langer, F.: Allotransplantation of partial joints in the treatment of osteoarthritis of the knee. In proceedings J. Bone Joint Surg. [Am.], *56:* 1540, 1974.
14. Kennedy, J.C., Grainger, R.W., and McGraw, R.W.: Osteochondral fractures of the femoral condyles. J. Bone Joint Surg. [Br.], *48:* 436, 1966.
15. Koch, W.: Ueber embolische Knochennekrosen. Arch. Klin. Chir., *23:* 315, 1879.
16. König, F.: Ueber freie Körper in den Gelenken. Dtsch. Z. Chir., *27:* 90, 1888.
17. Landells, J.W.: The reactions of injured human articular cartilage. J. Bone Joint Surg. [Br.], *39:* 548, 1957.
18. Lindholm, T.S., and Osterman, K.: Internal fixation of the fragment of osteochondritis dissecans in the hip

using bone transplants. J. Bone Joint Surg. [Br.], *62:* 43, 1980.

19. Lindholm, S., Pylkkanen, P., and Osterman, K.: Fixation of osteochondral fragments in the knee joint. Clin. Orthop., *126:* 256, 1977.

19a. Lipscomb, P.R., Jr., Lipscomb, P.R., Sr., and Bryan, R.S.: Osteochondritis dissecans of the knee with loose fragments. J. Bone Joint Surg. [Am.], *60:* 235, 1978.

20. Lotke, P.A., Ecker, M.L., and Abass A.: Painful knees in older patients. J. Bone Joint Surg. [Am.], *59:* 617, 1977.

21. Matthewson, M.H., and Dandy, D.J.: Osteochondral fractures of the lateral femoral condyle. J. Bone Joint Surg. [Br.], *60:* 199, 1978.

22. Milgram, J.E.: Tangential osteochondral fracture of the patella. J. Bone Joint Surg., *25:* 271, 1943.

23. Moran, T.J.: Cortisone-induced alterations in lipid metabolism morphologic and serologic observations in rabbits. Arch. Path., *73:* 300, 1962.

24. O'Donoghue, D.H.: Chondral and osteochondral fractures. J. Trauma, *6:* 469, 1966.

25. Paget, J.: On the production of some of the loose bodies in joints. St. Bartholomews Hosp. Rep., *6:* 1, 1870.

26. Paré A.: The Case Reports and Autopsy Records of Ambroise Paré, Hamby, W.B., ed. Springfield, Ill., Charles C Thomas, 1960.

27. Reiger, H.: Zur Pathogenese von Gelenkmausen. M.M.W., *67:* 719, 1920.

28. Rosenberg, N.J.: Osteochondral fractures of the lateral femoral condyle. J. Bone Joint Surg. [Am.], *46:* 1013, 1964.

29. Rozing, P.M., Insall, J., and Bohne, W.H.: Spontaneous osteonecrosis of the knee. J. Bone Joint Surg. [Am.], *62:* 2, 1980.

30. Smillie, I.S.: Osteochondritis Dissecans. Edinburgh, London, E. & S. Livingstone Ltd., 1960.

31. Watson-Jones, Sir R.: Fractures and Joint Injuries, 4th Ed. Edinburgh, E. & S. Livingstone Ltd., 1952, Vol. 1 p. 97.

32. Wershba, M., Dalinka, M.K., Coren, G.S., et al.: Double contrast knee arthrography in the evaluation of osteochondritis dissecans. Clin. Orthop., *107:* 81, 1975.

33. Wilson, J.N.: A diagnostic sign in osteochondritis dissecans of the knee. J. Bone Joint Surg. [Am.], *49:* 477, 1967.

11 Disorders of the Patella

John N. Insall

SYMPTOMS

Regardless of cause—and there are many—the symptoms of patellar dysfunction tend to be the same. In themselves, these symptoms are not distinctive and include pain, giving way, and catching or locking, all of which are produced by other internal derangements. However, the pattern of complaints in patients with patellar disorders is sufficiently specific to focus attention on the patellofemoral joint. Unfortunately, the menisci are usually assumed to be the major cause of mechanical derangement in the knee, and the patella is often ignored.

Typically, patients with patellar complaints have an aching pain situated behind the patella, on the medial side of the joint, and sometimes posteriorly in the popliteal fossa. The pain is aggravated by activity, particularly stair climbing[113] and sometimes by sitting with the knee in a flexed position (the so-called movie sign). Pain may be bilateral, and the onset of symptoms is usually gradual and unrelated to any significant traumatic episode. At times, however, a bout of strenuous activity or a minor injury may seem to have initiated the complaint, although questioning will usually demonstrate that such events merely served to worsen a preexisting disorder. Patellar dislocation or recurrent subluxation is an obvious exception to this rule and, although the diagnosis is usually fairly

obvious, there may be cases in which confusion can arise. Nevertheless, bilaterality and insidious onset are most characteristic of patellar pain.

The location of the pain can also produce diagnostic error, as the most common site is the anteromedial side of the knee (Fig. 11.1)—the same location of pain from meniscal pathology, a fact that has contributed to the removal of many a normal meniscus (Fig. 11.2). Less frequently, posterolateral pain may be felt and, when there is local tenderness in this region as well, the diagnosis of bicipital or popliteus tendinitis may be entertained. Popliteal pain is a frequent symptom of patellofemoral arthritis and, when there is an associated popliteal cyst, it may be assumed that the cyst is causing the pain, whereas in fact both are secondary to patellar arthritis.

Giving way or buckling is the second major symptom of patellar dysfunction. Sometimes the giving way represents an episode of dislocation or subluxation that can be documented by examination (objective instability), but sometimes exactly similar episodes occur in patients in whom it is impossible even under anesthesia to displace the patella passively from the femoral sulcus (subjective instability). For this reason, the boundaries between subjective instability, subluxation, and dislocation should not be too finely made, for there will be other patients with passively dislocatable patellae who do not complain of clinical

191

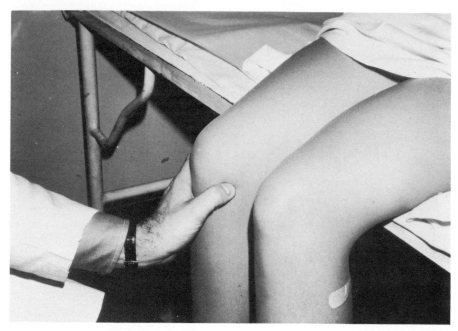

Fig. 11.1. Localized medial joint line tenderness usually at the midpoint is found in many patients with patellar pain.

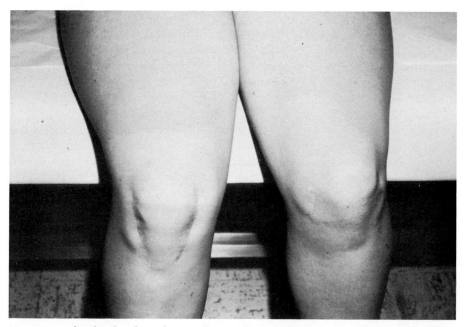

Fig. 11.2. This localized tenderness has, unfortunately, contributed to many unnecessary meniscectomies. Although all four menisci were removed, this young lady's symptoms remain unchanged. Fortunately, this sad occurrence should now be a thing of the past.

instability. Giving way of patellar origin may mimic the buckling caused by meniscal injury or ligamentous insufficiency, but most often it is a different sensation. Although the giving way may occur on pivoting or twisting movements such as occurs when "cutting" in sports, the patient is usually aware that it is the knee cap that has slipped. Otherwise, when the patient does not recognize the nature of the buckling, the event is described in such terms as the knee "collapsed" or "went forward." There is not the sensation of the joint "coming apart" or of "one bone sliding upon the other" that is so typical of ligament insufficiency. Episodes of patellar instability may or may not be followed by pain and swelling lasting for a few days to several weeks. Subluxation may occur with every motion of the knee with the patella subluxing laterally as the knee approaches full extension, and reducing again into the sulcus at about 30 degrees when the knee is flexed.

In habitual dislocation, which usually presents in late childhood or adolescence, the patella remains dislocated laterally throughout the range of motion (Fig. 11.3). The complaints then relate more to extensor mechanism weakness and inability to extend the knee fully. Green and Waugh[57] believe that habitual dislocation must be distinguished from congenital dislocation, which most often presents in infancy as a flexion contracture of the knee.

A grating sensation, particularly when the patellofemoral joint is loaded as in stair climbing or arising from a chair, is a fairly common complaint. Momentary "catching" may also be experienced, and interruption of smooth patellar gliding may precipitate buckling or giving way. Actual locking of the knee sometimes happens and, curiously, patellar locking is not always transient, but may give the impression of a true mechanical block. The mechanism for persistent locking is obscure, but most likely is related to

an alteration of the instant center of motion causing the surfaces to plow into one another rather than roll and glide smoothly. Secondary contracture of the posterior capsule is a feature of prolonged locking; a similar process probably accounts for the flexion contracture in some cases of patellofemoral arthrosis.

Many patients with patellofemoral disease complain of swelling. Sometimes this is a subjective sensation, for on examination an effusion is not found and circumferential measurement of the joint does not show an increase compared with the opposite side. Synovitis with distention by synovial fluid or blood occurs after an episode of patellar subluxation and sometimes with chondromalacia or arthritis. Cartilaginous or osteocartilaginous loose bodies may be generated from the articular surfaces and contribute to giving way and transient locking, although the patient is usually aware of a free body within the joint that also may be felt in the suprapatellar pouch.

The predominant signs of a patellar disorder are the following:
1. Crepitus
2. Tenderness
3. Malalignment
4. Subluxation

Examination should begin with the patient standing with the feet together. Genu varum or valgum can be readily observed as well as rotary malalignments such as the infacing or "squinting" of the patellae in patients with an increased quadriceps angle. The gait is observed and younger patients are asked to squat holding the halfway position briefly as pain in this position is usually patella in origin. Whenever possible, stair climbing should be observed, both going up and coming down as this activity also brings out patellar symptoms.

With the patient seated on the examining table, active extension is observed from the flexed position,

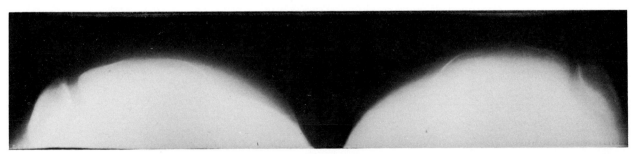

Fig. 11.3. In habitual dislocation, the patella remains permanently dislocated and cannot be reduced in any position.

from which patellar crepitus and painful catching as well as abnormal patellar tracking can be elicited.

Ficat and Hungerford[47] stress that it is particularly important to observe the entrance and exit of the patella into the sulcus at between 10 and 30 degrees of flexion. The more common abnormalities these workers have observed are the following:

1. An abrupt lateral movement at the termination of extension
2. A "bayonet" excursion characterized by an abrupt lateral translation just before full extension, and then full extension in a straight line
3. An atypical semicircular movement as if the patella were pivoting around the lateral trochlear facet
4. A motion in which there is a short medial displacement just before the final slight external movement associated with full extension

Hughston[71] has described a lateral position of the patella in the flexed knee for which he coined the term, "frog eye" patella. This seems to be associated with patella alta (Fig. 11.4), which can be suspected on clinical grounds if the patella is hypermobile and when the fat pad is unusually prominent. In fact, the fat pad may on inspection be mistaken for the patella because it occupies the femoral sulcus with the knee in extension while the patella is mostly situated in the supracondylar pouch.

Patellar tenderness can be elicited by the following maneuvers:

1. *Direct palpation of the patellar facet when the patella is displaced medially or laterally:* This method has a disadvantage in that synovium and capsule are of necessity intervening between the finger and articular surface. Misleading results are obtained when these tissues are inflamed.
2. *Compressing the patella against the femoral sulcus:* The knee must be sufficiently flexed to bring the patella from its resting and largely supracondylar position into the sulcus. The articular surfaces are then directly compressed by moving the patella from side to side. Direct compression combined with medial displacement is usually the most effective way of reproducing patellar pain (Fig. 11.5). Lateral displacement, on the other hand, evokes the well-known apprehension sign in which the patient's quadriceps contracts reflexly in an attempt to prevent subluxation; at the same moment, the patient may attempt to push away the examiner's hand.
3. *Pushing distally on the patella in the fully extended knee and asking the patient to contract the quadriceps:* Unfortunately in some knees, especially when there is a patella alta, this maneuver will entrap the synovium of the suprapatellar pouch

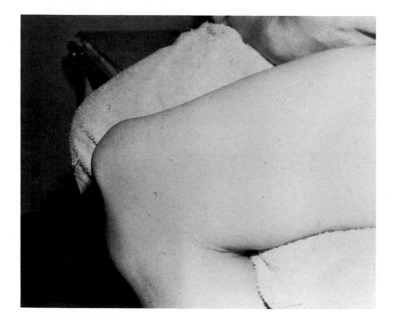

Fig. 11.4. Patella alta may be suspected clinically when, in extension, the fat pad is unusually prominent and in flexion the contour of the knee appears square.

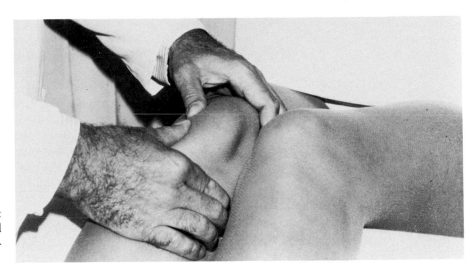

Fig. 11.5. Patellar pain is best elicited by flexing the knee and by compressing the patella medially in the femoral groove.

and produce exquisite pain even when the patellar surface itself is normal. Because of the frequency of false-positive results, this method is not recommended.

The quadriceps (Q) angle (Fig. 11.6) is measured by drawing an imaginary line connecting the center of the patella and the anterior superior iliac spine to produce a surface marking that approximates the line of pull of the quadriceps tendon. The direction of the ligamentum patellae is indicated by a second line drawn from the center of the patella to the center of the tibial tubercle. The intersection of these two imaginary lines forms the Q angle. In the normal knee, this measures 15 degrees; an angle exceeding 20 degrees is considered unequivocally abnormal. In fact, the surface marking of the Q angle is often an underestimation because in some conditions (particularly subluxing or dislocating patellae), the quadriceps tendon lies more laterally than the surface markings indicate.

RADIOLOGIC EVALUATION OF THE PATELLOFEMORAL JOINT

The anteroposterior view is of not much value, although arthrosis of the femorotibial joint and varus or valgus malalignment will be observed. These abnormalities may affect the patellofemoral articulation. In addition, as the outline of the patella is visible, anomalies such as patella magna or parva, bipartite patellae, and fractures can be seen.

Most information is obtained from the axial and lateral views. The lateral view is taken with the knee

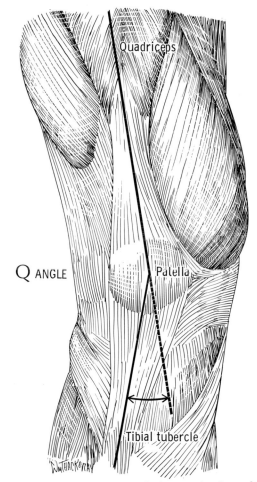

Fig. 11.6. The quadriceps angle (see text) is formed by the quadriceps tendon and patellar ligament.

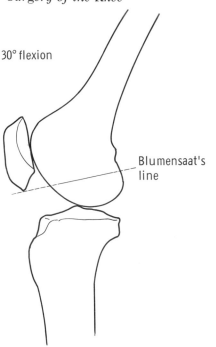

30° flexion

Blumensaat's line

Fig. 11.7. Blumensaat's line projects the intercondylar line of the femur to the lower pole of the patella.

in at least 30 degrees of flexion, avoiding excessive rotation, which obscures some of the bony landmarks such as the tibial tubercle and makes interpretation difficult. The patella is not visualized in the lateral view in rare cases of congenital absence of the patella and when the patella is completely displaced laterally as in habitual dislocation. In children under the age of 5, the ossific nucleus will not have appeared and thus the patella is invisible. Cartilage degeneration is often perceived in the lateral view, although not as well as in the axial views.

MEASUREMENT OF PATELLA ALTA AND INFERA

Patellar position is related to the length of the patellar ligament. Patella alta, in particular, is associated with patellar instability and dislocation and probably with sulcus development. There are several methods of identification:

1. Boon-Itt[15] derived a formula on the basis of 200

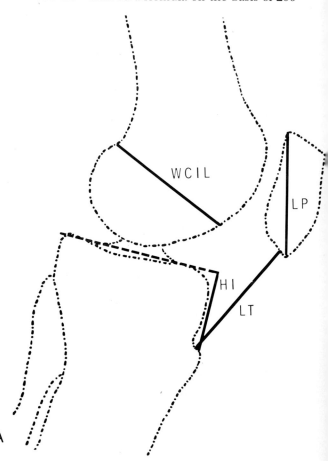

WCIL

LP

HI

LT

A

Fig. 11.8. (A) The Insall-Salvati measurements. (B) This patella is high riding, the notch on the tibia is clearly seen, and the measurement is not difficult to make. (C) In the immature knee, the tibial tubercle is not clearly visible and, although this patella appears high riding, it cannot be confirmed by measurement. (Part A from Insall, J., and Salvati, E.: Patella position in the normal knee joint. Radiology, *101:* 101, 1971, with permission.)

lateral radiographs of apparently normal adult knees which, although accurate, is too complicated for practical daily use.

2. Blumensaat[14] states that in a lateral radiograph with the knee flexed 30 degrees, the lower pole of the patella should lie on a line projected anteriorly from the intercondylar notch (Blumensaat's line) (Fig. 11.7). It is difficult to obtain routine radiographs with the knee flexed exactly the required degree, and this severely limits the usefulness of the method. Blumensaat's method is also inaccurate. In 44 radiographs of knees that were flexed exactly 30 degrees, in no case did the lower pole of the patella lie on Blumensaat's line; rather the patella was positioned above this line.

3. Insall and Salvati[78] sought a method that would fit the following requirements: (1) simple and practical as well as accurate, (2) applicable to the range of knee positions during routine radiography which in

the lateral view is usually 20 to 70 degrees of flexion, and (3) independent of the size of the joint and the degree of magnification of the radiograph. Because the ligamentum patellae is not elastic, its length determines the position of the patella, provided that the point of insertion into the tibia is constant.

Insall and Salvati describe an expression for normal patellar height in terms of the length of the patella tendon. Measurements were made on 114 knees in which the diagnosis of a torn meniscus was clearly established by a typical clinical history and examination, by a positive arthrogram, and by the finding of a meniscal tear at arthrotomy. Any case in which the slightest doubt existed was excluded, and the assumption was made that the joints examined were structurally normal before a traumatic episode produced a torn meniscus. All patients were adults and none showed radiologic evidence of osteoarthritis. The following measurements were made (Fig. 11.8A–C):

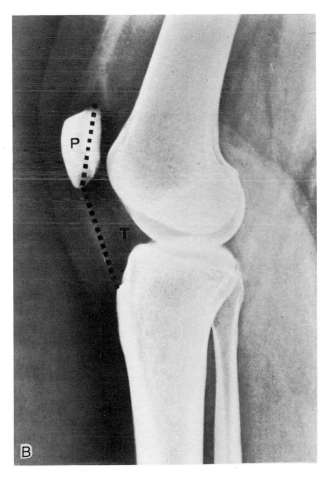

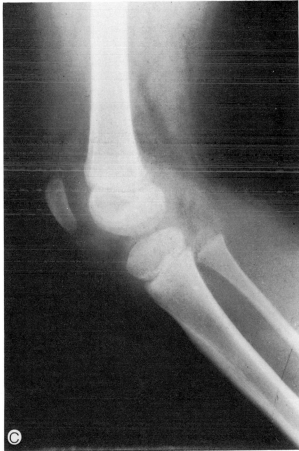

LT (Length of Tendon). The length of the patellar tendon was measured on its deep or posterior surface from its origin on the lower pole of the patella to its insertion into the tibial tubercle. The point of insertion is usually represented on the radiograph by a clearly defined notch.

LP (Length of Patella). The greatest diagonal length of the patella was measured.

WCBL (Width of the Femoral Condyles at Blumensaat's Line). Both condyles were measured at the level of Blumensaat's line and an average was obtained. This measurement was made to determine whether there was a great variation in patellar size. Patellar size was considered to be acceptably constant.

HI (Height of Insertion). The perpendicular distance from the level of the tibial condylar surface to the point of insertion of the patellar tendon was measured to determine whether there was a constant relationship between the level of the tibial tubercle and the tibial plateau. A great variation in the tendon insertion would have invalidated the measurements, but the insertion appeared to be acceptably constant. This measurement may, therefore, be disregarded for clinical evaluation.

The length of the patellar tendon (LT) was found to be approximately equal to the patellar length (LP) expressed as a ratio (because of variations in the size of individual knee joints and their projection on radiographs). The average value of the ratio LT/LP was 1.02, with a mean standard deviation of 0.13. It was concluded that in the normal knee, the length of the patellar tendon equals the diagonal length of the patella and, although some variation will naturally exist, the length of the patellar tendon should not differ from the patella by more than 20 percent (according to confidence limits ±20 percent falls within 98 percent limits of normal).

The measurements were repeated on bilateral knee roentgenograms in 50 asymptomatic volunteers by Jacobsen and Bertheussen,[83] who confirmed a similar degree of accuracy.

4. Blackburne and Peel[12] (Fig. 11.9) criticized the patella:tendon ratio on the basis of two observations:

    a. The radiographic marking of the tibial tubercle may be indistinct or even unrecognizable when the tibial tuberosity has been affected by Osgood-Schlatter's disease.

    b. The nonarticular portion of the lower pole of the patella varies considerably in size, and

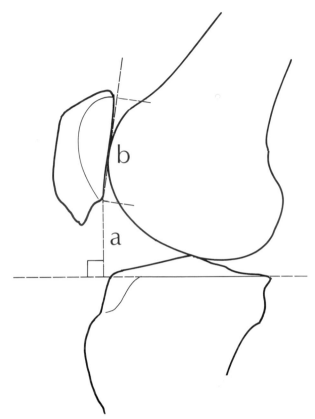

Fig. 11.9. The Blackburne and Peel measurements (see text). Distance *b* represents the articular surface of the patella; *a* is a vertical projection from a line drawn through the tibial articular surface.

these workers reason that it is the position of the articular surface that is of greatest clinical significance. To overcome these difficulties, they suggest a ratio between the perpendicular distance from the lowest articular margin of the patella to the tibial plateau (A) and the length of the articular surface of the patella (B) as measured in the lateral view of the knee taken with at least 30 degrees of flexion. The A:B ratio in 171 normal knees was 0.80 (SD, 0.14). There was no difference between the sexes.

AXIAL VIEWS

The axial or sunrise view of the patellofemoral joint adds considerably to our knowledge when performed in a correctly standardized manner. Unfortunately, all too often, this portion of the examination is either omitted or performed in a haphazard manner, so that much useful information is lost. There are various techniques available:

1. The method attributed to Settegast,[118] in which the patient lies prone with the knee acutely flexed (Fig. 11.10). The plate is placed beneath the knee with the tube directly above, so that the beam will be at right angles. This is the easiest examination for the technician to perform so that it is the most frequently done. Unfortunately, it is also the most uninformative because if the angle of flexion is poorly controlled, the image of the patella is often distorted and the patella lies on the femoral condyles rather than in the sulcus, which is the most important and functional position.

2. Hughston (Fig. 11.11) advocates a modification of the Jaroschy[85] technique. The patient is placed prone with the cassette beneath the knees. The knees are flexed 55 degrees and rest on the tube, which is angled at about 45 degrees. The disadvantages of this method are that images are distorted because the beam strikes the plate at an angle and the knees are also flexed more than is desirable.

3. Ficat[45] describes a technique in which the patient's knees are flexed over the end of the x-ray table. The tube is placed at the patient's feet and the cassette is held proximally against the anterior thigh. In this position it is perpendicular to the beam. Flexion views of 30, 60, and 90 degrees can be obtained. The technique is widely used in Europe, but seems less popular in the United States probably because of technical difficulties in obtaining the views.

4. Laurin et al.[92] describe a very similar method

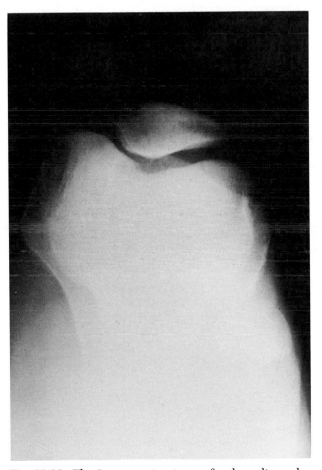

Fig. 11.10. The Settegast view is easy for the radiographer to take. Unfortunately, because the knee is acutely flexed, it is uninformative.

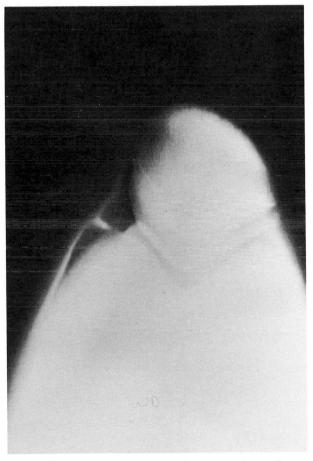

Fig. 11.11. The Hughston view taken at 45° shows the patella in a more functional position, but the images are distorted.

in which the x-ray tube is positioned distally between the feet and the cassette is held proximally against the anterior thighs (Fig. 11.12A–C). They recommend that the following details be observed:

    a. The patient should be seated with his or her feet at the very edge of the table. The x-ray

beam is directed parallel to the anterior border of the tibia and to the longitudinal axis of the patella. The x-ray beam is thus parallel to that specific proximal segment of the patellofemoral joint that must be visualized.

    b. The knees must be in a position of 20 degrees

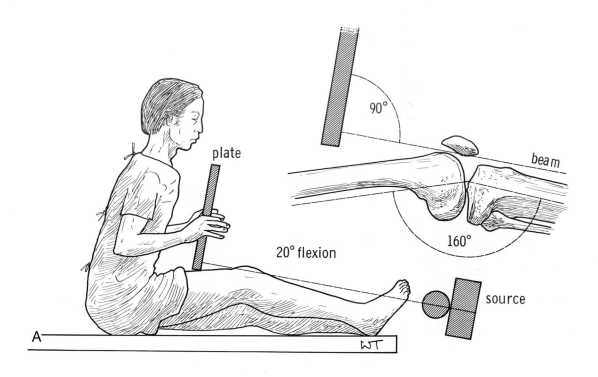

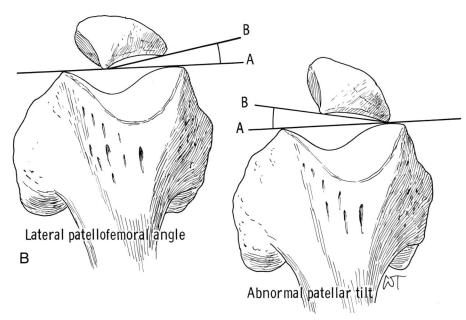

Fig. 11.12. (A) The Laurin technique. (B) In normal knees the angle formed between line A and line B is open laterally: in recurrent subluxation, the angle formed opens medially. (Figure continues).

of knee flexion, and the quadriceps must be relaxed. A special adjustable support under the knees is recommended to maintain the position of the relaxed knees.

c. The x-ray plate is held by the patient such that it is at 90 degrees to the proximal segment of the patellofemoral joint. The plate is

thus held at 90 degrees to the long axis of the tibia; it must not be laid flat against the thighs nor should it be at 90 degrees to the table top. The patient must forcibly press the lower edge of the plate against the thighs. Otherwise, especially, in muscular or obese patients, only the patella will appear at the

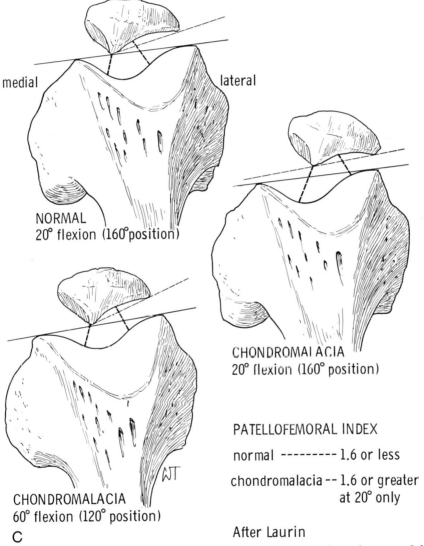

medial | lateral

NORMAL
20° flexion (160°position)

CHONDROMALACIA
20° flexion (160° position)

CHONDROMALACIA
60° flexion (120° position)
C

PATELLOFEMORAL INDEX

normal --------- 1.6 or less

chondromalacia -- 1.6 or greater
at 20° only

After Laurin

Fig. 11.12. (Continued). (C) The patellofemoral index corresponds to the ratio of the thickness of the medial patellofemoral interspace over the lateral patellofemoral interspace. In normal persons, the ratio is 1.6, since the medial patellofemoral interspace is equal to, or slightly less than, the lateral patellofemoral interspace. Patients with chondromalacia have a microtilt of the patella that is obvious only in the 20° position, with an increase in the medial patellofemoral interspace. (Redrawn from Lauria, C.A., Dussault, R., Levesque, H.P.: The tangential x-ray investigation of the patellofemoral joint. X-ray technique, diagnostic criteria, and their interpretation. Clin. Orthop., *144:* 16, 1979, with permission.)

bottom of the x-ray film and the patellofem-oral joint will not be included. Under such circumstances, the x-rays must be repeated and the technique modified either by pushing on the x-ray plate more forcibly or by holding the x-ray plate more proximal to the patella. The knees must not be flexed more than 20 degrees.

5. Merchant et al.[105] describe a technique whereby the patient is positioned supine with the knees flexed 45 degrees over the end of the table (Fig. 11.13). The knees are elevated slightly to keep the femora horizontal and parallel with the table surface. The x-ray tube is raised proximally over the patient and angled down 30 degrees from the horizontal. The film cassette is placed about 1 ft. (30 cm) below the knees resting on the shins and perpendicular to the x-ray beam. The legs are strapped together at about calf level to control rotation and both knees are exposed simultaneously. These investigators stress that it is important for the quadriceps muscle to be relaxed. They found that in a pilot group of 10 normal subjects

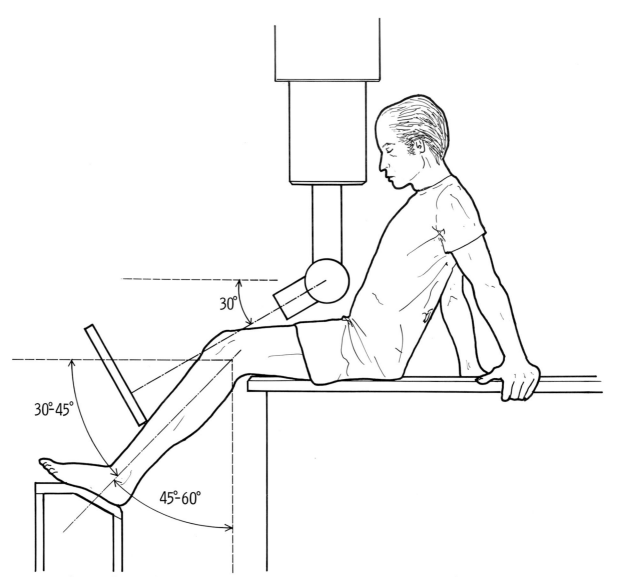

Fig. 11.13. The Merchant technique (see text). (From Merchant, A.C., Mercer, R.L., Jacobsen, R.H., et. al.: Roentgenographic analysis of patellofemoral congruence. J. Bone Joint Surg. [Am.], *56*:1391, 1974, with permission.)

there was no significant change in the shape of the intercondylar sulcus or in the relationship of the patella to the sulcus through a range of knee flexion from 30 to 90 degrees. They selected 45 degrees of knee flexion as the position of least flexion with which satisfactory results could be obtained. The congruence angle measures the relationship with the patella to the intercondylar sulcus. To make this measurement, the sulcus angle is bisected to establish a zero reference line. A second line is then projected from the apex of the sulcus angle through the lowest point on the articular ridge of the patella. The angle measured between these two lines is the congruence angle. If the apex of the patellar articular ridge is lateral to the zero line, the congruence angle is designated positive. If it is medial, the congruence angle is negative (Fig. 11.14A–D).

PATELLOFEMORAL MEASUREMENTS IN NORMAL AND ABNORMAL SUBJECTS

Aglietti et al.[3] measured the following parameters:
1. Quadriceps angle
2. Patellar height using the Insall/Salvati method

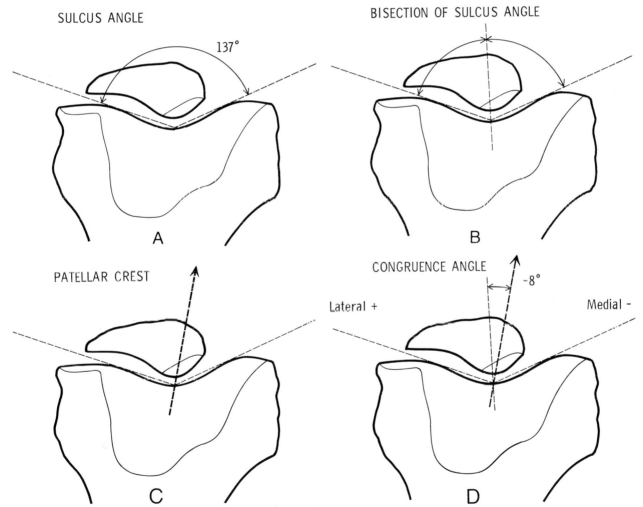

Fig. 11.14. The Merchant measurements. (A) The sulcus angle is measured taking the depth and highest points. (B) The sulcus angle is bisected. (C) A line is drawn from the apex of the sulcus angle to the lowest point of the patellar crest. (D) The angle formed by the bisection angle and the line through the patellar crest is the congruence angle. The normal is $-8°$.

3. Patellar height using the Blackburne and Peel method
4. Sulcus angle–Merchant method
5. Congruence angle–Merchant method

The measurement was made first in 150 normal persons with no history or physical findings of knee pathology. The control group was composed of 75 females and 75 males with an average age of 23, and only the right knee was measured.

Subjects younger than age 13 were excluded because x-ray measurements can be altered by the incomplete ossification of the knee. Also excluded from the study were subjects older than 35 in order to avoid asymptomatic early degenerative changes.

NORMAL VALUES

The Q angle was 15 degrees (range, 6 to 27 degrees; SD = 3 degrees). In the males it was 14 degrees (SD = 3 degrees) and in the females 17 degrees (SD = 3 degrees), with a statistically significant difference (p = 0.001).

TP ratio (of Insall–Salvati): 1.04 (range, 0.8 to 1.38; SD = 0.11). In the males it was 1.01 (SD = 0.09), and in the females 1.06 (SD = 0.12) with a significant difference (p = 0.05). The distance from plateau level to base of tibial tuberosity (average 24 mm) showed a significant variation only with sex, being 25 mm in males and 23.5 mm in females, but did not show any other variation with other parameters including the TP ratio.

AB ratio (of Blackburne and Peel): 0.95 (range, 0.65 to 1.38; SD = 0.13). The males have a ratio of 0.97 (SD = 0.12) and females of 0.94 (SD = 0.15), with an insignificant difference. The length of the articular surface of the patella showed a significant variation with sex, being larger in males but not with other parameters.

Sulcus angle: 137 degrees (range 116 to 151 degrees, SD = 6 degrees). There was no difference in the sulcus angle between males and females.

Congruence angle: −8 degrees (range, −24 to +8 degrees, SD = 6 degrees). It was −6 degrees (SD = 6 degrees) in males and −10 degrees (SD = 6 degrees) in females, with a significant difference (p = 0.001). Only four cases (males) had a positive congruence angle (2.6 percent), while 28 more cases (18 percent) consisting of 19 males and nine females had a congruence angle of 0 degrees. Only one male had a congruence angle above the upper limits of the 96 percent confidence interval (i.e., +6 degrees), while no females exceeded this limit (+2 degrees).

In terms of variance with age, there was no significant variation for all the parameters considered.

As far as correlation coefficients between the parameters, the quadriceps angle had a negative correlation with the congruence angle. The tendon:patella ratio had a positive correlation with the AB measurement of Blackburne and Peel and with the sulcus angle.

PATHOLOGIC VALUES

In addition to the normal group, Aglietti studied a pathologic group of 90 patients comprised of 56 females and 34 males, with an average age of 21. Excluded were patients older than age 35. A diagnosis of chondromalacia was made in 53 cases and recurrent subluxation in 37 cases. In the group of 53 patients with chondromalacia, the average age was 22 (minimum 13, maximum 34), 35 of whom were female and 18 male. Of the 37 patients with recurrent subluxation, the average age was 20 years (minimum 14, maximum 32), 21 were female and 16 male.

The diagnosis of chondromalacia was clinical and made on the basis of the well-recognized pattern of patellar pain. The natural history of these cases over a 4-year period was as follows: 45 percent underwent spontaneous partial or complete recovery with conservative measures such as reduction of activity, straight leg raising, isometric exercises, a patellar brace, and aspirin; 34 percent remained about the same; and 21 percent were eventually operated on.

The natural history of the 37 cases of recurrent subluxation was spontaneous recovery in 30 percent, no change in 43 percent, and surgical treatment in 27 percent.

The parameters in the 53 cases of chondromalacia were as follows:

Quadriceps angle: 20 degrees, significantly different from normal (p = 0.001), and the difference was significant both for females and for males. A quadriceps angle of 20° or above was present in 30 patients (56 percent).

TP ratio: 1.08, not significantly different in the females as compared with sex-matched controls but was significantly different in the males.

AB ratio: 0.91, insignificantly changed compared with controls.

Sulcus angle: 139 degrees, significantly different only for males, but not for females as compared with sex-matched controls.

Congruence angle: −2 degrees, a significant difference compared with controls both for males and females. Twenty-five percent of the patients had positive congruence angle values and 36 percent had a congruence angle of 0 degrees.

The 24 patients who recovered spontaneously showed as the only significant difference, compared with the rest of the group, an average quadriceps angle of 18 degrees (VS = 21 degrees).

RECURRENT SUBLUXATION

The parameters in these 37 cases (Fig. 11.15) were as follows:

Quadriceps angle: 15 degrees, not significantly changed from the controls.

Tendon:patella ratio: 1.23, significantly increased compared with controls. This held true for both males and females. A difference of more than 10

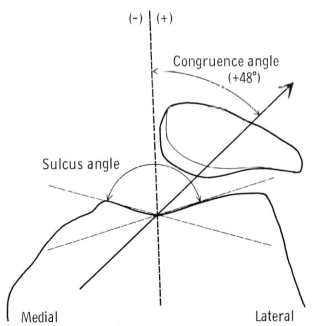

Fig. 11.15. In patients with recurrent subluxation, the patella is high riding, the sulcus angle is increased, and there is a marked abnormality of congruence.

mm in the values of LT and LP was present in 16 patients (43 percent).

AB ratio: 1.08, with a significant difference compared with controls only for females.

Sulcus angle: 147 degrees, significantly different from normal for both males and females.

Congruence angle: 16 degrees, significantly different from the normal for both males and females. Sixty-five percent of patients had a positive CA value and 13 percent had CA of 0°.

The 11 patients in this group who improved spontaneously showed, as the only significant difference from the rest of the group, a CA average value of 5 degrees.

Merchant's original observations indicated a range of values for patellar congruence that perhaps were too wide for significant clinical application. In this study of "normal" knees, there were also subjects with an increased quadriceps angle, a high-riding patella and patellar incongruence. This is perhaps not surprising, as there are numerous examples of asymptomatic anatomic variation, such as hip dysplasia and spinal abnormalities. However, in a sufficiently large group of patients it is possible to obtain an average measurement and a range within which most normal persons would fall. Thus, in the "normal" knees, the average quadriceps angle measured 15 degrees, the patellar length was equal to the patellar ligament length, and the average measurement of the congruence angle was −8 degrees.

Insall et al.[80] previously showed an association of patella alta with recurrent subluxation. Brattström,[17] using a rather complex radiologic technique, found a failure of sulcus development in patients with recurrent dislocation. Ficat and Hungerford,[47] on the other hand, state that the sulcus development is genetically determined. Both concepts may be true. Several investigators have commented on the familial nature of recurrent dislocation, while Aglietti's study confirmed that both a high-riding patella and shallow femoral sulcus were present in his patients. Perhaps the primary abnormality in recurrent dislocation is an excessively long patellar tendon, such that the resulting malposition of the patella causes failure of proper development of the femoral sulcus. However, the association of patella alta and a shallow sulcus does not rule out the possibility that both are part of a congenital dysplasia that may also include abnormalities of the quadriceps muscle attachments and an anomalous band of fibrous tissue between the patella and

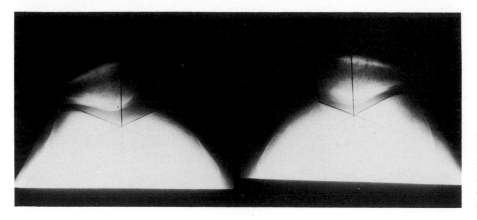

Fig. 11.16. Patients with a rotational malalignment and an increase in the quadriceps angle show a normal sulcus angle and a mildly abnormal congruence angle (left).

iliotibial band.[86] On the other hand, these soft tissue and muscular alterations may simply represent adaptive changes. Perhaps it is not profitable to speculate further on cause and effect because most probably genetically determined and acquired forms exist. Certainly patella alta is seen in cerebral palsy, and patellar dislocation has been reported in association with quadriceps fibrosis, an acquired condition in which multiple intramuscular injections were often given into the lateral aspect of the thigh in infancy.[59,69,97] Here it must be assumed that with growth, fibrosis in the vastus lateralis alters the quadriceps line of pull, ultimately resulting in dislocation. Likewise, in lateral malposition or permanent dislocation of the patella the lateral retinaculum contracts, perhaps giving the impression of an abnormal fascial band. Aglietti found that the congruence angle was grossly abnormal in recurrent dislocation whereas the quadriceps angle was not altered. This is perhaps not surprising because in habitual lateral malposition the quadriceps angle might in fact appear reduced.

In the patients clinically diagnosed as having chondromalacia, the major abnormality was an increase in the quadriceps angle, but the patella was not high riding and the femoral sulcus was normal. These patellae did not dislocate, and the average congruence angle was only mildly abnormal (Fig. 11.16).

PATELLOFEMORAL
CONTACT AREAS

The area of contact between patella and femur in normal knees has been studied by Goodfellow et al.,[54] who used a dye technique, and by Aglietti et al.,[4] who used a casting technique employing the injection of acrylic cement into the articulated joint.

Aglietti determined the normal contact areas in two specimens at different loads and degrees of flexion using a specially designed apparatus that permitted application of tension to the quadriceps tendon while making the castings.

Angles from 0 to 120 degrees of flexion were used (Fig. 11.17). The loads, which varied from 0 to 250 pounds, were applied to the conjoined vastus intermedius and rectus femoris tendons by means of a clamp, while the vastus medialis and lateralis were cut and disregarded. The retinacula were maintained and the cement was introduced into the joint from the previously opened suprapatellar pouch.

At 0 degrees of flexion, the patella was completely above the femoral articular surface for the full range of loads.

At 30 degrees of flexion, the inferior aspect of the patellar surface contacted the uppermost portion of the femoral condyles. Contact began between the lateral femoral condyle and the lateral facet of the patella but by 30 degrees contact was evenly distributed on both sides.

At 60 degrees of flexion, the contact was between the superior half of the patellar surface and part of the femoral groove slightly inferior to the contact area at 30 degrees. The area of contact was larger at 60 degrees than at 30 degrees of flexion.

At 90 degrees of flexion, the contact again was between the superior half of the patella and an area of the femoral groove just above the notch. The contact area was larger than at 60 degrees.

At 120 degrees of flexion, the contact was between the superior aspect of the patella and the areas on the

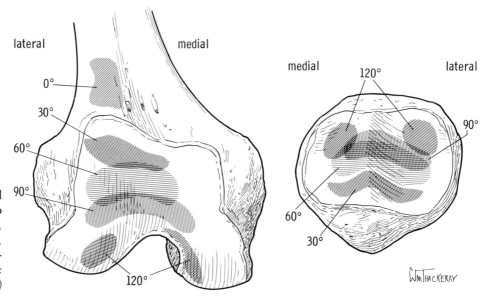

Fig. 11.17. Patellofemoral contact zones according to Aglietti. (From Aglietti, P., Insall, J.N., Walker, P.S., et. al.: A new patella prosthesis. Clin. Orthop., *107:* 175, 1975, with permission.)

femoral groove immediately surrounding the notch in a kidney-shaped fashion.

An increase in load did not significantly change the location of the contact and only slightly increased the area of contact.

The results obtained by Goodfellow[54] using a different dye technique were essentially the same. In addition, Goodfellow recorded the contact area at 140 degrees of flexion showing that in this position the odd facet of the patella came into contact with the lateral border of the medial femoral condyle. Beyond 90 degrees, the broad posterior surface of the quadriceps tendon also makes contact with the femur and the tendofemoral area is the more extensive of the two.

CLASSIFICATION OF PATELLAR DISORDERS

There are many well-recognized causes of the patellar syndrome. These categories are not mutually exclusive and will no doubt be added to in the future. They may be considered according to the amount and extent of articular damage present:

Presence of cartilage damage
  Chondromalacia
  Osteoarthritis
  Direct trauma and osteochondral fractures
  Osteochondritis
Variable cartilage damage
  Malalignment syndromes
  Synovial plicae
Usually normal cartilage
  Peripatellar causes: bursitis and tendinitis
  Overuse syndromes
  Sympathetic dystrophy
  Patellar anomalies

PRESENCE OF CARTILAGE DAMAGE

CHONDROMALACIA

As far as it is known, the first description of chondromalacic cartilage was given by Büdinger.[19,20] He described fissures that he believed were caused by trauma. The term chondromalacia however, was not used by Büdinger himself and is attributed to Aleman.[5] Owre[109] studied the anatomic location of the changes in the patella and reported that they were most frequently found straddling the patellar crest. Wiberg,[130] on the other hand, believed that chondromalacia was predominantly a disease of the medial facet and attributed this fact to its convex shape (Fig.

Wiberg shapes

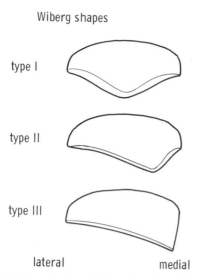

type I

type II

type III

lateral   medial

Fig. 11.18. Wiberg believed that chondromalacia occurred predominantly in type II patellae.

11.18). He believed that there was a localized increase in stress and that symptoms were dependent on the shape of the patella, being most common in those with small vertical and markedly convex facets. This finding is still unconfirmed, although many authors agree that chondromalacia is most frequently observed on the medial facet or the adjoining part of the patellar crest. The stages in the pathoanatomic changes in the articular cartilage described as chondromalacia are well known (Fig. 11.19A–C). Stage I is swelling and softening of the cartilage (closed chondromalacia). Stage II has fissuring within the softened areas, and in stage III there is a breakdown of the surface described as fasciculation. Stage IV should perhaps more properly be described as osteoarthritis, as it is characterized by erosive changes and exposure of the subchondral bone. The first three stages are usually confined to the patella, whereas stage IV commonly involves the opposite or mirror surface of the femur.

What is certainly true is that chondromalacia of the patella is generally regarded as an incidental finding being either a normal part of aging or a reaction of the articular cartilage to abnormal stress. In the latter instance (e.g., malalignment), it is probably not the cartilage damage itself that causes pain, but rather the hyperpressure that results from abnormal patellar tracking. Patellar realignment without regard for the

cartilage damage present is usually sufficient to relieve pain (see below).

Wiles et al.[131] state that "chondromalacia is a precursor of osteoarthritis." Certainly what Goodfellow calls age-dependent surface degeneration is seen with great frequency at autopsy, arthrotomy or arthroscopy. The incidence increases with age. In a study of 124 autopsies, Owre et al. found that in 32 subjects aged 20 to 29, edema occurred in 27 and fissuring in 18. The incidence of edema and fissuring increased thereafter until over the age of 60 all the subjects showed one or other change. Outerbridge,[107] observing the state of the medial facet at meniscectomy in 101 patients, found surface fissuring and fragmentation in 11 of 17 subjects aged 20 to 29. Emery and Meachim[43] found surface fibrillation of both medial and lateral facets at autopsy in most middle-aged subjects, which was increasingly common and severe with age (Fig. 11.20). The topographic distribution agreed closely with the necropsy studies of Owre. Both age changes and osteoarthritis were seen in the same areas. Insall et al.[80] studied the geographic distribution of chondromalacia found at surgery and plotted the findings on maps of the patella (Fig. 11.21). Knees with osteoarthritis were excluded from the study. The findings did not confirm the oft-repeated statement that chondromalacia is predominantly a lesion of the medial facet. Rather, the most frequently involved area was the midpoint of the patellar crest with extension equally onto the medial and lateral patellar facets. Seventy-one percent of the knees had a lesion located within an ellipse passing transversely across the central area of the patella, with the upper and lower thirds of the patellar articular surface being nearly always spared. The medial facet alone was involved in 21 percent and the lateral facet alone in 7 percent. Chondromalacia of the femur was never severe, and geographic distribution followed no particular pattern.

The widespread prevalence of the articular changes known as chondromalacia is beyond dispute. The lesions equally clearly are age dependent[53] and may be expected in most knees during and after the third decade of life. However, in most people, patellar chondromalacia is an incidental finding and not a cause of knee pain until the final stage of cartilage erosion and ulceration has occurred. A pain mechanism can be readily understood in osteoarthritis when the subchondral bone containing nerve endings is exposed, but it has always puzzled investigators how pain can be produced when the articular cartilage is intact or partially intact, as nerve fibers have never been demonstrated in either normal or abnormal cartilage.

Goodfellow et al.[55] have described a particular lesion of articular cartilage, which they have termed *basal degeneration* (Fig. 11.22). This disorder of the deep layers of the cartilage, in the early stages at least, does not involve the surface, which may appear intact. The involved area, however, is softened and can be detected with a probe. In later stages the lesion may appear as a localized blister on the surface or as fasciculation when the tangential surface fibers of the cartilage rupture and fronds of collagenous material protrude from the defect. If this disk of affected cartilage is surgically removed, it separates rather easily from the zone of calcified cartilage. Normal cartilage, on the other hand, can only be separated by the use of a sharp tool. The lesion of basal degeneration has two sites of predilection, the first being an area astride the junction of the medial and odd facets (Fig. 11.23) and the second straddling the inferior part of the patellar crest. These areas are close together and sometimes confluent.

Adding to the confusion over the significance of chondromalacic lesions is the fact that the characteristic syndrome of patellar pain and tenderness can occur when the patellar cartilage is intact, and no articular cartilage lesions of any kind can be demonstrated. It may be argued that in some cases this is attributable to overlooking a lesion of basal degeneration when the surface layer remains intact. Nonetheless, evidence is accumulating that patellar pain frequently occurs in an apparently normal patella. The paper by Darracott and Vernon-Roberts[35] is of interest in this regard. These workers describe the bony changes in 11 patellae with clinical chondromalacia. On examination of macerated patellae, they reported that "trabecular bone exhibited diffuse osteoporosis in three cases, and isolated foci of osteoporosis in the remaining eight patellae. A striking feature present in some patellae were discrete nodular aggregates of bone on trabeculae at the junction of normal and porotic areas. . . . In all cases the anterior surface of the patella appeared macroscopically normal and there was no evidence of trauma." Although the pathologic material cited by these investigators is probably unique, others have made similar clinical observations. Insall et al.[80] found eight of 87 knees treated by arthrotomy for "chondromalacia" to have a normal articular surface. Goodfellow et al.[55] reported a slightly higher

proportion (four of 27) in which this was the case. Larson et al.,[91] describing the results of lateral retinacular release operations, found that nearly 50 percent of the knees in which the synovium had been opened had a normal-appearing articular surface of the patellofemoral joint. Ceder and Larson,[26] in a later study of 64 knees done subsequently, found at arthrotomy normal articular cartilage in 24 knees, grade I chondromalacia in 26 knees, grade II chondromalacia in nine knees, and grade III chondromalacia in three knees. They stated that "the severity of chondromalacia did not correlate with the subjective and functional outcome following surgery." Arthroscopy now makes it possible to inspect the articular surfaces in many more cases in which the complaint is of knee pain than was previously possible, when arthrotomy was the only means of gaining direct visualization. Leslie and Bentley,[93] in an arthroscopic study of patients with clinical "chondromalacia," found that in fact only about one-half the patients showed objective evidence of this condition, a proportion that is hardly greater than what might be predicted were a similar arthroscopic examination conducted on an asymptomatic group of the same age. Casscells[24] offers the opinion that articular lesions and symptoms are usually unrelated. He states, "During the course of arthroscopic examination of many knees for other reasons it has been possible to identify many cases of asymptomatic chondromalacia." And later, in the context of painful knees in young girls, he states, "Having done arthroscopic examination of many such individuals I am convinced that chondromalacia is rarely the cause of these symptoms."

It seems, therefore, that one must look not only for a cause of chondromalacia, but for an explanation of patellar pain as well, recognizing that the two are not necessarily related and that chondromalacia used in a descriptive sense can exist without symptoms, and vice versa.

Some Causes of Chondromalacia

Surface Degeneration. According to Goodfellow et al.[55] the most frequently observed site of early surface fibrillation is the odd facet of the patella, which in Westerners is an area of habitual disuse. It has been observed in other joints, notably the hip and elbow, that similar changes occur in those areas least often subject to pressure[53]. The explanation offered by Harrison et al.[63] is cartilage malnutrition resulting

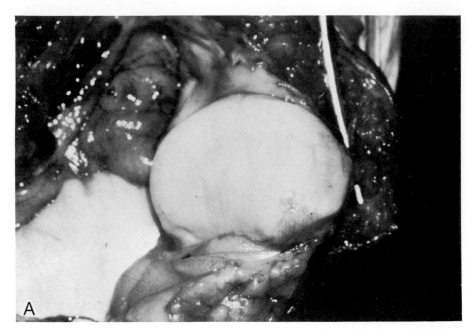

Fig. 11.19. Chondromalacia of the patella. (A) Stage I or closed chondromalacia shows an area of softening on both medial and lateral facets adjoining the patellar crest, as well as some very superficial fissures. (B) Stage II shows deeper fissures within the softened area (Figure continues).

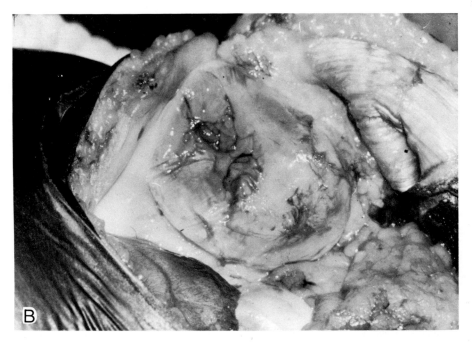

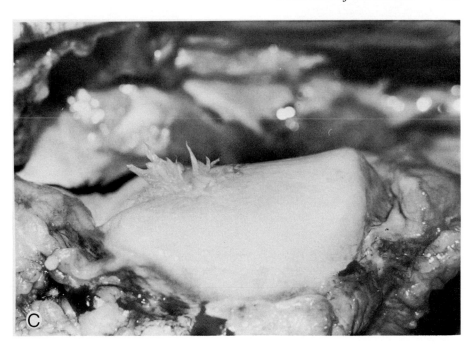

Fig. 11.19 (Continued.) (C) In Stage III the lower part of the patellar crest shows fasciculation.

from a lack of the intermittent pumping action of alternate pressure and rest.

If surface fibrillation on the odd facet is of no immediate clinical significance, it does not follow that this localized degeneration will be without long-range consequences. Bullough and Goodfellow[21] stress the unitary nature of articular cartilage, which is organized as a whole, so that a lesion in any part may prejudice the integrity of all of it. An interruption in the transmission of tension forces by a defect, even in an unloaded area, must lead to the setting up of abnormal stress patterns and predispose the adjacent loaded areas to mechanical breakdown. From autopsy studies, Heine-Rostock[66] found that these joints in the body that most frequently demonstrate surface changes in youth are those most susceptible to osteoarthritis in old age. This observation is supported because both chondromalacia and osteoarthritis of the knee are common in Westerners. However, according to Marar and Pillay,[102] the incidence of chondromalacia and osteoarthritis of the patella is considerably lower in orientals, possibly because the Chinese habitually squat with their knees in full flexion such that the odd facet is not an area of habitual disuse.

Basal Degeneration. Goodfellow considers basal degeneration traumatic in origin because that area between the middle and odd facets is subject to both heavy compression and the effects of shear as the patella glides onto the femoral condyles. He believes that the likelihood of its occurring in a particular individual is a function of minor variations in the anatomic shape of the patella. The odd facet of the patella contacts the medial femoral condyle in full flexion in that area in which osteochondritis dissecans is known to occur. One patient with basal degeneration had an osteochondritis dissecans at the classic site in his opposite knee.

An Abnormal Ridge on the Femur. Outerbridge[107,108] described an osteochondral ridge lying at the medial proximal margin of the femoral sulcus. Although this ridge is present in all knees, it is sometimes enlarged, and impingement may occur against the medial patellar facet at the initiation of flexion. This mechanism may exist in some knees, but it is not common. Marar and Pillay[102] found in 100 Chinese cadavers that in spite of a distinct ridge often seen at this site, it was well covered with overlying soft tissue and only became prominent after removal of this tissue. Moreover, there was no relationship between the ridge and chondromalacia of the patella.

Another objection to the theory is that at the beginning of flexion the patella enters the femoral sulcus from the lateral side, making impingement against even an enlarged ridge unlikely.

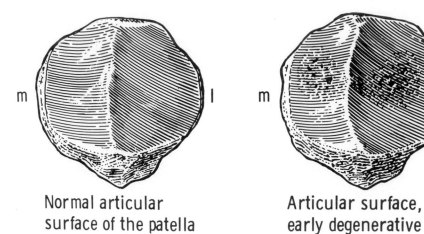

Normal articular
surface of the patella

Articular surface,
early degenerative
change

Fig. 11.20. Distribution of age-dependent changes found at autopsy by Emery and Meachim. (From Emery, I.H., and Meachim, G.: Surface morphology and topography of patellofemoral cartilage fibrillation in Liverpool necropsies. J. Anat., *116:* 103, 1973, with permission.)

Operative Findings in Chondromalacia

Patellae (n=105)

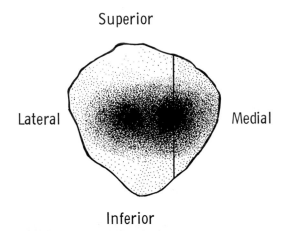

Superior

Lateral

Medial

Inferior

Fig. 11.21. Composite of patellar maps made at surgery showing the distribution of chondromalacia in a group of young persons. (From Insall, J., Falvo, K.A., and Wise, D.W.: Chondromalacia patellae: A prospective study. J. Bone Joint Surg. [Am.], *58:* 1, 1976, with permission.

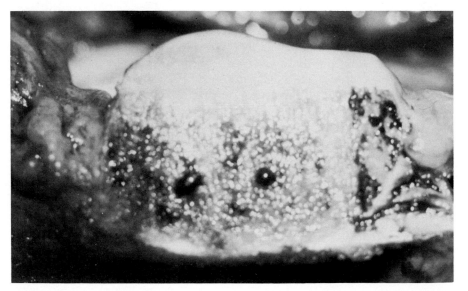

Fig. 11.22. Basal degeneration in the substance of the articular cartilage. The surface layer is softened but intact (this patient was treated by medial facetectomy providing the opportunity of obtaining this picture).

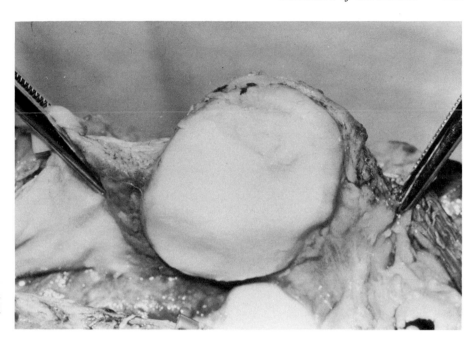

Fig. 11.23. A blister lesion on the ridge between the medial and odd facets.

Malalignment. The association between patellar subluxation and chondromalacia is well known (Fig. 11.24A,B).[98] More recently it has been shown that malalignment without actual dislocation is also associated with cartilage damage.

Direct Trauma. (see below)

Patellar Shape. Wiberg[130] describes three patellar types (Fig. 11.18):

Type I: Both facets are gently concave, symmetric, and roughly the same size.

Type II: The medial facet is smaller than the lateral, which remains concave, whereas the medial facet is either flat or slightly convex.

Type III: The lateral facet is much larger than the medial, which is short and has an almost vertical convexity.

It is tempting to assume that the decreased area of the medial facet, particularly when associated with convexity, might lead to increased local stress and therefore cartilage breakdown.[58] However, this association has not been demonstrated either by Wiberg himself or by subsequent investigators.

Biochemical Alteration. Chrisman[28] believes that some patients have a biochemical derangement in the cartilage and that "some families simply make a tissue which is more susceptible to wear." In his opinion, cartilage degradation is initiated by cathepsin, which splits protein polysaccharide bonds first, decreasing the elastic properties of cartilage. Shoji and Granda[119] investigated the acid hydrolases and chemical components of the articular cartilage of the patella from normal, chondromalacic and osteoarthritic patients. They concluded that (1) chondromalacia is a transitional form of osteoarthritis at the pathobiochemical level, and (2) degradation of the articular cartilage may begin with proteolysis and be further accelerated by depolymerization of glycosaminoglycans.

Although similar biochemical alterations are observed in both chondromalacic and osteoarthritic cartilage, it has not yet been shown that a primary abnormality of cartilage metabolism is responsible for initiating degeneration.

Postoperative Chondromalacia. The development of chondromalacia after arthrotomy or after prolonged immobilization for fracture healing is a well-known occurrence, probably resulting from a nutritional disturbance of the cartilage. Both arthrotomy and immobilization preclude normal use of the joint for a variable period; the patellar cartilage, being exceptionally thick, may be unusually vulnerable when the pumping action that supplies its nutrients is denied. Other factors may play a part; for example, (1) medial capsular incisions and postoperative quadriceps atrophy may produce a patellar imbalance akin to malalignment (Fig. 11.25), and (2) postoperative

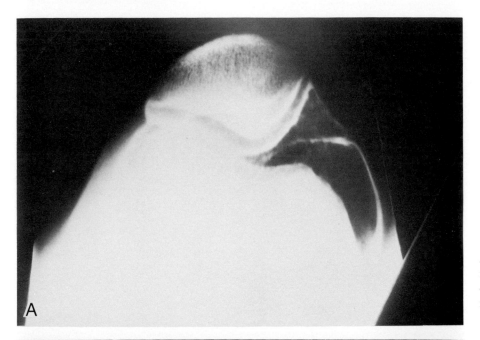

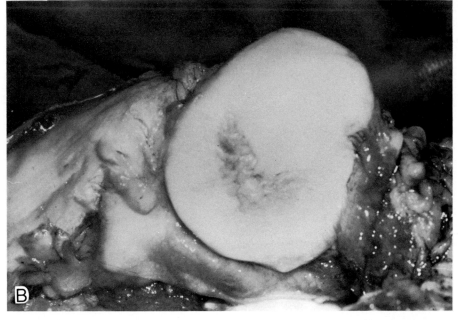

Fig. 11.24. (A) A patellofemoral arthrogram showing the contact area between lateral femoral condyle and lateral patellar facet. (B) The articular surface of the same patient showing scuffing of the articular cartilage in the same region with an adjoining extensive area of softening crossing the central ridge.

rehabilitation exercises done injudiciously with heavy weights applied to the flexed leg can produce enormous loads on the patella.

Bone Compliance.   Abernethy et al.[1] studied the articular cartilage of the patella in 100 knees at necropsy. The pattern of articular damage was consistent with that found by other observers. The earliest changes were observed in the periphery, then in the central medial facet, and finally in the central lateral facet. With increasing age the more advanced changes were generally found in the lateral facet. The bone underlying the medial facet was relatively less stiff than that of the rest of the contact area of the patella. Increased stiffness beneath the lateral facet was associated with more advanced articular damage. There was a fairly abrupt change between relatively com-

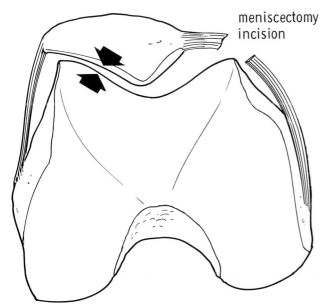

meniscectomy incision

Fig. 11.25. Medial parapatellar capsular incisions may precipitate lateral patellar tracking, even though this was not present before surgery.

pliant bone and stiff bone in the area of the central medial facet adjoining the patellar crest. This is the area in which the earliest cartilage changes were seen. Under load, the cartilage of the patella is subjected to considerable deformation, which to some extent is shared by the underlying bone. As the amount of bony deformation depends on the compliance of the bone, there will be a local shear stress within the cartilage overlying the junction of soft and hard areas.

Pain Pathways in Chondromalacia

Although chondromalacia is usually asymptomatic, it is possible that in some cases at least the articular changes themselves indirectly give rise to pain. Because of the absence of nerve fibers, the cartilage itself is insensitive; it is generally conceded that the source of pain is the subchondral bone. Two possible pain mechanisms exist.

Basal Degeneration. The fascicular lesion called basal degeneration disorganizes the fibrous structure of the intermediate zone of collagen fibers. Normal articular cartilage contains a latticelike framework in the intermediate zone that becomes compressed into a more or less tangential arrangement when the surface is loaded (Fig. 11.26). It may be argued that if this pattern is interrupted, the underlying bone plate must be subject to pressure variations from which it is normally protected by the cushioning effect of intact articular cartilage. Uneven loading may also transmit pressure to the subchondral plate that in some areas exceeds the pain threshold of the nerve endings. The site of the lesion of basal degeneration is such that this area is compressed against the femur when the knee is flexed,[55] which would account for the "movie sign" of pain evoked by prolonged sitting. It should be noted that while the foregoing hypothesis was constructed specifically for the lesion of basal degeneration, it may well have a wider implication.

Chemical Causes. Experimentally synovial inflammation can be caused by the injection of cartilage components,[30] in particular the proteoglycans, which are normally not found in the synovial fluid. When blister lesions rupture or damaged cartilage releases small pieces into the joint, degradative enzymes such as cathepsins are released, which in turn cause further cartilage softening and breakdown. However, this mechanism, although possibly pertinent to severe osteoarthritis, seems unlikely to play a major part in the pain of chondromalacia. Cases with an effusion containing joint debris are encountered, but they are distinctly uncommon, and most show no evidence of synovial reaction. Synovial biopsies done by us in chondromalacia patients invariably exhibit synovium devoid of inflammation.

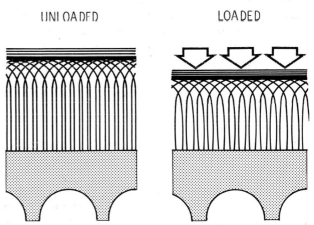

Fig. 11.26. Diagram showing the effect of loading of normal articular cartilage. (From Goodfellow, J.W., Hungerford, D.S., and Woods, C.: Patellofemoral mechanics joint and pathology. 2. Chondromalacia patellae. J. Bone Joint Surg. [Am.], *58:* 291, 1976, with permission.)

Natural History of Chondromalacia

Although it is widely believed that the pathologic changes of chondromalacia represent an early stage of osteoarthritis, it is also generally accepted that most patients displaying the clinical symptoms and signs attributed to this condition get better. If these viewpoints do not seem consistent, it may be attributed to (1) the poor correlation between chondromalacia and "the chondromalacia syndrome" of anterior knee pain and (2) the inclusion of patients with patellar pain attributable to another cause, who are assumed to suffer from chondromalacia.

Surprisingly, the untreated course of both the clinical syndrome and the pathologic changes has received little study. Chondromalacia of the patella sometimes progresses to osteoarthritis, although the course usually cannot be followed in a single patient. However, a possible sequence of events can be shown in a series. Emery and Meachim[43] found that age-related changes in the cartilage started on the periphery, then appeared on the central medial facet, and with increasing age tended to spread across the patellar crest to the lateral facet. The changes on the lateral facet, although appearing later, seem to progress more rapidly, and bony erosion first appears on the central part of the lateral facet; erosion to bone was unusual on the medial facet, even when the lateral is eburnated and almost devoid of cartilage.

Wiles et al.[132] gave follow-up results in 14 knees operated upon for other conditions in which fissuring was observed but the articular cartilage was left intact. After periods ranging from 1 to 5 years there were no symptoms in five knees, mild aching in another five, troublesome symptoms in two, and severe symptoms in another two. In general the 10 patients with minimal symptoms had only a small area of cartilage involved, whereas the remaining four had more extensive changes.

With reference to the clinical syndrome, Karlson[87] reexamined 71 men who had been diagnosed as having chondromalacia, but whose symptoms did not warrant operation. After a follow-up ranging from 1 to 20 years, 10 patients had no subjective complaints, 45 had mild symptoms such as stiffness and fatigue after exertion, and 16 had sufficient trouble to cause absence from work or a change of occupation. Radiographs were obtained in 35, and none showed advanced osteoarthritis.

Truly more definitive information is needed on this important point. It is hoped that the widespread use of arthroscopy will soon begin to provide more knowledge about the behavior of pathologic cartilage lesions. On an anecdotal level, I believe that most patients with the clinical syndrome do not get better, but rather become adjusted when symptoms are relatively mild. As they grow older, sports or other pain-producing activity may be discontinued, and with maturity comes better tolerance of chronic pain. In those patients with severe and persistent symptoms, the subsequent course of the condition is often altered by surgery.

OSTEOARTHRITIS

It will be obvious from the foregoing section that osteoarthritis defined as loss of articular cartilage is widely regarded as merely the end result of the progression of chondromalacia. As described by Wiles et al.[131] chondromalacic cartilage becomes flaky, pieces of cartilage break off, and an ulcerlike lesion develops at the base of which lies the subchondral bone (Fig. 11.27).

Histologic and biochemical assay from residual cartilage located at the margins of this ulcer is indistinguishable from cartilage removed from chondromalacic lesions elsewhere, so that the concept of chondromalacia progressing through various stages to osteoarthritis (stage IV chondromalacia) is a valid one. Nonetheless, there are important reasons for regarding patellofemoral arthritis as a separate entity. First, the patients are middle-aged or older and very seldom give a long history of knee pain beginning in adolescence. Rather, these patients usually have symptoms of relatively brief duration before presenting for examination, which typically indicates well-advanced changes of osteoarthritis (loss of cartilage space, sclerosis, and osteophyte formation) at that time (Fig. 11.28). Unquestionably these advanced findings did not suddenly occur and were preceded by the stages of development observed in autopsy studies by Bennett et al.[9] and more recently by Emery and Meachim.[43] On the assumption that the presenting stage of advanced osteoarthritis takes years rather than months to develop, the early stages of the process must have taken place without the awareness of the patient (the usual asymptomatic nature of chondro-

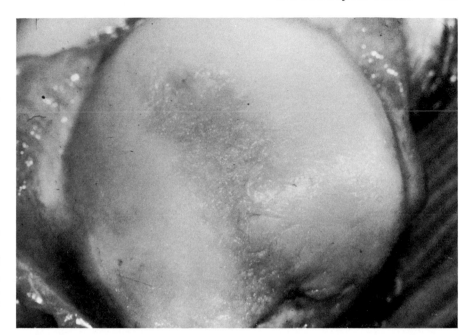

Fig. 11.27. Stage IV chondromalacia or osteoarthritis. Unlike the first three stages of chondromalacia this lesion, in which subchondral bone is exposed, does not occur in young people.

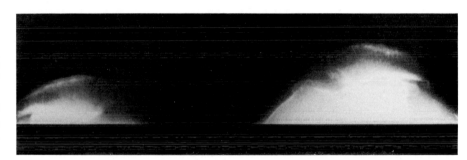

Fig. 11.28. This 51-year-old woman had symptoms for only a few months. Nevertheless, these advanced radiologic changes were present, which must have been many years in developing.

malacic lesions has already been discussed). In established osteoarthritis, there are nearly always similar lesions to be found in the femoral sulcus unlike the earlier stages in which this surface is usually normal. In osteoarthritis there is no difficulty in explaining the pain mechanism, as the sensitive subchondral bony surfaces are in contact with each other. The existence of a pain mechanism does not, however, explain why radiographically similar joints in different patients (or even in the same patient) may be painful in one and not in the other. Similarly, variation in the intensity of symptoms in the same joint occur from time to time, although the radiographic appearance remains unchanged.

Etiology

Ficat et al.[46] are of the opinion that the excessive lateral pressure syndrome (ELPS) is the most frequent cause of patellofemoral arthrosis (Fig. 11.29). Certainly in the established picture cartilage erosion is predominantly lateral, and the patella often appears laterally positioned if not laterally subluxed. However, whether this lateralization is a consequence of the loss of cartilage space or whether the cartilage erosion is caused by tight lateral structures remains unclear. Ficat[45] regards the ELPS as a separate entity, but others may prefer to regard it merely as a part of a more generalized quadriceps mechanism malalignment.

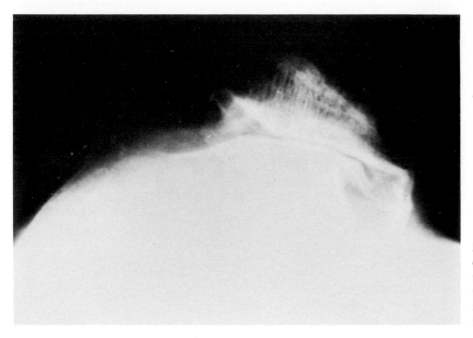

Fig. 11.29. According to Ficat,[45,46,47] patellofemoral arthrosis is often caused by a contracted band in the lateral retinaculum (in this case ossified).

In our experience it is unusual for patients with patellofemoral arthrosis to have experienced patellar dislocation in earlier life, and normally the stigmata of malalignment (increased quadriceps angle, patella alta, genu valgum, rotational abnormalities) are not seen.[23] In some cases, the arthrosis clearly follows a patellar fracture, other injury, or previous surgery. Medial facet arthrosis is seldom if ever seen as a primary entity, but may follow as the late result of a tibial tubercle transfer for patellar dislocation.

However, most often patellofemoral arthrosis seems to arise de novo in a structurally normal joint for which no obvious cause can be assigned. Most frequently there is also an associated femorotibial arthrosis. In a series of 600 cases of radiologically established gonarthrosis cases attending the knee clinic at The Hospital for Special Surgery, patellofemoral arthrosis was found to be associated with medial femorotibial narrowing in 65 percent, and with lateral femorotibial narrowing in 20 percent of cases. The characteristic lateral patellofemoral narrowing and lateral displacement was seen in all three types, even when the patellofemoral arthrosis was associated with medial compartment arthrosis and varus angulation. In our opinion, the predominance of lateral facet erosion merely reflects the normal valgus vector of the patellofemoral mechanism (Fig. 11.30).

Loose bodies are very common in patellofemoral arthrosis but generally do not cause symptoms. They are often situated out of the way in the posterior compartment and do not interfere with the mechanics of motion. Even anterior and suprapatellar loose bodies may remain permanently in the joint recesses, and it is only those of small and intermediate size that move about becoming interposed between the joint surfaces. The patient with symptomatic loose bodies is well aware of the fact and offers this information in the history. Loose bodies that are not causing locking or buckling are nearly always asymptomatic and in particular should not be regarded as a source of chronic pain.

DIRECT TRAUMA AND OSTEOCHONDRAL FRACTURES

Chaklin[27] described changes in the patellar cartilage that he believed were caused by direct application of force in the region of the patella. The usual mechanism was a fall on the knee or a contusion from a hard object, or sometimes a fall from a height. The patient usually states that after injury he noted a slight swelling and later instability and pain in the anterior portion of the knee joint. Chaklin described the *sartorius symptom* in order to differentiate chondropathy from meniscal injury. The patient is made to lift the

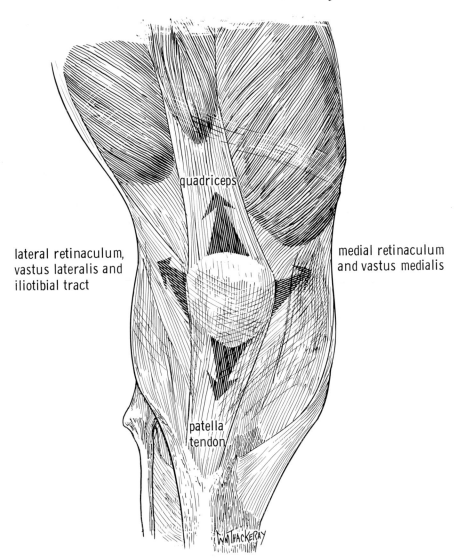

quadriceps

lateral retinaculum,
vastus lateralis and
iliotibial tract

medial retinaculum
and vastus medialis

patella
tendon

WMTHACKERAY

Fig. 11.30 Normal valgus vector of the patellofemoral mechanism may be the cause of predominantly lateral facet arthritis.

injured limb in an extended position and, when slight resistance is made, a contraction of the quadriceps and a compensatory tenseness of the sartorius will be noticed. This "symptom" is positive in injuries to the medial meniscus and negative in chondropathy. The changes in the patella caused by injury described by Chaklin seem characteristic of chondromalacia resulting from other causes, except for one variation, which consists of the appearance of a deep crack on the center of the patella. Chaklin also noted areas having the appearance of synovitis caused by irritation.

Soto-Hall[123] also described patellar lesions after acute trauma. The clinical pattern was similar to that de-

scribed by Chaklin. After the original injury, there was a short period of total disability followed by a quiescent period of several months, during which there were some mild symptoms. There was then a gradual development of more severe symptoms culminating in a marked disability. Pathologic changes described are initially of edema, softening, and fissuring, followed by fraying of the cartilage; in the late stages, ulceration with exposure of subchondral bone occurs. Also described were amputation specimens obtained after severe injury, in which linear fractures of the articular cartilage were found. Soto-Hall also described two patients with severe degeneration after

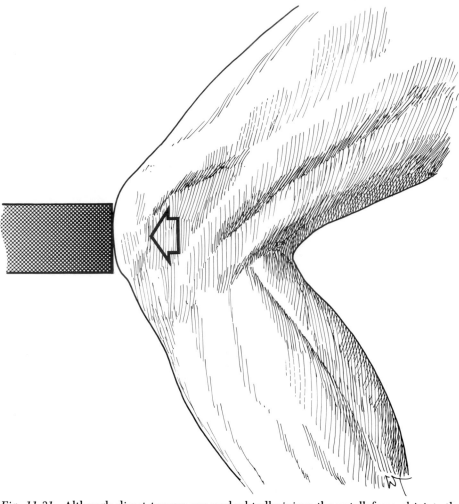

Fig. 11.31. Although direct trauma can undoubtedly injure the patellofemoral joint, the dashboard knee is difficult to assess.

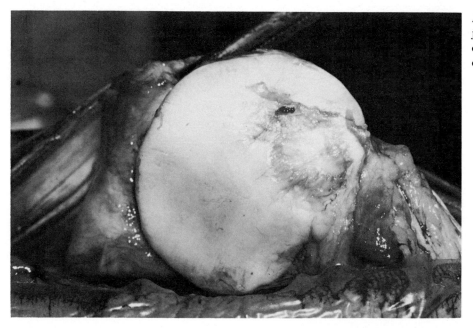

Fig. 11.32. Osteochondral injury to the medial patella facet caused by a forceful patellar dislocation.

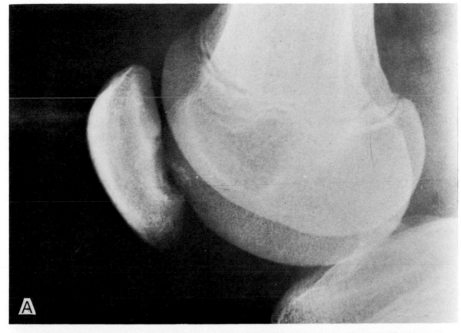

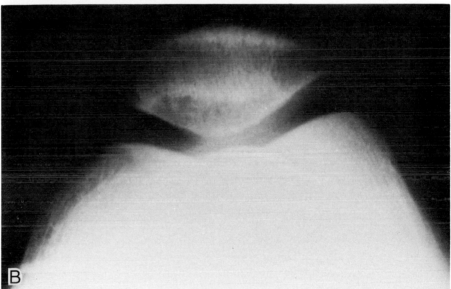

Fig. 11.33. (A,B) Lateral and skyline views of osteochondritis of the patella.

recurrent subluxation and emphasized the importance of quadriceps muscle imbalance in contributing to cartilage destruction.

Direct injury to the patella is common because of its exposed location, and articular damage can result (Fig. 11.31). The dashboard knee is a well-recognized example, although it must be said that the assessment of these cases is often complicated by litigation and compensation considerations.

Although patellar subluxation usually occurs in knees that already have abnormal patellar tracking, severe injury may damage a structurally normal knee. A severe twist causes a shearing injury to the patella, which may result in an osteochondral fracture and the formation of a loose body.

The osteochondral fracture caused by a forceful patellar dislocation is a tangential fracture of the medial patellar facet (Fig. 11.32) and sometimes of the lateral lip of the femoral sulcus. The location of these fractures suggests that they occur during repositioning of the patella rather than during displacement and may in part result from strong quadriceps contraction. Fractures are not often seen in recurrent subluxation because in this condition the patellofemoral joint is usually dysplastic and the bony anatomy offers little resistance to either displacement or return.

There is a severe reaction that follows the injury that caused the osteochondral fracture and the joint is filled with blood. The late outcome depends on the size of the articular defect, the fate of the loose body, and the adequacy of patellar tracking. The loose body may remain free in the joint and, particularly when relatively small, may cause repetitive mechanical derangements. Some loose bodies become attached to the synovium either in the suprapatellar pouch or in the intercondylar region anterior to the cruciates. Pedunculated loose bodies with a limited freedom of motion can also interfere with joint function.

OSTEOCHONDRITIS

A loose fragment may sometimes separate from the patella, usually in the region of the crest or inferior pole, which is readily diagnosable radiographically either on the lateral or skyline view (Fig. 11.33A,B). Although a history of causative trauma is usually lacking, the site of the lesion suggests a possible relationship to osteochondral fracture.[2,33] There is, however, no acute reaction, and no hemarthrosis occurs. Symptoms are generally mild or nonexistent until the osteochondritic fragment partially or completely separates. Complaints may then either be those typical of a patellar disorder or secondary to the loose fragment which when formed usually remains free in the joint and not attached to synovium. Smillie[122] considers osteochondritis dissecans of the patella a feature of dysostosis.

VARIABLE CARTILAGE DAMAGE

MALALIGNMENT SYNDROMES

Patellar subluxation and dislocation are well known to cause articular damage. However, although MacNab[98] suggested that the damage sustained is attributable more to the abnormal excursions of the patella that occur with normal flexion and extension of the knee than to the occasional episodes of dislocation, only recently has there been general acceptance that patellar tracking abnormalities may produce symptoms in the absence of actual mechanical instability.

The symptoms caused by malalignment can therefore be (1) patellar instability, subluxation, or dislocation; (2) pain; or (3) a combination of the two. Symptoms resulting from malalignment nearly always begin in adolescence or early adult life, and only occasionally do patients present for the first time over the age of 30. Although MacNab[98] found that untreated recurrent dislocation eventually resulted in severe osteoarthritis, Crosby and Insall[34] found that in their untreated cases this was seldom the case (Fig. 11.34). In older patients who already have established arthritis, the more readily measured features of malalignment so commonly seen in younger patients are not present. The lateral position of the patella associated with lateral facet patellofemoral arthritis was recognized by MacNab and is cited by Ficat as evidence for the excessive lateral pressure syndrome (ELPS). However, in our experience the counterpart of ELPS before the development of radiologic arthritis is not seen in younger patients in the absence of other abnormalities such as an increased quadriceps angle or patella alta. One would certainly expect chronic derangements of patellar tracking to lead eventually to osteoarthrosis;[129] it is surprising that there is no conclusive evidence that this is so, indicating the need for further investigation into the natural history of the condition.

Genu valgum, genu recurvatum, rotational abnormalities, and increased quadriceps angle, hyperlaxity,[22] patella alta, lateral position of the tibial tubercle, underdevelopment of the femoral sulcus, aberrant attachments of the iliotibial band,[86] and quadriceps dysplasia have all been implicated in patellar malalignment syndromes. Some of these factors may be familial and interrelated (e.g., patella alta and an underdeveloped sulcus). For practical purposes, clinical cases of malalignment fall into two distinct groups, although features of each can be found in the same patient.

Rotational Malalignment

Rotational malalignment is characterized by excessive femoral anteversion with internal rotation of the distal end of the femur and a compensatory external rotation of the tibia. The result is a limb in which the

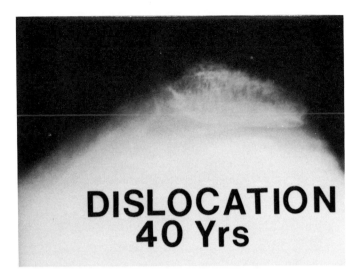

Fig. 11.34. Although this patient had a history of recurrent dislocation going back 40 years, changes caused by osteoarthritis were not pronounced.

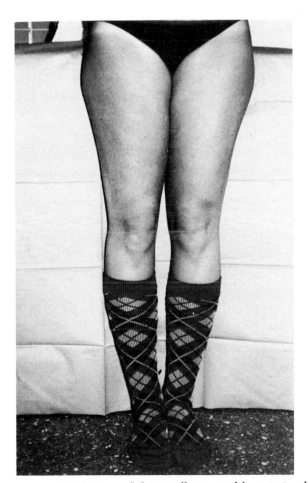

Fig. 11.35. Squinting of the patellae caused by rotational malalignment of the limb. This phenomenon is accompanied by an increase in the Q angle.

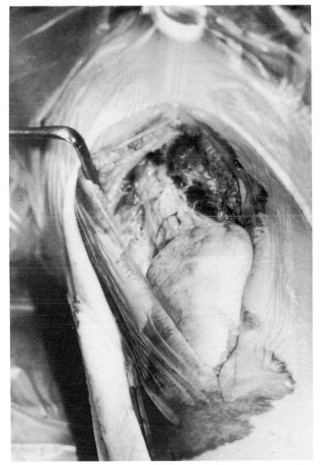

Fig. 11.36. The quadriceps tendon often lies more laterally than the surface marking of the Q angle predicts.

knee is internally rotated relative to the hip and ankle joints, so that when standing with the feet together the patellae appear to "squint" (Fig. 11.35). There is often a mild degree of genu varum. The quadriceps angle is increased and when the extensor mechanism is exposed at surgery the quadriceps tendon is found to lie even more laterally than predicted so that the surface measurement actually underestimates the Q angle (Fig. 11.36). The femoral sulcus is normal, and a mild degree of patellofemoral incongruence is found on the Merchant view. Patients with this type of malalignment typically complain of pain more than instability and on inspection the articular surfaces are either normal or show relatively mild chondromalacia.

Patella Alta

Patella alta is associated with an abnormal femoral sulcus, dysplasia of the vastus medialis, a lateral position of the patella, and a thickened lateral retinaculum. Sometimes in extreme cases the lateral patellar border is directly attached to the iliotibial band. It has been reported that patella alta may follow Osgood Schlatter's apophysitis.[84] In patients with patella alta, the primary complaint is usually of patellar instability, subluxation, or dislocation.[79] Severe examples of patellar chondromalacia[90] are found in this group, yet pain is often intermittent and mostly related to episodes of patellar instability.

A combination of patella alta and increased quadriceps angle is present in some knees and can be more difficult to recognize than the variants alone because each by itself is less pronounced. Cartilage lesions may be present.

Patella alta leads to gross disturbance of patellar tracking, which may be visible clinically as a lateral deviation of the patella when the knee is actively extended. Congruence views of the patella are also grossly abnormal.

Habitual lateral tracking may also produce adaptive changes, and in time the quadriceps tendon comes to lie more to the lateral side of the knee. The vastus medialis becomes stretched and the vastus lateralis contracted; these alterations can be accelerated by episodes of patellar dislocation. In its most advanced form, the condition results in habitual dislocation with an irreducible patella lying laterally (Fig. 11.37).

Along with lateral displacement of the quadriceps, the patellar retinacular structures undergo concomitant stretching and contracture. Shortening of the lateral patellar retinaculum gives rise to the concept of the excessive lateral pressure syndrome and provides the rationale for lateral patellar release.

Quadriceps dysplasia[50] is another term used to explain tracking abnormalities that may occur without patellar malposition. Dysplasia of the vastus medialis and abnormal attachments of the vastus lateralis are described; the term quadriceps dysplasia should be reserved for such cases. It should not be used indiscriminately to explain patellar pain when objective clinical evidence of dysplasia is lacking.

The anatomic variants are genetically determined

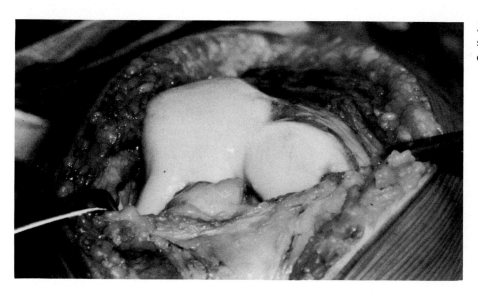

Fig. 11.37. A convex femoral sulcus in a patient with habitual dislocation of the patella.

and it is a common experience to have more than one child in a family present with the same symptoms and similar appearing knees on examination. Rubacky[115] has reported on a case of familial chondromalacia, and Miller[106] recorded a number of members of the same family presenting with recurrent dislocation of the patella in which the pattern of inheritance was consistent with the transmission of the predisposing factor as an autosomal dominant.

Goldthwait[52] said of recurrent dislocation, "This condition is seen almost entirely in girls or women"; most published series in the literature support a female predominance. If the concept of malalignment is broadened to include patients who have lateral patellar tracking but do not necessarily dislocate, the sex difference is not so obvious. Insall et al.[80] studied 80 patients who were equally divided according to sex; Hughston[71] reported a series of athletes, 72 percent of whom were male.

Pain Mechanism in Malalignment Syndromes

Tracking syndromes sometimes cause chondromalacia of the articular surface, but this does not necessarily mean that chondromalacia is the cause of the pain; in fact, in a study of our cases, the preoperative severity of pain correlated poorly with the severity and extent of patellar chondromalacia found at operation (Fig. 11.38). The worst examples of chondromalacia were found in patients with recurrent dislocation who had little or no pain in between the dislocations. It seems likely, therefore, that pain can occur independently of articular damage and cartilage failure in patients with the "chondromalacia" syndrome may either be coincidental or due to another cause (e.g., patellar malalignment) without itself being responsible for pain.

The pain associated with malalignment is probably explained by the particular and unique anatomy of the patella which in the region of the vertical crest possesses a convex bony surface covered by a thick layer (7 mm) of relatively soft articular cartilage. A soft convex surface is particularly sensitive to sideways loading such as would occur in patellar tracking abnormalities. The effect can be visualized by considering the analogy of an eraser on the end of an ordinary lead pencil. (Repetitive sideways loading soon causes the eraser to shear from its attachment to the pencil, whereas direct compression using much greater force has little effect.) In the same manner, defor-

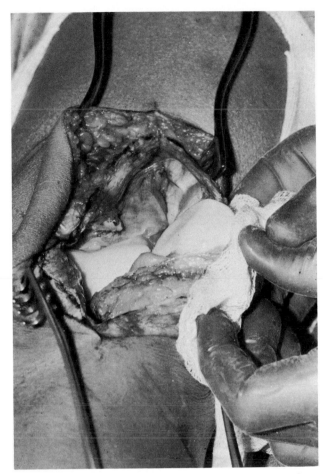

Fig. 11.38. Complaints of patellofemoral pain correlate poorly with articular damage. In this case with typical malalignment pain the patella was normal.

mation of the convex articular cartilage of the patella produces abnormal shear loading on the subchondral bone even when the cartilaginous surface is intact.[81] Repeated deformation of the vertical crest would also explain the softened and fissured areas that may be found in exactly this region as well as tangential fissures within the substance of the cartilage itself. According to this hypothesis, the pain threshold in the subchondral bone can be exceeded even when the cartilage is intact (1) when excessive stress or force is exerted (e.g., athletics or direct trauma), or (2) when normal stresses are applied in an abnormal direction (e.g., lateral loading) (Fig. 11.39A,B).

Thus the current view of malalignment[76] is that lateral tracking and lateral loading of the patella is the primary source of pain but may be incidently the cause of chondromalacia as well.

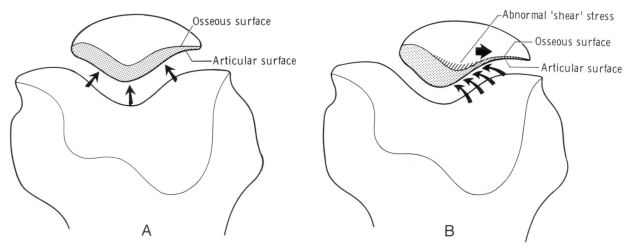

Fig. 11.39. In normal balance, forces across the patellofemoral joint are evenly distributed (A). In cases of excessive lateral loading (B) the articular cartilage in the region of the crest is deformed and excessive loads are transmitted to the subchondral bone.

SYNOVIAL PLICAE

In early intrauterine life the medial and lateral compartments as well as the suprapatellar pouch are separated from each other by thin membranes that later involute so that the knee becomes a single cavity. A plica represents persistence of an embryonic synovial septum into adult life, and the incidence in the general population is estimated at approximately 20 percent. The infrapatellar plica (ligamentum mucosum) is fan shaped and lies between the intercondylar notch of the femur and the fat pad. It is the most common plica but is not implicated in the plica syndrome. The *suprapatellar plica* separates the medial and lateral compartments from the suprapatellar pouch. When it persists into adult life, it usually does so as an incomplete septum or as a medially or laterally based synovial fold. Hughston et al.[73] described 49 knees in which this synovial layer became inflamed or scarred and caused symptoms of swelling, snapping, or instability. The *medial patellar plica* lies along the medial wall of the joint, originating near the suprapatellar plica and coursing obliquely downward to attach distally to the synovial membrane covering the infrapatellar fat pad (Fig. 11.40).

A suprapatellar or medial patellar plica slides over the femoral condyles during flexion and extension of

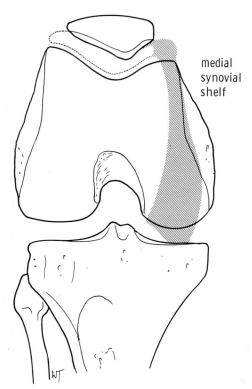

Fig. 11.40. Of the various folds or plicae projecting into the synovial cavity, it is the medial patellar plica that is most often the cause of symptoms.

the knee and may become inflamed during strenuous exercise. Alternatively, symptoms may follow blunt trauma to the front of the knee. Symptoms are often indistinguishable from those arising from other patellar disorders. According to Hardaker et al.,[62] effusion is an inconstant finding; some patients have tenderness over the irritated femoral condyle, while others have tenderness just medial or lateral to the superior pole of the patella. A symptomatic medial patellar plica can often be palpated as a tender band-like structure paralleling the medial border of the patella, and a palpable snap is often present when the knee is moved. In their series of 61 knees, a medial suprapatellar plica was found in 22, and a lateral suprapatellar plica in 13. Five knees had a suprapatellar plica with both lateral and medial components and six had a transverse suprapatellar plica spanning the entire pouch. The remaining 15 knees had a medial patellar plica. In 37 knees, synovitis and erosion of cartilage could be demonstrated and chondromalacia patellae was present in 35 knees.

Recognition of a symptomatic plica[110] is a comparatively recent event largely due to the increasing use of arthroscopy. Also, as the plica is often found in association with other internal derangements, it is perhaps too soon to assess its true pathologic significance.

USUALLY NORMAL CARTILAGE

PERIPATELLAR CAUSES: BURSITIS AND TENDINITIS

Bursitis

Numerous bursae are described around the knee that, under certain circumstances, can become infected or inflamed (Fig. 11.41). The prepatellar bursa is subcutaneous and present in most people. It usually covers the lower half of the patella and the upper half of the patellar ligament. Because it becomes chronically inflamed in those whose occupation involves much kneeling, inflammation of this bursa has been known as housemaid's knee. It is seldom difficult to recognize. The infrapatellar bursa lies between the lower part of the patellar ligament and the upper part of the tuberosity of the tibia. It is small and separated from the synovial membrane of the knee by the fat pad. The pain, tenderness, and swelling lo-

Fig. 11.41. Bursae around the knee that commonly become inflamed.

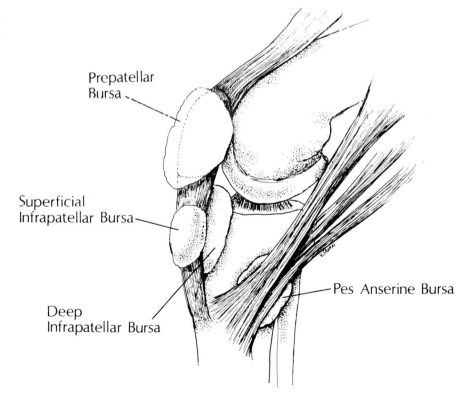

calized in this region are usually distinctive. Pes anserinus bursitis is overdiagnosed; the pain is often attributable to other causes (e.g., medial meniscal tears, degenerative arthritis, or osteonecrosis).

Tendinitis

Traction epophysitis of the patella is well established (Sinding-Larsen),[121] and a similar condition may effect the lower pole of the patella in athletes in the absence of radiographic evidence (jumper's knee). Both conditions can be recognized by localized point tenderness at the lower pole of the patella. Sometimes a similar condition affects the quadriceps tendon insertion at the upper pole of the patella. There may be local swelling and tenderness. Usually this is encountered, as the name suggests, in athletes who subject the extensor apparatus to excessive strain. Apart from the radiographically visible lesion at the lower pole of the patella, which may result in elongation of the lower pole, or even the formation of a separate ossicle, the pathology of this condition is unknown. Smillie[122] refers to it as tennis elbow of the knee.

Apart from these conditions, peripatellar tendinitis is an ill-defined diagnosis that should be used with caution in the absence of clear objective evidence.

In *lesions of the fat pad*,[70] according to Smillie,[122] the condition is primarily an enlargement of the fat pad. This may be caused by (1) trauma in the form of a direct injury, such as by the dashboard of a car; (2) edema in the premenstrual water-retention syndrome; (3) space-occupying lesions, such as a bucket-handle tear of the medial meniscus; and (4) recurvatum of the knee.

Enlargement of the fat pad results in synovial lesions with surface hemorrhages. There is swelling on either side of the patellar tendon as compared with the opposite side, particularly prominence occurring between the patellar tendon and iliotibial band. There is vague tenderness to deep pressure on the patellar tendon. Fat pad lesions are said to be most common in the female.

As with plicae, fat pad lesions have not been universally recognized as a frequent cause of anterior knee pain. Occasional cases that have indisputable pathologic significance are encountered, however. These include several cases of calcified hematoma and ossifying chondroma and a synovioma. In the latter case the synovioma had almost completely replaced

the fat pad and had been perforated during a diagnostic arthroscopy, but the lesion was not discovered until an arthrotomy was performed at a later date.

Overuse Syndromes

Even in structurally normal knees, habitual overloading caused by activity may cause pain, perhaps by causing microfractures in the subchondral bone.

The patellae studied by Darracott and Vernon-Roberts[35] showed diffuse or focal osteoporosis; nodular aggregates of trabecular bone termed bird's nest were found often at the margin of focal porosis. These aggregates could represent healing stress fractures, although the authors themselves did not think so. These patellae were excised from patients in the Royal Air Force with a clinical diagnosis of chondromalacia patellae. Further clinical details are not available but, as the overlying articular cartilage was virtually normal in all cases, perhaps these patients had an overuse syndrome or possibly a sympathetic dystrophy, as these investigators considered the changes suggestive of a derangement of the blood supply.

Overuse syndromes are usually related to occupation or athletics and the cause can often be readily identified (e.g., the association of patellar pain and jogging).

Overuse or occupational use syndromes are very common in one form or another, particularly in middle-aged persons when there may be early degenerative changes in the joint as well. In such cases the association with activity may not be as clear cut as in others because symptoms may persist after the initiating cause has passed. The same is true when excessive activity or stress precipitates symptoms in a younger patient with malalignment. A careful history and a cautious therapeutic approach will usually avoid misdiagnosis and possible ill-advised surgery.

SYMPATHETIC DYSTROPHY

Protracted patellar pain may follow minor injury. When the symptoms seem quite out of proportion to the lack of severity of injury, or when recovery after an uneventful operation is unduly delayed, reflex sympathetic dystrophy[38] should be considered.

Causalgia associated with peripheral nerve injuries, the painful phantom limb, Sudek's atrophy, and the shoulder–hand syndrome are well recognized if not well understood. These conditions are all characterized by burning or aching pain associated with trophic and vasomotor changes. The recognition of a similar syndrome in the knee joint can be attributed to the work of Ficat and Hungerford.[47]

Although the manifestations are protean and minor degrees of the condition very difficult to recognize, a typical case will show the following features:

1. *Intense pain:* Often described as burning or aching, such pain is out of proportion to any possible cause and often to the physical signs themselves. The joint is usually hypersensitive and for this reason examination is often difficult. The patient may complain of the pressure of bedclothes or clothing; even light touch on the skin provokes a reaction. For this reason when the knee bears a scar, a neuroma may be suspected.

2. *Stiffness:* Some loss of motion is the rule and may range from restriction of terminal extension or flexion to an almost complete ankylosis. There is often induration and thickening of the capsular tissues, which may extend into the thigh. In long-standing cases severe muscle atrophy is present.

3. *Vasomotor changes:* The skin of the region has a blotchy discoloration and is cold to the touch; there may be loss of hair. Radiologically the most striking feature is decalcification, which is most severe in or even restricted to the patella. In minor degrees of the condition it is important to obtain comparative views of the opposite knee. The skyline view is the most informative in this respect.

There is a tendency to regard this condition as psychogenically determined; indeed, many patients appear tense, anxious, and introspective. Whatever the truth, it is generally agreed that there is an autonomic disturbance with possible precapillary arterial venous shunting in the skin and reflex dilation of the intraosseous vascular bed leading to capillary stasis.

According to Ficat and Hungerford,[47] investigations include scintimetry, intramedullary pressure measurements, intraosseous phlebography, core biopsy, and thermography.

Scintigraphy is characterized by a marked increase in uptake; when this is not the case, a diagnosis of sympathetic dystrophy should be abandoned. *Thermography* is useful in documenting a vasodilator disorder and is helpful in distinguishing between a functional and an organic disorder.

The *intramedullary pressure* is usually elevated and *intraosseous phlebography* shows intramedullary stasis. Ficat and Hungerford[47] described difficulties in obtaining a good specimen by *core biopsy*; however, the usual finding was dilatation of the sinusoids, focal hemorrhage, and fibrosis, with a trabecular necrosis in some cases. They point out the similarity at both hemodynamic and cellular levels between sympathetic dystrophy and osteonecrosis.

Sympathetic ganglionic block with a local anesthetic will confirm the diagnosis in some cases by giving transient relief of pain.

Reflex sympathetic dystrophy in various forms is probably not that rare and, as with other conditions, is diagnosed more frequently with increased awareness of its existence. Although the results of treatment may be disappointing, recognition of the entity is of the utmost importance because the risk of therapeutic misdirection is great. Many of these patients have multiple operations on the assumption that the disorder is the result of mechanistic causes. Often in retrospect the original operation itself may seem suspect (e.g., removal of a hypermobile meniscus), and after each successive surgical procedure the patient's condition becomes worse.

PATELLAR ANOMALIES

A variety of congenital anomalies may be encountered, the most common of which are the bipartite and tripartite patellae.[6] According to Smillie,[122] the abnormality is not necessarily bilateral or symmetrical. The usual site for anomalous ossification is the superolateral pole of the patella. Occasional cases of sagittal or coronal reduplication of the patella have been reported, usually in patients with multiple epiphyseal dysplasia (Fig. 11.42).

The bipartite patella needs to be differentiated from a traumatic separation caused by a fracture; when the condition is bilateral, this distinction is not difficult (Fig. 11.43). Bipartite patellae are usually asymptomatic, but occasionally the movement of one fragment against the other causes pain that is relieved by excision of the ossicle.

Congenital absence of the patella[11] is extremely rare and is usually associated with the nail patellar syndrome (hereditary onycho-osteodysplasia),[40] in which knee symptoms may be the presenting complaint.

Fig. 11.42. A bipartite patella is usually bilateral. When there is a history of trauma, as in this case, it is difficult to distinguish a bipartite patella from a fracture.

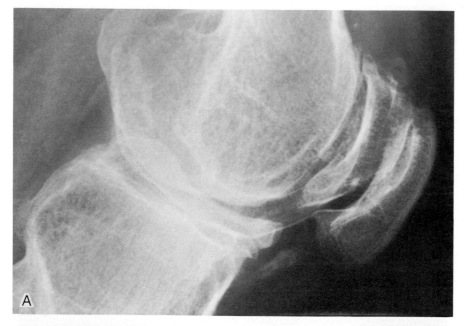

Fig. 11.43. (A,B) Sagittal reduplication of the patella.

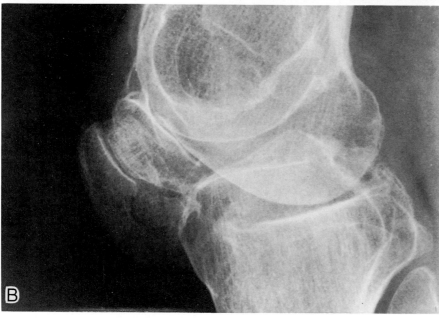

TREATMENT OF PATELLAR DISORDERS

Because of the significant differences in the response and in the method of treatment selected, it is not enough to simply identify a patellar disorder. The patient must also be categorized into the appropriate subgroup.

CONSERVATIVE TREATMENT

Although the response may vary according to the type of patellar syndrome involved, it is customary to recommend certain measures in the initial management of patients with patellar pain.

USUALLY HELPFUL

Activity

Rest is initially necessary when the syndrome is of acute onset, and particularly when there is effusion or hemarthrosis. A large effusion should be aspirated for diagnostic reasons and to make the patient more comfortable. Splinting may be necessary but should be for as short a time as possible to prevent muscle atrophy.

In subacute or chronic syndromes, when the patellar pain is clearly related to specific activity (such as running), either the elimination or the alteration of this activity can normally be expected to produce an improvement. The use of orthotics in runners has become popular and may be helpful to these patients. Activity change in the malalignment syndromes is much less helpful and the activity level can usually be left to the discretion of the patient, for there is little evidence that activity has any long-term harmful effects. Prohibiting normal physical activity in adolescent patients runs the risk of introducing unhealthy psychological elements and producing mental cripples. Clearly, common sense dictates that in some cases very strenuous sports should be avoided, but in general the less deviation there is from normal routine the better it is for the patient.

Exercises

An exercise program is recommended, taking care to avoid exacerbation of patellar pain. This usually means performing muscle-strengthening exercises with the knee in extension. Selective strengthening of the vastus medialis would seem desirable as this portion of the quadriceps muscle influences patellar tracking;[96] however, in practice this is difficult to achieve. Weight-lifting from the flexed position is usually contraindicated and, if done at all, must be attempted with extreme caution, moving the knee against resistance only so long as pain is not felt.

It is our experience that symptoms secondary to patellofemoral arthrosis respond best to exercise. A simple program of straight leg raising without weights done several hundred times a day often produces a dramatic improvement that may be continued indefinitely, particularly if the exercise program is maintained on a regular basis. The response to exercises in patients with a malalignment syndrome is less certain, and often no definite benefit is apparent.

Normally a physical therapist is not helpful, as quadriceps development can only be improved by active exercise. The exception is in patients with sympathetic dystrophy who require much encouragement in addition to other modalities, such as heat and cold, whirlpool baths, and transcutaneous electrical stimulation, which may be helpful. When the knee is stiff, active assisted exercises are needed. In some cases manipulation under anesthesia will be required but should be deferred as long as progress by more gentle means is being made. Sympathetic ganglion blocks with a local anesthetic may be helpful therapeutically but the beneficial effect is often dishearteningly brief.

Knee Braces

In malalignment syndromes an elastic patellar cutout brace with appropriate padding placed in a horseshoe fashion around the sides and upper pole of the patella is particularly helpful not only for improving stability but also for relief of pain. There is some objection to braces of this kind because of possible muscle atrophy but this has never seemed a problem to us particularly when the patient pursues a continuing exercise program.

Patellar bracing is less effective when used for patellar disorders not associated with malalignment, although it may be worth trying for patellofemoral osteoarthritis.

Anti-inflammatory Agents

Prolonged aspirin therapy[31] over a period of months has been recommended because of an inhibiting action against degradative enzymes such as cathepsins, which may play a part in the development of chondromalacia. Simmons and Chrisman[120] have shown that after the production of experimental chondromalacia in rabbits by scarification, moderate levels of salicylates had a definite protective effect against fibrillation. However, once fibrillation was established, the effect of salicylates was not marked. Chrisman et al.[31] also believe that salicylates may have an effect clinically in preventing the development of chondromalacia. In a small group of patients with recurrent dislocation of the patella, these workers found that chondromalacia was less pronounced in those treated preoperatively with aspirin.[31] However, the numbers were small and the findings inconclusive; our experience has been that aspirin is of doubtful value other than for its known analgesic properties.

Aspirin and other anti-inflammatory agents are most likely to be helpful in osteoarthritis and for peripatellar causes such as plicae. Their value is dubious in malalignment syndromes probably because the pain mechanism is not directly related to inflammation or cartilage degeneration.

Orthotics

Various kinds of orthotics designed to improve foot posture may be helpful for certain athletes and runners but are not appropriate for other conditions.

Not Advised

The use of plaster casts and splints is not recommended because of the rapid muscle atrophy produced. One of the objectives of treatment is to preserve good muscle tone; immobilization, except after acute injury, has no place in the management of patellar pain. The use of crutches is to a lesser degree open to the same objection and is rarely indicated.

Intra-articular injections with steroids may be helpful for patellofemoral arthritis, and judicious use in older patients is acceptable. However, steroid injections are to be condemned in the young and in athletes. In any event, they are ineffective in the malalignment syndromes.

SURGICAL TREATMENT

INDICATIONS

The indications for surgical treatment vary according to the etiology of the patellar disorder. In general, surgery gives the best results in malalignment syndromes and for the removal of loose bodies and is the least desirable alternative for other causes.

In the event that conservative management fails to give relief, the patient must consider tolerating and adjusting to the symptoms. It is widely believed that in younger patients pain eventually remits, but perhaps it is nearer the truth to state that most patients do not become progressively worse and in time find a certain level of pain acceptable in their daily lives. Be this as it may, it is certainly wise to postpone consideration of surgery until conservative measures have been tried for at least 6 months. In fact, most surgical patients will usually have had complaints for much longer than this and of an intensity that cannot be tolerated indefinitely. Aside from these generalities, more precise indications for surgery are difficult to define. It should also be borne in mind that whereas surgery is usually successful treatment for malalignment, the results are not nearly as good when patellar pain is attributable to other causes. Surgery is contraindicated for overuse syndromes and sympathetic dystropy. Finally, an operation should not be considered with the sole objective of returning the patient to sports. Instead, athletic activity should be discontinued; when this measure is sufficient to relieve symptoms, the situation must be accepted. In regard to recurrent dislocation of the patella, it has been said that surgery is indicated after the second dislocation, in part to prevent the development of osteoarthritis. This recommendation is unduly aggressive, as recent studies[34,61] have shown that late osteoarthritis is not inevitable and that certain techniques of patellar realignment may hasten rather than retard the development of patellofemoral degeneration.

MALALIGNMENT SYNDROMES AND PATELLAR INCONGRUENCE

There must be objective evidence of malalignment (an increased quadriceps angle, patella alta, lateral patellar tracking, or patellofemoral incongruence). Sometimes incongruence is observed in the absence of abnormal anatomy (e.g., when there is severe atrophy of the vastus medialis after a medial meniscectomy). The surgical approaches are therefore aimed at correcting patellar incongruence. Although multitudinous realignment procedures have been described, they may be classified into three basic groups: (1) lateral release of the patellar retinaculum and vastus lateralis, (2) proximal realignment, and (3) distal

Disorders of the Patella

realignment. A lateral release is common to most realignment techniques, and some workers recommend a combination of proximal and distal realignment.

LATERAL RETINACULAR RELEASE

The indications for an isolated lateral release are well defined by Merchant and Mercer,[104] "That group of patients with limiting patellar symptoms for whom a total surgical realignment is not justified or must be delayed." Ficat et al.[46] also recommend a lateral release for patients with established lateral facet patellofemoral arthritis.

Technique

The operation is performed through a 3-cm vertical lateral parapatellar incision centered on the upper pole of the patella. By dissecting skin flaps, the entire lateral retinaculum and the lower fibers of vastus lateralis can be visualized. The operation may also be per-

formed arthroscopically, that is, through a stab incision monitored intra-articularly by the arthroscope. As the arthroscopic method does not permit hemostasis of the important lateral retinacular vessels, infiltration with epinephrine is desirable to minimize bleeding. The open lateral release avoids opening the synovium (the patella may be inspected arthroscopically beforehand).

Ficat et al.[46] recommend careful inspection of the lateral retinaculum noting thickness, texture, and fiber direction, as well as abnormal fascia lata fibers. Abnormal insertion of the vastus lateralis should also be sought. The lateral retinaculum is divided longitudinally 1 to 2 cm from the patellar border, extending distally to the tibial tubercle and proximally into the lower fibers of vastus lateralis (Fig. 11.44A). The synovium should not be opened as a routine unless there are fibrous bands intimately adherent to it that cannot be freed without entering the joint. The synovium is most likely to be perforated anterosuperiorly, but when this happens, it is of no great consequence. Ceder and Larson[26] describe a Z-plasty lateral retin-

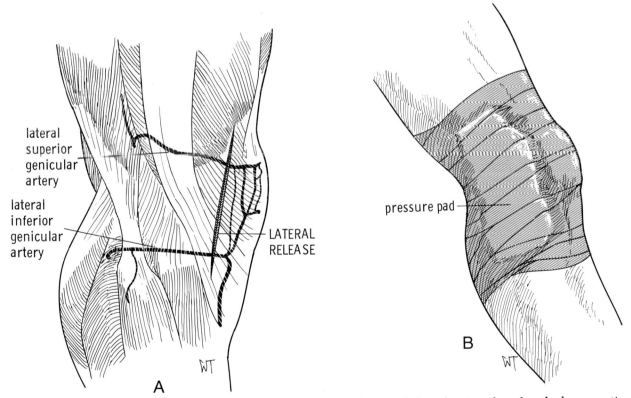

Fig. 11.44. (A) To be effective, lateral retinacular release must divide not only lateral retinaculum, but the lower portion of vastus lateralis as well. Inevitably, branches from the superior and inferior lateral genicular arteries are divided. (B) When the lateral release is done blind, a lateral pressure pad must be applied to control bleeding.

acular release designed to prevent synovial herniation. The superficial longitudinal fibers are incised vertically down to the deeper transverse fibers of the retinaculum. The superficial fibers are dissected free of the deeper layer in a posterior direction. The deeper fibers are then incised down to synovium and sharply elevated anteriorly from the synovium. Closure is by approximation of the posterior cut edge of the superficial layer to the anterior cut edge of the deep layer, which effects a lengthening of 1 to 3 cm. It seems questionable whether this refinement is worthwhile, as synovial herniation has not been observed by us. Conversely, Ficat[46] recommends excising 5 to 10 mm of the retinaculum to prevent reformation and scarring.

After the release, the tourniquet is deflated to allow coagulation of the major vessels. When the wound is closed, a bulky compression dressing is applied for a period of 1 to 2 days. The dressing is then removed and active motion is begun to prevent readherence of the divided lateral capsule. Alternatively, when performed by the arthroscopic technique, a lateral pressure pad is applied over the retinacular vessels; the pad is not removed for 1 week to 10 days, and the knee is exercised with it in place (Fig. 11.44B). Full activity is regained in 2 to 3 weeks regardless of the method used.

Results

Merchant and Mercer[104] reported the results of 20 lateral releases in 16 patients; seven were excellent, 10 good, and three poor. The best results were in five patients with a clinical history of dislocation or subluxation and radiologic evidence of patellar subluxation (Fig. 11.45A,B). All five had an excellent result and also showed a significant improvement of patellar alignment in the axial view. The worst group were those patients who had only pain without history of subluxation and no radiologic evidence of patella alta or lateral subluxation. Of the six knees in this category, there were one excellent, two good, and three poor results. The only complication reported was a bloody effusion 5 days after surgery.

Ceder and Larson[26] gave the results of 64 operations with a follow-up ranging from 1 to 43 months. The results were excellent in 26 knees, good in 26, fair in seven, and poor in five knees. These workers concluded that there is no specific symptom complex or physical or radiographic finding that delineates the patient who will benefit from an isolated lateral retinacular release.

Ficat[47] gives the result of 174 operated cases followed for at least 6 months. Seventy-six percent were excellent and good, and he concluded that those patients with stage 1 cartilage lesions tended to do better.

The Hospital for Special Surgery experience with lateral release has been less sanguine. The indications were those described by Merchant and Mercer[104] and, as in their series, most were under 20 years of age. Of 30 knees operated on, 20 had a follow-up of more than 2 years. Fifty percent were satisfactory, and in seven knees a subsequent proximal realignment was done (satisfactory in six). We agree with Merchant and Mercer that patients with subluxation do better than those with pain and, like Ceder and Larson,[26] we found the condition of the articular cartilage of no prognostic value.

Lateral release is a simple procedure and the temptation to overuse the operation must be resisted. The proportion of satisfactory results will clearly be higher when spontaneous improvement without surgery might have occurred.

PROXIMAL REALIGNMENT

Proximal realignment is in fact a rearrangement of the muscular attachments to the patella, and its purpose is to alter the line of pull of the quadriceps muscle. The quadriceps angle is not altered, nor is the length of the patellar tendon, but the realignment corrects the adverse affect of patellofemoral incongruence. The method can be applied both for patellar pain and patellar dislocation. It is a more major procedure than lateral release and is indicated only after a protracted period of conservative management.

Surgical Technique

The operation is done under tourniquet after exsanguinating the limb, either by elevation or with a bandage (Fig. 11.46A–E).[77,80] A midline skin incision is made extending proximally from the tibial tubercle for a distance of approximately 6 inches (15 cm). The skin edges are undermined sufficiently to expose the patella and quadriceps expansion; the incision should

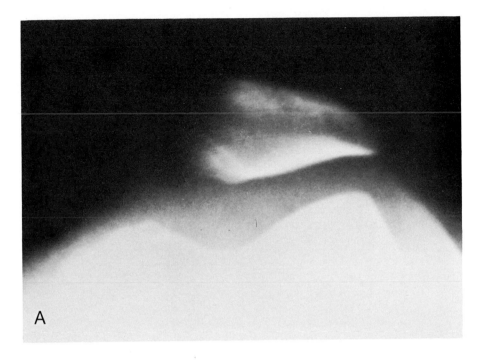

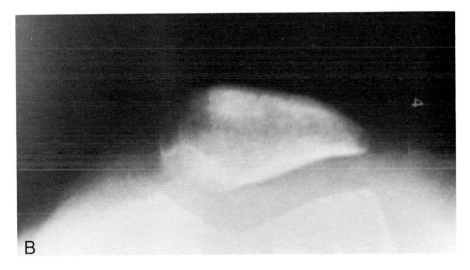

Fig. 11.45. (A) Merchant view of a knee with lateral patellar tracking. (B) After lateral release congruence is improved.

be sufficiently extensive so that the components of the quadriceps tendon are clearly seen. Both the vastus medialis and vastus lateralis must be exposed, as well as the proximal extent of the quadriceps tendon and the insertion of the fibers from rectus femoris. Arthrotomy is performed by an incision beginning proximally at the apex of the quadriceps tendon and placed within the tendon close to the border of vastus medialis. The incision is continued distally to the pa-

tella and extended across the medial border of this bone and then distally medial to the patellar ligament.[75] The incision described is therefore almost straight. The fibers of the quadriceps expansion medial to the incision are dissected from the bone with a scalpel. Because of the vertical ridges on the anterior surface of the patella, this can present difficulty and should be done with deliberation and care so as to preserve the expansion intact without lacerations.

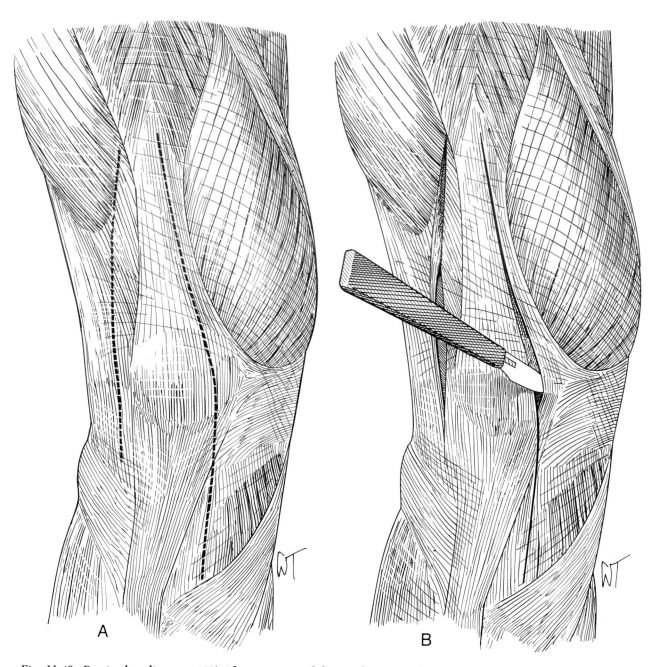

Fig. 11.46. Proximal realignment. (A) After exposure of the quadriceps mechanism, two incisions are made. The first enters the knee joint by a capsular incision placed at the margin of vastus medialis over the medial quarter of the patella and medial to the patellar tendon. The second is a lateral release extending into the fibers of vastus lateralis. (B) To preserve continuity of the medial flap the quadriceps expansion crossing the patella must be carefully preserved and separated by sharp dissection (Figure continues).

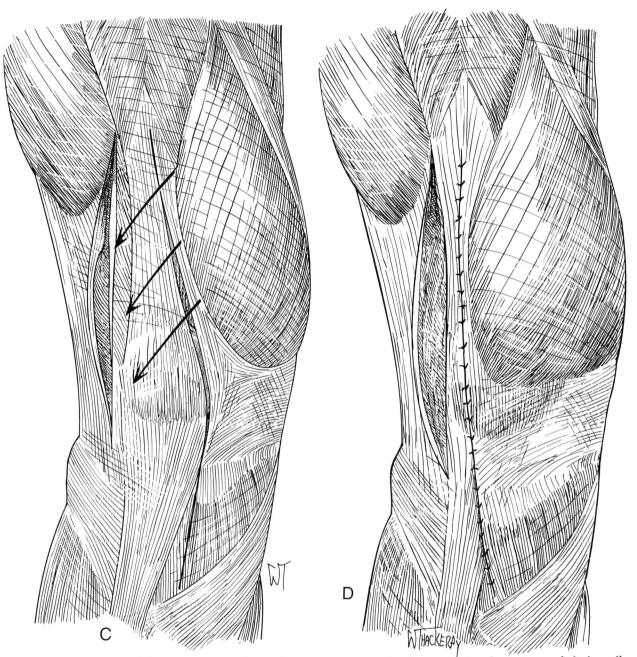

Fig. 11.46 (Continued). (C) Realignment is affected by advancing the medial flap containing the vastus medialis laterally and distally in the line of the fibers of the oblique portion of vastus medialis. (D) After suturing, the incision lies in a straight line across the front of the patella and the lateral release should open widely (Figure continues).

237

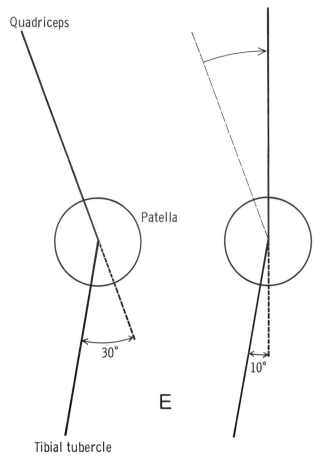

Quadriceps

Patella

30°

10°

E

Tibial tubercle

Fig. 11.46 (Continued) (E) The functional Q angle is thus decreased by altering the proximal limb (i.e., by changing the direction of pull of the quadriceps tendon). (From Insall, J.: Patellar pain syndromes and chondromalacia patellae. In Instructional course lectures. The American Academy of Orthopaedic. Surgeons. St. Louis, The C. V. Mosby Co., *30:* 342, 1981, with permission.)

This is necessary to obtain a secure closure when the quadriceps repair is completed. The fibers of the expansion can be easily separated from the bone if the dissection proceeds from above and below alternately thus forming a **V** and leaving the thinnest central part until last. When done in this manner, the central portion separates from the bone easily and can be fully preserved. Upon reaching the medial border of the patella, the synovial lining is incised; proceeding distally, the fat pad is divided in the line of the capsular incision until the patella can be everted for inspection of the joint.

A second capsular incision is now made on the lateral side beginning proximally in the fibers of vastus lateralis and extending distally to the tibial tubercle between 1 and 2 cm from the lateral border of the patella. It is desirable, but not essential, to maintain the integrity of the synovium. Sometimes this is not possible because of fibrous bands that appear to be in the substance of the synovium itself, and if holes are made no harm is done. A number of substantial vessels cross to the patella in the lateral retinaculum. There is a group of two or three vessels at the level of the upper pole of the patella that are usually the largest and that bleed profusely if not coagulated or ligated. A second group of rather smaller vessels runs beneath the retinaculum more distally at the lower pole of the patella, usually one or two in number. These also should be identified and coagulated.

The interior of the knee is thoroughly explored, and a selective debridement is done when necessary (see section on debridement). In the malalignment syndromes, regardless of the extent of the patellar lesions, the femoral sulcus is usually normal. (The exception is occasional evidence of an osteochondral fracture at the lateral border of the femoral sulcus caused by a patellar dislocation.) In older patients erosive changes may be seen in the sulcus (together with a similar lesion on the patella itself), and these should be characterized as degenerative arthritis. Usually some other type of surgical management is more appropriate than realignment.

The Quadriceps Reconstruction. At this stage of the operation, the tourniquet should be released to enable any bleeding points not previously identified to be coagulated. The tourniquet is reinflated and a thorough irrigation performed. The quadriceps must then be reconstructed in such a manner that the subsequent line of pull will be in a more medial direction (Fig. 11.46E). This is the purpose of the operative procedure and, by altering the direction of quadriceps action, patellar congruence is restored and patellar instability prevented. The first suture is placed in such a manner that the most distal part of the vastus medialis is brought laterally and distally overlapping the upper pole of the patella and adjoining quadriceps tendon. Before performing the overlap, the synovium should be removed from the deep surface of the medial flap which includes the vastus medialis, the medial part of the quadriceps expansion, and distally the medial capsule of the knee. The amount of overlap that can be achieved depends on the preoperative laxity of the tissues. In some knees the vastus medialis will be sutured as far across as the lateral border of the patella, but the more usual amount of overlap is 10 to 15 mm. A second suture is inserted at the lower pole of the patella, also bringing across the medial flap as tightly as the tissues will allow. The type of suture material used is not important and may be absorbable or nonabsorbable according to the surgeon's preference. The two initial sutures determine the remainder of the closure and, after placing them, the knee should flex to 90 degrees without the sutures breaking. The remaining closure is completed distally by suturing the flap as it lies and proximally with as much overlap of the vastus medialis over the quadriceps tendon as possible.

Occasionally in patients with recurrent dislocation and extreme lateral position of the patella, the medial flap is so stretched that overlapping to the lateral patellar border is still insufficient to hold the patella in the center of the femoral sulcus. In these circumstances, the medial flap including the vastus medialis should be everted and the free border rolled back on itself; a series of sutures are inserted so that in effect a tuck is made in the muscle. The reefed vastus medialis and quadriceps expansion are sutured anterior to the patella and quadriceps tendon. The tuck must be sufficient to keep the patella centralized. The resulting bulk of muscle and capsule lying anterior to the patella may appear esthetically unpleasing, but the tissue atrophies rapidly so that within a few weeks the enlargement will have disappeared.

Two features of the repair should be emphasized. First, the lateral incision into vastus lateralis must extend proximally almost as far as the medial incision. The most common error is a reluctance to make an adequate division of the vastus lateralis and, unless this is done, a proximal rearrangement of the quadriceps is not possible. It might be expected that extensive division of the muscle would cause quadriceps weakness, but in practice this has not been observed.

Second, the more distal part of the closure must be snug, but not excessively tight. In practice, it is almost impossible to overdo the overlapping in this area because this is prevented by soft-tissue tension and the anatomy of the femoral sulcus. Excessive tightness is revealed by observing the behavior of the patella when the knee is flexed.

After routine closure of the subcutaneous tissues and skin, a compression dressing is applied. A suction drain is not normally needed.

Aftercare

The patient is permitted to get out of bed on the second postoperative day and is allowed full weight-bearing as tolerated. Crutches are only needed for a few days, and the patient can go home within a week. The compression dressing is left in place for 2 full weeks, at which time the sutures are removed. Straight leg raises are then begun (if the quadriceps is not working by this time, side raises are done initially). Flexion is also allowed and encouraged; with normal progress, 90 degrees of flexion is reached 4 to 6 weeks after surgery, by which time the gait has returned to normal. Three hundred straight leg raises each day are done by the patient for several months. Often weights are avoided completely because they have not proved necessary to rehabilitate quadriceps strength and may provoke patellar pain if used too vigorously.

Results

Seventy-five proximal realignments performed between 1969 and 1979 for patellar pain and instability were recently studied.[125] Ten operations were bilateral. The procedures were done in 40 female and 25 male patients, and the average age was 20 years (range 13 to 32 years). Patients were selected for operation very carefully. All had extensor mechanism dysplasia and had serious complaints of pain or instability for a long time ranging from 1 to 5 years. All had lengthy conservative treatment. The symptoms were always severe enough to interfere with everyday activity, and not only with exercise or sports. Absence from school was a frequent problem in the younger patients.

Of the 75 knees, 36 had an increased quadriceps angle (at least 20 degrees), 21 had a high-riding patella (TP ratio 1.19 on average), and 18 had both conditions (quadriceps angle over 20 degrees, average TP ratio 1.23). Twenty knees had a preoperative Merchant view, and the findings for the sulcus angle and congruence angle were in accord with the measurements of Aglietti,[3] which have been previously described. Thus the ten knees with an increased quadriceps angle had an average sulcus angle of 138 degrees and an average congruence angle of 0 degrees. The six knees with a high-riding patella had a sulcus angle averaging 161 degrees and a congruence angle that averaged +25 degrees. The four knees with both variants had an average sulcus angle of 143 degrees and a congruence angle of +19 degrees.

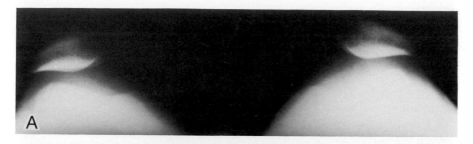

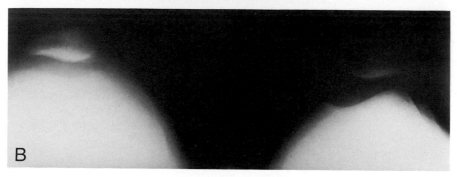

Fig. 11.47. (A) Radiograph showing marked patellofemoral incongruence bilaterally. (B) After proximal realignment of the right knee, the congruence angle on this side is now normal. The results of proximal realignment can be correlated with success in restoring patellofemoral congruence (see text).

The 75 knees were divided according to the primary symptoms into 40 knees with patellar pain (32 with increased quadriceps angle, three with a high-riding patella, and five with both), 29 knees with subluxation (18 with a high-riding patella, four with an increased quadriceps angle, and seven with both), and six knees with both pain and subluxation (all with increased quadriceps angle and a high-riding patella).

The findings at surgery for patellar surface lesions were normal or grade 1 in 76 percent, grade II in 12 percent, grade III in 4 percent, and grade IV in 8 percent of cases. Pain was moderate to severe in 32 of the 57 grade 1 lesions (56 percent), in seven of the nine grade II lesions (77 percent), in none of grade III lesions, and in four of the grade IV lesions (66 percent). Fourteen patellae were shaved at surgery and seven were shaved and drilled.

The grading system was similar to that described by Bentley.[10] At a follow-up ranging from 2 to 10 years and averaging 4 years, the results were as follows: excellent in 37 percent, good in 54 percent, fair in 5 percent, and poor in 4 percent. In stage 1 cartilage lesions, excellent and good results were obtained in 93 percent of cases. Excellent and good results were obtained in 100 percent of the stage II lesions, 33 percent of the stage III lesions, and 83 percent of the stage IV lesions. In the 21 knees in which the patella was shaved or drilled, 86 percent had a satisfactory result. Postoperatively only 14 patients could not participate in sports.

In 57 knees, a postoperative Merchant view was obtained. In the 52 satisfactory knees, the average congruence angle was −11 degrees (Fig. 11.47A,B). Thirty-five knees had a negative angle, five measured 0 degrees, and 12 had a positive congruence angle. Five knees were rated fair or poor, and in these the average congruence angle was 0 degrees. (Two knees had a positive congruence angle, two were 0, and one had a negative angle.) Naturally one must not put too much store in radiographic measurements of any kind, and some inconsistencies are to be expected. However, these findings suggested a trend in that correlation was shown between clinical improvement and correct alignment, whereas no such correlation existed with either the severity of chondromalacia or its treatment by patellar shaving.

Complications of proximal realignment were relatively few and minor. They included superficial phlebitis, hematoma, delayed wound healing, and culture negative drainage. Five knees required manipulation under general anesthesia to achieve a better range of motion. One subsequent patellectomy was performed because of persistent patellar pain.

DISTAL REALIGNMENT

Under this heading come all procedures in which the attachment of the patellar ligament to the tibial tubercle is detached and transferred in a medial and distal direction thereby reducing the quadriceps angle and to some extent correcting patella alta.[39] Many variations exist and the precise technique may consist of removal of a block of bone that is then locked into a slot cut distally and medially,[64] or more simply, by removal of the ligament insertion together with a sliver of bone which is then reattached with staples.[72] The latter method not only is simpler but allows greater precision in placement. A lateral release and sometimes an advancement of the vastus medialis obliquus are usually combined with a distal transfer.

Of the many variations that exist, two techniques that appear to have particular merit will be described.

PROXIMAL AND DISTAL RECONSTRUCTION[72]

Under tourniquet control, a lateral curved incision centered over the patella is made. Skin flaps are dissected to expose the medial and lateral aspects of the extensor mechanism. Release of the contracted lateral structures is first performed in a manner similar to that previously described. The release includes the vastus lateralis tendon. A medial parapatellar incision is next carried out above the patella and along the medial margin of the patellar tendon. The distal one-third of the fibers of the vastus medialis are released from the supramedial edge of the patella. An inspection of the entire joint is carried out, and lesions not related to the extensor mechanism are corrected.

In cases in which distal extensor mechanism reconstruction is indicated, particularly when the quadriceps angle is increased, the patellar tendon insertion is detached. An osteotome is placed in the infrapatellar bursa and directed distally so that the insertion is lifted with a thin wafer of bone. The deep surface of the patellar tendon is not detached from the fat pad. The soft tissues are next stripped from the tibia just medial to the original insertion and the cortex is fish-scaled. The patellar tendon is displaced a short distance medially, usually about 5 to 10 mm. With patella alta, it is also moved an appropriate distance distally so that 1 to 2 cm remain between the tibia and the lower pole of the patella (Fig. 11.48A,B). A medium-size staple is used to fix the patellar tendon through a full range of motion in order to ensure that this insertion is correct.

Chondromalacia of the patella is managed by superficial shaving or by full-thickness chondrectomy. Sclerotic subchondral bone is drilled.

The tourniquet is deflated and hemostasis is secured. The vastus medialis obliquus is advanced pulling the muscle directly in line with its fibers (Fig. 11.48C). The muscle should never be moved below the midpoint of the medial patellar edge. The advancement should be carried out with the knee flexed 45 degrees. The muscle is usually advanced only a few millimeters and is secured into the patella with a nonabsorbable suture. After every stitch or two, the knee is carried through a range of motion; if any abnormal motion of the patella can be observed, the sutures are removed to correct this, and the advancement is redone. Working proximally, the remainder of the vastus medialis is reattached onto the patella and quadriceps tendon. Below the starting point of the advancement, the medial capsule and retinaculum are not advanced but closed in a side-to-side fashion.

Aftercare

The knee is immobilized for 3 weeks, followed by active range of motion and physical therapy.

ELMSLIE-TRILLAT METHOD[42,126]

The preferred skin incision begins lateral parapatellar proximally and proceeding distally crosses the ligamentum patellae in a gentle curve ending toward the medial side (Fig. 11.49). After exposing the extensor mechanism, a lateral release is performed extending into the lower fibers of vastus lateralis. The lateral synovium may be opened and the joint explored through this route. The insertion of the patellar ligament is defined by making a second capsular incision medially. On the lateral side the incision used for the lateral release is extended distally. Using osteotomes, the insertion of the patellar ligament is partially separated together with a thin sliver of bone extending distally for 2 to 3 cm. At this level, a series of drill holes are made transversely. The proximal end of the tibial tubercle is now sufficiently mobile to allow a medial displacement of up to 1 cm pivoting at the distal base made more flexible by the drill holes. The tubercle is then fixed at its new and more medial site with a cancellous bone screw. Goutallier and Debeyre[56] have added an additional modification placing a bone graft taken locally beneath the medial edge of the transferred tubercle so that posterior displacement of the graft is prevented.

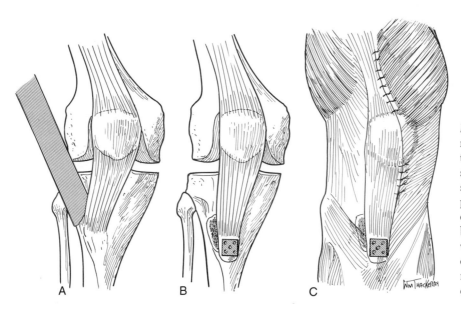

Fig. 11.48. Proximal and distal realignment by the Hughston technique. (A,B) The distal insertion of the patellar tendon is sometimes detached and displaced for a short distance medially and distally. Fixation is by a staple. (C) A careful advancement of vastus medialis is done, testing that the patella moves smoothly after placing each stitch.

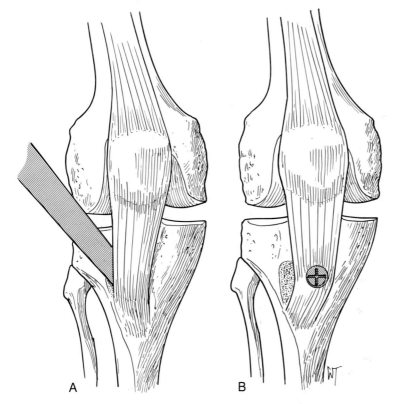

Fig. 11.49. The Elmslie-Trillat technique (see text). The distal periosteal attachments of the patellar ligament are undisturbed.

Aftercare

The knee is immobilized in extension for 2 weeks. At this time, provided secure fixation was obtained at surgery, an active range of motion is begun and rehabilitation exercises commenced.

Results of Distal Realignments

MacNab[98] gives the results in 33 operations followed for 6 months to 3 years. There were 22 excellent, six good, two fair, and two poor results, and one recurrence of dislocation. However, in 10 more cases, followed from 8 to 22 years after operation, there were no satisfactory results, four having a fair and six a poor rating. All these patients had clinical or radiographic evidence of osteoarthritis.

Heywood[68] used a combined subjective and objective grading similar to that of MacNab. He studied 53 knees and found a preponderance of good or excellent results even after 10 years. Overall, 71 percent were considered satisfactory; the major reasons for failure were pain, swelling, and tenderness, which came on gradually after operation in spite of the fact that the dislocations were relieved.

Heywood observed four cases of genu recurvatum when the operation was performed in children under the age of fourteen. MacNab also emphasized the danger of this operation before fusion of the epiphyses.

Hughston and Walsh[72] give their results of proximal and distal reconstruction in 96 patients with a range of follow-up from 2 to 21 years. Using very strict criteria, 21 were excellent, 47 good, 21 fair, and seven poor. Neither sex nor age affected the overall results. Only two patellectomies were later required.

Insall et al.[80] had 68 percent satisfactory results in 34 knees followed at least 2 years. This compared with 81 percent good or excellent results obtained by proximal realignment performed in 53 knees over the same period of time.

LATE OSTEOARTHRITIS

As shown by the preceding statistics, tibial tubercle transfer seems to be a satisfactory solution for the dislocating patella. It is unusual for the patella to dislocate again, and for the first few years after operation, most of the patients do well. However, follow-up for a longer period of time reveals a disturbing trend. The patients in whom osteoarthritis developed in MacNab's series have already been mentioned. He attributed this to the severity of chondromalacia that preexisted the surgery and suggested that it would be better if patellar realignment were carried out at an early stage of the disorder. Heywood was able to show that the incidence of osteoarthritis was related to the duration of the dislocations. He also felt that early operation was indicated and believed that the evidence showed adequate realignment would stop further degeneration.

Crosby and Insall,[34] in a retrospective study of the Hauser technique at The Hospital for Special Surgery, came to the opposite conclusion. Follow-up radiographs (average 7.3 years) after treatment by distal realignment were graded for osteoarthritic changes (Fig. 11.50). Nine knees showed no osteoarthritis, moderate changes were found in 19, and severe degeneration was present in three. By contrast, after an average follow-up of 19 years, radiographs of 23 untreated patients with recurrent dislocation showed very little evidence of osteoarthritis; in fact 22 showed no evidence of osteoarthritis at all and the one patient with severe changes had a dislocating patella for 54 years. These workers concluded that prevention of osteoarthritis should not be a reason for realignment of the unstable patella and believed that distal realignment may actually enhance the incidence of osteoarthritis.

Hampson and Hill[61] came to a similar conclusion after reviewing 44 knees surgically treated by a Hauser operation more than ten years previously. The average time from operation was 16 years, the range being from 10 to 25 years. At follow-up, 70 percent of the radiographs showed osteoarthritis. Moreover, the incidence was time related. One-half of the knees with a follow-up of less than 16 years showed osteoarthritis, whereas in those with a follow-up of more than 16 years, 18 of 20 knees were so affected. These investigators did not find the frequency of dislocation before operation to influence the long-term result.

In cross section, the shape of the upper tibia is roughly triangular and the patellar ligament is inserted into the apex. Transfer of the tibial tubercle medially is therefore of necessity also a posterior displacement (Fig. 11.51). Goutallier and Debeyre[56] observed that the effect of this adjustment would be to reduce the extensor moment arm and increase patellofemoral compression forces. This explanation prob-

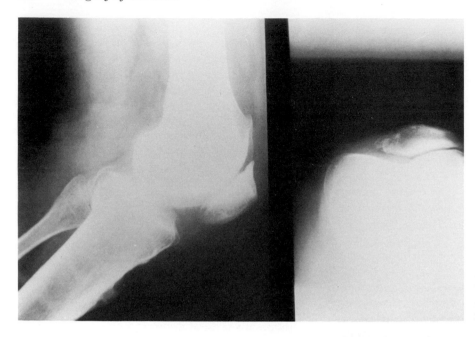

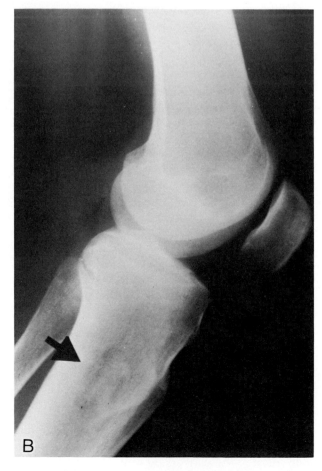

Fig. 11.50. Radiograph taken 10 years after a Hauser procedure. Although no further dislocations had occurred, the patient was now having symptoms attributable to osteoarthritis. (From Crosby, E. B., and Insall, J.: Recurrent dislocation of the patella. J. Bone Joint Surg. [Am.], *58:* 9, 1976, with permission.)

Fig. 11.51. Posterior displacement of the tibial tubercle must be avoided (see text). (A) Because of triangular shape of the tibia medial displacement is often posterior as well. (B) Radiograph showing posterior position.

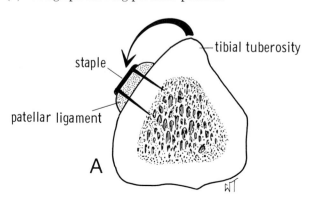

staple

tibial tuberosity

patellar ligament

A

B

ably accounts for the late osteoarthritic changes that occur after the Hauser operation. The techniques of Hughston and Elmslie-Trillat described above largely avoid this undesirable posterior shift, and the late results may therefore be better, although for the moment sufficient data on this point are lacking.

OTHER COMPLICATIONS OF TIBIAL TUBERCLE TRANSFER

Genu recurvatum may develop if a bone block is transferred in children less than 14 years old and corrective tibial osteotomy may be required. Distal migration of the tibial tubercle has been reported by MacNab, who suggests that this may result in a low patella. However, Fielding et al.[49] have demonstrated that distal migration resulting from growth can occur without affecting the ultimate patellar position.

Detachment of the patellar tendon may require reoperation. Chronic pain over the tibial tubercle has been noted after the transfer.

An anterior compartment syndrome after tibial tubercle transfer has been reported. This is apparently attributable to bleeding into the anterior myofascial space from minor arteries severed during the transfer, which then retract but continue to bleed.

Permanent loss of motion has also been recorded and sometimes manipulation is not successful in obtaining improvement.

CONCLUSIONS

The policy at The Hospital for Special Surgery is to perform proximal realignment in all cases as the initial operation; only when this operation fails should distal realignment be considered. When necessary our preferred technique is that of Hughston, moving the insertion distally to correct patella alta with only a few millimeters of medial displacement. Contrary to the deleterious effects of medial transfer, it has never been shown that distal transfer by itself is harmful, provided that the distal advancement is done moderately. The patella should not be pulled over the fat pad and thus excluded from normal articulation.

CHONDROPLASTY

In many cases of patellar malalignment, cartilage damage is found; most workers consider some degree of chondroplasty desirable in addition to realignment.

Wiles et al.[132] reported good results by excision of cartilage in 20 of 28 knees. Their follow-up was an average of 5.5 years. These workers found that (1) the amount of cartilage excised did not influence the end result, and (2) the poor results were evident early, within a few months of operation. Only one knee that initially did well subsequently deteriorated.

Chaklin[27] and Soto-Hall,[123] however, state that the best results are obtained in localized chondromalacia when only a limited excision of articular cartilage is carried out. Bentley[10] has recommended cartilage excision for lesions less than 13 mm in diameter, preferring patellectomy when the lesions are larger.

SHAVING VERSUS CARTILAGE EXCISION AND DRILLING

Wiles et al.[131] recommended shaving the cartilage with a scalpel, beveling the margin of healthy cartilage at the edge to leave a smooth surface. Bentley[10] found shaving unsatisfactory at all ages, in both sexes, and at all stages of the disease. He considered that shaving further damages the cartilage and alters the loading of the patellofemoral joint. An alternative to shaving is to excise the damaged cartilage completely and to drill the subchondral bone to encourage vascularization and a fibrocartilaginous repair. However, the fibrocartilage that does fill the defect may do so incompletely and have unsatisfactory functional properties. Animal experiments[116] and clinical experience have both shown regeneration to be unpredictable and often unsatisfactory. Insall et al.[80] found that in a series of 79 patients in which both methods were employed, the results were satisfactory in 84 percent when shaving was used and 60 percent when the cartilage was excised and drilled.

In fact, depending on the circumstance, both methods have an application. Our current recommendation is that the cartilage should be left untouched unless the expected result after shaving or repair cannot be worse than the surface that already exists. If in our judgment this is so, large areas of diffuse softening and fasciculation are conservatively smoothed by shaving so that protruding fronds and roughened areas are removed, without extensively exposing the subchondral bone. This type of shaving can be done with a knife or very conveniently by an arthroscopic shaver. The latter does not damage normal cartilage and thus readily trims shaggy tissue the required

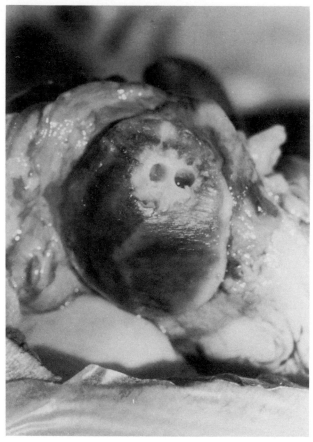

Fig. 11.52. Chondrectomy is suitable for circumscribed areas of damaged cartilage.

amount. Excision and drilling lends itself to sharply circumscribed lesions of small extent when circumstances are propitious for a good repair and shaving would extensively damage adjoining normal cartilage (Fig. 11.52). This type of lesion can be cored out leaving vertical edges; a few drill holes are placed in the base. Early motion during postoperative rehabilitation may improve the quality of the repair.[116]

PATELLAR PAIN CAUSED BY OTHER SYNDROMES

Surgery is not very satisfactory in the treatment of patellar pain caused by overuse, osteoarthritis, idiopathic cartilage degeneration, direct trauma, or other causes. For these other situations it is recommended that conservative treatment should be followed when-

ever possible, but when called for there are a number of surgical procedures to be considered, namely, debridement, tibial tubercle elevation, patellar replacement, and patellectomy.

DEBRIDEMENT

Debridement alone not associated with realignment has won a mixed reputation. Some investigators have reported success with the method, particularly when the subchondral bone is drilled (Fig. 11.53), while others have found the procedure both unpredictable and unreliable.[74] In the previous section, mention has already been made of the experience of Wiles et al.[131,132] and Bentley.[10] Pridie[111] suggested perforation of the subchondral bone plate to allow ingrowth of fibrous tissue. Ficat et al.[48] have recently carried this concept a stage further by performing what they term spongialization of exposed bone.

TECHNIQUE OF SPONGIALIZATION

A lateral parapatellar approach is used, elevating the posteroinferior border of vastus lateralis and dividing the lateral retinaculum.[48] This approach permits the patella to be tilted to expose the entire undersurface.

When the cartilage has lost all its functional value, the abnormal bone is circumscribed with a knife, leaving the edges of normal cartilage perpendicular to the surface. Degenerated cartilage is then detached from the subchondral bone. The bone is completely excised, either by making a series of drill holes and then removing the bridge between them with rongeur or by decorticating with a high-speed drill. When the cancellous bone surface is smooth, the wound is closed. The lateral retinaculum is left open after resecting about 1 cm so as to prevent reattachment by scarring.

Aftercare

A pressure dressing is applied. The patient is allowed to bear weight as tolerated, and movement is begun after the second postoperative day, depending on the state of the wound. After the third week, Ficat et al.[48] recommend jogging with very small steps as the best method of rehabilitating the quadriceps. They

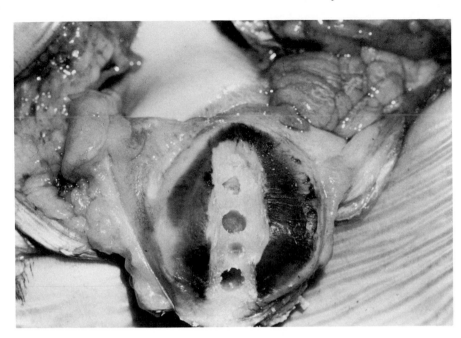

Fig. 11.53. Debridement and drilling of the patella after the method of Pridie.

believe that this small degree of flexion without resistance is an excellent means of improving the quality of regeneration.

Results

Ficat et al.[48] report on 85 patients of whom five also had an anterior advancement of the tibial tubercle. With a follow-up of 6 months to 3 years, 79 percent of the patients had a good or excellent result.

In this series four knees were reexplored and tissue was obtained for microscopy. The tissue was more cellular with less fibrous structure than normal cartilage, and the proteoglycans were less abundant.

A similar technique performed arthroscopically, termed "abrasion chondroplasty," is advocated by Johnson. In this method, the subchondral bone is removed with a mechanical burr; Johnson has demonstrated by repeat arthroscopy regeneration of a cartilage-like material over the abraded areas. He reports an impression that the results are good but has not so far offered a detailed follow-up.

The major indications for debridement are patellofemoral arthrosis and post-traumatic chondromalacia. The spongialization technique of Ficat seems an improvement on the Pridie operation, and particularly if his results can be duplicated using arthroscopic techniques, the operation will deserve greater consideration for the management of a most difficult clinical problem.

PATELLAR RESURFACING

McKeever[103] described a cobalt–chromium alloy (Vitallium) prosthesis for resurfacing the patella that was anatomic in shape having medial and lateral facets. The prosthesis was fixed to the bone with a transfixion screw and the patella was trimmed to fit the prosthesis (Fig. 11.54). McKeever reported generally good results in 40 knees. There were four failures attributable to infection, but no mechanical failures. DePalma et al.,[37] using McKeever's prosthesis, had a similar experience and gave results in 17 patients. Eight were rated excellent, six good, two fair, and one poor. However, Levitt[94] found that with longer follow-up, the results in the patients of DePalma et al. were not as satisfactory, although some patients remained pain free without evidence of progressive arthritis even after many years.

Encouraged by this report of such a satisfactory outcome in some patients, we were led to believe that the overall results might be helped by redesigning the shape of the prosthesis and improving fixation by the use of acrylic cement.

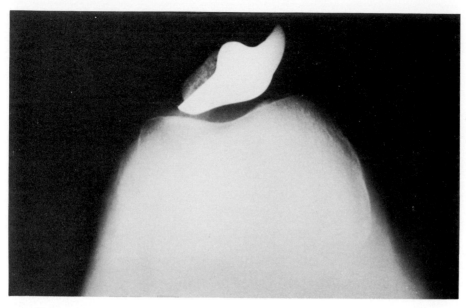

Fig. 11.54. The McKeever prosthesis was fixed with a screw. In spite of its anatomic shape, this prosthesis did not always fit as intended.

In 1973, a new cobalt–chromium patellar prosthesis[4] was designed at The Hospital for Special Surgery having a dome shape to the prosthetic articulating facet that obviated the need for special rotary alignment (Fig. 11.55). (Binding of the articular surfaces due to incorrect rotary fitting was thought to be a possible source of failure with the anatomic McKeever prosthesis.) The dome prosthesis was available in two sizes, and the anterior surface of the prosthesis had a stud for anchorage to the residual bone of the patella after excision of its articular facets.

Thirty-one patellar replacement operations using this prosthesis were done at The Hospital for Special Surgery between 1973 and 1976.[82] Two patients were lost to follow-up, and the remaining 29 knees (in 28 patients) were studied and reviewed. The diagnosis in 22 knees was patellofemoral osteoarthritis, in five knees chondromalacia patellae after patellar subluxation and realignment by the Hauser technique, and in two knees habitual dislocation with severe osteoarthritis. After a follow-up ranging from 3 to 6 years the results were excellent in two knees, good in 14, fair in three, and poor in 10 knees. The 10 poor results were all attributable to persistent pain, and in most cases the failure was evident within the first 6 months after surgery. In the osteoarthritic group, the results were better when there was no femorotibial involvement (67 percent satisfactory). Surprisingly, because the cartilage of the femoral sulcus was normal, the

five knees with patellar chondromalacia did not do better, but perhaps the abnormal patellar mechanics involving the previous tibial tubercle transfer adversely affected the result.

We have not completely given up this prosthesis and still use it in selected cases. We believe the indications are for (1) patellofemoral arthritis without evidence of femorotibial narrowing, and (2) young patients after failed patellar surgery. Unfortunately, most patients in this group have had a previous Hauser operation, and the patellofemoral mechanism has been permanently altered by medial and posterior displacement of the tibial tubercle. Patellar replacement is a hemiarthroplasty and the long-term results are consistent with the results of hemiarthroplasty in other joints. The cases of persistent pain no doubt arise partly from imperfect congruence between the implant and the opposing surface. One solution to this difficulty is to replace the femoral sulcus as well as the patella. Blazina et al.[13] recently reported on such a patellofemoral replacement, and their results seem slightly better than ours with replacement of the patella alone. However, a large number of their patients had secondary or revisionary procedures, and the follow-up time was relatively short. A major objection to complete patellofemoral replacement in younger patients is the extreme difficulty of salvage should the operation not succeed. In case of failure with patellar replacement alone, a patellectomy can be done and

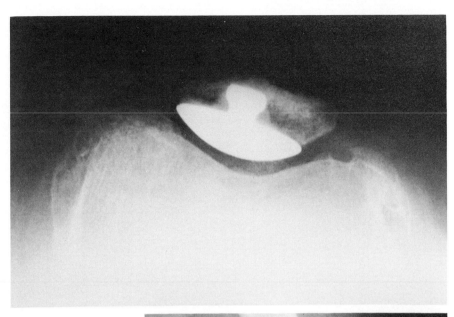

Fig. 11.55. The HSS dome prosthesis.

the patient is no worse than had patellectomy been the primary choice. On the other hand, patellectomy does not provide a solution after failure of patellofemoral replacement (Fig. 11.56), and revision is only possible by using a total knee prosthesis, clearly an unsatisfactory alternative in younger patients. For this reason, we think the concept of patellofemoral replacement is a bad one; it should not be used in younger patients, and in the elderly total knee arthroplasty gives better results than either patellofemoral replacement or patellectomy.

TIBIAL TUBERCLE ADVANCEMENT

Decompression of the patellofemoral joint by elevating the tibial tubercle was first proposed by Maquet,[99–101] who calculated that overall patellofemoral articular pressure is reduced by approximately one-half by a 2-cm anterior displacement of the tibial tubercle. Bandi and Brennwald[8] demonstrated in an experimental model a one-third reduction of patellofemoral force for a 10-mm anterior displacement. Ferguson et al.,[44] using miniature contact stress sensors embedded in the retropatellar cartilage, showed that progressive increase in tendon elevation caused progressive reduction in the contact stress. However, most of the contact stress relief occurred with a 12.5-mm tendon elevation and that further elevations were

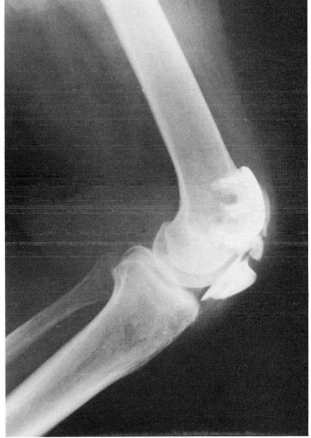

Fig. 11.56. With patellofemoral resurfacing, the polyethylene patella is likely to articulate with the femur at some point during movement. Salvage is extremely difficult.

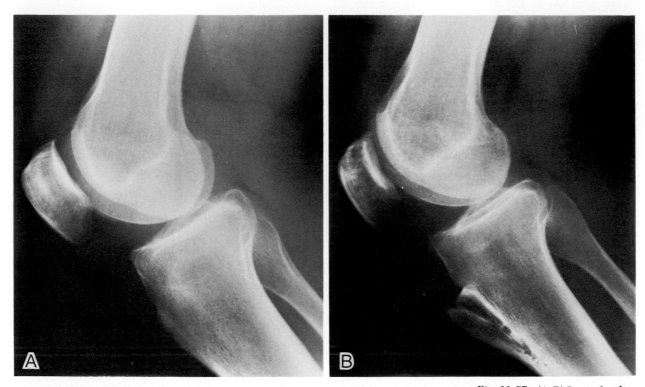

Fig. 11.57. (A,B) Lateral radiograph pre- and post-tibial tubercle elevation. Note vertical rotation of the patella and increased superior pole contact.

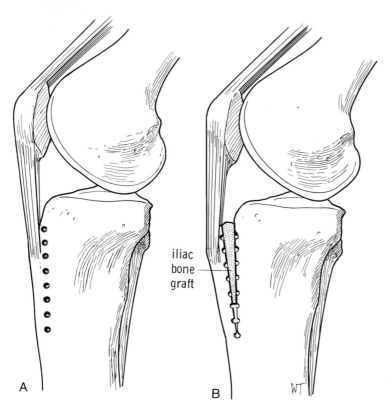

iliac
bone
graft

A   B

Fig. 11.58. The Maquet technique of elevating the tibial tubercle.

250

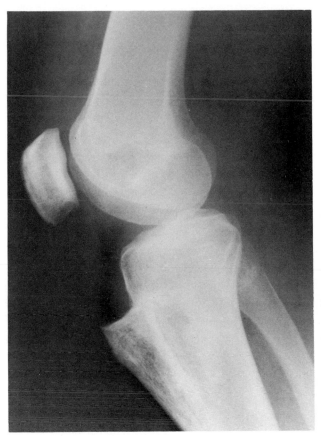

Fig. 11.59. Lateral radiograph showing correct position of the iliac graft which should be flush with the tip of the tubercle.

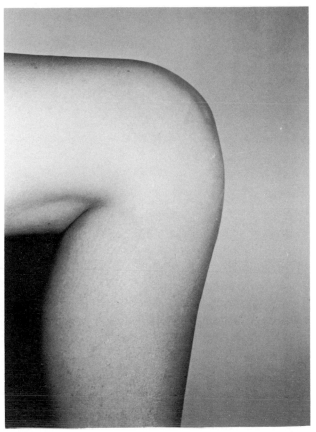

Fig. 11.60. The bump is not objectionable after a correctly performed Maquet procedure.

only marginally useful. In addition to reduction of overall contact stress, there was increased superior patellar pole contact caused by vertical rotation of the patella (Fig. 11.57A,B). As a result, the patellofemoral contact areas were altered so that the superior pole of the patella begins to make contact with the femoral sulcus at a smaller angle of flexion than would normally be the case.

Because Maquet and others have reported skin necrosis as a complication of large elevations of the tibial tubercle, Ferguson's recommendation of an optimal advancement of one-half inch (12.5 mm) seems appropriate.

Technique

A lateral parapatellar skin incision is made extending distally below the level of the tibial tubercle (Fig. 11.58). The extensor mechanism is exposed, and the joint is entered through a lateral parapatellar approach, dividing the lateral retinaculum and lower fibers of vastus lateralis. Appropriate debridement is carried out. The tibial tubercle is isolated by a second capsular incision placed medial to the patellar ligament and tubercle. An osteotomy is carried out with osteotomes, and the tibial tubercle and adjoining part of the tibial crest are split distally for a distance of 10 to 12 cm. Maquet[100,101] recommends that a series of drill holes be made first to outline the osteotomy: Bandi[7] makes a shorter osteotomy, using a single drill hole 3 cm below the tubercle to prevent extension of the osteotomy distally. The tibial tubercle is levered forward and held by a bone graft taken from the iliac crest. As the distal cortex is not broken, the graft is self-locking and is stable without internal fixation. The upper margin of the graft should extend slightly proximal to the tip of the tibial tubercle to prevent a fracture of the tip of the tubercle occurring later (Fig. 11.59). The skin is closed leaving the lateral retinaculum open. A pressure dressing is applied.

Aftercare

The knee is immobilized until wound healing has taken place, after which range of motion and rehabilitation exercises are begun. Weight-bearing is permitted as tolerated.

Results

Both Maquet[99] and Bandi[7] have reported good results in a small series of patients. Radin and Leach[112] observed a good result in 20 of 21 patients with patellofemoral arthrosis treated by the Maquet technique (Fig. 11.60).

At The Hospital for Special Surgery, 30 knees were studied after the procedure had been performed according to the Maquet technique.[114] The preoperative diagnosis was chondromalacia in 15 knees, patellofemoral arthrosis in 14 knees, and one case followed a patellectomy. The average age was 34 years (range: 16 to 38 years). The patients were followed from 1 to 5 years. Seventeen knees had various prior procedures, including five Hauser procedures and eight meniscectomies.

The initial amount of elevation of the tubercle averaged 1.75 cm, but some settling usually occurred, for an average elevation at the time of follow-up of 1.37 cm.

The operation was combined with tibial osteotomy in eight knees, proximal realignment in six knees, and patellectomy in four knees. In the remaining 12 knees, the tibial tubercle elevation was done as a solitary procedure.

There were a significant number of complications. Skin necrosis occurred in the region of the tibial tubercle in four knees, which in one case led to a subsequent deep infection, ultimately requiring debridement and skin grafting. A stress fracture through the tibial tubercle proximal to the graft occurred in three knees resulting in the formation of a separate small ossicle (Fig. 11.61A,B), and in all there was some residual tenderness and slight extension weakness. The ossicle was excised in one knee because of local tenderness. A fracture through the proximal tibia occurred in one case, an obese woman who fell 6 weeks after the operation. The fracture resulted in a nonunion that did not heal in spite of two bone-grafting procedures. There were two deep infections, one after skin necrosis.

Evaluation of the results was complicated by the varying etiologies and the additional procedures done at the same time as the tubercle elevation. However, these variables are also found in other comparable series for which the indication for the operation exists.

The major preoperative complaint was pain, and a subsidiary complaint in some cases was weakness and buckling. The success or failure of the procedure thus depended largely on relief of pain with the element of subjectivity that this always implies. Complications previously noted were not taken into account except in so far as they affected the end result at the time of review.

Because of the number of associated procedures, it was decided to evaluate the knees in two groups:
1. Tibial tubercle elevation alone (12 knees): Results were good in eight, fair in two, and poor in two knees.
2. Tibial tubercle elevation combined (18 knees): Results in this group were good in 10 knees, fair in seven knees, and poor in one knee.

From this it can be seen that about two-thirds of the patients gained satisfactory pain relief, whether the Maquet procedure was done by itself or combined with another operation. The remaining one-third were not improved, and three knees were actually worse. The poor rating in two knees was directly attributable to a complication; in one a persistent nonunion of a tibial fracture, and in the other an osteomyelitis following deep infection.

Our conclusion concerning the merits of the operation was that although the procedure did relieve pain in most cases, the significant number of serious complications and the unpredictability of the result must limit the indications to a few severely disabled cases.

TIBIAL TUBERCLE ELEVATION AFTER PATELLECTOMY

Kaufer[88,89] has shown that after patellectomy, full extension may require as much as a 30 percent increase in quadriceps force. Tibial tubercle elevation can lengthen the extension moment arm so that much

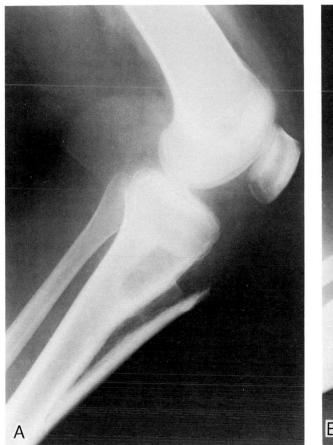
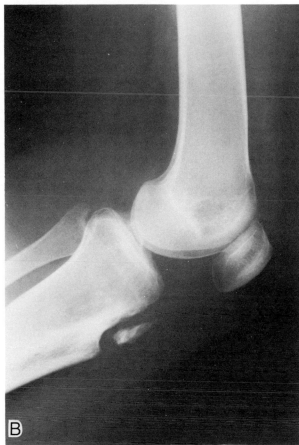

Fig. 11.61. (A) The bone graft was not sufficiently proximal. (B) The tip of the tibial tubercle fractured, forming a separate ossicle.

of the adverse affect of patellectomy is mitigated. Radin and Leach reported six good results in nine knees after a Maquet procedure had been done for a failed patellectomy. In the six patients with a good result, muscle strength increased significantly after the anterior displacement of the tibial tubercle.

PATELLECTOMY

Patellectomy has been the subject of controversy for many years. Brooke,[18] by means of a cadaver experiment, showed that excision of the patella actually improved the efficiency of the quadriceps muscle; Hey Groves[67] and Watson-Jones[127] subsequently supported this belief. More recently, the theoretical calculations of Maquet (Fig. 11.62) and experimental work by Haxton[65] have shown an important function in lengthening the quadriceps moment arm.[124] Kaufer[00] found that the force necessary to produce full extension after patellectomy was increased by 15 to 30 percent.

Clinical studies have been equally divergent in opinion. Scott[117] stated that only 5 percent of 101 cases considered that they had a normally functioning joint after patellectomy. DePalma and Flynn[36] found evidence of widespread degenerative arthritis after patellectomy in the knees of dogs.

Haliburton and Sullivan[60] found that 87 percent of patients with advanced degenerative joint disease were improved by patellectomy. West,[128] in a series of cases that included chondromalacia, osteoarthritis, comminuted fractures, and recurrent dislocation of the patella, found that 82 percent were satisfactory after

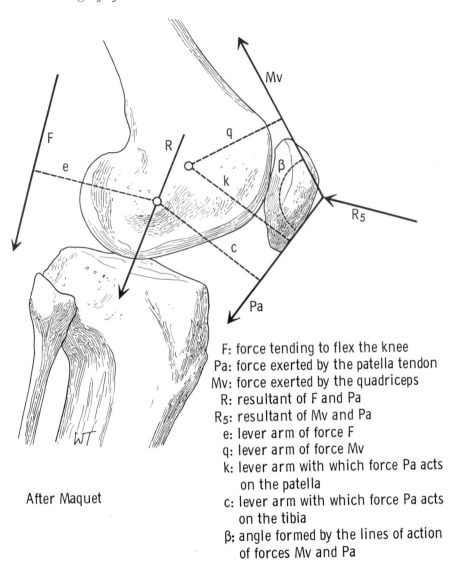

F: force tending to flex the knee
Pa: force exerted by the patella tendon
Mv: force exerted by the quadriceps
R: resultant of F and Pa
R_5: resultant of Mv and Pa
e: lever arm of force F
q: lever arm of force Mv
k: lever arm with which force Pa acts
   on the patella
c: lever arm with which force Pa acts
   on the tibia
β: angle formed by the lines of action
   of forces Mv and Pa

After Maquet

Fig. 11.62. Patellectomy decreases the lever arm C and increases the angle B, and the force PA exerted by the patellar tendon. (From Maquet, P.: Advancement of the tibial tuberosity. Clin. Orthop., *115:* 225, 1976, with permission.)

patellectomy. Some weakness and quadriceps atrophy was noted, but he found no evidence that patellectomy caused generalized arthritis.

Geckeler and Quaranta[51] performed a long-term review of the results of treatment of osteoarthritis of the knee by patellectomy. Their three failures were attributed to improper selection of patients in that these knees had a generalized degenerative arthritis. The results were good or excellent in three-fourths of patients and no evidence of progressive joint degeneration attributable to the patellectomy was evident. Duthie and Hutchinson[41] also found no evidence that arthritic changes in the femoral condyles were a se-

quel of patellectomy, but believed that there was a direct relationship between the postoperative symptoms and the extent of ossification in the quadriceps tendon (Fig. 11.63A,B). In an attempt to prevent symptomatic ossification of this type from occurring, Compere et al.[32] have described a "tube" technique of patellectomy; they report 90 percent good or excellent results with this method.

Boucher[16] described the operation for fracture, chondromalacia, and recurrent dislocation. The results were good in almost all cases, but some aching of the knee was a common complaint. He believed that bone forming within the tendon might cause pain.

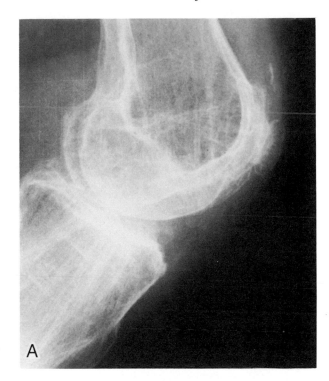

Fig. 11.63. (A,B) Ossification in the patellar tendon after patellectomy.

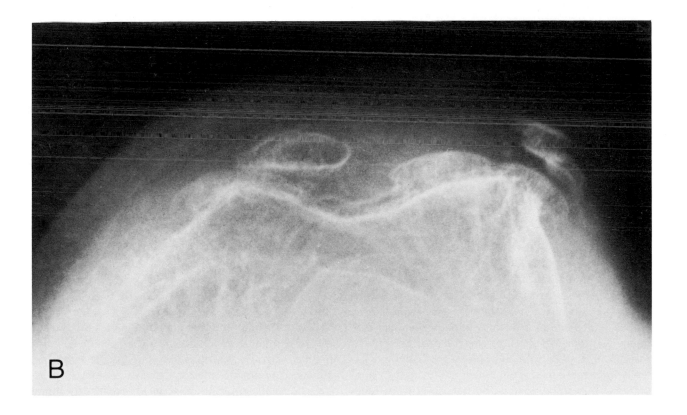

Bentley[10] stated that for chondromalacia the results of primary patellectomy are better than when secondary patellar excision is done after other operations such as shaving and drilling have failed. Partial patellectomy after the manner of Cave and Rowe[25] has its adherents, but Chrisman and Snook[29] found the method unpredictable in the relief of pain; our experience has been similar.

With regard to technique, Kaufer recommends end-to-end suture of the quadriceps tendon and patellar ligament, but West[128] recommended a simple longitudinal incision whenever possible, and Duthie and Hutchinson[41] also found no disadvantage in excising the intact patella through a vertical split in the aponeurosis.

Notwithstanding the good results found in these series, the majority opinion today is that excision of the patella should be an "end of the road" solution to the problem of patellar pain. Most published series have contained a mixed group of patients and the indications have included rheumatoid arthritis, osteoarthritis, chondromalacia, and patellar fractures. This and the association of arthritis in the femorotibial joint has made evaluation difficult. The Hospital for Special Surgery experience is probably representative. In a recent study of 100 patellectomies,[95] the result was considered good in 72 knees. Failure was nearly always attributable to unrelieved pain, in some cases with additional complaints of weakness and instability. The age of the patient, range of motion, extension lag, and the postoperative appearance of the knee were not important factors. Calcification in the patellar tendon[41] was not related to complaints of pain in this series, and the type of surgical technique also did not seem to influence the outcome.

TECHNIQUE OF PATELLECTOMY

LONGITUDINAL EXCISION

A midline skin incision is used, exposing the patella. A vertical incision is made in the midline through the lower part of the quadriceps tendon crossing the patella and extending distally into the patellar ligament. By sharp dissection, the quadriceps aponeurosis is separated from the patella medially and laterally until the bone is completely enucleated. In most patients this can be done without perforating the aponeurosis, but it does not seem of great consequence even if this happens. After removal of the patella, the resulting vertical split is approximated by side-to-side suture with a slight overlap in the central portion. The suture line is tested by flexing the knee through 90 degrees.

Aftercare

Simple immobilization in a pressure dressing is sufficient, allowing weight-bearing as tolerated. When the wound is healed, knee flexion and quadriceps rehabilitation are begun.

"TUBE" TECHNIQUE

Compere[32] advocates a transverse skin incision, but a vertical incision is equally acceptable (Fig. 11.64). The patella is exposed. The knee joint is entered through a medial parapatellar capsular incision. The capsule is also incised through a lateral parapatellar incision. The patella is everted and carefully enucleated from the quadriceps expansion, taking care to preserve the thin dorsal fibers. After removal of the patella, the medial border of the quadriceps aponeurosis is brought underneath and sutured to the lateral border of the expansion. When the sutures are cut the knots lie in the midline in the femoral sulcus and the tendon is now in the form of a tube. The medial capsule is closed with advancement of the vastus medialis distally and slightly laterally. The passive range of motion is tested through 90 degrees; adjustments to the tension of the closure of the capsule may be done if desired.

Aftercare

As for a patellectomy done through a vertical incision.

SURGERY OF SOFT TISSUE LESIONS

Removal of chronically inflamed bursae from around the knee may occasionally be necessary. The infrapatellar bursa is sometimes irritated by the residual effects of Osgood-Schlatter disease. A separated ossicle is usually present and excision of this through a vertical split in the patellar tendon effects a cure.

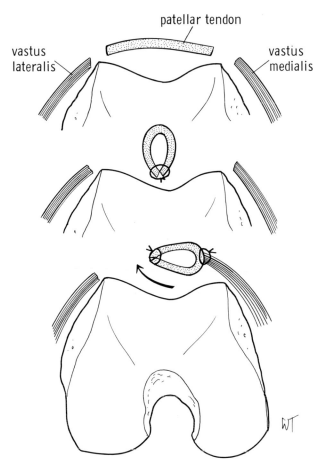

patellar tendon

vastus
lateralis

vastus
medialis

WT

Fig. 11.64. Compere's technique for patellectomy (see text). Ossification will occur within the tube.

Scarification of the patellar tendon adjoining the lower pole of the patella has been advocated for the treatment of jumper's knee when this condition is chronic and resistant to conservative treatment.

Partial or subtotal excision of the fat pad is recommended by Smillie through either a medial or lateral parapatellar skin incision; the capsule is incised and a wedge of tissue is removed from the fat pad between the capsule and synovial membrane. Synovial tags are not excised but invaginated into the synovium with a suture. I have had no experience with this operation.

PARTIAL SYNOVECTOMY FOR ABNORMAL PLICAE

When symptoms are attributed to a suprapatellar or medial patella plica, a partial synovectomy including the plica may be indicated. This can be done through an arthrotomy incision, or the synovial band may be divided and removed under arthroscopic control. I have had little experience with the excision of plicae as an isolated procedure; because the synovial folds are seen with such frequency, I do not know in how many cases symptoms may genuinely be attributed to them.

REFERENCES

1. Abernethy, P.J., Townsend, P.R., Rose, R.M., et al.: Is chondromalacia patellae a separate clinical entity? J. Bone Joint Surg. [Br.], *60:* 205, 1978.
2. Aichroth, P.: Osteochondral fractures and their relationship to osteochondritis dissecans of the knee. J. Bone Joint Surg. [Br.], *53:* 448, 1971.
3. Aglietti, P., Insall J.N., and Cerulli, G.: Patellar pain and incongruence. I: Measurements of incongruence. Clin. Orthop. *176:*217, 1983.
4. Aglietti, P., Insall, J.N., Walker, P.S., et al.: A new patella prosthesis. Clin. Orthop., *107:* 175, 1975.
5. Aleman, O.: Chondromalacia post-traumatica patellae. Acta Chir. Scand., *63:* 149, 1928.
6. Andersen, P.T.: Congenital deformities of the knee joint in dislocation of the patella and achondroplasia. Acta Orthop. Scand., *28:* 27, 1959.
7. Bandi, W.: Chondromalacia patellae and femoro-patellare arthrose actiologie, klinik und therapie. Helv. Chir. Acta, *39*(suppl. 11): 1, 1972.
8. Bandi, W., and Brennwald, J.: The significance of femoropatellar pressure in the pathogenesis and treatment of chondromalacia patellae and femoro-patellar arthrosis. In Ingwersen, O.S., et al., eds.: The Knee Joint. New York, American Elsevier, p. 63, 1974.
9. Bennett, G.A., Waine, H., and Bauer, W.: Changes in the Knee Joint at Various Ages. New York, The Commonwealth Fund, 1942.
10. Bentley, G.: Chondromalacia patellae. J. Bone Joint Surg. [Am.], 52: 221, 1970.
11. Bernhang, A.M., and Levine, S.A.: Familial absence of the patella. J. Bone Joint Surg. [Am.], 55: 1088, 1973.
12. Blackburne, J.S., and Peel, T.E.: A new method of measuring patellar height. J. Bone Joint Surg. [Br.], 59: 241, 1977.
13. Blazina, M.E., Fox, J.M., DelPizzo, W., et al.: Patellofemoral replacement. Clin. Orthop., *144:* 98, 1979.
14. Blumensaat, C.: Die Lageabweichungen und Verrenkungen der Kniescheibe. Ergeb. Chir. Orthop., *31:* 149, 1938.
15. Boon-Itt, S.B.: The normal position of the patella. J. Roentgen Soc., *24:* 389, 1930.
16. Boucher, H.H.: Patellectomy in the geriatric patient. Clin. Orthop., *11:* 33, 1958.

17. Brattström, H.: Shape of the intercondylar groove normally and in recurrent dislocation of patella: A clinical and x-ray anatomical investigation. Acta Orthop. Scand., 68(suppl.): 1964.

18. Brooke, R.: The treatment of fractured patella by excision. A study of morphology and function. Br. J. Surg., 24: 733, 1937.

19. Büdinger, K.: Uber Ablösung von Gelenkteilen und verwandte Prozesse. Dtsch. Z. Chir., 84: 311, 1906.

20. Büdinger, K.: Ueber Traumatische Knorpelrisse in Kniegelenk. Dtsch. Z. Chir., 92: 510, 1908.

21. Bullough, P., and Goodfellow, J.: The significance of the fine structure of articular cartilage. J. Bone Joint Surg. [Br.], 50: 852, 1968.

22. Carter, C., and Sweetnam, R.: Familial joint laxity and recurrent dislocation of the patella. J. Bone Joint Surg. [Br.], 40: 664, 1958.

23. Casscells, S.W.: Gross pathological changes in the knee joint of the aged individual. A study of 300 cases. In proceedings J. Bone Joint Surg. [Am.], 57: 1033, 1975.

24. Casscells, S.W.: The arthroscope in the diagnosis of disorders of the patellofemoral joint. Clin. Orthop., 144: 45, 1979.

25. Cave, E.F., and Rowe, C.R.: The patella. Its importance in derangement of the knee. J. Bone Joint Surg. [Am.], 32: 542, 1950.

26. Ceder, L.C., and Larson, R.L.: Z-plasty lateral retinacular release for the treatment of patellar compression syndrome. Clin. Orthop., 144: 110, 1979.

27. Chaklin, V.D.: Injuries to the cartilages of the patella and the femoral condyle. J. Bone Joint Surg., 21: 133, 1939.

28. Chrisman, O.D.: Biochemical aspects of degenerative joint disease. Clin. Orthop., 64: 77, 1969.

29. Chrisman, O.D., and Snook, G.A.: The role of patelloplasty and patellectomy in the arthritic knee. Clin. Orthop., 101: 40, 1974.

30. Chrisman, O.D., Fessel, J.M., and Southwick, W.O.: Experimental production of synovitis and marginal articular exostoses in the knee joints of dogs. Yale J. Biol. Med., 37: 409, 1965.

31. Chrisman, O.D., Snook, G.A., and Wilson, T.C.: The protective effect of aspirin against degeneration of human articular cartilage. Clin. Orthop., 84: 193, 1972.

32. Compere, C.L., Hill, J.A., Lewinnek, G.E., et al.: A new method of patellectomy for patellofemoral arthritis. J. Bone Joint Surg. [Am.], 61(5): 714, 1979.

33. Cox, F.J.: Traumatic osteochondritis of the patella. Surgery, 17: 93, 1945.

34. Crosby, E.B., and Insall, J.: Recurrent dislocation of the patella. J. Bone Joint Surg. [Am.], 58: 9, 1976.

35. Darracott, J., and Vernon-Roberts, B.: The bony changes in "chondromalacia patellae." Rheumatol. Phys. Med., 11: 175, 1971.

36. DePalma, A.F., and Flynn, J.J.: Joint changes following experimental partial and total patellectomy. J. Bone Joint Surg. [Am.], 40: 395, 1958.

37. DePalma, A.F., Sawyer, B., and Hoffman, J.D.: Reconsideration of lesions affecting the patellofemoral joint. Clin. Orthop., 18: 63, 1960.

38. De Takats, G.: Sympathetic reflex dystrophy. Med. Clin. North Am., 49: 117, 1965.

39. Devas, M., and Golski, A.: Treatment of chondromalacia patellae by transposition of the tibial tubercle. Br. Med. J., 1: 589, 1973.

40. Duncan, J.G., and Souter, W.A.: Hereditary onychoosteodysplasia. The nail-patella syndrome. J. Bone Joint Surg. [Br.], 45: 242, 1963.

41. Duthie, H.L., and Hutchinson, J.R.: The results of partial and total excision of the patella. J. Bone Joint Surg. [Br.], 40(1): 75, 1958.

42. Elmslie, R.C.: Unpublished work at St. Bartholomew's Hospital, London, 1912–1932. Quoted by I.S. Smillie. In Diseases of the Knee Joint, 5th Ed., p. 90. Edinburgh, Churchill Livingstone, 1978.

43. Emery, I.H., and Meachim, G.: Surface morphology and topography of patello-femoral cartilage fibrillation in Liverpool necropsies. J. Anat., 116: 103, 1973.

44. Ferguson, A.B., Jr., Brown, T.D., Fu, F.H., et al.: Relief of patellofemoral contact stress by anterior displacement of the tibial tubercle. J. Bone Joint Surg. [Am.], 61(2): 159, 1979.

45. Ficat, P.: Pathologie femoro-patellaire. Paris, Masson, et. cie, 1970.

46. Ficat, P., Phillippe, J., Cuzacq, J.P., et al.: Le syndrome d'hyperpression externe de la rotule. J. Radiol., Electrol. Med. Nucl. 53: 845, 1972.

47. Ficat, P., and Hungerford, D.S.: Disorders of the patellofemoral joint. Baltimore, Williams & Wilkins, 1977.

48. Ficat, P., Ficat, C., Gedeon, P., et al.: Spongialization: A new treatment for diseased patellae. Clin. Orthop., 144: 74, 1979.

49. Fielding, J.W., Liebler, W.A., and Tambakis, A.: The effect of a tibial-tubercle transplant in children on the growth of the upper tibial epiphysis. J. Bone Joint Surg. [Am.], 42: 1426, 1960.

50. Fox, T.A.: Dysplasia of the quadriceps mechanism. Surg. Clin. North Am., 55: 199, 1975.

51. Geckeler, E.O., and Quaranta, A.V.: Patellectomy for degenerative arthritis of the knee. Late results. J. Bone Joint Surg. [Am.], 44: 1109, 1962.

52. Goldthwait, J.E.: Slipping or recurrent dislocation of the patella: With the report of eleven cases. Boston Med. Surg. J., 150: 169, 1904.

53. Goodfellow, J.W., and Bullough, P.G.: The pattern of ageing of the articular cartilage of the elbow joint. J. Bone Joint Surg. [Br.], 49: 175, 1967.

54. Goodfellow, J., Hungerford, D.S., and Zindel, M.: Patellofemoral joint mechanics and pathology. I.

Functional anatomy of the patello-femoral joint. J. Bone Joint Surg. [Br.], *58*: 287, 1976.

55. Goodfellow, J., Hungerford, D.S., and Woods, C.: Patello-femoral joint mechanics and pathology. 2. Chondromalacia patellae. J. Bone Joint Surg. [Br.], *58*: 291, 1976.

56. Goutallier, D., and Debeyre, J.: Le recentrate rotulien dans les arthroses fémoro-patellaires latéralisées. Rev. Chir. Orthop., *60*: 377, 1974.

57. Green, J.P., and Waugh, W.: Congenital lateral dislocation of the patella. J. Bone Joint Surg. [Br.], *50*: 285, 1968.

58. Gritzka, T.L., Fry, L.R., and Cheesman, R.L., et al.: Deterioration of articular cartilage caused by continuous compression in a moving rabbit joint. J. Bone Joint Surg. [Am.], *55*: 1698, 1973.

59. Gunn, D.R.: Contracture of the quadriceps muscle. J. Bone Joint Surg. [Br.], *46*: 492, 1964.

60. Haliburton, R.A., and Sullivan, C.R.: The patella in degenerative joint disease. A clinicopathologic study. Arch. Surg., *77*: 677, 1958.

61. Hampson, W.G.J., and Hill, P.: Late results of transfer of the tibial tubercle for recurrent dislocation of the patella. J. Bone Joint Surg. [Br.], *57*: 209, 1975.

62. Hardaker, W.T., Whipple, T.L., and Bassett, F.H.: Diagnosis and treatment of the plica syndrome of the knee. J. Bone Joint Surg. [Am.], *62*: 221, 1980.

63. Harrison, M.H.M., Schajowicz, F., and Trueta, J.: Osteoarthritis of the hip: A study of the nature and evolution of the disease. J. Bone Joint Surg. [Br.], *35*: 598, 1953.

64. Hauser, E.D.W.: Total tendon transplant for slipping patella. Surg. Gynec. and Obstet., *66*: 199, 1938.

65. Haxton, H.: The function of the patella and the effects of its excision. Surg. Gynecol. Obstet., *80*: 389, 1945.

66. Heine-Rostock: Über Primäre Kronische Gelenkerkrankungen. Verh. Dtsch. Orthop. Ges., *22*: 7, 1927.

67. Hey Groves, E.W.: A note on the extension apparatus of the knee joint. Br. J. Surg., *24*: 747, 1937.

68. Heywood, A.W.B.: Recurrent dislocation of the patella. J. Bone Joint Surg. [Br.], *43*: 508, 1961.

69. Hněvkovský, O.: Progressive fibrosis of the vastus intermedius muscle in children. J. Bone Joint Surg. [Br.], *43*: 318, 1961.

70. Hoffa, A.: The influence of the adipose tissue with regard to the pathology of the knee joint. J.A.M.A., *43*: 795, 1904.

71. Hughston, J.C.: Subluxation of the patella. J. Bone Joint Surg. [Am.], *50*: 1003, 1968.

72. Hughston, J.C., and Walsh, W.M.: Proximal and distal reconstruction of the extensor mechanism for patellar subluxation. Clin. Orthop., *144*: 36, 1979.

73. Hughston, J.C., Stone, M., and Andrews, J.R.: The suprapatellar plica: Its role in internal derangement of the knee. In Proceedings of The American Academy of Orthopaedic Surgeons. J. Bone Joint Surg. [Am.], *55*: 1318, 1973.

74. Insall, J.N.: Intra-articular surgery for degenerative arthritis of the knee. A report of the work of the late K.H. Pridie. J. Bone Joint Surg. [Br.], *49*: 211, 1967.

75. Insall, J.: A midline approach to the knee. J. Bone Joint Surg. [Am.], *53*: 1584, 1971.

76. Insall, J.: "Chondromalacia patellae": patellar malalignment syndrome. Orthop. Clin. North Am., *10*(1): 117, 1979.

77. Insall, J.: Patellar pain syndromes and chondromalacia patellae. In Instructional Course Lectures. The American Academy of Orthopaedic Surgeons. St. Louis, The C.V. Mosby Co., *30*: 342, 1981.

78. Insall, J., and Salvati, E.: Patella position in the normal knee joint. Radiology, *101*: 101, 1971.

79. Insall, J., Goldberg, V., and Salvati, E.: Recurrent dislocation and the high-riding patella. Clin. Orthop., *88*: 67, 1972.

80. Insall, J., Falvo, K.A., and Wise, D.W.: Chondromalacia patellae: A prospective study. J. Bone Joint Surg. [Am.], *58*: 1, 1976.

81. Insall, J., Bullough, P.G., and Burstein, A.H.: Proximal "tube" realignment of the patella for chondromalacia patellae. Clin. Orthop., *144*: 63, 1979.

82. Insall, J., Tria, A.J., and Aglietti, P.: Resurfacing of the patella. J. Bone Joint Surg. [Am.], *62*: 933, 1980.

83. Jacobsen, K., and Bertheussen, K.: The vertical location of the patella. Acta Orthop. Scand., *45*: 436, 1974.

84. Jakob, R.P., von Gumppenberg, S., and Engelhardt, P.: Does Osgood-Schlatter disease influence the position of the patella? J. Bone Joint Surg. [Br.], *63*: 579, 1981.

85. Jaroschy, W.: Die Diagnostische Verwertbarkeit der Patellaraufnahmen. Fortschr. Roentgenstr., *31*: 781, 1924.

86. Jeffreys, T.E.: Recurrent dislocation of the patella due to abnormal attachment of the iliotibial tract. J. Bone Joint Surg. [Br.], *45*: 740, 1963.

87. Karlson, S.: Chondromalacia patellae. Acta Chir. Scand., *83*: 347, 1940.

88. Kaufer, H.: Mechanical function of the patella. J. Bone Joint Surg. [Am.], *53*: 1551, 1971.

89. Kaufer, H.: Patellar biomechanics. Clin. Orthop., *144*: 51, 1979.

90. Lancourt, J.E., and Cristini, J.A.: Patella alta and patella infera. Their etiological role in patellar dislocation, chondromalacia and apophysitis of the tibial tubercle. J. Bone Joint Surg. [Am.], *57*: 1112, 1975.

91. Larson, R.L., Cabaud, H.E., Slocum, D.B., et al.: The patellar compression syndrome: Surgical treatment by lateral retinacular release. Clin. Orthop., *134*: 158, 1978.

92. Laurin, C.A., Dussault, R., and Levesque, H.P.: The

tangential x-ray investigation of the patellofemoral joint: X-ray technique, diagnostic criteria and their interpretation. Clin. Orthop., *144*: 16, 1979.

93. Leslie, I.J., and Bentley, G.: Arthroscopy in the diagnosis of chondromalacia patellae. Ann. Rheum. Dis., *37*(6): 540, 1978.

94. Levitt, R.L.: A long-term evaluation of patellar prostheses. Clin. Orthop., 97: 153, 1973.

95. Lewis, M.M., Fitzgerald, P.F., Jacobs, B., et al.: Patellectomy: An analysis of one hundred cases. In proceedings J. Bone Joint Surg. [Am.], 58: 736, 1976.

96. Lieb, F.J., and Perry, J.: Quadriceps function. An anatomical and mechanical study using amputated limbs. J. Bone Joint Surg. [Am.], *50*: 1535, 1968.

97. Lloyd-Roberts, G.C., and Thomas, T.G.: The etiology of quadriceps contracture in children. J. Bone Joint Surg. [Br.], *46*: 498, 1964.

98. MacNab, I.: Recurrent dislocation of the patella. J. Bone Joint Surg. [Am.], *34*: 957, 1952.

99. Maquet, P.: Biomechanische Aspekte der Femur-Patella Beziehungen. Z. Orthop., *112*: 620, 1974.

100. Maquet, P.: Advancement of the tibial tuberosity. Clin. Orthop., *115*: 225, 1976.

101. Maquet, P.G.J.: Biomechanics of the Knee With Application to the Pathogenesis and the Surgical Treatment of Osteoarthritis. Berlin, Springer, 1976.

102. Marar, B.C., and Pillay, V.K.: Chondromalacia of the patella in Chinese. A postmortem study. J. Bone Joint Surg. [Am.], 57: 342, 1975.

103. McKeever, D.C.: Patellar prosthesis. J. Bone Joint Surg. [Am.], *37*: 1074, 1955.

104. Merchant, A.C., and Mercer, R.L.: Lateral release of the patella: A preliminary report. Clin. Orthop., *103*: 40, 1974.

105. Merchant, A.C., Mercer, R.L., Jacobsen, R.H., et al.: Roentgenographic analysis of patellofemoral congruence. J. Bone Joint Surg. [Am.], 56: 1391, 1974.

106. Miller, G.F.: Familial recurrent dislocation of the patella. J. Bone Joint Surg. [Br.], *60*(2): 203, 1978.

107. Outerbridge, R.E.: The etiology of chondromalacia patellae. J. Bone Joint Surg. [Br.], *43*: 752, 1961.

108. Outerbridge, R.E.: Further studies on the etiology of chondromalacia patellae. J. Bone Joint Surg. [Br.], *46*: 179, 1964.

109. Owre, A.: Chondromalacia patellae. Acta Chir. Scand., 77 (suppl. 41): 1936.

110. Pipkin, G.: Knee injuries: The role of the suprapatellar plica and suprapatellar bursa in simulating internal derangements. Clin. Orthop., *74*: 161, 1971.

111. Pridie, K.H.: A method of resurfacing osteoarthritic knee joints. In proceedings J. Bone Joint Surg. [Br.], *41*: 618, 1959.

112. Radin, E., and Leach, R.: Anterior displacement of tibial tubercle for patello-femoral arthrosis. Orthop. Trans., *3*: 291, 1979.

113. Reilly, D.T., and Martens, M.: Experimental analysis of the quadriceps muscle force and patello-femoral joint reaction force for various activities. Acta Orthop. Scand., 43: 126, 1972.

114. Rozbruch, J.D., Campbell, R.D., and Insall, J.: Tibial tubercle elevation (the Maquet operation): A clinical study of 31 cases. Orthop. Trans., 3: 291, 1979.

115. Rubacky, G.E.: Inheritable chondromalacia of the patella. J. Bone Joint Surg. [Am.], *45*: 1685, 1963.

116. Salter, R.B., and Simmonds, D.F.: The biological effect of continuous passive motion on the healing of full thickness defects in articular cartilage. J. Bone Joint Surg. [Am.], 62: 1232, 1980.

117. Scott, J.C.: Fractures of the patella. J. Bone Joint Surg. [Br.], *31*: 76, 1949.

118. Settegast: Typische Roentgenbilder von normalen Menschen. Lehmanns Med. Atlanten, 5: 211, 1921.

119. Shoji, H., and Granda, J.L.: Acid hydrolases in the articular cartilage of the patella. Clin. Orthop., 99: 293, 1974.

120. Simmons, D.P., and Chrisman, O.D.: Salicylate inhibition of cartilage degeneration. Arthritis Rheum., 8: 960, 1965.

121. Sinding-Larsen, C.: A hitherto unknown affection of the patella in children. Acta Radiol., *1*: 171, 1921.

122. Smillie, I.S.: Injuries of the Knee Joint, 2nd Ed. Baltimore, Williams & Wilkins, 1951.

123. Soto-Hall, R.: Traumatic degeneration of the articular cartilage of the patella. J. Bone Joint Surg., 27: 426–431, 1945.

124. Sutton, F.S., Thompson, C.H., Lipke, J., et al.: The effect of patellectomy of knee function. J. Bone Joint Surg. [Am.], 58: 537, 1976.

125. Tria, A.J., Insall, J., and Aglietti, P.: Anatomic basis of patellar pain. Presented at the American Academy of Orthopaedic Surgeons Meeting, Atlanta, Georgia, 1980.

126. Trillat, A., Dejour, H., and Couette, A.: Diagnostic et traitement des subluxations recidivantes de la rotule. Rev. Chir. Orthop., *50*: 813, 1964.

127. Watson-Jones, R.: Fractures and other bone and joint injuries. Baltimore, William Wilkins, 1940.

128. West, F.E.: End results of patellectomy. J. Bone Joint Surg. [Am.], *44*: 1089, 1962.

129. West, F.E., and Soto-Hall, R.: Recurrent dislocation of the patella in the adult. J. Bone Joint Surg. [Am.], *40*: 386, 1958.

130. Wiberg, G.: Roentgenographic and anatomic studies on the femoropatellar joint. With special reference to chondromalacia patella. Acta Orthop. Scand., *12*: 319, 1941.

131. Wiles, P., Andrews, P.S., and Devas, M.B.: Chondromalacia of the patella. J. Bone Joint Surg. [Br.], 38: 95, 1956.

132. Wiles, P., Andrews, P.S., and Bremner, R.A.: Chondromalacia of the patella. J. Bone Joint Surg. [Br.], 42: 65, 1960.

12 Acute Ligament Injuries

Russell F. Warren

During the past decade, considerable controversy has been reflected in the orthopedic literature regarding the significance and treatment of acute ligamentous injuries of the knee. Treatment varies widely from a complete nonsurgical approach to the repair of all ligament injuries of the knee.

In the sports medicine clinic at The Hospital for Special Surgery, we advocate early repair of cruciate ligament injuries in active and athletic patients with isolated or combined lesions. In contrast, we seldom use surgery for treatment of injuries to the medial collateral ligament (MCL) and lateral collateral ligament (LCL).

Whether a surgical or a nonsurgical approach is taken depends on a group of variables, including activity levels, associated pathology, and patient goals, that vary with each patient.

The key to treatment is accurate recognition of the problem. Unfortunately, the responsibility for the initial diagnosis often rests with an emergency room staff whose training in the evaluation of acute knee injuries may be scant. Not uncommonly, injuries are missed or passed off as a mild sprain when in fact there is significant damage. As a result, optimal treatment is delayed or is no longer possible. We strongly believe that the history and examination will generally permit a diagnosis of ligament damage with a high degree of accuracy. A roentgenographic examination should be obtained but is generally not helpful except in ruling out associated bone injury. Arthrography and arthroscopy are important diagnostic aids that usually confirm the clinical impression while adding information about the menisci and articular surfaces.

RISK FACTORS

Ligament injuries are most common during the second and third decades, with males predominating in a 2:1 ratio.[24] In the growing child, ligament damage of the knees is less likely, as epiphyseal separation rather than collateral ligament damage occurs. However, it is important to consider ligament damage, particularly of the cruciate ligaments.

Ligament injuries of the knee are usually a result of athletic injury. Seventy-nine percent of our patients had been involved in some type of sports activity with football (31.75 percent) and skiing (29.9 percent) the most common. Automobile and motorcycle accidents accounted for most of the remainder. The average age of our athletic population was 25.5 years, while the average age of nonathletic patients was 37.5 years.

These figures vary with the physician's location and interest. They will probably change considerably over the ensuing years as sex and age become less of a deterrent to athletic activity. It appears that female injury rates in athletics are similar to males in noncontact sports except for the knee, where they appear to be at a greater risk.

In creating an environment in which injuries to knee ligaments may be decreased or minimized, a variety of factors must be considered. These include rule changes,[4,18,21] equipment changes, and improved preseason conditioning. The high incidence of knee injuries in football associated with crack back blocking and downfield blocking below the waist has resulted in a series of rule changes at both the scholastic and collegiate levels that has had a significant effect in decreasing the incidence of knee injuries.

A reduction in knee and ankle injuries followed the use of multiple short cleats on football shoes. In contrast, knee injuries in skiing have not decreased.[9] A 71 percent decrease in tibial shaft fractures and ankle sprains has been noted, but the rate of knee injuries has continued at about 20 percent. This is related to the mechanics of the binding which, when it fails to release, places the knee at risk to rotational and valgus–varus stresses. In a long-term study[6] of football injuries, it was found that 41 percent of all knee injuries occurred before the first game, with 78 percent occurring by the third game. After the institution of a 6-week preseason conditioning program, there was a 68 percent reduction of all injuries up to the third game, with no change in the incidence over the remainder of the season. Nonsurgical knee injuries were decreased 35 percent and surgical knee injuries 63 percent. Although other factors were undoubtedly involved, the study appears to demonstrate that athletic conditioning reduces knee injuries. Similarly, a West Point study showed that poor rehabilitation after injury leads to a high rate of reinjury. Adequate rehabilitation before resuming athletic competition at any level reduces the incidence of reinjury. Thirty-one percent of our patients had a knee injury before the one leading to surgery. Although some of those patients undoubtedly had undiagnosed knee ligament injury, the lack of proper rehabilitation after nonsurgical or surgical treatment was a significant and correctable factor.

LIGAMENT HEALING

Understanding the nature of ligament healing is essential to treatment of acute ligamentous injuries of the knee. The ability of a ligament to heal depends on the blood supply, the approximation of the tissue, the stress placed across the ligament, and the timing of this stress.

The collateral ligaments receive their blood supply mainly from the overlying and adjacent soft tissues. The superficial portion of the medial collateral ligament is encased in well-vascularized loose areolar connective tissue, which provides an incomplete sheath for the ligament.[8] The deep portion of the medial collateral ligament receives most of its blood supply from the capsular and synovial vessels. The lateral collateral ligament lying within the deep capsule is encased in a loose areolar connective tissue that is rich in vessels.[17]

The blood supply of the cruciate ligaments is more tenuous than that of the collateral ligaments because of their intra-articular, extrasynovial location. Terminal branches of the middle genicular and inferior genicular arteries contribute vessels to the synovial covering of the ligaments and the infrapatellar fat pad. Vessels from the synovial sheaths and the infrapatellar fat pad then supply the ligaments (Fig. 12.1). It has been demonstrated experimentally that after injury to the anterior cruciate ligament, there is an extensive vascular response within the ligament that is markedly decreased if the soft tissues (infrapatellar fat pad and synovium) are removed before injury. As with the collateral ligaments, the bony attachments of the cruciate ligaments do not contribute vessels to the vascular network.[2]

Ligament healing has been studied in animal models.[5,17] After injury to the collateral ligament, a defect is created. It is initially filled with blood. During the first week, vessels from the adjacent areolar tissue penetrate the hematoma to form a fibrovascular scar. Fibroblastic proliferation starts by the fifth day, followed by collagen production. If the ligament ends are approximated, scarring is significantly reduced; if separated, the scar is increased and organization is poor.

By 2 weeks, the fibroblasts are aligned in a parallel fashion; after 3 weeks, there is good tensile strength. Gradually the number of cells decreases and the fiber bundle size increases. By 8 weeks, the ligament appears normal, except for increased thickness.[17]

O'Donoghue[16] and Clayton[5] have separately studied collateral ligament healing and have noted that strength improvements are related to surgical repair. The repaired ligaments demonstrated less scar pro-

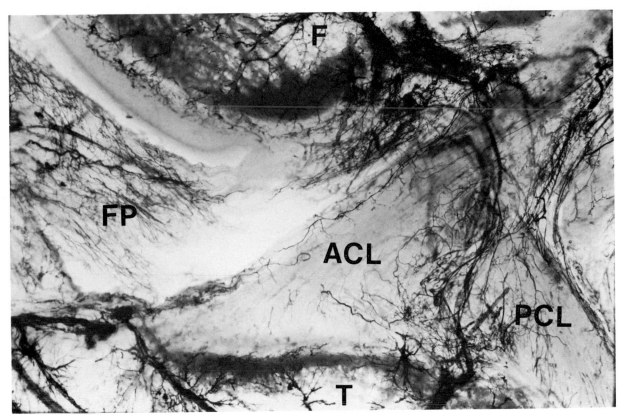

Fig. 12.1. Sagittal section (5 ml thick) of a human knee joint (Spalteholz technique) showing the vascularity of the ACL. Branches of the middle genicular artery (arrow) supply the ACL as well as the distal femoral epiphysis. F, femur; PCL, posterior cruciate ligament; FP, infrapatellar fat pad. (From Arnoczky, S.P.: The anatomy of the ACL. Clin. Orthop., *172:* 19, 1983, with permission.)

duction, better fiber orientation, and increased tensile strength. Using relatively slow methods of tissue loading, the controls generally sustained bony avulsion. Ligaments permitted to heal without repair failed at the original site of injury. In contrast, the repaired ligaments when tested at 4 to 6 weeks did not fail at the suture line but sustained bony avulsions similar to the control. Repair leads to (1) less scar formation, (2) better collagen orientation in the scar, (3) closure of the gap to restore ligament length and geometry, and (4) more rapid return of ligament strength.[13]

KNEE LIGAMENT EVALUATION

In evaluating ligament injuries, a sound understanding of the functional anatomy combined with a careful history and examination allows the physician to arrive at an accurate diagnosis in most patients. Standard anteroposterior and lateral roentgenograms play a role in evaluation of injury to exclude fractures. Arthrography is often confirmatory and will provide information on the status of the menisci. The role of arthroscopy has increased but should not be performed in lieu of an accurate physical examination.

HISTORY

The history provides information that indicates possible ligament damage. Approximately 40 percent of anterior cruciate ligament injuries are associated with a "pop" at the time of injury. The forces applied to the knee, whether or not the leg was weighted, and the position of the knee at the time of injury should be noted. Although contact is often involved in injury, its absence does not ensure the integrity of the ligament structures as a patient may be injured simply by applying a high torque to the knee and rapidly changing direction. Tennis players who change direction in attempting to make a backhand may tear their anterior cruciate ligament, as they internally rotate the tibia while externally rotating the femur. At the time of injury, did the patient notice instability of the knee? Often a patient describes a sense of movement between the bones or the feeling of the leg letting go while attempting to stand. Do not be fooled by the patient who walks into the office with minimal discomfort. A ligament that is completely disrupted may produce little in the way of pain. Conversely, a partial tear may be acutely painful. Similarly, the absence of significant swelling, although important, does not ensure the integrity of the ligaments. The synovial sleeve surrounding the cruciate ligament can remain intact despite rupture of the ligament. Massive knee ligament injury may disrupt the capsule peripherally, allowing the hemarthrosis to drain into the soft tissues. It is important to ascertain whether there have been previous knee problems. In some patients an acute injury is suspected, but the patient actually has had a long history of cruciate damage and has sustained a new episode of giving way. This is important if primary repair is contemplated.

MECHANISM OF INJURY

In evaluating the status of patients, a careful history regarding the mechanism of injury provides important clues as to the forces involved and the ligaments at risk. Thus in skiers who sustain valgus and external rotation injury, medial collateral and anterior cruciate ligament ruptures are found. Similar mechanisms exist in football and soccer.

Varus with internal rotation of the tibia on the femur combined with hyper-extension commonly occurs as skis cross and a skier falls forward or a basketball player jumps for a rebound landing with a foot internally rotated and the knee in extension. A tear of the anterior cruciate ligament often results. Pure hyperextension may occur as players are tackled from the front or the person falls forward with the foot fixed to the ground. Damage may occur to the anterior cruciate ligament as well as to the posterior capsule and the posterior cruciate ligament.[10,11]

Hyperflexion injuries, although rare, may occur if a player has his leg pinned under him resulting in stress on the anterior cruciate ligament. A pure valgus force without rotation places the medial collateral ligament at risk; when combined with rotation, the anterior cruciate ligament is stressed.

Direct posterior displacement in which a blow is applied to the proximal tibia accounted for 57 percent of our posterior cruciate ligament injuries, while hyperextension accounted for 23 percent, and valgus with external rotation for 20 percent. Pure varus forces are less common causes of severe injury, and they are most likely to occur in the person with genu varum. Complete disruption of the lateral collateral ligament progresses to dislocation and damage to the cruciate ligaments and peroneal nerve. An understanding of the mechanism of injury thus provides a clue to the involved ligament.

EXAMINATION

After acute knee injury, look for obvious deformity such as a dislocated knee or patella. Often, before the emergency room evaluation, a dislocated knee may have reduced spontaneously; hence the leg should be checked distally for intact neurocirculatory function before evaluating the knee. Ecchymosis and abrasions may give a clue as to the site of damage or the direction of injury (Fig. 12.2). In addition, abrasions may preclude early surgical intervention. Before actually examining the injured knee, evaluate the normal knee to gain the patient's confidence and to note the degree of movement on various clinical tests. In an acute injury, tenderness along the origins of the medial collateral ligament and the lateral collateral ligament, joint line, and patella is fairly reliable in localizing the site of damage. Joint tenderness may be associated with ligament damage or with meniscal damage. In injuries to the anterior cruciate ligament, as a result of internal rotation, tenderness may be appreciated at the posterolateral corner of the knee. In palpating the patella, any defects in the soft tissue suggesting possible displacement should be noted. Lateral pressure on the patella with the knee flexed 30 degrees may indicate patellar instability in association with medial collateral–anterior cruciate ligament injury. If possible, the joint should be placed through a range of motion to discover any recurvatum, limited flexion,

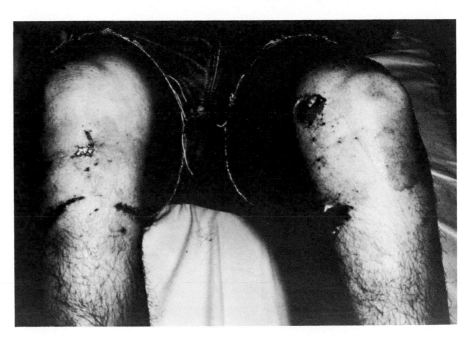

Fig. 12.2. Abrasions sustained in a motorcycle accident that resulted in a ruptured PCL in the right knee and lateral ligament injury on the left.

or lack of extension. Joint effusion should be palpated and speed of development noted. An acutely injured knee is not routinely aspirated unless a large effusion interferes with the examination or causes great discomfort. If the knee is aspirated, the fluid should be examined. A bloody effusion is often associated with intra-articular ligament damage, particularly of the anterior cruciate ligament, while the presence of fat suggests bony injury. Although rarely required for ligament evaluation, 10 ml of 1 percent lidocaine (Xylocaine) may be injected after aspirating the knee of blood or before arthrography to allow the patient to relax during your examination and ensure a more reliable examination.

The primary area of interest in acute knee ligament injury is in the performance of tests for specific ligament damage. In the acute situation a straight plane examination will provide the necessary information required to establish a program of treatment. Additional rotational tests, although important, are often inaccurate because of muscle guarding and anesthesia will generally be required to make them reliable. The cruciates are the key to a functioning knee. With the cruciates intact, the knee can tolerate considerable medial or lateral ligament laxity without symptomatic instability. If there is cruciate damage, many patients will develop significant symptoms, and when combined with collateral ligament injury the symptoms

are more severe. The first stability test to be performed is the Lachman test for evaluating the competence of the anterior cruciate ligament. It is highly accurate even in the acute situation. In essence, it is an anterior drawer test performed at 20 to 30 degrees of knee flexion. If the knee is extended further, the excursion decreases yielding a false-negative test result. To perform the Lachman test, the femur is held firmly with one hand while an anteriorly directed force is applied to the posterior surface of the tibia with the other hand (Fig. 12.3). The examiner should note the degree of anterior excursion as well as the end point. The end point is the resistance felt at the end of excursion, as play is taken out of the anterior cruciate ligament and the stiffness increases rapidly.

In addition, the degree of displacement and obliteration of the sulcus anteriorly should be observed. The Lachman test has nearly complete reliability. False-negative results may occur if a bucket-handle tear of a meniscus is displaced and prevents anterior tibial excursion or alters the end point. Rarely a bucket-handle tear of a meniscus may alter the end point with a normal anterior cruciate ligament, suggesting a false-positive Lachman test. In performing this and other stability tests, the normal knee should be used as a control and evaluated before testing the injured knee. After the Lachman test, the knee, if the effusion permits, is flexed to 80 degrees with the hips at

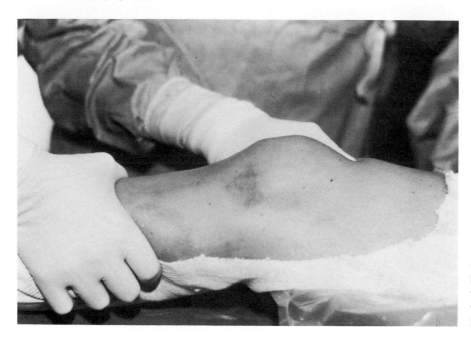

Fig. 12.3. Lachman test, performed by holding the femur with one hand and pulling forward on the tibia with the knee flexed to 30 degrees.

45 degrees, and a posterior dropback associated with complete posterior cruciate injury can be noted. This is often absent in partial lesions of the posterior cruciate ligament.

Next, the posterior drawer test is performed by placing the hand on the proximal tibia and applying a posteriorly directed gradual force (Fig. 12.4). Again, excursion and end point should be noted. In an acute injury to the posterior cruciate ligament, the end point is lost, but in chronic posterior cruciate ligament injury a sharp end point is observed as the secondary restraints have stretched out over time, permitting gross posterior displacement.

Testing for posterior-lateral instability is similar to the posterior drawer except that in addition to the posterior force an external rotational force is applied to the proximal tibia; increased external rotation and dropback of the tibia on the femur are appreciated if laxity is present. Anterior drawer testing is then performed with the knee in a similar position (Fig. 12.5). Before performing this test, hamstring spasm must be noted and eliminated if the test is to be reliable. In performing this test excursion and end point should be observed. In the acute situation the loss of the end point as in the Lachman test is a more sensitive indicator of anterior cruciate ligament injury than laxity. The anterior drawer test, although accurate in chronic injury, has a high level of false negatives (50

percent) in the acutely injured, even under general anesthesia. Grading of these injuries has been suggested but has little value or reliability after acute injury with current testing methods. Recently a device has become available whereby the actual excursion of the tibia on the femur can be measured both passively and actively (KT-1000). Our experience to date with this device is limited, but it may provide a way of grading the degree of excursion as well as diagnosing complete anterior cruciate ligament disruption by a noninvasive method.

After the anterior and posterior stability tests, the knee is tested for medial and lateral stability first in extension and then in flexion. With the knee in extension, the examiner holds the tibia medially and the femur laterally to create a valgus stress. The knee is then flexed to 30 degrees and the test is repeated. If the medial side opens in extension, there has been combined damage to the superficial medial ligament and the anterior cruciate ligament. If the opening is grossly positive in extension, damage to the posterior cruciate ligament should also be suspected. If instability is noted only with the knee flexed 30 degrees, the damage is mainly to the superficial medial ligament, although tearing of the deep and posterior oblique fibers may certainly be present.

In evaluating knee ligament sprains, a classification based on the severity of the injury is useful.[13] In es-

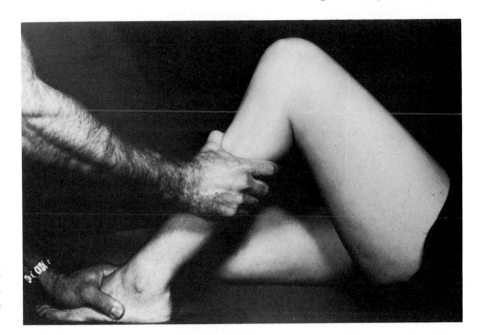

Fig. 12.4. Posterior drawer test, performed with the knee flexed to 90 degrees and the hip at 45 degrees. Note the tibial drop-back indicating injury to the PCL.

Fig. 12.5. Anterior drawer test for ACL injury, performed with the knee flexed 90 degrees.

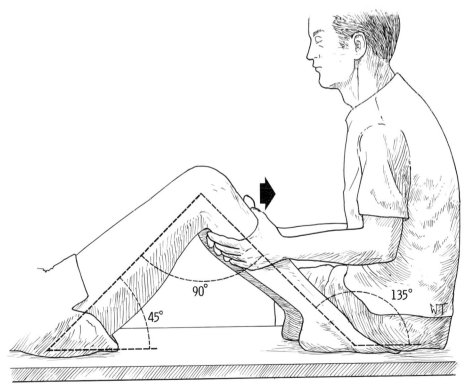

sence, a mild sprain (first-degree, or grade I) has local tenderness minimal swelling and no instability. A moderate sprain (second-degree or grade II) has mild to moderate instability with local tenderness along the ligament. A third-degree or grade III sprain has marked instability with complete ligament disruption. It is in the grading of those injuries that some confusion in treatment arises. It is useful to break grade II sprains into two groups: IIa with mild opening of less than 5 mm and IIb with an opening of 5 to 10 mm but without complete ligament disruption.

Interpretation of the tests for the lateral side is more difficult. In essence, with the knee in extension and lateral opening, there is usually damage to the lateral collateral ligament and the anterior cruciate ligament. If there is marked instability laterally in extension, then damage to the posterior cruciate ligament and posterior corner is probably present. If instability is present on varus testing in flexion, there is damage to the lateral collateral ligament and often the capsule and popliteus tendon.

Additional tests for lateral and medial instabilities are difficult in the acute situation, but can be performed readily under anesthesia.[14]

The external rotation recurvatum test is performed by extending the knee from 10 degrees of flexion to extension and noting the degree of tibial rotation and recurvatum. Hughston performs this test by holding the large toe and bringing the knee into extension (Fig. 12.6). If this test is positive, the knee goes into recurvatum with some external tibial rotation and implies damage to the posterior-lateral corner of the knee capsule including the lateral collateral ligament, popliteus tendon, and arcuate ligament. Often there is associated posterior cruciate ligament damage, and the lateral instability may place stress on the peroneal nerve.

The pivot shift test is a distinct indicator of anterior cruciate ligament injury. Initially described by Palmer, it has been tested in a variety of positions and methods by several investigators. The test combines anterior displacement of the tibia on the femur with internal rotation of the tibia; both of these motions are checked by the anterior cruciate ligament.

If the anterior cruciate ligament is intact, the shift will be negative, although rarely a mild shift is seen bilaterally in patients with ligamentous laxity. Unfortunately in the acutely injured patient guarding will often give a negative test, but under general anesthesia this test is positive in nearly 100 percent of anterior cruciate ligament ruptures. In order to perform this test, a valgus stress is applied with the foot in a mildly internally rotated position (Fig. 12.7). The knee is moved from flexion to extension. A positive shift represents a transient subluxation of the tibia on the femur. At about the 30 degrees position, the tibia

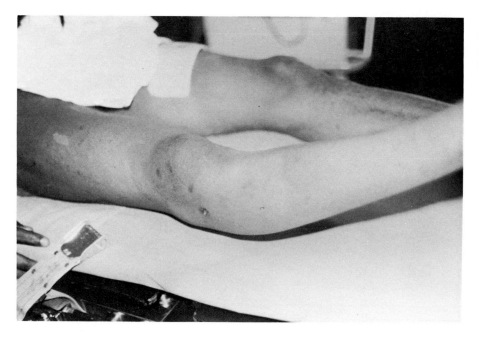

Fig. 12.6. External rotation recurvatum test for posterolateral corner damage, often including the PCL and ACL.

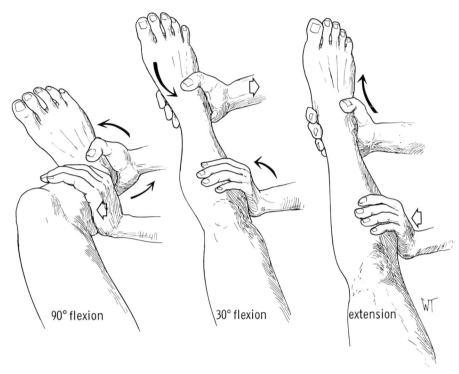

90° flexion   30° flexion   extension

Fig. 12.7. Pivot shift test, performed with the foot held in mild internal rotation and applying a valgus force to the proximal tibia as the knee is brought from a flexed position of 45 degrees to extension. A sudden jump is noted as the tibia subluxes anteriorly.

subluxes forward from a reduced position to an unreduced position. The iliotibial band can be best observed as it jumps forward. This sign can be graded on a I to III basis. Grade I is a subtle shift perceptible only with marked valgus. In a grade III, minimal pressure can produce a gross subluxation forward. Grade II is obtained with a moderate valgus force

The test should be performed gently as excessive force will result in marked pain. The key to noting a pivot shift is to apply an adequate valgus force on the knee.

Factors that may produce a false-negative shift include insufficient valgus force, holding the leg externally rotated or forced into maximum internal rotation. In addition, medial collateral ligament injury

Fig. 12.8. The crossed hand method of performing a pivot shift test facilitates the detection of a shift in large patients.

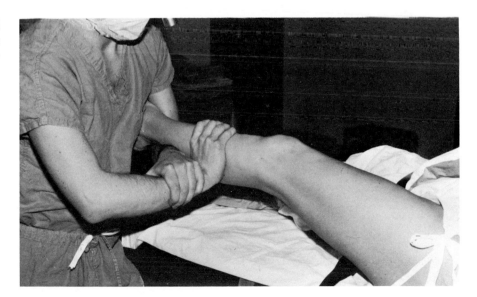

may markedly decrease this test as well as a previous lateral meniscectomy. In a large patient some difficulty may be encountered in performing this test. We have found that a crossed hand method facilitates the application of a valgus force (Fig. 12.8) and permits less experienced examiners to note the presence of a shift more frequently.

In performing the pivot shift test, one must be careful not to misinterpret posterolateral instability. In this situation, a reverse pivot shift manuever will be noted that can be marked at times. This test is performed with the foot externally rotated rather than internally, and the knee is moved from a flexed to an extended position. Minimal valgus force is required: as the knee is brought into extension a jump will be noted. This represents the posteriorly positioned tibia suddenly moving into a reduced position on the femur. It signifies damage to the posterolateral corner of the knee and is generally associated with PCL, LCL, and popliteus tendon injury.

The use of these tests is outlined in Table 12.1.

RADIOLOGIC EVALUATION

In evaluating knee injuries, standard anteroposterior and lateral views are required with Merchant and tunnel views providing additional information if knee

Table 12.1 Tests Associated with Specific Ligament Injuries.

Test	Tissue
Lachman	ACL
Anterior drawer	ACL
Posterior drawer	PCL
Valgus	
0 degrees	MCL, ACL
Grossly positive	MCL, ACL, PCL
30 degrees	MCL
Varus	
0 degrees	LCL, ACL
Grossly positive	LCL, ACL, PCL
30 degrees	LCL
Pivot shift	ACL
Slocum	ACL, MCL, usually with posterior medial capsule
Posterior lateral drawer and reverse pivot shift	Posterior lateral instability with damage to the PCL

Abbreviations: ACL, anterior collateral ligament; LCL, lateral collateral ligament; MCL, medial collateral ligament; PCL, posterior collateral ligament.

motion is sufficient to allow these radiographs to be taken. It is interesting how often patients with knee injuries have been told that the films are negative, the assumption being that there is no significant damage. It should be obvious that radiographs will not generally indicate ligament injury. Stress films for knee instability are frequently mentioned as being important, but we have generally not found them necessary in evaluating either cruciate or collateral ligament injuries.

Standard films should be evaluated for avulsion injuries at the attachment sites of each ligament. This is particularly true for children, in whom cruciate injuries are frequently of an avulsion type. An interesting lateral tibial avulsion injury termed a Sicund fracture may be noted on the anteroposterior view. This fracture is invariably associated with an anterior cruciate ligament injury and represents an avulsion of the mid-third of the lateral capsule from the tibial plateau. It is generally 1 or 2 cm in length, with minimal displacement. At surgery we have found this fragment lying slightly posterior to the mid-third of the tibia deep to the posterior edge of the iliotibial band. In viewing these radiographs, loose bodies or osteochondral fragments should be carefully searched for, as patellar dislocation may occur particularly in combined anterior cruciate/medial collateral ligament injuries. In children the epiphysis should be closely evaluated for injury if instability has been noted. While ligament injuries do occur in children, epiphyseal injury is more frequent. Generally, though, the clinical examination will find that the movement on stressing the knee is occurring at the growth plate rather than the joint line. Gentle stress views may be helpful in confirming this diagnosis.

ARTHROGRAPHY

In evaluating patients with known or suspected anterior cruciate ligament injury, we have found arthrography helpful. If performed well, important additional information regarding the status of the menisci and the possibility of reattaching them may be gained. In addition, the status of the anterior cruciate ligament may be confirmed, as we have noted a 96 percent accuracy of diagnosis in acute knee injuries.

ARTHROSCOPY

The necessity and benefit of early arthroscopy in evaluating patients with acute knee injuries have been disputed, because hemorrhage makes visualization difficult. The use of a large trocar and application of vigorous irrigation, however, will clear the blood from the joint. In more than 90 percent of cases, the status of the ligaments can be ascertained on an outpatient basis, but if a classic history of cruciate damage has been obtained, and the examination is equivocal, arthroscopy aids in the diagnosis. Generally examination under anesthesia will have already noted the instability; the Lachman test has been found to be nearly 100 percent accurate and the pivot shift to be positive in 99 percent of patients with acute tears of the anterior cruciate ligament. Thus, the functional integrity of the cruciate ligament should be known before insertion of the arthroscope. We are currently using arthroscopy when the examination is equivocal or when additional information regarding the status of the menisci is required before making a decision regarding the need for surgery. We do not use it as a routine procedure in the acutely injured knee.

If arthroscopy is performed, considerable care in evaluating the cruciates is required (Fig. 12.9). After flushing the joint adequately to remove all blood, excellent visualization in the acutely injured knee is possible. The joint is examined in an orderly manner taking particular care in evaluating the menisci for vertical type tears in the posterior horns of the menisci. In evaluating the menisci, a decision about the significance of the tear and whether it requires resection or possibly reattachment must be made.

Evaluation of the anterior cruciate ligament is carried out by direct observation and palpation while stressing the ligament. At times the synovial sleeve will be intact, making it appear that the anterior cruciate ligament is competent; however, careful palpation while stressing the ligament will generally indicate significant ligament damage. Whereas midportion tears are most common, proximal avulsions do occur and may easily be missed. In addition, a persistent vertical septum is present in about 4 percent of patients and may make visualization of the anterior cruciate ligament difficult.

In evaluating the posterior cruciate ligament, a posterior medial portal is required. This will allow ex-

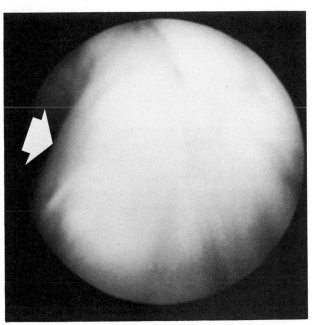

Fig. 12.9. Arthroscopic view of intact ACL (arrow).

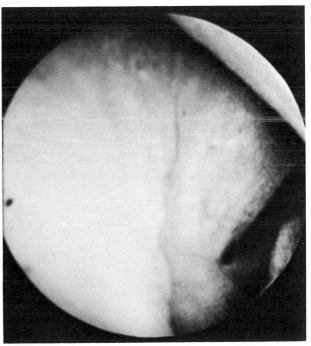

Fig. 12.10. Intact PCL (arrow) viewed from the posteromedial portal.

cellent visualization of the posterior cruciate ligament from the side. It can then be stressed under observation and palpated from an anterior portal (Fig. 12.10).

TREATMENT

The key to proper treatment is early and accurate diagnosis. Most studies of surgical and nonsurgical treatment[6,7,16,24] are retrospective, with diagnostic accuracy often in doubt. Not until prospective studies on completely diagnosed cases are done will an accurate comparison of surgical and nonsurgical results be possible.

MEDIAL COLLATERAL LIGAMENT INJURIES

In managing injuries of the medial collateral ligament, the degree of injury has been considered an important factor in determining surgical treatment. However, medial collateral ligament injuries with intact cruciates, regardless of degree, can be treated nonsurgically. The degree of injury does determine the amount of immobilization and how soon an exercise program may be started. In a 1976 study we did not find symptomatic instability in any patient in whom injury had been confined to the medial collateral ligament, regardless of degree, whether they had been treated surgically or nonsurgically. It was only when the anterior cruciate ligament was also injured that giving way developed. Even those knees that open widely on a valgus stress in flexion, but that are stable in extension and have a negative Lachman test, have done well with nonsurgical treatment. Protecting the ligament with bracing for a longer period than the standard 6-week interval appears to permit the ligament to achieve sufficient strength in spite of not having the ends surgically approximated.

GRADE I INJURY

In a grade I injury with pain along the medial collateral ligament with some associated swelling and no instability, the patient can be placed on crutches with minimal or no weight-bearing. Some patients with slight pain and good muscle control will not require

crutches, but will need only a protective splint initially. Range of motion should be carried out daily with straight leg raising and isometric exercises. Within 4 to 5 days, as weight-bearing is progressively tolerated, a splint can be used. Isotonic exercises using Universal or Nautilus equipment can be started after 4 to 5 days. The program is initiated with light weights, progressing on to heavy weights, in an attempt to reach a goal of 50 percent of body weight in the quadriceps and 60 to 70 percent of this value for hamstrings. The patient can discard the crutches and be fully ambulatory after 5 to 7 days. Running is resumed at this stage, with return to sports activity dependent on the degree of symptoms and the requirement of the sport. Many players are able to return to sports activity 7 to 10 days after injury, wearing a light knee brace initially. Before resumption of activity, a player should be able to demonstrate no strength deficit on Cybex isokinetic testing, run at full speed without a limp, and perform agility drills. It is important that the rehabilitation program continue throughout the season.

GRADE IIA AND IIB INJURIES

A grade IIa or IIb injury represents various degrees of disruption of the ligament, but not complete disruption. Group IIa includes those with a slight opening medially (less than 5 mm). In grade IIb, there is more opening, but a good end point is observed. Pain is more prominent, and an effusion may be present with tenderness along the ligament. Those with slight opening and possessing good muscle control are treated like grade I injuries. The patient may be placed on crutches and a program of range of motion exercises begun. A Jordan splint provides some protection during progressive weight-bearing. Crutches can generally be discontinued about the fifth day or as soon as the patient feels comfortable. During the next 5 days, the splint should be maintained to provide protection, as any slight twist or valgus force on the knee may aggravate the injury. Isometric and straight leg raising exercises can be started, followed by isotonic exercises at 5 to 7 days. Cybex (isokinetic exercises) may be instituted earlier, allowing the patient to apply only a mild force in the midranges of speed, gradually increasing both speed and force. Soccer or football players may be able to return to competition by the end of the third week with a knee-hinge brace. A patient with poor musculature, or whose sports activity requires a greater degree of risk may require a slower rate of return to athletic activity. In a grade IIb injury, there may be a disruption of a portion of the ligament but a component is intact. Grade IIb injuries are considerably more unstable than are grade IIa and should be immobilized for about 4 to 5 weeks in 30 degrees of flexion to relax the posterior capsule and medial collateral ligament. Range of motion is begun during the fifth week by means of a hinged brace. Crutches are used initially, but weight-bearing is started as pain decreases, usually in about a week. During the immobilization phase isometric straight leg raises are emphasized. Once motion is started, and 90 degrees of flexion is achieved, isotonic and isokinetic exercises are added. Later, swimming and bicycling are beneficial, but running may not be resumed until quadriceps strength is approximately 80 percent that of the normal knee and motion is about 100 to 110 degrees. Generally these patients are off sports activity for about 8 to 10 weeks. Nonathletic patients may progress more slowly with their program, but full rehabilitation should be attempted. Subsequently at follow-up patients with medial collateral ligament grade IIb injury may have a slight jog of motion on valgus stretching but do not have symptoms of instability.

In treating patients with grade I and II medial collateral ligament injury, the possibility of meniscal damage should be explained to the patient. However, we have not noted a significant incidence of meniscal lesions if the ligament injury is confined to the medial collateral ligament. This is in contrast to the 30 to 40 percent incidence associated with anterior cruciate ligament injury.

How aggressively to go about making the diagnosis is open to debate. With the changing concept of meniscal repair, if meniscal damage is strongly suspected an arthrogram or arthroscopy is performed although the need for early meniscal repair has yet to be established. In grading injuries to the medial collateral ligament, the important question is whether the cruciate ligaments are intact. Thus in those knees tested at 30 degrees of flexion that open in a "barn door" fashion, invariably the anterior cruciate ligament is torn as well as the medial collateral ligament. If the knee starts to hinge open more than 10 mm but an end point is perceived without gross opening, the

anterior cruciate ligament is intact. When tested in extension, no instability is noted. In these patients, surgery is not indicated. The key, though, is to perform an adequate Lachman test to confirm that the anterior cruciate ligament is intact. Overall, there are few patients who fall within this class, as most complete grade III medial collateral tears have also torn anterior cruciate ligaments.

During the early 1970s isolated medial collateral ligament grade III injuries were operated on. Distal tears tended to stay approximated to the tibia and, other than reattaching the superficial medial collateral ligament to the tibia, little was done. Proximal transverse tears were repaired but had not retracted significantly allowing easy repair. A case could be made for reattaching the proximal origin, as there may be some decreased vascularity of the medial collateral ligament with slower healing usually resulting. Over the past 7 years, however, we have not operated on any patients with a pure medial collateral ligament injury regardless of the degree of instability nor have we found to date that any patient has developed symptoms of instability or required reconstructive surgery.

In treating grade III injuries nonsurgically, an approach similar to that for grade IIb is used, except that the leg is immobilized for 6 weeks. Hinges may be applied at 4 weeks allowing a limited arc of motion. Protection against valgus stress should be continued for an additional 2 months. Reconditioning including strength, flexibility, and agility is required before permitting the patient to return to athletic activity.

MEDIAL COLLATERAL LIGAMENT SURGERY

Grade III medial collateral ligament ruptures in association with a torn anterior or posterior cruciate ligament usually require surgical repair (Fig. 12.11) which is recommended for patients even in the fifth to sixth decade, unless there are medical problems that preclude surgery or the patient is willing to wear a brace and limit activity. If a conservative approach is followed, casting at 30 degrees of flexion for 6 weeks with the application of a hinge at 4 weeks is necessary. Unfortunately, even if the medial collateral ligament heals in a functional position, the patient is left with an anterior cruciate ligament insufficiency that is ag-

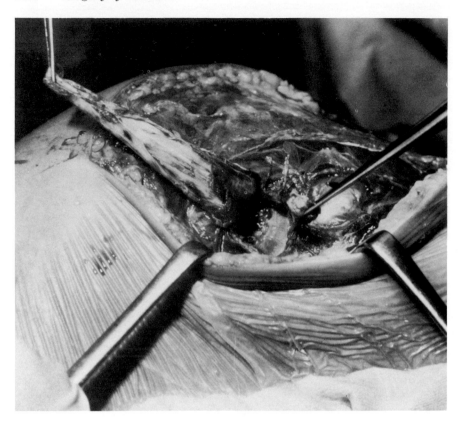

Fig. 12.11. Left knee: medial view of disruption of the superficial medial collateral ligament from the tibia while the deep portion is torn from the femur.

gravated by the loss of the secondary restraining effects of the superficial medial collateral ligament. As a result, even in older patients, symptomatic giving way is likely to occur with daily activities.

MEDIAL ANATOMY

In performing surgery for medial collateral tears, careful attention to the anatomy of the three individual layers of the medial side of the knee is critical (Fig. 12.12).[22] Layer 1 includes the deep fascia or crural fascia and invests inferiorly the sartorius muscle and tendon. Posteriorly the fascia is thin and overlies the two heads of the gastrocnemius. Proximally it is continuous with the fascia overlying the vastus medialis. Anteriorly, layer 1 blends with layer 2, 1 to 2 cm anterior to the edge of the superficial medial collateral ligament. Thus to view the superficial medial collateral ligament, an incision in layer 1 must be made directly over its fibers. If the cut is anterior to the medial ligament, it is not possible to dissect posteriorly and find the ligament.

Layer 2 consists of the superficial medial collateral ligament and soft-tissue attachments anterior to this ligament. It also extends posteriorly to the medial corner of the knee, where the fibers become more oblique. At the posteromedial corner of the knee, layer 2 joins layer 3. Layer 3 consists of the capsule of the joint and the deep medial ligament. It is attached directly to the femur and the tibia. Anteriorly it is thin and does not appear to have any stabilizing effect. Deep to the superficial medial ligament, a thickening in the capsule is called the deep medial ligament. It extends from the meniscus to the femur. Posteriorly layer 3 joins layer 2.

Thus in entering the knee to view the posterior horn of the medial meniscus, a vertical incision incises both layers simultaneously. The superficial medial ligament is the prime static stabilizer of the medial side of the knee.[23] It is because of its proximal attachment site close to the instant center of motion of the knee that its fibers maintain some tension throughout the arc of knee flexion. As the knee flexes, the anterior fibers tighten and the posterior fibers relax. The reverse occurs as the knee extends. If the

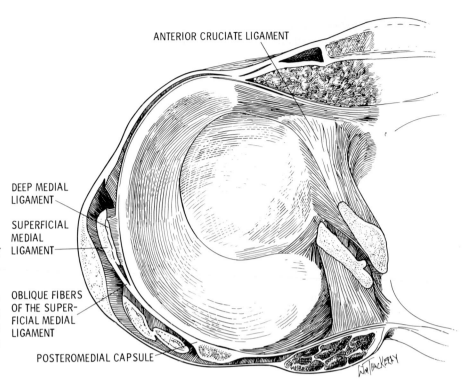

Fig. 12.12. Cross section of medial side of knee demonstrating three-layer concept. (From Warren, L.F., and Marshall, J.L.: The supporting structures and layers on the medial side of the knee. J. Bone Joint Surg. [Am.] *61:* 56, 1979, with permission.)

ANTERIOR CRUCIATE LIGAMENT

DEEP MEDIAL LIGAMENT

SUPERFICIAL MEDIAL LIGAMENT

OBLIQUE FIBERS OF THE SUPERFICIAL MEDIAL LIGAMENT

POSTEROMEDIAL CAPSULE

Fig. 12.13. Attaching the MCL proximally is critical, as an abnormal insertion site will create high stresses within the ligament during flexion and extension.

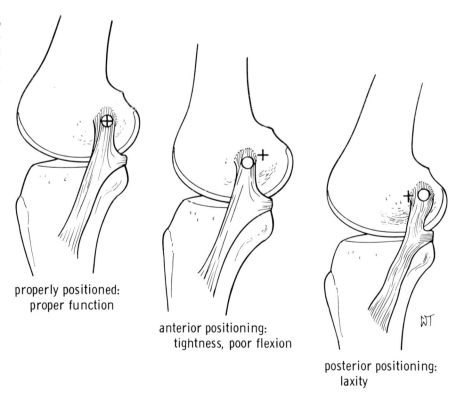

properly positioned: proper function

anterior positioning: tightness, poor flexion

posterior positioning: laxity

medial collateral ligament is reattached too far anteriorly or posteriorly, the balance will be disturbed, resulting in high tension in the ligament and subsequent failure of the repair (Fig. 12.13). Thus in reattaching the avulsed ligament, the reattachment site should be tested by flexing and extending the knee to determine the proper site.

COMBINED ANTERIOR CRUCIATE/MEDIAL COLLATERAL LIGAMENT INJURIES

In combined anterior cruciate/medial collateral ligament injuries, a longitudinal incision running from the tibial flare to the adductor tubercle is used (Fig. 12.14). Serpentine incisions are avoided to minimize devascularizing the margin of the flap. Dissection is carried out down to layer 1 exposing the anterior and posterior margins as indicated. The infrapatellar branch of the saphenous nerve should be avoided if possible, but if injured should be excised proximally up to the exit from the sartorius muscle.

Before opening the joint, an incision is made in layer 1 overlying the superficial medial collateral ligament (Fig. 12.15). Local tenderness often provides a guide to the site of suspected damage, and at surgery hemorrhage is noted. If a tear is suspected distally, the pes tendons must be elevated to permit visualization of the long superficial insertion. In the mid-ligament, transverse tears may extend posteriorly. When dissecting posteriorly, remember that the semimembranosus tendon lies at the medial corner with an anterior extension. Proximally, the origin of the medial collateral ligament lies deep to the vastus medialis and must be explored if damage is suspected. Sometimes damage is at more than one site or is incomplete at one site and complete more proximally.

Deep to the superficial medial collateral ligament lies the deep medial collateral ligament. It is the attachment for the medial meniscus and plays a minor role in knee stability. It is important for meniscal stability and may tear proximally or distally in transverse lesions of the superficial medial collateral ligament.

Once the damage to the medial structures has been evaluated, a plan for repair must be created. A medial parapatellar incision extending from the quadriceps tendon to the tibial plateau is used. A careful joint inspection for loose bodies, osteochondral defects, and meniscal lesions is followed by inspection of the cruciates. Repair of either the anterior cruciate or posterior cruciate ligament is carried out before collateral ligament repair. A markedly disrupted medial ligament, as seen in a knee dislocation, facilitates cruciate repair. Multiple loops of nonabsorbable sutures are used with reinforcement added to the repair in about 20 percent of cases. If there is associated meniscal damage, reattachment versus resection must be decided.

For healing to occur, the meniscus must have access to the capsular circulation.[3,18] It has been well demonstrated (Fig. 12.16) that the peripheral 10 to 30 percent of the meniscus has adequate circulation for healing to take place, if the tear communicates with the vascular region. If the tear is within the body at the inner edge, a partial meniscectomy may be performed. Peripheral tears are reattached using Dexon sutures in a serial fashion along the rim of the meniscus (Fig. 12.17). If the tear is within the body of the meniscus, healing will occur if vascular access channels are created. If the tear is in the posterior horn of the meniscus, an incision must be made posterior to the medial collateral ligament at the posterior medial corner of the knee. This is accomplished by making a vertical incision running from the femoral condyle to the proximal tibia, avoiding the semimembranosus tendon. Layers 2 and 3 are incised and excellent visualization of the posterior compartment obtained (Figs. 12.15 and 12.17). Medial collateral ligament repair is then performed using No. 0 Dexon sutures. If there is detachment from the bone distally the bone is roughened to create a bleeding surface. Drill holes are made to permit suture placement, or a staple is used. In proximal tears, the position of reattachment should be over the instant center of knee motion because if placed forward of this point, it tightens on flexion and results in laxity (Fig. 12.13). Before reattaching the superficial medial collateral ligament, the deep medial collateral ligament should be repaired. Drill holes along the edge of the femur may facilitate this repair if an avulsion has occurred.

Transverse tears in the medial collateral ligament are repaired with No. 0 Dexon sutures extending from an anterior to posterior direction. Occasionally the tissue of the superficial medial ligament is of such poor quality and holds sutures so inadequately that a Bosworth-type procedure using the semitendinosus

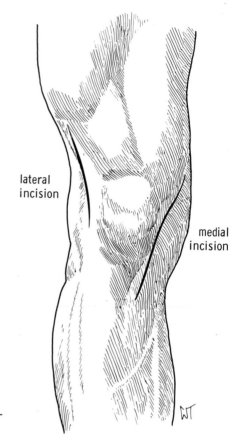

Fig. 12.14. Medial and lateral incisions are used in combined ACL/MCL injuries.

Fig. 12.15. Approaches to the medial side of the knee to expose the MCL. An incision made at position 1 will not allow visualization of the superficial MCL because layers 1 and 2 are joined together; therefore, the incision must be at position 2 directly over the MCL; position 3 represents the posterior medial approach to the posterior horn of the medial meniscus.

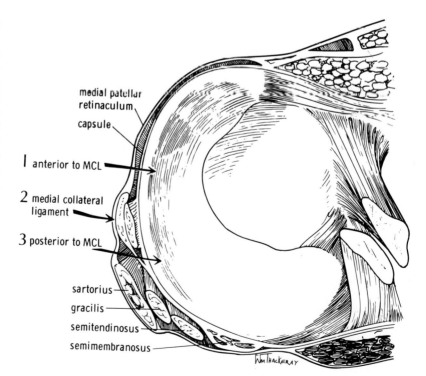

277

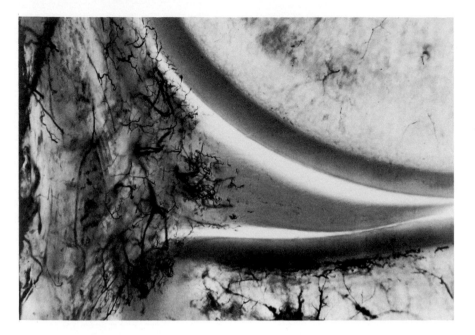

Fig. 12.16. Frontal section of the medial compartment of the knee demonstrating vessels from the perimeniscal capillary plexus penetrating the peripheral border of medial meniscus. (From Arnoczky, S.P., and Warren, R.F.: The microvasculature of the human meniscus. Am. J. Sports Med., *10*: 90, 1982, with permission. © 1982 Am. Orthopedic Society for Sports Medicine.)

tendon may be helpful. This procedure may be considered for patients in whom primary repair has been delayed for 3 to 4 weeks. The tissues at that stage are often edematous and hold the sutures with difficulty. The semitendinosus tendon is identified by lifting the pes tendons up and dissecting proximally. The tendon is then dissected out proximally to the muscle origin. A Penrose drain is placed about it, and the tendon is pulled forward to the femoral attachment of the medial collateral ligament (Fig. 12.18). It is stapled in place after a bony bed is created in which the tendon can be attached.

The knee should be placed through a full arc of motion, noting tension within the graft. The goal is to have it mimic the function of the anterior fibers of the superficial medial ligament. It is important that the bony surface be prepared down to bleeding bone to permit attachment of the graft to the femur. With this method, the remaining portion of the superficial medial collateral ligament can be reattached to the graft to reinforce it.

Attention is then directed toward the posterior medial corner of the knee if the tear extends in this direction. In combined anterior cruciate/medial collateral ligament injuries there is often a peripheral tear of the meniscus as well as damage to the posterior portion of the medial collateral ligament. Before plicating the posterior medial capsule, the meniscus is

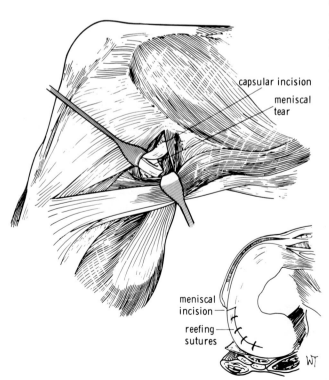

Fig. 12.17. Posteromedial approach for meniscal repair.

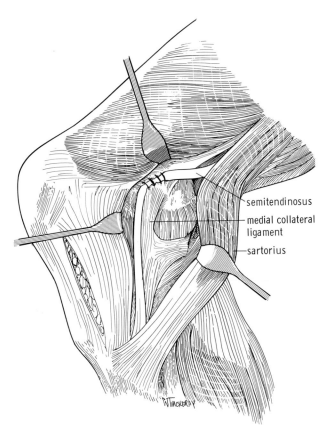

Fig. 12.18. Bosworth procedure utilizing the semitendinosus tendon.

reattached. The fat pad is attached to the anterior cruciate repair, and the anterior arthrotomy incision must be closed before completing the posterior repair to avoid difficulty in closing the retinaculum properly.

In closing the retinaculum, careful reattachment of the vastus medialis is performed, as patellar pain after surgery will occur if there is muscle detachment. After the anterior closure, the posterior medial corner is repaired. The key is to reattach the deep layer to the meniscus and to plicate the capsule at this site if it has been stretched out. The tibia is internally rotated and the layers advanced anteriorly over the posterior portion of the medial collateral ligament.

After completion of the repair, the tourniquet is released to coagulate any major bleeders. A Hemovac drain is placed in the soft tissues overlying layer 1, but not in the joint. The skin is closed with subcuticular Dexon and the leg is then immobilized in a Jones dressing with lateral and medial plaster splints.

POSTOPERATIVE PROGRAM

After surgery, patients are placed on bed rest for 24 hours with the leg elevated in a fixed sling. Intravenous antibiotics are continued for 24 hours and then stopped. The day after surgery, isometric exercises are attempted and an electrical muscle stimulator may be applied. The patient moves to a chair with the leg elevated on the second day, followed by crutch-walking and non-weight-bearing on day 3. On days 4 to 5, the dressing is removed and a cylinder cast is applied with the knee flexed 30 degrees. Straight leg raising exercises are increased and the patient discharged on day 5 or 6. At 3 to 4 weeks, the cylinder cast may be converted to a hinge cast, as knee stiffness is more likely to occur in combination injuries and can be lessened by motion. At 6 weeks, the cast is removed and a limited motion brace applied (Fig. 12.19). Initially, motion from 30 to 60 degrees is allowed. This is increased to a minus 10 degree extension stop at 12 weeks. The brace is removed three to four times a day for active assisted range of motion. Isotonic or isokinetic exercises are slowly instituted but should avoid the last 30 degrees of extension if the anterior cruciate ligament has been repaired, as quadriceps contraction at 30 degrees or less will create significant tension within the anterior cruciate ligament.

After repair, it is important to emphasize that the goal is to restore range of motion. A therapist may be necessary but should be cautioned to avoid overloading the ligament too soon. Patients are provided with a flow sheet indicating their expected progress. As a rule, by 6 weeks after the cast is removed they should have regained 90 degrees of flexion. If this has not been achieved, a therapist should be employed three times a week. Swimming activity is started in the early period after cast removal and by 8 to 9 weeks postinjury an exercise bicycle with a low torque setting is used to aid in knee motion. Passive assisted movements may be required to restore motion.

Once having achieved 90 degrees of flexion, isotonic or isokinetic exercises are added. Free weights attached to the leg are avoided initially, as excessive forces may be placed on the collaterals when the muscles are relaxed. Universal or Nautilus equipment may be used at the 3-month mark avoiding full extension at first. Isokinetic exercises at both low speeds of 5 rpm and high speeds of 32 rpm are helpful, as there

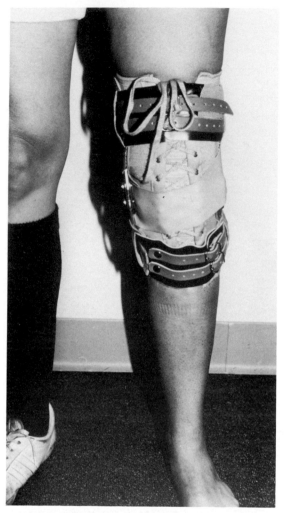

Fig. 12.19. Limited motion brace used postoperatively. Hinges are usually set for a 30- to 60-degree arc of motion which is subsequently increased.

is greater atrophy in fast twitch fibers than in slow twitch fibers. It is important to exercise the muscle group that is least likely to stress the repair. In anterior cruciate ligament injury, this is the hamstrings. While it is true that the anterior cruciate is maximally stressed by quadriceps activity in the terminal 30 degrees of extension, extension up to that point may be safely used. In anterior cruciate ligament injuries hamstring strength deficits are often significant: hamstring exercises are performed throughout a full arc of flexion.

After posterior cruciate ligament injury, quadriceps exercises are the main component of therapy. As mo-

tion and strength improve, activities may be increased. Initially bike riding is resumed at 4 months. Light interval jogging is started at 5 months. Fifty yards of jogging are followed by 50 yards of walking, with a gradual increase of the jogging over a month. If at the end of the month the patient has strength of 90 percent and motion of 120 degrees, agility drills may be added to the program. These consist of running in a large circle followed by progressively smaller circles and then reversing the direction. Figure-eight running is helpful in learning to change direction quickly. Use a large figure-eight pattern and progress to a tighter and quicker turn, and then reverse the direction. Jumping rope and stair running are additional ways of adding stress to the knee and building confidence.

Throughout the training period a brace is worn. It is discontinued at 6 months if the knee is clinically stable. Sports activity is resumed at 6 to 8 months, initially starting with sports in which the patient is in control of the environment and gradually resuming sports in which contact is involved.

It takes time to rebuild confidence and unless the patient is so informed, full potential will not be achieved. If the rehabilitation is incomplete in terms of strength or mobility, or if the repair is less than optimal, contact sports should be avoided.

ANTERIOR CRUCIATE INJURY

Controversy had existed regarding the function of the anterior cruciate ligament, but it has been well demonstrated that the anterior cruciate ligament provides the primary restraint against anterior tibial displacement on the femur. As to the clinical significance of injury to the anterior cruciate ligament, debate still exists regarding the treatment of isolated injuries, but in combined injuries surgical repair is advocated.

In developing a concept for or against repair of the anterior cruciate ligament, several questions must be addressed. First, what is our ability to perform repair and are the results repeatable? Second, if repair is not performed, what are the consequences and are the reconstructive efforts comparable? Third, what are the consequences regarding knee deterioration if primary repair is postponed temporarily or indefinitely? Fourth, what are the factors that may make the patient more likely to have problems?

It is quite apparent that the symptom complex of giving way is associated with anterior cruciate ligament insufficiency and not with collateral ligament damage.[24] This symptom may be described as the sensation of one bone slipping on another associated with variable pain and swelling. It is actually a pivot shift, and the patient will recognize it as such when the test is performed. After anterior cruciate ligament insufficiency, all patients examined under anesthesia will have a positive pivot shift test varying from mild to severe. Although it may be mild initially, it often increases over time. In addition, meniscal degeneration occurs with time, as attested to by the high incidence (60 to 70 percent) of meniscal injury by the time reconstruction is decided on, as compared with the incidence (25 to 33 percent) in acute injury. Joint degeneration is also seen in most patients.

A variety of factors appear to influence the course of these symptoms. The patient's age, activity level, specific sports, and motivation are important in considering primary repair. Patients who are past their fourth decade and willing to forego activities likely to produce symptoms are generally treated conservatively. Younger patients who are obese, inactive, and poorly motivated are not candidates for primary repair in isolated anterior cruciate ligament injury. In contrast, young athletes whose sports require changing direction quickly, decelerating rapidly, and jumping are candidates for primary repair of anterior cruciate ligament injuries. If the patient is markedly loose jointed with recurvatum of the knee, a primary repair with reinforcement offers the best opportunity of salvaging the knee, as late reconstructions often fail in these patients. Regarding late reconstruction versus early primary repair, our results indicate that those with primary repair are more active in sports, have less subsequent meniscal damage, and score better on our follow-up examinations. Using The Hospital for Special Surgery (HSS) scoring system, primary repairs in isolated injuries score 44 versus 40 for later reconstructions of isolated anterior cruciate ligament injuries.

Concerning our ability to carry out primary repair, we have continued to advocate this with fascial reinforcement predicated on the quality of the repair. About 20 percent of our primary repairs require reinforcement at surgery. In a follow-up study averaging 29 months in 70 patients, giving way was not noted nor had meniscal surgery been required in any pa-tient. One patient had been reinjured and required surgery at 1 year, at which time the disrupted repair was noted. We are currently carrying out a 5-year follow-up study and have noted no further deterioration.

Primary repair in properly selected patients will significantly decrease the likelihood of developing symptoms. In the event that the patient is willing to accept certain limitations and a possible reconstruction later, primary repair is not advised. The loss of secondary restraints makes primary repair of the anterior cruciate ligament more imperative. Both the collateral ligaments and the menisci act as significant restraints to anterior tibial displacement if the anterior cruciate ligament is not present.[3,12] Thus if collateral ligament damage is associated with anterior cruciate ligament injury, repair is generally advised. Meniscal damage occurs in 25 to 30 percent of cases and is equally important. We have demonstrated that after anterior cruciate ligament injury, medial meniscectomy will result in an 18 to 58 percent increase in tibial displacement on the femur with the knee at 0 degrees and 90 degrees of flexion. Thus any significant meniscal damage should increase the need for

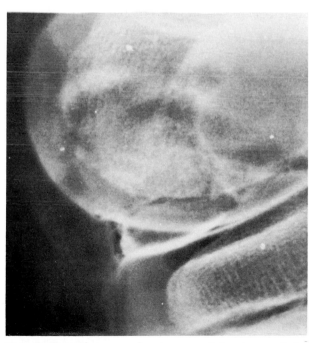

Fig. 12.20. Arthrogram showing a peripheral tear of the medial meniscus that was reattached in a 12-year-old patient.

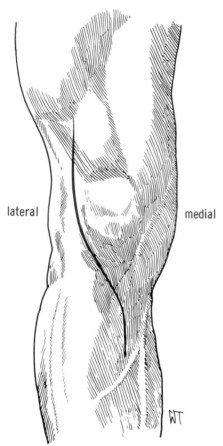

lateral

medial

WT

Fig. 12.21. Lateral incision, which allows visualization of the joint medially and reattachment of the ACL laterally through the same incision.

anterior cruciate ligament repair. In many anterior cruciate ligament injuries, the meniscal tears are peripheral or vertical tears that lend themselves readily to reattachment (Fig. 12.20). If the tear is in the inner margin, partial excision is performed.

Thus in evaluating the patient in whom doubt exists regarding the need for primary anterior cruciate repair we will perform arthroscopy or arthrography to substantiate that the menisci are intact. Generally primary anterior cruciate ligament repair should be performed within 1 to 2 weeks after the injury has occurred. If the interval is longer, arthroscopy can indicate the quality of the tissues. If cruciate tissue is poor and the menisci are intact, a period of observation with subsequent reconstruction, if required, would be advised. In performing repair after 1 to 2 weeks, reinforcement should generally be added to the repair.

ANATOMY

The anterior cruciate ligament consists of two main bundles that reciprocally tighten on flexion and extension.[1] The anterior medial band is the smaller of the two and tightens as the knee flexes, while the posterior lateral bulk tightens as the knee extends. Overall, the anterior cruciate ligament is 38 mm long and 11 mm wide. The tibial insertion is located anteriorly and is 30 mm long, while the femoral attachment is 23 mm long and located well posterior on the femur.

The circulation to the anterior cruciate ligament is precarious, as it is mainly supplied by the soft tissues including the synovium, fat pad and middle genicular artery. Little or no circulation enters through the bone.[2]

REPAIR TECHNIQUE

In injury restricted to the anterior cruciate ligament, the incision is a straight medial approach running from the femoral condyle to 2 inches (5 cm) below the joint line. More recently we have used a lateral incision crossing the infrapatellar tendon, which allows ligament repair and lateral reattachment through one incision. In addition, it is less likely to injure the infrapatellar branch of the saphenous nerve (Fig. 12.21). The vastus medialis is identified and a parapatellar capsular incision made extending from the tibial plateau to the quadriceps tendon. A long retractor is inserted to pull the infrapatellar tendon laterally, but in most cases the patella is not dislocated. Orderly evaluation of the joint is carried out noting cartilage defects and meniscal lesions. If the meniscus is deemed reparable, this is carried out, or a partial meniscectomy is performed. In posterior rim tears of the meniscus, the reattachment is performed via a second posterior capsular incision (Fig. 12.17) at the posteromedial corner of the knee (see medial collateral ligament section). Lateral meniscectomy can be performed through the medial incision by using a figure-8 position. Often arthroscopic instruments will aid in this technique.

In evaluating the cruciates, the knee should be flexed to about 90 degrees. The anterior cruciate ligament is identified and probed. Tension is placed on the ligament via a drawer test, and its ability to take up tension is assessed. Usually the damage is obvious, but at times, the synovial sleeve remains intact, making assessment more difficult. The synovial sleeve of the anterior cruciate ligament is connected to the posterior cruciate ligament, and it should be separated with a periosteal elevator. If the pivot shift and Lachman tests are positive but the sleeve is intact, open the sleeve with a longitudinal incision. The proximal and distal stumps must be identified. Proximally this requires dissecting well back into the intercondylar notch to expose the entire femoral attachment.

In most athletic injuries the tear is spiral, with a longer stump anteriorly attached to the tibia and a shorter proximal stump posteriorly (Fig. 12.22). Distal avulsions are rare (fewer than 2 percent) and midportion mop-end tears account for 80 percent of such injuries. Variable-sized proximal tears account for the remainder, with occasional avulsions seen.

In violent high-velocity automobile injuries, avulsions are more frequent, particularly from the femur, whereas in children anterior cruciate ligament injuries usually occur distally with bone and cartilage attached. In dissecting out the ligament, attempt to preserve the soft tissues; the intercondylar notch should be carefully assessed, as a prominent lateral wall may impinge on the anterior cruciate ligament making disruption more likely. In some patients the anterior cruciate ligament is abnormally thin, placing it at greater risk. If the lateral wall of the intercondylar notch is unusually prominent, an osteotome is used to trim the condyle 1 to 2 mm. Repair of the ligament is then carried out proximally and distally. The concept is to place multiple sutures at varying depths in the ligament to distribute the tension throughout the repair. Nonabsorbable sutures on a small KHT3 needle of 0 Polydec are used. A head lamp facilitates the procedure. Initially sutures are placed at the end of the stump and then progressively deeper until reaching the bony attachment site. Six to eight sutures are generally required. Attention is then directed toward the distal stump, and the suturing procedure is repeated. In placing the sutures, an anterior–posterior orientation is made as the posterior portion attaches to the femur and anterior sutures are brought out over the top of the lateral femoral condyle (Fig. 12.23). The tibial drill holes are placed medial and lateral to the anterior cruciate ligament attachment site with a 7/64 nonthreaded pin (Fig. 12.24).

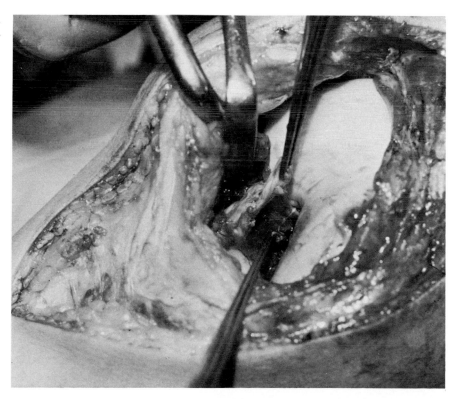

Fig. 12.22. Arthrotomy demonstrating typical spiral tear through the ACL.

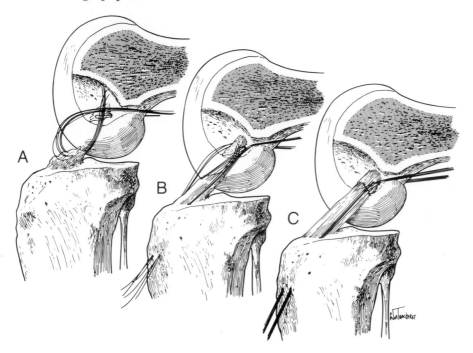

Fig. 12.23. Primary repair of the ACL.

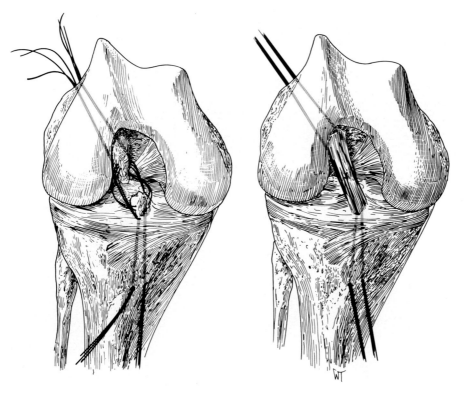

Fig. 12.24. Anterior view of primary repair of the ACL.

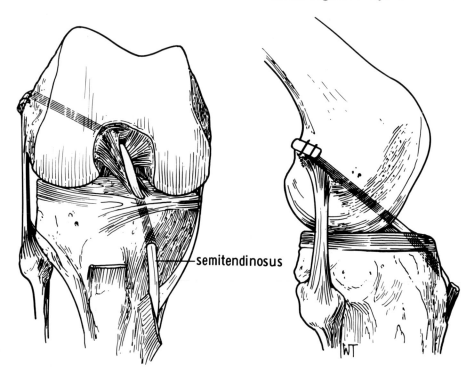

Fig.   *12.25.* Semitendinosus
reinforcement of the ACL.

A lateral incision 5 cm long at the superior edge of
the lateral femoral condyle is made down to the iliotibial band. A longitudinal incision at the edge of the
iliotibial band is made and the vastus lateralis elevated off the femur.

The superior-lateral genicular artery is identified
and coagulated. The periosteum is incised longitudinally and a tunnel created entering the joint over the
top of the lateral femoral condyle. A drill hole (7/64)
is placed in the lateral femoral condyle exiting at the
anterior edge of the femoral attachment of the anterior cruciate ligament. Following this, 22-gauge wires
are placed through all the holes and the sutures pulled
through the tibia first. Next, the distal sutures are
advanced to the femur pulling the posterior ends
through the drill hole and the anterior sutures over
the top. The sutures are pulled tight and the joint
placed through an arc of motion noting tension within
the anterior cruciate ligament. The knee is flexed to
45 degrees and displaced posteriorly as the sutures
are tied in place. Again, joint motion is checked and
joint stability assessed.

If, during the repair, the tissue appears inadequate
or the sutures do not hold well, reinforcement is carried out, but it is important to perform a complete

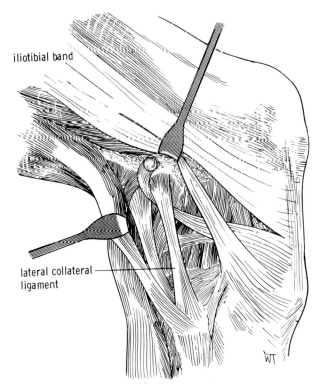

Fig. 12.26. Lateral sling procedure as used in primary ACL
repair.

primary repair initially. The drill hole distally is enlarged to one-quarter inch. The semitendinosus tendon is dissected proximally and incised at the muscle tendon junction but is left attached distally. A Bunnell suture is placed in the proximal end and is then passed through the tibia and out over the top of the lateral femoral condyle, where it can be stapled to the femur (Fig. 12.25).

Next, an absorbable suture is passed through the ligament or graft and the fat pad incised and attached to the anterior cruciate ligament. This may aid revascularization of the tissue. Reinforcement is necessary in about 20 percent of such repairs. Over the past year, we have added a lateral sling procedure to augment our acute repairs. This should be particularly helpful in patients with a 3+ pivot shift. This procedure is performed by dissecting free a strip of iliotibial band aproximately 9 cm long and 1 cm wide leaving it attached to Gerdy's tubercle. A Bunnell suture (Fig. 12.26) is then placed in the graft. Following this, the leg is placed in a figure-8 position to identify the lateral collateral ligament. The graft is passed deep to the lateral collateral ligament at its femoral attachment and should be positioned before tying the anterior cruciate ligament sutures. After the anterior cruciate ligament sutures are tied, the foot is externally rotated and the sling stapled to the femur in a bony bed.

Before wound closure, the tourniquet is released and hemostasis obtained. Closure over a Hemovac drain in the soft tissues is performed. The leg is placed in a Jones dressing with two plaster slabs holding the knee at 30 degrees of flexion.

The postoperative progression is similar to that described under the medial collateral/anterior cruciate ligament sections.

LATERAL SIDE INJURY

Damage to the lateral collateral ligament and the posterolateral corner of the knee is relatively uncommon, but postinjury symptoms can be marked. Isolated injury to the lateral collateral ligament is extremely rare, as nearly all patients have associated damage either to the anterior cruciate ligament or the posterior cruciate ligament. The lateral collateral ligament is the primary supporting structure on the lateral side of the knee, accounting for 55 percent of the resistance to a varus force at 5 degrees of flexion and for more than 69 percent of the resistance at 25 degrees. The cruciates are important secondary restraints providing 22.4 percent of the resistance at 5 degrees and 14.4 percent at 25 degrees of flexion. In both positions, it was mainly the anterior cruciate ligament that contributed to the resistance.[23]

Posterolateral instability is important in evaluating and treating patients with lateral side injury. Generally it is associated with damage to the posterior cruciate ligament. Although not prominent initially, it may become obvious with time as secondary restraints fail. In lateral side injuries, anterolateral instability is noted, but it is a reflection of anterior cruciate ligament injury rather than lateral side injury. Peroneal nerve damage may accompany lateral side injury and should be looked for prior to examining the knee. In 46 patients with lateral collateral ligament injury, five had sustained injury to the peroneal nerve.

ANATOMY

The lateral structures are divided into three anatomic layers (Fig. 12.27).[20] Superficially, layer 1 extends from the prepatellar bursa to the lateral retinaculum, including the iliotibial band and posteriorly, the biceps tendon. Just behind this lies the peroneal nerve. Layer 2 originates anteriorly and arises from the vastus lateralis fascia and the patella. It includes the more proximally located patellofemoral ligament, which runs in a posterior direction reaching the fabella in some specimens. Distally lies the patellomeniscal ligament, which runs in a distal posterior direction. The deep layer 3 has some variations. In the anterior third, it is a thin, apparently weak structure. In the middle third, it is firmly attached to the tibial plateau and may avulse with a fleck of bone, as seen in the midcapsular sign associated with anterior cruciate ligament injury. Posteriorly (Fig. 12.28), the deep capsule divides into two layers divided by the inferior-lateral genicular artery.

Phylogenically, there has been an evolution from a one-capsule layer in lower mammals to a two-layer system as the fibula has migrated distally from its direct involvment with the femur. As a result, a new capsular layer has formed. The more superficial portion of the deep layer 3 contains the lateral collateral

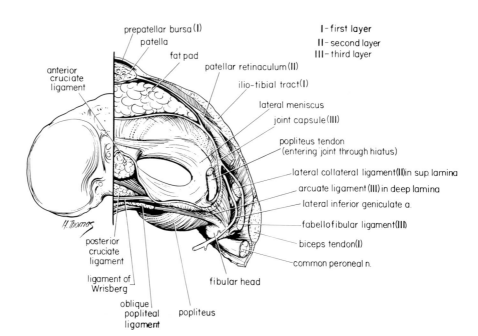

Fig. 12.27. Three-layer approach to lateral side anatomy. (From Seebacher, J.R., Inglis, A.E., Marshall, J.L., et al.: The structure of the posterolateral aspect of the knee. J. Bone J. Surg. [Am.], *64:* 536, 1982, with permission.)

I – first layer
II – second layer
III – third layer

prepatellar bursa (I)
patella
fat pad
patellar retinaculum (II)
ilio-tibial tract (I)
lateral meniscus
joint capsule (III)
popliteus tendon (entering joint through hiatus)
lateral collateral ligament (II) in sup. lamina
arcuate ligament (III) in deep lamina
lateral inferior geniculate a.
fabellofibular ligament (III)
biceps tendon (I)
common peroneal n.
fibular head
popliteus
oblique popliteal ligament
ligament of Wrisberg
posterior cruciate ligament
anterior cruciate ligament

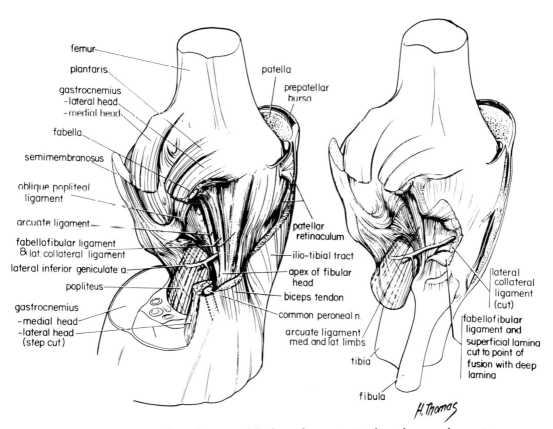

femur
plantaris
gastrocnemius
 -lateral head
 -medial head
fabella
semimembranosus
oblique popliteal ligament
arcuate ligament
fabellofibular ligament & lat. collateral ligament
lateral inferior geniculate a.
popliteus
gastrocnemius
 -medial head
 -lateral head (step cut)
patella
prepatellar bursa
patellar retinaculum
ilio-tibial tract
apex of fibular head
biceps tendon
common peroneal n.
arcuate ligament med. and lat. limbs
tibia
fibula
lateral collateral ligament (cut)
fabellofibular ligament and superficial lamina cut to point of fusion with deep lamina

Fig. 12.28. Posterior lateral corner of the knee demonstrating how the capsule consists of those layers separated by the interior geniculate artery. (From Seebacher, J.R., Inglis, A.E., Marshall, J.L., et al.: The structure of the posterolateral aspect of the knee. J. Bone J. Surg. [Am.], *64:* 536, 1982, with permission.)

ligament, and just posteriorly lies the short collateral or fabellofibular ligament, a structure of variable size. The deep layer is a thin, capsular layer of tissue through which the popliteus tendon enters and crosses the meniscus to attach to the femur deep to the lateral collateral ligament. A bare area is created on the lateral meniscus, which accounts for its poor circulation at this site. Running in the deep layer from the fibula to the fabella lies the arcuate ligament. In addition to this vertical limb, the arcuate ligament fans medially to join the fibers of the oblique ligament of Winslow. This structure varies in size inversely with the size of the fabella and the short collateral ligament.

In testing for ligament function, the knee is tested in extension and flexion with the application of a varus force. Opening in extension implies marked damage laterally, including the lateral collateral and anterior cruciate ligaments and often the posterior cruciate ligament if the knee opens widely. If the knee opens in flexion, damage to at least the lateral collateral ligament must be present, and injury to the iliotibial band, popliteus, and biceps is often present.

In performing the posterior drawer test, an attempt should be made to see whether the tibia subluxates posterolaterally on the femur in association with posterior cruciate ligament injury. It implies injury to the popliteus and arcuate complex. If the knee is brought into extension, the tibia swings into varus and rotates externally, again implying damage to the posterolateral corner. A third test is the reverse pivot shift test performed by holding the foot in external rotation as a standard pivot shift maneuver is performed (see Examination, above). Generally, these are massive injuries involving all the lateral side structures, often including the peroneal nerve.

In milder injuries, the crossed-leg position with the application of a varus force permits the examiner to palpate the lateral collateral directly noting any deficiency or local tenderness.

TENDERNESS

In those patients with incomplete injury of a grade I or grade II type with intact cruciate ligaments, conservative management similar to that for medial collateral ligament injuries grade I and II would be followed. Grade III injuries are nearly always associated with cruciate lesions and, if present, surgery is indicated in most active patients.

SURGICAL TECHNIQUES

In operating on lateral side injuries, the skin incision must be planned to permit adequate treatment of associated cruciate damage. If only the anterior cruciate ligament is torn, a longitudinal incision running from the lateral femoral condyle distally crossing the infrapatellar tendon allows good visualization of both the anterior cruciate ligament and the lateral structures (Fig. 12.20). If there is associated medial side injury, two straight incisions are best, if care is taken to avoid undermining the skin over the patella. Generally if the posterior cruciate ligament is torn, a medial side view is preferred, but if there is only lateral side damage, the lateral approach is taken.

Initially the dissection is over the most obvious area of injury identifying the structures in layer 1: the iliotibial band, biceps, and posteriorly the peroneal nerve. The nerve is not routinely dissected free unless there is associated nerve damage or reattachment of the soft tissues, including the biceps, and lateral collateral ligament to the fibular head is required. If there is gross transverse destruction of all structures down to the joint, as is frequently seen in complete dislocations, the iliotibial band and the capsule deep to this must be identified to allow reattachment. If the lesion enters the joint and the meniscus is detached, it should be carefully evaluated for the possibility of reattachment. Posterolaterally, the lateral collateral ligament and the short collateral ligament are identified within the superficial layer of the deep capsule superficial to the inferior genicular artery. Deep to this lies the popliteus tendon, which must be identified and its attachment to the femur noted. Avulsion may occur from the femur or there may be disruption within its muscle tendon junction. Generally the arcuate ligament, lying over the popliteus is a thin, weak structure. Having identified the pathology laterally, the joint is then opened and the cruciates and menisci inspected via a medial parapatellar incision. Cruciate repair is carried out, followed by meniscal reattachment. If the posterior cruciate ligament is torn distally or in its midportion, dissection posterolaterally over to the intercondylar notch is required. Before this procedure is carried out, the status of the lateral meniscus must be noted; if a peripheral tear is present, reattachment is carried out before lateral side repair. The technique consists of inserting absorbable No. 0 Dexon sutures in a vertical mattress fashion through the meniscus and peripheral capsule. In posterior horn tears, three to four sutures should be placed no more than 1 cm apart. If the meniscus is grossly unstable, a stabilization suture to the popliteus tendon may be placed, but this structure is relatively avascular. If the capsule posteriorly has been torn from the tibia, reattachment using pull through sutures may be necessary.

If the entire posterolateral capsule, including the lateral collateral ligament, the popliteus tendon, and the arcuate complex, has been stretched or avulsed proximally, it is best to advance this entire region as a unit. The tissue is advanced in a superior and anterior direction while pulling the tibia forward and internally to correct a posterolateral dropback. A raw bleeding surface on the femur must be prepared for the insertion of a staple to reattach the soft tissues to this site (Fig. 12.29).

It is imperative that a functioning lateral collateral ligament be obtained, as it is the most important lateral support. Its proximal and distal attachments must be identified within the superficial capsule of layer 3. Usually by placing the foot on the opposite leg and

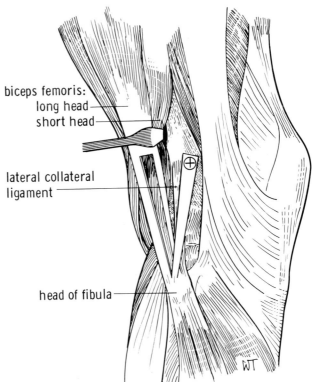

Fig. 12.30. Biceps tendon reinforcement of LCL. The deficit in the biceps tendon can be easily closed after transfer.

flexing the knee to 90 degrees while stressing the lateral side, it can be easily palpated within the capsule and its integrity noted. If the tear is distal at the fibular head with detachment of the biceps tendon as well, the peroneal nerve should be dissected free to allow reattachment without fear of nerve damage. Drill holes are placed in the proximal fibula to facilitate attachment of both the biceps and the lateral collateral ligament. Usually a short Bunnell suture is placed through the ligament and pulled through the drill holes. If the lateral collateral ligament is torn in its midportion and an adequate repair cannot be obtained, it should be reinforced primarily with a portion of the biceps tendon. A slip of biceps tendon approximately 6 to 7 mm in width and 7 cm in length (Fig. 12.30) is created and then rerouted proximally to the femoral attachment site of the lateral collateral ligament. It may be sutured in a drill hole, or a staple is applied.

After repair of the lateral structures and cruciate ligament(s), a meticulous closure is done after releasing the tourniquet to obtain hemostasis. Closure is

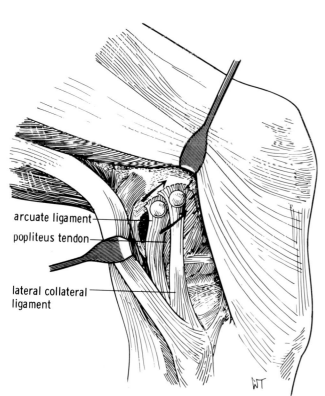

Fig. 12.29. Reattachment or advancement of posterolateral capsule containing avulsed LCL and popliteus tendon.

similar to that discussed for medial collateral ligament repair. The leg is held in a valgus or neutral position depending on the associated ligament damage, and a Jones dressing with plaster slabs is applied. Postoperative care is similar to that for medial side injuries, with the exception being that bracing may require a posterolateral strap to hold the tibia in an internally rotated direction if there was posterolateral instability.

POSTERIOR CRUCIATE LIGAMENT INJURY

In a recent review of ligament injuries we found that posterior cruciate ligament injury represented 8.1 percent of our knee ligament surgery performed over the past 15 years. However, this incidence probably underemphasizes the true incidence of posterior cruciate ligament injury, as it is frequently missed or lesions may be incomplete.

MECHANISM OF INJURY

In a review of 64 posterior cruciate ligament injuries, 48 percent of the injuries were athletic, 41 percent were vehicular accidents including motorcycles, and 11 percent were industrial and household accidents. Three mechanisms of injury were noted with posterior tibial displacement, accounting for 57 percent of the injuries.

Hyperextension injures the anterior cruciate ligament initially and, if continued, will damage the posterior capsule and the posterior cruciate ligament. This occurred in 23 percent of the patients. An extreme valgus or varus stress damages the collaterals initially, followed by the cruciates. Twenty percent of patients described this mechanism.

ANATOMY

The posterior cruciate ligament is larger and stronger than the anterior cruciate ligament, averaging 38 mm in length and 13 mm in width. It consists of two main components, a smaller posterior portion that tightens as the knee is brought into extension and a larger, bulkier component located anteriorly that tightens on

flexion. In repairs and reconstruction it is the function of the larger component that is sought. The posterior cruciate lies within the synovial sleeve and is an extra-articular structure, but with its more posterior location it has a closer relationship to the vascular structures of the posterior capsule, which may favorably affect repair.

EXAMINATION

In evaluating patients for posterior cruciate ligament instability, it is critical to note the presence of a small posterior sag when viewed from the side. If the knee cannot be flexed 75 to 90 degrees, the excursion of the tibia on the femur is diminished, making evaluation more difficult. Aspiration of the joint may be required to permit adequate flexion. If the examination is still inadequate, and there is a strong suspicion of posterior cruciate ligament injury, an examination under anesthesia and arthroscopy is required. If there is no posterior sag initially on posterior drawer testing, but there is some increased excursion, then a partial lesion not requiring repair may be present. If a sag is associated with an increased excursion and a loss of end point on drawer testing, the posterior cruciate ligament is completely torn or incompetent. The posterior drawer test is highly accurate in chronic cases of posterior cruciate ligament injury and even in acute injuries in which there is no other ligament damage. When there is associated damage to the anterior cruciate ligament, the accuracy rate falls because of failure to center the tibia on the femur.[19] In each patient whose posterior cruciate ligament injury was missed preoperatively, there was associated anterior cruciate ligament injury. If the sag is not appreciated before the drawer test is performed, a false-positive anterior drawer test implies that there is damage to the anterior cruciate ligament, when in fact the posterior cruciate ligament or both the posterior and anterior cruciate ligaments may be damaged. In evaluating acute knee injuries, an accurately performed Lachman test will indicate the status of the anterior cruciate ligament. If the examiner notes significantly increased anteroposterior motion with an excellent end point, disruption of the posterior cruciate ligament should be suspected. It can be confirmed by the posterior drawer test.

In patients with gross instability to varus or valgus

stress in extension, it is likely that damage to both the posterior cruciate and the anterior cruciate ligaments will be found. For either of these tests to be positive, the anterior cruciate ligament must also be torn. We have seen patients with complete tears of the posterior cruciate and the medial collateral ligaments in whom the abduction stress test in extension was negative because the anterior cruciate ligament was intact. In combined anterior cruciate and posterior cruciate ligament damage, hyperextension is apparent. A posterolateral dropback is also associated with posterior cruciate injury. If the integrity of the posterior cruciate ligament is in question and surgery is contemplated, examination under anesthesia combined with arthroscopy is indicated. Arthroscopy is performed through an anterior-lateral portal. Probing of the ligament is important, but with an intact anterior cruciate ligament, evaluation of the posterior cruciate ligament may be difficult. However, the posteromedial portal permits excellent visualization of the ligament. At the same time, a probe may be passed through a lateral portal to permit evaluation of the stress that the ligament takes up as the posterior drawer is applied.

In deciding on surgery, such factors as activity level, associated ligament damage, and degree of instability are important. In our review, patients with chronic collateral and posterior cruciate ligament insufficiency without anterior cruciate ligament injury scored poorly at follow-up averaging only 28 of 50 points on the HSS ligament scoring system.[19] In addition, 95 percent of our patients with chronic deficiency complained of chronic pain, in contrast to those with anterior cruciate ligament insufficiency. Complaints of instability, particularly notable while descending stairs, were present in 86 percent of patients, with 48 percent having instability on daily activity and 38 percent associated with stress and sports activity. The results with reconstruction seem significantly poorer than those of primary repair; hence primary repair is advocated in complete posterior cruciate ligament disruption in isolated as well as combined lesions. However, the results of primary ligament surgery appear to be inferior to those for anterior cruciate ligament injury.[15] Thus reinforcement is a routine component of the repair in all midportion posterior cruciate lesions.

In contrast to anterior cruciate ligament injury, our study found that partial lesions of the posterior cruciate ligament were present in 28 percent of cases. It appears that many of these lesions may be treated by closed methods. In this situation, damage has occurred, but examination shows no dropback or sag. If the posterior drawer sign demonstrates increased excursion with an end point, arthroscopy should be performed to demonstrate the integrity of some fibers of the posterior cruciate ligament. If it is greater than 40 to 50 percent, conservative treatment is indicated. The patient with partial injury is non-weight-bearing initially in a protective splint or cast. A hinge allowing limited motion of 30 to 60 degrees is applied at 3 weeks and is converted to a minus 10-degree extension stop at 6 weeks. The ligament should be protected from high stresses for a minimum of 2 months, as significant additional damage is possible. With this program, we have noted that some patients have been able to return to high levels of activity, including collegiate football, with mild but asymptomatic instability.

REPAIR TECHNIQUE

Having concluded that surgery is indicated, the approach is predicated on the associated instabilities. Generally repair from a posteromedial approach is preferred. The exception is when there is marked lateral damage without medial instability, or when there is isolated avulsion of the posterior cruciate ligament from the tibia. If the radiograph demonstrates a large tibial fragment and the clinical (Fig. 12.31) examination demonstrates no associated ligament damage, arthroscopy should be performed to delineate any associated intra-articular injuries. If no abnormal findings are observed, and the posterior cruciate ligament is intact proximally, a posterior approach may be used to reattach the avulsed fragment of the bone with a cancellous screw. We have seen patients in whom this was not done because of the mistaken impression that there was minimal displacement when in fact the fragment had migrated superiorly and anteriorly over 1 cm, rendering the posterior cruciate ligament incompetent. The posterior cruciate ligament attaches well distal to the articular surface and runs over the posterior prominence of the tibia.

In most patients, repair is performed using a medial approach. Often, arthroscopy has been performed to evaluate the site of damage. The damage

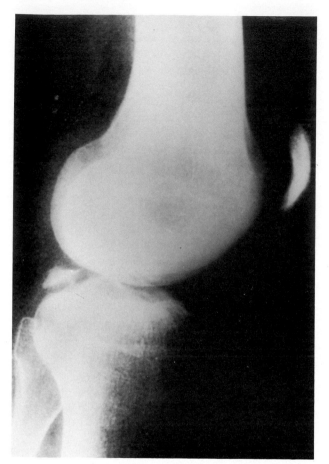

Fig. 12.31. Tibial avulsion fracture seen in PCL injury.

margin. The holes should be separated by at least 1 cm to provide a wider attachment site. The sutures are then pulled through the drill hole using a 22-gauge wire loop. If the tear is midportion or distal without a bone fragment, a posterior medial approach is required. It is performed by completing the exposure of the posterior medial corner of the knee, creating a capsular incision as in viewing the posterior horn of the medial meniscus. A vertical incision is created running from the femur to the tibia in the weak area of the capsule. Viewing medially, the posterior cruciate ligament can be seen. A peripheral rim tear of the meniscus greatly facilitates repair; otherwise, partial detachment at the posterior horn of the medial meniscus is performed. To facilitate exposure, the semimembranosus tendon is divided to be repaired later. A second approach is to dissect outside of the capsule and lift the medial head of the gastrocnemius in order to approach the posterior tibial surface, opening the capsule vertically. This approach is

to the posterior cruciate ligament is proximal in one-third, midportion in one-third (Fig. 12.32), and distal in one-third of cases. If the damage is proximal with an avulsion, simple reattachment can be carried out using the multiple-loop suture technique. A straight medial incision permits access to the joint anteriorly and posteriorly if necessary. If there is marked proximal injury or avulsion, the multiple-loop sutures are performed as in anterior cruciate ligament repair using a series of No. 0 nonabsorbable sutures passing through progressive depths of the ligament (Fig. 12.33).

In reattaching the proximal site of the posterior cruciate ligament, an incision is made over the medial femoral condyle, avoiding the vastus medialis obliquus and medial collateral ligament. In placing the drill holes in the medial femoral condyle, the normal attachment site of the posterior cruciate ligament should be recalled, as it is quite close to the articular

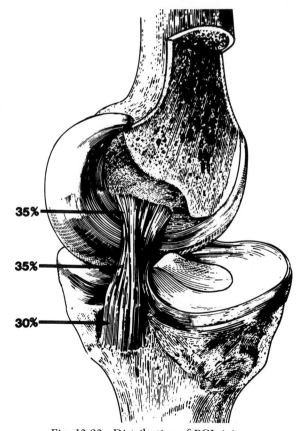

Fig. 12.32. Distribution of PCL injury.

more difficult and does not permit easy suturing of the ends of the ligament.

Once the distal end of the posterior cruciate ligament has been located, several sutures are placed at a progressive depth in the ligament. Next, two drill holes are placed in the proximal tibia in an anterior to posterior direction, taking care to protect the neurovascular structures posteriorly (Fig. 12.33).

Midportion tears of the posterior cruciate ligament present the most difficulty. Multiple-loop sutures are used first in the proximal stump and then in the distal stump. They are then passed through their appropriate drill holes. Because of the difficulty of performing the repair adequately and the greater strength required of the posterior cruciate ligament, augmentation of the midportion tears of the posterior cruciate ligament should be routine. It may be accomplished by using a free stump of the semitendinosus tendon or a portion of the medial head of the gastrocnemius tendon. In using the semitendinosus tendon, one of the drill holes proximally and distally is enlarged to one-quarter inch to accept the tendon (Fig. 12.33).

The tendon is then detached proximally. A drill hole is placed from anterior to posterior in the tibia to accept the graft. A Bunnell suture is placed in the graft and is pulled through the tibia and then to the femur. Next, the tibia is displaced anteriorly on the femur and the sutures and graft are secured. If collateral ligament repair is required, the knee is held flexed while completing it and tying the posterior cruciate ligament sutures. Closure is as described above.

Proper positioning of the knee after repair has spurred debate. We recommend that the knee be placed in extension, but not hyperextension, which stresses the posterior fibers of the posterior cruciate ligament. It appears to be an easier position to control anteroposterior translation of the tibia on the femur, particularly in combined anterior cruciate/posterior cruciate ligament injuries, in which it is difficult to find the true center position. In this situation, we generally place the knee in the 90-degree position pulling the tibia forward on the femur before tying the PCL sutures followed by the anterior cruciate ligament sutures. The goal is to avoid a fixed posterior

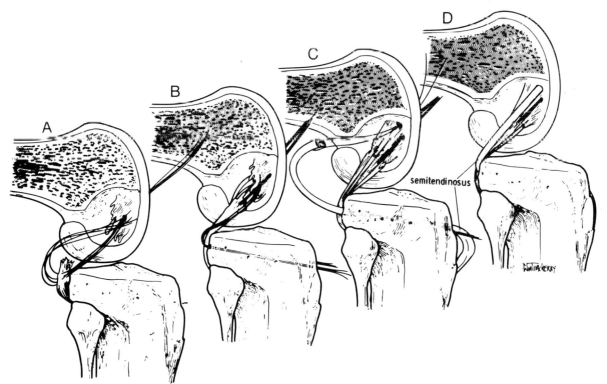

Fig. 12.33. PCL repair with multiple-loop sutures technique combined with semitendinosus reinforcement.

subluxation, which will result in chronic pain and limited extension. A Steinmann pin across the joint to hold the tibia forward was found unsatisfactory. Our postoperative program is similar to that for anterior cruciate ligament injuries except that the posterior cruciate ligament is held slightly longer, averaging about 7 weeks. After that, the knee is placed in a limited motion brace to avoid hyperextension or full flexion (Fig. 12.19). The brace is removed three times a day for range of motion exercises. At 12 weeks the brace is converted to a full range of motion brace except for the final 10 degrees of extension.

Rehabilitation efforts follow. Posterior cruciate repairs seem to have poorer results than those for anterior cruciate ligament. Return to activity is poorer and less predictable with motion at times difficult to regain. Manipulation may be required at about 4 months to regain flexion. Extension lag is not a problem, but we have seen some patients in whom the primary repair was performed with the knee subluxed posteriorly, for whom it is extremely difficult to regain extension. One of the reasons for failure appears to be that damage to the posterolateral corner of the knee was not recognized and repaired primarily, as a result of which instability symptoms developed. It is imperative that a complete repair be performed initially if optimal results are to be obtained.

REFERENCES

1. Abbott, L.C., Saunders, J.B., Bost, F.C., et al.: Injuries to the ligaments of the knee joint. J. Bone J. Surg., *26*: 503, 1944.
2. Arnoczky, S.P., Rubin, R.M., and Marshall, J.L.: Microvasculature of the cruciate ligaments and its response to injury. J. Bone J. Surg. [Am.], *61*: 1221, 1979.
3. Butler, D.L., Noyes, F.R., and Grood, E.S.: Ligamentous restraints to the anterior-posterior drawer in the human knee. J. Bone J. Surg. [Am.], *62*: 259, 1980.
4. Cahill, B.R.., and Griffith, E.H.: Effect of preseason conditioning on the incidence and severity of high school football knee injuries. Am. J. Sports Med. *6*: 180, 1978.
5. Clayton, M.L., and Weir, G.J.: Experimental investigations of ligamentous healing. Am. J. Surg., *98*: 373, 1959.
6. Ellsasser, J.C., Reynolds, F.C., and Omohundro, J.R.: The non-operative treatment of collateral ligament injuries of the knee in professional football players. J. Bone J. Surg. [Am.], *56*: 1185, 1974.
7. Feagin, J.A.: The syndrome of the torn anterior cruciate ligament. Orthop. Clin. North Am., *10(1)*: 81, 1979.
8. Jack, E.A.: Experimental rupture of the medial collateral ligament of the knee. J. Bone J. Surg. [Br.], *32*: 396, 1950.
9. Johnson, R.J., and Pope, M.H.: Ski binding biomechanics. Physician Sportsmed. *10* (2): 49, 1982.
10. Kennedy, J.C., Hawkins, R.J., Willis, R.B., et al.: Tension studies of human knee ligaments. J. Bone J. Surg. [Am.], *58*: 350, 1976.
11. Kennedy, J.C., Roth, J.H., and Walker, D.M.: Posterior cruciate ligament injuries. Orthop. Dig., 19, 1979.
12. Levy, I.M., Torzilli, P.A., and Warren, R.F.: The effect of medial meniscectomy on anterior-posterior motion of the knee. J. Bone J. Surg. [Am.] *64*: 883, 1982.
13. Marshall, J.L., and Rubin, R.M.: Knee ligament injuries—a diagnostic and therapeutic approach. Orthop. Clin. North Am., *8(3)*: 641, 1977.
14. Marshall, J.L., Warren, R.F., and Wickiewicz, T.L.: Primary surgical treatment of anterior cruciate ligament lesions. Am. J. Sports Med., *10(2)*: 103, 1982.
15. Moore, H.A., and Larson, R.L.: Posterior cruciate ligament injuries. Am. J. Sports Med. *8(2)*: 68, 1980.
16. O'Donoghue, D.H.: An analysis of end results of surgical treatment of major injuries to the ligaments of the knee. J. Bone J. Surg. [Am.], *37*: 1, 1955.
17. O'Donoghue, D.H., and Rockwood, C.A.: Repair of knee ligaments in dogs. J. Bone J. Surg. [Am.], *43*: 1167, 1961.
18. Peterson, T.R.: The crossbody block, the major cause of knee injuries. J.A.M.A., *211*: 449, 1970.
19. Savatsky, G., Marshall, J.L., Warren, R.F., et al.: Posterior cruciate ligament injury. Orthop. Trans., *4*: 293, 1980.
20. Seebacher, J.R., Inglis, A.E., Marshall, J.L., et al.: The structure of the posterolateral aspect of the knee. J. Bone J. Surg. [Am.], *64*: 536, 1982.
21. Torg, J.S., Quedenfeld, T.C., and Landau, S.: The shoe-surface interface and its relationship to football knee injuries. Am. J. Sports Med. *2(5)*: 261, 1974.
22. Warren, L.F., and Marshall, J.L.: The supporting structures and layers on the medial side of the knee. J. Bone J. Surg. [Am.], *61*: 56, 1979.
23. Warren, L.F., Marshall, J.L., and Girgis, F.: The prime static stabilizer of the medial side of the knee. J. Bone J. Surg. [Am.], *56*: 665, 1974.
24. Warren, R.F., and Marshall, J.L.: Injuries of the anterior cruciate and medial collateral ligaments of the knee. Clin. Orthop., *136*: 191, 1978.

13 Chronic Instability of the Knee

John N. Insall

No aspect of knee surgery is as controversial as chronic ligamentous laxity.[1] Cadaver experiments and clinical measurements of injured knees at surgery have yielded findings that are confusing, ambiguous, or even contradictory. This observation is not new, as Brantigan and Voshell[11] made similar comments in the 1940s.

The foundation of modern anatomic study (discussed in the anatomy section) was made by Palmer[74] in Sweden and by Brantigan and Voshell[11] in America. These workers described lesions in anatomic terms as single-plane laxities. Rotary laxity is a comparatively recent concept based on descriptions by Slocum and Larson,[77] Hughston,[38] Kennedy,[51] Nicholas,[70] and others. Single-plane laxity is recognized by all, but rotary instability is debated. Does rotary instability result from a combination of cruciate and collateral ligament injury,[63] or is it possible for rotational instability to occur when the prime static stabilizers are intact? For example, Hughston et al. state that anterolateral rotary instability is caused by a tear of the middle one-third of the lateral capsular ligament, although these investigators recognize that this instability is accentuated by a tear of the anterior cruciate.

METHODS OF MEASUREMENT

Several methods of determining instability exist, and all have built-in limitations and sources of error.

CLINICAL OBSERVATIONS

The degree of instability in a given direction is usually expressed as mild (1+), indicating that the joint surfaces separate ≤5 mm; moderate (2+), with a separation of 5 to 10 mm; and severe (3+), with a separation of ≥10 mm, according to the recommendations of the Committee on the Medical Aspects of Sports of the American Medical Association.[17]

In a handbook entitled *Standard Nomenclature of Athletic Injuries,* a sprain is defined as an injury limited to ligament and a strain as a stretching injury of muscle or its tendinous attachment to bone. A first-degree sprain of a knee ligament is defined as a tear of minimum number of fibers of the ligament with no instability. A second-degree sprain is a disruption of more fibers with generalized tenderness but no instability, and a third-degree sprain is a complete disruption of the ligament with instability. These definitions are probably inadequate today because they do not account for interstitial failure[15] of the ligament giving rise to stretching and elongation, but without loss of continuity and disruption (Fig. 13.1). Interstitial failure occurs before disruption with all ligaments subject to excessive stress, but the late result varies from one ligament to another. Therefore, the result of a medial ligament sprain (even in most cases of complete disruption) is healing with elongation, so that stress testing shows some instability with a firm end point. A similar mode of failure is seen with pos-

295

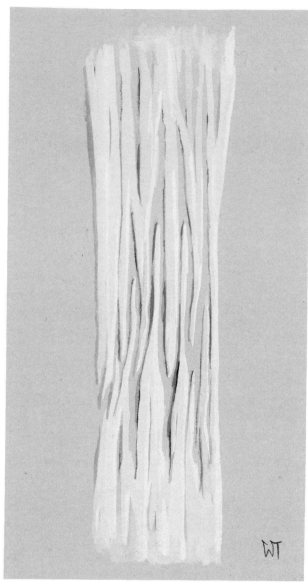

Fig. 13.1. Interstitial ruptures within the substance of the ligament produce elongation without much visible surface alteration.

terior cruciate injury and after healing there is a ligament that to inspection and palpation appears in continuity (Fig. 13.2). In contrast, after anterior cruciate injury, there is often total loss of continuity so that to passive stress testing the anterior drawer has no end point. It is therefore relatively easy to diagnose anterior cruciate ligament (ACL) incompetence by inspection but more difficult to make the same judgment concerning the posterior cruciate ligament (PCL),

although Lysholm and Gillquist[60] claim success using arthroscopy to make a direct inspection of the posterior portion of this ligament. However, the assessment of direction in anteroposterior instability usually depends on a judgment of the resting or neutral position made by flexing both knees to 90 degrees and comparing one with the other (Fig. 13.3). Therefore, with PCL stretching injuries, unless the dropback in the resting position is recognized, an apparent anterior drawer may be misinterpreted as attributable to an ACL injury (Fig. 13.4). Even when 2+ or 3+ anteroposterior laxity is present, both cruciate ligaments appear in continuity to inspection.

This difference in behavior after injury between the cruciate ligaments has for some reason not received wide attention, but clearly provides an important source of error in any assessment of ligament function based upon clinical observations. A second limitation of clinical observation is that knee injuries often produce lesions of several supporting structures, so that in a combination injury the wrong structure may be blamed for the instability. (Selective cutting experiments on cadaver knees are more accurate in this respect because the lesion causing laxity is known beyond doubt.) On the other hand, clinical observations have an advantage that follows from their major drawback: most clinical injuries are multistructural in a way difficult to emulate in the laboratory. Moreover, living tissues heal and other supporting structures hypertrophy. This is impossible to duplicate in any experimental model, which is why rotary laxities that compare with clinical lesions are particularly difficult to create and evaluate experimentally.

CLINICAL DATA SUPPORTED BY STRESS RADIOGRAPHY

Kennedy and Fowler,[51] Jacobsen,[45] and Torzilli et al.[84] have used stress radiographs to determine abnormal motion, particularly in an anteroposterior direction. All these investigators used a basically similar technique, although the sophistication of the equipment varied. In all an adjustable seat was used so that the knee could be positioned at 90 degrees with the foot held in a foot plate. The thigh was immobilized with tourniquets and after the jig had been adjusted for patient size, stress was applied to the tibia by calf and shin slings in both anterior and posterior direc-

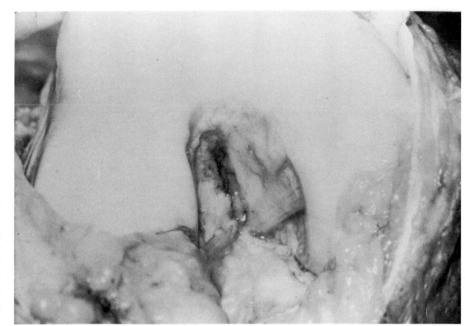

Fig. 13.2. Interstitial failure occurred in the posterior cruciate ligament of this knee. The fibers of the ligament are clearly visible, although the bulk is somewhat less than normal. The anterior cruciate is lax but, on applying an anterior draw, was observed to be normal.

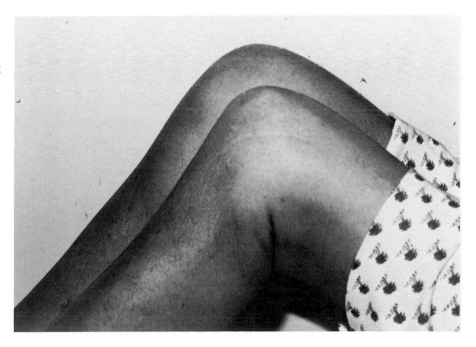

Fig. 13.3. The neutral position or starting point must be assessed by examination for any tibial dropback in the resting position.

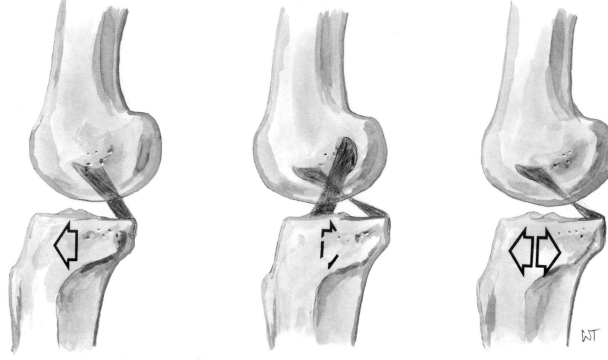

Fig. 13.4. Diagram showing the possibilities when anteroposterior stability is found. (Left) The direction may be purely anterior and due to an anterior cruciate rupture. (Center) The direction may be purely posterior and due to a posterior cruciate attenuation. (Right) Abnormal motion may be present in both directions and associated with anterior cruciate rupture and posterior cruciate attenuation.

tions. The slings were attached to a constant tension spring (Torzilli) (Fig. 13.5A,B), pulley weights (Jacobsen), and a piston motivated by Freon gas (Kennedy). The amount of force applied was (15 and 30 lb) (Torzilli), 20 kg (44 lb) (Jacobsen), and not given (Kennedy). Jacobsen and Kennedy assessed laxity in an anterior direction only while Torzilli attempted to assess the resting position (by comparison with the normal knee) and measured abnormal laxity in both anterior and posterior directions. On the lateral radiographs obtained, movement of the medial and lateral femoral condyles was measured separately with respect to the corresponding posterior margins of the tibial plateaus (Fig. 13.6). Kennedy used templates to simplify the measurement.

Using the stress machine, both Jacobsen and Kennedy reported increased accuracy over clinical methods alone. However, Torzilli et al. were unable to reduplicate their results because immobilization of foot and thigh was insufficient to prevent other movements from occurring (Fig. 13.7). Tibial rotation was the most frequent out-of-plane motion observed, followed by femoral rotation and femoral abduction and adduction (Fig. 13.8). The cumulative error from these motions observed while testing normal knees was as much as 10 mm with the major contribution coming from unwanted femoral motion. Torzilli et al then attempted to measure out-of-plane motion and compensate for it using a formula derived from an experimental cadaver model into which the unwanted motions could be precisely introduced and measured. Many reference points on both femur and tibia were required to make the measurements, some of which could not always be identified with precision on the radiograph. Probably because of this, compensatory calculations were not only cumbersome but did not always improve the accuracy of the method. Stress radiography is useful (1) to determine the neutral or

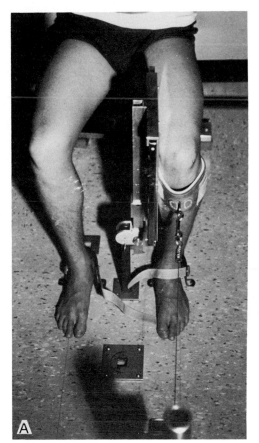

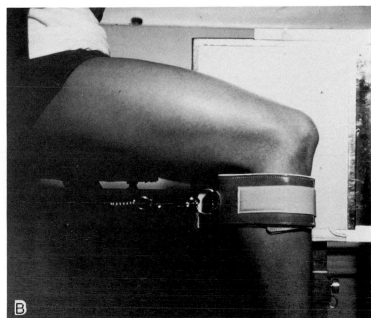

Fig. 13.5. A simple stress machine testing the knee at 90 degrees of flexion. A neutral film is taken of both knees to assess the starting point. Further films are taken with anterior traction (A) and posterior traction (B) using a constant tension spring.

Fig. 13.6. Using Jacobsen's method, both femoral condyles and both tibial plateaus are measured separately.

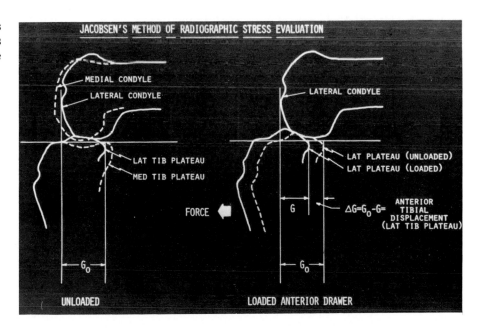

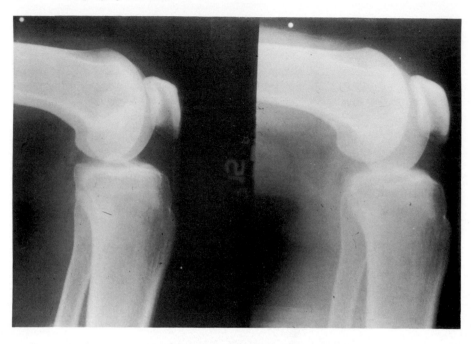

Fig. 13.7. Radiograph of a normal knee in the resting position (left) with posterior traction applied (right). Note that the position of the femoral condyles relative to one another has changed.

resting point by comparison with the normal side, so that the method can be used to detect whether abnormal laxity is anterior or posterior in direction, and (2) to confirm the diagnostic accuracy of the clinical examination.

CADAVER EXPERIMENTS AND SELECTIVE CUTTING

Cadaver experiments generally require fixation of the bones in a rig so that laxity after cutting ligamentous structures is measured in a single plane; in this respect, the result cannot be compared with clinical observations. In most experiments the muscular at-

tachments are excised from the preparation. An exception is the popliteus tendon, which usually remains attached to the muscle belly and therefore may be affected by postmortem changes. Specimens are either fresh or frozen, and it can be assumed that the ligamentous structures perform much as they do in life.

Selective cutting experiments have been done by many investigators.[11,12,27,30,33,34,51,62,89] The laxities created have been measured by visual and manual assessments, strategically placed marking pins,[89] especially designed goniometer linkages,[62] and the Instron machine.[12] Most investigators assessed increase in laxity after a cutting procedure. Butler et

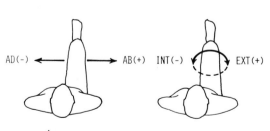

Fig. 13.8. Out-of-plane motions, such as femoral abduction and adduction, can greatly influence Jacobsen's measurements and thereby contribute to inaccuracy.

Femoral AB/ADduction

(mm)

$-3.00 \leq \Delta G_a \leq +7.00$
$-6.00 \leq \Delta H_a \leq +7.50$

Femoral Rotation

(mm)

$-1.00 \leq \Delta G_a \leq +1.50$
$-1.00 \leq \Delta H_a \leq +0.50$

Tibial Rotation

(mm)

$-2.25 \leq \Delta G_a \leq +3.00$
$-2.50 \leq \Delta H_a \leq +2.25$

al. used a new testing method based on the force provided by each ligament in resisting anterior and posterior drawer. The advantage of this method is that results do not depend on the cutting order. The investigators were generally in agreement in regard to the abnormal mobility of the joint produced by division of the various ligaments. There is a difference of opinion over certain aspects, notably the following: (1) Brantigan and Voshell[11] state that their experiments on dissected specimens and fresh intact joints fail to show any increase of lateral movement when the collateral ligaments were divided provided that the cruciate ligaments were intact; (2) Markolf et al[62] found significant left-to-right laxity differences in intact knees; (3) Markolf et al found that with the anterior cruciate intact, large increases in anteroposterior laxity were observed when the medial collateral ligament and posterior capsule were sectioned in combination, while other investigators found no increase in anterior laxity when the anterior cruciate was intact; and (4) Kennedy and Fowler[51] found that isolated section of the medial capsular ligament (deep medial ligament) caused moderate instability. Other investigators consider the superficial medial ligament more important as a medial stabilizer, and Warren et al.[89] specifically state that they could not confirm Kennedy and Fowler's observations in their experiments.

With these exceptions, the findings may be summarized as described below.

Medial Stability. The long fibers of the superficial medial collateral ligament are the primary stabilizers of the medial side of the knee against valgus and rotary stress.

Warren et al.[89] found that ablation of the deep capsular ligament and posterior capsule had no effect on stability to valgus stress but when the long fibers were divided, 5 to 7 mm of medial opening occurred throughout the entire range of motion. When the sequence of cutting was altered, significant opening occurred after section of the long fibers, although the deep fibers and posterior capsule remained intact. Division of the latter structures did not then give rise to further opening. There is a consensus that valgus instability in a position of full extension must indicate damage to the cruciate ligaments as well as the medial stabilizers. Hallen and Lindahl[34] considered their specimens extended "when there was resistance to further extension." Warren et al.[89] made their measurements in a position described as 0 degrees of flexion, stating that although the joint appeared fully extended they had made no attempt to gain the last few degrees of extension. They therefore agree that clinical instability to valgus stress in full extension is a reliable indicator of cruciate damage.

All agree that the medial collateral ligament forms a check against external rotation. Most investigators consider the ligament as a whole without distinguishing between the superficial and deep portions. Hallén and Lindahl found a significant increase in total rotation of the tibia after sectioning the superficial ligament but did not test the effect of cutting the deep ligament alone. Kennedy and Fowler[51] sectioned the deep portion of the ligament in otherwise intact specimens. They noted instability but did not measure it. Warren et al.[89] found

> In our experiments the remarkable resistance to external rotation of the tibia was retained after the deep ligament and the oblique fibers of the posterior capsule were cut. In no specimen with the long fibers still intact was a total increment of more than one degree of external rotation allowed. This was true in all positions of knee flexion from 0 to 90 degrees. In contrast, the permissible degree of external rotation in flexion increased as soon as the long fibers were sectioned.

These workers found that in the intact specimen there was an average 6 degrees of external rotation possible with the knee in extension, increasing slightly to an average of 9 degrees of external rotation at 90 degrees of flexion. With the long fibers of the superficial medial ligament divided, there was a slight increase in extension (average 8 degrees), increasing as the knee was progressively flexed until at 90 degrees there was on average 19 degrees of external rotation.

These anatomic findings seem at variance with the clinical concepts of Slocum and Larson,[77] who have stated that "rupture of the medial capsular ligament [deep medial ligament] is the basic lesion which permits abnormal external rotation of the tibia."

Lateral Instability.[35,49,50,87] On the lateral side of the knee, single-plane lateral stability against varus stress is provided by the iliotibial tract, the lateral collateral ligament, the lateral capsule and arcuate ligament, the popliteus tendon and muscle, and, when present, the fabellofibular ligament. In extension, intact cruciate ligaments contribute as well. In flexion, the fibers of the iliotibial tract come to lie almost parallel to the articular surface of the tibia, and its contribution to lateral stability is limited to the retinacular fibers that extend to the patella. The lateral collateral ligament is relaxed in flexion. Thus in the normal knee, greater single plane as well as rotary laxity are permitted in flexion, and there is more backward rolling of the lateral femoral condyle with flexion than on the medial side.

Anterior Stability.   The anterior cruciate ligament is the prime restraint of single-plane anterior displacement of the tibia on the femur. According to Furman et al.,[30] when the entire ligament is ruptured there is an increased anterior drawer in both flexion and extension, perhaps some hyperextensibility and increased internal and external rotation in all positions. When the anteromedial band alone is ruptured, there is an anterior drawer in flexion but not in extension and increased internal rotation at 45 degrees of flexion. With rupture of the posterolateral bulk alone, the anterior drawer is positive with the knee extended but negative with the knee flexed 90 degrees; there is increased hyperextensibility and increased external rotation with the knee flexed 45 degrees. Resistance to the anterior drawer after rupture of the entire ligament was provided by the superficial portion of the medial collateral ligament. The other portions of the medial collateral ligament, the lateral collateral ligament, the posterior part of the joint capsule, and the posterior cruciate ligament have no effect on the anterior drawer in flexion.

Posterior Stability.   Single-plane laxity can only occur when there is stretching or rupture of the posterior cruciate ligament. According to Butler et al.[12] this ligament provides 95 percent of the total restraining force. Secondary restraint is provided by the postero–lateral capsule and popliteus complex, and the medial collateral ligament.

Hyperextension.   The femoral condyles that are in relation to the tibial plateaus are less curved than the anterior portions that normally articulate with the patella. The abrupt change in the curve of the condyles wedges the tibial portion of the femoral condyles away from the tibial condyles. Thus hyperextension is resisted by both collateral ligaments, both cruciate ligaments, and posterior capsule and posterior oblique ligaments of the knee. The menisci become compressed between the joint surfaces anteriorly and the medial and lateral femoral condylar grooves prevent the menisci from sliding forward.

Rotational Instability.   In the intact knee, the axis

of rotation is through the medial femoral condyle[74] (Fig. 13.9), illustrated by the greater mobility of the lateral meniscus, the relaxation of the lateral collateral ligament in flexion, and the change in orientation of the iliotibial tract.

In the normal knee, the anterior drawer is associated with internal tibial rotation and the posterior drawer with external rotation. Laxity of the superficial medial ligament with intact cruciate ligaments may shift the axis of rotation toward the center of the joint by allowing greater mobility of the medial femoral condyle. "Isolated" anterior cruciate laxity[26] increases both internal and external rotation in all positions of the joint, although when the superficial medial ligament is intact, the axis of rotation continues to be the medial femoral condyle. Posterior cruciate laxity also causes rotational instability, particularly in external rotation. Isolated lateral laxity when the cruciates are intact has little effect on rotational stability because the lateral ligament is always relaxed in flexion and the lateral capsule allows considerable rotation as part of normal knee motion. Evidence gleaned from selective cutting experiments strongly suggests that rotational laxity cannot occur when the superficial medial ligament and both cruciate ligaments are intact. Secondary capsular stretching increases the laxity following injury to the prime stabilizers. In terms of diagnosis, it is simpler to think in anatomic terms and

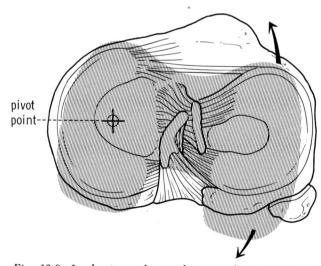

pivot point-- - -

Fig. 13.9. In the intact knee, the axis of rotation is the medial femoral condyle. Rotation is accentuated by damage to the cruciate ligaments, and the pivot point is shifted laterally by injury to the superficial medial ligament because its tethering effect is lost.

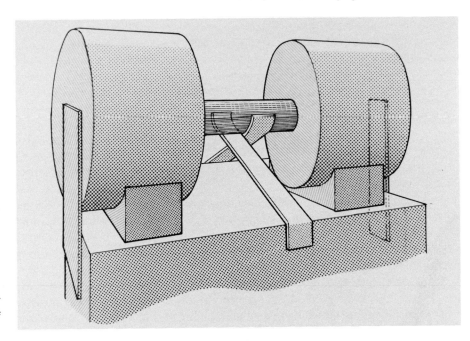

Fig. 13.10. Diagram illustrating the concept of single-plane laxity. (Redrawn from Palmer)

assess instability in single planes (Fig. 13.10). Rotary tests can reinforce the information obtained from the primary examination (Table 13.1).

CLINICAL DIAGNOSIS OF CHRONIC INSTABILITY[5,18,41]

VALGUS STRESS

Opening of the medial compartment should be tested in full extension and at 30 degrees of flexion. Laxity in full extension indicates injury to the superficial me-

dial ligament and both cruciate ligaments. Laxity only at 30 degrees of flexion indicates a lesion of the superficial medial ligament with at least one cruciate intact.

VARUS STRESS

In full extension any laxity in the lateral stabilizing structures will be masked by intact cruciate ligaments. Therefore, laxity in this position indicates concomitant cruciate damage.

Table 13.1. Restraints to Knee Instabilities

Instability	Knee Position	Prime Restraint	Secondary Restraints
Medial (valgus stress)	Flexion	Superficial MCL	ACL, PCL
	Extension	Superficial MCL	ACL, posterior capsule deep MCL, PCL
Lateral (varus stress)	Flexion	ACL, PCL, popliteus, arcuate lig.	PCL
	Extension	LCL, IT Band, arcuate lig.	
Anterior		ACL	MCL
Posterior		PCL	
Hyperextension		ACL	Posterior capsule, PCL
Rotational Internal	Flexion	ACL, PCL	LCL, popliteus, IT band
	Extension	ACL	LCL, popliteus, IT band, PCL
External	Flexion	MCL	ACL, LCL, popliteus, medial capsule

Abbreviations: ACL, anterior cruciate ligament; LCL; lateral collateral ligament; MCL; medial collateral ligament; PCL; posterior cruciate ligament. IT band; iliotibial band.
(From Marshall, J.L., and Rubin, R.M.: Knee ligament injuries—A diagnostic and therapeutic approach. Orthop. Clin. North Am., 8:641, 1977, with permission.)

Some laxity at 30 degrees of flexion is normal as relaxation of the lateral structures increases with the flexion angle. Excessive laxity only in this position indicates lesions of the arcuate complex and iliotibial tract with intact cruciates. The integrity of the lateral ligament cannot be assessed because it is normally relaxed in this position.

ANTEROPOSTERIOR TESTING[38]

The starting point must be determined by inspection and radiologic assessment of both knees flexed 90 degrees. Dropback of the tibia in this position is diagnostic of posterior cruciate laxity, and a positive anterior drawer test is to be expected. However, injury to both cruciate ligaments is probably more common than clinically suspected, so that the anterior drawer must be assessed for the extent and quality of "end point." When there is a dropback, an excessive anterior drawer and no end point, both cruciate ligaments are damaged.

The anterior drawer tested near full extension (Lachman test)[83] is often more informative than the test done in flexion because it is in the nearly extended position that functional instability occurs more commonly. A positive anterior drawer in flexion and a negative test in extension suggest a lesion of the anteromedial band alone.

The assessment of anteroposterior instability is the most difficult part of the knee examination, and it is sometimes impossible to be sure of the starting point from clinical observation alone. In these cases, stress radiography in both flexion and extension may be helpful. When laxity of both cruciate ligaments is suspected, stress tests become mandatory despite their limitations.

Rotational tests are extremely useful when used in conjunction with single-plane anteroposterior testing.

TESTS FOR ROTARY INSTABILITY

PIVOT SHIFT[31,32] AND REVERSE PIVOT SHIFT

In 1972, Galway et al.[32] described the pivot shift test as a sign of symptomatic anterior cruciate insufficiency, which accentuates the normal hypermobility of the lateral tibial plateau (Fig. 13.11A,B). The knee is brought from extension into flexion while the foot is held internally rotated, and a gentle valgus pressure is applied to the region of the fibular head. In extension, the lateral tibial plateau is subluxed anteriorly with respect to the femur, and at or about 30 degrees of flexion a sudden reduction occurs that can be both seen and felt. This test, or one of its variants as performed by Slocum,[82] Hughston[41] or Losee,[59] is an extremely valuable and reliable index of anterior cruciate insufficiency. Although sometimes not reproducible in tense patients, it is positive under anesthesia when the anterior cruciate is absent. When there is a significant anterior drawer and the pivot shift is negative, the laxity found clinically is almost certainly caused by posterior and not by anterior cruciate laxity. In the reverse pivot shift[46] test the tibia subluxes in flexion and reduces in extension. The maneuver is performed by beginning with the knee in flexion and carrying it through into extension, while holding the foot in external rotation. The reduction can be seen and felt at about 30 degrees of flexion.

In combined posterior and anterior cruciate lesions it is sometimes possible to see both types of pivot shift occurring sequentially. Bringing the knee from flexion to extension, reduction occurs first; then, as the foot is changed from external to internal rotation, a further shift can be seen as the tibial plateau subluxes anteriorly.

Anteromedial rotary instability measured by the Slocum test[77] is found with lesions of the superficial medial ligament and the anterior cruciate ligament. The anterior drawer is performed at 90 degrees of flexion with the foot in three positions. Initially with the foot straight ahead, the anterior drawer is assessed. The foot is then internally rotated 15 degrees when a reduction of excursion is found, indicating tightening of the lateral capsule and lateral ligament. Failure of the anterior drawer to reduce in amount when the foot is externally rotated 15 degrees is said to indicate incompetence of the posteromedial capsule.

HYPEREXTENSION

Hyperextension, resisted by both cruciate ligaments, is found when both are damaged. Genu recurvatum is seldom seen when the anterior cruciate

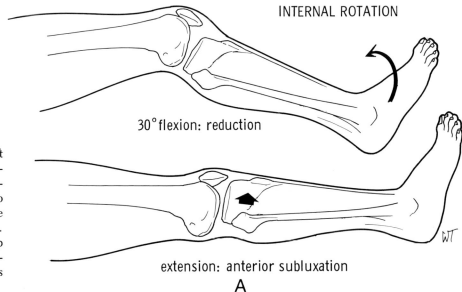

INTERNAL ROTATION

30° flexion: reduction

extension: anterior subluxation

A

Fig. 13.11. (A) In the pivot shift test, the foot is internally rotated and the tibia subluxes forward as the knee is brought into extension. (B) In the reverse pivot shift, the opposite occurs. There is a normal relationship between the bones in extension, but the tibia subluxes posteriorly with flexion.

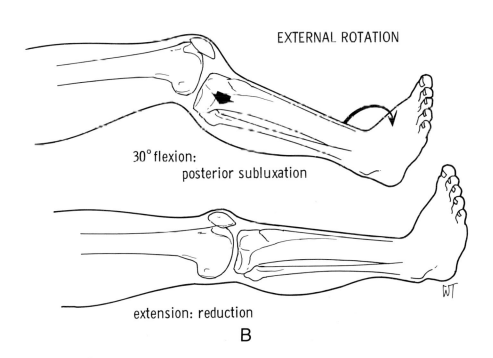

EXTERNAL ROTATION

30° flexion: posterior subluxation

extension: reduction

B

alone is torn but is encountered when the posterior cruciate is damaged by itself. In Hughston's external rotation recurvatum test,[41] the limb is suspended in extension by the big toe alone, and both recurvatum and external rotation can be seen.

INCIDENCE OF VARIOUS LIGAMENT INJURIES

Although the type and extent of ligamentous injury at the knee varies considerably, anterior cruciate and medial collateral ligament instabilities predominate in general orthopaedic practice. In reporting on 129 knee ligament injuries over a period of 17 years, Pickett and Altizer[75] noted that 115 (89 percent) involved the anterior cruciate ligament, the medial collateral ligament or a combination of the two. Posterior cruciate injuries are incurred most frequently in road accidents or football. Lateral side injuries are also relatively uncommon but are caused by severe trauma of the same nature.

Therefore, although the possible combinations of ligament injury are great, in practice most chronic instabilities of the knee, require reconstruction of the anterior cruciate ligament and superficial medial ligament.

CONSERVATIVE MANAGEMENT

Exercise

The most effective way to strengthen a muscle is the progressive resistance principle advocated by DeLorme.[19] Beginning with a light weight, a set number of repetitions are performed, gradually increasing the weight but not the number of repetitions as the strength of the muscle increases. The purpose is to exercise the muscle to the point of fatigue and then allowing a rest period before the next set of exercises is performed. The weight can be a sandbag, an exercise shoe with provision for adding weights or more sophisticated equipment such as the universal gym, Cybex, or Nautilus machines. The equipment offers one major advantage over simpler forms of weights, in that the load can be kept constant throughout the range of motion. With conventional weights applied to the foot and lifted from flexion to extension the resistance is least in flexion and greatest

in extension. This is a disadvantage when degenerative change in the patellofemoral joint causes pain as full extension is approached (Fig. 13.12). The use of a machine allows the knee to be exercised against maximum resistance in any chosen position so that the muscles can be exercised through a range of motion that is painless, for example, from 90 to 45 degrees of flexion. The athlete with powerful musculature often lifts 50, 60, or even 70 pounds, and the forces generated at the patellofemoral joint amount to several thousand pounds per square inch. Loads at this level may be beyond the capacity of normal articular cartilage to withstand and may cause further deterioration when the cartilage is already damaged.

According to a study performed at The Hospital for Special Surgery,[64] athletes rehabilitated with traditional straight leg raising and nonspecific weight lifting had significant deficits in strength (measured as maximal isometric contraction), power (measured as speed of force development), and endurance (measured as the number of repetitions performed at a fixed rate until peak force per repetition fell below 50 percent of the maximum) on the affected side. Deficits in power were much greater than deficits in strength for both quadriceps and knee flexors. Speed of muscle force development (power) and endurance were the most important parameters for competitive function and injury prevention. Measurements of overall muscle function correlated closely with indices of clinical function of the patient. Knees with medial collateral ligament injuries showed the greatest deficit in strength and power of the quadriceps. Knees with anterior cruciate ligament lesions had relatively the greatest deficit in the knee flexors. In normal knees the strength and power of extensors and flexors are greatest in the midrange of flexion.

Strength is developed with low-speed weight-lifting techniques and power with low weight at high rates of repetitive contractions. Both types of exercises are performed through the functional or mid-flexion range of motion. In addition to the knee extensors, for anterior cruciate ligament injuries, knee flexors are emphasized.

In exercising the knee after surgery, the same principles are followed, but first motion in the knee must be regained. Isometric exercises with straight leg raising and lateral leg raising are emphasized. When 90 degrees of motion has been achieved, isotonic exercises are begun in the seated position with light weights

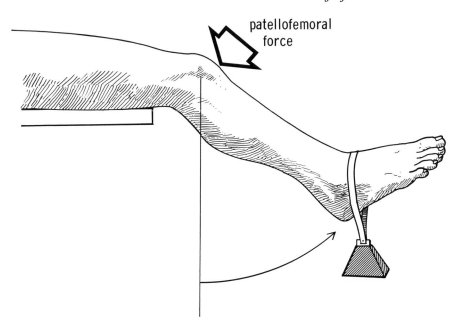

Fig. 13.12. Exercising the quadriceps with weights can lead to tremendous forces being transmitted through the patellofemoral joint.

on the foot (about 5 lb). The knee is slowly extended and lowered. Three sets of 10 repetitions are performed with a one-minute rest between sets. Muscle fatigue at the end of each set is the objective, and weights are increased when the patient can easily do

three sets. Knee flexors are performed with weights on the foot and the patient prone or standing (Fig. 13.13). As motion increases, rapid repetitions with light weights are added to build power capacity. Pain or muscle fatigue is the end point of each session.

Fig. 13.13. Hamstring exercises are important in anterior cruciate insufficient knees.

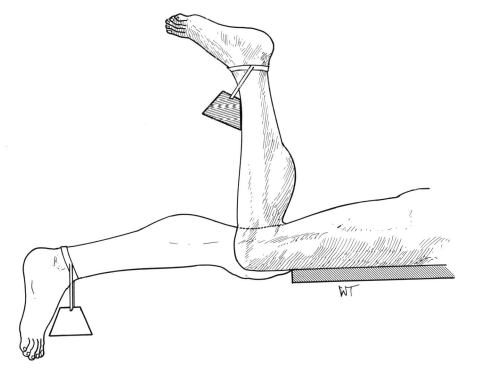

Chondromalacia of the patella can prevent or limit the ability to exercise in this manner. In all cases, the exercises should be performed through a painless range (Fig. 13.14), or if not, rehabilitation is done with isometric exercises alone using straight leg raises and lateral leg raises. An isokinetic device may be used in lieu of weights and effectively works the extensors and knee flexors simultaneously.

Later, jogging, bicycling, and swimming are added to the program, followed by patterned running, figure eights, start/stop, and cutting maneuvers.

Marshall and Rubin[64] recommend allowing full participation in a sport when the patient can perform certain functional tests, when manual estimates of strength in quadriceps and hamstrings are nearly equal, and when thigh circumference is within 1 to 2 cm of the normal side. The functional tests are running symmetrically in place, hopping on the affected leg, running figure-eight circles in either direction and doing start and stop tests confidently and quickly.

BRACING

Simple elastic braces with patellar cutouts and side bars give the subjective feeling of stability and are helpful in the treatment of patellar disorders but cannot be relied on for support of ligamentous instability.

The Lenox Hill derotation brace[70] can be effective for anterior and medial instabilities. It does not help posterior instability and may aggravate patellar disorders. Some patients, particularly recreational athletes, do not tolerate the brace well because it is cumbersome and uncomfortable; it can also cause skin irritation and is expensive. The brace is not appropriate for use in cases in which the instability occurs during the course of everyday activity, as it is certainly not suitable for continuous use. The brace is made at the Lenox Hill Hospital Brace Shop in New York City and can be obtained by sending a plaster mold of the patient's leg together with a description of the instabilities present. Although the brace is most effective for the control of anterior and medial instabilities, it can be modified for lateral instability.

After surgical reconstruction, some techniques optimally require prolonged support and protection. It has been demonstrated that ligamentous tissue does not regain normal strength for approximately 1 year. Recovery is delayed by prolonged immobilization but is hastened by carefully controlled and protected motion.[71] The cast brace that incorporates stops to limit range of motion is the best way of providing functional stresses while preventing reinjury.

INDICATIONS FOR SURGICAL RECONSTRUCTION

Not every case of chronic knee laxity requires a reconstruction.[24] In fact, most do not, and can be managed successfully with a combination of exercises and bracing. Sometimes a patient is better advised to give up the sports activities that cause symptoms of instability rather than to undergo a major surgical procedure. This is particularly true for older people and for patients with double-jointedness. In hyperextensible joints, the surgical result is not always predictable because of a propensity for stretching. Each case is an individual one, and the age, sex, body build, frequency of instability, and the expected objectives from surgery must be carefully assessed. Any potential surgical candidate must participate in a period of muscle rehabilitation lasting several months before any decision is made.

Clear-cut indications for surgery exist in some circumstances.

First, unpredictable buckling that occurs during the course of the everyday activity and does not respond to an exercise program. The most common cause of this instability is an old rupture of the anterior cruciate ligament. Bracing is seldom appropriate for this type of instability because most effective braces are too uncomfortable to be worn continuously. When a person cannot step off a curb or turn in the shower without fear of the knee giving way, a reconstruction is justified.

Second, for many young persons, the desire to resume playing a sport is strong and a completely sedentary existence unacceptable. Most chronic laxities found in young people are caused by various athletic injuries. A high school football player should not be encouraged to return to the same sport after a severe ligament injury, but should probably be directed toward another sport in which the risk of reinjury is less. For professional athletes, this argument does not apply, and a whole career may depend on a successful reconstruction. Such a consideration is not valid for amateur or recreational athletes. Nonetheless, the

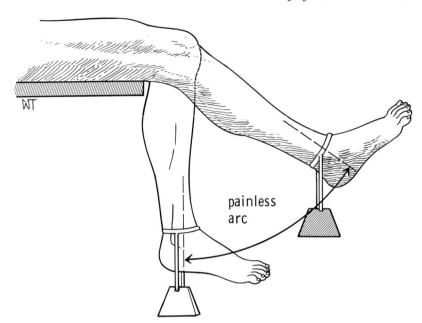

painless
arc

Fig. 13.14. In cases of chondromalacia of the patella, weight-lifting must be done only through a painless range of motion. When this is not possible, straight leg raising alone is done.

ability to perform at some level, in some kind of sport is highly desirable and must be recognized as a true indication for ligament reconstruction.

Third, clinical evidence shows that long-standing ligament instability leads to meniscal tears and later to osteoarthritis of the knee in some people,[28] although there is no way of predicting who will be affected (Fig. 13.15). One question that patients frequently ask is "What will happen if I do not have my knee operated upon?" In answering, the risk of osteoarthritis must be mentioned. There is no hard evidence that surgical reconstruction can prevent osteoarthritis, but it does seem that if frequent painful episodes of instability are occurring, especially when accompanied by an effusion, late osteoarthritis is a likely end result. It also seems reasonable that if these episodes can be eliminated, deterioration of the joint should occur more slowly. The risk of osteoarthritis is not an indication by itself but should be linked with symptoms and the desire to improve the present function of the knee. In this context it is interesting that most patients undergoing total knee replacement for severe osteoarthritis are female with no history of past injury, and in most the anterior cruciate ligament is present (Fig. 13.16). In view of the frequency of anterior cruciate injury, one must assume that severe degenerative arthritis as a late sequel is relatively uncommon.

Fourth, the indications for surgery are more subjective than objective. In most cases the patient seeks the doctor's advice because of instability or insecurity, or in some cases of posterior cruciate injury, pain. Simply because laxity is found on clinical examination is not sufficient reason for a reconstruction. Subjective symptoms and the objective signs usually bear some relationship to each other, but this is by no means always the case. I have seen patients present with the typical syndrome of anterior cruciate insufficiency after recent injury and on examination have the expected findings of positive anterior drawer and pivot shift tests. However, on examining the other presumably normal knee, even greater laxities are found. The patient then recalls an ancient injury to this knee as well, but believes it to have fully recovered. In a unique and very important study, McDaniel and Dameron[69] examined 50 patients with surgically verified but untreated ruptures of the anterior cruciate ligament. After an average follow-up of 10 years, 72 percent had returned to strenuous sports, although most of the knees had anterior and rotary laxity on examination. The incidence of radiographic arthritis was low. The information given in this study serves as a baseline for evaluation of the results of primary repair of the anterior cruciate ligament.

The discrepancy between symptoms of instability

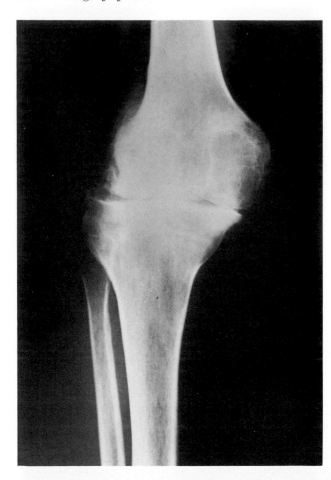

Fig. 13.15. Radiograph of a 40-year-old athletic man who injured the knee 20 years before (probably an anterior cruciate ligament injury). The appearance of severe panarthritis with lateral subluxation without malalignment is typical of the arthritis that follows ligament injuries.

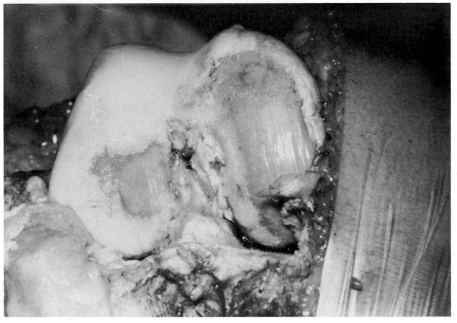

Fig. 13.16. Photograph of the knee of a 68-year-old woman undergoing total knee replacement. Characteristically in this type of case, the anterior cruciate ligament is present and there is no history of previous injury.

and objective findings of laxity also complicates assessment of the results of reconstruction. Some tests are more significant than others and, for example, the pivot shift probably correlates better with symptoms of instability than does the anterior drawer test. However, no correlation is absolute; one must remember that surgery is not indicated to cure a physical sign without symptoms nor should the end result be judged solely on the basis of the stability examination alone.

SURGICAL TECHNIQUES

Having decided that a patient who has undergone rehabilitation can be helped further only by surgery, specific techniques must be considered. It is recommended that just as the diagnosis should be made in terms of single-plane laxities, the concepts of ligament reconstruction should be similarly guided. For example, if the patient has anterior and medial laxities, the reconstruction should be directed toward restoring continuity and function of the anterior cruciate ligament and the superficial medial ligament. Similarly, posterior instability requires posterior cruciate reconstruction and single-plane lateral laxity, reconstruction of the complex of structures that in normal anatomy provide for lateral stability.

The key to successful reconstruction of the knee for chronic ligament instability is the control of abnormal anteroposterior motion. Medial or lateral reconstruction is seldom necessary as an isolated procedure, and is usually combined with either an anterior or a posterior reconstruction. Medial laxity alone with intact cruciate ligaments seldom seems to cause clinical instability, and lateral laxity with intact cruciates, if it exists at all, is rare. Collateral ligament laxity when combined with cruciate laxity does not always require reconstruction. For example, when faced with the most common combination of instabilities (anterior and medial), cruciate reconstruction alone without making any attempt to tighten the medial structures will often restore subjective stability. Successful cruciate reconstruction may also diminish laxity of the medial ligament to passive testing illustrating the effect of cruciate integrity on varus and valgus laxity. As a rule of thumb, 1+ and 2+ laxities of the medial ligament (up to 10 mm of medial joint opening) can be ignored when anterior cruciate reconstruction is done (at least when using the method of bone block iliotibial band

transfer). Greater laxities require a separate medial reconstruction.

During the last decade, substitution procedures have been designed to compensate for cruciate insufficiency by either extra-articular capsular tightening or the use of tendon or fascial slings. Examples are the pes anserinus transfer of Slocum and Larson[78-81] for anteromedial instability and the lateral fascial sling procedures of MacIntosh,[61] Ellison et al.,[22] and Losee[59] for anterolateral instability. At The Hospital for Special Surgery, both on the Knee Service and Sports Medicine Service, this type of procedure has not been entirely satisfactory as a form of primary reconstruction. We believe that extra-articular capsular reinforcement is best employed as an ancilliary procedure in conjunction with direct reconstruction of the anterior or posterior cruciate ligament (Fig. 13.17).

However, an extra-articular reinforcement should not be done in conjunction with every case of cruciate

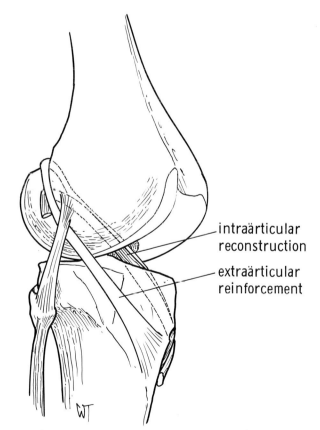

intraärticular
reconstruction

extraärticular
reinforcement

Fig. 13.17. Intra-articular reconstruction with extra-articular backup.

reconstruction, because there are serious practical disadvantages to this approach. For a combined intra- and extra-articular reconstruction, the skin incisions required are more difficult to plan than for the intra-articular reconstruction alone; therefore, the risks of wound-healing difficulties and skin necrosis are higher. In addition, some of the techniques for cruciate reconstruction obviate the need for postoperative cast immobilization, and this important advantage is lost when an ancilliary extra-articular substitution is added. There is some evidence that routine extra-articular substitution improves the result of intra-articular reconstruction,[14,91] and as this approach is becoming more widely practiced, more information should soon be available. Meantime, the "braces-and-belt" approach seems most justified in treating high-level or professional athletes for whom the disadvantages of longer rehabilitation and increased complication risk may be less important than they are for the recreational athlete.

The surgical techniques are described under the headings of the four primary single-plane laxities with substitution procedures as a separate section. The list of techniques is not intended to be comprehensive, but rather to represent methods in widest use. The most-used techniques at The Hospital for Special Surgery are described in detail. With regard to which are best, it is not possible to say. As discussed below under Results, different investigators express their results in different terms and often use different terminology to express the lesions they were reconstructing in the first place. The greatest body of information is available for the syndrome of anterior cruciate insufficiency, although not all workers have specifically used this term. Also, the follow-up time of published series is often short and cases are included that have had less than the customary 2-year minimum follow-up generally considered necessary. In addition, techniques are continually modified so that by the time any long-term follow-up study is published, the technique described for that series may no longer be practiced by that investigator.

With these reservations in mind, a compilation of techniques must have a personal bias toward what has worked best in our experience.

ANTERIOR INSTABILITY

The primary lesion is anterior cruciate insufficiency.

BONE BLOCK ILIOTIBIAL BAND TRANSFER[43]

Contraindications

Single-plane lateral laxity or previous surgery that would impair the use of the iliotibial band as a graft. When both cruciates have been injured, the posterior should be reconstructed first.

Technique

The operation is done with tourniquet hemostasis. The knee is exposed by a lateral parapatellar skin incision 20 to 25 cm in length. A lateral flap is dissected to expose the distal portion of the iliotibial band. The medial skin flap is dissected to the medial border of the patella so that the joint can be entered through a longitudinal, straight midline utility capsular incision. To prevent skin necrosis, which occurs predominantly in the lateral flap, the skin incision should be C shaped with the apex two fingerbreadths lateral to the patellar margin.

The lateral intermuscular septum is identified and the outline of the portion of the band anterior to the septum is marked, including its point of insertion into the tibia. It is desirable to obtain as large a graft as possible; on the other hand, the posterior fibers of the iliotibial band must remain, with 3 to 4 mm being quite sufficient (Fig. 13.18A). However, the demarcation of the posterior margin of the band is not always clear, so that choosing the correct placement of the posterior incision can be difficult. The extent of the iliotibial band is best appreciated with the knee at 40 degrees of flexion and the foot in full internal rotation. The anterior incision is made at the lateral border of the patella and extends proximally into the lower fibers of vastus lateralis and distally to the tibia along the lateral border of the patellar tendon. The attachment of this portion of the band to Gerdy's tubercle is then outlined providing a rectangle of bone 1 cm in width and 2 cm in length. A drill hole, using a Steinmann pin rather than a drill bit (because the bone block is weakened less), is made in the proximal third of the block. The bone block, removed with an osteotome, is composed of cortical bone and a small amount of underlying cancellous bone. The bone block with the attached iliotibial band is then dissected proximally to a point just proximal to the lateral femoral condyle. Branches of the lateral superior genicular artery run into the graft from a posterior direction and should be preserved. The fascial strip obtained is somewhat triangular being wider proximally and is converted into a tube by folding it longitudinally and suturing the edges together (Fig. 13.18B).

The periosteum along the postero-lateral border of the femoral shaft is incised and stripped posteriorly with an elevator until the posterolateral joint capsule is reached. The origin of the lateral head of gastrocnemius and a portion of the arcuate ligament may be partially reflected in continuity with the periosteum. If the medial capsular incision has not yet been made, the joint is entered through this route, as the patella is dislocated laterally. A clamp is passed posteriorly above, behind, and around the lateral femoral condyle (the so-called over-the-top method of MacIntosh)[62] (Fig. 13.18C). The point of the clamp is located from the lateral side and a hole made in the posterior capsule at this point. It may be difficult to pass the bone block through this hole into the intercondylar notch because of its size; forcible traction of the bone block may result in fragmentation of the bone and loss of subsequent fixation. It is necessary to enlarge the hole progressively so that the bone block will pass easily. For this purpose, a series of urethral dilators are useful until the hole is large enough to admit a No. 36 to 40 plastic chest tube (Fig. 13.18D). The plastic tubing, which is of sufficient size to take the bone block within its lumen (Fig. 13.18E), is passed through the hole. During this stage, osteophytes that may have formed in the intercondylar notch should be removed. The bone block with the attached graft is drawn into the end of the plastic tubing using a suture passed through and over the bone block. The block and the surrounding tubing are then drawn forward together into the intercondylar notch (Fig. 13.18F).

The final step is to fix the bone to the tibia. The orientation of the fascial graft must approximate the line of the normal anterior cruciate ligament as closely as possible. The direction of the graft is adjusted by trial and error until the femoral condyles do not impinge on the graft when the knee is in extension. The fixation point established by these trials usually lies just medial to the tibial tubercle and adjoins the medial articular surface of the tibia. A vertical slot large enough to accommodate the bone block is cut in the anterior aspect of the tibia at the fixation point. The vertical slot should be between 1 and 1.5 cm deep so that the attachment of the graft to the tibia approxi-

mates the normal attachment of the anterior cruciate ligament. *The tourniquet is released before fixing the graft to obtain extra length.* The knee is flexed to 90 degrees and the tibia is displaced posteriorly. An AO cancellous bone screw and washer are passed through the hole in the bone block (Fig. 13.18G); using the tip of the screw as a lever, the bone block is drawn into the vertical slot on the tibia and fixed with the screw. The bone block and screw are therefore recessed below the anterior surface of the tibia, and with the knee in flexion the bone block is held at an almost 90-degree angle to the direction of the graft itself (Fig. 13.18H).

This procedure provides a substantial band of tissue that passes from the posterolateral to the anteromedial part of the knee on a line very close to that of the original cruciate ligament and which is thicker than the normal ligament. Once in place, the band is continuous locally with the vastus lateralis and lateral intermuscular septum and proximally with the tensor fascia lata and gluteus maximus and its tension does not vary much during flexion and extension of the knee.

Intraoperative examination after fixation of the graft should show completely negative Lachman and pivot shift signs and no change in lateral stability. The anterior drawer sign is always reduced but not always completely eliminated. The wound is closed, repairing the medial capsular incision, but leaving the graft site on the lateral aspect open. The defect is much too large to approximate side to side. The tourniquet should be released before closure and any large vessels coagulated.

Postoperative Care

A bulky Robert Jones dressing is applied in the operating room to provide firm but not rigid support. The fixation of the bone block is so solid that no other form of immobilization is required. On the second postoperative day, the patient is allowed out of bed and begins to stand and walk using crutches and putting partial weight on the leg. Full weight-bearing using crutches is possible on the fourth or fifth day and the patient is allowed to go home at about this time. The use of crutches is discontinued at about 3 weeks or as soon as the patient is able to walk without them. After 14 days, the dressing is removed and if the wound has healed, the sutures are removed. At this time, straight leg raising exercises are started and the number performed is increased until the patient

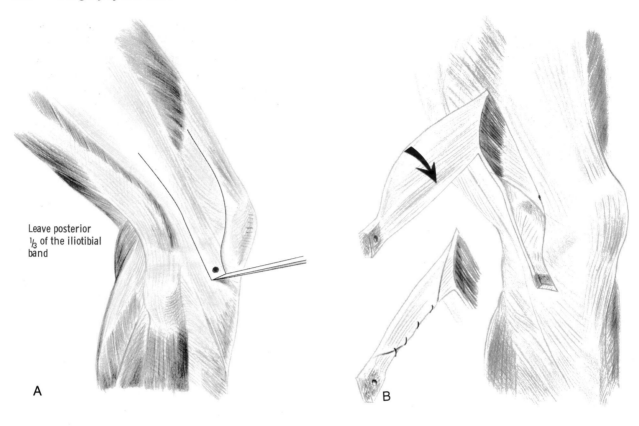

Leave posterior
¹⁄₃ of the iliotibial
band

A

B

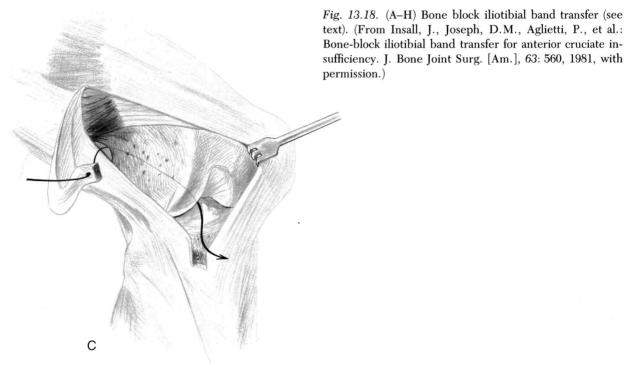

Fig. 13.18. (A–H) Bone block iliotibial band transfer (see text). (From Insall, J., Joseph, D.M., Aglietti, P., et al.: Bone-block iliotibial band transfer for anterior cruciate insufficiency. J. Bone Joint Surg. [Am.], *63*: 560, 1981, with permission.)

C

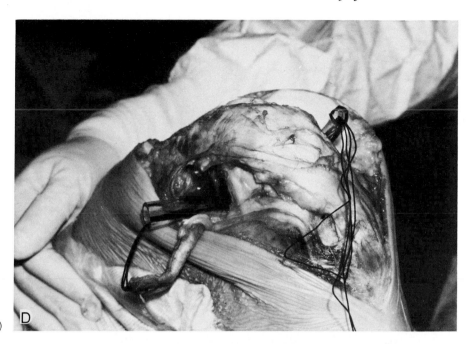

Fig. 13.18. (Continued.)

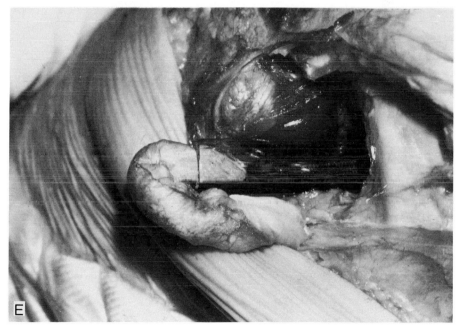

can do 300 or more per day. Unrestricted knee flexion is permitted after the wound has healed, and no external splinting is used. Progressive weight-lifting exercises are instituted after the knee can be flexed to 90 degrees and when straight leg raising can be done with ease. Recovery usually is rapid and most patients can resume normal everyday activities at 4 to 6 weeks after operation. Running in a straight line is started at 3 months and activities involving pivoting movements at 6 months. Patients who wish to participate

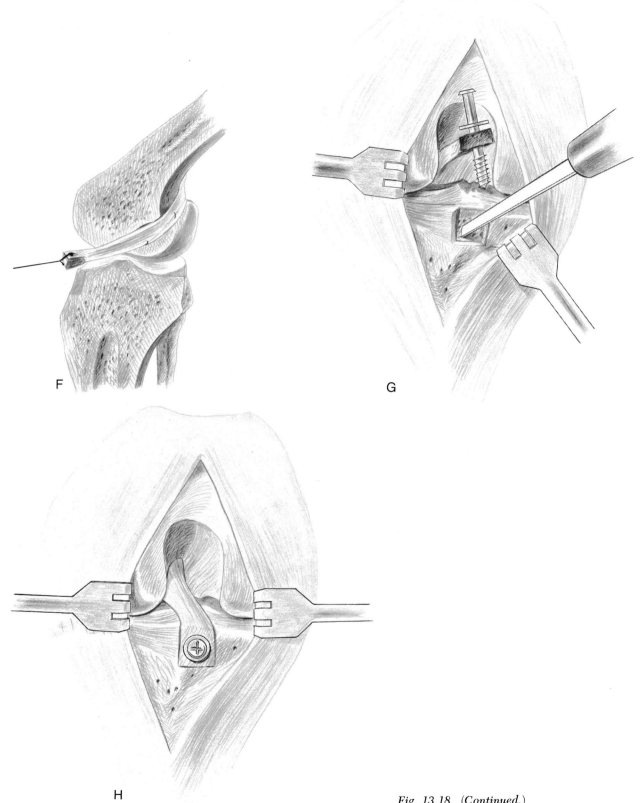

F

G

H

Fig. 13.18. (Continued.)

in strenuous or contact sports are given a Lenox Hill brace for protection, which is usually discontinued after 1 year.

THE MODIFIED JONES[47,48] TECHNIQUE OF QUADRICEPS TENDON SUBSTITUTION (Marshall)[66,67,88]

A medial parapatellar approach to the knee is used. Skin flaps are developed for visualization of the quadriceps tendon. In addition, a second incision is used to expose the lateral femoral condyle. Incidental meniscectomies, if required, are carried out before cruciate ligament reconstruction.

Harvesting the graft is then carried out (Fig. 13.19). Starting proximally at a point 5 or 6 cm above the superior pole of the patella, a rectangular-shaped graft 2 cm wide is outlined. At the level of the patella, this spans out over the entire length of the patella and then narrows down over the infrapatellar tendon extending to the level of the tibial tubercle.

At the level of the patella the tendon can be taken in either of two ways. It can be dissected cleanly off the patella using sharp dissection, or it can be taken with a thin sliver of bone from the entire patellar surface using an osteotome. During dissection, care must be taken not to slip off the edge of the patellar surface, which would disrupt the retinacular attachment to the patella. The graft is then taken full thickness at the level of the infrapatellar tendon. The thin prepatellar portion of the graft is reinforced by turning down part of the more robust portion from the quadriceps tendon. The graft is then tubed over itself. After this, a Bunnell suture of zero silk on two Keith needles is passed through the length of the graft starting at the level of the tibial tubercle. A Thompson stitch is also used at the proximal end of the graft. The ends of the sutures are left long. The Thompson stitch prevents the graft from acting in an accordion-like manner on the Bunnell stitch.

At this time, drill holes are placed. For the proximal attachment of the graft, sutures can be brought out through bone in the lateral femoral condyle, or using a more recent procedure they can be brought out over the top, as in the MacIntosh method (Fig. 13.20).

If the graft is to be brought out through bone, a drill hole must be made in the lateral femoral con-

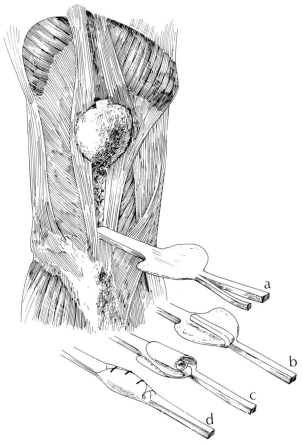

Fig. 13.19. The Marshall modification of the Jones technique of quadriceps tendon substitution. Development of the graft from the central third of the patellar ligament, the prepatellar expansion, and the quadriceps tendon. (From Marshall, J.L., Warren, R.F., Wickiewicz, T.L., et al.: The anterior cruciate ligament: A technique of repair and reconstruction. Clin. Orthop., *143*: 97, 1979, with permission.)

dyle. If the surgeon is experienced, free hand drilling can be accurate. In order to get proper femoral attachment of the cruciate graft, the hole must be made from the outside (laterally) into the knee joint. Drilling from the inside out does not permit a posterior position for the attachment site. If the drill hole is placed too far anteriorly or inferiorly, excessive tension is placed on the repair because of the abnormal lengthening; as the knee goes into extension, the repair will pull off the bone. A C-shaped drill guide that accepts variable bore-size drill bits facilitates drilling from outside into the intercondylar notch. A narrow drill is passed first to ensure the proper position pos-

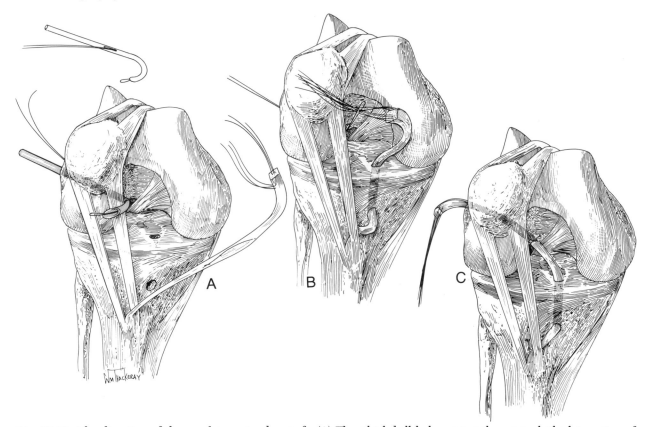

Fig. 13.20. The direction of the quadriceps tendon graft. (A) The tibial drill hole exist at the original tibial insertion of the A.C.L. The hollow tube with wire passer is in place around the lateral femoral condyle. (B) The graft goes under the intrapatellar tendon. (C) The final position of the graft. (From Marshall, J.L., Warren, R.F., Wickiewicz, T.L., et al.: The anterior cruciate ligament: A technique of repair and reconstruction. Clin. Orthop., *143*: 97, 1979, with permission.)

teriorly and superiorly for the cruciate origin. This is then drilled again to obtain a hole of adequate diameter.

To bring the graft out over the top, the dissection is carried down to the intermuscular septum to permit visualization of the superior border of the lateral femoral condyle. A clamp is then passed around the lateral femoral condyle in the same manner used for iliotibial band transfer.

The tunnel thus formed is deepened using a curved rasp shaped like a hollow tube passer. This provides a groove with a bleeding bone bed for the graft to lie in and removes any osteophytes at the condylar margin that form secondary to the instability. The rasps are passed in both directions (outside in and inside out) to ensure an adequate groove. In addition, the groove is extended over the outside of the lateral femoral condyle with a Cobb gouge to accept the graft.

Most knees that suffer from chronic anterior cruciate insufficiency will have marginal osteophytes deep in the intercondylar notch. These must be removed so the graft can pass without impingement (Fig. 13.21).

A ³⁄₈- to ½-inch drill hole is made free handed. The drill enters the tibia just medial to the infrapatellar tendon and exists at the the site of the original anterior cruciate origin. This placement assures that the tendon graft will have an orientation similar to that of the normal cruciate. The margins of the drill holes should be smooth so that no rough edges can abrade the graft.

Before passing the graft, three or four sutures of No. 3–0 Dexon are placed in the remaining stump of the cruciate distally if present and also in the fat pad and ligamentum mucosum. Similar sutures are also placed in the posterior synovial sheath but are left untied for later attachment to the graft. The graft is

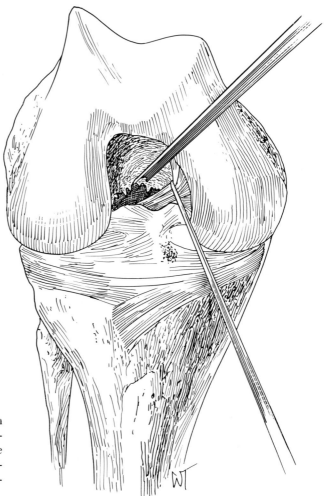

Fig. 13.21. Marginal osteophytes in the intercondylar notch must be removed before passage of the graft. (From Marshall, J.L., Warren, R.F., Wickiewicz, T.L., et al.: The anterior cruciate ligament: A technique of repair and reconstruction. Clin. Orthop., *143*: 97, 1979, with permission.)

now ready to be passed. It is brought out medially under the remaining medial strip of the infrapatellar tendon through a groove made subperiostally, all sharp edges being smoothed. Using No. 21 wires as guides and the Bunnell and Thompson stitches as traction devices, the graft is pulled up into the joint through the tibial drill hole.

The graft is then passed through either the femoral condylar drill hole or over the top of the condyle, lies in the groove made earlier and is secured to the lateral aspect of the lateral femoral condyle by using a staple (Fig. 13.22). In addition, the periosteum is sutured to cover the graft. When securing the graft in place, an assistant must keep firm tension on the graft by means of the traction stitches. Placement and tension can be checked as the knee is taken through a

range of motion ensuring that the graft is secure without rolling or stripping occurring.

When stapling the graft, the knee is flexed about 80 degrees while an assistant applies a posterior force on the proximal tibia to ensure complete reduction. Once secured with a staple, the excess graft may be excised.

The anterior and posterior fat pad and cruciate stump, if present, are sutured to the graft by means of the previously placed sutures. The purpose of this is to encourage revascularization of the graft.

The knee is then carefully taken through a full range of motion to ensure proper placement and that impingement does not exist. The ligament should be tight enough through the full range of motion without acute angular deviations to its course of motion.

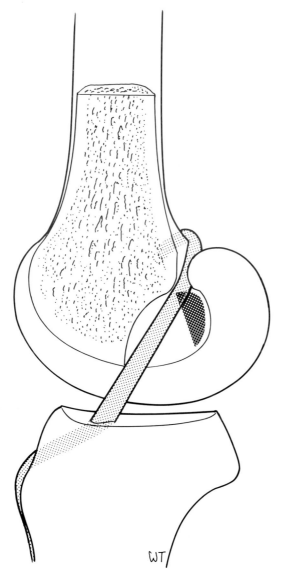

Fig. 13.22. The final alignment of the quadriceps tendon graft.

The leg is placed in a large, soft, bulky dressing at 35 to 40 degrees of flexion.

Postoperative Care

About 6 days postoperatively, the dressing is removed and a cylinder cast is applied with the knee in approximately 20 degrees of flexion. The immobilization is held for 5 weeks. The patient may progress to full weight-bearing over a 3- to 4-week period in the cast.

After cast removal, the knee is protected for 2 months by using a brace. The brace uses stops to limit range of motion over the first month, which are then removed for the second month. A rehabilitation program is begun while the patient is in the brace and continues for at least 1 year postoperatively.

QUADRICEPS TENDON SUBSTITUTION
(Eriksson)

Eriksson's modification of the Jones procedure differs from that described above (Fig. 13.23A,B).[3,4,25] The graft consists of the medial third of the patellar tendon, dissecting off two-thirds of the part of the ligament covering the patella. A drill hole is made from the tibial tubercle into the knee joint close to the normal tibial attachment of the anterior cruciate ligament, and the tendon flap is pulled into the knee joint. Through a separate incision over the outside of the lateral femoral condyle, two drill holes are made into the knee for sutures (Palmer's method). A shallow hole is excavated in the lateral femoral condyle at the normal posterior insertion of the anterior cruciate ligament. The sutures through the ligament are put at varying sites on the ligament in order to facilitate stretching of the ligament flap when the sutures are tied one by one.

Instead of reflecting the tendon proximally from the patella, a layer of bone from the patella may be taken instead. The most medial part of the patellar tendon covering the patella is not used in order to prevent lateral subluxation of the patella from developing. This has been used as an argument against taking the medial third as a graft rather than the central part of the patellar tendon.

Eriksson stresses the need to suture the graft under tension as it never becomes tighter by itself only looser. To stretch the ligament the two drill holes for the sutures must be placed over and under each other at the posterior insertion of the anterior cruciate ligament.

QUADRICEPS TENDON SUBSTITUTION
USING A FREE GRAFT (Clancy)[14]

One argument against the quadriceps tendon substitution method is that in order to obtain adequate length at least a part of the thinner expansion crossing

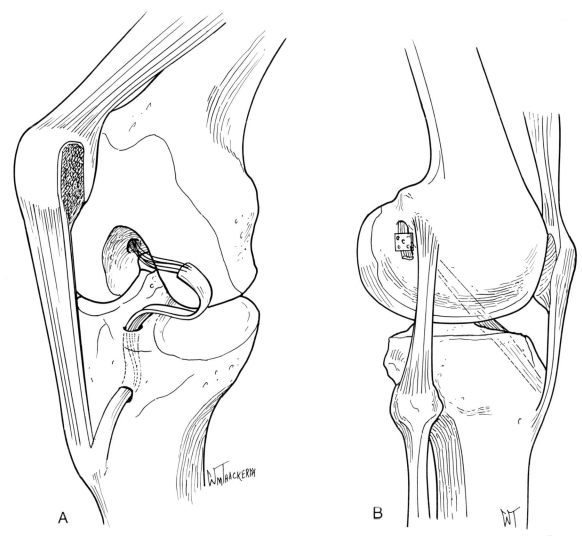

Fig. 13.23. (A) The Eriksson quadriceps tendon substitution takes the graft from the medial third of the patella, sometimes with a bone graft from the patella. (B) As the graft is usually of insufficient length, two drill holes for sutures must be made through the lateral femoral condyle to anchor the proximal end of the graft. (From Eriksson, E.: Reconstruction of the anterior cruciate ligament. Orthop. Clin. North Am., *7(1):* 167, 1976, with permission.)

the patella must be used. By making a free graft and taking blocks of bone from the patella and tibial tubercle, this difficulty can be overcome. This technique is described in Chapter 14.

FASCIA LATA (modified Hey Groves)[36,37]

Through a long anteromedial approach, the knee joint is exposed, and through another longitudinal incision on the lateral aspect of the thigh ending distal to the head of the fibula the fascia lata is exposed.

The knee is flexed and the joint explored. Then through the lateral incision a strip of fascia lata, 8 inches long and 3 inches wide is reflected distally leaving it attached distally to the tibia (Fig. 13.24A). A ⅜-inch drill hole is made obliquely through the lateral femoral condyle, beginning on its lateral surface and emerging as far posteriorly as possible in the intercondylar notch. Alternatively an over-the-top route above and around the lateral femoral condyle may be chosen (Fig. 13.24B). A drill hole of similar size is made obliquely through the tibia beginning anteromedial, just anterior to the superficial medial liga-

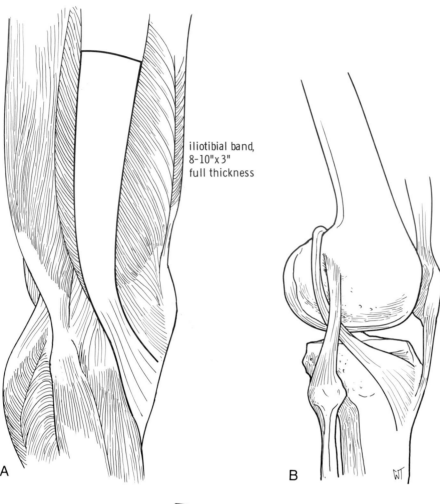

iliotibial band,
8-10"x 3"
full thickness

A

B

Fig. 13.24. Hey Groves fascia lata graft (modified). (A) A large fascia lata graft is harvested. (B) The graft is passed beneath the lateral collateral ligament and over the top of the lateral femoral condyle. (C) The graft is brought into the intercondylar notch, passed through a drill hole in the tibia, and turned proximally along the anterior border of the superficial medial ligament. It is fixed with a staple to the medial femoral condyle.

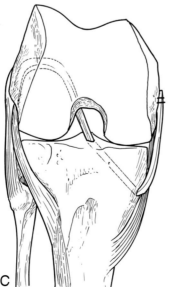

C

ment and emerging within the knee just anterior to the tibial spine. These two holes make a passage for the new ligament which, when the knee is extended, will be as oblique as possible in the sagittal plane. A strip of gauze is passed through each hole to remove any particles of bone. The openings are beveled. The graft is passed beneath the lateral ligament and the fascial strip is then passed via stay sutures through the holes and pulled taut with the knee flexed 90 degrees. The free end is pulled proximally in line with the anterior border of the superficial medial ligament and fixed to the medial femoral condyle with sutures and staples (Fig. 13.24C). This method therefore combines a reconstruction of the anterior cruciate ligament and the superficial medial ligament.

Postoperative Care

The knee is immobilized in 10 degrees of flexion in a pressure dressing reinforced with splints. At 1 week, a long leg cast is applied that is changed at 6 weeks to a cast brace permitting limited motion. A cast brace is worn for another 2 months.

SEMITENDINOSUS OR GRACILIS TENDON TRANSFER (Lindemann)[20,58]

Through a medial parapatellar skin incision, the insertion of the semitendinosus or gracilis tendon into the tibia is identified and detached, and the tendon is dissected proximally until the muscle belly is reached (Fig. 13.25). The tendon is rerouted and brought within the knee through the posterior capsule. To do this, a short lateral incision is made, the fascia lata split and the posterior–distal aspect of the femur exposed immediately proximal to the posterior capsule of the joint. The dissection continues to connect with the medial incision so that the popliteal vessels are retracted posteriorly. The tendon is passed through to the lateral incision. The knee is entered by making an aperture through the posterolateral capsule, and the tendon is brought to the front of the knee. An oblique drill hole is made through the tibia emerging anterior to the tibial spine through which the tendon is passed and sutured on its emergence to the periosteum and pes anserinus. Cast immobilization in flexion for 6 weeks is required.

Fig. 13.25. Lindemann transfer of the semitendinosus tendon.

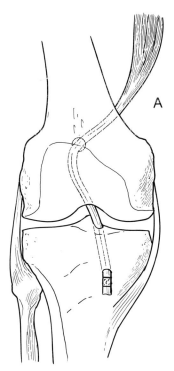
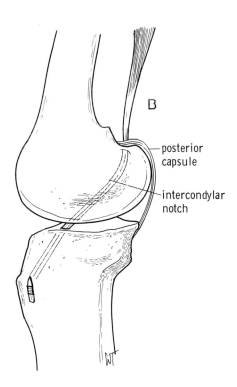

Because the tendon remains attached to its muscle belly, a dynamic function is claimed in addition to the tendon's function as a static stabilizer.

SEMITENDINOSUS TENODESIS (Cho)[16]

Through a medial parapatellar incision, the semitendinosus tendon is identified and freed proximally to its muscle belly where it is divided, the muscle being sutured to the adjoining gracilis. The free tendon is then withdrawn to its distal insertion and an oblique hole made through the tibia through which the tendon is passed. A hole through the lateral femoral condyle, emerging as far posterior as possible, is made and the tendon passed through it to be sutured to the lateral border of the lateral femoral condyle. Cast immobilization for 6 weeks is required.

COMBINED SEMITENDINOSUS AND FASCIA LATA GRAFT (Zarins and Rowe)[91]

This method is a combination of the Hey Groves fascia lata graft and semitendinosus tenodesis. Medial and lateral incisions are made and through the medial incision the semitendinosus tendon is identified and detached from its muscle belly. Through the lateral incision the fascia lata graft is harvested as for the Hey Groves procedure. An oblique drill hole is made through the tibia emerging anterior to the tibial spine. The fascia lata graft is dissected distally to the head of the fibula and rerouted beneath the lateral collateral ligament, similar to the method of MacIntosh. The free end of the graft is then passed over the top of the lateral femoral condyle into the knee joint and out through the oblique drill hole in the tibia. The free end can be sutured locally or brought up to the medial femoral condyle and reattached at that site. The semitendinosus tendon is brought in the reverse direction and sutured proximally to the fascia lata graft and adjoining soft tissue of the lateral femoral condyle. This reconstruction produces a massive intra-articular graft, incorporates lateral extra-articular substitution and allows a medial reconstruction as well. On the other hand, the surgery is extensive, with lengthy medial and lateral scars, and cast immobilization for 6 to 8 weeks is required.

POSTERIOR INSTABILITY

The lesion is due to posterior cruciate insufficiency. The posterior cruciate is the strongest, and perhaps the most important stabilizing ligament in the knee.[41,52,54] Because of its strength it is less commonly injured in sports, and most chronic laxities are the result of road and industrial accidents. Because of the chronic posterior subluxation of the tibia that results, the extensor mechanism is placed at a mechanical disadvantage and anterior knee pain due to patellofemoral arthrosis is often a major presenting complaint, overshadowing the accompanying instability. Posterior cruciate insufficiency is a difficult surgical problem. Most methods of reconstruction involve tendon transfers using gastrocnemius, popliteus,[8] semitendinosus or ligamentum patellae, although other structures such as menisci have been recommended.

MEDIAL HEAD OF GASTROCNEMIUS[39] WITH BONE BLOCK[42]

The tendinous part of the medial head of gastrocnemius provides a massive graft and is perhaps the most widely used tissue. However, obtaining adequate length is a problem[52] and the use of a "leader" of braided Dacron,[40] nonabsorbable suture[7] or proplast[90] has been recommended. The method to be described takes a bone block contiguous with the tendon insertion to increase length and aid fixation (Fig. 13.26A–G).

A medial parapatellar skin incision is used, and the medial skin flap is dissected to expose the medial capsule and medial femoral condyle. The knee joint is entered anteriorly through the straight midline utility approach, crossing the medial border of the patella. The diagnosis may not be immediately apparent upon inspection, and although there is obviously excessive anteroposterior laxity, both cruciate ligaments may appear present. In fact, because of the tibial dropback, the anterior cruciate is relaxed and lies flat upon the tibial surface creating the illusion that it is perhaps the anterior that is deficient. However, with anterior drawer the anterior cruciate comes into prominence and the presence of a taut anteromedial band should leave no doubt about its integrity. When both cruciates are damaged, this confirmation is not present.

Closer inspection of the posterior cruciate shows attenuation, but unlike similar anterior cruciate lesions, some continuity of the ligament normally persists. In this respect, chronic posterior cruciate laxity resembles chronic laxities of the medial ligament in which interstitial stretching and healing with lengthening is the rule. Presumably the size and bulk of the posterior cruciate and its relatively retrosynovial position favor this response rather than the reabsorption found after anterior cruciate rupture. Because of difficulty in diagnosis by inspection, unusually careful preoperative evaluation is needed, including lateral radiographs for comparison with the opposite knee.

The femoral attachment of the posterior cruciate is cleared from the bone; the remaining fibers of the ligament should not be excised, but should rather remain to become reattached to the inferior surface of the graft. Associated meniscal tears are appropriately removed.

Turning attention again to the medial aspect of the joint, the femoral attachment of the superficial medial ligament is identified and the interval between the posterior border of the ligament and the medial head of gastrocnemius is developed. Following the medial head proximally, its attachment of bone is outlined and a bone block 1 cm wide by 1.5 cm in length is outlined in continuity with the tendinous origin (Fig. 13.26A). Fleshy fibers of the muscle arise directly from the capsule and adjoining part of the medial femoral condyle superior and posterior to the tendinous portion. The bone block to be removed is outlined with osteotome cuts and the bone block is predrilled with a Steinmann pin for eventual AO cancellous bone screw fixation. The bone block is then removed and the tendinous portion of the muscle separated both from the posterior capsule of the knee and the adjoining fleshy fibers for some distance into the calf; some fairly firm fascial bands also connect it to the semimembranosus tendon sheath. Good mobilization at this stage is necessary to obtain the required length for the graft. Once the tendon has been exposed, removed, and retracted, the posterior capsule comes into clear view, and by blunt dissection the posterior upper tibia is exposed. The middle genicular artery, which enters the posterior capsule to provide the blood supply for the cruciate ligaments, tethers the popliteal artery to the capsule and should be ligated (Fig. 13.26B). The attachment of the posterior cruciate to

the tibia is identified by a groove on the surface of the bone that can be felt through the capsule. With a Bennett retractor protecting the popliteal vessels, an incision is made through the capsule at this point from inside the knee. The hole is enlarged with dilators until a No. 36–40 plastic chest tube will pass through. A stay suture is passed through the bone block and three other stay sutures of heavy silk are passed through the tendon at a more distal level, the most inferior being at least 2 cm distal to the bone block. These sutures will be used at a later stage for applying traction to the graft. The bone block is then delivered with the plastic tube into the intercondylar notch of the knee (Fig. 13.26C). A drill hole is made through the medial femoral condyle emerging within the joint as closely as possible to the original site of cruciate attachment (Fig. 13.26D). The hole is progressively enlarged up to $\frac{1}{2}$ inch (12.5 mm) diameter. A rectangular recess is made into the cortex of the medial femoral condyle on its medial aspect adjoining the superior border of the drill hole. The bone block is then brought into the drill hole, and using the previously placed stay sutures, the tendon is advanced until the bone block can be turned superiorly into the recess. The bone block is quite fragile, and only gentle traction must be applied to avoid fragmentation. When the bone block is in position, it is transfixed with an AO cancellous bone screw with a washer attached; the screw is driven transversely across the femur (Fig. 13.26E). Very firm fixation should ensue; the tendinous graft represents a substantial band of tissue in the line of the posterior cruciate ligament.

After the wound is closed, a Robert Jones compression bandage is applied reinforced by splints and the knee held in 45 degrees of flexion. The immobilization is continued for three weeks when the sutures are removed and the knee is allowed to extend. Weight-bearing with crutches is permitted and the crutches are discarded when the patient is able to do without them. The standard rehabilitation program is applied.

QUADRICEPS TENDON SUBSTITUTION[13]

An anteromedial parapatellar approach is used and the quadriceps mechanism exposed. The quadriceps tendon graft is harvested in the same manner as for anterior cruciate substitution. The drill hole is made

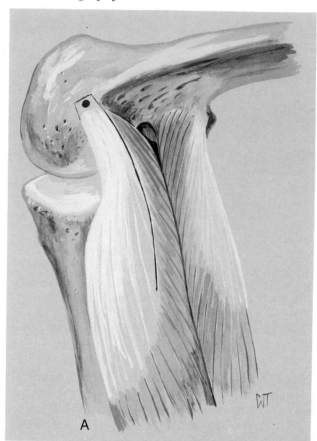

A

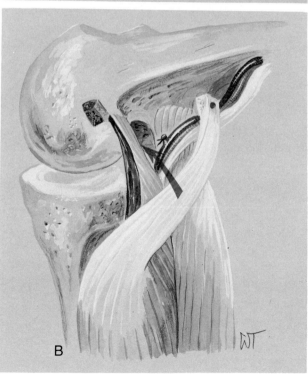

B

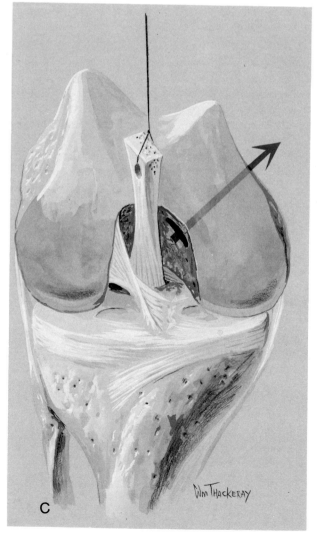

C

Fig. 13.26. Transfer of medial head of gastrocnemius with bone block for posterior cruciate insufficiency. (A) The tendinous part of the medial head of gastrocnemius with a bone block is detached and separated into the calf. (B) The middle genicular artery is ligated and the popliteal vessels retracted posteriorly. A hole is made through the posterior capsule of the knee in line with the posterior cruciate attachment. (C) Using a No. 36–40 plastic chest tube, the bone block is drawn to the front of the knee (Figure continues).

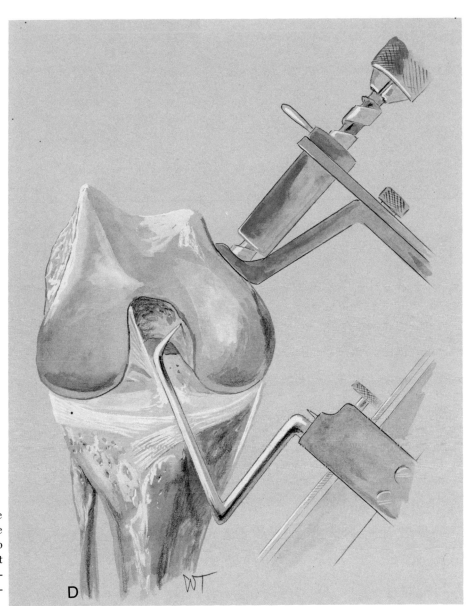

Fig. 13.26 (Continued). (D) The drill hole is made through the medial femoral condyle to emerge on the median aspect as close as possible to the posterior cruciate attachment (Figure continues).

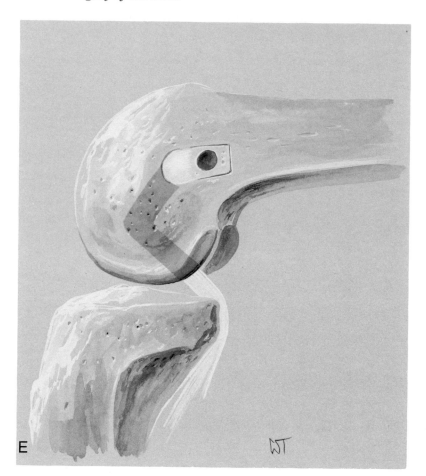

Fig. 13.26 (Continued). (E) The bone block is carefully drawn through the hole in the medial femoral condyle and turned into a recess adjoining the medial exit of the bony tunnel (Figure continues).

through the tibia from front to back after reflecting the skin flap and exposing the posterior capsule by blunt dissection. The graft is brought out through the drill hole and passed back into the knee through an adjoining hole in the posterior capsule. A second drill hole, ⅜ of an inch in diameter, is made through the medial femoral condyle, through which the graft is passed and brought out medially where it is sutured and stapled. A Steinmann pin is driven through the joint, holding the tibia in the anterior reduced position because the cast cannot be relied upon to hold the reduction by itself. Alternatively, the Steinmann pin can be passed transversely across the tibia at the level of the tibial tubercle and then incorporated in the cast to fulfill the same function (Fig. 13.27). The knee is immobilized at 30 degrees of flexion and held for 6 to 8 weeks.

SEMITENDINOSUS TENODESIS

The semitendinosus tendon is harvested. Leaving its distal insertion intact, the graft is used in the same manner as that described for quadriceps tendon substitution (Fig. 13.28). Steinmann pin fixation is required.

MEDIAL INSTABILITIES

Instability is caused by laxity of the superficial fibers of the medial ligament. Medial laxity rarely requires reconstruction as an isolated procedure and is nearly always done in combination with a cruciate substitution procedure. A choice must be made be-

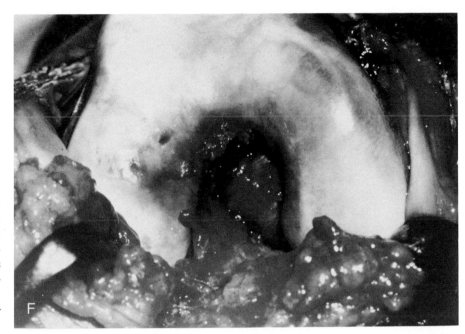

Fig. 13.26 (Continued). (F) The completed graft. (G) Screw fixation of the bone block. (From Insall, J.N., and Hood, R.W.: Bone-block transfer of the medial head of the gastrocnemius for posterior cruciate insufficiency. J. Bone Joint Surg. [Am.], *64*: 691, 1982, with permission.)

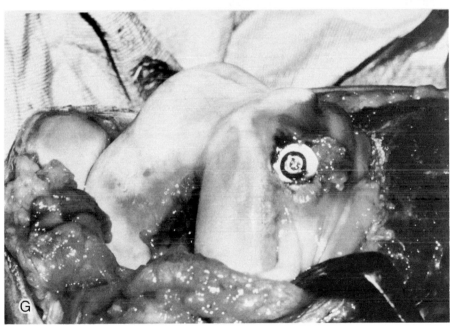

tween procedures that (1) tighten the ligament without disturbing its continuity, and (2) those that tighten by detaching either the proximal or distal end of the ligament. Both methods may be used in conjunction with a reinforcement by a tissue graft.

Operations that detach one end or other of the ligament have an inherent disadvantage. If the fixation fails at the site of reattachment, the instability may be worse than it was before. For this reason, reattachment of the ligament should be reserved only for the most severe cases of instability, so that if the ligament does pull free, or fail to heal with adequate strength, the state after surgery will not be noticeably worse.

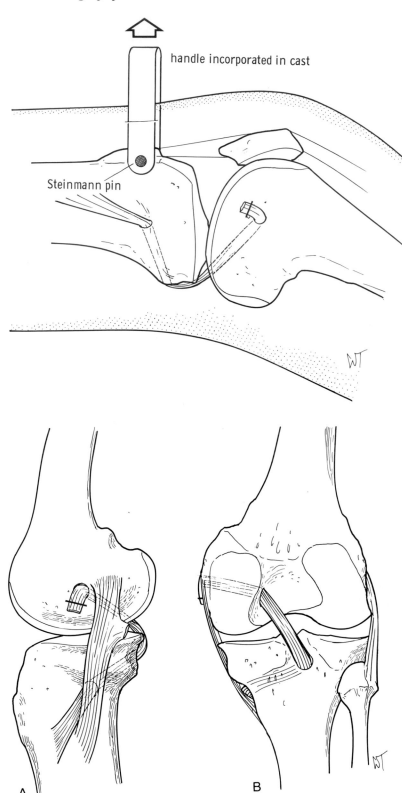

handle incorporated in cast

Steinmann pin

Fig. 13.27. It is often impossible to hold the tibia that is reduced after posterior cruciate reconstruction. One method of doing this is to pass a Steinmann pin through the tibial tubercle and, while applying anterior traction, to incorporate the pin and the bow in the cast.

Fig. *13.28.* Semitendinosus tenodesis for posterior cruciate reconstruction. Steinmann pin fixation is required in order to perform this technique.

A

B

REATTACHMENT OPERATIONS

According to Bartel et al.[9] there is better restoration of normal anatomical function when the repositioning of the ligament attachment is done distally rather than proximally. When the femoral attachment is advanced proximally the resulting changes in length of the anterior and posterior borders differ significantly from normal. Proximal relocation is also influenced by the position of the knee. If the ligament is relocated when the knee is at full extension, the anterior border becomes increasingly slack as the knee is flexed. It will be much looser than a normal knee at flexion angles greater than 45 degrees, which would probably result in an increased medial laxity at these angles. If the ligament is relocated proximally when the knee is flexed, then as the knee is extended the anterior border will become increasingly tight. For example, if the ligament is tightened at a knee flexion angle of 90 degrees, the anterior border must stretch about 8 mm as the knee extends to 20 degrees of flexion. With proximal reattachment, ligament deformation is very sensitive to antero–posterior placement.

The relative deformation is not affected significantly by distal advancement or antero–posterior placement when tibial reattachment is used. Changes in length of the anterior border of the superficial medial ligament that occur as the knee is flexed are most like those of normal knees when the tibial attachment is advanced distally and anteriorly. The changes are least like those of the normal knee when the femoral attachment is advanced proximally and posteriorly. For an optimal result, the medial collateral ligament should be advanced distally and anteriorly with the knee in 30 degrees of flexion.

From this study it must be clear that proximal reattachment should be avoided whenever possible. However, at times this may be unavoidable, for example, when the instability has been caused by femoral avulsion and the medial meniscus remains intact. For such cases the reattachment point should be as close as possible to the original insertion of the ligament. In particular posterior placement should be avoided.

TECHNIQUE OF DISTAL REATTACHMENT

MODIFIED MAUCK[68]

An incision is made vertically 1 cm medial to the tibial tubercle, through the periosteum and insertion of the pes anserinus, which is then reflected medially by subperiosteal dissection until the long fibers of the medial ligament are encountered. The distal insertion is identified and removed together with a rectangle of bone approximately 1 centimeter square. A similar-size rectangle is removed from a distal and anterior position at the site of relocation. This piece of bone is added to fill the first defect and the ligament is reattached in its new position by a washer and bone screw. To avoid making two defects in the tibia, Vigliani's method[86] may be used (Fig. 13.29). The distal attachment is raised by subperiosteal dissection, leaving the ligament in continuity with the surrounding periosteum. At the original site of attachment, a bone block somewhat more than 1 cm square is removed. The ligament is pulled tight and inserted into the defect with the bone block placed on top of it. The

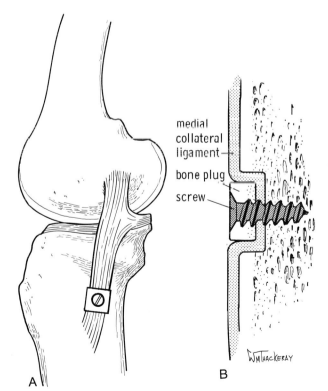

Fig. 13.29. The Vigliani method for distal reattachment of the superficial medial collateral ligament.

medial
collateral
ligament

bone plug

screw

A   B

attachment is then secured by driving the bone block back into the tibia with a bone screw. A modification of the Vigliani method may also be used to tighten the long fibers without removing the distal insertion (see below).

O'DONOGHUE

The principle, according to O'Donoghue,[73] is to detach the whole medial capsular and ligamentous mass from the tibia beginning at the midline in front and extending around the midline posteriorly. A cuff is thereby developed without making any effort to identify particular ligaments, because their identity is often lost in scar. This cuff is then advanced downward on the tibia. O'Donoghue often combines this procedure with reconstruction of the anterior cruciate ligament using the iliotibial band (see Hey Groves technique).

PROXIMAL REATTACHMENT

In some cases, an intact medial meniscus may make the less desirable proximal reattachment necessary. An anterior incision is made in the capsule to expose the medial femoral condyle through which the entire capsular mass, including the long fibers of the medial ligament, is elevated in continuity with the proximal periosteum. Proximal reattachment is by staples. Alternatively, at the site of normal attachment of the medial ligament, a block of bone 1 cm wide and 1.5 cm in an anteroposterior direction is raised, exposing the underlying cancellous bone. The capsular structures are placed into the defect under tension. The bone block is placed on top of them and fixed with a cancellous bone screw and washer.

PRESERVING THE CONTINUITY OF THE LONG FIBERS OF THE MEDIAL LIGAMENT

Some procedures are preferred for lesser degrees of medial instability, as they are less extensive, require less immobilization, and cannot make the instability any worse than it was originally.

REEFING

A continuous reefing stitch of heavy suture material (e.g., No. 2 chromic catgut) is placed in the medial capsule beginning posteriorly and extending to the margin of the patellar tendon (Fig. 13.30). The suture is placed at the level of the joint line and is locked with each stitch. An intact medial meniscus does not preclude this method. A reefing stitch is perhaps the simplest method of treating medial laxity but should only be used in combination with another procedure, for example, semitendinosus or fascia lata reinforcement or together with anterior cruciate reconstruction.

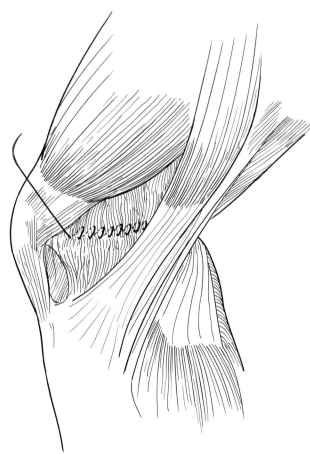

Fig. 13.30. A single continuous reefing stitch of heavy catgut is the simplest method of tightening the medial capsular structures. The balance of the medial meniscus if present must not be disturbed.

POSTEROMEDIAL CAPSULE ADVANCEMENT (Slocum)[81]

The medial capsule of the knee is exposed from the medial margin of the patella to the posterior margin of the medial femoral condyle. The medial meniscus must have been excised. The posterior incision is made in the interval between the posterior capsule and the posterior oblique fibers of the superficial medial ligament. When the posterior capsule is lax, the bone of the posterior tibia is roughened and two or three drill holes are placed front to back emerging at the posterior margin of the tibia. The posterior capsule is then drawn tight against the bone by sutures passed through the drill holes and tied anteriorly. This step can be omitted when the posterior capsule is not unusually lax. The oblique fibers of the medial ligament are then sutured under tension to the direct head of the semimembranosus tendon insertion into the tibia. The free anterior margin of the posterior capsule is then carried forward and sutured through the trailing edge of the long fibers of the medial ligament. The

repair is further reinforced by dividing the conjoint tendon of the semimembranosus from the tibia and using the direct insertion as a pivot point suturing this part of the semimembranosus tendon to the medial ligament superficial to the previous repair. A pes anserinus transfer (described under substitution procedures) is usually done in conjunction with this posteromedial repair.

ADVANCEMENT OF POSTERIOR OBLIQUE LIGAMENT (Hughston)[40]

Hughston originally described this technique for repair of acute medial ligament injury but has since adapted it for use in recontructive procedures (Fig. 13.31). The posterior oblique ligament is a thickening of the capsular ligament attached proximally to the adductor tubercle of the femur and distally to the tibia and posterior aspect of the capsule. As described by Hughston, the distal attachment has three arms: (1) the central or tibial arm which attaches to the pos-

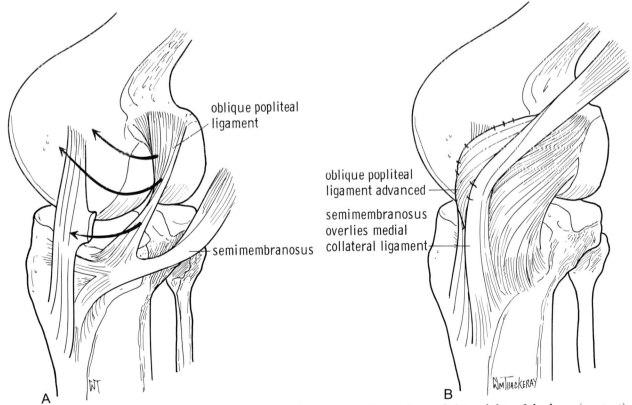

Fig. 13.31. (A,B) Advancement of the posterior oblique ligament (Hughston) for medial instability of the knee (see text).

terior surface of the tibia medial to the semimembranosus tendon; (2) the superior arm which is continuous with the posterior capsule and the proximal part of the oblique popliteal ligament, and (3) the inferior arm which attaches distally to the sheath covering semimembranosus tendon and to the adjoining part of the tibia. For the reconstruction of chronic instability, the posterior oblique ligament is separated from its attachment to the superficial medial ligament by a vertical incision through the capsule. Three sutures of nonabsorbable material are then placed. The superior suture advances the posterior oblique ligament toward the adductor tubercle and overlaps the medial collateral ligament attachment.

The central suture advances the posterior oblique ligament over the central position of the superficial medial ligament. The distal suture advances the inferior arm over the more distal part of the medial collateral ligament. The repair is reinforced by sutures passed through the sheath of the semimembranosus tendon, which is brought anteriorly and proximally to be sutured into the trailing edge of the superficial medial ligament. The knee is immobilized postoperatively in 60 degrees of flexion with the foot in internal rotation.

VIGLIANI (MODIFIED)

The Vigliani bone block method of reattaching the medial collateral ligament has already been described. A modification of the method may be used without detaching the insertion into the tibia. The medial collateral ligament is exposed throughout its length by a subperiosteal resection of the periosteum and pes anserinus insertion. Immediately proximal to the distal insertion, a block of bone rather more than 1 cm in size is removed. The long fibers of the medial ligament are placed into the defect and the piece of bone inserted on top. By using a bone screw and washer, the long fibers can be tightened to a desired degree. This method shortens the medial ligament somewhat and therefore may reduce postoperative flexion to some degree. The fixation is remarkably secure and no form of external support is needed postoperatively; the method is thus particularly attractive when used in conjunction with the iliotibial band reconstruction of the anterior cruciate ligament.

TENDON TRANSPOSITION[10]

In addition to medial reconstruction reinforcement using a pes anserinus tendon may be of value (Fig. 13.32). Usually either semitendinosus or gracilis tendon is chosen because the natural direction of these tendons make them most suitable, but the sartorius tendon may also be used. The tendon is left attached distally and mobilized proximally avoiding the saphenous nerve until the tendon can be transposed to the medial femoral condyle. A trough is created in the soft tissues, which are then closed over the tendon, which, if not itself sutured, may preserve a dynamic function.

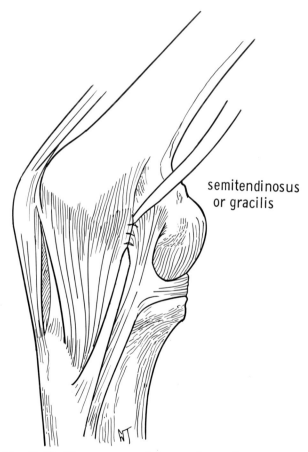

semitendinosus or gracilis

Fig. 13.32. Transposition of the gracilis tendon (see text). (From Bosworth, D.M.: Transplantation of the semitendinosus for repair of laceration of medial collateral ligament of the knee. J. Bone Joint Surg. [Am.], 34:196, 1952, with permission.)

LATERAL INSTABILITIES[53,56,57,85]

Single plane lateral stability is provided by the iliotibial band, the lateral ligament, the arcuate ligament and the popliteus tendon. As in the case of medial laxity, collateral instability is made worse by cruciate insufficiency, and for practical purposes lateral reconstruction will always be done in conjunction with cruciate reconstruction. This type of instability is rare and the literature on it sparse.

MODIFIED HEY GROVES TECHNIQUE USING THE FASCIA LATA

Long lateral and shorter medial parapatellar skin incisions are required (Fig. 13.33). Through the lateral incision a strip of fascia lata 8 to 10 inches in length and 2 to 3 inches in width is harvested. Dissection extends distally toward the insertion of the iliotibial band, which may be damaged and scarred from the injury. The proximal end of the graft is passed beneath the lateral ligament and then over the top of the lateral femoral condyle and brought into the intercondylar notch. A drill hole is made through the lateral tibial plateau from a point immediately posterior to Gerdy's tubercle emerging anterior to the tibial spine at the approximate insertion of the anterior cruciate ligament. The fascia lata graft is passed through this hole, pulled tight, and stapled to the lateral femoral condyle. In order to reach the site of attachment, the graft passes superficial to the iliotibial band and may be sutured to it. Excess graft that remains may be turned distally again to reinforce the repair.

EN BLOC ADVANCEMENT OF THE LATERAL CAPSULE AND RELATED STRUCTURES[21]

The lax lateral capsule with the popliteus tendon, lateral ligament, arcuate ligament, and the origin of the lateral head of gastrocnemius are separated from the bone of the lateral femoral condyle (Fig. 13.34). The bony surface proximal to the original attachment

Fig. 13.33. (A,B) The Hey Groves fascia lata technique can also be used for lateral reconstruction (see text).

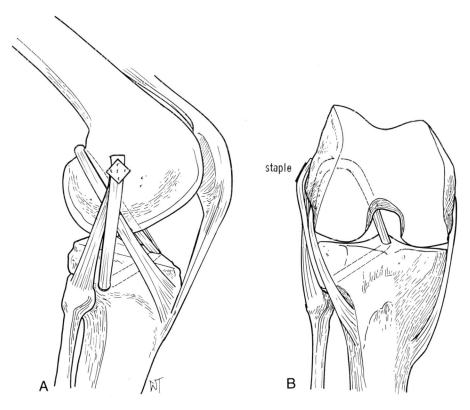

staple

A   B

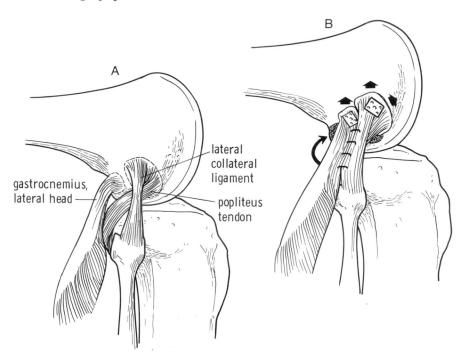

Fig. 13.34. En bloc advancement of popliteus tendon, lateral collateral ligament, arcuate ligament, and lateral head of gastrocnemius for lateral instability.

is freshened and the cuff of tissue obtained is advanced anteriorly and proximally to be reattached, either by stapling or by a series of drill holes placed through the bone through which sutures can be passed. This repair may be supplemented by the fascia lata graft as described above.

BICEPS FEMORIS TENDON

The biceps tendon is split and the anterior two-thirds detached from the head of the fibula; this portion is brought forward and attached to the tibia in the region of Gerdy's tubercle.

Most lateral reconstructions, depending on circumstances and the availability of suitable tissue, consist of a combination of these repairs.

SUBSTITUTION PROCEDURES

In addition to reconstruction intended to replace the function of the prime supporting ligaments, other methods have other purposes. Used mainly for the control of rotary instability, these are extra-articular capsular reinforcements, which restrain rotary movement of the knee without regard to its specific cause.

At The Hospital for Special Surgery, substitution procedures are used primarily as ancilliary or backup methods in combination with cruciate reconstruction.

PES ANERINUS TRANSFER
(Slocum and Larson)[56,57,78,80]

The pes anserinus is exposed from the sartorius above to the semitendinosus tendon below (Fig. 13.35). Dissection is carried anteriorly to expose the medial face of the tibia, the tibial tubercle, and the lower one-half of the patellar tendon, and posteriorly to just above the joint level. The upper and lower borders of the pes anserinus are clearly identified. A 1-inch incision is now made through the gastrocnemius fascia at the lower margin of the semitendinosus just posterior to the tibia. The semitendinosus is grasped and lifted forward and upward. A knife is used to separate the distal, fascial, and tibial attachments of the semitendinosus, avoiding damage to the underlying distal insertion of the medial collateral ligament and the medial inferior genicular vessels that lie at the posteromedial aspect of the tibia at this level.

Severance of the distal 90 percent of the tibial attachments of the pes from the tibia is now carried out by sharp dissection. The fascial attachments to the

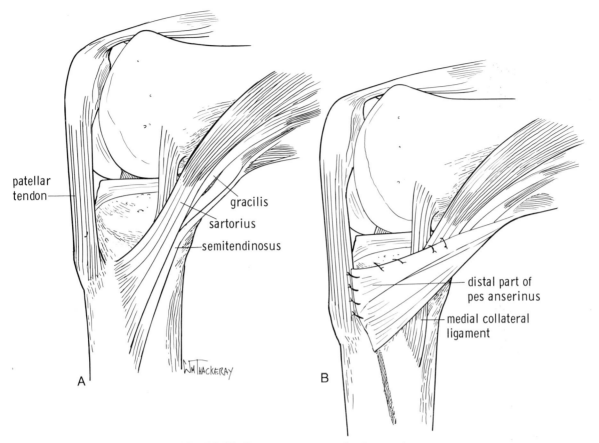

Fig. 13.35. Pes anserinus transfer (see text).

lower border of the pes are dissected posteriorly to the point where the distal free end of the pes can be approximated to the tibial tubercle and lower medial margin of the patellar tendon. There are two layers of fascia that must be freed. Superficially, the deep fascia is attached to the sartorius. Care should be taken in dissecting this layer to avoid severing the sartorial branch of the saphenous nerve, which emerges below the distal muscular fibers of the sartorius and lies in the fatty areolar tissues just beneath the superficial fascia. The point of emergence of this nerve appears to vary considerably depending on how far distally the fleshy fibers of the muscle extend. Occasionally it is necessary to dissect this nerve free if it appears compressed by the upward reflection of the pes. More deeply, the gastrocnemius fascia is attached to the semitendinosis tendon. Frequently strong tendinous bands extend from the main tendon into the gastrocnemius fascia and must not be confused with the main

body of the tendon, which attaches to the tibia. The fascia should only be dissected from the tendon far enough posteriorly to permit easy insertion of the pes to its newly transplanted level. If dissected above the supracondylar level, it may permit upward luxation of the pes tendons with loss of medial support and rotational control of the tibia. Once the pes is free of its fascial and bony moorings, the lower portion is folded upward so that it overlies the upper portion to form a double layered tendinous mass. Starting distally so that tension can be adjusted with each successive suture, the free end of the pes anserinus is sewn to the periosteum overlying the tibial tubercle and distal one-half inch of the medial border of the patellar tendon. The transplanted pes forms a sling beneath the medial flare of the tibial metaphysis; if it lies above this level, the supporting action is lost. The free border of the reflected semitendinosus tendon now lies proximally and it is sutured to the perios-

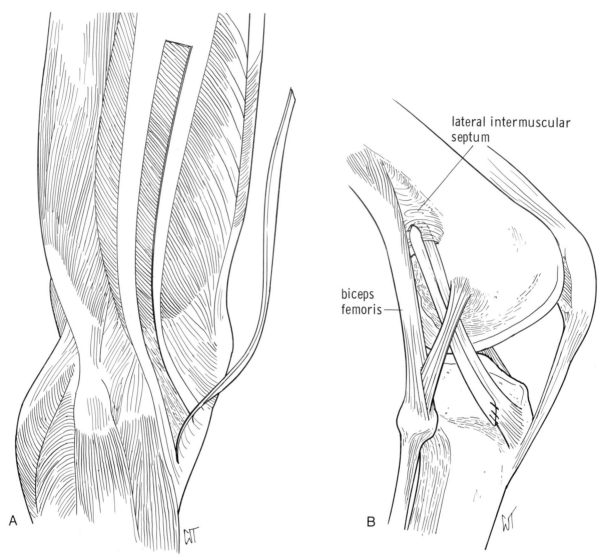

Fig. 13.36. (A,B) MacIntosh fasciodesis (see text).

teum adjacent to the patellar tendon and to the fascia overlying the medial collateral ligament to prevent upward displacement when the knee is extended. Sometimes release of the tourniquet is necessary before the free end of the pes can be approximated to the tibial tubercle and patellar tendon.

MACINTOSH FASCIODESIS

The MacIntosh operation was originally performed as follows. A one-half inch strip of the fascia lata was freed proximally, leaving the distal attachment to Gerdy's tubercle intact. The free proximal end of the fascia was looped around the lateral collateral ligament and pulled back on itself to be sutured to the surrounding tissue and the fascia overlying Gerdy's tubercle. To prevent anterior subluxation of the lateral tibial plateau, the foot was held in external rotation while the fasciodesis was tightened; afterward the knee was immobilized in full external rotation and at 90 degrees of flexion.

MacIntosh has modified the procedure (Fig. 13.36) so that instead of folding the free end of the fascial graft distally, it is brought around the lateral femoral condyle into the intercondylar notch to be aligned

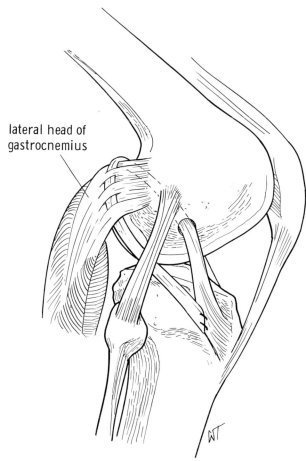

lateral head of gastrocnemius

Fig. 13.37. Losee sling and reef lateral reconstruction (see text). (From Losee, R.E., Johnson, T.R., and Southwick, W.O.: Anterior subluxation of the lateral tibial plateau. A diagnostic test and operative repair. J. Bone Joint Surg. [Am.], *60:* 1015, 1978, with permission.)

and passed through a tibial drill hole to act as a substitute for the anterior cruciate ligament. The MacIntosh procedure is now both an extra-articular and an intra-articular reconstruction for an absent anterior cruciate ligament.

THE SLING AND REEF PROCEDURE
(Losee)

The incision for the lateral repair starts 15 cm proximal to the joint, follows the lateral intermuscular septum to the level of the joint line, continues anteriorly along the lateral joint line, and then curves

distally along the lateral margin of the tibial tubercle to a point 3 cm distal to it (Fig. 13.37). Parallel incisions 2.5 cm apart are made in the iliotibial tract. The landmarks for these incisions are the anterolateral tubercle of the tibia (Gerdy's tubercle) and the bifurcation of the iliotibial tract, where it divides to a posterior branch going to Gerdy's tubercle and an anterior branch running superficially toward the patella. The iliotibial tract is incised from the bifurcation proximally for a distance of 12 to 14 cm and then the same incision is extended distally as far as the joint line. The second incision is made parallel and about 2.5 cm posterior to the first one, beginning at the posterior edge of the iliotibial tract at Gerdy's tubercle. The resulting 16 cm strip of iliotibial tract is transected at its proximal end and dissected off the vastus lateralis and intermuscular septum down to its attachment at Gerdy's tubercle. A tunnel is then made through the lateral femoral condyle. An incision is made in the periosteum just anterior and inferior to the femoral attachment of the fibular collateral ligament. This incision should be located at the center of rotation for the arc traversed by Gerdy's tubercle as the knee is flexed and extended.

Before making the incision, the correct location can be determined by trial placement of the strip at various loci on the condyle just anterior to the fibular collateral ligament. The tunnel's entrance must be close to the margin of the joint surface yet not so close that flexion and extension will be obstructed. To create the tunnel a 0.9-cm curved osteotome is driven in a posteromedial direction and guided beneath the cortex of the lateral femoral condyle so that it emerges in the substance of the tendon of origin of the lateral head of the gastrocnemius muscle. The ribbon of iliotibial tract is threaded through a Gallie needle and passed through the tunnel from front to back. To verify the correct placement of the tunnel, the lateral tibial plateau is subluxed anteriorly. Then if the tunnel is properly placed, pulling on the transferred portion of the fascial strip should reduce this subluxation and maintain stable reduction when the test for anterior subluxation of the lateral tibial plateau is performed. The knee should also be flexed to 90 degrees to make sure that the sling does not pull loose.

If the strip does not function properly, either it was not placed correctly or the indications for surgery were not fulfilled. When the indications for surgery are correct but anterior subluxation is not prevented by the sling or if the sling becomes lax during flexion of the knee, the ribbon of iliotibial tract may be passed in a more horizontal direction beneath the fibular collateral ligament.

Once the strip has been passed and its position is satisfactory, it is sutured at the points of entrance and exit from the tunnel or to the fibular collateral ligament. The strip is next passed through the tendon of origin of the lateral head of the gastrocnemius entering it at a point 1 cm distal and 0.5 cm medial to the posterior opening of the tunnel and then running horizontally and laterally, thus encircling at least a 1-cm strip of the gastrocnemius tendon of origin. A second reefing stitch is then passed through the gastrocnemius, starting at a point 1.5 cm medial and 0.5 cm distal to the point of emergence of the previous reefing stitch. From here it is directed distally and laterally so that it comes out through the substance of the arcuate ligament posterior to the fibular collateral ligament just above the level of the joint line. The strip is then passed beneath the fibular collateral ligament just distal to the joint line, and it is established that tension on this strip pulls the gastrocnemius and posterolateral capsular structures into close approximation with the fibular collateral ligament. Before the strip is sutured in place, it is pulled posteriorly around the fibular collateral ligament and, while tension is maintained, the tibia is held in external rotation and the knee is held in 45 degrees of flexion. The displaced gastrocnemius tendon and posterolateral part of the capsule are sutured to the fibular collateral ligament and the strip of fascia lata is carefully sutured to the fibular collateral ligament. The remaining portion of the fascia is then sutured to Gerdy's tubercle and any excess fascia is used to reinforce the repair.

It is wise to test for anterior subluxation of the lateral tibial plateau at appropriate stages during the repair to be sure that stability is maintained. A defect in the fascia lata persists at the completion of the repair in which the vastus lateralis is exposed, but this defect causes only a harmless and asymptomatic muscle hernia.

A padded plaster cast is applied from groin to the toes with the knee flexed and the tibia held in external rotation. The knee is flexed 20 degrees beyond the position at which anterior subluxation of the lateral tibial plateau is demonstrated; 30 to 45 degrees of flexion is the usual position. At 7 weeks, the cast is removed and the patient then wears a long brace with either a pelvic band or a quadrilateral socket and the foot maintained in 10 degrees of external rotation for an additional 3 months.

THE ELLISON PROCEDURE[23]

A one-half inch strip comprising the central portion of the iliotibial band is removed with a sliver of bone from its attachment to Gerdy's tubercle. The strip is dissected free proximally for about 3 inches. The bone block with its attached fascia is then threaded around the fibular collateral ligament from posterior to anterior and, with the knee flexed and the foot held in external rotation, is reattached to the tibia distal and anterior to its point of original attachment. It is held with a staple. Ellison recommends closing the resulting fascial defect. With the knee in flexion and the foot in external rotation, the limb is immobilized in a plaster cast for 6 weeks.

ASSESSMENT OF RESULTS

It has been exceptionally difficult to assess the results of various ligament reconstruction procedures. Indeed inherent difficulties are involved, and added to these are the continuous technical modifications that have been applied to many techniques. Thus to quote Slocum et al., "A given procedure often becomes obsolete before long-range evaluation can be accomplished."[81]

Basically, the results of ligament reconstruction can be assessed in two ways: (1) by static stability testing, and (2) by functional assessment in terms of the patient's subjective feelings of security, the absence of "giving way," and the ability to run, cut, and participate in vigorous sports. Unfortunately, patients who appear excellent in one of these categories may rate poorly in the other. In an experimental and clinical study of injuries to the ligaments of the ankle joint, Freeman et al.[29A] have shown that techniques that best restored objective static stability often failed to relieve the subjective feelings of instability. These workers concluded that this discrepancy was attributable to imperfect restoration of proprioceptive sense.

On the other hand, to express results purely in

terms of patient satisfaction has its drawbacks, and care must be taken in recommending a procedure that gives high patient satisfaction but negligible improvement on objective clinical examination. Whereas these difficulties do exist, they should not be used either as an excuse for poorly performed surgery or to denigrate the ideal objective of improving the patient's condition equally in both categories.

Furthermore, when it comes to clinical signs, there is no agreement as to what to look for, owing largely to conflicting methods of terminology and classification. As an example, consider the most common knee instability of all. Anteromedial rotary instability was the term used by Slocum and Larson[77,78] to describe abnormal anterior and medial motion, which allowed the medial tibial plateau to ride forward on the femur to an excessive degree. Medial capsular laxity was considered an important factor, and reconstruction of the posteromedial capsule was an essential part of the procedure.

In 1972, Galway et al.[32] recognized that a similar type of rotary laxity occurred laterally when the anterior cruciate ligament was absent. These investigators termed this condition anterolateral rotary instability and described a maneuver that reproduces the anterior subluxation of the lateral tibial plateau. The pivot shift test has subsequently become widely accepted as a means of assessing the anterior cruciate insufficient knee. Slocum and Larson and Galway et al. recognized that anterior cruciate injury was involved in the production of both anteromedial and anterolateral instabilities, but on the surface at least, their descriptions seemed to be of two entirely different entities. In fact, it now appears that they were describing different manifestations of the same injury.

While it may certainly be true that the pivot shift phenomenon has more functional significance than does the anterior drawer test, results of the surgical reconstruction should not be judged in terms of its affect on the pivot shift alone. It is surely better if the improvement in the anterior drawer and Lachman tests are given as well, in addition to recording residual medial, lateral, or posterior single-plane laxities. The patient's functional state, the subjective sense of stability, and the ability to participate in sports or other strenuous activities must be known. The correlation between objective static stability and functional stability is also necessary information. Certain functional tests are of value in assessing the injured knee.[18]

Hopping on one leg, a standing broad jump performed with the affected leg (Fig. 13.38A,B), and running in figure eights are three examples of such functional tests. When this information is collected routinely and presented in a comparable manner with meaningful long-term follow-up, it will then be possible to assess the merits of various reconstructive procedures. Probably some form of numerical grading[65] (Fig. 13.39) that takes into account all factors is the most satisfactory rating system. Finally, it takes time to assess the worth of any operative procedure, particularly a ligament reconstruction, because of the lengthy rehabilitation process. Short-term or preliminary reports of a new surgical procedure are of very questionable value and any data with a follow-up time of under 2 years should be set aside.

LIGAMENT INSTABILITY

RESULTS

The results to be discussed are not comprehensive for every technique previously described but rather are intended as a guide as to what can be expected after ligament reconstruction.

O'Donoghue[73] has reported on the results of 60 medial reconstructions using a technique whereby the medial capsular structures are advanced distally as a flap. Twenty-six cases also showed absence of the anterior cruciate ligament in addition to medial instability. Instability and disability were rated according to a five-point grading system.

INSTABILITY

0: No abnormal motion

1+: Demonstrable but not disabling abnormal motion; abnormal motion not appreciated by the patient

2+: Definite somewhat disabling abnormal motion; abnormal motion recognized by the patient

3+: Obvious moderately disabling abnormal motion, quite apparent to the patient

4+: Gross very disabling instability without end point; the knee gives way and support is required during ordinary activity

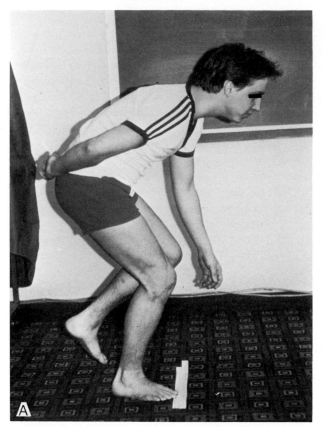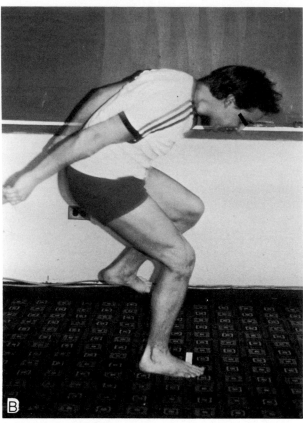

Fig. 13.38. (A,B) The standing broad jump provides a good objective evaluation before and after ligament reconstruction. This patient, who has had a bone block iliotibial band ACL reconstruction, takes off and lands confidently on the operated leg and can jump a distance equal to that performed with the other normal side.

DISABILITY

None: Patient able to engage in all activities

Grade 1: Patient able to participate with reduced proficiency in organized athletics; patient not conscious of instability during regular activities

Grade 2: Patient unable to engage in vigorous sports; experiences episodes of discomfort or swelling

Grade 3: Patient unable to participate in any sports; has pain and swelling

Grade 4: Patient severely restricted in all activities, including walking, climbing stairs, and the like, often requiring a brace, cane or crutches

According to O'Donoghue[73] instability was improved by one grade in 14 knees, by two grades in 22, by three grades in 20, and by four grades in three knees.

In terms of improvement in disability, two knees failed to improve, and 15 improved by one grade, 23 by two grades, 16 by three grades, and four by four grades. In only two patients was disability not decreased after medial reconstruction.

Nicholas[70] gives the result of the five-one reconstruction in 52 consecutive cases. The five-one reconstruction involves a proximal advancement and tightening of the medial ligament with a medial meniscectomy, posterior capsular tightening, vastus medialis advancement and a pes anserinus transfer.

In no patient was complete stability restored, but this failure did not necessarily preclude participation in sports. All told, 43 of the 52 patients were thought to have gained some measurable improvement in rotary laxity or a decrease in the valgus or anteroposterior displacement demonstrable by testing. Nine patients were listed as failures and were not improved in any component of instability.

Forty-three patients returned to their sport, 26 without a brace, and the other 17 wearing a derotation brace. Twelve of the 17 patients had some type of mild buckling that made continued use of the brace necessary.

The minimum follow-up in Nicholas's cases was 3 years; he noted a tendency toward improvement with the passage of time, both objectively and subjectively. Nicholas emphasizes the importance of muscle rehabilitation after reconstructive surgery. He notes that instability is a rather indefinite entity that can vary from time to time, even during the same examination. For this reason he regards the ability to perform sports after reconstruction the most important evidence that the surgery has been effective.

The results of extra-articular reconstructions for so-called rotary instability are conflicting. It would appear that the fundamental lesion for knees requiring this type of reconstruction is insufficiency of the anterior cruciate ligament. Therefore it is probable that the indications are the same as for intra-articular anterior cruciate reconstructions.[29]

Losee et al.[59] in describing the sling and reef operation, give their results on 50 operations with results described as good in 41, fair in six and poor in three knees. Subjectively, however, all 50 patients were satisfied and said that they would have the operation again. Thirty-five patients returned to their preinjury athletic activity, such as basketball, baseball, handball, skiing, tennis, and horseback riding. In 47 of the 50 knees, the pivot shift test was negative at postoperative examination. These results appear very satisfactory, but as some of the patients had a short follow-up, it is possible that there may be some deterioration at some future time. Losee et al. cite 15 of the 50 knees as showing a mild degree of laxity and speculate that these loose repairs may eventually stretch out and fail.

Ireland and Trickey,[44] in describing results of the MacIntosh operation, also found mostly satisfactory results. On the other hand, Kennedy et al.[55] in using the somewhat similar Ellison procedure, found the results to be disappointing. After follow-up as short as 6 months, the pivot shift remained positive in 12 of 15 knees. Subjective results were described as excellent in three, good in four, fair in five, and poor in three knees.

Warren and Marshall,[89] in a retrospective study, give the results of 19 pes anserinus transfers. The pes transfer was often combined with capsular repair for medial instability. The results were excellent in one knee, good in four knees, fair in nine knees, and poor in five knees. These workers concluded that as a general rule, extra-articular surgery without attention to the cruciate ligaments often results in failure.

Although the principle of pes anserinus transfer is biomechanically sound,[72] Freeman et al.[29] found that the clinical results deteriorated with time and that associated anterolateral instability was made worse by the procedure. After an average 9-year follow-up of 48 patients using a modified Hospital for Special Surgery knee rating system, 38 percent of the patients had no limitation of function and only two knees had a good result. One-half the knees had significant radiologic changes and more than one-third had saphenous nerve damage.

Recent reports suggest that long-standing pessimism concerning intra-articular reconstructions of the cruciate ligaments must be reevaluated.[2,7] Late failure is probably a consequence of inadequate technique and the failure of an intra-articular graft to revascularize; in particular, it seems unlikely that any action of the synovial fluid is a cause of graft absorption. Arnoczky et al.[6,7] have shown that vascularization of a patellar tendon graft occurs with vessels derived from the infrapatellar fat pad.[76] Our own observations with intra-articular grafts fashioned from the distal portion of the iliotibial band confirm that grafted material can remain intact within the synovial cavity for long periods.[43] With some techniques (distal iliotibial band or semitendinosus tendon), the graft may retain at least partial vascularity. Arthrotomy performed 2 years after an anterior cruciate graft with distal iliotibial band has shown no loss of substance in the graft, which was covered with synovium in which prominent vessels were visible (Fig. 13.40).

A similar appearance was found in six other cases with a shorter follow-up time of 1 to 2 years (the arthrotomy was done for the purpose of removing a fixation screw). With other methods, such as the patellar tendon graft, presumably a creeping substitution process occurs, as has been demonstrated in experimental animal studies.[7] For optimal results prolonged postoperative protection is desirable. Noyes et al.[71] claim that maximal ligament healing takes between 6 and 12 months and occurs most predictably

THE HOSPITAL FOR SPECIAL SURGERY SPORTS MEDICINE SERVICE
KNEE INJURIES DISCHARGE SUMMARY FOLLOW-UP SCORE SHEET

.NAME	TEL: HOME ( ) -	WORK: ( ) -
CHART NO.: HSS# PVT# AGE: SEX:		
DATE OF INJURY:	DATE OF SURGERY:	
DIAGNOSIS:		
TREATMENT: NON-OP:		
SURGICAL FINDINGS:		
SURGICAL PROCEDURES:		

INSTRUCTIONS: NORMAL PERSON HAS HIGHEST SCORE. AWARD POINTS WHEN NO PATHOLOGY.									
DATE OF EXAMINATION:									
TIME: POST INJURY/POST SURGERY:									

A. PATIENT'S OWN EVALUATION.
  N= NORMAL   I= IMPROVED
  S= SEVERE W= WORSE									

B. PAIN: 0= YES, 1= NO
  SWELLING: 0,1
  STAIRS DIFFICULTY: 0,1
  CLICKING-NUMBNESS: 0,1
  GIVING WAY: 0–4
    4= NORMAL, NONE
    2= WITH STRESS ONLY
    1= WITH STRESS UPON
       DAILY ACTIVITY
    0= REGULARLY UPON
       DAILY ACTIVITY									

RETURN TO SPORTS OR WORK: 0–3
    3= FULL RETURN
    2= RETURN TO ORIG. WITH
       LIMITATIONS
    1= RETURN TO DIFFERENT
    0= NO RETURN									

C. (1)FUNCTIONAL TESTS
    DUCK WALK:*   0,1,2
    RUN IN PLACE: 0,1
    JUMP ON ONE LEG:* 0,1,2
    HALF SQUAT: 0,1
    FULL SQUAT: 0,1									

```
* FOR C1   0 = CAN NOT PERFORM
           1 = CAN PERFORM BUT WITH DISCOMFORT
           2 = CAN PERFORM
```

Fig. 13.39. Numerical grading of knee function after knee surgery. Hospital for Special Surgery sample form. (From Marshall, J.L., Fetto, J.F., and Botero, P.M.: Knee ligament injuries. A standardized evaluation method. Clin. Orthop., *123*: 115, 1977, with permission.)

(2) SPECIFIC KNEE EXAM

TENDERNESS	0,1									
JOINT EFFUSION	0,1									
SWELLING (SOFT TISSUE)	0,1									
CREPITATION	0,1									
MUSCLE POWER	0–3									
3= NORMAL 2= DIMINISHED FLEX. OR EXT. 1= DIMINISHED FLEX. & EXT. 0= VERY WEAK										
THIGH SIZES 0–2 2= EQUAL 1= 1–2CM DIFFERENCE 0= >2CM DIFFERENCE										
RANGE OF MOTION 0–3 3= NORMAL DEGREES 2= LIMITED FLEX. OR EXT. 1= LIMITED FLEX. & EXT. 0= >90°										
STABILITY: INCLUDE FOR EACH EXAM: A= HARD END POINT B= SOFT END POINT LCL 0–5 (A/B) 5= NORMAL 4= MILD INST. IN FLEXION 3= MODERATE INST. IN FLEX. 2= INST. IN FLEX. & EXT. 0= GROSS INSTABILITY										
MCL 0–5 (A/B) 5= NORMAL 4= MILD INST. IN FLEX. 3= MODERATE INST. IN FLEX. 2= INST. IN FLEX. & EXT. 0= GROSS INSTABILITY										
ACL 0–5 (A/B) 5= NORMAL (= OPP. LEG) 4= SLIGHT JOG 3= MODERATE JOG 2= SEVERE IN NEUTRAL 0= SEVERE IN NEU. & ROT. PIVOT SHIFT: NEG., 1+, 2+, 3+ LACHMAN: EXCURSION (NL/ ↑) END POINT (A/B)										
PCL 0–5 (A/B) 5= NORMAL (= OPP. LEG) 4= SLIGHT JOG 3= MODERATE JOG 2= SEVERE IN NEUTRAL 0= POSTEROLATERAL DROPBACK										

D.   TOTAL SCORE: MAX. 50 PTS.

E.   PHYSICIAN'S INITIALS

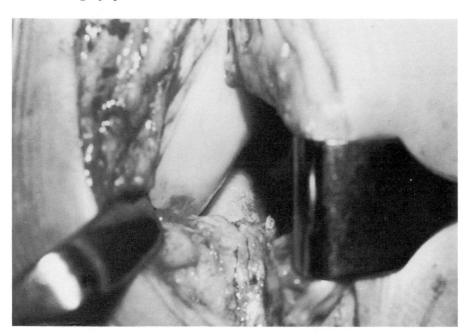

Fig. 13.40. The viability of an anterior cruciate ligament graft (see text). (From Insall, J., Joseph, D.M., Aglietti, P., et al.: Bone-block iliotibial-band transfer for anterior cruciate insufficiency. J. Bone Joint Surg. [Am.], *63:* 560, 1981, with permission.)

when the ligaments are subject to mild functional stresses insufficient to cause damage. Cast bracing, which permits a limited range of motion but protects against reinjury, thus seems better than prolonged immobilization in a rigid cast.

Quadriceps tendon substitution by the Jones[47] technique or a modification thereof is probably the most widely performed intra-articular reconstruction. Jones[48] reported that after an average follow-up of 110 weeks on 46 patients who were recreational athletes, 27 had slight restrictions. Three had a slight loss of terminal extension and 13 had lost more than 20 degrees of flexion. The anterior drawer sign was positive postoperatively in 29 of the 46 patients. Marshall et al.[66] recently reported on 40 patients treated by a modification of the Jones technique, 15 of whom were followed for more than 2 years. All 40 had a positive anterior drawer test when last seen, but this laxity was judged to be severe in only four cases. Twenty-two of the 40 patients had a positive pivot shift test postoperatively. Not all the patients had had the pivot shift tested preoperatively, but in one-half of those who did, the sign was negative at the time of their last follow-up examination. Those with a persistent pivot shift did not score lower or complain of giving way. The Lachman test was the only clinical stability test that correlated with the end result score. Those

with an anterior excursion with the knee near extension averaged 38.6 points (out of a possible 50 points), while those with a negative Lachman test averaged 45 points. All but one patient were able to return to some sports involvement postoperatively, and 18 were able to describe their return to sports as essentially complete.

At The Hospital for Special Surgery, the results of the bone block iliotibial band transfer have been recently evaluated. Twenty-four patients had a follow-up of more than 2 years; 13 were rated excellent, eight good, and three fair. The 13 patients with excellent results stated that the knee felt completely stable for any activity they wished to undertake. None was using a brace. The pivot shift was negative in all cases, the Lachman negative in eight and 1+ in five, and the anterior drawer 2+ in one patient and negative or 1+ in the remainder.

The eight patients with good results had no complaints of instability, and six engaged in strenuous sports without a brace. Five patients were placed in this category because of occasional complaints of pain, one because of occasional effusions, one because of limitation of flexion, and one because of a positive pivot shift. The static stability testing showed the Lachman sign was negative in three and 1+ in five, the anterior drawer was 1+ in four and 2+ in four, and the pivot shift was positive in two and negative in six. Three cases with fair results were so rated because of recurrent instability in two, and progressive osteoarthritis in one. In all three cases, the clinical instability was less than before operation, and the patients considered the operation a success.

There is virtually no information on the results of lateral reconstruction and very little on posterior cruciate reconstruction. In a small personal series of eight posterior cruciate reconstructions[42] using the medial head of gastrocnemius with a bone block, the three patients with excellent results had normal stability on the posterior drawer test, had no complaints whatsoever, and were fully active in sports. The three patients with good results had 1+ or 2+ posterior laxity, but no subjective complaints of instability. All were fully active but complained of intermittent swelling and pain after activity. One of the patients rated as fair was put in this category because of a reinjury 9 months after the initial operation; she later underwent a medial and anterior cruciate reconstruction. The other fair result was a consequence of severe pain caused by patellofemoral arthritis that was not relieved by patellectomy. It takes a severe injury to damage the posterior cruciate ligament, and these knees seem more susceptible to early osteoarthritis than after any other ligamentous injury. The patellofemoral joint works at a mechanical disadvantage when the tibia is displaced backward and seems particularly likely to undergo degeneration. Residual pain from osteoarthritis was a major reason for results that were less satisfactory after posterior cruciate reconstruction.

Recent clinical evidence suggests that combined intra- and extra-articular reconstruction may give better results than either alone. Clancy et al.[14] have used a patellar tendon graft augmented by medial and lateral extra-articular tendon transfers (pes anserinus and biceps tendon, respectively). They report that 48 of 50 patients had a satisfactory result after a follow-up ranging from 2 to 5 years. This is a higher rate of success than reported using any other method and if these remarkable results can be maintained and duplicated by others, the combined procedures may prove the best solution for anterior cruciate insufficiency. However, these workers do caution that their patients were not in the main highly competitive athletes, and the procedure has not yet been tested under the most stressful circumstances.

COMPLICATIONS OF LIGAMENT RECONSTRUCTION

INFECTION

Deep infection should not be masked by the prolonged use of postoperative antibiotics. Two days of intravenous therapy is certainly adequate prophylaxis, and oral antibiotics should not be given beyond this time. Prolonged temperature elevation sometimes lasting 7 to 10 days is not unusual, presumably caused by the absorption of hematoma. More suspect is a progressive temperature elevation occurring a few days after surgery, especially when the fever swings up and down and the patient looks toxic. Aspiration of the joint should give the diagnosis, provided antibiotics are not being given; intra-articular sepsis, once confirmed, should be treated by immediate debridement followed by primary closure over suction drainage. The drain may be removed after 36 hours, and the patient is treated with a suitable antibiotic given intravenously for 3 to 6 weeks. Consultation with an infectious disease specialist is strongly recommended to monitor the antibiotic therapy. Fortunately, deep sepsis is rare, but provided that the complication is recognized and treated aggressively, the reconstruction and the knee joint can be preserved. Procrastination, inadequate drainage, and inappropriate antibiotic therapy can lead to at best disruption of the reconstruction and at worst fibrous ankylosis or severe postseptic arthritis. Drainage by aspiration and oral antibiotic therapy are seldom advisable.

HEMATOMA

Postoperative hematoma formation can be minimized by release of the tourniquet before wound closure in order to control major bleeding. Reinflation and subsequent irrigation avoid the problem of prolonged oozing during the time it takes to close the wound. In spite of this precaution, considerable loss of blood can occur into the surgical area postoperatively, sometimes accompanied by an alarming drop in the hematocrit. These patients often run a high fever but appear to be relatively well. The drop in hematocrit is particularly disturbing to those surgeons who do ligament reconstructions infrequently. However, the blood loss does not indicate major arterial injury unless there are additional signs that indicate otherwise. On inspection the wound usually appears relatively benign, although the leg is of course swollen. Treatment consists of replacing the blood loss and observation. Aspiration is usually ineffective and is done mostly for the purpose of eliminating the possibility of infection. Surgical removal of the hematoma is not often necessary. Apart from slightly prolonging convalescence, the end result is not adversely affected.

SKIN NECROSIS

Most ligament reconstructions require extensive exposure, particularly when combined procedures are done; often there are previous incisions on the knee that in themselves predispose to skin necrosis. Surgeons should remember that subsequent procedures may be required after their own and should plan their skin incisions accordingly. Curly or S-shaped incisions are those most likely to cause future difficulty. Most knee surgery can be done through a single straight anterior or slightly curved lateral parapatellar skin incision, and subsequent surgery can then be easily done through the same scar. "Railroad" incisions, in which the new incision parallels an old scar, are particularly hazardous, albeit sometimes unavoidable (Fig. 13.41). Skin necrosis, if it occurs, should be treated initially by immobilization and watchful neglect. Debridement instituted too early can lead to disastrous widening of the area of necrosis and to infection of the underlying tissues. All but the most severe cases of necrosis heal given time and do not prejudice the ligament reconstruction. Skin necrosis is probably the most common major complication of this type of surgery and, given the nature of the techniques described, is to some degree unavoidable. Proper placement of skin incisions minimizes the frequency and extent of necrosis. The potential for this complication must feature in the planning of the ligament reconstruction and is an argument against routine combined intra- and extra-articular reconstruction.

KNEE STIFFNESS

Extensive intra- and extra-articular soft tissue surgery followed by prolonged immobilization would seem a recipe for adhesions and loss of motion. In fact it is remarkable that prolonged or permanent knee stiffness does not occur more often. Slow recovery of full extension is the rule, particularly when the knee has been immobilized in flexion. However, recovery does

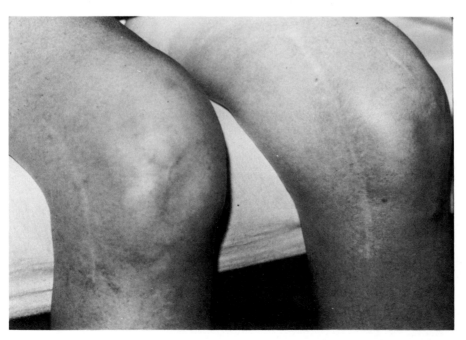

Fig. 13.41. The placement of these scars is unfortunate, as often a second parallel scar is required for subsequent surgery, bringing with it the risk of skin necrosis.

occur aided by quadriceps rehabilitation and, if necessary, by hamstring stretching exercises. The loss of terminal flexion (sometimes as much as 20 degrees) may be permanent, but this loss is of trivial importance and does not trouble the patient.

Occasionally motion is not regained to normal extent; sometimes in these cases an element of sympathetic dystrophy may exist. The tissues themselves develop a wooden texture, and muscle atrophy is often marked. The bones may appear osteoporotic on radiographic examination.

When flexion does not return after several months of therapy, a manipulation under anesthesia may be required. In addition to general anesthesia, a muscle relaxant should be given and adhesions overcome by firm, steady pressure on the tibia. Careful manipulation by an experienced surgeon is a safe enough procedure, and the risk of doing damage is minimal. The keys to success are (1) adequate relaxation, and (2) constant pressure until adhesions give way. Sudden jerky movements should be avoided.

When there is a suspicion of sympathetic dystrophy, manipulation may still be needed and, in fact, may need to be repeated several times, motion being regained in small increments rather than all at once. Other measures for sympathetic dystrophy may also be required, such as systemic cortisone therapy, sympathetic block, as well as prolonged and persistent physical therapy.

Manipulation of the knee for extension loss is less rewarding than for the more usual failure to regain flexion. Fortunately flexion contractures are rarely permanent and tend to correct themselves with therapy.

EFFUSION

Prolonged swelling beyond the early postoperative period may be attributable to several causes:

1. Low-grade infection: Although repeated aspiration of the knee is not recommended, diagnostic aspiration in these circumstances should be done to exclude infection.
2. Muscle atrophy and weakness: Failure to rehabilitate the musculature makes the knee susceptible to repeated minor injury, especially when the patient attempts such activities as running before the knee is ready for it. The treatment is to reduce

activity and intensify muscle exercises. However, sometimes the exercises themselves may be partly responsible, such as weight-lifting from the flexed position when there is patellar chondromalacia.
3. Degenerative changes as a result of long-standing chronic instability: Severe arthrosis is a contraindication to ligament reconstruction, but many borderline cases exist in which restoration of stability seems worthwhile in spite of preexisting articular damage. Arthrosis may contribute to postoperative effusions, even after a successful reconstruction, and may limit the patient's recovery. Palliative treatment consists of modifying activity, using a flexible knee support, and undergoing intensive muscular rehabilitation.

TENDINITIS

Persistent soreness and tenderness in the soft tissues may occur either at the site of an extra-articular reconstruction, or at the donor site of the graft. Patellar tendinitis after the removal of the graft for a quadriceps tendon substitution is one example and tenderness over a staple is another. When the tenderness is clearly related to a fixation device removal is indicated, but often the cause is not self-evident and must be treated with restraint and reassurance. In most cases the local soreness and tenderness gradually subside.

MUSCLE HERNIA

Muscle hernia may occur as a result of the removal of a fascial graft from the lateral side. Although the resulting bulge is seldom of more than cosmetic significance, the possibility of a troublesome muscle hernia is a disadvantage to techniques that use the proximal fascia lata as the source of graft material. In contrast, the distal part of the fascia lata and the iliotibial band may be used without fear because even large defects in the lateral retinacular structures of the knee do not cause trouble of any kind. Closure of the lateral retinaculum has been recommended, but in my opinion is quite undesirable, because even when possible it will result in lateral hyperpressure of the patellofemoral joint.

REFERENCES

1. Abbott, L.C., Saunders, J.B., Bost, F.C., et al.: Injuries to the ligaments of the knee joint. J. Bone Joint Surg., *26*: 503, 1944.
2. Alm, A.: Survival of part of patella tendon transposed for reconstruction of anterior cruciate ligament. Acta Chir. Scand., *139*: 443, 1973.
3. Alm, A., and Gillquist, J.: Reconstruction of the anterior cruciate ligament by using the medial third of the patellar ligament. Acta Chir. Scand., *140*: 289, 1974.
4. Alm, A., Liljedahl, S., and Stromberg, B.: Clinical and experimental experience in reconstruction of the anterior cruciate ligament. Orthop. Clin. North Am., *7(1)*: 181, 1976.
5. Apley, A.G.: Instability of the knee resulting from ligamentous injury. A plea for plain words. J. Bone Joint Surg. [Br.], *62*: 515, 1980.
6. Arnoczky, S.P., Rubin, R.M., and Marshall, J.L.: Microvasculature of the cruciate ligaments and its response to injury. An experimental study in dogs. J. Bone Joint Surg. [Am.], *61*: 1221, 1979.
7. Arnoczky, S.P., Tarvin, G.B., and Marshall, J.L.: Anterior cruciate ligament replacement using patellar tendon. An evaluation of graft revascularization in the dog. J. Bone Joint Surg [Am.], *64*: 217, 1982.
8. Barfod, B.: Posterior cruciate ligament—Reconstruction by transposition of the popliteus tendon. In proceedings Acta Orthop. Scand., *42*: 438, 1971.
9. Bartel, D.L., Marshall, J.L., Schieck, R.A., et al.: Surgical repositioning of the medial collateral ligament. An anatomical and mechanical analysis. J. Bone Joint Surg. [Am.], *59*: 107, 1977.
10. Bosworth, D.M.: Transplantation of the semitendinosus for repair of laceration of medial collateral ligament of the knee. J. Bone Joint Surg. [Am.], *34*: 196, 1952.
11. Brantigan, O.C., and Voshell, A.F.: The mechanics of the ligaments and menisci of the knee joint. J. Bone Joint Surg., *23*: 44, 1941.
12. Butler, D.L., Noyes, F.R., and Grood, E.S.: Ligamentous restraints to anterior–posterior drawer in the human knee. J. Bone Joint Surg. [Am.], *62*: 259, 1980.
13. Clancy, W.: Posterior cruciate ligament reconstruction. Preliminary report of a new technique. Orthop. Trans., *5*: 487, 1981.
14. Clancy, W.G., Jr., Nelson, D.A., Reider, B., et al.: Anterior cruciate ligament reconstruction using one-third of the patellar ligament, augmented by extra-articular tendon transfers. J. Bone Joint Surg. [Am.], *64*: 352, 1982.
15. Clendenin, M.B., DeLee, J.C., and Heckman, J.D.: Interstitial tears of the posterior cruciate ligament of the knee. Orthopedics, *3*: 764, 1980.
16. Cho, K.O.: Reconstruction of the anterior cruciate ligament by semitendinosus tenodesis. J. Bone Joint Surg. [Am.], *57*: 608, 1975.
17. Committee on the Medical Aspects of Sports: Standard Nomenclature of Athletic Injuries. pp. 99, 101. Chicago, American Medical Association, 1968.
18. Daniel, D., Malcom, L., Stone, M.L., et al.: Quantification of knee stability and function. Contemp. Orthop., *5(1)*: 83, 1982.
19. DeLorme, T.L.: Restoration of muscle power by heavy-resistance exercises. J. Bone Joint Surg., *27*: 645, 1945.
20. DuToit, G.T.: Knee joint cruciate ligament substitution, the Lindemann (Heidelberg) operation. South Afr. J. Surg., *5(1)*: 25, 1967.
21. Edmonson, A.S., and Crenshaw, A.H.: Campbell's Operative Orthopaedics, 6th Ed., pp. 42–44. St. Louis, C.V. Mosby, 1980.
22. Ellison, A.E., Wieneke, K., Benton, L.J., et al.: Preliminary report. Results of extra-articular anterior cruciate replacement. J. Bone Joint Surg. [Am.], *58*: 736, 1976.
23. Ellison, A.E.: Distal iliotibial-band transfer for anterolateral rotatory instability of the knee. J. Bone Joint Surg. [Am.], *61*: 330, 1979.
24. Ellsasser, J.C., Reynolds, F.C., and Omohundro, J.R.: The nonoperative treatment of collateral ligament injuries of the knee in professional football players. J. Bone Joint Surg. [Am.], *56*: 1185, 1974.
25. Eriksson, E.: Reconstruction of the anterior cruciate ligament. Orthop. Clin. North Am., *7(1)*: 167, 1976.
26. Feagin, J.A., Abbott, H.G., and Rokous, J.R.: The isolated tear of the anterior cruciate ligament. J. Bone Joint Surg. [Am.], *54*: 1340, 1972.
27. Fetto, J.F., and Marshall, J.L.: Injury to the anterior cruciate ligament producing the pivot-shift sign. An experimental study on cadaver specimens. J. Bone Joint Surg. [Am.], *61*: 710, 1979.
28. Fetto, J.F., and Marshall, J.L.: The natural history and diagnosis of anterior cruciate ligament insufficiency. Clin. Orthop., *147*: 29, 1980.
29. Freeman, B.L., Beaty, J.H., and Haynes, D.B.: The pes anserinus transfer. A long-term follow-up. J. Bone Joint Surg. [Am.], *64*: 202, 1982.
29a. Freeman, M.A.R., Dean, M.R.E., and Hanham, I.W.F.: The etiology and prevention of functional instability of the foot. J. Bone Joint Surg. [Br.], *47*: 678, 1965.
30. Furman, W., Marshall, J.L., and Girgis, F.G.: The anterior cruciate ligament. A functional analysis based on postmortem studies. J. Bone Joint Surg. [Am.], *58*: 179, 1976.
31. Galway, R.D.: The pivot shift syndrome. Proceedings of the New Zealand Orthopaedic Association. J. Bone Joint Surg. [Br.], *54*: 558, 1972.
32. Galway, R.D., Beaupré, A., and MacIntosh, D.L.: Pivot

shift: a clinical sign of symptomatic anterior cruciate insufficiency. Proceedings of the Canadian Orthopaedic Association. J. Bone Joint Surg. [Br.], *54:* 763, 1972.

33. Girgis, F.G., Marshall, J.L., and Al Monajem, A.R.S.: The cruciate ligaments of the knee joint. Anatomical, functional, and experimental analysis. Clin. Orthop., *106:* 216, 1975.

34. Hallen, L.G., and Lindahl, O.: Rotation in the knee joint in experimental injury to the ligaments. Acta Orthop. Scand., *36:* 400, 1965.

35. Hallen, L.G., and Lindahl, O.: The lateral stability of the knee joint. Acta Orthop. Scand., *36:* 179, 1965.

36. Hey Groves, E.W.: Operation for the repair of the crucial ligaments. Lancet, 2: 674, 1917.

37. Hey Groves, E.W.: The crucial ligaments of the knee joint. Their function, rupture, and the operative treatment of the same. Br. J. Surg., 7: 505, 1920.

38. Hughston, J.C.: The posterior cruciate ligament in knee joint stability. In proceedings J. Bone Joint Surg. [Am.], *51:* 1045, 1969.

39. Hughston, J.C., and Degenhardt, T.C.: Reconstruction of the post cruciate ligament. Clin. Orthop., *164:* 59, 1982.

40. Hughston, J.C., and Eilers, A.F.: The role of the posterior oblique ligament in repairs of acute medial (collateral) ligament tears of the knee. J. Bone Joint Surg. [Am.], *55:* 923, 1973.

41. Hughston, J.C., Andrews, J.R., Cross, M.J., et al.: Classification of knee ligament instabilities. Part I and II. J. Bone Joint Surg. [Am.], *58:* 159, 1976.

42. Insall, J.N., and Hood, R.W.: Bone-block transfer of the medial head of the gastrocnemius for posterior cruciate insufficiency. J. Bone Joint Surg. [Am.], *64:* 691, 1982.

43. Insall, J., Joseph, D.M., Aglietti, P., et al.: Bone-block iliotibial-band transfer for anterior cruciate insufficiency. J. Bone Joint Surg. [Am.], *63:* 560, 1981.

44. Ireland, J., and Trickey, E.L.: MacIntosh tenodesis for anterolateral instability of the knee. J. Bone Joint Surg. [Br.], *62:* 340, 1980.

45. Jacobsen, K.: Stress radiographical measurement of the anteroposterior, medial and lateral stability of the knee joint. Acta. Orthop. Scand., *47:* 335, 1976.

46. Jakob, R., and Staübli, H.U.: The reversed pivot shift sign—a new diagnostic aid for posterolateral rotatory instability of the knee. Its distinction from the true pivot-shift sign. Orthop. Trans., 5: 487, 1981.

47. Jones, K.G.: Reconstruction of the anterior cruciate ligament. A technique using the central one-third of the patellar ligament. J. Bone Joint Surg. [Am.], *45:* 925, 1963.

48. Jones, K.G.: Reconstruction of the anterior cruciate ligament using the central one-third of the patellar liga-

ment. A follow-up report. J. Bone Joint Surg. [Am.], *52:* 1302, 1970.

49. Kaplan, E.B.: The iliotibial tract. Clinical and morphological significance. J. Bone Joint Surg. [Am.], *40:* 817, 1958.

50. Kaplan, E.B.: The fabellofibular and short lateral ligaments of the knee joint. J. Bone Joint Surg. [Am.], *43:* 169, 1961.

51. Kennedy, J.C., and Fowler, P.J.: Medial and anterior instability of the knee. An anatomical and clinical study using stress machines. J. Bone Joint Surg. [Am.], *53:* 1257, 1971.

52. Kennedy, J.C., and Grainger, R.W.: The posterior cruciate ligament. J. Trauma, 7: 367, 1967.

53. Kennedy, J.C., and Swan, W.J.: Lateral instability of the knee following lateral compartment injury. J. Bone Joint Surg [Br.], *54:* 763, 1972.

54. Kennedy, J.C., Hawkins, R.J., Willis, R.B., et al.: Tension studies of human knee ligaments. Yield point, ultimate failure, and disruption of the cruciate and tibial collateral ligaments. J. Bone Joint Surg. [Am.], *58:* 350, 1976.

55. Kennedy, J.C., Stewart, R., and Walker, D.M.: Anterolateral rotatory instability of the knee joint. An early analysis of the Ellison procedure. J. Bone Joint Surg. [Am.], *60:* 1031, 1978.

56. Larson, R.L.: Part 2. Dislocations and ligamentous injuries of the knee. In Rockwood, Jr., C.A., and Green, D.P., eds.: Fractures, vol. 2, pp. 1182. Philadelphia, J.B. Lippincott, 1975.

57. Larson, R.L.: Combined instabilities of the knee. Clin. Orthop., *147:* 68, 1980.

58. Lindemann, K.: Über den plastichen Ersatz der Kreuzbänder durch gestiette Schnenverpflanzung, Ztschr. Orthop., *79:* 316, 1950.

59. Losee, R.E., Johnson, T.R., and Southwick, W.O.: Anterior subluxation of the lateral tibial plateau. A diagnostic test and operative repair. J. Bone Joint Surg. [Am.], *60:* 1015, 1978.

60. Lysholm, J., and Gillquist, J.: Arthroscopic examination of the posterior cruciate ligament. J. Bone Joint Surg. [Am.], *63:* 363, 1981.

61. MacIntosh, D.L.: The anterior cruciate ligament. Over-the-top repair. Annual Meeting of The American Academy of Orthopaedic Surgeons, Dallas, Texas, January 1974.

62. Markolf, K.L., Mensch, J.S., and Amstutz, H.C.: Stiffness and laxity of the knee. The contributions of the supporting structures. J. Bone Joint Surg. [Am.], *58:* 583, 1976.

63. Marshall, J.L., and Baugher, W.H.: Stability examination of the knee: A simple anatomic approach. Clin. Orthop., *146:* 78, 1980.

64. Marshall, J.L., and Rubin, R.M.: Knee ligament in-

juries—A diagnostic and therapeutic approach. Orthop. Clin. North Am., 8(3): 641, 1977.

65. Marshall, J.L., Fetto, J.F., and Botero, P.M.: Knee ligament injuries. A standardized evaluation method. Clin. Orthop., 123: 115, 1977.

66. Marshall, J.L., Warren, R.F., Wickiewicz, T.L., et al.: Reconstruction of functioning anterior cruciate ligament. Preliminary report using quadriceps tendon. Orthop. Rev. 8(6): 49, 1979.

67. Marshall, J.L., Warren, R.F., Wickiewicz, T.L., et al.: The anterior cruciate ligament: A technique of repair and reconstruction. Clin. Orthop., 143: 97, 1979.

68. Mauck, H.P.: A new operative procedure for instability of the knee. J. Bone Joint Surg., 18: 984, 1936.

69. McDaniel, W.J., Jr., and Dameron, T.B., Jr.: Untreated ruptures of the anterior cruciate ligament. A follow-up study. J. Bone Joint Surg [Am.], 62: 696, 1980.

70. Nicholas, J.A.: The five-one reconstruction for anteromedial instability of the knee. Indications, technique, and the results in fifty-two patients. J. Bone Joint Surg. [Am.], 55: 899, 1973.

71. Noyes, F.R.: Functional properties of knee ligaments and alterations induced by immobilization. Clin. Orthop., 123: 210, 1977.

72. Noyes, F.R., and Sonstegard, D.A.: Biomechanical function of the pes anserinus at the knee and the effect of its transplantation. J. Bone Joint Surg. [Am.], 55: 1225, 1973.

73. O'Donoghue, D.H.: Reconstruction for medial instability of the knee. J. Bone Joint Surg. [Am.], 55: 941, 1973.

74. Palmer, I.: On injuries to the ligaments of the knee joint. Acta Chir. Scand. (Suppl.): 53, 1938.

75. Pickett, J.C., and Altizer, T.J.: Injuries of the ligaments of the knee. A study of types of injury and treatment in 129 patients. Clin. Orthop., 76: 27, 1971.

76. Rubin, R.M., and Marshall, J.L.: Vascular anatomy of the cruciate ligaments in the dog. Normal and injured states. Trans. Orthop. Res. Soc., 1: 148, 1976.

77. Slocum, D.B., and Larson, R.L.: Rotatory instability of the knee. Its pathogenesis and a clinical test to demonstrate its presence. J. Bone Joint Surg. [Am.], 50: 211, 1968.

78. Slocum, D.B., and Larson, R.L.: Pes anserinus transplantation. A surgical procedure for control of rotatory instability of the knee. J. Bone Joint Surg [Am.], 50: 226, 1968.

79. Slocum, D.B., Larson, R.L., and James, S.L.: Late reconstruction procedures used to stabilize the knee. Orthop. Clin. North Am., 4(3): 679, 1973.

80. Slocum, D.B., Larson, R.L., and James, S.L.: Pes anserinus transplant: Impressions after a decade of experience. J. Sports Med., 2: 123, 1974.

81. Slocum, D.B., Larson, R.L., and James, S.L.: Late reconstruction of ligamentous injuries of the medial compartment of the knee. Clin. Orthop., 100: 23, 1974.

82. Slocum, D.B., James, S.L., Larson, R.L., et al.: Clinical test for anterolateral rotary instability of the knee. Clin. Orthop., 118: 63, 1976.

83. Torg, J.S., Conrad, W., and Kalen, V.: Clinical diagnosis of anterior cruciate ligament instability in the athlete. Am. J. Sports Med., 4: 84, 1976.

84. Torzilli, P.A., Greenberg, R.L., and Insall, J.: An in vivo biomechanical evaluation of anterior-posterior motion of the knee. Roentgenographic measurement technique, stress machine, and stable population. J. Bone Joint Surg. [Am.], 63: 960, 1981.

85. Trillat, A.: Posterolateral instability. In Schultz, K.P., Krahl, H., and Stein, W.H., eds.: Late Reconstructions of Injured Ligaments of the Knee, pp. 99–105. New York, Springer, 1979.

86. Vigliani, F., Martinelli, B., and Tagliapietra, E.A.: The early surgical treatment of rupture of the tibial collateral ligament of the knee. Italian J. Orthop. Traumat., 1: 151, 1975.

87. Wang, J.B., and Marshall, J.L.: The popliteus tendon as a static lateral stabilizer of the knee. Trans. Orthop. Res. Soc., 2: 172, 1977.

88. Warren, R.F., and Marshall, J.L.: Injuries of the anterior cruciate and medial collateral ligaments of the knee. Clin. Orthop., 136: 191, 1978.

89. Warren, L.F., Marshall, J.L., and Girgis, F.: The prime static stabilizer of the medial side of the knee. J. Bone Joint Surg. [Am.], 56: 665, 1974.

90. Woods, G.W., Homsy, C.A., Prewitt, J.M., III, et al.: Proplast leader for use in cruciate ligament reconstruction. Am. J. Sports Med., 7: 314, 1979.

91. Zarins, B., and Rowe, C.R.: Anterior cruciate ligament reconstruction: Combined method using semitendinosus tendon and illiotibial tract. Orthop. Trans., 4(3): 291, 1980.

14 Ligamentous Surgery of the Knee

Henri Dejour
Pierre Chambat
and
Paolo Aglietti

The problems of reconstruction of ligamentous lesions of the knee must be considered differently, depending on the age of the lesion—whether recent or old.

In the case of a recent lesion, the diagnostic and therapeutic features depend on anatomic physiologic alterations. Such alterations can be tested immediately, by thorough clinical examination and paraclinical tests, allowing a precise evaluation of both the type of ligamentous rupture, as well as the potential evolution of the lesion. The information obtained allows us to decide whether conservative or operative treatment is more suitable for the return of normal knee function.

In the case of an old lesion, the picture is more or less complicated by disorganized healing, initial tissue necrosis, and retraction, and completed by secondary degenerative changes with ligamentous stretching and meniscal tears. This process often demands that we abandon the anatomic ideal and limit ourselves to a less satisfactory reconstructive surgery, with less predictable results. It is often difficult to satisfactorily correlate instability (an essentially functional phenomenon) and ligamentous laxity, (an objective clinical finding).

STABILITY OF THE KNEE

In order for the stability of the knee to be perfect for the most variable demands, the whole capsuloligamentous unit must be preserved. The rupture of one of the ligaments will therefore have different functional and anatomic consequences according to the physiologic role of each of the ligaments and its healing potential, spontaneously or after surgery. It is important to separate (1) the two cruciate ligaments, considered together, and which we call "central pivot," and (2) the capsuloligamentous systems at the periphery on the medial and on the lateral sides.

The central pivot is able to give perfect stability by itself when the knee is in internal or neutral rotation. When there is external rotation the central pivot cannot prevent some opening of the articular surfaces.

The medial capsuloligamentous system controls the valgus stresses, protecting the central pivot as well, and above all external rotation, when the knee is in flexion. Its specific and irreplaceable role is completed by the posteromedial corner, which is actively controlled by the semimembranosus tendon expansions. The large posterior horn of the medial meniscus is the passive element of this posteromedial cor-

353

ner, with its attachments to the capsular layer. The posterior horn of the medial meniscus prevents anterior translation of the medial tibial plateau in external rotation.

The peripheral lateral capsuloligamentous system is more complex. It has two roles. It prevents on one hand varus laxity in extension, and on the other internal rotation in flexion, while protecting the central pivot. The anatomic elements that participate in this function are the fascia lata, the capsule anterior to the popliteus hiatus, and finally the lateral collateral ligament. The motor element is the biceps femoris muscle. The ligamentous formation anterior to the lateral collateral ligament is called the preligamentous system.

The specific and irreplaceable function of the lateral capsular ligamentous system is also to limit external rotation in extension. This function is particularly important at the moment of single-leg weight-bearing. A lesion of the posterolateral corner including the retroligamentous formations situated posterior to the lateral collateral ligament (popliteus tendon and muscle, capsule and arcuate ligament) would allow a varus–recurvatum–external rotation of the tibia with posterolateral subluxation of the lateral tibial plateau, which would considerably worsen the varus laxity in single-leg weight-bearing, particularly if there is a constitutional varus of the knee. If the lesion includes the lateral collateral ligament and the pre- and retroligamentous structures, the knee becomes varus in single-leg weight-bearing. The natural and physiologic mobility of the lateral femorotibial compartment gives this system a relative degree of constitutional laxity both in varus and in external rotation–recurvatum. Constitutional hyperlaxity, when it exists, increases the functional importance of these lesions.

The healing potential of the cruciate ligaments is poor. The intra-articular situation, with poor vascularity, makes spontaneous healing, even with cast immobilization, impossible. It is particularly true for the anterior cruciate ligament no matter what type of rupture. In every case this ligament either retracts or becomes necrotic. The posterior cruciate ligament, which is better vascularized and less intra-articular, at least partially avoids this unfavorable evolution, except when the rupture is located in the middle third, where healing, even incomplete, is unlikely. We can therefore say that every unrepaired lesion of the central pivot will leave some sequelae.

The vascular supply of the peripheral structures is good. Particularly if there is cast immobilization and avoidance of stresses during the phase of healing, there is practically complete healing of the lesion provided there was not a significant separation at the level of the rupture. The separation is a function of the articular opening at the time of the trauma; it varies in degree when there are no lesions of the central pivot or when only one cruciate ligament is ruptured. By contrast, the separation is very large in cases of dislocation of the knee or in ruptures of both cruciates.

DIAGNOSIS

HISTORY

The diagnostic approach, the preliminary stage of every therapeutic discussion, begins with the clinical history and identification of the mechanism of injury, the patient's subjective symptoms, and the immediate and long-term sequelae.

CLINICAL EXAMINATION

The clinical examination must be very precise with the goal of determining the type of acute or chronic ligamentous lesion involved, as well as the accompanying intra-articular degenerative changes that may already exist or that may appear later due to the evolution of the lesion.

This examination begins with the morphotype study of preexisting alignment and torsion, and identification of the points of ligamentous tenderness, meniscal tenderness, and patellar tenderness; however, only specific tests of the knee will allow us to progress in the assessment of laxity. These tests are not equally important; for the purposes of this discussion, we shall start off with those that permit evaluation of the elements of the central pivot as rupture of the anterior or posterior cruciates is the condition necessary and sufficient for their presence.

There are two specific tests for the anterior cruciate lesion and one specific test for the posterior cruciate lesions.

SPECIFIC TESTS FOR THE
ANTERIOR CRUCIATE LIGAMENT

Anterior Drawer in Extension (Fig. 14.1). The knee is slightly unlocked in slight flexion; only anterior subluxation of the tibia is tested relative to the femur, and not the full anterior–posterior mobility of the tibia, which can be also increased in cases of lesions of the posterior cruciate ligament or of the posterolateral corner. This differentiation might seem difficult, but we believe that sufficient experience permits differentiation of cases in which the anterior cruciate is absent (soft end point) from those in which the anterior cruciate is present (hard end point). This test is very important, particularly in cases of acute lesions, but it is sometimes difficult to show the translation, which is more a feeling of direct touch than a visual sensation. This test is almost impossible if the muscular masses are too large.

Dynamic Tests. Dynamic tests add a visual aspect to the anterior drawer in extension, making it easier for the examiner to appreciate. A number of these tests (e.g., pivot shift, Slocum, jerk test) have been described in the literature.

The "jerk in extension" is the test we prefer (Fig. 14.2). It consists of the knee unlocked near extension, with an anteroposterior and a valgus stress applied. It is the progressive flexion that causes, as with the other tests, a jerk. This demonstrates a rupture or insufficiency of the anterior cruciate ligament. The magnitude of the dynamic test and the degree of flexion where it occurs is variable depending on the association of peripheral lesions to the total or partial absence of the anterior cruciate ligament.

The greater the anterior laxity, the larger the anterior subluxation of the tibia; this causes a retarded jerk upon flexion, which occurs at 20 or sometimes 30 degrees of flexion, when the fascia lata becomes a flexor moving behind the instant center of rotation of the knee.

SPECIFIC TESTS FOR THE
POSTERIOR CRUCIATE LIGAMENT

The posterior direct drawer is always positive when the posterior cruciate ligament is ruptured. This posterior drawer may sometimes be difficult to test at 60 degrees of flexion in cases of recent ligamentous lesions because of hemarthrosis. One needs to know how to test it at 30 degrees of flexion, where it has

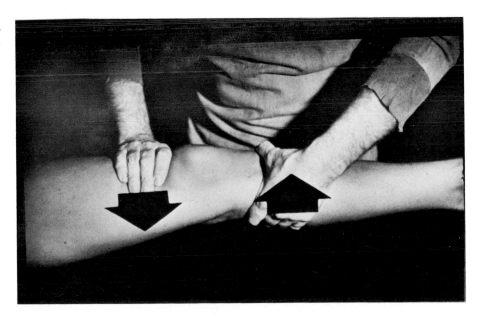

Fig. 14.1. Anterior drawer in extension (Trillat-Lachman test).

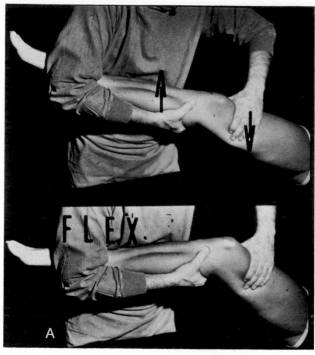

Fig. 14.2. (A) Extension jerk test. (B) Mechanism of the jerk test (see text).

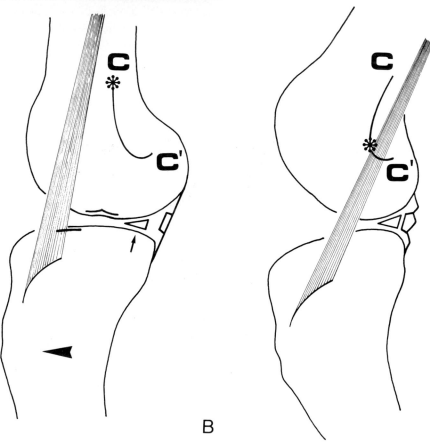

the same diagnostic significance. The sensitivity of this test is attributable to the fact that nothing but the quadriceps muscle can oppose the posterior drawer.

All the other clinical laxity tests are different in the sense that they evaluate the peripheral structures often injured with lesions of the central pivot.

VARUS OR VALGUS LAXITY

In extension or in the position of the physiologic screw-home mechanism and maximum stability of the knee, laxity of 10 or 15 degrees, without rotation, implies not only a peripheral lesion, but equally a lesion of the central pivot, which by itself normally prevents opening of the surfaces. This test is only positive in the recent acute ligament lesions, because peripheral healing usually would negate it in chronic laxity.

Valgus at 30 Degrees of Flexion. In valgus, when the foot is in external rotation, laxity indicates a rupture of the medial collateral ligament and of the posteromedial corner. This causes an anterior subluxation of the tibia associated with opening of the medial joint space, because of the unlocking caused by external rotation at the level of the central pivot. This test diminishes or becomes negative with the same peripheral lesions when the knee is in internal or neutral rotation if the cruciates are normal.

Varus at 30 Degrees of Flexion. Normally there is a certain laxity that is difficult to differentiate from a pathologic laxity if it is moderate. This permits testing the midthird of the external compartment (and the lateral collateral ligament) no matter what the rotation of the foot.

ANTERIOR AND POSTERIOR DRAWER SIGNS

The drawers must be tested in external rotation, neutral rotation, and internal rotation of 10 degrees, keeping in mind the tibial torsion, which determines the neutral position (compare with other side).

Anterior Drawer Signs

Drawer Sign in External Rotation. There is a 1+ laxity with an insufficiency of the collateral ligament and of the posteromedial corner. There is an in-creased external rotation with advancement of the medial tibial plateau greater than is found with a true anterior drawer. This is the case particularly in the acute laxities but can be encountered as well in chronic cases after medial meniscectomy, because the function of the posterior horn of the medial meniscus is lost. Obviously the anterior drawer in external rotation is greatly augmented if there is an associated lesion of the anterior cruciate ligament.

Direct Drawer Sign. It can only be positive if there is a rupture of the anterior cruciate ligament, plus an associated lesion of the posteromedial corner to allow anterior subluxation of the tibia; the lateral tibial plateau has enough physiological laxity to permit this movement. The extent of the anterior drawer is often variable during the same examination or from one examiner to the other; indeed it changes with force application on the tibia, because this force must overcome the restraint represented by the medial meniscus against the medial femoral condyle and the flexor muscles, which are often slightly contracted.

Anterior Drawer Sign in Internal Rotation of 10 Degrees. An insufficiency of the lateral ligamentous structures is shown in association with a lesion of the anterior cruciate ligament. Normally the anterolateral capsular structures are useful for the stability of the knee in internal rotation; they help the central pivot. In fact, it is an advancement of the lateral tibial plateau, in neutral position, more than an anterior drawer in internal rotation that shows the presence of this type of lesion.

Posterior Drawer Sign

External Rotation Posterior Drawer Sign. As a posterior movement of the lateral tibial plateau, this backward movement can be moderate; in this case, it is only a posterior subluxation of the lateral tibial plateau without a posterior drawer and without posterior movement of the tibia below the femur. This means an isolated insufficiency of the posterior lateral corner, which can be present to a moderate extent even if the posterior cruciate ligament is intact. Obviously posterior cruciate ligament rupture increases this external rotation posterior drawer, which then corresponds to a posterior translation of the entire proximal tibia associated with an increased posterior subluxation of the lateral compartment.

Posterior Drawer Test. The direct posterior drawer (see above) corresponds to a rupture of the posterior cruciate ligament. If there is an isolated rupture, the posterior drawer in external rotation is not increased over the direct posterior drawer. One has to consider all the possible small and subtle differences, as we will see in the classifications.

RECURVATUM

There are two recurvatums. The first corresponds to a direct recurvatum, without any rotation, a true hyperextension; this condition is possible only if there is a rupture of the posterior cruciate in association with a bilateral lesion of the posterior capsule.

The second recurvatum, the varus recurvatum external rotation, points to an insufficiency of the posterolateral corner, which can be associated with a cruciate rupture. The functional correspondence of this varus recurvatum external rotation found during physical examination is the "thrust" during single leg weight bearing which reproduces the same deformity.

As mentioned earlier, all the tests described do not have the same importance, depending on whether the lesion is acute or chronic.

The presence of hemarthrosis and muscular spasm makes the tests more difficult, even if they have been preceded by a puncture of the hemarthrosis with the goal of lessening intra-articular tension. The tests that the patients can best tolerate are those done at 10, 20, or 30 degrees of flexion, the capacity of the capsule being then at its maximum. Testing of varus or valgus at 30 degrees of flexion, and the anterior drawer in extension, meet such criteria. At 60 degrees of flexion the flexor muscles, by acting in this position, make the search for anterior drawers quite difficult. All the tests requiring excessive force as well as those with rather abrupt movements such as those performed during dynamic tests are often very poorly tolerated by the patient when there are peripheral ruptures. For this reason we attach great importance to the search for an anterior drawer in extension, which is fundamental in the search for anterior laxities. This test is accurate in more than 95 percent of anterior cruciate lesions, making general anesthesia unnecessary.

On the other hand, in chronic laxities, even though they are less evident because of the peripheral healing that limits joint opening and anterior and posterior displacement of the tibial plateau under the femur, the knee tests done in the form of a gentle examination, repeated several times, give the possibility of making a precise diagnosis with all the possible variations, as we shall see below under the classifications.

ANCILLARY TESTS

The clinical examination, however precise, cannot obscure the need for subsidiary tests, such as simple roentgenograms, dynamic roentgenograms, arthrography, or arthroscopy.

Roentgenographic Examination

The roentgenographic examination consists of a simple anteroposterior projection, if possible with single-leg weight-bearing, a lateral projection at about 30 degrees of flexion, and a skyline view of the patellae. This standard knee series permits appreciation of several possible findings:
1. Osteochondral loose fragments in the joint, sometimes not visible in the immediate period after the injury
2. Osseous fragment detachments at the level of the ligamentous insertions (medial collateral ligament at the femoral insertion, lateral collateral ligament at the head of the fibula) or detachment of the capsule (Fig. 14.3) (the edge of the lateral tibial plateau)
3. Degenerative joint changes, in the form of narrowing of the joint space with mild osteophytosis in the medial compartment, or the modification of the morphology of the tibial spines which are remodeled like a hockey stick.

Dynamic Radiographs

Dynamic films are obtained applying moderate force particularly in cases of recent acute ligamentous ruptures. We do not consider them a routine diagnostic aid for the study of the laxities, except in cases in which there are combined lesions of the anterior and posterior cruciate ligaments. In these cases, dynamic films enable study of the contribution of the anterior

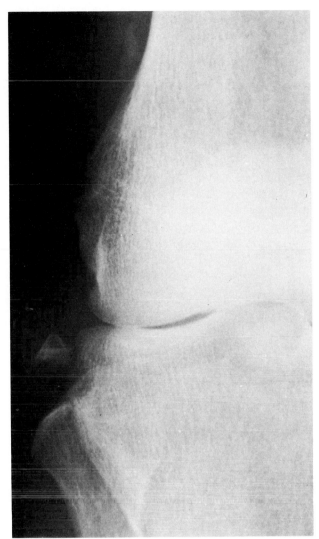

Fig. 14.3. Detachment of the lateral capsule from the lateral tibial plateau with a bony fragment.

ditions. Its main value is in detecting the presence of lesions of the menisci. Arthrography can be performed almost without risk and, if technically well done, permits accuracy of diagnosis for meniscal lesions on the medial side of about 80 percent and on the lateral side of about 75 percent. It is particularly useful in detecting peripheral tears of the posterior horn of the medial meniscus, for which other tests, particularly arthroscopy, are less accurate. Now that meniscal repairs for peripheral meniscal lesions are more widely used, it is possible by means of arthrography to demonstrate the presence of lesions amenable to suture.

Arthrography can also be used in the acute phase. With specific attention to technical details, this technique may show the presence not only of peripheral capsular lesions through which the dye escapes, but also the presence of lesions of the cruciates, particularly of the anterior cruciate. This examination must be done using double-contrast methods (air and radiopaque materials) after thorough aspiration of the effusion and hemarthrosis. The anterior cruciate studies must be done at the beginning of the procedure before carrying out studies of the menisci and the other structures. Epinephrine is added in order to slow the reabsorption of the contrast material, and stress is applied to the knee to isolate the cruciate in the central pivot. In the best hands, this study has permitted a high percentage of accuracy, but unfortunately this experience has not been reproduced by all.

Arthroscopy. Arthroscopy is an important diagnostic element for the problems of ligamentous surgery of the knee, but its use is not the same for fresh ruptures as for chronic laxities. In fresh ruptures it permits a complete diagnosis with appreciation of the site and type of the rupture when the lesion has been already diagnosed during the clinical examination. In chronic laxities, it permits an intra-articular evaluation with demonstration of the meniscal lesions responsible for part of the instability and of any chondral lesions. These are important factors for the prognosis.

Arthroscopy for Fresh Ruptures. Technically, arthroscopy is possible in fresh ruptures only if it is done after a profuse lavage of the joint with an isotonic fluid in an effort to diminish the synovial swelling and to clean the joint cavity perfectly. This lavage must be done with weak pressure in order to mini-

and posterior components to the laxity. These films can be particularly important at follow-up in attempting to judge the quality of the objective results. But, as we have said for the examination, if the posterior drawer has an almost constant significance, it is not the same for the anterior drawer, which may appear secondarily, due to stretching. An exception is the anterior drawer in extension, a position in which the dynamic films must be taken.

Arthrography. Arthrography of the knee, with single (air) or double-contrast method, is an examination still widely used, particularly in chronic con-

mize extra-articular diffusion of the fluid, which may cause compression in the popliteal region of the knee or in the anterior compartment of the leg. Arthroscopy may allow a complete evaluation of the articular surfaces and the appreciation of the rare intrameniscal lesions. It gives the possibility of exploring the peripheral ligamentous systems at the level of the joint line above or below the menisci and of diagnosing a peripheral detachment of the menisci. One can find ruptures of the meniscal attachment at the level of the meniscofemoral or meniscotibial "coronary" ligaments; arthroscopy may help evaluate the clinically suspected site of rupture of the posteromedial corner. One can find a detachment of the meniscus at the periphery, without horizontal interruption of the capsular femorotibial ligament. In these cases, arthroscopy gives very interesting information, sometimes not clinically suspected. This type of lesion usually has a very mild clinical manifestation, without valgus laxity but still with a true lesion of the posteromedial corner.

The chief use of arthroscopy is its ability to verify the condition of the central pivot. In this case the purpose of arthroscopy is not to confirm a lesion diagnosed by clinical means but, with the help of the probe, to determine the level of rupture of both anterior and posterior cruciates. There may be a proximal rupture at the level of the femoral condyles or a distal rupture at the level of the tibia or an intraligamentous "mop-end" rupture at different levels in the cruciate fascicles. In other cases it may show a rupture with an intact synovial layer that may represent an interesting manifestation of spontaneous healing.

This topographic precision is important in making a decision concerning surgery immediately after arthroscopy. In our statistics of 50 knees with acute lesions in which arthroscopy was done, we were able to find in three cases the presence of an old rupture of the anterior cruciate that had occurred several months earlier after a minor injury that had been of little consequence and that had been forgotten. In these cases, the injury that had brought the patient to medical attention was an episode of giving way caused by a chronic insufficiency of the anterior cruciate ligament.

This finding, probably attributable to an inaccurate collection of the clinical data, is fundamental in making decisions regarding acute versus chronic lesions, which are managed quite differently.

Arthroscopy in Chronic Laxities.   In chronic laxity, arthroscopy may give us supplementary information, allowing us to confirm the meniscal lesions diagnosed by arthrography (peripheral detachments, intracartilaginous ruptures, and the existence of a partial bucket handle or flap tears), but, above all, arthroscopy can give key information about the nature and location of the chondral lesions that may influence the long term prognosis.

In the intermediate phase between acute and chronic lesions, arthroscopy has allowed us to diagnose in eight cases of flexion contracture that had lasted for more than 15 or 20 days after the injury a rupture of the anterior cruciate ligament; this had formed a flap that had become interposed between the femoral condyle and the tibial plateau and was preventing extension. In these cases, without examination under general anesthesia, diagnosis has been difficult, and arthroscopy has given us crucial information.

CLASSIFICATION OF THE LESIONS

Classification of the laxities of the knee is critical for adequate treatment and for a comparison of the results (Fig. 14.4).

As there is no precise relationship between fresh and chronic laxities, to include both in the same classification requires an explanation. Fresh lesions are secondary to trauma in a certain direction and, depending on the exact position and rotation of the knee, the ligamentous structures will tear in the order in which they are stretched.

Whether referring to acute ruptures or chronic insufficiencies our classification is based on anatomic lesions. Every word of the classification (e.g., anteromedial) appears in an isolated fashion but the word rupture for the acute lesion and insufficiency for the chronic one is omitted.

In acute lesions, in which there are peripheral tears, the tests are positive for the peripheral structures (varus or valgus at 30 degrees) alone or associated with lesions of the central pivot (anterior drawer in external rotation, direct anterior drawer, or posteroexternal drawer). What happens in chronic laxity is different because there is more or less perfect healing of the initial lesion and progressive degradation of certain other structures due to alteration of the stresses in the tissues caused by the initial rupture.

If we use the same classification for acute and chronic

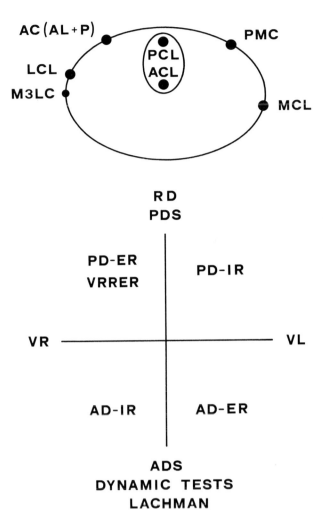

RD
PDS

PD-ER
VRRER

PD-IR

VR ——————————————— VL

AD-IR

AD-ER

ADS
DYNAMIC TESTS
LACHMAN

Fig. 14.4. Graphic representation of pathologic anatomical lesions (above) and clinical tests of instability (below). PCL, posterior cruciate ligament; ACL, anterior cruciate ligament; M3LC, midthird lateral capsule; LCL, lateral collateral ligament; AC (AL + P), arcuate complex (arcuate ligament plus popliteus tendon); PMC, posteromedial capsule; and MCL, medial collateral ligament. Filled black dots represent normal structures, open circles are ligament lesions. RD, recurvatum direct; PDS, posterior drawer sign; PD-ER, posterior drawer external rotation; VRRER, varus recurvatum external rotation; PD-IR, posterior drawer internal rotation; VR, varus test; VL, valgus test; AD-IR, anterior drawer internal rotation; AD-ER, anterior drawer external rotation; ADS, anterior drawer sign (direct). Dynamic tests include jerk, pivot shift; Lachman, anterior drawer in extension.

lesions we must remember that in fresh lesions the different tests for the peripheral structures are rather obvious, while in the chronic laxities they are less evident and sometimes even difficult to find.

ISOLATED PERIPHERAL LESIONS

One type of peripheral ligamentous rupture can be isolated, without rupture of the central pivot. This is possible only if at the time of the injury the central pivot was not under tension, that is, if the knee was in external rotation, or "unlocked." In this condition of rotation, the peripheral structures participate in the stability of the knee; their tension makes them susceptible to the excessive stresses caused by trauma. In the same way, if the central pivot is intact, the clinical expression of a peripheral insufficiency is essentially found on external rotation, while its expression is attenuated in neutral rotation and may sometimes even disappear in internal rotation because of the tightened surfaces caused by torsion of the anterior cruciate ligament over the posterior cruciate ligament.

It is therefore possible to distinguish several types of lesions.

MEDIAL (FIG. 14.5)

1. Medial lesions are secondary to valgus injuries of the knee in external rotation. The lesions occur in the posteromedial corner and radiate anteriorly towards the medial collateral ligament.
2. In a fresh rupture, the clinical examination shows tests of valgus in flexion and external rotation of 1+ and anterior drawer in external rotation of 1+; this last test may be absent or limited by the posterior horn of the medial meniscus if this has remained attached to the tibia in cases of lesions above the meniscus.
3. The natural evolution is toward healing, which minimizes the clinical tests. The only remaining problem may be that of the medial meniscus that has been detached. But in some cases an insufficiency of the medial compartment may persist and, in the chronic phase, cause problems of clinical instability.

LATERAL (FIG. 14.6)

1. Caused by injuries in varus and recurvatum with the foot in neutral or external rotation, the lesions are located over the popliteus–arcuate complex and over the lateral collateral ligament.

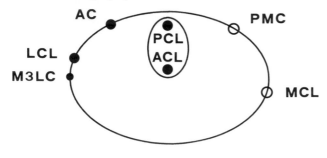

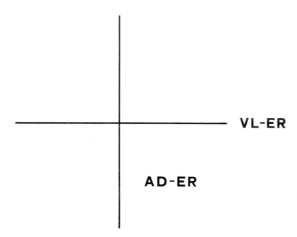

Fig. 14.5. Medial peripheral instability.

2. Clinically, such lesions are manifested by a positive varus test at 30 degrees and a positive recurvatum–external rotation test.

3. The healing of such lesions is often imperfect because of the varus stresses at the time of single-leg weight-bearing, and often there are positive tests in the chronic phase with a tendency to become progressively worse with longer follow-up. This is most likely in cases of constitutional varus.

COMBINED PERIPHERAL
(FIG. 14.7)

1. Combined peripheral lesions may occur with movements of severe tibial rotation, without varus or valgus stress. They may be diffuse, involving both medial, and lateral structures, but the absence of joint line opening minimizes the importance of the lesions, which are often of the interstitial type, at least on the lateral side. Although these lesions are rare, we have observed them occasionally. The tests in varus and valgus are very

weakly positive; healing is the rule, making the signs disappear. Only meniscal problems may remain.

LESIONS WITH RUPTURE
OF THE CENTRAL PIVOT

Most laxities of the knee involve a rupture of the central pivot, which may be any of the following:

1. Anterior cruciate ligament, which is primarily responsible for the dynamic control of the knee.

2. Posterior cruciate ligament, which has an important role in the static control of the knee.

3. Both the anterior and posterior cruciates in association.

These ruptures of one of the two elements of the central pivot or of the two elements in association are the fundamental characteristics of the classification. They permit differentiation of the anterior laxities, the posterior laxities, and the anteroposterior laxities that will be subsequently subdivided in relationship to the association with peripheral lesions. It is an anatomic classification.

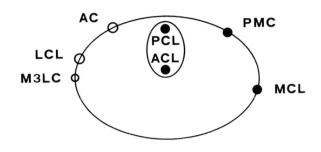

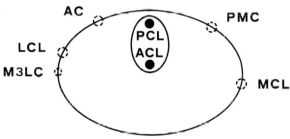

Fig. 14.6. Lateral peripheral instability.

Fig. 14.7. Combined peripheral instability (interrupted open circles represent incomplete lesions).

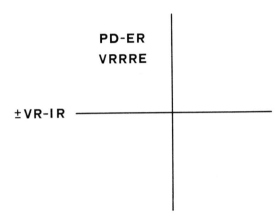

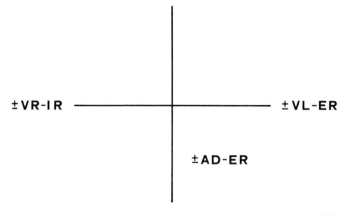

ANTERIOR LESIONS

Isolated Anterior (Fig. 14.8)

1. These laxities are caused by isolated rupture of the anterior cruciate ligament. They occur with forced internal rotation (landing from a jump in internal rotation, with contracture of the quadriceps to absorb the deceleration) or with a hyperextension force in internal rotation (empty air kicking).
2. Clinically, these laxities have an anterior drawer in extension, as well as positive dynamic tests, which are sufficient to diagnose an anterior cruciate lesion.
3. In our experience, there is no spontaneous healing of the anterior cruciate ligament, hence there is an insufficiency of the anterior cruciate in the chronic phase with persistently positive dynamic tests and a drawer sign in extension.

ANTERIOR CRUCIATE LIGAMENT AND PERIPHERAL LESIONS

Anteromedial (Fig. 14.9)

1. This instability corresponds to a ruptured anterior cruciate ligament in association with rupture of the posteromedial corner and sometimes of the medial collateral ligament.
2. There is a positive drawer in extension and positive dynamic tests clinically in the acute phase, but the latter may sometimes not be too evident because of the difficulty in obtaining locking of the internal compartment necessary for the jerk. Such lesions also have an anterior drawer in external rotation of 2+ and a direct anterior drawer of 1+ (anterior cruciate ligament in association with the posteromedial corner). There may be a positive valgus–flexion–external rotation test of 2+ (medial

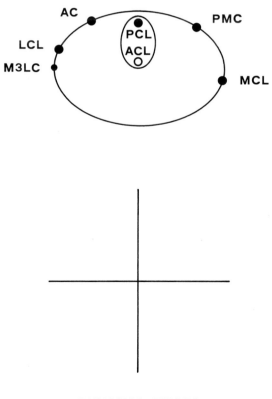

DYNAMIC TESTS
LACHMAN

Fig. 14.8. Isolated anterior instability.

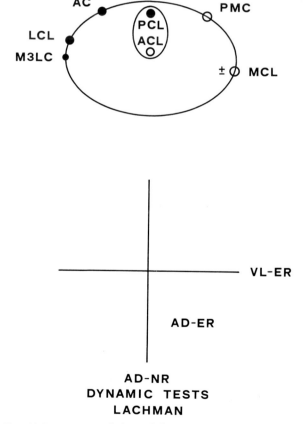

DYNAMIC TESTS
LACHMAN

Fig. 14.9. Anteromedial instability. AD-NR, anterior drawer in neutral rotation, usually 1+.

collateral ligament with more medial compartment opening because of the ruptured anterior cruciate).

3. Chronic anteromedial laxity may represent the evolution of the acute lesions. In these cases, the dynamic tests are always positive, and only the valgus laxity is attenuated. However, this type of laxity may also be caused by degenerative evolution of an isolated lesion of the anterior cruciate ligament with secondary involvement of the medial meniscus, which is the most important element of the posteromedial corner. The medial meniscus may also have been surgically removed.

ANTEROLATERAL

Anterolateral instability represents a rupture of the anterior cruciate ligament associated with a rupture of the lateral ligamentous structures, which control forward and backward movement of the lateral tibial plateau in its two sections, the border of which is the lateral collateral ligament. One must therefore distinguish between the anterolateral preligamentous instabilities and the anterolateral retroligamentous instabilities.

Anterolateral Preligamentous
(Fig. 14.10)

1. This instability corresponds to a rupture of the midthird lateral capsular ligament, which may also involve the lateral collateral ligament. It is produced by varus injuries in internal rotation. These lesions increase the signs of insufficiency of the anterior cruciate ligament and decrease control of the anterior subluxation of the lateral tibial plateau.
2. Clinically there is a positive anterior drawer in extension and positive dynamic tests or very positive dynamic tests (anterior cruciate ligament plus preligamentous structures), a laxity in varus at 30 degrees (if there is rupture of the lateral collateral ligament), and a positive internal rotation drawer (anterior cruciate ligament plus lateral structures in the preligamentous area).
3. In the chronic phase these lesions are characterized by similar clinical tests. The internal rotation drawer tends to become less evident, and the same applies to the varus laxity at 30 degrees.

Anterolateral Retroligamentous
(Fig. 14.11)

1. This instability corresponds to a rupture of the popliteus–arcuate complex, and perhaps a rupture of the lateral collateral ligament. It is caused by varus and recurvatum injuries with the foot in internal rotation. This posterolateral insufficiency does not in itself amplify the rupture of the anterior cruciate ligament, at least in its dynamic component, hence the clinical signs of anterior cruciate ligament rupture are not increased. On the other hand, this posterolateral insufficiency is increased by the absence of the anterior cruciate ligament because the knee does not lock in extension thereby increasing the posterior subluxation of the lateral tibial plateau.
2. In the acute phase there is a positive anterior drawer in extension and a positive 2+ dynamic test, a positive varus laxity at 30 degrees (lateral collateral ligament), and a positive varus recurvatum external rotation (attributable to the popliteus complex).
3. The evolution of the lesion because of this anterior cruciate–posterolateral insufficiency is aggravated by the varus stresses normally present in the single leg weight-bearing position, which does not permit correct healing at the posterolateral level, so that the clinical expression in the chronic phase remains evident. In the chronic phase, however, this type of laxity can also be of secondary or degenerative type in patients with a varus morphotype and with a ruptured anterior cruciate ligament that augments the stresses on the posterolateral corner, which stretches progressively. In the long term, such a laxity is severe because it causes rapid wear of the internal compartment and of the medial meniscus producing wear of the cartilage surfaces and femorotibial medial osteoarthritis.

ANTERIOR COMBINED
(FIG. 14.12)

1. These instabilities correspond to a rupture of the anterior cruciate ligament in association with rupture of the medial and lateral ligamentous structures. They are caused by injuries in internal rotation—axial loading (landing after a jump) or in hyperextension (empty kick). These mechanisms

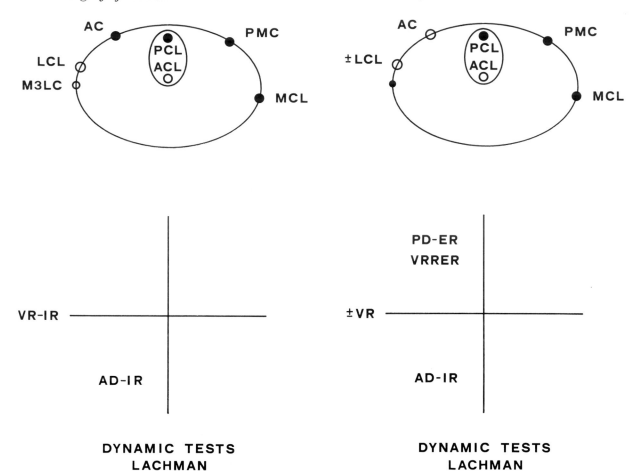

Fig. 14.10. Anterolateral preligamentous instability.

Fig. 14.11. Anterolateral retroligamentous instability.

are the same as those which cause an isolated rupture of the anterior cruciate ligament but of greater magnitude, that is to say more internal rotation and more hyperextension.

2. Anatomically there is an association of an anteromedial laxity and an anterolateral laxity clinically demonstrating an anterior drawer in extension, positive dynamic tests (anterior cruciate ligament), anterior drawer in external rotation of 2+, and a direct drawer of 2+ (anterior cruciate ligament plus the posteromedial corner), valgus flexion external rotation of 1+ (medial collateral ligament), a varus internal rotation of 1+ (lateral collateral ligament),

and varus recurvatum external rotation (if there is a lesion of the posterolateral corner).

3. Therefore these are major laxities, the prognosis of which is poor because of the rapid onset of meniscal and bicompartmental articular surface lesions.

POSTERIOR LESIONS

ISOLATED POSTERIOR
(FIG. 14.13)

These laxities represent an isolated rupture of the posterior cruciate ligament caused by a direct blow to the upper tibia in a flexed knee. Clinically there is

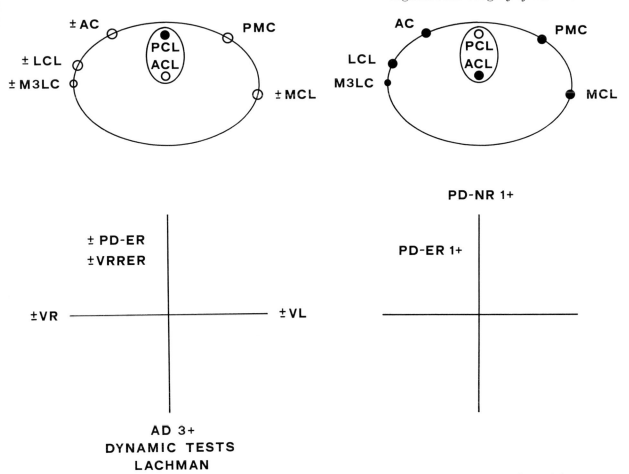

Fig. 14.12. Anterior combined instabilities.

Fig. 14.13. Posterior isolated instability.

a posterior drawer 1+ that is not increased in external rotation; the test remains the same in the chronic phase because there is a poor chance of healing of this ligament.

POSTERIOR CRUCIATE LIGAMENT AND PERIPHERAL LESIONS

POSTEROMEDIAL (FIG. 14.14)

1. This instability is due to a rupture of the posterior cruciate ligament in association with a rupture of the posteromedial capsular structures sometimes radiated to the medial collateral ligament. It occurs with valgus and hyperextension injuries with the foot in external or in neutral rotation (skiing).
2. Clinically, there is a posterior drawer of 1+ (posterior cruciate ligament), an anterior drawer in external rotation of 1+, and a positive valgus flexion external rotation test of 1+; these two latter signs are attributable to the lesion of the posteromedial corner.
3. The associated lesions of the posteromedial corner and the posterior cruciate ligament do not augment each other. There is a parallel progression of the two lesions. The posteromedial corner tends

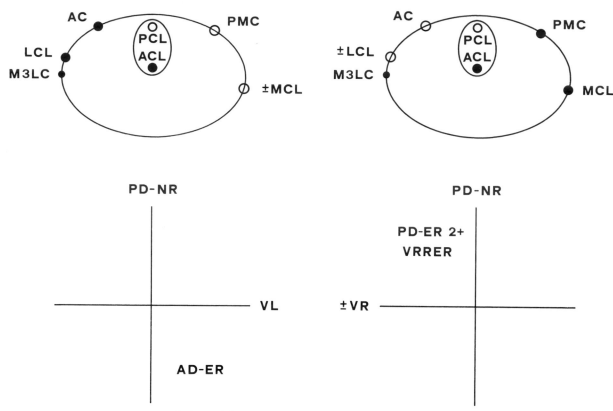

Fig. 14.14. Posteromedial instability.

Fig. 14.15. Posterolateral instability.

to show healing capacities that make both the anterior drawer in external rotation and the valgus flexion external rotation test disappear, explaining the relative rarity of chronic posteromedial laxities which most often become a pure posterior laxity.

POSTEROLATERAL (FIG. 14.15)

1. This instability is due to a rupture of the posterior cruciate ligament and of the posterolateral capsular structures (popliteus complex ± lateral collateral ligament). It occurs most often in flexion–external rotation injuries with anteroposterior trauma.
2. Clinically, there is a posterior drawer of 2+ (posterior cruciate ligament), a posterolateral drawer of 2+ (posterior cruciate ligament plus posterolateral corner), and a positive varus recurvatum external rotation test (posterolateral corner augmented by the posterior cruciate ligament).
3. These two lesions augment each other and have a

very poor prognosis with potential chronic deterioration and positive clinical tests only slightly different from those shown in the acute phase. In the long term, the deterioration and the insufficiency of the posterior and lateral ligaments will show laxity in the weight-bearing lower extremity with varus and recurvatum, and sooner or later medial compartment osteoarthritis will appear.

POSTERIOR COMBINED (FIG. 14.16)

1. This instability represents a rupture of the posterior cruciate ligament associated with a rupture of the posterior parts of the medial and lateral compartments and sometimes the posterior capsule. It occurs with a hyperextension injury in the load-bearing extremity, with the foot in external or neutral rotation.
2. Clinically there is a positive posterior drawer of

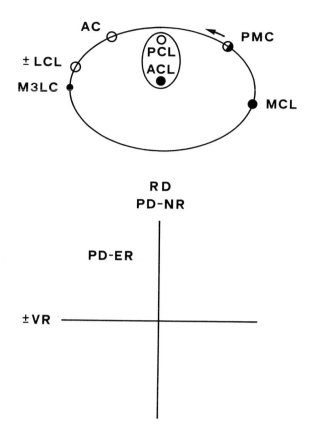

Fig. 14.16. Posterior combined instability. The half-empty PMC dot represents extension of the lesion toward the posteromedial capsule.

2+ (posterior cruciate ligament plus posterior capsule), a positive posterolateral drawer of 2+ (posterior cruciate ligament plus posterolateral corner), and a direct recurvatum of 2+ (posterior cruciate ligament plus the posterior capsule).

3. The healing of this lesion is less than perfect because of the continuing stresses in varus and recurvatum, particularly over the posterolateral aspect; in the chronic phase the clinical examination remains the same.

ANTEROPOSTERIOR LESIONS

An anteroposterior laxity involves a major lesion caused by severe trauma with significant opening of the joint surfaces that can be medial, lateral, or posterior. It can be associated with lesions of the tibial plateau caused by compression.

ANTEROPOSTERIOR MEDIAL (FIG. 14.17)

1. This instability corresponds to a rupture of the two cruciate ligaments and of the entire medial compartment ligamentous structures.
2. Clinically there is a posterior drawer of 2+, a direct anterior drawer, a positive valgus flexion external rotation sign, and a positive anterior drawer in external rotation of 2+. The dynamic tests are positive, but they are performed with difficulty because of the absence of the medial hinge.
3. In the chronic phase, healing can occur; hence the group of tests we have mentioned are still positive. Furthermore, if the test of valgus external rotation in flexion is less, the dynamic tests can become more positive because healing has recreated the medial hinge.

ANTEROPOSTERIOR LATERAL (FIG. 14.18)

1. This instability corresponds to a rupture of the two cruciate ligaments and of the entire external compartment.
2. Clinically there is a positive posterior drawer, a positive external rotation posterior drawer of 2+, and a positive direct anterior drawer of 1+, varus internal rotation of 2+, varus recurvatum external rotation of 1+, and dynamic tests of 1+ if the fascia lata is intact. Nerve lesions are frequently associated.
3. The evolution of such lesions is both ominous and rapid, and lateral healing is unlikely because of the stresses in varus.

ANTEROPOSTERIOR COMBINED (FIG. 14.19)

1. These instabilities correspond to a rupture of the two cruciates with compartmental posterior lesions caused by hyperextension of the load-bearing extremity.
2. Clinically there is a posterior drawer of 2+, a positive anterior drawer of 1+, and a positive direct recurvatum test. The anterior drawer in extension is positive, while the other tests are only mildly positive.

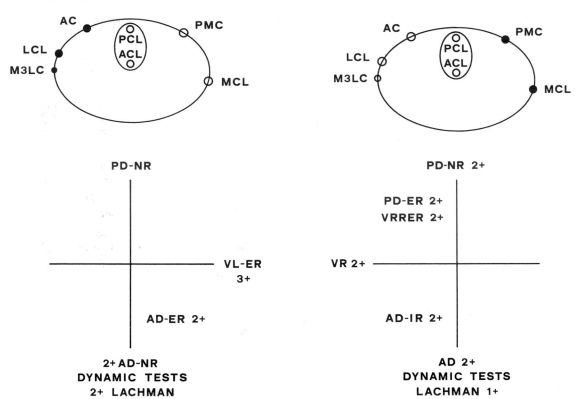

Fig. 14.17. Anteroposterior medial instability.

Fig. 14.18. Anteroposterior lateral instability.

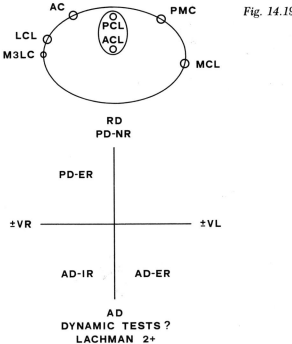

Fig. 14.19. Anteroposterior combined instability.

KNEE DISLOCATIONS

When trauma continues after rupture of the two elements of the central pivot, there may be a translation and a dislocation of the knee, as characterized by the existence of bicompartmental lesions (rupture caused by joint opening on one side and capsular periosteal detachment on the other side). However, detachment may take place on the same side as the impact (translocation without joint opening); and will take place at the level of the femur if the femur is translated above the tibia (Fig. 14.20) and at the level of the tibia if the tibia is translated below the femur (Fig. 14.21). Therefore, one must distinguish among lateral dislocations (with lateral translation of the tibial plateau below the femur), medial dislocations, anterior dislocations, and posterior dislocations.

LIGAMENTOUS REPAIR IN ACUTE LESIONS

OSSEOUS DETACHMENT AT THE LEVEL OF THE INSERTION OF THE LIGAMENTS

Detachment of bone at the point of ligament insertion is the most favorable situation; it can be treated by one of several methods (Figs. 14.22–14.24):
1. Direct fixation with screws, (A) if there is a detachment at the level of the insertion of the posterior cruciate ligament in the posterior intercondylar eminence, or (B) "retrograde" screw fixation in the case of a detachment of the anterior cruciate ligament at the level of the anterior intercondylar eminence
2. A staple may be used at the insertion of the tubercle of Gerdy. A staple may also be used to fix the superior insertion of the lateral collateral ligament provided that the synovial recess is not occluded.
3. Transosseous stitches are good, no matter what site, if the osseous fragment is particularly small.

INTRALIGAMENTOUS RUPTURES

An intraligamentous rupture presents difficult problems of reconstruction. At the level of the central pivot, all repairs must be done with transosseous

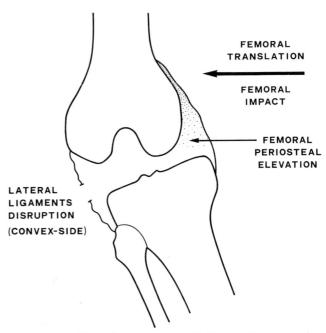

Fig. 14.20. Knee dislocation type I. Femoral impact.

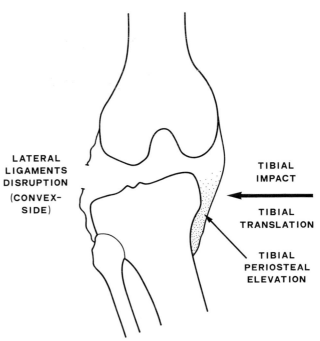

Fig. 14.21. Knee dislocation type II. Tibial impact.

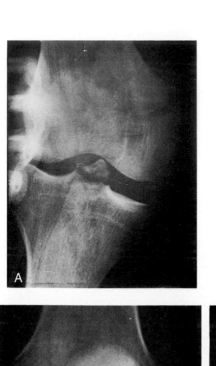

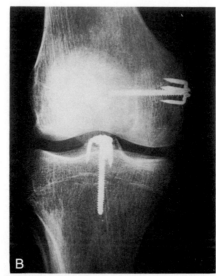

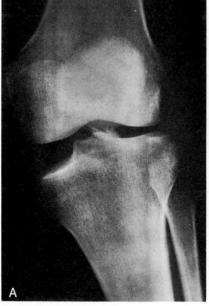

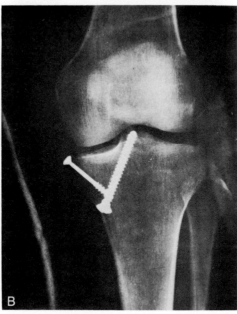

Fig. 14.22. (A.B.) Bony avulsion of the medial epicondyle and anterior intercondylar eminence treated with screw-staple fixation.

Fig. 14.23. (A.B.) Bony avulsion from the anterior intercondylar eminence and medial tibial margin treated with screw fixation. The spine fixation is *en rappel.* (retrograde)

stitches, and the site of reinsertion must be as precise as possible.

ANTERIOR CRUCIATE LIGAMENT
(FIG. 14.25)

In the case of rupture of the anterior cruciate ligament in the proximal third, the technique consists (Fig. 14.26) of passing multiple stitches in a U fashion (without zig-zagging) and without shortening the ligament. These sutures permit reinsertion of the ligament into the femoral condyle. A series of stitches is passed in a transosseous tunnel, and another series is passed over the top of the lateral femoral condyle. The two series are then sutured together over the posterolateral aspect of the lateral femoral condyle.

In cases of rupture near the lower end, the same technique is applied, but if the lesion is at the level of the midthird, or if there is a "mop-end" type of lesion at different levels, the fascicles of the cruciate ligament must be sutured by means of double tunnels, one in the tibia and one in the femur.

This is somewhat theoretical because even though the repair may appear satisfactory, it is very rare that one can produce a true continuity of the anterior cruciate ligament. This ligament may have value as far as proprioceptive functions are concerned, but its mechanical value is modest and the repair should be augmented.

A frequently used anterolateral extraarticular reconstruction (Fig. 14.27) uses a strip of fascia lata of 0.5 cm in width, detached at its proximal superior portion, and left attached at the level of the tubercle of Gerdy. This strip is passed beneath the superior end of the lateral collateral ligament and then from distal to proximal through a tunnel in the lateral femoral condyle. The inferior orifice is situated just behind the origin of the lateral collateral ligament, and the superior orifice is situated 1 cm higher and slightly posterior. The strip of fascia lata is returned beneath the collateral ligament and is then fixed in a bony tunnel prepared at the level of the tubercle of Gerdy.

This technique has been used to protect the direct repairs of the anterior cruciate ligament by suture in order to diminish the anterior hypermobility of the lateral compartment. This can only be used when there is an isolated rupture of the anterior cruciate ligament and when the peripheral structures are apparently healthy. By contrast, if there is a peripheral posterolateral lesion there is a significant risk of a permanent posterolateral subluxation of the tibia.

Augmentation reconstructions (Fig. 14.28) of the anterior cruciate ligament designed to reinforce the sutured anterior cruciate ligament are also frequently used. This is done intra-articularly with the semitendinosus, which is dissected as high as possible and sectioned at the level of its musculotendinous junction. The distal insertion is not detached. This new ligament is then passed in a tibial tunnel, which exits at the anterior insertion of the anterior cruciate ligament. The graft parallels the resutured anterior cruciate ligament and is passed over the top of the lateral femoral condyle and is sutured to the posterolateral capsular structures.

POSTERIOR CRUCIATE LIGAMENT

The problems with the posterior cruciate ligament are very similar. When there is a rupture (Fig. 14.29) at the upper third near the level of the femoral condyle, surgical repair is possible with precise sutures and with stitches passed in two bony tunnels at the level of the lateral aspect of the medial femoral condyle in the notch. For the rupture at the level of the middle third, one must do a double type of suturing with tibial and femoral tunnels. The rupture at the inferior third requires only a transtibial tunnel.

If the preparation of the femoral tunnels for reinsertion of the posterior cruciate and the subsequent suture does not present particular problems, this is not the case for the tibial tunnels when there is no possibility of opening of the joint in varus or valgus, because there are no associated peripheral laxities. In these cases it is possible to work in the intercondylar notch and to reinsert the posterior cruciate into the tibia. Alternatively we recommend a posterior or posteromedial approach. Apart from the rupture in the upper third, which may allow a good repair even if we do not find the stump of the proximal insertion of the posterior cruciate ligament, the other types of ruptures, particularly those in the middle third, are usually mechanically insufficient and require an augmentation reconstruction (Fig. 14.30) according to the technique of Lindemann (modified) using only one tendon (semitendinosus).

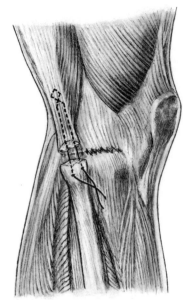

Fig. 14.24. Metallic wire fixation of the tip of the head of the fibula.

PERIPHERAL STRUCTURES

The repairs must be direct. This implies a simple end-to-end suture without excessive tension on the ruptured formations having precisely identified all the different anatomic structures. In cases of rupture near the insertion, some transosseous or capsuloperiosteal stitches permit a correct repair. In the case of rupture with laceration of the anatomic tissues, it is some-

times necessary to use other structures to reinforce the direct sutures.

For the medial collateral ligament we have used the semitendinosus tendon, which is redirected (Fig. 14.31) in order to duplicate the superficial fibers of the medial collateral ligament, according to the technique described by Helfet. For the lateral collateral ligament, the superficial tendon of the biceps can be used. A strip of tendon is prepared from the main tendon of the biceps and is left attached distally to the fibular head. It duplicates the lateral collateral ligament from the fibular head toward the superior condylar insertion.

Finally, if the meniscus is healthy, as it is in most cases, meniscal disinsertion with a horizontal interruption of the capsular ligament will require a reinsertion and suture (Fig. 14.32) of both the meniscofemoral and meniscotibial ligaments. Meniscectomy should not be done in fresh ligamentous ruptures.

SURGICAL APPROACH

With a few exceptions we use a medial parapatellar approach permitting us to make a medial arthrotomy. This examination is very important because it will determine the means used to treat the lesions.

If necessary, the internal compartment exploration is facilitated by three surgical steps: (1) freeing the inferior border of vastus medialis, (2) detaching the tendons of the pes anserinus at the anterior insertion

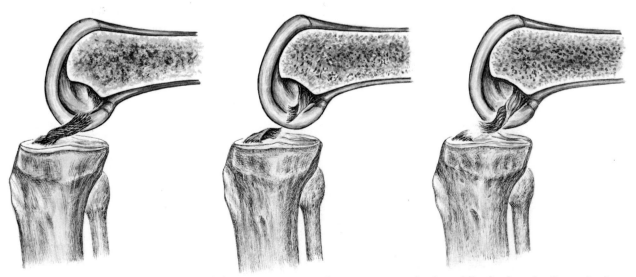

Fig. 14.25. Three levels of rupture of the anterior cruciate ligament: upper third, middle third, and inferior third.

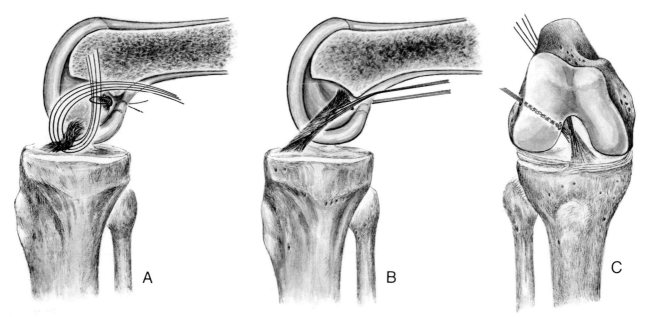

Fig. 14.26. (A–C) Technique of direct suture of acute upper third lesion of the anterior cruciate ligament with multiple U sutures (see text).

and reflecting them posteriorly together with the skin flap, and (3) making an incision in the fascia superficialis. In cases of doubt, a posteromedial exploration of the knee is done through a separate capsular incision.

For the lateral compartment, the incision starts between the tubercle of Gerdy and the head of the fibula and it bends gently to follow the inferior border of the vastus lateralis. The exploration is facilitated by a longitudinal incision of the fascia lata. A posterolateral exploration is possible with a posterolateral arthrotomy behind the lateral collateral ligament and above the popliteus tendon.

Both on the medial and the lateral sides, the lesion must be thoroughly evaluated with a methodical progression and by means of a simultaneous intra- and extra-articular evaluation that will give a complete picture. The dissection is guided by the ecchymotic infiltration; the dissection must be performed gently and carefully to prevent damage to healthy fibers and thereby worsening the extent of the lesion(s).

The repair begins with the central pivot, followed by extra-articular repairs or intra-articular augmentation procedures. All the central pivot stitches are prepared but are only tied after all the peripheral lesions have been repaired.

Rupture of the posterior cruciate ligament at its lower third with osseous detachment must be ap-

proached differently in our experience if the lesion is isolated. In these cases we use the posterior approach described by Trickey (Fig. 14.33).

The patient is in the prone position; the knee is opened with a posterior approach to permit partial detachment of the medial border of the medial head of gastrocnemius. We then perform a posterior arthrotomy centered over the lateral border of the medial femoral condyle, which can easily be appreciated through the posterior approach and which permits visualization of the distal portion of the posterior cruciate ligament. This is sometimes repaired with a screw or sometimes with a screw staple directly fixing the bony fragment to the tibia.

POSTOPERATIVE TREATMENT

IMMOBILIZATION

Postoperative treatment requires immobilization for 45 days.

For ruptures of the anterior cruciate ligament, the cast is full length including the foot with the knee in 20 to 30 degrees of flexion. This position relieves excessive tension on the peripheral lesions and anterior cruciate repair.

For the posterior cruciate ligament, the problem is

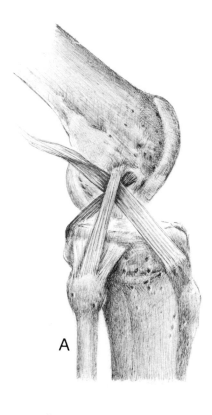

A

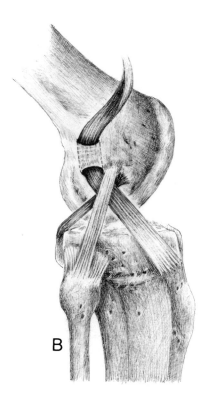

B

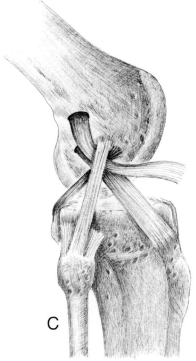

C

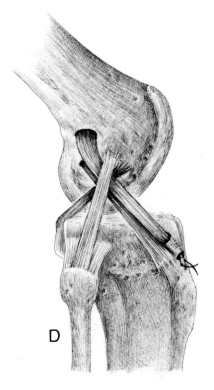

D

Fig. 14.27. (A–D) Technique of anterolateral extra-articular reconstruction. The strip of fascia lata anchors the lateral tibial plateau to the lateral femoral condyle as a tenodesis (see text).

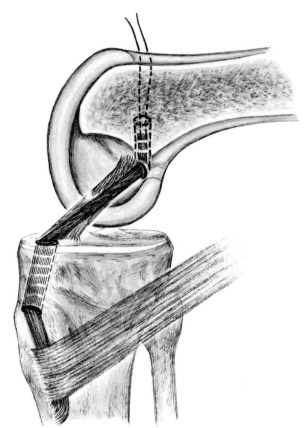

Fig. 14.28. Augmentation (intra-articular) of the anterior cruciate ligament, using the semitendinosus tendon.

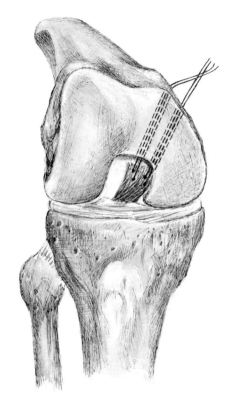

Fig. 14.29. Direct suture of the posterior cruciate ligament to the medial femoral condyle.

more complex, as the force of gravity by itself would tend to sublux the tibia posteriorly. In our experience immobilization in flexion always results in posterior subluxation which is not improved by the use of femoro-tibial pins. We have therefore decided on a position very close to full extension so that the posterior ligamentous structures are in tension to provide an anteroposterior stabilization of the knee.

REHABILITATION

Rehabilitation is a fundamental phase of ligamentous surgery of the knee. During the period of cast immobilization, the patient is not allowed to bear weight for 45 days. During this period, it is important and useful to do static contraction of the muscles.

Electrotherapy is used with specific windows in the cast for the different muscular groups, and vertical and transverse passive mobilization of the patella is done through an anterior window centered over the knee.

After cast removal, the work phase will begin regaining motion, and muscular force, and allowing progressive weight-bearing.

Regaining the range of motion is done progressively (Fig. 14.34). One must remember to avoid two mistakes: too rapid gain in flexion may stretch the suture line and a too rapid gain in extension may cause recurvatum. This may distend the repair as well as the extra-articular posterolateral reinforcement, which we believe must be protected by keeping a certain degree of flexion contracture, particularly if there is a congenital or constitutional varus. This risk of progressive stretching exists either because of the insufficiency of the anterior cruciate ligament or be-

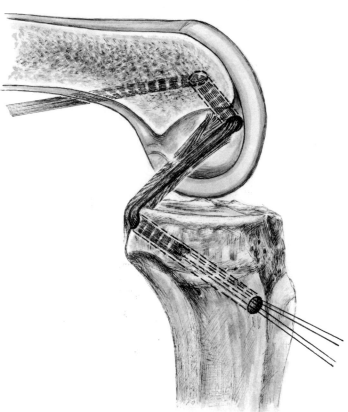

Fig. 14.30. Augmentation (intra-articular) of the posterior cruciate ligament, using the semitendinosus tendon.

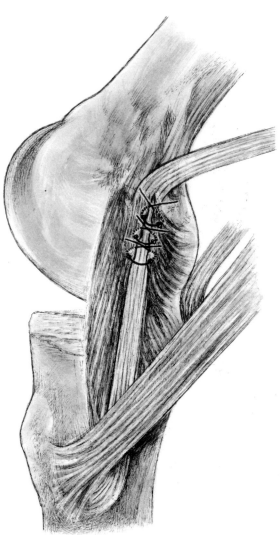

Fig. 14.31. The semitendinosus can be redirected in order to reinforce the long fibers of the medial collateral ligament.

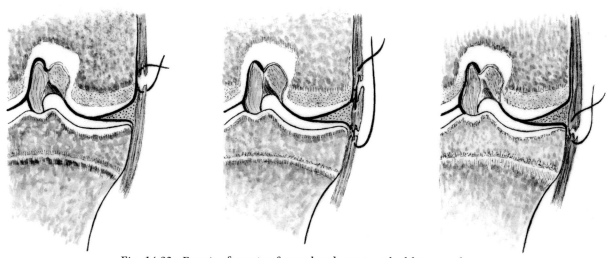

Fig. 14.32. Repair of meniscofemoral and meniscotibial ligament lesions.

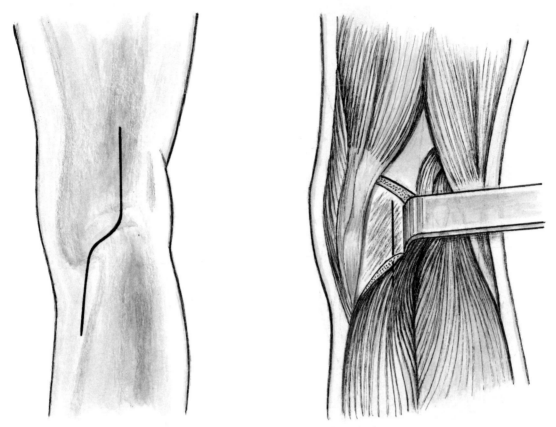

Fig. 14.33. Trickey posterior approach to the knee (see text).

Fig. 14.34. Progression of re-habilitation after ligamentous repair (acute lesions) of the anterior cruciate ligament.

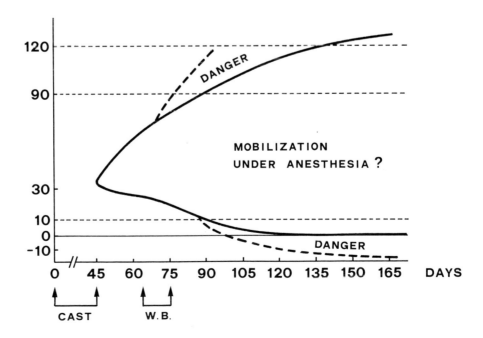

cause of the insufficiency of the posterior cruciate ligament with which the posterolateral corner contributes to the control of the posterior drawer.

On the other hand, one must always remember that the other risk is too slow rehabilitation and mobilization, which may lead to a manipulation under general anesthesia. This is done when necessary at the third month.

This range-of-motion work is done manually, without excessive stresses, both passively and actively assisted. It must be done by applying force at the superior end of the tibia, trying to obtain the sliding movements of the knee and avoiding the range-of-motion gains obtained by anterior joint opening, when the knee works like a simple hinge.

Recuperation of the muscular force is obtained by working on the quadriceps, and the hamstrings, acting as flexors and rotators.

The work of the quadriceps can be dangerous in cases of rupture of the anterior cruciate ligament because of the anterior force it exerts. It is mandatory that the quadriceps works with resistance at the level of the anterior tibial tuberosity. This type of work can begin as static contraction and then as dynamic contraction from the 75th day if the patellar cartilage will permit.

The work of the hamstrings is variable according to the lesion. For the anterior cruciate ligament, these muscles are not detrimental and in fact are important because in the first few degrees of flexion they decrease the anterior drawer. They also decrease the risk of recurvatum. The work of the flexors in cases of rupture of the anterior cruciate ligament can therefore be intense and begin early in rehabilitation.

By contrast, for the posterior cruciate ligament, there is a significant risk of stressing the suture line by the work of the hamstrings; in our opinion, this risk contraindicates all work in flexion.

The rotators of the knee do not create particular problems. The only thing to remember is that work must be isometric and without insisting on internal rotation which, because of the torsion of the central pivot, may excessively stress the anterior cruciate ligament.

Weight-bearing is allowed between the 60th and 75th days according to the quality of the muscular rehabilitation.

After this, physical therapy enters the phase of proprioceptive rehabilitation without particular precau-

tions, except that the patient should not return to sports activity too soon.

SURGICAL INDICATIONS

Having discussed the problems of diagnosis and surgical technique, it is now important to discuss the surgical indications for acute lesions. The fundamental issue is the integrity of the central pivot.

If there is no rupture of the anterior or posterior cruciate ligaments, and only peripheral tears, we consider these "benign" lesions. In such cases, peripheral healing is the rule, because the integrity of the central pivot has not caused a significant separation at the level of the rupture.

In cases of benign lesions, one may find an intraligamentous or "interstitial" rupture involving a certain number of fibers without total interruption of the ligament (clinical disability, ligamentous tenderness, and negative, or very weakly positive tests). Here, it is only necessary to stop the activities and to unload the joint for 3 weeks; after this, a short period of rehabilitation is necessary.

A true interruption of the ligaments may be the case, as shown by the presence of a certain number of tests (valgus–flexion–external rotation, anterior drawer in external rotation, and posterolateral drawer) that demonstrate the presence of a peripheral rupture even if the central pivot is intact. This is possible because of the unlocking caused by the external rotation. In these cases, healing requires strict immobilization in a cast at 30 degrees of flexion for 45 days. This period of immobilization is followed by rehabilitation.

When there is a rupture of the central pivot, the clinical situation is more serious. When there is a rupture of the anterior cruciate ligament every lesion, in high-level athletes, or occasionally athletic young patients, must be operated upon even if the lesion is isolated, and without regard to the site of the rupture. There is no sport requiring load-bearing and pivoting that is possible without an anterior cruciate ligament. On the other hand, if the case involves a patient who indulges in sports occasionally and who is older, the surgical indication must be considered together with the patient, because the morbidity following the operation may be a handicap for the professional life of the patient.

Surgical indication in these cases must be discussed according to certain parameters. These include the association with peripheral lesions, which can be more or less well tolerated according to the morphotype of the patient. For example, a lateral lesion, even if minimal, can decompensate very quickly in cases of varus and recurvatum, and medial lesions may be poorly tolerated when knee alignment is valgus.

The site of rupture of the anterior cruciate ligament is also important because a lesion in the upper third, as well as avulsion of the bony insertions, suggests operation: in these cases, the chances of success are best.

For a rupture of the posterior cruciate ligament, surgery is not always indicated. In cases of an isolated lesion with a moderate (1+) posterior drawer and without radiologic evidence of bone avulsion, we tend towards non operative treatment because we believe that in such cases of intraligamentous rupture, the posterior drawer never becomes totally negative after surgical repair. On the other hand, surgery is indicated if the laxity is above 1+, or if there are peripheral lesions, particularly posterolateral lesions, which potentiate the insufficiency of the posterior cruciate ligament. Also when there is a varus morphotype, the surgical option is used more often, because the risk of decompensation is significant.

We believe that a rupture of both cruciate ligaments is a definite indication for surgery; the same applies to dislocations of the knee, for which surgery is indicated under the age of 50.

SURGICAL RECONSTRUCTION IN CHRONIC INSUFFICIENCY

A chronic laxity is a consequence of incomplete healing of the initial lesions and of secondary progressive stretching. The surgical techniques currently in use cannot solve all these problems, yet certain techniques, even if imperfect, tend to reconstruct the normal anatomy. This is the case with intra-articular reconstructions of the central pivot. Other techniques are palliative operations, that is to say, they are designed to diminish the functional consequences of the insufficiency of one of the ligaments. This is the goal with anterolateral extra-articular reconstructions in cases of anterior cruciate ligament insufficiency.

ANTERIOR INSUFFICIENCY

INTRA-ARTICULAR RECONSTRUCTION OF THE ANTERIOR CRUCIATE LIGAMENT

We make a new ligament using a free graft prepared from the midcentral third of the patellar tendon with two bone blocks at each end taken from the patella and the tibial tubercle (Fig. 14.35). Metallic wires are passed through holes drilled in each of the two osseous blocks of the transplant. The lateral femoral condyle is then prepared for positioning of the patellar fragment. Through an anterior approach, a crater is produced at the level of the posterior insertion of the anterior cruciate ligament on the lateral femoral condyle. After this, using a cruciate **C** guide, a bone tunnel is drilled from the crater to the lateral aspect of the lateral femoral condyle. The patellar end of the graft is held in the crater with the metallic wire, which goes through the condylar tunnel and is fixed over a screw and washer on the lateral femoral metaphysis.

The tibial tunnel is then drilled, exiting just anteromedial to the tibial insertion of the anterior cruciate ligament. The tibial bone block of the free graft is passed through the tunnel and the graft is appropriately tensioned, fixing the wire over a screw and washer with the knee flexed at about 20 degrees. This is done after checking the range of motion, which must be free from 0 to 90 degrees of flexion and after observing possible impingement between the new ligament and the lateral aspect of the intercondylar notch. In certain cases the notch has to be enlarged. Sometimes it is difficult to have a ligament that will be equally tensed both in extension and at 90 degrees of flexion. We prefer to have perfect tension in the range between 10 to 20 degrees of flexion, a range in which it is most important that anterior cruciate function be reproduced. Precise positioning and preparation of the crater and bony tunnels is required (Fig. 14.36AB).

ANTEROLATERAL RECONSTRUCTION

This reconstruction is identical to the one described for augmenting acute ligamentous ruptures. It must allow a free range of motion between 0 and 90 degrees of flexion. This operation is very often done in association with the above described intra-articular reconstruction.

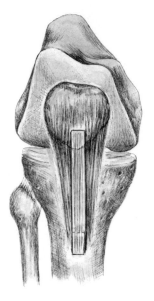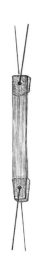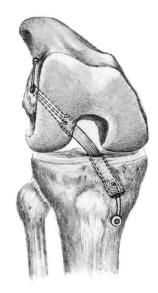

Fig. 14.35. Free graft reconstruction of the anterior cruciate ligament (see text).

Meniscal Suture And Posteromedial Reconstruction

Meniscal suture corresponds to a reconstruction of the posteromedial corner, as the medial meniscus is a fundamental stabilizer of this corner. The reconstruction is only possible if there is a peripheral lesion of the meniscus without a lesion in the meniscal body. The reinsertion is done through a retroligamentous posteromedial incision (Fig. 14.37) after a thorough freshening of the meniscal wall. Six or seven reabsorbable vertical sutures are passed in the meniscal wall and then through the capsule. The sutures are first passed and later tied. It is important not to create an imbalance with too high or too low a suture in the capsule. At the end of the operation, there must be a range of motion of 0 to 90 degrees.

Theoretically, *posteromedial reefing* has two goals. It must correct medial laxity, and it must permit better control of external rotation, particularly when there is a lesion of the anterior cruciate ligament.

One must remember the often transient benefit of this type of reconstruction. Fortunately persistence of a certain amount of medial laxity generally does not prevent a good functional result.

Having used several different reconstructions proposed in the literature (O'Donohue, Nicholas, Hughston, Slocum), we have developed our own technique. The principle is that one must respect the points of insertion of the superficial medial collateral ligament, as well as the capsular equilibrium above and below the meniscus. If these principles are not adhered to, the results will be recurrence of laxity or limited range of motion, particularly a flexion contracture (which is not a disaster if less than 5 degrees).

Posteromedial reefing is considered only if there is no medial meniscus. The goal of the operation is to diminish advancement of the medial tibial plateau below the femoral condyle. This is obtained by a sort of cerclage (Fig. 14.38) of the femoral condyle at the level of the joint line. The arthrotomy exposes the superficial medial collateral ligament, from the medial epicondyle to the reflected tendon of the semimembranosus. The reconstruction starts with a stitch at the level of the previous meniscal wall, which is sutured *en paletot* to the medial collateral ligament. This first stitch is a reference stitch and prevents excessive tension toward the upper or lower direction and imbalance of the corner. The remaining arthrotomy flap is equally sutured over the medial collateral ligament without excessive traction upward toward the femur or downward toward the tibia. Remember that full extension must still be possible at the end of the reconstruction. The tendons of the pes anserinus are lifted in bulk without eversion to cover the reefing.

When there is also valgus laxity the posteromedial capsule is treated as described above.

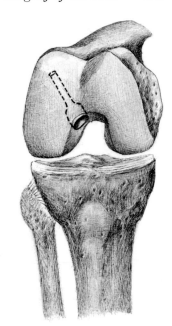
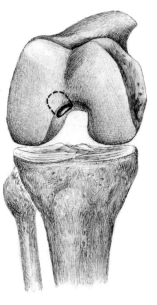

Fig. 14.36. (A,B) Positioning and preparation of the crater in the lateral femoral condyle and of the femoral and tibial tunnels.

A

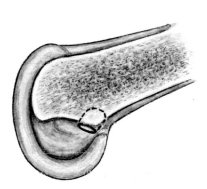

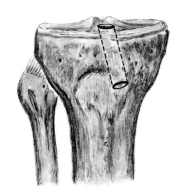
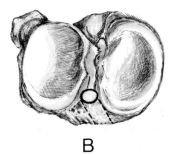
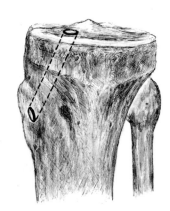

B

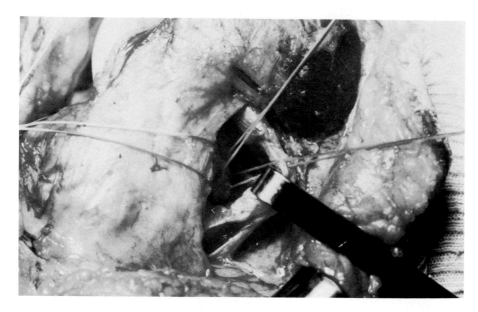

Fig. 14.37. Medial meniscus reinsertion (suture) at the posteromedial corner.

MEDIAL RECONSTRUCTIONS

Once the reconstruction is done, it should demonstrate, during the operation, a range of motion from −5 to 90 degrees.

Repositioning and reattachment of the medial collateral ligament is only desirable if there is an osseous detachment, usually condylar, of the superficial medial collateral ligament. In other cases, which occur more often, we prefer not to disinsert the ligament, but to reinforce it with one of tendons of the pes anserinus following Helfet's technique. This gives an almost anatomic doubling of the ligament, if the positioning of the condylar attachment is performed well. In the case of a significant laxity above the meniscus, some mop-end stitches along the transplant may serve to shorten the ligament without sectioning it.

At the level of the posteromedial corner the crucial element is the meniscus, hence the great value that we attribute to meniscal suture, when this is possible.

POSTEROLATERAL RECONSTRUCTIONS

The goal is to diminish the posterolateral hyperrotation of the lateral tibial plateau with a posterolateral subluxation. An osseous block including the insertion of the lateral collateral ligament and the popliteus tendon is detached and is then fixed using a staple after translation in a superior and forward direction. Even if this type of reconstruction lessens the posterior subluxation of the lateral tibial plateau, it usually does not prevent decompensation into varus in single-leg weight-bearing. This is a fundamental element of the prognosis and we therefore believe it preferable to aim for a degree of flexion contracture during the postoperative period in order to avoid recurvatum. This is functionally equal to a reconstruction operation of the posterolateral corner.

POSTERIOR INSUFFICIENCY

RECONSTRUCTION OF THE POSTERIOR CRUCIATE LIGAMENT (FIG. 14.39)

We have used the semitendinosus and the gracilis tendons as transplants in this reconstruction. They are dissected and freed at the distal insertion and passed through a tunnel in the medial femoral condyle emerging just anterior to the insertion of the posterior cruciate ligament. The grafts are then passed backwards and enter from a posterior direction one or two tunnels in the tibia. The transplants are then put under tension in extension and fixed to the anteromedial tibia with stitches. The two tibial tunnels can be prepared through the intercondylar notch, be-

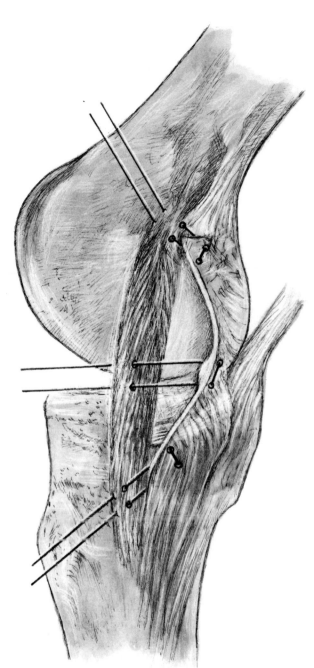

Fig. 14.38. Technique of posteromedial reefing.

the tunnel and the passage of the wire is done through a wide posteromedial arthrotomy.

The review of our patients operated on according to the method described above has shown that only one-half were significantly improved after the operation. Therefore we have since tried to reconstruct the two fascicles (anteromedial and posterolateral) of the posterior cruciate ligament. For the anteromedial fascicle, we have used the semitendinosus, which is positioned according to the technique described above. For the posterolateral fascicle, we have used a free graft taken off the midthird of the patellar tendon as described for the anterior cruciate ligament. This free graft is fixed to the medial femoral condyle through the anterior approach. The fixation to the tibia is done through the posterior approach described by Trickey, having turned the patient to the supine position. We still find it difficult to recommend this operation because the surgical technique is prolonged and our follow-up is insufficient. At this point we can state that this operation has improved significantly the signs of insufficiency of the posterior cruciate ligament.

POSTEROLATERAL RECONSTRUCTION

This reconstruction is practically identical to the one described for the anterior laxity. It involves a superior and anterior translation of the femoral insertion of lateral collateral ligament and popliteus tendon.

THE ROLE OF OSTEOTOMY IN CHRONIC INSUFFICIENCY

This problem stems directly from the fact that the insufficiency of the central pivot causes progressive ligamentous stretching at the periphery, aggravated by the patient's morphotype. Of particular importance is stretching of the posterolateral corner in cases of constitutional varus. This posterolateral instability in itself may be a factor causing signs of hyperpressure in the medial compartment of the knee. In our experience, this is imperfectly controlled by the posterolateral reconstruction, which does not prevent the decompensation in single-leg load-bearing. For this reason in major forms of instability we propose an

cause the posterior cruciate ligament is absent in a chronic lesion. The passage of the anchoring stitches (Fig. 14.40) is done with the aid of a soft wire passer. In cases of a narrow intercondylar notch, this technique is technically impossible and the preparation of

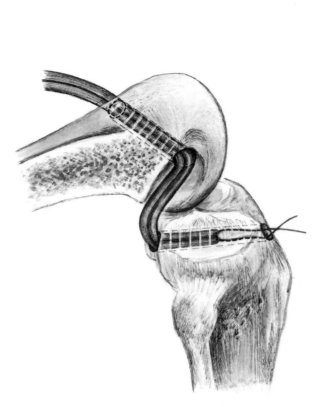
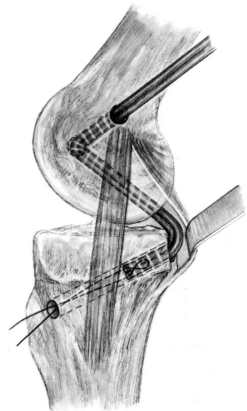

Fig. 14.39. Reconstruction of the posterior cruciate ligament using the semitendinosus and the gracilis tendons.

osteotomy to obtain valgus and prevent this evolution (a normal correction is ideal). This osteotomy is done in the same surgical setting as the ligament reconstruction.

POSTOPERATIVE TREATMENT

We do not immobilize knees that we reconstruct for chronic instability. These patients come out of the operating room with a splint holding the knee in slight flexion for the anterior cruciate ligament and in extension for the posterior cruciate ligament.

From the third postoperative day after pain has diminished, patients begin to work to minimize atrophy and obtain range of motion.

For problems of atrophy, we have used electrotherapy, isometric contraction of the different muscle groups, and transverse and longitudinal mobilization of the patella. For the recovery of range of motion and muscular force, physical therapy follows the same pattern presented for the acute ligamentous ruptures (Fig. 14.41) except there is no period of cast immobilization.

Weight-bearing is permitted between the 45th and 60th postoperative days; this also signals the date of the beginning of the proprioceptive rehabilitation up until the return to sports activities.

SURGICAL INDICATIONS

The indication for ligamentous reconstruction is based on the type and severity of the instability and must correspond with the patient's request, as well as the long-term potential of the laxity towards a progressive degeneration. The latter aspect must be discussed with the patient.

These two factors, the symptoms and the potential evolution of the lesion, must be considered along with certain other factors, such as age, particular sport, and morphotype.

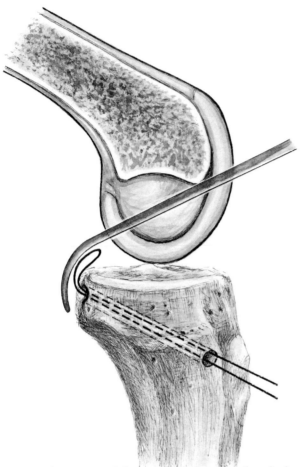

Fig. 14.40. Intercondylar notch approach to the tibial attachment point during reconstruction of the posterior cruciate ligament.

ANTERIOR INSUFFICIENCY

Each case of anterior laxity responsible for an instability must be treated by a surgical operation in an attempt to reconstruct the central pivot. This reconstruction of the central pivot in the intercondylar area can be associated, in our opinion, with peripheral operations, such as the anterolateral extra-articular reconstruction, with the goal of protecting the new ligament, and diminishing the anterior hypermobility of the lateral tibial plateau. The posteromedial reconstruction is done with the goal of providing better control of rotation of the medial tibial plateau. This is done only in cases of absence of the medial meniscus, because the meniscus by itself creates this type of stability. In the same way, if there is a peripheral

disinsertion of the medial meniscus, a reattachment of this important structure is advisable. An exception to the reconstruction of the central pivot is the case of a patient who is not very active in sports or who is relatively old. In these conditions, we use a palliative anterolateral reconstruction with the goal of decreasing the anterolateral jerk. A point of particular interest is the eventual necessity of reconstruction of the posterolateral area in cases of anterior laxity with a retroligamentous component. In cases of less severity, during physical therapy we avoid at all times genu recurvatum. In the most marked severe cases we perform an osteotomy of the proximal tibia to obtain valgus (to a normal correction), thereby decreasing the posterolateral ligament stresses.

POSTERIOR INSUFFICIENCY

The indication for reconstruction of the posterior cruciate is more difficult than that of the anterior cruciate because the problems of static degeneration are greater than problems of dynamic instability (apart from the dynamic problems caused by associated meniscal lesions). In the case of an isolated lesion with a posterior drawer of 1+ that does not increase in external rotation, the indication is debatable because the prognosis is relatively good and the operations we can offer do not completely negate the posterior drawer.

If the posterior laxity is more significant, we believe it is justified to advise a reconstruction that can be associated, after the intra-articular stage, with a posterolateral reconstruction, particularly in cases of insufficiency of the posterolateral corner. Posterolateral reconstruction is not enough in certain cases, for which we propose a tibial osteotomy to obtain valgus and normal correction.

RESULTS:
ACUTE LIGAMENTOUS LESIONS

It is crucial to differentiate in a very precise manner those cases in which there is an isolated rupture of the anterior cruciate ligament, those in which there is a rupture of one of the two cruciates associated with peripheral lesions, and those in which both cruciates are ruptured.

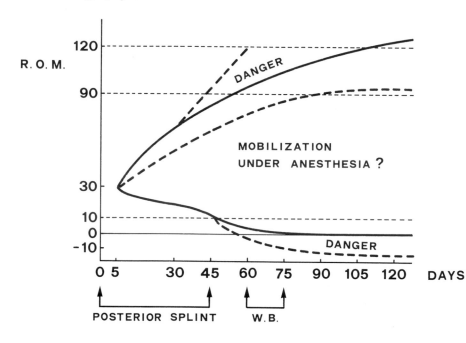

Fig. 14.41. Progression of rehabilitation after reconstruction of chronic anterior cruciate ligament insufficiency.

LESIONS OF THE ANTERIOR CRUCIATE LIGAMENT

Cases of isolated rupture of the anterior cruciate ligament are those without clinically detectable peripheral lesions, even if surgically some ecchymosis on the medial or lateral side is found.

Ten patients have had a simple direct suture for a high rupture of the anterior cruciate. The postoperative period, after 45 days of immobilization, has been uncomplicated, with easy gain of range of motion.

Functionally, the results have been judged good (return to sport at the same or higher level) in one-half of cases, fair (sports to an inferior level or only recreational sports) in four patients, and poor (sports given up) in one patient.

The clinical examination has also been very reassuring; the dynamic tests, which were constant preoperatively, were present in three knees, but attenuated and not disturbing the patients in recreational sports. However persistent dynamic tests may cause eventual progressive deterioration (among these three patients, there has been one medial meniscectomy for peripheral disinsertion of the meniscus 1½ years after the surgical repair).

Seventeen patients have had repair of the anterior cruciate ligament associated with an anterolateral reconstruction. This reconstruction was initially done per primum because a weak repair had been obtained in cases of rupture of the mid- or lower thirds (five cases). After this, this reconstruction became a routine for the 12 following patients. The postoperative treatment has been more difficult than for simple suture, because after 45 days of immobilization we have noted in four patients difficulty in regaining range of motion. Three patients have had manipulation under general anesthesia to correct limited flexion.

Functionally, the results have been good in 12 patients, fair in four patients, and poor in one patient, who has been unable to return to sports and still has pain and fatigue attributable to difficulty in regaining the correct range of motion.

Clinically, the dynamic tests were absent in 13, present but to a low degree in three, and very positive in one patient. One must note that the positive tests were found twice in the good results and twice in the fair results.

Six patients have had a direct suture and repair of the anterior cruciate ligament reinforced with an intra-articular augmentation reconstruction with the semitendinosus tendon. We decided to use this augmentation to avoid difficulty in regaining motion.

The only problem has been for one patient, for whom pain persists on the medial aspect of the knee, probably related to the section of the semitendinosus.

Functionally, there have been four good results and two fair results. Clinically, five patients have had negative positive dynamic tests.

ANTERIOR CRUCIATE AND MEDIAL COMPARTMENT LESIONS

Thirty-five patients had such a lesion. The bad results were related to the magnitude of the medial lesions. These patients have had a direct suture of the anterior cruciate ligament associated in five cases with an augmentation reconstruction using the semitendinosus and a direct suture of the medial ligament.

The postoperative treatment in these patients has been relatively simple with recovery of the range of motion in all except three cases (one requiring manipulation under general anesthesia).

Functionally in the 35 patients the results have been judged as good in 26 patients, fair in seven and poor in two patients.

In 17 percent of cases, there was persistent laxity in valgus at 30 degrees of 1+, with a positive drawer in external rotation in 60 percent of cases and the dynamic tests were positive in seven patients.

LESIONS OF THE ANTERIOR CRUCIATE AND THE LATERAL COMPARTMENT

Eight patients with such a lesion had a suture of the anterior cruciate ligament and of the lateral compartment structures.

Recovery of motion has been difficult in two instances, requiring manipulation under general anesthesia.

Functionally, the results have been good in five and fair in three. These patients have, particularly if there is varus of the tibia, positive laxity in varus at 30 degrees of 1 to 2+, and the dynamic tests were positive in two.

LESIONS OF THE ANTERIOR CRUCIATE, MEDIAL AND LATERAL COMPARTMENTS

Twelve patients had this type of lesion. The rupture of the lateral compartment was preligamentous in two cases, retroligamentous in six cases, and both pre- and retroligamentous in four cases.

We find this to be one of the most difficult lesions to treat. After a peripheral repair, performed as carefully as possible, the anterior cruciate ligament was sutured directly in nine and reinforced with an intraarticular reconstruction in three.

After cast immobilization, the postoperative treatment has been simple, with recovery of range of motion, except in two patients. These patients had a flexion external rotation contracture due to scarring of the posterolateral corner.

Functionally, there were seven good results, three fair results, and two poor results.

Clinically, three patients had positive dynamic tests laxity in varus at 30 degrees and a varus recurvatum sign with external rotation; these were all cases of retroligamentous laxity and demonstrates the difficulty in obtaining good healing of such lesions. In contrast, lesions of the medial compartment have a better prognosis, with only five patients showing laxity in valgus at 30 degrees.

LESIONS OF THE POSTERIOR CRUCIATE LIGAMENT

ISOLATED RUPTURE OF THE POSTERIOR CRUCIATE LIGAMENT

We have followed up eight patients with an intraligamentous rupture and 14 patients with a posterior bony detachment of the posterior cruciate ligament. Of the eight patients with intraligamentous rupture, three had a direct suture plus a Lindemann reconstruction with the semitendinosus. The rehabilitation of the knees immobilized in flexion (three patients) has been difficult owing to the problems in regaining the anterior gliding of the tibia. In fact, posterior retraction caused a permanent posterior subluxation, making the knee function like a hinge, with absence of gliding, in two patients.

The functional results have been satisfactory, with five good, two fair, and one poor result, but all showed at least a 1+ positive posterior direct drawer sign.

For the 14 patients with a detachment of a bone fragment from the posterior intercondylar eminence and operated on using the Trickey approach and immobilized in extension, the results have been far more satisfactory, with 11 good results and three fair results. Only two patients have a posterior drawer, both of whom had inadequate fixation of the bony fragment.

RUPTURE OF THE POSTERIOR CRUCIATE LIGAMENT AND OF THE MEDIAL STRUCTURES

We have had eight patients with this type of lesion after ski injuries. The posterior cruciate ligament had a direct suture and a reconstruction using the semitendinosus. We had four good results, three fair results, and one poor result. The medial structures obtained good healing in three cases. Five knees had laxity in valgus at 30 degrees of 1+. There was at follow-up a posterior drawer of 1+ (five times) and 2+ (one time). The condition of these knees was similar to those that had only an isolated rupture of the posterior cruciate ligament.

RUPTURE OF THE POSTERIOR CRUCIATE LIGAMENT AND OF THE LATERAL STRUCTURES

We have had three patients with this type of lesion. They have been casted in flexion; the postoperative course has been difficult with a posterior subluxation and difficulty in regaining the anterior gliding motion of the tibia below the femoral condyle. We consider these severe lesions producing one good result and two fair results. All patients had a positive posterior drawer of between 1 and 2+, a positive posterior drawer in external rotation of 2+, and a laxity in varus of 1+ and a positive varus–recurvatum–external rotation test.

RUPTURE INVOLVING BOTH CRUCIATE LIGAMENTS

We must distinguish between a lesion of the two cruciate ligaments associated with rupture of the peripheral structures on the medial side and those associated with rupture of the peripheral structures on the lateral side.

For medial lesions, in 18 cases followed up in 1978 we found seven good results; these patients were capable of returning to their sport normally or at the same level they had before the injury. Five patients had a fair result and six patients had a poor result, with muscle wasting, pain, and instability.

Fourteen patients had anteroposterior laxity, with seven showing a prevalence of anterior cruciate ligament insufficiency and seven a prevalence of insufficiency of the posterior cruciate ligament. Only four patients do not have laxity in valgus at 30 degrees of flexion.

In 12 cases associated with lateral peripheral lesions followed up in 1978, the etiology was more frequently a motor vehicle or work accident rather than a sports injury. The peroneal nerve had been injured in four cases (three permanently). We had three good results, four fair results, and five poor results. In 11 patients there was a persistent anteroposterior laxity. The posterior cruciate ligament laxity was always predominant. Ten patients had very apparent varus of the knee; this shows the unsatisfactory evolution of posterolateral and lateral laxity, which remained present in 11 patients.

Even if there are residual problems particularly concerning the healing of the central pivot and the posterolateral structures, suture and repair of the ligamentous structures as soon as possible after the injury has given us a better percentage of satisfactory results than obtained by reconstruction of chronic laxities.

RESULTS: CHRONIC

ANTERIOR CHRONIC

For the anterior chronic laxities, we present the results of anterolateral reconstructions and of intra-articular anterior cruciate ligament reconstructions.

Anterolateral Reconstruction

We have followed up 25 patients 20 of whom had an intra-articular operation (medial meniscectomy in 15 cases, lateral meniscectomy in three cases, double meniscectomy in two cases) and all had an anterolateral extra-articular reconstruction for an old rupture of the anterior cruciate ligament.

Recall that this patient population is one showing little motivation for sports and/or of relatively older age.

Functionally, we have noted 13 good results, seven fair results, and five poor results.

Clinically, the anterolateral reconstruction does not

totally control the anterolateral subluxation of the lateral tibial plateau and therefore does not negate the dynamic tests, which were negative in only 10 patients. These last cases were those with a residual portion of the anterior cruciate, which was detached from the femur and was found to be adherent to the posterior cruciate, leading us to consider the possibility of some retained function. We have seen, in some patients, a return of the dynamic tests, which became positive again, leading us to conclude that there might have been a progressive deterioration of the reconstruction.

Objectively (by varus testing at 30 degrees) we have not found a deterioration of the lateral ligamentous complex caused by this type of anterolateral reconstruction. But the radiographic alterations in the medial compartment with joint space narrowing, and marginal tibial and femoral remodeling probably represent a prearthritic condition. This is clearly more noticeable than the situation found after intra-articular reconstructions of the central pivot.

These medial compartment changes probably have multiple causes: medial meniscectomy, anterior cruciate ligament insufficiency, and a functional deterioration of the active and passive lateral compartment system of the knee.

RECONSTRUCTION OF THE ANTERIOR CRUCIATE LIGAMENT

We have followed 99 patients operated on with more than 17 months of follow-up. The technique was as described for reconstruction of the anterior cruciate ligament, using the middle third of the patellar tendon as a free graft.

Eighty patients had a rupture of the anterior cruciate ligament while playing sports, and 33 patients had been operated upon previously (19 meniscal surgery and 14 ligamentous reconstructions).

Four patients had an isolated anterior cruciate ligament laxity, 34 patients had an anteromedial laxity, three had an anterolateral retroligamentous laxity, and 55 patients had an anterior combined laxity.

Functionally, we had 49 good results, 40 fair results, and 10 poor results (those unable to perform any type of sport). As far as range of motion is concerned, we did four manipulations under general anesthesia, with three good and one poor result. We

also did four arthrolyses with two good results, one fair result, and one poor result.

When reconstruction of the central pivot was the first operation on the knee, the results were definitely better (66 percent good, 30 percent fair, 4 percent poor), but when the operation was a reoperation, we had inferior results (19 percent good, 60 percent fair, and 21 percent poor).

Clinically, only 11 patients had positive dynamic tests and the direct anterior drawer was positive in 39 instances (39 percent).

The anterior drawer in external rotation was positive in 89 cases (89 percent), clearly showing the difficulty we have had in regaining a functionally satisfactory posteromedial corner after a medial meniscectomy.

In the same way, the laxity in valgus at 30 degrees has not been modified by the operation, being positive in 24 knees preoperatively and in 18 knees postoperatively.

POSTERIOR CHRONIC

RECONSTRUCTIONS FOR THE POSTERIOR CRUCIATE LIGAMENT

Twenty-eight of the 48 patients who had this type of operation have been followed up for a minimum of 18 months.

Twenty-one of these patients had had a motor vehicle accident, which explains the associated lesions (three pelvic fractures, two femoral shaft fractures, five patellar fractures, and four tibial fractures).

The laxity can be classified as an isolated posterior in 11 cases, a posterolateral in eight, a posteromedial in three, and an anteroposterior in six. Seven patients had had a previous operative procedure for the anterior cruciate ligament and four had had a meniscectomy. The intra-articular reconstruction of the posterior cruciate was associated in six cases with a posterolateral reconstruction and in four with a posteromedial reconstruction.

The results have been judged as good in 15 instances, fair in nine, and poor in five. There was an average improvement of 50 percent of the posterior drawer as measured on dynamic films. There was minor loss of range of motion.

Radiologically, reconstruction of the posterior cruciate ligament does not seem to have modified the natural history of the knee, with single-leg weight-bearing radiographs showing the presence of changes in the femoral tibial joint in 10 knees.

Apart from the reconstruction of the anterior cruciate ligament, which we believe to be a truly effective operation, one must recognize that other reconstructions are not totally satisfactory, leading us to conclude that it is necessary to treat lesions of the ligaments in the acute stage, before the occurrence of degenerative phenomena.

SUMMARY

The surgical indication is based on the diagnosis of the type of ligamentous laxity, but recognizing two totally different problems. One is static and degenerative (posterior cruciate ligament and lesions of the posterolateral corner), the other dynamic with functional instability and giving way (anterior cruciate ligament and associated intra-articular pathology both meniscal and cartilaginous).

The static problems can be treated with ligamentous reconstructions and with bone operations, such as tibial osteotomy, to obtain alignment and correct torsions.

The dynamic phenomena have several origins. One is intra-articular such as meniscal or articular lesions following insufficiency of the anterior cruciate ligament. Another is the laxity itself which is reproduced by the dynamic tests. The dynamic tests are directly influenced by two aspects: (1) the convexity of the lateral tibial plateau, and (2) impingement between the anteromedial tibial spine and the medial femoral condyle. It is important to determine in a given knee the role attributable to meniscal or cartilaginous lesions and the instability attributable to insufficiency of the anterior cruciate ligament. There may be a role for isolated arthroscopic partial meniscectomies in some cases. Reconstruction of the anterior cruciate ligament can be limited to cases showing a high risk of future determination.

A precise diagnostic effort is very important; one must recognize the different types and subtypes of laxities and should keep in mind all the subtleties of the peripheral insufficiencies even if they do not go in the same direction as the lesions of the central pivot (e.g., posterolateral corner and anterior cruciate; posteromedial corner and posterior cruciate). This is important to prevent performing the wrong technical procedure (e.g., reconstruction of the posterolateral corner in cases of anterolateral instability).

Finally, study of the patients' morphotype in the frontal, sagittal, and rotational planes is very important. This has recently been made easier and more precise with computerized tomography.

REFERENCES

1. Cho, K.O.: Reconstruction of the anterior cruciate ligament by semitendinosus tenodesis. J. Bone Joint Surg. [Am.], 57:608, 1975.
2. DeHaven, K.E., and Collins, H.R.: Diagnosis of internal derangements of the knee. The role of arthroscopy. J. Bone Joint Surg. [Am.], 57:802, 1975.
3. Dejour, H., and Chambat, P.: La chirurgie ligamentaire du genou. Encycl. Med. Chir., Paris, Techniques chirurgicales orthopédie. 4.2.06, 44790.
4. Dejour, H., et al: Résultat à 5 ans du traitement des laxités antérieures. Symposium 56 ème réunion de la SOFCOT. Paris, 1981.
5. Eriksson, E.: Reconstruction of the anterior cruciate ligament. Orthop. Clin. North Am., 7(1):167, 1976.
6. Frankel, V.H., Burstein, A.H., and Brooks, D.B.: Biomechanics of internal derangement of the knee. Pathomechanics as determined by analysis of the instant centers of motion. J. Bone Joint Surg. [Am.], 53:945, 1971.
7. Girgis, F.G., Marshall, J.L., and Al Monajem, A.R.S.: The cruciate ligaments of the knee joint. Anatomical, functional and experimental analysis. Clin. Orthop., 106:216, 1975.
8. Hughston, J.C., Eilers, A.F.: The role of the posterior oblique ligament in repairs of acute medial (collateral) ligament tears of the knee. J. Bone Joint Surg. [Am.], 55:923, 1973.
9. Hughston, J.C., Andrews, J.R., Cross, M.J., et al: Classification of knee ligament instabilities. Part I. The medial compartment and cruciate ligaments. J. Bone Joint Surg. [Am.], 58:159, 1976.
10. Hughston, J.C., Andrews, J.R., Cross, M.J., et al: Classification of knee ligament instabilities. Part II. The lateral compartment. J. Bone Joint Surg. [Am.], 58:173, 1976.
11. Jones, K.G.: Reconstruction of the anterior cruciate ligament. A technique using the central one-third of the patellar ligament. J. Bone Joint Surg. [Am.], 45:925, 1963.

12. Jones, K.G.: Reconstruction of the anterior cruciate ligament using the central one-third of the patellar ligament. A follow-up report. J. Bone Joint Surg. [Am.], 52:1302, 1970.

13. Kennedy, J.C., Hawkins, R.J., Willis, R.B., et al: Tension studies of human knee ligaments. Yield point, ultimate failure, and disruption of the cruciate and tibial collateral ligaments. J. Bone Joint Surg. [Am.], 58:350, 1976.

14. Marshall, J.L., and Rubin, R.M.: Knee ligament injuries—a diagnostic and therapeutic approach. Orthop. Clin. North Am. 8(3):641, 1977.

15. Nicholas, J.A.: The five-one reconstruction for anteromedial instability of the knee. Indications, technique and the results in fifty-two patients. J. Bone Joint Surg. [Am.], 55:899, 1973.

16. Noyes, F.R., DeLucas, J.L., and Torvik, P.J.: Biomechanics of anterior cruciate ligament failure: An analysis of strain-rate sensitivity and mechanisms of failure in primates. J. Bone Joint Surg. [Am.], 56:236, 1974.

17. Norwood, L.A., Jr., and Cross, M.J.: The intercondylar shelf and the anterior cruciate ligament. Am. J. Sports Med., 5:171, 1977.

18. O'Donoghue, D.H.: An analysis of end results of surgical treatment of major injuries to the ligaments of the knee. J. Bone Joint Surg. [Am.], 37:1, 1955.

19. O'Donoghue, D.H.: Reconstruction for medial instability of the knee. Technique and results in sixty cases. J. Bone Joint Surg. [Am.], 55:941, 1973.

20. Prudhon, J.L., and Chambat, P.: Arthroscopie et ruptures ligamentaries fraiches du genou. J. Med. Lyon. 1362, 1981.

21. Rigal, F., Chambat, P., Prudhon, J.L., et al: Protocole de rééducation des plasties ligamentaires du genou. Ann. Med. Phys., 24:3, 1981.

22. Slocum, D.B., and Larson, R.L.: Rotatory instability of the knee. Its pathogenesis and a clinical test to demonstrate its presence. J. Bone Joint Surg. [Am.], 50:211, 1968.

23. Trickey, E.L.: Rupture of the posterior cruciate ligament of the knee. J. Bone Joint Surg. [Br.], 50:334, 1968.

15 Fractures of the Knee

Paolo Aglietti
and
Pierre Chambat

Part I   Fractures of the Patella

Fractures of the patella occur very frequently. They often require surgical treatment involving one of several methods: osteosynthesis, partial patellectomy, and total patellectomy. Some surgeons have a radical attitude and prefer one or the other technique, while others use different techniques in different types of fracture. The consequences of a patellar fracture as they affect joint function, mobility, muscle power, and development of osteoarthritis can be significant, as the functional role of the patella is needed to obtain a successful result.

ANATOMY AND FUNCTION

The patella is a triangular-shaped bone with rounded edges. It has a rounded point on its anteroinferior margin, the patellar apex, so that the anterior height exceeds the height of the posterior articular surface. The anterior surface is gently convex and lies deep to the fascia and the tendinous fibers of the rectus femoris as they pass distally to the tibial tubercle.

The average dimensions[2,75] are: anterior surface height 40 to 45 mm, articular surface height 30 to 35 mm, total width 40 to 47 mm, and thickness 20 to 23 mm. The articular surface is divided into medial and lateral facets by a major vertical ridge. A second vertical ridge near the medial border of the medial facet divides the latter from the odd facet, which is quite small. Often a transverse ridge can be found dividing the main facets into a larger superior and a smaller inferior area.

Wiberg[98] divided the patellae into three types according to the relative size of the medial and lateral facets:

Type I The medial and lateral facets are of equal size and both are slightly concave (24 percent of cases).

Type II The medial facet is concave but is smaller than the lateral facet; this is the most frequent type, accounting for 57 percent of cases.

Type III The medial facet is definitely smaller and convex, and accounts for 19 percent of cases.

Baumgartl[7] considered a type II–III with a small, flat medial facet, a type IV with a very small, steeply sloped facet with a medial ridge still present and a type VI (Jaegerhut) having no ridge and no medial

395

facet. This classification takes into account various degrees of patellar dysplasia. The lateral facet is consistent in contour and dimensions,[51] while the medial facet shows progressive dysplasia, hypoplasia, and a vertical medial facet. This can also be expressed in terms of the patellar index.[24]

The contact area between patella and femur begin at the distal part of the patella around 15 degrees of flexion (surface area $\pm$ 2 cm^2). It then moves proximally and reaches the maximum surface area as flexion proceeds (around 60 to 80 degrees $\pm$ 5 cm^2). At maximum flexion the patella lies deep between the femoral condyles: the upper facets articulate with the two femoral condyles.[2,36]

The rectus femoris becomes tendinous at a distance of 6 to 8 cm above the patella. The tendon enlarges as it approaches the patella; its fibers continue over the anterior surface of the patella and into the patellar tendon.[75]

The vastus medialis can be divided into vastus medialis obliquus,[52] which makes an angle of 50 to 75 degrees with the rectus femoris (60 degrees on average), and vastus medialis longus. The vastus medialis obliquus usually becomes tendinous a few millimeters from the superomedial margin of the patella. Some aponeurotic fibers continue distally to contribute to the medial retinaculum.

The vastus lateralis makes an angle of 31 degrees on average with the rectus and becomes tendinous at approximately 2.8 cm from the superolateral border of the patella. Some aponeurotic fibers contribute to the lateral retinaculum, and infrequently to the infrapatellar tendon. Those fibers are connected to the iliotibial tract.

The vastus intermedius inserts with most of its fibers directly into the superior pole of the patella. According to classic descriptions, the quadriceps insertion into the superior pole of the patella is trilaminar.[50,55,79] The rectus femoris is anterior or superficial; the two vasti form the middle layer, and the vastus intermedius is the deepest. However, the actual structure is more complex and extremely variable; beneath the superficial layer are a variable number of fiber bundles.

The fascia lata spreads over the anterior aspect of the knee. Its medial and lateral extensions contribute to the patella retinacula; laterally it thickens to form the iliotibial tract, which inserts into Gerdy's tubercle. Deep to the fascia the patellofemoral ligaments[44] which are thickenings in the capsule connect the patella to the medial and lateral epicondyles.

The infrapatellar tendon is a flat, strong structure originating in the central fibers of the rectus femoris and inserting into the tibial tubercle. Its average length[75] is 4.6 (3.5 to 5.5) cm.

The vascular supply to the patella comes from the superior and inferior genicular arteries, which form the peripatellar plexus. The genicular artery supreme contributes to the plexus. The plexus penetrates the lower pole and the central anterior surface; the upper pole is supplied by a central penetrating artery.[23,81]

The patella increases the extension moment arm.[45] The maximum torque in isokinetic conditions[90] is found at approximately 60 degrees, and this is related to lengthening of the quadriceps fibers,[39] as well as the lever arm. The quadriceps tension increases with flexion, and can reach six to seven times body weight.[46] Patellofemoral compression force also increases with flexion and is related to the type of activity.[76] It is very low for isometric contraction in extension, becoming high when climbing stairs or squatting.[72] Patellofemoral pressures vary with activity[57] from approximately 25 kg/cm^2 when walking to 80 kg/cm^2 when climbing stairs, and to higher values when jumping or landing from a jump.

MECHANISMS OF INJURY AND TYPES OF FRACTURES

Fractures of the patella account approximately for 1 percent of all skeletal injuries.[13,64] The injury is most frequent between 40 and 50 years. The average age is 48, with a range of 16 to 82 years in our series of surgically treated cases.[1] There is a slight dominance of males (averaging in our series 56.5 percent). The average age is usually lower in men and older in women (42 years and 52 years, respectively, in our series). In another study,[13] the peak incidence is in the fourth decade for men and in the sixth decade for women. There is usually no predominance of side, and bilateral fractures are rare.[66]

In our series the most frequent cause is an accidental fall or a fall from a height (59 percent), followed by traffic accidents[1,64] (25 to 35 percent). Work injuries account for the rest of the causes (6 percent). Road traffic accidents were not the most frequent cause, as has been found by other workers.[13,66,85]

In terms of specific mechanism of injury, fractures of the patella can be the result of a direct trauma (blow to the front of the knee), an indirect trauma, or a combination of both. The powerful force exerted by the quadriceps is transmitted to the quadriceps tendon, the patella, and the patellar tendon. When the patient suddenly stops or lands from a jump with the knee bent, the patella is compressed and is bent over the femur. The forces increase with knee flexion and at 45 to 65 degrees of flexion the central area of the patella is forced against the femur. A mixed type of injury (direct plus indirect) can occur frequently.

While in the past[12,94] fractures of the patella were divided into two main types according to the mechanism of trauma, with transverse fractures caused by an indirect trauma and comminuted fractures caused by a direct trauma, it is now recognized that other factors can be important: the degree of flexion of the knee at the moment of injury, age of the patient, presence of osteoporosis, and the velocity of injury.

It is generally recognized that while these mechanisms are the usual, different types of fractures can be caused by the same injury.[13,66,85] Furthermore, longitudinal fractures are not as uncommon as previously reported and are caused by direct forces against the knee.[49] In recent studies,[66] it was shown that transverse and comminuted fractures occur more frequently in older patients and in about equal proportions. While in certain older studies[22] transverse fractures accounted for about 70 percent of the cases, an increasing number of fractures from direct trauma is now found. In half of our surgically treated cases,[1] the reported injury was indirect and the typical fracture was transverse, with little anterior comminution.[41] Although sometimes it involved the extreme upper or lower pole, more frequently the fracture was in the central part of the patella. The patella is usually already fractured when the patient falls to the ground because he or she is unable to maintain knee extension during deceleration. After the fracture, the quadriceps tension lacerates the quadriceps expansions and the retinacular structures, and the bony fragments separate.

Although the fractures from direct trauma are usually stellate or comminuted, direct injuries can cause longitudinal marginal fractures and occasionally transverse fractures. In our series a purely direct injury was found in only 18 percent of cases, while more frequently a mixed injury was reported (30 percent).

In the event of a direct trauma, there is usually an abrasion or contusion on the anterior aspect of the knee. Displacement of the fracture is less important than in fractures from indirect trauma because the retinacular structures are often spared. Open fractures are frequent; they have been found in 7 percent of our patients and in 21 percent in another series.[77]

We believe that most often, although it is difficult to reconstruct the events, a combination of muscle contraction, direct trauma, and joint collapse causes the fracture and the separation. In our series of surgically treated cases, 84 percent were transverse fractures (pure transverse or with some marginal comminution of one of the fragments) and 16 percent were comminuted fractures. Our series does not include longitudinal fractures which we treated conservatively, but for which some favor surgical treatment, particularly when displaced.[4,17] The transverse fractures were located in the middle third (Fig. 15I.1) (31 percent), in the inferior third (Fig. 15I.2), including those called "apical" fractures (31 percent), at the junction between middle and inferior thirds (27 percent), and at the superior third, the so-called basal fracture (3 percent). The distal fragment in transverse fractures may show some comminution (8 percent) (Fig. 15I.3). Severely comminuted fractures were encountered in 16 percent (Fig. 15I.4).

In the series of Ricard and Moulay,[77] type I fractures, (simple transverse) account for 25 percent of cases, type II, (complex transverse, with comminution of one of the fragments, more often the inferior) account for 45 percent of cases, and type III, (totally comminuted) for 20 percent. Two other types can be described (10 percent); fracture of the base, near the quadriceps tendon, which in rare instances can assume the form of an enucleation of the base when the periosteum with some surrounding bone is detached and fracture of the apex when the fracture isolates a distal extra-articular fragment of small dimensions.

Our series as well as others does not include osteochondral fractures of the patella described by Milgram[59] and termed tangential osteochondral fractures. These fractures are usually located at the medial aspect of the patella,[25,91] and although sometimes may follow direct trauma[8] are frequently associated with sports activities[65,67] and acute lateral dislocation of the patella.[25,73,80] During athletic activity, the superolateral pole of the patella may be fractured by uncontrolled muscular activity (vastus lateralis) in a

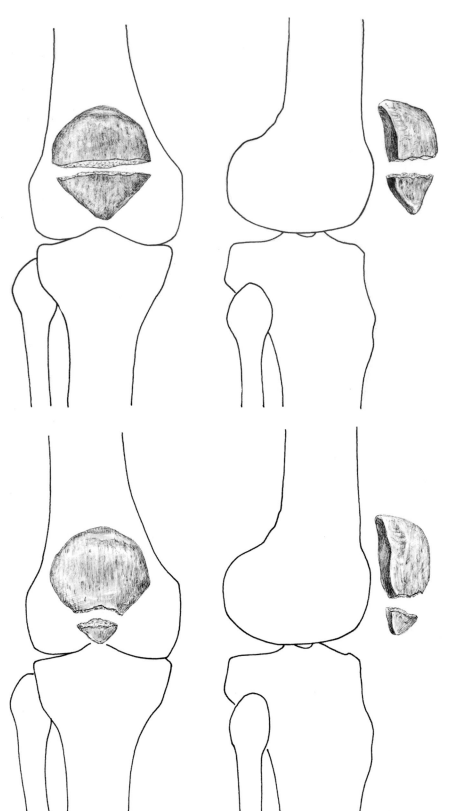

Fig. 151.1. Transverse fracture of the patella in the middle third.

Fig. 151.2. Apical fracture of the patella.

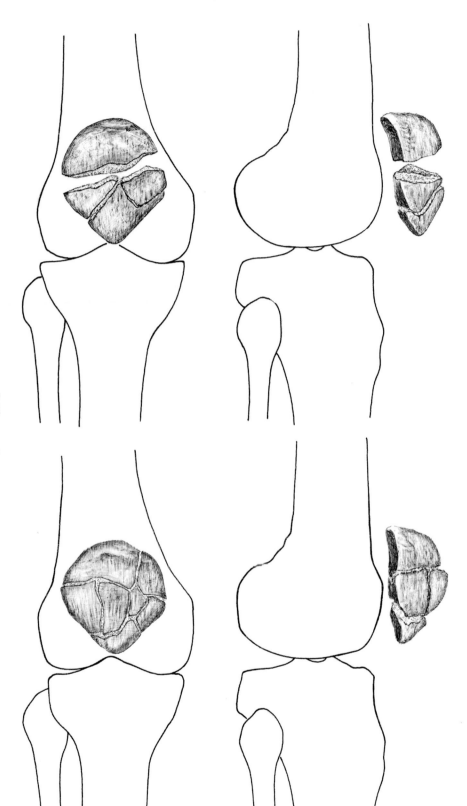

Fig. 151.3. Transverse fracture with comminution of the distal fragment.

Fig. 151.4. Comminuted fracture of the patella.

normal patella, but are more frequently in the presence of a superolateral accessory nucleus.[74,95]

CLINICAL FINDINGS

Usually the clinical diagnosis of fracture of the patella is easy. The joint is swollen by the hemarthrosis. Blood containing fat globules can be aspirated.[37] Sometimes the knee is less distended because of diffusion of the hemorrhage into the soft tissues around the knee. If the fragments are separated, a gap can be clinically appreciated. The patient is usually unable to lift the leg up off the table because of discontinuity of the extensor mechanism. After 1 or 2 days, when the pain has subsided, the patient may be able to lift the leg if the fracture has little displacement and if the quadriceps expansions and retinacular structures are spared.

The diagnosis of certain fractures, like the marginal fractures, osteochondral fractures, longitudinal fractures, and fractures without displacement of the distal nonarticular pole, can be more difficult and require radiologic examination and sometimes arthroscopy.[65]

RADIOLOGIC EVALUATION

Standard anteroposterior and lateral views of the knee are sufficient for the common transverse or comminuted fractures. However, for diagnosis of more difficult fractures, such as marginal or longitudinal ones, oblique and skyline views are necessary. At times, diagnostic techniques such as arthrography[5] are necessary, particularly for osteochondral fractures.

Flexion views may be helpful in deciding the need for surgical treatment in cases of doubt. In fact, the indication is mainly based on clinical findings (e.g., the patient, after the hemarthrosis has been aspirated and pain has subsided, cannot lift the leg). A separation of more than 3 mm and a step-off of more than 2 mm in the articular surfaces of the main fragments are also indications for surgery.

Longitudinal marginal fractures are most often located laterally. As they produce few symptoms and signs, good-quality films, including skyline views, are needed. These fractures are usually located at the junction between the middle and lateral third of the patella. This location differs from the purely supero-

lateral location of the accessory ossification center of the bipartite patella. In this condition, the fracture line is regular and the finding is often bilateral.

CONSERVATIVE TREATMENT

In fractures with minimal displacement, with little or no separation, (including stellate and comminuted fractures) and in many longitudinal fractures, with intact extensor mechanism, conservative treatment gives satisfactory results.

After aspiration of the hemarthrosis, the leg is placed in a plaster cylinder with the knee in a few degrees (5 degrees) of flexion. The plaster should be well molded over the femoral condyles with special felt protection applied over the ankle (to prevent discomfort from the cylinder sliding down).

The plaster cylinder is kept for 3 to 6 weeks. The patient is allowed to walk with two crutches with partial weight-bearing after various intervals of time (1 to 3 weeks), according to the type of fracture and displacement. After removal of the plaster cylinder, joint motion is started, in a gradual, active manner.

SURGICAL TREATMENT

INTERNAL FIXATION

The goal of treatment is to obtain continuity of the extensor mechanism with as normal a patellofemoral congruence as possible. If the treatment is not successful, patellofemoral arthritis,[86] stiffness[41] and quadriceps weakness are common sequelae. Exact anatomic restoration of the fragments and secure fixation to permit early motion must be achieved.

Cameron performed the first open operation on a patellar fracture in 1877 (quoted by Lister[53]). Berger and Quenu first used a metal wire cerclage in 1892.[9] Many surgical techniques are employed for patellar fractures since open reduction and internal fixation was shown to give better results and have several advantages over conservative treatment in displaced fractures of the patella.

Cerclage is recommended by many workers.[3,6,13,26,56,58,70] Magnuson[56] and Payr[70] described the technique of passing wires through vertical longitudinal holes, Anderson[3] the standard circumferential equatorially wiring, and Böhler[12] recommended the transverse drill-hole technique. All three methods employ cast immobilization ranging from 4 to 6 weeks.

Thomson[88,89] introduced the partial patellectomy method and Blodgett and Fairchild[11] and Brooke[14] the total patellectomy. Some use a longitudinal screw in certain cases of transverse or longitudinal fractures.[27,62,85]

During the last 15 years, the Association for the Study of Internal Fixation (ASIF) school has diffused and popularized the technique of tension cerclage either alone or associated with longitudinal K wires. This technique does not usually require cast immobilization. This technique and the results of tension cerclage have been studied by many investigators.[10,33,48,61,62,69,92]

The two stainless-steel wires (1.2 mm) are introduced anteriorly through the quadriceps and patellar tendons. One of them can be placed in a figure 8 fashion (Fig. 151.5). This method ensures that the wire is anterior to the patella. Tightening of the wires overreduces the transverse fracture, but when the knee is flexed the pressure of the femoral condyles against the patella transforms the traction or tension into interfragmentary compression. Two twisting sites of the wires allow greater compression.[82] This technique (Fig. 151.6) can be used in association with two longitudinally inserted and parallel K wires to avoid tilting of the distal fragment. The same technique has also been used (with K wires) in comminuted fractures with more difficulty.

The knee is mobilized very early and usually no cast is needed. It is kept in a position of flexion of 20 to 25 degrees and further flexion is encouraged toward 70 degrees; no extension beyond 20 degrees is allowed for the first 3 weeks. Partial weight-bearing is allowed after 4 weeks. Cast immobilization is needed only in case of insufficient reduction and fixation.

The efficacy of various forms of fixation of transverse fractures of the patella was tested in cadavers with experimentally produced fractures.[96] Four fixation techniques were tested; standard circumferential wiring,[3] vertical wiring through drill holes,[56,70] standard tension band wiring anterior to the patella,[62] and "modified" tension band wiring, with two longitudinal K wires across the fracture.[62] In this latter case, the wire loop was passed behind the tips of the K wires and over the anterior surface of the patella. The behavior of the fracture was observed and measured

in terms of separation between the fragments through the arc of motion against resistance, from 90 degrees of flexion to extension and vice versa, with the different techniques and with or without retinacular repair.

In circumferential wiring there was separation from 90 to 30 degrees; from 30 to 0 degrees there was a posterior angulation with an articular surface gap, even after the quadriceps was relaxed. When the retinaculum was repaired, the extent of the gap was reduced. In vertical wiring only a small articular surface gap that increased toward full extension was observed. This decreased after retinacular repair. In tension band wiring, at 90 degrees of flexion, with the quadriceps relaxed, the articular surface was distracted by posterior angulation. Moving toward extension, this tended to decrease, to a complete closure at 60 degrees. From 30 to 0 degrees there was again posterior angulation. At full extension this angulation reached its maximum. This was lessened somewhat by retinacular repair, but there was considerable variability. In the "modified" tension band wiring no separation was measured through the entire range of motion.

Thus, with knee motion, there are stresses at the fracture site, particularly toward extension. Tension band wiring, for which early motion has been widely suggested, did not entirely prevent separation of the fragments. The Magnuson technique (vertical wiring)[56] was actually better, at least from 90 to 10 degrees, with minimum separation from 10 to 0 degrees. The circumferential technique was not effective in fixation. The modified tension band wiring with the wire loop anchored to K wires was best; there was no separation from 90 to 0 degrees after repetitive cycles of flexion–extension.

PARTIAL PATELLECTOMY

Partial patellectomy, with removal of the usually distal small fragment or fragments, can be used as an alternative to internal fixation, particularly when there is one large and one or more small fragments. The large fragment can be saved. This operation requires the suturing of the patellar tendon with nonabsorbable sutures to the patella through vertical bone tunnels. Care should be taken to prevent tilting of the remaining patellar fragment. The bone should be nes-

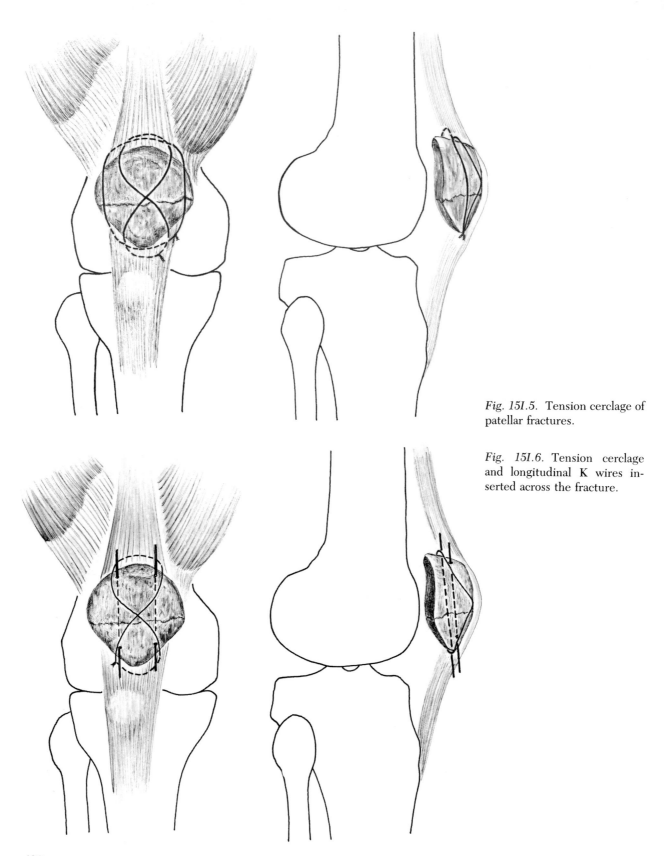

Fig. 151.5. Tension cerclage of patellar fractures.

Fig. 151.6. Tension cerclage and longitudinal K wires inserted across the fracture.

tled within the tendon. Multiple drill holes are bored and the tendon fixed to the fragment, nestling the bone into the tendon in a layered fashion. An overlapping repair of the aponeurosis is done after the surface of the bone has been denuded and the tendon is sutured near the articular cartilage of the main fragment, to avoid tilting.[31] A special technique, requiring the saving of a small fragment with the attached patellar tendon and the placement of it inside a crater in the proximal large fragment, has also been studied.[63,77] In most cases, partial (distal) patellectomy has been used as an alternative method to internal fixation, but some use it routinely, claiming better results than osteosynthesis.[4,17,26] After partial patellectomy, cast immobilization is needed for 3 to 4 weeks.

TOTAL PATELLECTOMY

Only in severely comminuted fractures with no large fragments can total patellectomy be recommended.[18,27,28,34,41,42,85] The quadriceps tendon is sutured to the patellar ligament. Patellectomy, with removal of all the fragments, is usually done by an extraperiosteal method; the repair is end to end or *en paletot* to avoid laxity. An overlapping suture reinforced with a triangular flap created from the quadriceps tendon[19,84] or a vastus medialis advancement,[97] can be used. The suture must allow immediate flexion to 80 to 90 degrees on the operating room table. A cast or removable splint is applied for an average of 3 weeks. We believe that total patellectomy should be used only when it is impossible to achieve anatomic or near-anatomic repositioning of all the multiple fragments.

In fact, considerable controversy exists as to the results of patellectomy for fractures. Some report good results.[11,14,16,18,19,20,30,54,60,71,94,97] The frequently observed calcifications are believed to be the origin of problems by some workers,[31,93] but have not proved to be the cause of pain and osteoarthritis by others.[19,60] Still others believe these calcifications are actually advantageous because they simulate a new patella.[30] All the investigators underline the need for prolonged physical therapy. Others report frequent unsatisfactory results.[27,32,83] Experimentally it has been shown that the patella has its own important functions in the knee[43,44]; in animal studies its removal has been shown to cause degeneration.[15,21,29,35] A partial pa-

tellectomy produces a slight reduction in the extension force, but a total patellectomy might reduce extensor apparatus power beyond the limits of compensation.[45,87] The patella is an important component of the extensor mechanism of the knee, designed to increase its mechanical advantage.[68,72] We therefore believe that fractured patellae should be repaired rather than excised, whenever possible.

The surgical incisions employed for patellar fracture surgery can be longitudinal or transverse. We find that longitudinal incisions heal better, although transverse incisions are more cosmetic. We have never used the lateral parapatellar incision,[4] but believe it can be advantageous. An essential step of all surgical procedures is repair of the quadriceps expansions and retinacular structures on both sides of the patella.[3,13,38,40,41,47,62,83,86]

COMPLICATIONS

In our series of surgically treated patellar fractures,[1] 80 were treated with internal fixation, 26 with partial patellectomy, and nine with total patellectomy.

In the 80 cases treated with *osteosynthesis*, the complications were four infections (5 percent), four pseudoarthroses (5 percent), two loss of reduction with redisplacement of the fragments (2.5 percent), and two clinically diagnosed deep vein thromboses (2.5 percent). Of the four infections, two healed without sequelae, one required patellectomy for an infected pseudoarthrosis (poor result), and one healed with a fair functional result. The four aseptic pseudoarthroses were caused by insufficient fixation in cases of distal fragment comminution, one case with circumferential wiring, two cases with tension cerclage without K wires and one with cerclage and thin 1-mm wires. The final result after partial patellectomy was poor in two, fair in one, and good in the other. The two cases with displacement of the fragments were caused by insufficient fixation, one after a tension cerclage with thin wires and one after a circumferential wiring. In both cases, the cerclage lost tension and the fragments were displaced. Both required reoperation with good functional results. A late breakage of the wires is a frequent possibility after union, but has no relevance on the result.

For the *partial patellectomy* group, the complications were: two with early failure of the sutures (8 percent); both required reoperation with one good and one fair result attributable to stiffness. The proximal fragment tilted in two (8 percent) with reoperation required in both, one for patellectomy with a fair final result and one for a new surgical repair of the suture with a poor result. One deep infection (4 percent) healed conservatively, but with a poor functional result, and there was one deep vein thrombosis (4 percent).

In the *total patellectomy* group, the complications were one infection (11 percent), in a case of open fracture that obtained a fair result after debridement, and one deep vein thrombosis (11 percent).

RESULTS

Our 115 cases were treated with osteosynthesis, partial patellectomy, or total patellectomy.

Of the 80 cases treated with *osteosynthesis*, a traditional circumferential cerclage was used in 14 with chromic catgut (Fig. 15I.7) or metal wiring, followed by a cast for 5 to 6 weeks. Most were treated by tension cerclage with metal wiring (Figs. 15I.8–10), by one or two simple anterior cerclages in 42 (15 of which also had a posterior splint), and by a modified anterior cerclage (Figs. 15I.11 and 15I.12) anchored over two K wires in 24 (a posterior splint was used in 16 knees). In one exceptional case, a screw was used for fixation (Fig. 15I.13).

The partial patellectomy done in 26 cases was used as an alternative method in cases of comminution of the distal fragment with one large proximal fragment. The tendon (usually without bony fragments) was sutured to the proximal fragment with nonabsorbable material through transosseous drill holes. The total patellectomy done in nine cases of comminuted fracture was performed with the end-to-end technique or the *en paletot* overlapping suture. This was done in six cases of severe comminution or in cases of comminution and severe open wounds (three cases). After partial patellectomy a cast was applied for 4 weeks and after the total patellectomies for 5 weeks, on average.

The results were evaluated using a modified Hospital for Special Surgery (HSS) knee score.[78] An excellent result has 95 to 100 points, good 85 to 94, fair 75 to 84, and poor below 75. The follow-up ranges from 1 to 4 years, and is 2 years on average.

Osteosynthesis. Results were 32 excellent (40 percent), 36 good (45 percent), eight fair (10 percent), and four poor (5 percent). The four poor results were attributable to infected pseudoarthrosis (one case), pseudoarthrosis (two cases), and pain and stiffness (one case).

Pain was absent or slight and occasional in 63 cases (79 percent), and present to a varying degree, usually moderate, in 17 cases (21 percent). It was severe only in one case, with early patellofemoral osteoarthritis and suspected reflex sympathetic dystrophy. Muscle atrophy was absent in 48 cases (60 percent), in 20 (25 percent) there was 1-cm atrophy, and in 10 (12.5 percent) 1 to 2 cm atrophy. Only in two cases (2.5 percent) was there an atrophy of more than 2 cm. Muscle strength (clinical evaluation) was normal in 58 cases (72 percent), good (slight weakness) in 11 cases (14 percent) and fair (quadriceps could be broken) in 11 cases (14 percent). Fast extension (clinically evaluated) was found to be slower in eight cases in which the muscle strength had been found excellent or good. In only three cases was there a slight (5-degree) extension lag.

As far as arc of motion, full extension was present in 71 cases (89 percent) and in nine cases there was up to 10 degrees of flexion contracture (11 percent). Maximum flexion was complete and normal (greater than 135 degrees) in 47 cases (59 percent), greater than 90 degrees in 25 (31 percent), and less than 90 degrees in eight (10 percent).

As far as degree of reduction and maintenance of reduction, a "perfect" reduction was achieved at surgery in 71 cases (89 percent) and an incomplete reduction (greater than 2 mm of step-off or gap) in nine knees (11 percent). At follow-up in six additional cases (three of the six with traditional circumferential wiring), reduction was not maintained. Time to union as seen radiologically took 45 days in 68 cases (85 percent) and 60 days in the remaining eight.

Osteoarthritis was absent in most cases (67 knees, or 84 percent). It was slight in 12 knees (15 percent), but in five of these patients it was already present before operation. It was severe only in one case. We could not find a precise relationship between degree of reduction and degree of osteoarthritis.

Calcifications or ossifications were seen in 51 cases (64 percent). Most were located in the peripatellar areas, but some were in the patellar or quadriceps tendons. There was no relationship of calcification with degree of flexion, pain or osteoarthritis. The longi-

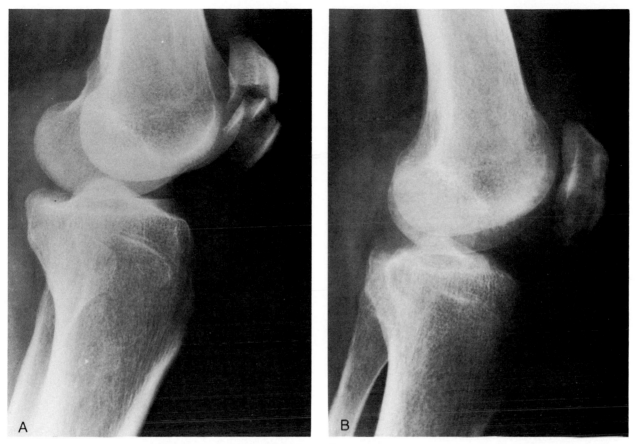

Fig. 151.7. (A) Transverse patellar fracture. Treated with traditional circumferential cerclage with chromic catgut; (B) showing good result after 6 weeks of cast immobilization.

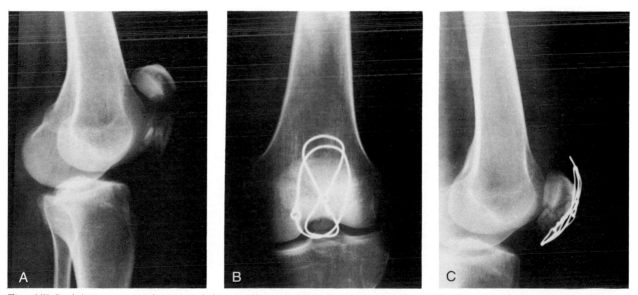

Fig. 151.8. (A) Transverse fracture of the patella with some distal fragment comminution. (B,C) Treated with tension band cerclage with two wires; after 1 month, the fracture shows good healing, with a little step on the articular surface.

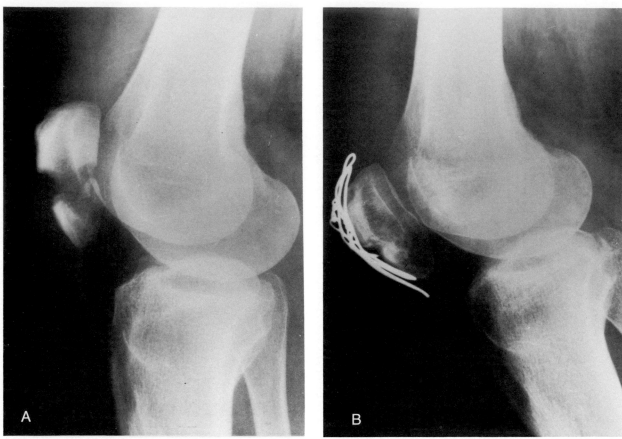

Fig. 151.9. (A) Transverse fracture of the patella at the middle-distal third with some interfragmentary comminution. (B) Treated with tension band cerclage; showing excellent result at 6 months. (From Aglietti, P., and Scarfi, G.: Trattamento chirurgico delle fratture di rotula. Archivio Putti, *30*: 301, 1980, with permission.)

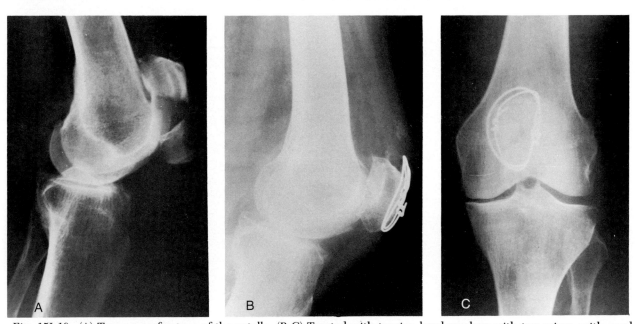

Fig. 151.10. (A) Transverse fracture of the patella. (B,C) Treated with tension band cerclage with two wires; with good result at 2 years. (From Aglietti, P., and Scarfi, G.: Trattamento chirurgico delle fratture di rotula. Archivio Putti, *30*: 301, 1980, with permission.)

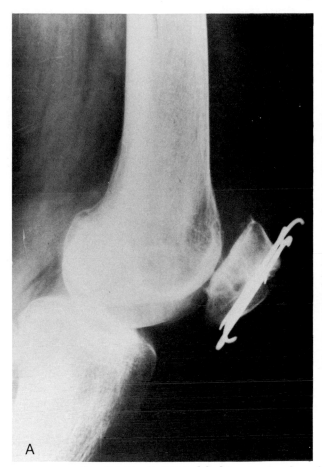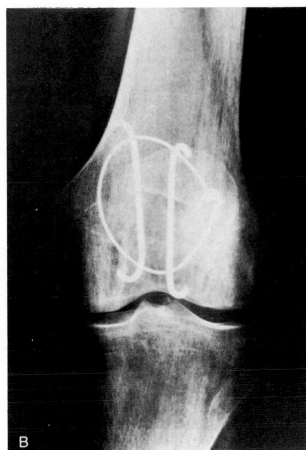

Fig. 151.11. (A,B) Modified tension band cerclage with one cerclage wire and two K wires.

tudinal length of the patella was increased in 12 cases (15 percent); there was again no relationship with osteoarthritis.

Age did not seem to influence the results, as excellent or good results were obtained in 87 percent below 48 years and in 83 percent above this age. If the trauma was from a vehicular accident or a fall from a height or when there were associated fractures, excellent or good results were obtained in 78 percent. Open fractures had 81 percent excellent or good results. The level of fracture influenced the prognosis with 90 percent excellent or good in the basal or apical fractures. The best results were obtained by the tension band wiring technique (88 percent excellent or good) as compared with traditional circumferential wiring (79 percent).

In conclusion, the results of our osteosynthesis operations were similar to those found in other statistics.[6] Ricard and Moulay[77] reported 82 percent excellent and good results (mainly after classic cerclage) and quote other series as having 79 to 86 percent acceptable results.

Partial Patellectomy.   All cases were treated with the "nestling" technique described earlier (Fig. 151.14). The results were eight excellent (31 percent), 12 good (46 percent), four fair (15 percent), and two poor (8 percent). The two poor results were attributable to one infection and one tilting of the proximal fragment.

Pain was absent or slight in 21 cases (80 percent), present in the remaining five cases (20 percent), but severe in only one. Muscular atrophy was absent in 13 cases (50 percent), in seven cases there was 1-cm atrophy (27 percent), and in six (23 percent) atrophy was up to 2 cm. Muscle strength was normal in 17 cases (65 percent), good in five (20 percent), and fair in four (15 percent). In three cases with normal

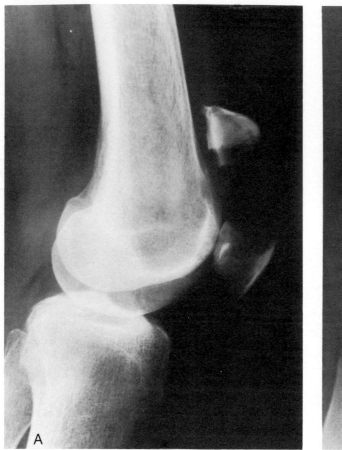
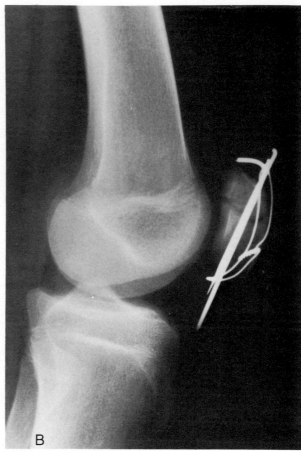

Fig. 151.12. (A) Transverse fracture of the patella. (B) Treated with modified tension cerclage. The K pins were too long and had to be removed at 3 months after secure healing of the fracture. (From Aglietti, P., and Scarfi, G.: Trattamento chirurgico delle fratture di rotula. Archivio Putti, *30*: 301, 1980, with permission.)

strength, extension was slower. In two cases there was a slight (5-degree) extension lag.

In three cases (11.5 percent) there was a flexion contracture (up to 10 degrees). Complete maximum flexion was present in 14 cases (54 percent), while in eight (31 percent) it was incomplete but greater than 90 degrees, and in four (15 percent) less than 90 degrees.

Slight osteoarthritis was present in four cases (15 percent) and in two it was there before operation. Only one case had severe osteoarthritis.

Radiologically observed calcifications were found in 15 cases (57 percent), but they did not have any relationship with the quality of result. The same applied to a slight patellar tilting present in four cases (15 percent).

Age did not influence the results, as excellent or good results were obtained in 76 percent of cases above and 78 percent of cases below age 48. In cases of open fractures there were 75 percent excellent or good results, with associated fractures 73 percent. Apical extra-articular fractures carry the best prognosis after this operation (82 percent excellent or good).

Comparing our results with those of others, Thomson found 81 percent of excellent or good results, in Burny's series the results were better than osteosynthesis, and in Ricard and Moulay's series excellent or good results were obtained in 79 percent of the cases (approximately the same as after osteosynthesis).

Total Patellectomy. The results have been two excellent (22 percent), three good (33 percent), three fair (33 percent), and one poor (12 percent). Residual

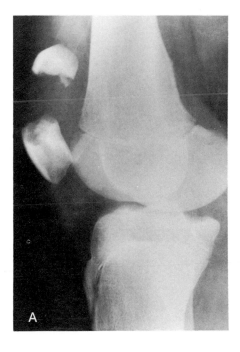
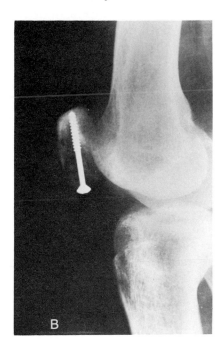

Fig. 151.13. (A) Transverse fracture of the upper third of the patella. (B) Treated with a screw; showing good result at 1 year. (From Aglietti, P., and Scarfi, G.: Trattamento chirurgico delle fratture di rotula. Archivio Putti, *30*: 301, 1980, with permission.)

pain was present in two cases and was classified as moderate. Muscle atrophy was present in six cases (66.5 percent), in four up to 1 cm and in two up to 2 cm, and absent in three cases (33.5 percent). Muscle strength was normal in four cases (44 percent), good in four (44 percent), and fair in one (12 percent). Ex-

tension was slower in four cases (44 percent), and an extension lag was present in two cases (22 percent).

No knees had a flexion contracture, and maximum flexion was normal in seven cases (78 percent) and greater than 90 degrees in the remaining two cases.

There were no cases of osteoarthritis; calcifications

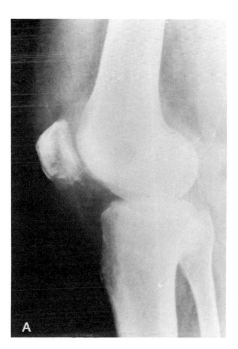
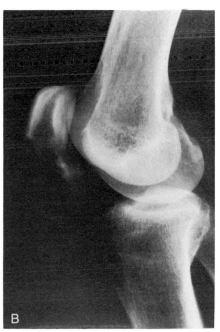

Fig. 151.14. (A) Distal patellar fracture of the apex. (B) Treated with partial patellectomy. Good result at 1 year. (From Aglietti, P., and Scarfi, G.: Trattamento chirurgico delle fratture di rotula. Archivio Putti, *30*: 301, 1980, with permission.)

were observed in four cases without apparent influence on the result. Age seemed to have an influence on the results, as most of the unsatisfactory results were after 50 years.

Comparing our results with other statistics, West[97] reported 69 percent of acceptable results, Castaing[19] 82 percent, and Ricard and Moulay[77] 69 percent.

CONCLUSIONS

We believe that the best form of surgical treatment for patellar fractures is the tension cerclage suture. It has the advantage of allowing early motion. Not all fractures can be treated in the same manner. The indications of the tension cerclage method can be expanded if the modified technique, with vertical K wires, is used. When this method is not applicable, we suggest the use of partial patellectomy for fractures with comminution of the distal third and total patellectomy for severe comminution.

REFERENCES

1. Aglietti, P., and Scarfi, G.: Trattamento chirurgico delle fratture di rotula. Arch. Putti, *30:* 301, 1980.
2. Aglietti, P., Insall, J.N., Walker, P.S., et al.: A new patella prosthesis. Design and application. Clin. Orthop., *107:* 175, 1975.
3. Anderson, L.D.: Fractures, pp 477–691. In Crenshaw, A.H. (ed.): Campbell's Operative Orthopaedics, 5th Ed. St. Louis, C.V. Mosby, 1971.
4. Andrews, J.R., and Hughston, J.C.: Treatment of patellar fractures by partial patellectomy. South. Med. J., *70:* 809, 1977.
5. Ashby, M.E., Shields, C.L., and Karmy, J.: Diagnosis of osteochondral fractures in acute traumatic patellar dislocations using air arthrography. J. Trauma, *15:* 1032, 1975.
6. Assennato, G.: Fratture della rotula. Giorn. Ital. Ortop. Traum., *III:* 145, 1977.
7. Baumgartl, F.: Das Kniegelenk. Berlin, Springer Verlag, 1964.
8. Beltrami, P., and Travaglini, F.: Le fratture sotto condrali della regione femororotulea. Arch. Ortop., *81:* 331, 1968.
9. Berger, and Quenu, B.: Suture de la rotule par un procédé nouveau (cerclage de la rotule). Soc. Chir. Paris, *18:* 523, 1892.
10. Bianchi Maiocchi, A., Bombelli, R., and Benedetti, G.B.: Le osteosintesi. A. Gaggi, ed. Bologna, Tecnica ica AO. 1971.
11. Blodgett, W.E., and Fairchild, R.D.: Fractures of the patella. J.A.M.A., *106:* 2121, 1936.
12. Boehler, L.: Die technik der Knochenbruchbehandlung. Vien, 12–13th ed. Vol 2 Part 2 Wein Maudrich, 1957.
13. Boström, A.: Fracture of the patella. Acta Orthop. Scand. (Suppl.), *143:* 1, 1972.
14. Brooke, R.: The treatment of fractured patella by excision. A study of morphology and function. Br. J. Surg., *24:* 733, 1937.
15. Bruce, J., and Walmsley, R.: Excision of the patella. Some experimental and anatomical observations. J. Bone Joint Surg., *24:* 311, 1942.
16. Boucher, H.H.: Patellectomy in the geriatric patient. Clin. Orthop., *11:* 33, 1958.
17. Burny, F.: Résultats éloignés du traitement des fractures récentes de la rotule. Acta Orthop. Belg., *35:* 392, 1969.
18. Cabanac, J.: La place de la patellectomie dans les fractures récentes de la rotule. S.O.F.C.O.T. XLVI réunion annuelle. Rev. Chir. Orthop., *58(Suppl 1):* 388, 1972.
19. Castaing, J., Castellani, L., Plisson, J.L., et al.: La patellectomie totale: Technique et résultats. Rev. Chir. Orthop., *55:* 259, 1969.
20. Castaing, J., El Hasar, S., Burdin, Ph., et al.: Etude de 113 cas de fractures de la rotule (ostéosynthèse ou patellectomie?). Ann. Orthop. Ouest, *8:* 33, 1976.
21. Cohn, B. N.E.: Total and partial patellectomy. Surg. Gynecol. Obstet., *79:* 526, 1944.
22. Corner, E.M.: Figures about fractures and refractures of the patella. Ann. Surg., *52:* 707, 1910.
23. Crock, H.V.: The arterial supply and venous drainage of the bones of the human knee joint. Anat. Rec., *144:* 199, 1962.
24. Cross, M.J., and Waldrop, J.: The patella index as a guide to the understanding and diagnosis of the patellofemoral instability. Clin. Orthop., *110:* 174, 1975.
25. Dejour, H., and Chambat, P.: Les fractures ostéochondrales. pp. 139–146. In Duparc J. et al. (eds.): Les fractures du genou. Paris, Expansion Scientifique Française, 1975. (Cahiers d'enseignement de la S.O.F.C.O.T: I)
26. Delplace, J., and Hussenstein, J.: Avantages de l'ostéosynthèse adaptée dans les fractures de la rotule. Ann. Chir., *26:* 1225, 1972.
27. DePalma, A.F.: Diseases of the Knee. Philadelphia, J.B. Lippincott, 1954.
28. DePalma, A.F.: The management of fractures and dislocations. Philadelphia, W.B. Saunders, 1959.
29. DePalma, A.F., and Flynn, J.J.: Joint changes follow-

ing experimental partial and total patellectomy. J. Bone Joint Surg. [Am.], *40:* 395, 1958.

30. Dobbie, R.P., and Ryerson, S.: The treatment of fractured patella by excision. Am. J. Surg., *55:* 339, 1942.

31. Duthie, H.L., and Hutchinson, J.R.: The results of partial and total excision of the patella. J. Bone Joint Surg. [Br.], *40:* 75, 1958.

32. Fairbank, H.A.T.: Excision of the patella. Br. Med. J., *2:* 62, 1945.

33. Ferrini, L., and Pecorelli, F.: Osteosintesi delle fratture di rotula con la tecnica del "tirante". Arch. Putti, *29:* 299, 1978.

34. Flinchum, D.: Patellectomy: When, why and how. South. Med. J., *59:* 897, 1966.

35. Garr, E.L., Moskowitz, R.W., and Davis, W.: Degenerative changes following experimental patellectomy in the rabbit. Clin. Orthop., *92:* 296, 1973.

36. Goodfellow, J., Hungerford, D.S., and Zindel, M.: Patellofemoral joint mechanics and pathology, I: Functional anatomy of the patellofemoral joint. J. Bone Joint Surg. [Br.], *58:* 287, 1976.

37. Gregg, J.R., Nixon, J.E., and DiStefano, V.: Neutral fat globules in traumatized knees. Clin. Orthop., *132:* 219, 1978.

38. Griswold, A.S.: Fractures of the patella. Clin. Orthop., *4:* 44, 1954.

39. Haffajee, D., Moritz, U., and Svantesson, G.: Isometric knee extension strength as a function of joint angle, muscle length and motor unit activity. Acta Orthop. Scand., *43:* 138, 1972.

40. Hipps, H.E.: Surgical repair of patellar fractures. Comparative analysis of various techniques. Am. J. Surg., *101:* 198, 1961.

41. Hohl, M., and Larson, R.L.: Fractures and dislocations of the knee. P. 1131. In Rockwood, C.A., Jr., and Green, D.P. (eds.): Fractures (Vol II). Philadelphia, J.B. Lippincott, 1975.

42. Horwitz, T., and Lambert, R.G.: Patellectomy in the military service. Surg. Gynecol. Obstet., *82:* 423, 1946.

43. Jensenius, H.: On the results of excision of fractured patella. Acta Chir. Scand., *102:* 275, 1952.

44. Kaplan, E.B.: The lateral meniscofemoral ligament of the knee joint. Bull. Hosp. Joint Dis., *17:* 176, 1956.

45. Kaufer, H.: Mechanical function of the patella. J. Bone Joint Surg. [Am.], *53:* 1551, 1971.

46. Kettelkamp, D.B., and De Rosa, G.P.: Biomechanics and functional role of the patellofemoral joint. In Instructional Course Lectures. The American Academy of Orthopedic Surgeons. St. Louis, The C.V. Mosby Co., *25:* 27, 1976.

47. Kopell, H.P., and Thompson, W.A.: Patellar fracture and repair of the patellar retinacula. Gen. Pract.: *26:* 112, 1962

48. Labitzke, R.: Laterale Zuggurtung. Arch. Orthop. Unfallchir., *90:* 77, 1977.

49. Lapidus, P.W.: Longitudinal fractures of the patella. J. Bone Joint Surg., *14:* 351, 1932.

50. Last, R.J.: Some anatomical details of the knee joint. J. Bone Joint Surg. [Br.], *30:* 683, 1948.

51. Laurin, C.A., Levesque, H.P., Dussault, R., et al.: The abnormal lateral patellofemoral angle. A diagnostic roentgenographic sign of recurrent patellar subluxation. J. Bone Joint Surg. [Am.], *60:* 55, 1978.

52. Lieb, F.J., and Perry, J.: Quadriceps function. An anatomical and mechanical study using amputated limbs. J. Bone Joint Surg. [Am.], *50:* 1535, 1968.

53. Lister, J.: An address on the treatment of fracture of the patella. Br. Med. J., *2:* 855, 1883.

54. MacAusland, W.R.: Total excision of the patella for fracture. Report of fourteen cases. Am. J. Surg., *72:* 510, 1946.

55. Madigan, R., Wissinger, H.A., and Donaldson, W.F.: Preliminary experience with a method of quadricepsplasty in recurrent subluxation of the patella. J. Bone Joint Surg. [Am.], *57:* 600, 1975.

56. Magnuson, P.B.: Fractures, 2nd ed. Philadelphia, J.B. Lippincott, 1933.

57. Matthews, L.S., Sonstegard, D.A., and Henke, J.A.: Load bearing characteristics of the patellofemoral joint. Acta Orthop. Scand., *48:* 511, 1977.

58. McConnell, B.E.: An operation for fractures of the patella using the temporary patellar tendon substitution technic. South. Med. J., *69:* 87, 1971.

59. Milgram, J.E.: Tangential osteochondral fracture of the patella. J. Bone Joint Surg., *25:* 271, 1943.

60. Mishra, U.S.: Late results of patellectomy in fractured patella. Acta Orthop. Scand., *43:* 256, 1972.

61. Mordente, G., and Ceffa, A.: L'osteosintesi mediante doppio cerchiaggio epirotuleo nelle fratture trasversali diastasate di rotula. Minerva Ortop., *27:* 185, 1976.

62. Müller, M.E., Allgöwer, M., and Willenegger, H.: Manuel d'ostéosynthèse. Masson, Paris, 1970.

63. Neidhardt, J.H., Morin, A., Barbe, Ch., et al.: L'encastrement des fragments dans le traitement des fractures de la rotule. Lyon Chir., *69:* 391, 1973.

64. Nixon, J.E., and DiStefano, V.J.: Injuries of the knee; fractures of the patella. P. 745. In Heppenstall, R.B.: Fracture Treatment and Healing. Philadelphia, W.B. Saunders, 1980.

65. Noyes, F.R., Bassett, R.W., Grood, E.S., et al.: Arthroscopy in acute traumatic hemarthrosis of the knee. Incidence of anterior cruciate tears and other injuries. J. Bone Joint Surg. [Am.], *62:* 687, 1980.

66. Nummi, J.: Fractures of the patella. A clinical study of 707 patellar fractures. Ann. Chir. Gynaecol. Fenn., *179(Suppl.):* 1, 1971.

67. O'Donoghue, D.H.: Chondral and osteochondral fractures. J. Trauma, *6:* 469, 1966.

68. O'Donoghue, D.H., Tompkins, F., and Hays M.B.: Strength of quadriceps function after patellectomy. West. J. Surg. Gynecol. Obstet., *60:* 159, 1952.

69. Pauwels, F.: Le Hauban. Son rôle dans las sollecitation des os longs. Son emploi dans l'osteosynthèse de compression. In La Fization Externe en Chirugie, 5–30. Symposium du 19 novembre 1965, Université de Bruxelles.

70. Payr, E.: Zur operativen behandlung der kniegelenksteife nach langdauernder ruhigstellung. Zentralb. Chir., *44:* 809, 1917.

71. Peeples, R.E., and Margo, M.K.: Function after patellectomy. Clin. Orthop., *132:* 180, 1978.

72. Perry, J., Antonelli, D., and Ford, W.: Analysis of knee joint forces during flexed knee stance. J. Bone Joint Surg. [Am.], *57:* 961, 1975.

73. Puddu, G., and Mariani, P.: Le fratture osteocondrali del giocchio. Giorn. Ital. Ortop. Traum. Suppl., *I:* 135, 1977.

74. Puddu, G., Mariani, P., and Alzani, R.: La sindrome da mobilizzazione del nucleo accesorio della rotula. Giorn. Ital. Ortop. Traum., *4:* 193, 1978.

75. Reider, B., Marshall, J.L., Koslin, B., et al.: The anterior aspect of the knee joint. An anatomical study. J. Bone Joint Surg. [Am.], *63:* 351, 1981.

76. Reilly, D.T., and Martens, M.: Experimental analysis of the quadriceps muscle force and patellofemoral joint reaction force for various activities. Acta Orthop. Scand., *43:* 126, 1972.

77. Ricard, R., and Moulay, A.: Les fractures de la rotule. P. 75. In Duparc J., et al. (eds.): Les Fractures du Genou (Cahiers d'enseignement de la Expansion Scientifique Française, Paris, 1975, SOFCOT, I.)

78. Rinonapoli, E., and Aglietti, P.: Confronto tra casistiche omogenee di fratture articolari del l'estremo prossimale della tibia trattate incruentemente e cruentemente. Giorn. Ital. Ortop. Traum., Suppl., *III:* 105, 1977.

79. Roberts, J.M.: The surgical knee. Surg. Chir. North Am., *54:* 1313, 1974.

80. Rorabeck, C.H., and Bobechko, W.P.: Acute dislocation of the patella with osteochondral fracture. J. Bone Joint Surg. [Br.], *58:* 237, 1976.

81. Scapinelli, R.: Blood supply of the human patella. Its relation to ischaemic necrosis after fracture. J. Bone Joint Surg. [Br.], *49:* 563, 1967.

82. Schauwecker, F.: The Practice of Osteosynthesis. Stuttgart, Georg Thieme, 1974.

83. Scott, J.C.: Fractures of the patella. J. Bone Joint Surg. [Br.], *31:* 76, 1949.

84. Shorbe, H.B., and Dobson, C.H.: Patellectomy. Repair of the extensor mechanism. J. Bone Joint Surg. [Am.], *40:* 1281, 1958.

85. Smillie, I.S.: Injuries of the knee joint. 4th ed. Edinburgh, Livingstone, 1970.

86. Sorensen, K.H.: The late prognosis after fracture of the patella. Acta Orthop. Scand., *34:* 198, 1964.

87. Sutton, F.S., Thompson, C.H., Lipke, J., et al.: The effect of patellectomy on knee function. J. Bone Joint Surg. [Am.], *58:* 537, 1976.

88. Thomson, J.E.M.: Comminuted fractures of the patella. Treatment of cases presenting one large fragment and several small fragments. J. Bone Joint Surg., *17:* 431, 1935.

89. Thomson, J.E.M.: Fracture of the patella treated by removal of the loose fragments and plastic repair of the tendon. A study of 554 cases. Surg. Gynecol. Obstet., *74:* 860, 1942.

90. Thorstensson, A., Grimby, G., and Karlsson, J.: Force–velocity relations and fiber composition in human knee extensor muscles. J. Appl. Physiol., *40:* 12, 1976.

91. Trillat, A., Dejour, H.: Les fractures chondro-osseuses du versant articulaire interne de la rotule. Rev. Chir. Orthop., *53:* 331, 1967.

92. Vasciaveo, F.: L'osteosintesi a compressione secondo Pauwels nel trattamento delle fratture dell'olecrano e della rotula. Atti SERTOT, *16:* 35, 1974.

93. Wass, S.H., and Davies, E.R.: Excision of the patella for fracture with remarks on ossification in the quadriceps tendon following the operation. Guys Hosp. Rep., *91:* 35, 1942.

94. Watson Jones, R.: Fractures and Joint Injuries. 4th ed. Baltimore, Williams and Wilkins, 1952.

95. Weaver, J.K.: Bipartite patellae as a cause of disability in the athlete. Am. J. Sports Med., *5:* 137, 1977.

96. Weber, M.J., Janecki, C.J., McLeod, P., et al.: Efficacy of various forms of fixation of transverse fractures of the patella. J. Bone Joint Surg. [Am.], *62:* 215, 1980.

97. West, F.E.: End results of patellectomy. J. Bone Joint Surg. [Am.], *44:* 1089, 1962.

98. Wiberg, G.: Roentgenographic and anatomic studies on the femoropatellar joint. Acta Orthop. Scand., *12:* 319, 1941.

Part II Fractures of the Distal Femur

Fractures of the distal femur are defined as fractures involving the distal 10–15 cm of the femur and may involve the condyles and the articular surfaces. Stiffness is the most important problem associated with these fractures, occurring more frequently than with fractures of the proximal tibia. The reduction and the fixation of the frequently multiple fragments can be very difficult as well as restoration of correct limb alignment. Sir Watson-Jones[87] noted that "few injuries present more difficult problems" than fractures of the distal femur.

ANATOMY

Most fractures of the distal femur are of the split type, with separation, while the osteochondral crush or compression characteristic of the tibial plateau fracture is rarely seen.[30] The "weakness points" in the distal femur are located in a sagittal plane through the intercondylar notch, where the patella can act as a wedge. The area of transition between the cortical bone and the trabecular bone is another point of weakness. Because of the linea aspera and the resistance of the anterior cortex of the shaft, critical or weakness points are also located in a frontal plane oblique from proximal to distal and from posterior to anterior.

In the condyles of the femur the critical points start at the condylotrochlear (or patellar) groove, which is at the junction of the trochlea with the medial or lateral condyles. From this typical location the fracture follows a frontal, sagittal, or oblique plane in each condyle.[79] The groove on the lateral femoral condyle is more pronounced than on the medial condyle. This groove divides the articular surface of the lateral condyle in half. On the medial condyle a less prominent groove separates the anterior one-third of the articular surface from the posterior two-thirds.[22]

Two forces produce the deformities: the initial trauma and the imbalance of muscle action. Four large muscle groups are important: the quadriceps, the adductors, the hamstrings, and the gastrocnemius. It is well known that the distal fragment may be flexed by the gastrocnemius, but this is usually more pronounced in high fractures. The flexion can be augmented by the overriding of the proximal fragment caused by the quadriceps and hamstrings. If the fracture heals with a posterior angulation at the supracondylar level, limitation of flexion of the knee will result.

The heads of gastrocnemius can rotate and spread the condylar fragments in intercondylar fractures. Valgus or varus deformity can be produced by the adductors. Most of the fibers of the adductors magnus and longus insert into the proximal fragment and only a few into the distal fragment. This usually causes a valgus deformity and an external rotation of the proximal fragment. If, on the other hand, the supracondylar fracture line is oblique from just proximal to the lateral epicondyle to well above the medial epicondyle, the adductors displace the distal fragment medially, into varus and internal rotation. In T, Y, or V fractures of the supracondylar and intercondylar region, the proximal fragment may be driven into the distal fragment, wedging the condyles apart.

Certain anatomic configurations of the articular surfaces may explain some of the problems encountered with this type of fracture. The knee has a relatively flat component (tibial plateau) and a convex component (the femoral condyles). The ligaments are attached close to the articular surface of the plateaus, but away from the articular margins of the convex component. During knee flexion, the ligaments move little in relationship to the plateaus, but to a great extent in relationship to the condyles of the femur. The articular capsule, the quadriceps, and the ligaments may form adhesions with the intra-articular

413

fractures, and this complication is more likely to occur when the fracture involves the femoral component of the joint. The adhesions may limit range of motion. Architectural malunion of the femoral condyles may block the movement of the flat (tibial) component in its course around the convex (femoral) component.

Reduction of fractures of the distal femur, both closed and open, requires restoration of the anatomy and of the axis in the sagittal and frontal planes. The femoral shaft axis makes an angle of approximately 83 degrees in the frontal plane with the knee joint or 7 degrees with a vertical line. This angle is less in tall patients with a narrow pelvis (5 degrees) and larger in short patients with a wider pelvis (9 degrees). This phenomenon is explained by the normal configuration of the femur, as the medial femoral condyle is lower than the lateral. The knee joint line is horizontal and the tibial shaft axis is vertical.

The femur, at the level of its middle and distal thirds, has an anterior curvature in the sagittal plane. Therefore, reposition of the fractures of the distal femur requires correction of the common posterior angulation (recurvatum) at the supracondylar level, to give a mild anterior curve.

The relative vulnerability of the popliteal artery de-pends on two factors.[41] First, the close anatomic relationship with the osteoarticular elements; in fact the artery is in almost direct contact with the bone at the level of the popliteal surface, protected only by the capsule and ligaments. At the tibial level the popliteus muscle separates the artery from the bone. The second factor is the relative immobility of the artery in the adductor canal superiorly and the soleus canal inferiorly. In fractures of the distal femur, the artery can be injured at the level of the adductor canal (if the fracture is high) or in the popliteal space (usually by the posterior angulation of the inferior fragment).

MECHANISM OF INJURY, AGE, AND SEX

Most patients are injured by high-velocity motor vehicle accidents, as shown in Table 15II.1. The knee can be injured by a dashboard trauma, with violent force exerted on the anterolateral part of the flexed knee, or by a violent direct force exerted on the lateral aspect of the extended leg, such as when a pedestrian is struck by an automobile. Motorcycle accidents account for an increasing amount of high-

Table 15II.1.   Mechanism of Injury, Age, Sex

Investigators	No. of Cases	Type of Injury	%	M (%)	F (%)	Age (years)
Stewart et al.[73]	442	Vehicular accidents Accidental falls Miscellaneous	45 34 21	53	47	6–65 5 percent < 6 10 percent > 65 peaks 6–15 and 46–65
Neer et al.[53]	110	Traffic accidents (the majority) Trivial falls (the minority)		59	41	23–86 peak 50–59
Chiron et al.[18]	137	Vehicular accidents Skiing Falls Miscellaneous	50 30 10 10	60	40	5–91 (10–80) peak 50–70 > 50% over 51
Trojan[80]	378	Traffic accidents	60	62	38	1/3 50–70
Stringa et al.[75]	123	Traffic accidents Falls and miscellaneous Occupational injuries	66 19 15	69	31	16–91 > 50% less than 50
Palazzi et al.[57]	75	Vehicular accidents Falls and occupational injuries Miscellaneous	55 41 4	54	46	10–70
Della Torre et al.[25]	54	Traffic accidents Falls occupational injuries	62 24 14	53	47	17–89 mean 53
Seinsheimer[68]	47			42	58	Average age 53 (18–91) for men 41, for women 63

velocity trauma with a direct force exerted on a flexed knee (usually anterolaterally). Trauma to the anterior and medial aspects of the flexed knee may occur, although more rarely.

The second most frequent cause is a fall on the flexed knee. The injured patient is usually older and osteoporotic (frequently female), and the low-velocity force is usually caused by a trivial fall at home or at work. Sometimes the trauma is indirect, rotational, or twisting, and it can cause a supracondylar spiral fracture, particularly in osteoporotic patients or in those with arthritis, vascular disease, or paralysis.

Falls from a height are responsible for a limited number of fractures. There is axial load combined with an angular force. In occupational lesions the mechanisms are various: falls from a height, accidental falls, direct forces such as the knee being hit by an object or vehicle. The most frequently associated sport is skiing.

CLASSIFICATIONS

A classification is useful only if it helps the management of the fractures. Table 15II.2 reports in detail the various classifications used by investigative groups to help the reader understand the frequency of the different types of fractures and the results obtained. A simple classification, including all the fractures based on fracture anatomy, is the most useful. The fractures can essentially be divided into three classes:

1. Pure supracondylar: Undisplaced (Fig. 15II.1); displaced, simple (Figs. 15II.2 and 15II.3); and comminuted (Fig. 15II.4)
2. Supra- and intercondylar: Undisplaced (Fig. 15II.5); displaced, simple (Fig. 15II.6); and comminuted (Figs. 15II.7 and 15II.8)
3. Monocondylar: Sagittal (Fig. 15II.9); medial, lateral, frontal (Figs. 15II.10 and 15II.11); combination.

ASSOCIATED LESIONS

Other lesions are common: Palazzi et al.[57] found an incidence of associated lesions of 50 percent, we found an incidence of 80 percent[25] (including craniofacial lesions).

Associated Fractures. These are relatively common. Fractures of the same extremity (tibial fractures, including tibial plateau fractures; patellar fractures; foot and ankle fractures; hip fracture-dislocations) are listed with incidences of 28 percent,[53] 6 percent,[44] 23 percent,[57] and 26 percent.[25]

Open fractures were found in 27 percent[53] 10 percent,[44] 9 percent,[57] 8 percent,[66] and 20 percent[25] of cases.

Vascular Damage. This is fortunately unusual, but the possibility must always be considered because of the proximity of the popliteal vessels. Injury requires immediate diagnosis and treatment within 6 hours. Stewart et al.[73] reported two amputations (out of 442 cases) for severe vascular damage, Neer et al.[53] one amputation (in 110 cases). More recently, Schatzker and Lambert[66] reported a high incidence of 10 percent vascular damage (not necessarily leading to amputation).

The popliteal artery can be injured at various levels, usually at a high level near the adductor magnus arch. The mechanism of injury varies from compression to traction, detachment, or perforation. Pathologically, there can be sectioning or penetrating types of injuries, but most are contusions. False aneurysms have been observed.[59]

Despite major advancements in the management of arterial trauma, popliteal artery lesions caused by fracture-dislocations about the knee continue to be associated with significant limb loss, and the amputation rate is still on the order of 30 percent.[5,23,35,55]

Nerve Injuries. Nerve injuries, particularly of the peroneal nerve, are rare. Stewart et al.[73] and Neer et al.[53] reported none, although there were a few cases of secondary transient peroneal nerve lesions due to positioning. Palazzi et al.[57] report an incidence of 1.2 percent and Schatzker and Lambert[66] of 4 percent.

RADIOLOGY

The two standard views of the knee and supracondylar area are usually sufficient to show the fracture anatomy and displacement. Occasionally other views—oblique or tunnel—will be necessary to show the penetration of the fracture into the intercondylar area or into the joint, particularly if open reduction is to be undertaken, because accurate reduction and rigid internal fixation is required.

In the case of unicondylar fractures, the antero-posterior view often shows very little; it will be necessary to look for a double-contour image at the level of the joint line, or a supracondylar spur indicating a sagittal direction of the fracture. The lateral views are much more demonstrative; it is necessary to obtain a perfect film to show the line of Blumensaat, normally corresponding to the projection of the condylotrochlear grooves, which will be divergent in the case of fracture. Tomography in the lateral projection and skyline views of the patellofemoral joint are sometimes useful.

Particular attention should be paid to radiographic studies while the patient is in traction, in order to achieve good alignment.[53] A false-radiographic appearance of flexion of the distal fragment can be produced by rotation. In the case of a supracondylar fracture (particularly of the type IIA of Neer), with some medial and posterior displacement of the distal fragment, a distal internal rotation deformity caused by

Table 15II.2.   Classifications of Fractures

Investigators	Classification	Frequency (%)	Remarks
Stewart et al.[73]	Middle-distal femur	20	Classification based on fracture anatomy
	Supracondylar	48	
	Supraintercondylar	18–19	
	Monocondylar	14	
Neer et al.[53] (also used by Olerud[56] and by Mize[47])	Group I: Minimum displacement, impacted	31	Trivial violence; associated intercondylar T = 50%; porotic bone (50% > 65 years); no quadriceps damage; more frequent in females
	Group IIA: Condyles displaced medially, fracture line higher laterally	29	Often violent force to lateral flexed knee, associated intercondylar T > 50%; often lateral laceration of quadriceps; open in one-third of cases; 40% > 65 only
	Group IIB: Condyles displaced laterally, fracture line higher medially	21	Violent force to lateral extended knee, rarely a blow on medial flexed knee; quadriceps spared. Open in one-third; 25% > 65
	Group III: Comminuted supracondylar and shaft	19	Violent force to anterior flexed knee; often associated intercondylar; open > 50%; minority > 65; sex equal; often damage to quadriceps
Hohl[34]	Supracondylar		Supracondylar: undisplaced, impacted, displaced (transverse, oblique, comminuted); see Neer et al.[53] for supraintercondylar. Sagittal, frontal, combination for unicondylar.
	Supraintercondylar		
	Unicondylar		
Chiron et al.[18]	Pure supracondylar	54	
	Supraintercondylar	36	See Neer et al.[53] (for supraintercondylar)
	Unicondylar	9	
Trillat et al.[79]	Unicondylar fractures		Rare; may pass undiagnosed; blow on flexed knee, with angular force
	Lateral	75	Frontal (Hoffa), sagittal (Trelat) or intermediate in direction, begin at condylopatellar groove; soft tissues remain attached to the fragment
	Medial	25	More often of Trelat type; posterior cruciate often not attached to fragment (avascular changes); lateral ligament complex lesions often associated

(Continued)

external rotation of the hip joint and femoral shaft will show an apparent posterior angulation of the condylar fragment on the lateral view. This may lead to excessive flexion of the knee with resultant increased varus angulation and forward displacement of the shaft.

A true anteroposterior view is also difficult because of the flexed position of the knee. A 20-degree angulation of the x-ray beam to either side of the true anteroposterior or lateral view can distort the image enough to show considerable displacement. It is necessary to obtain consistent standard views of the distal femur, and no attempt should be made to show the tibia on the anteroposterior view.

CONSERVATIVE TREATMENT[13]

PLASTER CAST OR SPLINTS

Undisplaced, minimally displaced, stable or impacted supracondylar or supraintercondylar fractures can be treated with cast immobilization. This can also (Text continued on page 423.)

Table 15II.2.   *(continued)*

Investigators	Classification	Frequency (%)	Remarks
Stringa et al.[75]	Supracondylar	41	A simple and useful anatomic classification, based on Hohl[34]
	Supraintercondylar	33	
	Unicondylar	26	
Palazzi et al.[57]	Type I: Epiphyseal injuries	5	Based on Vidal and Marchand (1966)[83]
	Type II: Unicondylar	26	
	Type III: Supracondylar	65	
	Type IV: Supraintercondylar	13	
	Type V: Diaphysometaphysoepiphyseal	11	
Della Torre et al.[25]	Type A: Extra-articular		A simplified ASIF classification; no type A1 or B fractures observed in the reported series of cases
	1. Partial supracondylar	—	
	2. Simple supracondylar	20.9	
	3. Comminuted supracondylar	12.9	
	Type B: Monocondylar		
	1. Lateral	—	
	2. Medial	—	
	3. Tangential	—	
	Type C: Bicondylar		
	1. Simple intercondylar	16.6	
	2. Intercondylar plus comminuted supracondylar	31.5	
	3. Comminuted supraintercondylar	18.6	
Seinsheimer[68] (also used by Giles[31])	Type 1: Nondisplaced	10.6	Fractures up to 9 cm above the articular surface (on AP roentgenograms); classification enables to distinguish fractures into groups of patients of different ages, with mechanism of injury and prognoses; older patients with osteoporosis are included in type 1 or 2A. Articular disruption is the basis of this classification.
	Type 2: No extension into the intercondylar notch or into the condyles, simple (A) or comminuted (B)	A: 12.7 B: 34	
	Type 3: Involving the notch, medial condyle separated (A), lateral condyle (B), both (C)	A,B: 4.2 C: 32	
	Type 4: Involving the articular surface of one condyle, medial (A), lateral (B), comminuted (C)	17	Average age of type 4, 33 years; of type 3C, 52 years; of types 3A,B, 63; of type 2B, age 41 years for men and age 69 years for women
Shelbourne and Brueckmann[69]	Type 1: T or Y intercondylar	27	Other classifications found not to aid in treatment
	Type 2: Transverse	25	
	Type 3: Oblique	24	
	Type 4: Spiral	14	
	Type 5: Comminuted	8	

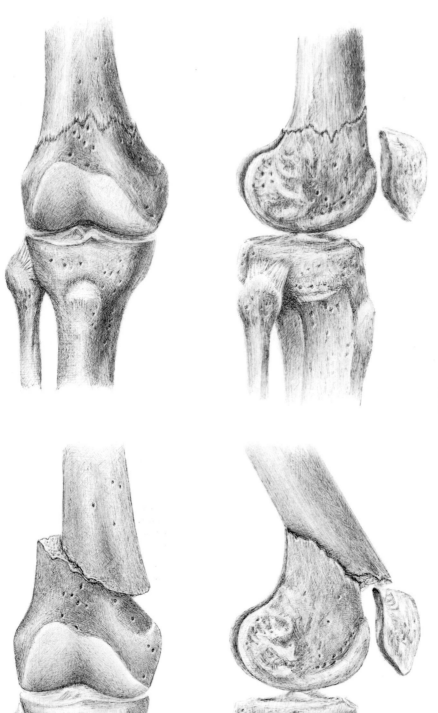

Fig. 15II.1. Pure supracondylar fracture, undisplaced.

Fig. 15II.2. Pure supracondylar fracture, displaced simple (lateral displacement).

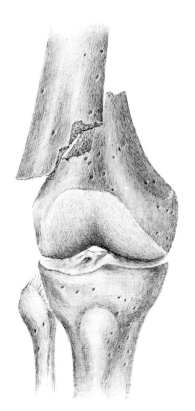
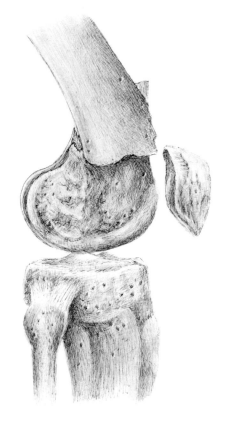

Fig. 15II.3. Pure supracondylar fracture, displaced simple (medial displacement).

Fig. 15II.4. Pure supracondylar fracture, displaced comminuted.

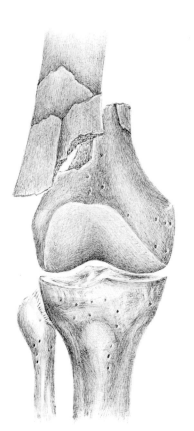
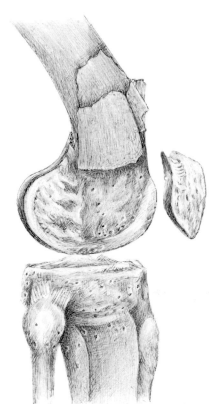

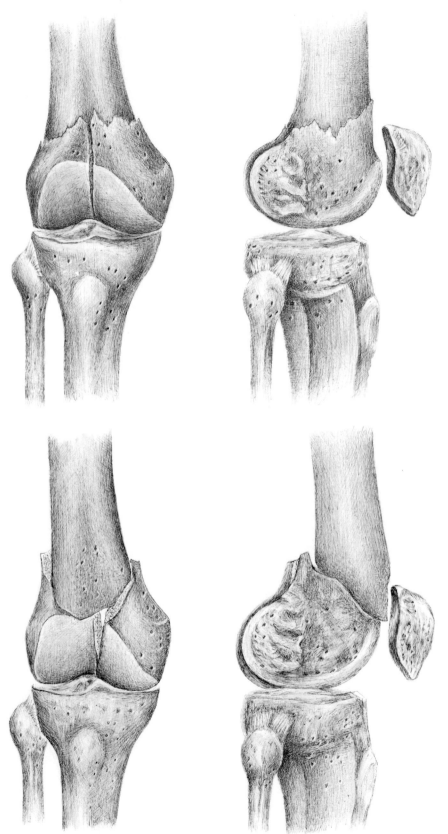

Fig. 15II.5. Supraintercondylar fracture, undisplaced.

Fig. 15II.6. Supraintercondylar fracture, displaced simple.

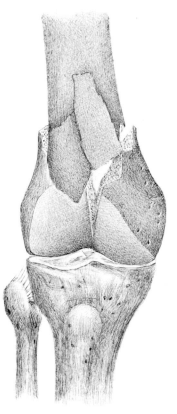
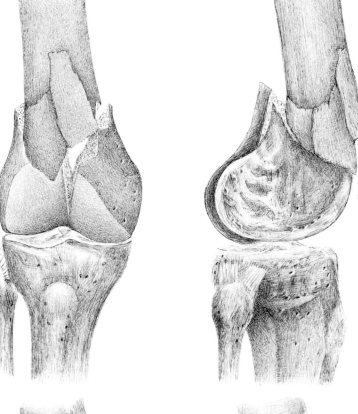

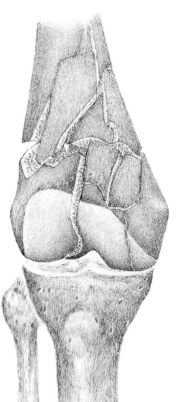
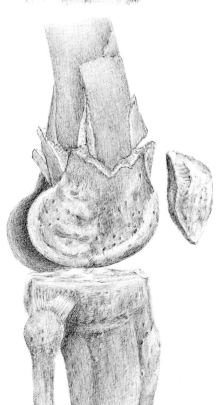

Fig. 15II.7. Supraintercondylar fracture, displaced with supracondylar comminution.

Fig. 15II.8. Supraintercondylar fracture, displaced with supracondylar and condylar comminution.

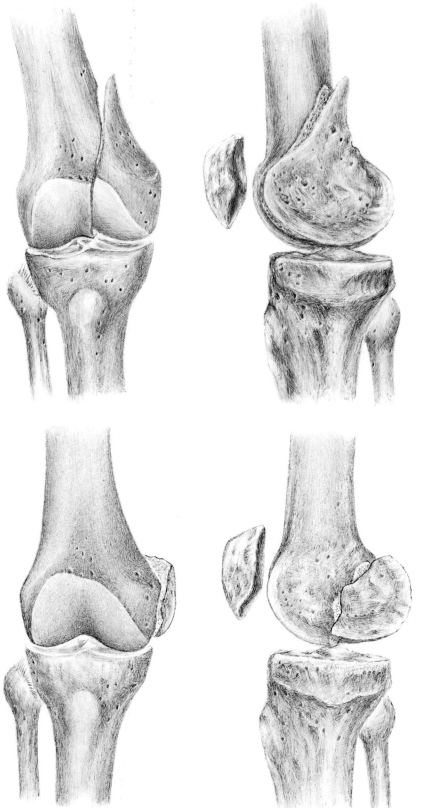

Fig. 15II.9. Monocondylar fracture, medial sagittal.

Fig. 15II.10. Monocondylar fracture, medial frontal.

422

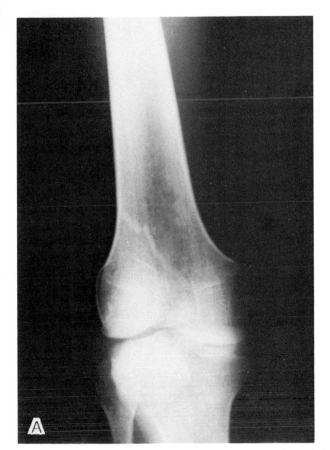
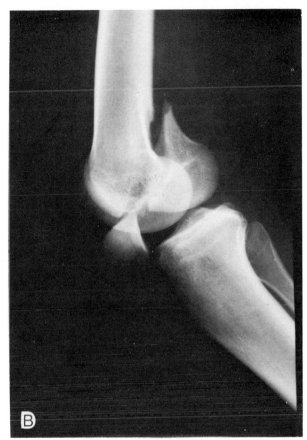

Fig. 15II.11. Monocondylar fracture, lateral–frontal, (A) anteroposterior, and (B) lateral view.

be done when the condition of the patient does not suggest other forms of treatment, such as operation or traction. We believe that this method should be used only on rare occasions, as patients tend to achieve less motion than with other methods. Other workers believe that immobilization should never be used.[68]

Cast or splint immobilization can be applied after joint aspiration and attempts at closed manipulation to correct minimal displacement or minor alignment deviations. Persistence of even minor joint surface irregularities (even if seen in only one projection) or of angular malalignment should lead to other forms of treatment. A particular problem occurs in very obese patients, in whom it is difficult to apply the cast.

Most of the time a well-molded plaster cylinder or a long leg cast from groin to ankle can be used. This is worn for 4 to 6 weeks and allows the patient to get up without weight-bearing or with toe touching. Roentgenograms should be taken at regular intervals to show that reduction is being maintained because

the powerful thigh muscles can cause angulation or displacement. The best position of the knee in the cast is that of almost full extension.

One of the advantages of this treatment is that the patient need not be hospitalized for more than a few days. The main disadvantage is the risk of joint stiffness, particularly in elderly patients. To limit the chance of this occurring, the cylinder cast can be changed to a cast-brace after a period of about 3 weeks, to allow weight-bearing and active knee motion.[54]

TRACTION, CLOSED REDUCTION, AND SPICA CAST

Skeletal traction through the tibial tuberosity or on occasion through the femoral condyles is applied in the emergency room; it is maintained for 7 to 8 days with the extremity on a Braun frame with the purpose of achieving gross alignment, preventing muscle contractures, helping decrease edema, and observing the circulation. Then, with the patient under general anesthesia on a fracture table, the fracture is manipulated and reduced with radiographic control and image intensifier. A spica cast is applied on the fracture table with adequate molding and compression to avoid displacement. The spica is maintained for an average of 2 months, but the patient can be discharged home after a few days. After this, a cylinder cast often needs to be applied for an additional 4 to 6 weeks. Partial weight-bearing can then be allowed in most cases. Range of motion is started only after about 3 months' immobilization.

This method has been used in the past,[26] while it has been used only on rare occasions by others.[53,73]

The advantage of this method is that it is not necessary to follow the patient every day for a long period of time and the hospitalization is short (15 to 20 days). There are numerous disadvantages, namely, the discomfort for the patient, the possibility of general complications particularly in the elderly, and severe joint stiffness caused by prolonged immobilization and muscle atrophy.

We believe that this form of treatment should seldom be used in the treatment of these fractures.

TRACTION

Traction is the most widely known conservative method.[90] It has been used for a long time in the forms of skin traction,[12,43,62,76] a single tibial skeletal pin[8,17,42,72,87] and double tibial and femoral skeletal pins.[32]

Treatment with continuous traction and early exercises described by Böhler is popular in Europe as reported by Trojan.[80] It can be successfully applied to supracondylar fractures that can be reduced by closed manipulation. It can also be applied to supraintercondylar fractures of the T or Y type, provided the condyles are only minimally displaced and the articular surfaces spared, and to the spiral supraintercondylar types without significant displacement.

This treatment cannot be used for the unicondylar articular fractures. In cases in which surgery is contraindicated, split, sagittal, unicondylar fractures are better treated by a cylinder cast after closed reduction.

Under local anesthesia the leg is placed on a Braun frame, and a Steinmann pin is inserted in the tibial tuberosity approximately 2 cm posterior to its anterior border. Care should be taken to place the pin exactly perpendicular to the long axis of the tibia to avoid traction into varus or valgus. The tibial tuberosity is preferred to the femoral condyles because the pin is close to or through the fracture, with possible risks of low-grade infection and stiffness. A traction bow is applied and with gentle traction the shortening and lateral angulation are corrected. After completion of these maneuvers, weights of approximately one-eighth to one-tenth body weight are applied.

Precise determination of the amount of traction depends on the strength of the thigh muscles and radiographic monitoring. Minimal residual displacements can be accepted because the continuous traction can often progressively reduce them. It is necessary to correct any recurvatum at the fracture site. Recurvatum is partly a consequence of the gastrocnemius action, and to prevent this the angle of the Braun frame is placed at the level of the supracondylar fracture and not at the knee joint. A small pillow can be used under the fracture site. The Braun frame should be fixed to the bed in order to maintain the correct position.

The direction of the traction is another important factor: in the case of femoral shaft fractures, the direction is parallel to the femur, whereas in supracondylar fractures this would not correct the recurvatum. If the direction of the traction is elevated, the recurvatum tends to increase. It is correct if the traction is lowered until it corresponds to the bisecting line between femoral axis and tibial axis with the knee in gentle flexion (25 degrees). In this situation, the traction cord usually touches the foot or the toes; to avoid this unpleasantness the cord is interrupted by a second traction bow encompassing the foot.

Radiographs are taken after 2 days; excessive traction should be avoided to prevent intercondylar or interfragmentary separation. The weights are reduced over time.

It is important to instruct the patient on early exercises. The first week the patient should be advised to move the ankle and toes frequently. Radiographs are again taken at the end of the first week, and residual varus or valgus deviation can be corrected by moving the direction of traction. Radiographs are repeated every week. During the second week the patient begins to contract the muscles of the thigh, particularly the quadriceps. Limited range-of-motion exercises can be started after the first month.

The traction is usually maintained for an average of 8 weeks. After this period most fractures have sufficient callus for partial weight-bearing. In the event of delayed callus formation, traction can be maintained for an additional 4 weeks, or the leg can be placed in a hinged cylinder cast for 4 weeks. The knee usually regains sufficient motion in about 4 to 8 weeks, after completion of treatment, provided intensive physical therapy and exercises are done.

The most commonly used traction methods in the United States are the two-wire technique described by Stewart et al.[73] and the one-wire technique, described by Neer et al.[53]

Preferably in the operating room or in the emergency room, using strict aseptic technique, a Kirschner wire ($\frac{3}{32}$ inch) is introduced from lateral to medial into the tibial tuberosity, and a second K wire is introduced from medial to lateral into the distal femur at the level of the adductor tubercle, corresponding to the upper pole of the patella with the knee extended.

The second wire through the distal femur is considered necessary to overcome the flexion position of the distal fragment. Through the tibial wire, a traction of 7 kg ± 5 is applied in line with the femur. Through the second femoral wire, traction is exerted upward, at right angles to the femoral shaft,[90] with a force of 1 to 3 kg. Stewart et al.[73] do not hesitate to pass this second wire through a comminuted fracture or even through an open fracture, provided the skin is clean and sterile technique is used. Penetration of the wire into the supracondylar pouch or synovium has resulted in no harm, according to Stewart, but every effort is made to avoid this. The second wire is not necessary in all cases, and we believe it should be used only when there is a tendency toward severe recurvatum. The leg is placed in a Thomas splint with a Pearson attachment to maintain moderate (15 to 35 degrees) flexion.

Neer et al.[53] emphasize some technical points of importance with the traction method. To avoid internal rotation–varus deformity at the fracture site, the threaded wire is placed more posteriorly on the medial side of the proximal tibia, such that it lies parallel to the floor when the tibia is externally rotated 15 to 20 degrees to align with the proximal fragment, which is usually held in external rotation. The Pearson at-

tachment is applied with a 20-degree angle to the Thomas splint at the level of the fracture, such that the distal fragment, patella, and tibia are lifted forward. Excessive weight on the proximal ring of the Thomas splint is avoided to prevent anterior displacement of the shaft.

Prolonged immobilization of the knee joint should be avoided. Clinical union should occur before starting knee motion, but once the fracture is clinically stable, progressive mobilization of the knee should be started. Complete consolidation as seen on the radiographs requires several months, but clinical union (early callus posteriorly, and absence of tenderness) is usually established at 5 weeks in most instances. When stability is present traction weights are reduced and passive motion is begun. Traction can usually be removed at 7 weeks and exercises permitted without suspension at 8 weeks, without weight-bearing. Borgen and Sprague[9] emphasize the importance of early exercises, first isometric but soon isotonic, in order to obtain at least a controlled active range of motion from full extension to 30 degrees of flexion after 4 weeks of traction.

The traction-suspension system described by Rienau[61] is used in Europe, particularly in France and Spain.[57] It involves the use of a pin in the proximal tibia, through which traction is applied along the axis of the femur; a second traction pin through the femur works vertically for suspension. No splints or frames are used and the thigh is kept in a balanced suspension sling.

In our unit we have limited experience with traction methods. We have used the Böhler system particularly for cases in which we found that an operation was contraindicated for general conditions or for local conditions such as osteoporosis, extreme comminution, and open wounds. We believe that the prolonged bed confinement in the hospital is a major disadvantage. We therefore usually prefer to use internal fixation.

CAST-BRACES

Functional cast-braces have been used successfully for supracondylar fractures, and also for supraintercondylar fractures.

Mooney et al.[48] were the first to publish the cast-brace treatment of fractures of the distal third of the femur in a prospective and controlled study of 150 patients. The fractures were treated in skeletal traction until they were determined to be firm, that is, when tenderness was no longer present and no shortening occurred when the traction was removed. The average time in traction was 7.2 weeks. After this period in traction a plaster of Paris cast-brace was applied. Proximally an adjustable plastic quadrilateral socket was used, not to provide ischial weight-bearing, but mostly for total contact support. This has the same characteristics of the quadrilateral socket of the above knee prosthetic socket. Foot and leg were then incorporated in the cast-brace, with joints at the knee. Single axis, posterior offset hinges were used parallel with the knee axis roughly corresponding to the level of the adductor tubercle. The mean time in the cast-brace determined empirically on the basis of function was 7.2 weeks. The patients were instructed on progressive weight-bearing with crutches and quadriceps setting and range of motion exercises.

Connolly et al.[19] showed that rotation and translation were less in a cast-brace with weight-bearing than traction in bed with routine exercises. There was no apparent advantage in prolonged traction prior to cast-brace application. Rotation and translation do occur to a certain extent during the early phases of healing with any form of conservative treatment. A weight bearing cast-brace permits controlled motion of the fracture fragments and promotes healing by the formation of periosteal callus.

The fracture must first be reduced in skeletal traction; then, with the patient sedated, after 1 to 3 weeks of traction, the cast-brace is applied. The thigh portion is prepared and molded first. The top of the plaster cylinder reaches to within 2.5 cm from the ischial tuberosity, but no attempt is made to produce an ischial weight-bearing effect. A 2.5-cm distance is also allowed medially to prevent impingement on the perineum and to enable the patient to sit and walk.

The thigh portion is trimmed inferiorly to allow 0 to 70 degrees of flexion at the knee. The traction is removed, and the rest of the cast is applied below the knee. The ankle and foot can be included to suspend the cast-brace, or the ankle can be left free and suspension can be obtained by incorporating the tibial traction pin. Preferably polycentric joints are then applied at the knee. If the radiographs show satisfactory alignment of the fragments, the patient begins gait training, advancing to partial weight-bearing on crutches. The cast-brace is kept until the fracture is healed. Time to healing varies considerably, but in approximately 57 percent of patients the fracture was healed at 14 weeks if the cast-brace was applied within 4 weeks of injury. No advantage from prolonged traction was evident. Some limited shortening was felt to be necessary to achieve union for fractures at the distal femoral level.

Borgen and Sprague[9] maintain traction for 3 to 6 weeks. Controlled active knee motion of at least 0 to 30 degrees at 2 to 3 weeks should be present. When there is no tenderness and a feeling of "reliability" at the fracture site and early callus formation on radiographs, the cast-brace is applied by the method of Mooney, but using polycentric hinges. The patient is then instructed on knee motion and partial weight-bearing. The time in traction can be shortened with increasing experience, but usually the minimum is 3 weeks. The average time to healing in the Borgen and Sprague series was 11.5 weeks.

The details of the application of this technique can be found in recent works.[28,64] Recently[77] the cast-brace treatment applied at 5 to 7 weeks has been shown to be advantageous over traction in a Thomas splint and also over intramedullary nailing for fractures of the distal half of the femur including fractures of the distal third. It has been demonstrated that the load through the fracture increases progressively as union proceeds, because of the physiologic feedback mechanism from the fracture site.[86] In supracondylar fractures and fractures of the distal third treated first with traction and then with cast-braces, the load carried on the limb soon after the brace was applied was 38 percent of body weight and at union it was 98 percent. The brace is a mechanism by which the patient reduces the forces on the fracture by a variable amount, depending on the degree of union, while alignment is maintained. The cast-brace functions as an antibuckling hinged tube, and for a distal femoral fracture a modified knee-hinge cylinder brace was designed[45] with supporting straps from the waist belt without an ankle and foot section.

In our unit we have limited experience with cast-brace treatment. We believe that the main advantage of this form of treatment is the possibility of range of motion exercises and early weight-bearing. This should be particularly evident for nondisplaced simple and comminuted supracondylar fractures for which cast-braces were shown to give better motion than internal fixation.[68] The main disadvantage of cast-braces is the continuous care required on an ambulatory basis to control the cast and avoid displacement. Experienced personnel are required.

SURGICAL TREATMENT

We believe that the treatment of choice for most fractures of the distal end of the femur is surgical. It is clear that open reduction and internal fixation of this type of fracture, which is often comminuted and multifragmented, is very difficult and time consuming. Obviously an orthopedic surgeon who decides on open treatment must accept the risks of complications, above all, infection. Therefore this surgery, which "does not tolerate mediocrity," can be done only by experienced surgeons[75] and in the best environmental conditions.[74] Poor or unsatisfactory results, often reported in the past, result from poor technique or inexperience. Before deciding in favor of surgical treatment, a surgeon must critically consider personal experience and the feasibility of using this technique properly at his or her institution.

The history of internal fixation for fractures of the distal end of the femur begins with the Blount blade plate.[1,80] In Italy the first report is from the Rizzoli Institute, where plates and screws had been used successfully with limited indications.[6] White and Russin[89] believed that internal fixation, particularly Blount plates, should have been the standard method, although their results did not substantiate that statement. Other reports favored surgical treatment with different devices, such as screws, Rush nails, and bolts.[21] Two reports decreased the enthusiasm for surgery, the one by Stewart et al.,[66] in which bolts, plates, blade-plates, and Rush nails were used, and the one by Neer et al.,[53] using the same devices. Rush pins were found to be a good method by others,[88] offering the possibility of early motion. Many reports at the end of the 1960s or the beginning of the 1970s favored internal fixation.[2,15,46,51,65,81,83,84] Most of the literature of the last decade deals with internal fixation after open reduction, which is believed by many to be the treatment of choice to allow rigid fixation, early motion, short hospital stay, and best results. In the early 1970s a survey done by mail[60] in the United States revealed that two-thirds of surgeons still were in favor of nonsurgical traction treatment for supracondylar fractures. More recently the advent of cast-braces has not modified the trend, which is toward surgical treatment.

Many internal fixation devices are available. Some are of mediocre design and in part responsible for the unsatisfactory results achieved in the past. This applies to some blade plates, like the Blount, the Milch, the Neufeld, the Zimmer, the Wright, and the Elliot.[27] These blade plates have a thin, pointed blade that can be relatively easily introduced into the condyles, but are weak because the plate is thin and can bend or fracture. The flexibility of these devices makes their insertion easier, but there may be mistakes in orientation, or the fixation of the fragments can be incomplete, necessitating external protection, braces, and traction. The Huchet plate, with two epiphyseal teeth, is an improvement over the Milch plate, and has been used in France.[37] Other devices, used mostly in the past, are the McLaughlin nail plates, and the Brown-D'Arcy,[11] which is provided with a medial compression plate connected to the triflanged nail. There are also screw plates (Fig. 15II.12), such as the Strycker, the Shelton,[70] and the Mancini.[26] Their advantage is the ease of adaptation and insertion, but there are many disadvantages, including instability of the screw plate junction, which does not allow rigid fixation, weakness with frequent breakages, and protuberance into soft tissues. The Shelton plate is a relatively new and stronger plate.

Other types of implants have been used with frequency, particularly for special cases such as open fractures requiring a fixation *a minima*. In the case of open fractures, for instance, external fixation devices have been used.[38] One or two intramedullary pins, such as Rush nails, introduced through each condyle (*en Tour Eiffel*), allowed only partial fixation, usually not enough for early mobilization. The single- and double-split diamond intramedullary nails,[82] directed toward each condyle, provide insufficient immobilization of the fragments, particularly when there is an intercondylar fracture. Substantial improvement in fixation has been reported with the Zickel intramedullary fixation device for the supracondylar region.[91] These are inserted like the Rush pins, and are usually two in number. They have a flexible diaphyseal stem and a strong curved condylar part through which compression screws are applied to anchor the rods to prevent backing out and to provide intercondylar fixation. However, a recent report[69] shows good results

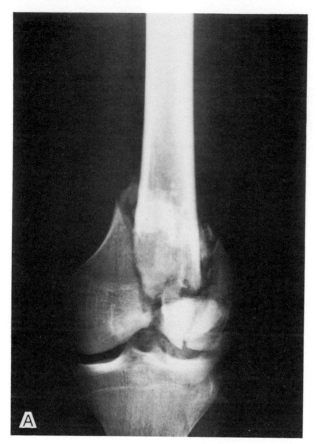
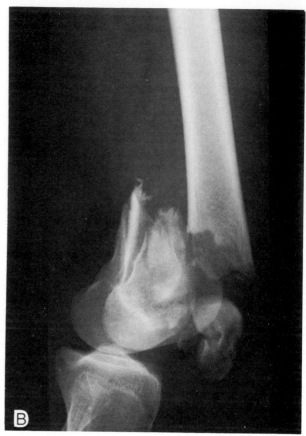

Fig. 15II.12. Male age 40. (A,B) Supraintercondylar fracture with condylar comminution and associated fracture of the patella. Surgical treatment with old design screw plate (C,D.). See page 427.

with regular and properly modified Rush (condylar) pins in a large series of cases. The importance of proper surgical technique and patient positioning at surgery is emphasized. The method has a wide application.

Three devices have gained wide popularity throughout the world: the ASIF 95-degree L-shaped condylar blade plate, the Judet screw plate, and the Richards condylar compression screwplate.

The ASIF blade plate (Fig. 15II.13) is the most widely and commonly used implant in Europe. This is the implant that we currently use. Accumulated experience[18,25,49,51,52,56–58,66,71,75] has shown the advantages as well as the difficulties encountered with this device.

The ASIF blade plate is very strong, with breakage or bending occurring very rarely. It permits rigid fixation, compression, and early mobilization. Great

precision is required. The site of introduction of the blade should be carefully selected in the lateral condyle; the same applies to the direction, in three planes, of the blade itself. It is impossible to make adjustments or to change the position of the blade because the implant is very rigid, the blade is at a fixed angle with the plate, and the bone of the condyles, is often porotic with several fragments, and does not tolerate the preparation of the canal for the blade more than one time. If orientation is not correct, there may be deformities (varus, valgus, rotational or recurvatum). The blows necessary to prepare and to introduce the blade may dislocate the condylar fragments. The Staca blade plate, a modification of the ASIF version, has the blade perforated along its length to enable the use of a guiding K wire.

A few technical points are important: (1) the site of

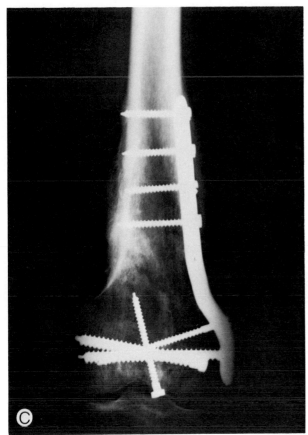
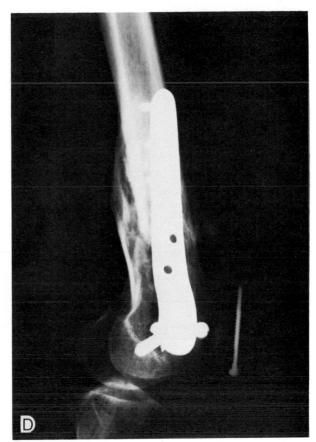

Fig. 15II.12. (Continued).

introduction of the blade in the lateral femoral condyle is in the line of the shaft, and therefore more anterior than the middle of the condyle; (2) the lateral collateral ligament insertion should be carefully avoided; (3) the blade should be close to the articular surface in order to fix the condyles properly, at a distance of no more than .5–2 cm; (4) its direction should be parallel to the joint surface in the frontal plane and with some "flexion" to accommodate the plate in line with the shaft in the sagittal plane; (5) the plate length should be long enough to have a good hold with at least 4 screws in the proximal fragment; (6) the blade should arrive at the opposite cortex without protruding.

The angle of the plate is 95 degrees, but with tension the angle increases to ± 97 degrees, corresponding to the normal medial angle between the femoral shaft and the knee joint. To determine the position of the plate, three K wires are used. One is placed into the knee parallel to the femoral condyles, a sec-

ond wire is placed under the patella, and a third wire is driven into the bone 1 cm proximal to the joint and parallel to the two previous wires; this third wire serves as a guide for the condylar plate, which is driven just proximal to it. In comminuted fractures cancellous screws are placed anterior or posterior to the projected entrance of the plate. The position of the third K wire is checked with the condylar template; the special condylar chisel is then hammered in at a distance of approximately 1.5 cm from the joint; the chisel guide must have the proximal arm parallel to the shaft of the femur.

The Judet screwplate (Figs. 15II.14 and 15II.15) has its main advantage in the good fixation of the condyles obtained with three large screws, which are less traumatic for the epiphysis than the blades. These are placed in different planes at a fixed angle and provide solid fixation of the fragments. Sometimes it is difficult to introduce extra screws into the epiphysis, but it is seldom necessary. The plate is relatively

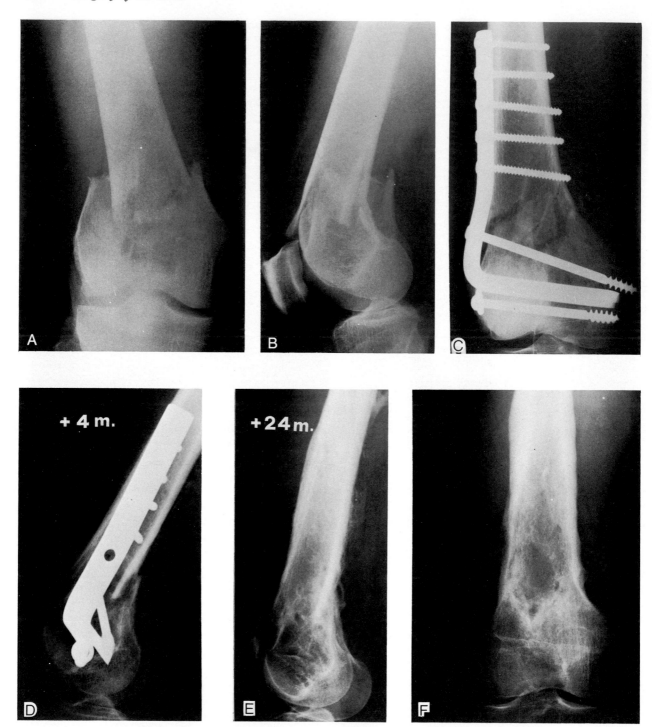

Fig. 15II.13. (A,B) Male age 48. Supraintercondylar fracture with some supracondylar comminution. (C,D) Surgical treatment with AO blade plate, (E,F) roentgenograms at 4 months, and at 24 months after removal of the internal fixation device (E,F). (From Della Torre, P., Aglietti, P., Altissimi, M.: Results of rigid fixation in 54 supracondylar fractures of the femur. Arch. Orthop. Traumat. Surg., 97: 177, 1980, with permission.)

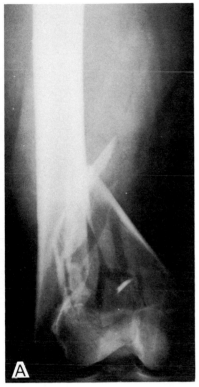
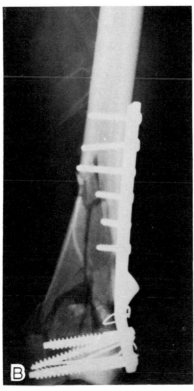
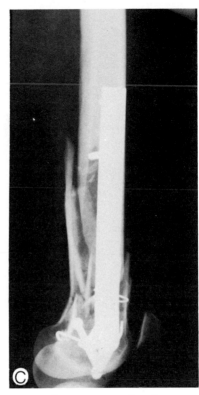

Fig. 15II.14. Female age 54. Severely comminuted supraintercondylar fracture (A). Surgical treatment with Judet screw plate (B,C), roentgenograms at 2 weeks.

bulky but has a curvature to adapt to the curve of the distal femur. There are right and left plates. This plate has been used with good results, not only by Judet,[36,39,40] but also by others,[10,63] although in a limited series of cases.

The Richards compression screw plate (Fig. 15II.16) has been used mostly in the United States.[31,54,92] The simplicity of a classic compression hip screw for intertrochanteric fractures of the femur has led some surgeons to apply the same method to the treatment of fractures of the distal femur. The screw makes a fixed angle of 80, 90, 95 or 100 degrees with the plate, which has a special distal barrel to accommodate the sliding cannulated screw, introduced first along a prepositioned Steinmann pin. Introduction of the compression lag screw takes place after careful preparation and tapping of its canal and is less traumatic to the condyles than the blade plates. Although the Richards screw plate is reported to have two disadvantages (it is difficult to adjust to the contours of the femur, and the distal fragment may rotate unless two

point fixation is obtained) recent reports[31,92] demonstrate the advantages of this screw-plate with stable fixation and without non union.

Positioning of the patient on the operating room table is important. Most surgeons prefer to use a regular operating room table with the patient supine and the injured extremity draped free so that the assistant controls the position and the amount of flexion of the knee. To maintain adequate knee flexion, sterile supports such as folded drapes are often necessary, and the radiographs are taken using sterile bags for the cassettes. Others leave the leg in traction and use a fracture table. There must be a radiolucent support under the knee to take films or to use the image intensifier.[50,58] Some prefer to have the x-ray tube under the knee (posterior–anterior direction) and to place the cassette in front of the knee.[92]

The operation is preferably done under tourniquet control; and the most widely used incision (and the one we prefer) is the lateral.[7,11,40,46,50–52,58,75,78] The skin incision is lateral and longitudinal at the lateral

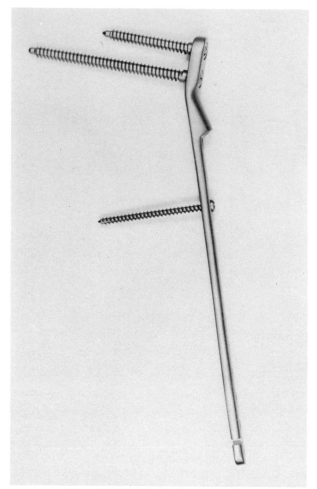

Fig. 15II.15. The Judet screw plate.

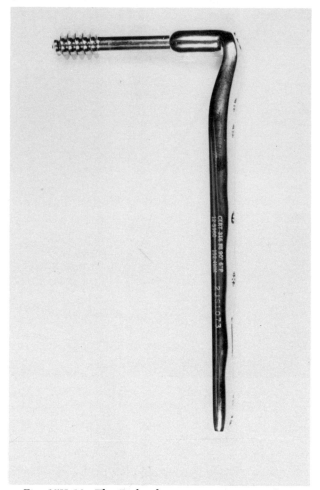

Fig. 15II.16. The Richards compression screw plate.

distal third of the thigh and bends forward distally toward the anterior tibial tuberosity. After incision of the fascia lata, the vastus lateralis is elevated from the intermuscular septum and is displaced forward and medially. The lateral retinaculum is incised and the patella is subluxed medially. In articular fractures, it is necessary to open the joint to check the reduction of the condylar fragments accurately.

The anterolateral approach is used less frequently. The skin incision is approximately the same as described above, although slightly more anterior, and the deep layers are approached going between vastus lateralis and rectus femoris. Distally the lateral retinaculum is incised at the side of the patella, which is dislocated medially. The medial exposure is better than with the posterolateral incision, but the extensor

mechanism is probably more damaged and the formation of adhesions is believed to be more frequent.

For better exposure in selected cases of severely comminuted intraarticular fractures a **Y** shaped incision through which the entire extensor mechanism is elevated with a block of bone from the tibial tuberosity has been recommended.[56] This provides wide access to both medial and lateral aspects of the distal end of the femur but the problem of skin sloughs or wound infection exists. More recently[47] a large J laterally placed incision has been recommended with a distal transverse portion located halfway between patella and tuberosity and with a distal vertical limb along the lateral border of the tuberosity which can be elevated. No retractors should be used to avoid skin necrosis.

An anterior-medial approach is also rarely electively used.[16] A limited medial approach is used for unicondylar fractures or it is rarely used in association with the posterolateral approach. Similarly, a limited lateral approach is used for lateral unicondylar fractures. More frequently, and safely, the anteromedial approach, between vastus medialis and rectus, is used today, after the experience with knee arthroplasties. This certainly gives superb intra-articular exposure, although there can be more problems with exposure of the proximal lateral fragment.

The principles of the surgical technique are essentially two: anatomic reconstruction of the fragments and rigid internal fixation. The fracture is opened, with the known risks, only if adequate reduction can be achieved. All the fragments, and particularly the intra-articular ones, should be carefully reduced. An adequate reconstruction is important for rapid healing and good function. Rigid fixation should also be ob-

tained as this is needed for early mobilization. The only person who knows exactly the rigidity of fixation is the surgeon who has done the operation. If any doubt exists, early mobilization should be protected (traction, cast-brace). Therefore, before attempting to operate on these difficult fractures, the surgeon should carefully assess his personal skill, the institution's capabilities, and the patient. The operation cannot be performed in an operating room that has limited equipment.

For unicondylar fractures with a sagittal or oblique fracture line, internal fixation with one (Fig. 15II.17), two, or three compression screws is often enough. This can be done through a limited medial or lateral incision over the nonarticular portion of the condyle. But if adequate reduction is in doubt, the joint should be widely opened. In the case of frontal fractures of the posterior condyles (Hoffa), the screws should be perpendicular to the fracture plane and therefore

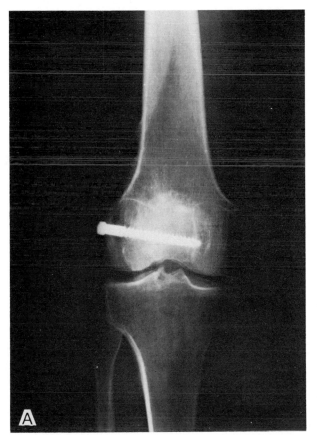 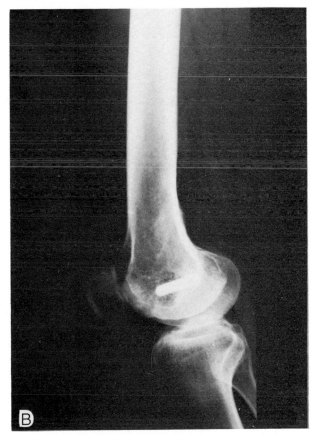

Fig. 15II.17. (A,B) Lateral unicondylar oblique fracture treated with single cancellous screw. Result at 3 years in a 25-year-old male.

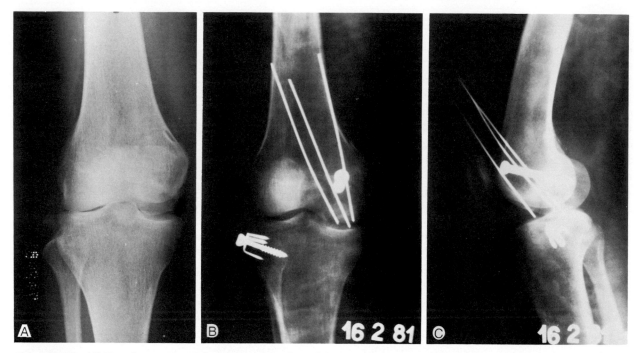

Fig. 15II.18. (A) Female age 28. Medial unicondylar frontal fracture with associated lateral compartment ligament lesion. (B,C) Surgical treatment with lateral compartment reconstruction and reduction, and internal fixation of the unicondylar fracture. Note the screw staple over the tubercle of Gerdy, the sagittal cancellous screw, and the K wires. Radiographs taken after two weeks.

should be inserted in the sagittal plane if possible from the outer surface of the condyle, which is not covered with cartilage. Sometimes screws must be inserted from posterior to anterior. If they have to go through articular cartilage they must be buried and removed early. Small additional articular fragments often associated with Trelat or Hoffa fractures can be fixed with K wires (Fig. 15II.18) introduced from the joint inside out, to go through the soft tissues of the front of the knee. Their ends can be left under the skin for easy early removal.

Supracondylar fractures without condylar or intercondylar fragments are relatively easy to reduce and fix rigidly with a blade plate like the ASIF version (Fig. 15II.19), which we prefer, or other devices like the Judet screw plate or the Richards compression screw plate. Interfragmentory compression can be applied.

The problem is more difficult in the case of supraintercondylar fractures (Figs. 15II.20–22). Reconstruction should begin from the articular portion; subsequently, the epiphysis should be fixed to the shaft. First, condylar fractures in the frontal plane, if present,

are reduced and fixed with compression screws perpendicular to the fracture plane. Then the two condyles must be reduced and fixed. A temporary fixation with K wires is often useful. Preliminary intercondylar compression screws should be introduced anteriorly or posteriorly in the condyles where they cannot interfere with the introduction of the blade. The epiphysis should then be fixed to the shaft after adequate reduction. Metaphyseal fragments should be reduced at this time, if possible. The plate should have a good hold on the proximal fragment (at least four screws having a firm grip on eight cortices).

If the fracture is comminuted, with many fragments, reduction and fixation is really complex. Again the condyles should be reconstructed first. It is almost impossible to reconstruct and reduce all the fragments, particularly in the metaphyseal region. It is important not to free them from the periosteum, to avoid necrosis. The surgeon should try to reduce the epiphysis with the diaphysis, leaving metaphyseal segments more or less as they are. The exact positioning of the plate is difficult (Fig. 15II.22) because of the intermediary metaphyseal fracture lines. The metaphyseal area often requires generous bone grafting (Fig. 15II.23) usually from the iliac crest as we know that gaps will not be filled. Others recommend acceptance of some shortening.[78]

A particular problem is created by severe osteoporosis, particularly in the elderly. In these cases, reduction and fixation are both difficult.[29,66] Unless there is an intra-articular fracture that cannot be reduced adequately by manipulation, closed reduction and traction treatment or cast-braces are a reasonable alternative to internal fixation. If operation is definitely needed, one must consider in selected cases the use of bone cement as an adjunct to internal fixation.[4,15,66] Bone cement of doughy consistency is inserted into the medullary cavity after the blade plate is inserted. The cement should remain strictly intramedullary. After the cement has set, holes can be drilled through it and tapped for cortical screws. The use of cement does not necessarily prevent callus healing, although periosteal callus formation can be weak[4] unlike intertrochanteric fractures.[33] According to Cameron et al.,[14] the strength of the cement–screw complex is higher when screws are placed into soft cement but this is more difficult. The incidence of infection is not found to be higher after the use of cement. In our opinion this method should only be used in desperation.

Open fractures also present difficult problems. Their results are usually inferior to those of closed fractures, with more complications, more pseudoarthroses, and more stiffness.[44] If there is a small puncture, it does not require immediate surgery. It is enough to close the wound after careful cleaning and to place the patient in traction. The operation can then be done after a few days, when the wound is healed. In the event of a large open wound with severe lesions of the soft tissues and with real risk of septic complications, some workers think that it is better to do an open fixation after complete debridement within a matter of hours from the injury (6 hours). The rigid internal fixation is the best condition for avoiding infection.[44,58] The wound is closed over drainage tubes and the patient is given high doses of IV antibiotics for 3 to 6 weeks.

This method decreases the incidence of pseudoarthrosis and stiffness and does not increase the risks of infection according to its proponents. If an infection is manifest, the pathogens must be isolated and the antibiotics selectively chosen. Often a second operation for debridement, incision and drainage is needed.

The internal fixation device should be maintained if possible in cases of sepsis.

Although emergency early fixation in open fractures seems to be the treatment of choice, it must be mentioned that some surgeons[31] including ourselves prefer to debride and delay the definitive operation. Others prefer to treat the cases conservatively (traction) and still others use external fixation[38] or internal fixation *a minima* (e.g., the Rush pins).

When the fracture of the distal third of the femur is associated with other features of the same extremity, the quality of the result is adversely affected, particularly when there is a fracture of the tibial plateaus, the patella, or the proximal tibia. Usually it is necessary to operate on all the levels to have the advantages of fixation of the supracondylar fracture and to avoid the complications of conservative treatment. Surgical treatment is also necessary in the case of vascular impairment in order to achieve stability of the fracture before vascular surgery is done. This can be done through a wide posteromedial approach with or without section of the medial head of the gastrocnemius. The medial route allows both operations, (osteosynthesis and vascular surgery) to be performed using the same approach.

A particular problem is the surgical treatment of a supracondylar pseudoarthrosis, which is usually at the metaphyseal level. Osteomuscular decortication with careful "petaling" is needed. Associated bone (iliac crest) grafting must be employed. The osteosynthesis device must often be changed for a more rigid one. Good results with blade plates have been reported.[67] In cases of infected pseudoarthrosis, external fixation devices have been used, sometimes with a double frame. But if the distal fragment is small and devascularized, an arthrodesis of the knee is necessary, with tibiofemoral nailing or with external fixators placed below the knee and in the proximal and distal fragments of the pseudoarthrosis.[85] Sacrifice of the knee was needed to obtain union, and this was achieved with a femorotibial plate.[31] The transarticular rod fixation as a salvage procedure in the treatment of supracondylar pseudoarthrosis does not necessarily cause definitive arthrodesis of the knee.[3] As an alternative solution to this problem we have on occasion performed total knee replacement using a specially constructed intramedullary rod attached to the femoral component (Chapter 20).

(Text continued on page 441.)

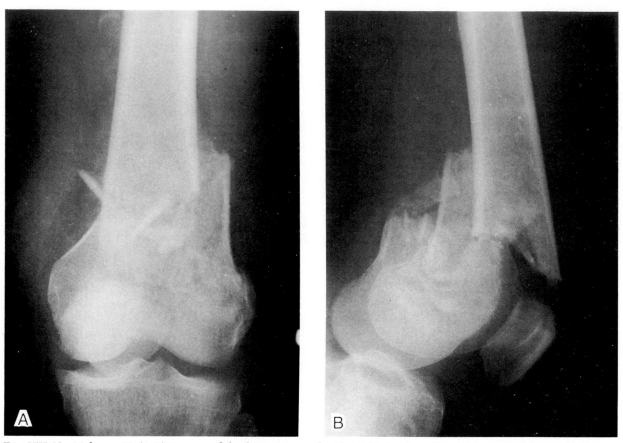

Fig. 15II.19.   Male age 40. (A,B) Supracondylar fracture treated with AO blade plate. (C,D) Roentgenograms at 32 months.

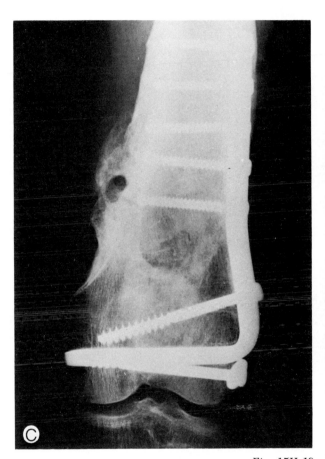
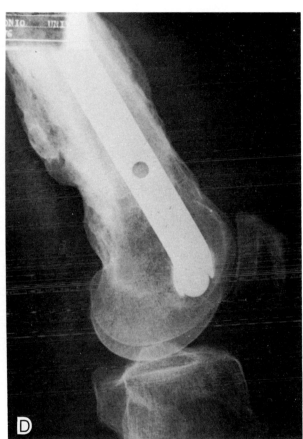

Fig. 15II.19. (Continued).

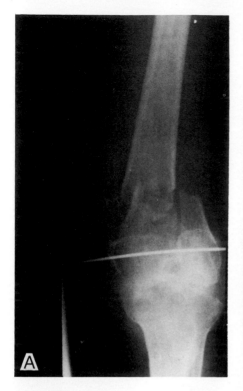

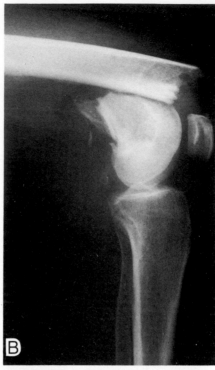

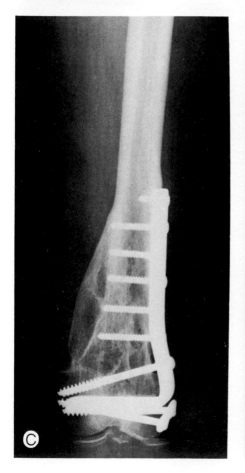

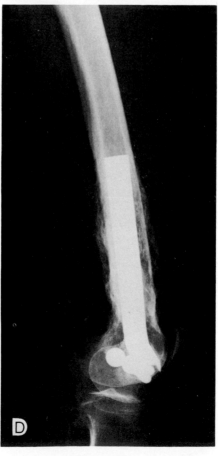

Fig. 15II.20. (A, B) Female age 52. Supraintercondylar fracture with severe displacement. (C, D) Treatment with AO blade plate. Roentgenograms at 27 months. (From Della Torre, P., Aglietti, P., Altissimi, M.: Results of rigid fixation in 54 supracondylar fractures of the femur. Arch. Orthop. Traumat. Surg., 97: 177, 1980, with permission.)

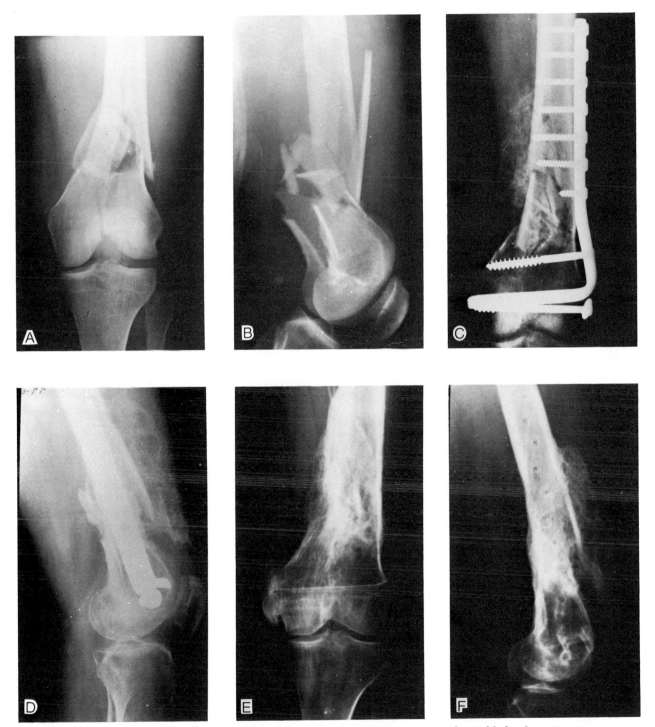

Fig. 15II.21. Female age 31. (A,B) Supraintercondylar fracture. (C,D) Treatment with AO blade plate. Roentgenograms at 1 year (E,F) and after removal of the devices. Note the myositis ossificans in the supracondylar anterior area and the ossification at the level of the medial epicondyle (blade too long). (From Della Torre, P., Aglietti, P., Altissimi, M.: Results of rigid fixation in 54 supracondylar fractures of the femur. Arch. Orthop. Traumat. Surg., 97: 177, 1980, with permission.)

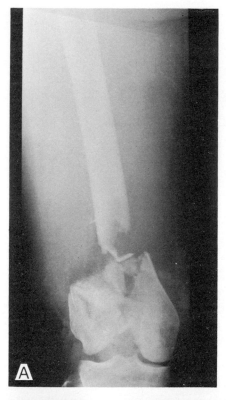

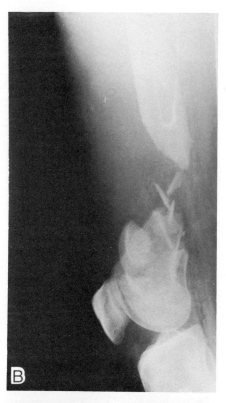

Fig. 15II.22. Female age 20. (A,B) Supraintercondylar open fracture with severe supracondylar comminution and loss of bone substance at the metaphyseal level. (C,D) Good result at 26 months after internal fixation with AO blade plate and iliac crest bone grafting. (From Della Torre, P., Aglietti, P., Altissimi, M.: Results of rigid fixation in 54 supracondylar fractures of the femur. Arch. Orthop. Traumat. Surg., 97: 177, 1980, with permission.)

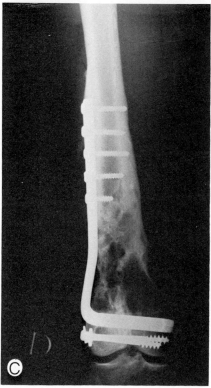

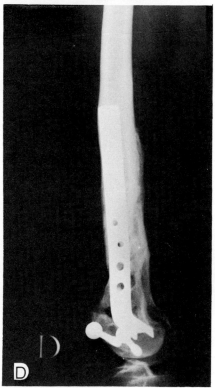

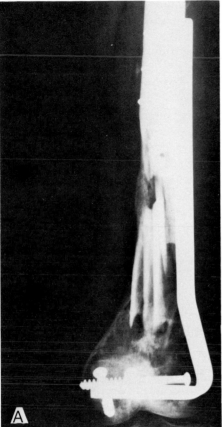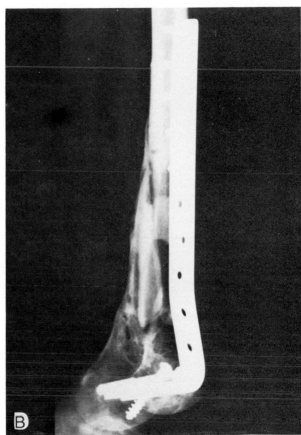

Fig 1511.23. (A,B) Severely comminuted supraintercondylar open fracture with bone loss. Treatment with AO blade plate and cortical bone grafting. Result roentgenograms at 1 year.

Associated ligament laxity is a rare but difficult problem. Diagnosis is difficult preoperatively. At the end of the reconstructive surgical procedure it is useful to check knee stability as gently as possible. There can be associated lesions of the collateral ligaments or of the cruciates, particularly in unicondylar fractures. They must be surgically repaired if severely disrupted, particularly on the lateral side. Their incidence varies from 5 percent[58] to 15 percent.[66] Associated ligament lesions, whether surgically repaired or conservatively treated, carry an adverse effect on the results because of the longer cast immobilization needed (usually 5 to 6 weeks).

In terms of postoperative management, a position of flexion of the knee is suggested by many. Some workers use a soft splint; others use traction through the tibial tuberosity. A flexion position of 70–80° is useful to avoid suprapatellar pouch adhesions; also, if the extremity is suspended, early motion can be encouraged.[31] After a few days the position of flexion is alternated with extension in a passive manner. After 1 week active movements are begun. The progression of exercises and the initiation of partial protected weight-bearing (usually not before the 10th to 12th week) should be carefully monitored by the surgeon who alone knows precisely the degree of stability achieved.

COMPLICATIONS

Death. Death is a rare complication and is usually related more to the severity of trauma, shock, head injuries, associated lesions, and other fractures, rather than to the fracture or its treatment. Stewart et al.[73] reported a mortality incidence of 2.5 percent, Neer et al.[53] an incidence of 3.6 percent, within 30 days of admission, in a large series of cases most of which were treated conservatively. In more recent series of patients treated surgically the mortality rate, within 3 months of admission, is 3 percent[18] and 3.7 percent.[25]

Deep Vein Thrombosis.   The incidence, on the basis of a clinical diagnosis, is relatively low. Neer et al.[53] reported 7 percent, while Blaimont et al.[7] believed that after internal fixation the thromboembolic complications are lower than after closed treatment because of earlier mobilization. The problem is not mentioned in some relatively large series.[18,25,57,66,73] Certainly we believe that deep vein thrombosis and pulmonary embolism can occur after fracture, whether conservatively or surgically treated.

Infection.   Postoperative infection is certainly the most important risk of open surgery. Data on infections are difficult to compare, as some operate on open fractures and others do not routinely use antibiotic prophylaxis. There is a recent trend to the use of antibiotics started at surgery or immediately before, and continued for a short period at high doses IV. The incidence of pin tract infection is reported to be low (2.5 percent) by Neer et al.[53]

Peroneal Nerve Palsy.   Attributable to positioning or splinting and rarely to the surgical intervention, the incidence of peroneal nerve palsy is 3 percent,[53] 1 percent,[18] and 0 percent in our series[25] and in Schatzker's series.[66]

Delayed Union.   Delayed union (4 months) after conservative treatment is relatively low, even with early mobilization of the knee. Creyssel et al.[21] report 12.5 percent, Stewart et al.[73] 7.3 percent, Neer et al.[53] 2.5 percent in cases mostly treated by traction, and DiMuria and Sartori[26] 12 percent in cases mostly treated by cast immobilization. After cast-brace treatment no delayed unions are reported: the cast-brace is usually removed at about 14 weeks[19] and only in a few patients is it kept longer. The patient carries 100 percent body weight on the affected limb after 14 to 16 weeks.[77,86]

After surgical treatment, the delayed union rate varies considerably. Stewart et al.[73] report 14.5 percent, Neer et al.[53] 11.5 percent, Chiron et al.[18] 0 percent, DiMuria and Sartori[26] 5 percent, Schatzker and Lambert[66] 17 percent (usually in the group not treated according to the principles of accurate reduction and rigid fixation), and Della Torre et al.[25] 2 percent after 5 months. The time to clinical and radiographic union averaged 4 months with the su-

pracondylar plate and leg screw,[31] and took 3 to 5 months with the ASIF blade plate in a recent series.[47]

Pseudoarthrosis (Nonunion).   After closed treatment, pseudoarthrosis is not very high. Stewart et al.[73] reported 13 percent, Neer et al.[53] 2.5 percent, DiMuria and Sartori[26] 1.5 percent, Mooney et al.[48] and Borgen and Sprague[9] 0 percent, and Connolly et al.[20] 2.3 percent after cast-brace.

After open treatment, nonunion was frequent in the older series. Stewart et al.[73] reported 19.5 percent, Neer et al.[53] 14 percent. It is less frequent in recent series with the ASIF implant. Olerud[56] reports 6 percent, Chiron et al.[18] 0 percent, Schatzker and Lambert[66] 5 percent, and Della Torre et al.[25] 4 percent. It is more frequent in the complex multifragmented fractures, particularly with open wounds. Trenz et al.[78] report a high 33 percent in these particularly difficult cases.

Malunion.   Certainly malunion is one of the major problems of closed treatment. Creyssel et al.[21] and Deburge[24] quote an incidence of more than 50 percent. Merle d'Aubigné and Alnot[46] reported 20 percent, but Neer et al.[53] only 5 percent (defined as 15 degrees angulation and/or 2 cm displacement). After cast-brace treatment, the malpositions accepted in the phase of traction tend to remain but usually do not increase in the cast-brace.[48] Shortening and angulation are believed to be minor problems.[19]

After surgical treatment the reported incidence varies considerably. Neer et al.[53] reported 31 percent, Chiron et al.[18] 4 percent (defined as more than 10 degrees angulation and/or 1.5 cm displacement). Della Torre et al.[25] reported 11 percent incidence of varus more than 10 degrees and an incidence of 11 percent recurvatum more than 10 degrees. Schatzker and Lambert[66] in a series also treated with ASIF implants found a six percent incidence of malunion affecting joint congruity. All malunions were in the group not treated strictly according to the principles of accurate reduction and rigid internal fixation. No malunions are reported in a series when a supracondylar plate and leg screw was used.[31]

RESULTS

Comparison of the results of different series is extremely difficult and should be attempted with great care. Different fracture types, levels, anatomy, patient age, and violence of injuries clearly have an important bearing on the prognosis and on the results. One other problem is the method of evaluation. This can include only functional criteria or radiologic criteria. It can be influenced to a predominant degree by a single parameter of knee function, such as mobility or pain. It can also be numerical (point score).

Stewart et al.[73] used a clinicoradiographic method wherein for a satisfactory result a range of motion of at least 130 degrees is required. Chiron et al.[18] used a similar method.

Neer et al.[53] introduced a numerical system that considered both clinical and radiographic parameters. Olerud[56] used the same system, including an evaluation of stability.

Schatzker and Lambert[66] and Mize[47] used only clinical criteria. A satisfactory result has no more than one of the following features: loss of length 1.2 cm, loss of flexion 20 degrees, 10 degrees varus or valgus, and minimal pain. Palazzi et al.[57] followed the method of Vidal and Marchand,[83] whereby clinical and radiographic criteria are separated. A result can be satisfactory with 90 degrees of flexion.

Della Torre et al.[25] used the clinical evaluation method devised at The Hospital for Special Surgery (Chapter 20).

To show the differences in the overall results according to the various methods of evaluation, the following example is illustrative. A supraintercondylar

Table 15II.3. Results: Cast Immobilization

Investigators	No. of Cases	Follow-up	Results	Remarks
Bianchi[6]	130	Average 3 years	50% good, 31% fair	A good result had no shortening, flexion at least 80 degrees; all types of fractures included
Lasi	45	Average 3 years	71% excellent, good	Evaluation with Vidal method;[83] comminuted intra- and extra-articular fractures included
Merle d'Aubigné and Alnot[46]			40% excellent, good	At least 90 degrees of motion required for satisfactory result
DiMuria and Sartori[26]	40	1–7 years	70% excellent, good	Articular fractures, evaluation with method of Neer et al.[53] modified by Olerud;[56] results better in sagittal monocondylar, or simple intercondylar than in comminuted or complex; age had negative influence: 35% < 90 degrees flexion
Palazzi et al.[57]	85	2 10 years	82% excellent, good	Conservative treatment used for less severe fractures; 70% good anatomic results
Seinsheimer[68]	18	Average 2 years		Nonunion 22%; range of motion average was better than 100 degrees; age had negative effect on range of motion

Table 15II.4. Results: Traction Mobilization

Investigators	No. of Cases	Follow-up	Results	Remarks
Stewart et al.[73]	144	1–20 years	67% excellent, good	Evaluation with Stewart method; excellent: no pain, no limp, no deformity or arthritis, and normal ROM
				Good: Occasional pain, slight limp, mild radiograph arthritis and deformity, ROM 0–130 degrees
				Fair: Pain with moderate activity, moderate limp, arthritis, deformity, ROM to 90 degrees
				Poor: Pain, limp, marked arthritis and deformity, marked restriction of ROM
Neer et al.[53]	48	1–29 years	90% excellent, good (84% in displaced supracondylar)	Evaluation with numerical score points system; functionally 70 degrees of motion seemed sufficient for satisfaction of the patient and working capacity, loss of motion more significant in groups III or IIA because of the concomitant extensor mechanism lesion

Abbreviation: ROM, range of motion.

fracture, healed with some intermittent pain, normal walking capacity without limp and without limitation, range of motion of 0 to 80 degrees without anatomic or radiographically significant alterations (e.g., incongruity, malalignment), and without instability. This fracture would be classified as excellent, according to Neer et al.[53] or Olerud,[56] Palazzi et al.,[57] Vidal and Marchand,[83] and Merle d'Aubigné and Alnot.[46] It would be fair according to Schatzker and Lambert[66] Mize[47] and Della Torre et al.,[25] and it would be poor

according to the classification system of Stewart et al.[73] or Chiron et al.[18]

As an aid to an understanding of the results of many published series, refer to Table 15II.3 for a review of cast treatment, to Table 15II.4 for traction, to Table 15II.5 for cast-braces, to Table 15II.6 for old internal fixation devices, to Table 15II.7 for ASIF blade-plates, and to Table 15II.8 for the Judet screw plate. These tables present the evaluation method used and the principal findings.

Table 15II.5.   Results: Cast-Braces

Investigators	No. of Cases	Follow-up	Remarks
Mooney et al.[48]	150	Short term	70% of the 150 fractures were of the distal third of the femur; there were no intra-articular fractures; no nonunions or refractures; ROM at 6 weeks after removal of cast-brace normal 30%; 90–135 degrees in 19%, 45–90 degrees in 21%, less than 45 in 9%, not recorded in 21%
Connolly et al.[20]	44	Short term	Fractures of the distal third of femur, not intra-articular. Shortening 2+ cm 8%, angulation not a problem, full ROM in 36%, 90–110 degrees in 30%, less than 90 degrees in 16 percent; brace applied after a very short period of traction
Thomas and Meggitt[77]	26	Short term	Fractures of the distal third of femur; average hospital stay 7 weeks; time to union 15 weeks (12–18); 89% of patients had full motion; brace applied at 5–7 weeks (like Mooney); no cases of delayed union; only four cases with significant angulation
Seinsheimer[68]	6	2 years average	No nonunions; average knee flexion 109 degrees; better results than with internal fixation for types 1, 2A, 2B

Table 15II.6.   Results: Old Internal Fixation Devices

Investigators	No. of Cases	Follow-up	Results	Remarks
Bianchi[6]	57	Average 3 years	88%, good or fair	Screws, plates; all types of fractures; good result with at least 80 degrees flexion
White and Russin[89]	46	Average 2 years	22%, poor results	Blount blade plate; 50% had errors in fixation
Stewart et al.[73]	69	1–20 years	54%, excellent, good	Blade plates, screws, bolts, Rush nails; Stewart evaluation method; 10 delayed union, 10 nonunions; limitation of motion frequent, caused by the trauma of surgery
Neer et al.[53]	29	1–29 years	52%, excellent, good	Rush nails, plates, blade plates, bolts; the treatment of choice was thought to be conservative; 23% flexion less than 60 degrees
DiMuria and Sartori[26]	45	1–7 years	75%, excellent, good	Olerud (Neer) evaluation method; variety of internal fixation devices; age was a negative factor on results; 35% had less than 90 degrees motion
Shelbourne and Brueckmann[69]	98	1–17 years; mean 3.5 years	84%, excellent, good	Rush pins. Evaluation method places emphasis on obtaining full extension more than full flexion; in severely comminuted fractures some shortening was encouraged for better contact; good or excellent equal no pain, < 2.5 cm shortening, > 90 degrees flexion, full extension, < 5 degrees deformity

Table 15II.7.   Results: ASIF Blade Plate

Author	Cases	Follow-up	Results	Remarks
Müller[51,52]	36	Average 1–2 years	95% satisfactory	Blade plate designed in 1959; Satisfactory results include medium results: with > 5 degrees recurvatum and > 10 degrees varus–valgus deformity; only four poor results
Chiron et al.[18]	72	Average 14 months	75% excellent, good	Evaluation similar to that of Stewart; 75% obtained 0–135 degrees motion; 14% at least 90 degrees; 11% less than 90 degrees; all fractures united, 60% healed at 3 months; 42% fair caused by inadequate fixation; 33% poor caused by medial protrusion of blade
Stringa et al.[75]	41	Average 2 years	76% excellent, good	Olerud evaluation method
Mordente and Gaeta[49]	45	1–7 years	78% excellent, good	At least 90 degrees flexion, occasional pain, less than 10 degrees malalignment
Schatzker and Lambert[66]	35	Average 22 months	71% excellent, good	Schatzker criteria; Excellent: Flexion loss 10 degrees, no deformity, no pain; Good: One of the following: length > 1.2 cm, > 10 degrees deformity, flexion loss 20 degrees. Fair: Two of the good criteria. Poor: Any of the following: flexion to 90 degrees, angular deformity > 15 degrees, pain. If rigid fixation had not been achieved, only 21% had good or excellent results; fracture involving articular surfaces had poor prognosis. Velocity of trauma had negative influence; osteoporosis had negative influence
Palazzi et al.[57]	69	2–10 years	79% excellent, good	Vidal criteria; 75% good results anatomically
Della Torre et al.[25]	48	1–10 years	71% excellent, good	Supraintercondylar fractures, no unicondylar; modified Hospital for Special Surgery rating system (excellent 95–100 points, good 85–94, fair 75–84, poor < 75); age had no influence; Success 100% in supracondylar, 87.5% in simple intercondylar, 43% in intercondylar and comminuted supracondylar, 50% in comminuted supraintercondylar; 78% had more than 90 degrees of flexion
Mize et al.[47]	30	Average 28.5 months	80% excellent, good	Schatzker criteria. Extensile approach used in 8 cases. Union in all knees. 2 malunions in valgus (elderly osteoporotic patients). Only 7 patients had 20–45° loss of flexion. 4 knees had unexplained mild lateral collateral laxity.

Abbreviation: ASIF, Association for the Study of Internal Fixation

Table 15II.8.   Results: Judet Screw-Plate

Investigators	No. of Cases	Follow-up	Results	Remarks
Honnart[36]	55	1–8 years	—	Considered mostly ROM; 67% > 100 degrees, 22% at least 80 degrees
Borroni[10]	22	1 year average	36% excellent 41% good	Excellent: Good alignment, no pain, > 120 degrees motion. Good: 90–120 degrees motion, good alignment and no pain

Abbreviation: ROM, range of motion.

CONCLUSIONS

Supracondylar fractures of the femur are severe lesions that are very difficult to treat. A good reduction is difficult, as many fractures are comminuted. Orientation of the distal fragments in the absence of a precise reduction of all the intermediary fragments is based solely on the experience of the surgeon. There can be residual deformities, and the quality of reduction significantly influences the final result. Although difficult, we believe that surgical treatment is best, particularly with the ASIF blade plate, the Judet screw-plate and the supracondylar-lag screw plate (Richards).

REFERENCES

1. Altenberg, A.R., and Shorkey, R.L.: Blade-plate fixation in non-union and in complicated fractures of the supracondylar region of the femur. J. Bone Joint Surg. [Am.], *31*: 312, 1949.
2. Balen, B.: Fracturas recientes del tercio distal del femur en el Adulto. Rev. Ortop. Traum., *11*: 259, 1967.
3. Beall, M.S., Jr., Nebel, E., and Bailey, R.W.: Transarticular fixation in the treatment of non-union of supracondylar fractures of the femur: A salvage procedure. J. Bone Joint Surg. [Am.], *61*: 1018, 1979.
4. Benum, P.: The use of bone cement as an adjunct to internal fixation of supracondylar fractures of osteoporotic femurs. Acta Orthop. Scand., *48*: 52, 1977.
5. Bergan, F.: Traumatic initial rupture of the popliteal artery with acute ischemia of the limb in cases with supracondylar fractures of the femur. J. Cardiovasc. Surg., *4*: 300, 1963.
6. Bianchi, G.: Le fratture del segmento inferiore del femore. Minerva Ortop., *6*: 49, 1955.
7. Blaimont, P., and Simmons, M.: Le traitement des fractures bases du femur chez l'adulte. Etude clinique Acta Orthop. Belg., *36*: 159, 1970.
8. Böhler, L.: The Treatment of Fractures. Bristol, John Wright and Sons, 1935.
9. Borgen, D., and Sprague, B.L.: Treatment of distal femoral fractures with early weight bearing. Clin. Orthop., *111*: 156, 1975.
10. Borroni, M., and Bottelli, G.C.: Il trattaurento delle fratture delle estremo distale del femore con vite-placca di judet. Ital. J. Orthop. Traumatol., *1*: 99, 1975.
11. Brown, A., and D'Arcy, J.C.: Internal fixation for supracondylar fractures of the femur in the elderly patient. J. Bone Joint Surg. [Br.], *53*: 420, 1971.
12. Buck, G.: An improved method of treating fractures of the thigh illustrated by cases and drawing. Trans. N.Y. Acad. Med., *2*: 232, 1861.
13. Burny, F., and Simons, M.: Traitement des fractures basses du femur chez l'adulte. Traitements conservateurs. Acta Orthop. Belg., *36*: 61, 1970.
14. Cameron, H.U., Jacob, R., Macnab, I., et al.: Use of polymethylmethacrylate to enhance screw fixation in bone. J. Bone Joint Surg. [Am.], *57*: 655, 1975.
15. Cauchoix, J., and Deburge, A.: Recent fractures of the lower end of the femur. Reconstr. Surg. Traumatol., *11*: 183, 1969.
16. Celoria, F.: Fracturas diaphyso-metaphyso-epiphysarias de la extremidad inferior del femur. Bol. Trab. Soc. Argentina Ortop. Traumatol. *38*: 348, 1973.
17. Charnley, J.: The Closed Treatment of Common Fractures. Edinburgh, Livingstone, 1961.
18. Chiron, H.S., Tremoulet, J., Casey, P., et al.: Fractures of the distal third of the femur treated by internal fixation. Clin. Orthop., *100*: 160, 1974.
19. Connolly, J.F., and King, P.: Closed reduction and early cast-brace ambulation in the treatment of femoral fractures. Part I. An in vivo quantitative analysis of immobilization in skeletal traction and a cast-brace. J. Bone Joint Surg. [Am.], *55*: 1559, 1973.
20. Connolly, J.F., Dehne, E., and Lafollette, B.: Closed reduction and early cast-brace ambulation in the treatment of femoral fractures. Part II. Results in 143 fractures. J. Bone Joint Surg. [Am.], *55*: 1581, 1973.
21. Creyssel, J., Lafaure, A., and Bobillon, J.L.: Sur le traitement des fractures de l'extrémité inférieure du femur. Lyon Chir., *61*: 785, 1965.
22. Danzig, L.A., Newell, J.D., Guerra, J., Jr., et al.: Osseous landmarks of the normal knee. Clin. Orthop., *156*: 201, 1981.
23. Dart, C.H., and Braitman, H.E.: Popliteal artery injury following fracture or dislocation at the knee. Arch. Surg., *112*: 969, 1977.
24. Deburge, A., Hy, X., and Machas, A.: Traitement des fractures récentes de l'extrémité inférieure du fémur. Presse Med., *75*: 527, 1967.
25. Della Torre, P., Aglietti, P., and Altissimi, M.: Results of rigid fixation in 54 supracondylar fractures of the femur. Arch. Orthop. Trauma. Surg., *97*: 177, 1980.
26. DiMuria, G.V., and Sartori, E.: Fratture articolari del terzo inferiore del femore. Arch. Putti Chir. Organi Mov., *29*: 111, 1978.
27. Elliot, R.B.: Fractures of the femoral condyles. Experiments with a new design femoral condylar blade-plate. South. Med. J., *52*: 80, 1959.
28. Fernandez Esteve, F.: Tratamiento biologico de les fracturas. Symposium, Valencia, 1980.
29. Gallannaugh, S.C.: Supracondylar fractures of the fe-

mur in the elderly: Treatment by internal fixation. Injury, 5: 259, 1974.

30. Gallinaro, P., and Crova, M.: Eziopatogenesi e classificazione delle fratture del ginocchio. Ital. J. Orthop. Traumatol., 3(Suppl. I): 23, 1977.

31. Giles, J.B., DeLee, J.C., Heckman, J. et al.: Supracondylar-intercondylar fractures of the femur treated with a supracondylar plate and lag screw. J. Bone Joint Surg. [Am.], 64:864, 1982.

32. Hampton, O.P.: Wounds of the Extremities in Military Surgery. St. Louis, C.V. Mosby, 1951.

33. Harrington, K.D.: The use of methylmethacrylate as an adjunct in the internal fixation of unstable comminuted intertrochanteric fractures in osteoporotic patients. J. Bone Joint Surg. [Am.], 57: 744, 1975.

34. Hohl, M.: Fractures of the distal femur. P. 1131. In Rockwood, C.P., and Green, D.P. (eds.): Fractures. Philadelphia, J.B. Lippincott, 1975.

35. Hoover, N.W.: Injuries of the popliteal artery associated with fractures and dislocations. Surg. Clin. North Am., 41: 1099, 1961.

36. Honnart, F.: La vis-plaque (Judet) dans le traitement des fractures de l'extrémité inférieure du fémur. A propos de 105 cas. In Systeme vis-plaque du Prof. Judet. Paris, Masson, 1975.

37. Huchet, C.A.: Osteosynthèse des fractures de l'extrémité inférieure du fémur. Ann. Orthop. Ouest, 1: 11, 1969.

38. Hurter, E.: Traitement de la fracture basse du fémur par fixateur externe. Acta Orthop. Belg., 36: 620, 1970.

39. Judet, R.: Fractures de l'extrémité inférieure du fémur. Acta Orthop. Belg., 36: 596, 1970.

40. Judet, R., Honnart, F., Suharso, T., et al.: La vis-plaque dans le traitement des fractures de l'extrémité inférieure du fémur. J. Chir. (Paris), 105: 235, 1973.

41. Kempf, I., Grosse, A., and Nonnenmacher, J.: Les traumatismes vasculaires au cours des fractures du genou. P. 153. In Duparc, J. et al (eds.): Les Fractures du genou. Paris, Expansion Scientifique Française, 1975. (Cahiers d'enseignement de la SOFCOT: I)

42. Kirschner, M.: Ueber nagelextension. Beitr. Z. Klin. Chir. Tübeng, 64: 266, 1909.

43. Mahorner, H.R., and Bradburn, M.: Fractures of the femur. Report of 308 cases. Surg. Gynecol. Obstet., 56: 1066, 1933.

44. Mazas, F., Capron, M., and De la Caffinière, J.Y.: Les éléments de gravité dans les fractures de l'extrémité inférieure du fémur. Rev. Chir. Orthop., 59: 415, 1973.

45. Meggitt, B.F., Juett, D.A., and Smith, J.D.: Cast bracing for fractures of the femoral shaft: A biomechanical and clinical study. J. Bone Joint Surg. [Br.], 63: 12, 1981.

46. Merle d'Aubigné, R., and Alnot, D.: Vingt-cinq ans de traitement des fractures de l'extrémité inférieure du femur. Acta Orthop. Belg., 36: 576, 1970.

47. Mize, R.D., Bucholz, R.W., and Grogan, D.P.: Surgical treatment of displaced, comminuted fractures of the distal end of the femur. J. Bone Joint Surg. [Am.], 64:871, 1982.

48. Mooney, V., Nickel, V.L., Harvey, J.P., et al.: Cast-brace treatment for fractures of the distal part of the femur. J. Bone Joint Surg. [Am.], 52: 1563, 1970.

49. Mordente, G., and Gaeta, V.: Le fratture del terzo distale del femore. Minerva Ortop., 28: 385, 1977.

50. Mouquin, F.: L'osteosynthèse de l'extrémité inférieure du femur. Osteosynthese, 8: 86091, 1970.

51. Müller, M.E.: Fractures basses du fémur. Acta Orthop. Belg., 36: 566, 1970.

52. Müller, M.E., Allgöwer, M., and Willenegger, H.: Manual of Internal Fixation. New York, Springer-Verlag, 1970.

53. Neer, C.S., Grantham, S.A., and Shelton, M.L.: Supracondylar fractures of the adult femur. A study of 110 cases. J. Bone Joint Surg. [Am.], 49: 591, 1967.

54. Nixon, J.E. and DiStefano, V.J.: Fractures of the distal femur. P. 709. In Heppenstall, R.B. (ed.): Fracture Treatment and Healing. Philadelphia, W.B. Saunders, 1980.

55. O'Donnel, T.F., Brewster, D.C., Darling, C.R., et al.: Arterial injuries associated with fractures and/or dislocations of the knee. J. Trauma, 17: 775, 1977.

56. Olerud, S.: Operative treatment of supracondylar-condylar fractures of the femur. Technique and results in fifteen cases. J. Bone Joint Surg. [Am.], 54: 1015, 1972.

57. Palazzi, C.S., Palazzi, C.C., and Soria Duran, I.J.: Fracturas de la extremidad inferior del femur classification, tecnica y resultados. Rev. Ortop. Trauma, 23IB: 71, 1979.

58. Perreau, M.: Traitement chirurgical des fractures de l'extrémité inférieure du fémur de l'adulte. P. 25. In Duparc, J. et al (eds). Les Fractures du genou. Paris, Expansion Scientifique Française, 1975. (Cahiers d'enseignement de la SOFCOT: I).

59. Rao, J.P., and Lapilusa, S.J.: An unusual complication of fracture of the lower femur. J. Trauma, 17: 889, 1977.

60. Riggins, R.S., Garrick, J.G., and Lipscomb. P.R.: Supracondylar fractures of the femur. A survey of treatment. Clin. Orthop., 82: 32, 1972.

61. Rienau, G.: Manuel de Traumatologie. 3rd ed. Paris, Masson, 1970.

62. Russell, R.H.: Theory and method in extension of the thigh. Br. Med. J., 2: 637, 1921.

63. Sanchez, R.J., and Quiles, M.Y.: Placa premodelada de judet: Empleo en la osteosintesis de fracturas de femur. Rev. Ortop. Traumatol. 20IB: 377, 1976.

64. Sarmiento, A., and Latta, L.: Fracture Bracing. New York, Springer-Verlag, 1980.

65. Scarfi, G.: Il trattamento delle fratture sovracondilo-idee di femore. Clin. Ortop., *23*: 59, 1971–1972.

66. Schatzker, J., and Lambert, D.C.: Supracondylar fractures of the femur. Clin. Orthop., *138*: 77, 1979.

67. Scuderi, C., and Ippolito, A.: Nonunion of supracondylar fractures of the femur. J. Int. Colloq. Surg., *17*: 1, 1952.

68. Seinsheimer F., III: Fractures of the distal femur. Clin. Orthop., *153*: 169, 1980.

69. Shelbourne, K.D., and Brueckmann, F.R.: Rush-pin fixation of supracondylar and intercondylar fractures of the femur. J. Bone Joint Surg. [Am.], *64*: 161, 1982.

70. Shelton, M.L., Grantham, S.A., Neer, C.S. et al.: A new fixation device for supracondylar and low femoral shaft fractures. J. Trauma., *14*:821, 1974.

71. Slätis, P., Ryöppy, S., and Huittinen, V.: AOI osteosynthesis of fractures of the distal third of the femur. Acta Orthop. Scand., *42*: 162, 1971.

72. Steinmann, F.R.: Eine neue extensiosmethode in der frakturenbehandlung. Zentralbl. f. Chir. Leipz., *34*: 938, 1907.

73. Stewart, M.J., Sisk, T.D., and Wallace, S.L.: Fractures of the distal third of the femur: a comparison of methods of treatment. J. Bone Joint Surg. [Am.], *48*: 784, 1966.

74. Stringa, G.: Fratture dia e sovracondiloidee del femore: Trattamento chirurgico. Acta Chir. Ital., *27*: 13, 1971.

75. Stringa, G., diMuria, C.V., and Sartori, E.: Il trattamento della fratture articolari dell'estremo distale del femore. Ital. J. Orthop. Traumatol., *3*(Suppl. I): 35, 1977.

76. Tees, F.J.: Fractures of the lower end of the femur. Am. J. Surg., *38*: 656, 1937.

77. Thomas, T.L., and Meggitt, B.F.: A comparative study of methods for treating fractures of the distal half of the femur. J. Bone Joint Surg. [Br.], *63*: 3, 1981.

78. Trenz, O., Tscherne, H., and Muhr, G.: Operationtechnik und ergebnisse bei distalen femurfrakturen mit supracondylären und condylären trummerzonen. Hefte Unfallheilkd., *126*: 402, 1975.

79. Trillat, A., Dejour, H., Bost, J., et al.: Les fractures unicondyliennes du fémur. Rev. Chir. Orthop., *61*: 611, 1975.

80. Trojan, E.: Traitement orthopedique des fractures de l'extrémité inférieure du fémur. P. 47. In Duparc, J. et al. (eds.): Les fractures du genou. Paris, Expansion Scientifique Française, 1975. (Cahiers d'enseignement de la SOFCOT: I)

81. Umansky, A.L.: Blade plate internal fixation for fracture of the distal end of the femur. Bull. Hosp. Joint Dis., *9*: 18, 1948.

82. Vesely, D.G.: The single and double split diamond femoral intramedullary nail. Clin. Orthop., *92*: 235, 1973.

83. Vidal, J., and Marchand, L.: Les fractures de l'extrémité inférieure du fémur. Traitement et resultats. Rev. Chir. Orthop., *52*: 533, 1966.

84. Vidal, J., Allieu, Y., Goalard, C., et al.: Notre conception actuelle du traitement chirurgical des fractures de l'extrémité inférieure du fémur. Acta Orthop. Belg., *36*: 586, 1970.

85. Vidal, J., Allieu, Y., Goalard, C., et al.: Arthrodèse du genou. Fixateur externe et enclouage fémoro-tibial. Rev. Chir. Orthop., *60*(Suppl. II): 308, 1974.

86. Wardlaw, D., McLauchlan, J., and Pratt, D.J. et al.: A biomechanical study of cast-brace treatment of femoral shaft fractures. J. Bone Joint Surg. [Br.], *63*: 7, 1981.

87. Watson-Jones, R.: Fractures and joint injuries. Baltimore, Williams & Wilkins, 1957.

88. Wertzberger, J.J., and Peltier, L.F.: Supracondylar fractures. J. Kansas Med. Soc. *68*: 328, 1967.

89. White, E.H., and Russin, L.A.: Supracondylar fractures of the femur treated by internal fixation with immediate knee motion. Am. Surg., *22*: 801, 1956.

90. Wiggins, H.E.: Vertical traction in open fractures of the femur. U.S. Armed Forces Med. J. *4*: 1633, 1953.

91. Zickel, R.E., Fietti, V.G., Lawsing, J.F., et al.: A new intramedullary fixation device for the distal third of the femur. Clin. Orthop. *125*: 185, 1977.

92. Zimmerman, A.J.: Intraarticular fractures of the distal femur. Orthop. Clin. North Am., *10*: 75, 1979.

Part III   Tibial Plateau Fractures

Articular fractures of the proximal tibia involve the articular cartilage, the epiphysis, and the metaphysis. Fractures of the intercondylar eminence, epiphyseal plate injuries, and anterior tibial tuberosity lesions are not included in this chapter.

Tibial plateau fractures occur in one of the most important load-bearing joints and are of uncertain prognosis. Many surgeons favor surgical management, but a nearly equal number prefer closed treatment. The goal of treatment is to achieve a stable, well-aligned, mobile joint with minimum surface irregularities and with adequate soft tissue healing. Prevention of late degenerative changes is also a purpose of treatment.

ANATOMY

The proximal upper tibia flares out from the shaft in the subcondylar area. Posterolaterally there is the articulation for the upper end of the fibula; superiorly one finds the medial and lateral tibial plateaus or condyles, with the nonarticular intercondylar eminence in between.

The upper surface of the lateral tibial plateau is saddleshaped, convex in the sagittal plane, slightly concave in the coronal plane. The medial tibial plateau is larger than the lateral, particularly in the sagittal dimension, and more uniformly and gently concave in both planes. In the frontal plane the articular surfaces of the proximal tibia are almost perpendicular to the long axis of the tibial shaft. In the sagittal plane the upper surface of the tibia slopes posteriorly and inferiorly 10 to 15 degrees from the horizontal. In addition, the tibia projects backward beyond the shaft in the sagittal plane.

In the normal individual even if the mechanical axis passes through the center of the tibial spines, with a corresponding femorotibial complementary angle of 6 to 7 degrees of valgus, the load is predominantly medial, as determined experimentally.[70,78,89]

This is reflected by the stronger trabecular pattern of the cancellous bone of the medial tibial condyles.[38,105] There are medial, lateral, anterior, and posterior pylons with vertical (compression) trabeculae, transverse and oblique (traction) trabeculae in a coronal section of the proximal tibial epiphysis.[29] Both the longitudinal and transverse trabeculae are weaker laterally, particularly in the anterior two-thirds, in front of the tibiofibular condensation.

The structural "points of weakness" of the proximal end of the tibia, resulting from the distribution of the trabecular pattern,[53] are located in a horizontal plane crossing the metaphyseal area. Two additional planes which, from each side of the intercondylar eminence, like an inverted V, are direct toward the medial or lateral aspects of the metaphysis. The location of these planes explains the direction of some of the main fracture lines.

The intercondylar eminence provides attachments to the menisci and the cruciate ligaments and is predominantly a nonarticular area facing the femoral intercondylar notch. From anterior to posterior the anterior intercondylar eminence provides attachment to the medial meniscus, the anterior cruciate ligament, and the lateral meniscus, and the posterior eminence provides the posterior attachments of the lateral and medial menisci, and the posterior cruciate ligament. Two bony prominences are encountered: the medial (anterior) spine, which is higher than the lateral and which gently slopes anteriorly, and the lateral (posterior) spine, which slopes posteriorly. The medial aspect of the medial spine and the lateral aspect of the lateral spine are articular contact areas under load.

The femorotibial weight-bearing areas have been studied by arthrographic methods[79] and cement casting methods[127] under loads. By one method[79] the total area measures 20 cm² in extension and 11.6 cm² in flexion (90 to 110 degrees). The contact area moves progressively backward with flexion. The contact area is evenly distributed between medial and lateral plateaus. The menisci increase the contact area. Without them the total area is reduced and varies between 12 and six cm², for both plateaus.

The role of the menisci in force transmission across the knee has been investigated[126] using casting techniques under high loads. Without load most of the contact is over the menisci and the medial aspect of the medial spine. With load the area extends over the plateaus. The contact areas in flexion are approximately 2 cm² for each condyle without menisci and 6 cm² with menisci. The lateral meniscus bears most of the load on that side of the joint. Medially, the load is shared almost equally between meniscus and exposed cartilage.[35]

The menisci are therefore clearly load-bearing structures; this was suggested many years ago by Fairbank[47] and has recently been documented.[115,117,126] At least 65 percent of the load in the standing position is transmitted by the menisci, which act as shock absorbers.[15] If they are removed, the pressure in the articular cartilage is increased. Removing the meniscus decreases the contact areas and increases the stresses in both cartilage and subchondral bone.[73] Meniscectomy sequelae are well documented.[68,71,75,82,121]

The transverse width of the femoral condyles is smaller anteriorly than posteriorly. In the flexed position, the posterior convex part of the femoral condyles is in contact with the tibial plateaus, but when the knee is extended the narrower but flatter anterior surface of the condyles comes into contact. In the last few degrees of extension the femur rotates internally, leaving uncovered a portion of the articular surface of the lateral plateau, which projects in the anteroposterior plane a few millimeters (0.5 cm) outside the condyle.[123] The medial femoral condyle is more or less uniformly rounded in its contour while the lateral condyle has an anterior flattened portion that articulates with the anterior horn of the lateral meniscus in extension. These anatomic details may explain some of the characteristics of plateau fractures.

MECHANISMS OF INJURY

It is sometimes difficult to understand the mechanisms of injury, as the conditions of fractures are multiple and often the patients do not remember the exact mechanisms.

Kennedy and Bailey[72] studied experimental plateau fractures. The forces were abduction (valgus) alone or combined with a compression force, compression force alone or combined with valgus force, in different positions of flexion of the knee.

When a predominantly *abduction* force was applied there were 10 typical split or wedge-type fractures of the lateral plateau, five typical crush or compression fractures and five mixed split-compression fractures.

When a predominantly *compression* force was applied, nine typical compression fractures were obtained in the lateral plateau, in three specimens no plateau fractures were obtained, and in the remaining knees, where accessory forces were applied before the application of the predominant compression force, a mixed type of fracture resulted. Increasing flexion tended to move the fracture site posteriorly.

There were some knees in which a mixed fracture was produced: the forces were combined valgus and compression. No comminuted bicondylar fractures were seen; however, in two cases, after the lateral plateau fracture, the compressive force was continued to a very high level and a bicondylar fracture was observed.

The forces that produce the fractures of the tibial plateaus are valgus or compression, or both. In abduction the mechanical center of rotation is medial and the hinge is the medial collateral ligament ("nutcracker" theory). With hinging in extension the prominent anterolateral part of the lateral femoral condyle is forced like a wedge into the lateral tibial plateau (Fig. 15III.1). When the knee is flexed the hinging action of the collateral ligament is weak, the posterior convex femoral condyles contact the tibia, and a wedge-type fracture cannot be predictably produced. With some flexion the abduction force can be dissipated elsewhere because the medial ligament is less taut and more rotation is allowed. In flexion the compressive loads tend to produce compression fractures of the lateral plateau or mixed fractures particularly if combined with an abduction force. Stronger compression forces produce a bicondylar fracture.

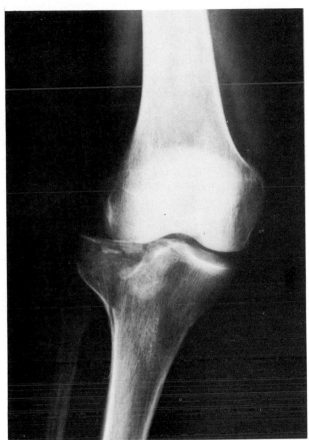

Fig. 15III.1. Mechanism of injury. The prominent antero-lateral part of the lateral femoral condyle is forced like a wedge into the lateral tibial plateau, producing a mixed split-compression fracture.

In only two of the 44 knees in the Kennedy and Bailey study were associated gross lesions of the medial collateral ligament or of the anterior cruciate ligament found. The mechanical role of the ligaments in the production of the plateau fractures is complex. Theoretically, as the distance between center of rotation (medial femorotibial contact area) and the medial collateral ligament is much shorter than the distance between the medial and lateral femorotibial contact areas,[9] the lateral depression would be much greater than the correspondent medial ligament elongation. This is known as the Bistolfi[9]-Hultén[65] law of inverse proportion of ligament and bony lesions. Practically, the problem is much more difficult.

Stretching of the collateral mechanism often exists as shown by the frequency of later calcification. True lesions of the collateral or cruciate ligaments can occur, particularly in some fracture types, as continuing angular or twisting forces of different velocities occur.

We believe that most condylar fractures are produced by the prominent anterior part of the lateral femoral condyle in extension.[2,10,21,39,101] In extension, owing to the screw home mechanism and the tension of the ligaments, the knee is vulnerable.

The mechanisms producing lateral, medial, and bicondylar fractures are similar.[101] The force is directed primarily distally, but may proceed in a medial or lateral direction splitting off one or both of the two condyles. The fractures usually involve the lateral plateau first; the main damage to the articular surface is lateral, and the surface of the medial plateau is rarely damaged. The size of the wedge depends on the location of the impact, while the extent of the depression depends on the sex and age of the patient, osteoporosis, the resistance of the subchondral bone, the amount of axial force, and the amount of flexion. With the knee toward extension, the intercondylar notch of the femur impinges on the intercondylar eminence after a few millimeters of depression. In flexion, the fracture would be predominantly of the compression type and would occur more posteriorly, where there is no such limit to depression because the intercondylar notch is much deeper. The degree of rotation is also important. In internal rotation, with tight ligaments, little hinging or wedging can occur and the valgus forces tend to be transmitted as compressive loads on the lateral plateau.

The presence of osteoporosis is important not only because it facilitates the crushing or depression of subchondral bone, but also because it explains, with the velocity of injury, the production of certain types of fractures. Split fractures usually occur in younger people without osteoporosis as a result of high-velocity trauma. Compression fractures occur in older people with osteoporosis and usually involve less severe trauma. Naturally the osteoporosis adversely affects the outcome because it is associated with increased comminution, and increased depression.

The lateral condyle is fractured more often than the medial. This is because of the physiologic valgus of the knee, the weaker trabeculation under the lateral tibial plateau, and the increased frequency of valgus injuries as the knee is protected medially by the contralateral side. The anatomic square shape of the lateral femoral condyle is also important in this respect.

Varus forces can occur, although infrequently.[39, 41,53] The hinge must be lateral. The medial condyle is fractured first, but usually there is no depression element and the plateau is split *en bloc*.

The fracture line in the medial fractures often begins close to the lateral side of the intercondylar eminence, (perhaps because of trabecular weakness) and there can be an element of depression of the lateral plateau. This can be explained by the superolateral subluxation of the tibia that occurs after the fracture. In fact the compressed fragment of the lateral plateau

is hinged laterally and not medially, as in the usual lateral plateau fractures, and there can be lateral ligamentous lesions. Other investigators[32, 101] explain this type of "spinotuberosity" fracture by the same wedge action of the lateral femoral condyle that occurs in valgus-compression trauma, because the fracture always begins laterally, but can then proceed in a medial or lateral direction.

A varus force associated with flexion and external rotation of the tibia has been suggested as the mechanism of production of the posterior split fractures of the medial condyle.[100] For the same fracture a purely hyperflexion mechanism has been proposed[88] on the basis of the movement of the fragment with knee position (reduction in extension).

Table 15III.1.   Mechanism of Injury to the Tibial Plateau

Investigators	No. of Cases	Mechanisms	%
Roberts[105]	230	Falls	44
		Automobile drivers	26
		Hit by cars	13
		Other	18
Porter[99]	138	Falls, twists	61
		Bumper	29
		Automobile drivers	8.6
		Sports	1.9
Rasmussen[102]	260	Traffic accidents	45
		Other	55
Bakalim and Wilppula[4]	197	Falls, twists	47
		Automobile and automotor drivers	28
		Bumper	25
Hohl[63]	900	Bumper	52
		Falls from heights	17
		Other	31

Table 15III.2.   Age and Sex as Factors in Tibial Plateau Fractures

Investigators	No. of Cases	Age (Years)	M	F	Remarks
Roberts[105]	230	49	52	48	Patients with local compression are older than the rest.
Porter[99]	138	47	53	47	Preponderance of women in 6th and 7th decades; only "crush" fractures included
Rasmussen[102]	260	55	55	45	Males have lower average age; medial plateau fracture average age 49 years, bicondylar 53 years, men more frequent in those two groups (69%); patients with lateral fractures are older (61 years for posterior compression) and predominantly women (61% for posterior compression)
Bakalim and Wilppula[4]	197	52	46	54	
Rinonapoli and Aglietti[104]	128	49	66.5	33.5	
Burri et al.[16]	278	49	67	33	
Schatzker[111]	94	57	40.5	59.5	

Table 15III.3.　Fracture Types

Investigators	No. of Cases	Lateral (%)	Medial (%)	Bicondylar (%)
Roberts[105]	230	61.5	14.3	24.3
Courvoisier[23]	200	55	14	31
Bakalim and Wilppula[4]	197	64	19.2	18
Rasmussen[102]	260	70	12	18
Rinonapoli and Aglietti[104]	128	60.5	8	31.5
Duparc[38,39]	200	60	10	30

In clinical practice, the fractures are caused by the following: pedestrians being hit by a car, causing fender fractures[21] or bumper fractures,[14] pedestrians being hit by a motorcycle or bicycle; injuries to car occupants; falls from a height; accidental falls or twists; and direct application of force to the knee (Table 15III.1).

Table 15III.2 gives information about the average age and the sex ratio of a number of published series.

CLASSIFICATION

Tibial plateau fractures can be divided into fractures of the lateral plateau, bicondylar fractures, and fractures of the medial plateau. Table 15III.3 reports the various incidence found in different series.

Morphologically three fracture types are defined: split, split-compression, and compression. A split fracture (Fig. 15III.2) (wedge, cleavage, or separa-

Fig. 15III.2. Split fracture.

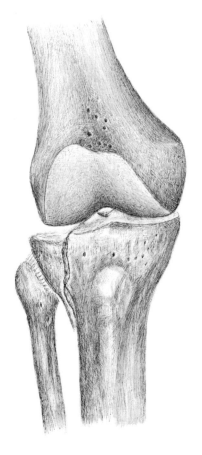
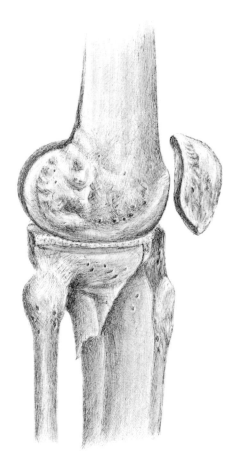

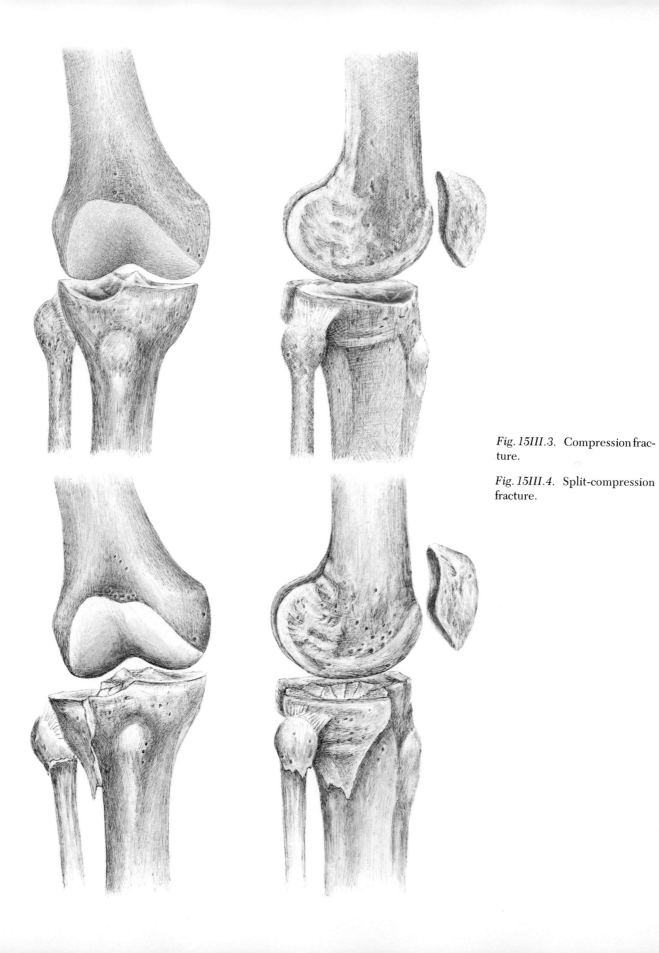

Fig. 15III.3. Compression fracture.

Fig. 15III.4. Split-compression fracture.

tion) is one in which the margin of the tibial plateau is separated from the rest of the plateau with little if any crushing of the bone at the borders of the fracture line. A compression fracture (Fig. 15III.3) shows crushing of the subchondral bone with the margins of the plateau usually spared, there is a mosaic pattern on the articular surface and vertical depression of fragments. A mixed fracture (Fig. 15III.4) shows split and compression.

The characteristics of the fractures may vary, from clear-cut split to marked compression with or without marginal associated fragments. Lateral, medial, and bicondylar fractures can occur with or without compression, but compression is more frequent laterally, and practically all pure compression fractures are lateral.

RASMUSSEN CLASSIFICATION

One of the most important and widely used classifications is that of Rasmussen.[102] This is the classification we routinely use. In parentheses are the figures given by Rasmussen; without parentheses are our figures using the same classification.[104]

Lateral plateau fracture (70%) 60.5%
   Split (14%) 11.5%
   Split-compression (25%) 28%
   Compression (31%) 21%
      Anterior (7%)
      Posterior (13%)
      Central (10%)
      Total (1%)
Medial plateau fracture (12%) 8%
   Split (6%)
   Split-compression (5%)
   Compression (1%)
Bicondylar fracture (18%) 31.5%
   Split (7%)
   Split-compression (11%)

HOHL CLASSIFICATION

The classification of Hohl[62,63] is based on a study of more than 900 fractures and is widely known in the United States:

I   Undisplaced (24%)
II   Local compression (26%)
III Split compression (26%)
IV   Total-condylar depression (11%)
V   Split (3%)
VI   Comminuted (10%)

Type I: Undisplaced Fracture. This fracture shows less than 4 mm of depression or separation (condylar widening); very few of these fractures tend to displace further in the first few weeks, particularly those extending from the intercondylar area to the medial or lateral tibial cortex.

Type II: Local Compression Fracture. This fracture has a plateau depression shaped like the condyle that has caused it. A few millimeters of depression of the lateral plateau causes a minimal valgus deformity that can be well tolerated.

Type III: Split-Compression Fracture. This fracture has a compressed area in the middle of the plateau and a peripheral split fragment.

Type IV: Total-Condylar Depression Fracture. This type of fracture usually affects the medial plateau without articular surface damage. The fracture line begins near the intercondylar eminence area. Closed reduction of the fragment is easy, for its capsular attachments to the femur remain, but maintaining the reduction can be difficult and loss of reduction can occur in the cast. Manipulative reduction is less easy in the laterally located fractures of this type.

Type V: Split Fracture. This fracture is uncommon, but it differs from the split-compression type in that there is no articular surface compression. Usually the posterior articular margin of the medial plateau is split with a portion of its articular surface. Displacement shows separation and distal migration. Posteromedial frontal fractures tend to reduce in extension; the femoral condyle tends to dislocate into the split fragment with flexion.

Type VI: Comminuted Fracture. This fracture shows involvement of both plateaus. There can be articular surface damage, particularly in the lateral condyle; there are usually fracture lines extending from the intercondylar area to the medial and lateral cortices. They can be very difficult to reconstruct surgically and often realign satisfactorily in traction.

SCHATZKER CLASSIFICATION

The classification of Schatzker et al.[111] is based on the study of 94 fractures:

I   Pure cleavage fracture (6%)
II   Cleavage combined with depression (25%)

III   Pure central depression (36%)
IV   Fractures of medial condyle (10%)
    Split or wedge (one-third)
    Depressed and comminuted (two-thirds)
V   Bicondylar fractures
VI   Tibial plateau fractures with dissociation of the tibial metaphysis and diaphysis (20%)

Type I: Pure Cleavage Fracture.   This type occurs in younger patients, average age 32, usually without osteoporosis, as a result of high-velocity trauma.

Type II: Cleavage Combined with Depression.   In this fracture, there is lateral cleavage combined with depression; it occurs in older patients (average age 57 years) usually as a result of high-velocity trauma.

Type III: Pure Central Depression of the Lateral Plateau.   In this, the commonest fracture in the series, there is no wedge fragment and the lateral cortex is intact. It occurs in the older age group with osteoporosis (average age 63 years) or is the result of less severe low-velocity trauma.

Type IV: Fracture of the Medial Condyle.   This fracture has two subtypes. The medial plateau can be split off as a wedge of various sizes (type A), or it may be compressed and depressed (type B). Type A occurs in younger patients as the result of severe violent trauma and is probably an unrecognized knee dislocation or subluxation which reduced spontaneously. Type B is rare and occurs in older patients with osteoporosis as the result of minor trauma. Type IV fractures have the worst prognosis, probably because of associated ligament injuries.

Type V: Bicondylar Fracture.   This type usually occurs in old persons. Both tibial plateaus and diaphysis are in continuity.

Type VI: Tibial Plateau Fracture with Dissociation of the Tibial Metaphysis and Diaphysis.   This fracture shows the characteristics of a transverse fracture of the proximal tibia, which separates metaphysis from diaphysis. In addition, there is compression or comminution of one or both plateaus, resulting from high-velocity trauma (average age 56 years).

MOORE CLASSIFICATION

The classification of Moore[86] is based on the observation of 132 fracture-dislocations:
I   Split (37%)
II   Entire condyle (25%)

III   Rim avulsion (15%)
IV   Rim compression (12%)
V   Four-part (11%)

In a tibial plateau fracture, there is involvement of the articular surface, usually without concomitant significant injury to capsule or ligaments. In a knee dislocation there are severe soft tissue injuries to ligaments and capsule, as well as frequent neurovascular involvement, but without fractures.

The term *fracture-dislocations* describes a group of lesions much more serious than plateau fractures and characterized by the marked joint instability due to soft tissue injuries and with a high incidence of neurovascular lesions, especially the peroneal nerve, and popliteal artery. The incidence of instability and neurovascular injuries increases from type I to V. The associated ligament injuries are either intraligamentous or bony avulsions at the site of attachment of the ligaments. According to the studies of Noyes and Grood,[94] fast loading causes intraligamentous failure and slow loading causes bone failure by an avulsion fracture. The average age for the fracture-dislocations was 39, less than the average age for tibial fractures and more than the usual age for pure knee dislocations. There were twice as many men as women.

Type I: Split Fracture.   This type is the most common and has been considered a classic tibial plateau fracture. It corresponds to Hohl type V, to Schatzker type IVA, and to the posterior fracture-separation of Postel et al.[100]

The fracture can be recognized in the lateral view, as it is placed in the coronal plane and is directed posteroinferiorly at an angle of 30 to 45 degrees with the axis of the tibia. It usually contains about one-half the articular surface of the medial plateau or the posteromedial tibial plateau. The fragment is unstable, and in flexion displaces distally with posteromedial subluxation of the femoral condyle. In the frontal view it presents as a vertical fracture line beginning at the intercondylar eminence or occasionally in the lateral compartment: it continues as an oblique medial metaphyseal fracture line with a 45-degree angle. When there is displacement, two levels may be observed at the medial joint line.

The medial capsule is avulsed from the posteromedial fragment but the rest of the medial or posterior structures are intact. Associated avulsion fractures of the fibular styloid or of the anteromedial tibial spine are frequent. Varus alignment results frequently. There are no significant intraligamentous injuries and neurovascular complications are rare. Instability clinically is found in 58 percent of cases. This lesion is interpreted as the result of a fall with hyperflexion or varus-external rotation in flexion.[100]

Type II: Entire Condyle Fracture. Here the entire condyle, medially or laterally, is fractured. This fracture is different from the classic Hohl type IV in that there is a fracture of all or part of the intercondylar eminence usually as part of the plateau, but occasionally separate. The fracture usually starts in the opposite plateau, crosses the tibia in a sagittal plane at an angle of 45 degrees to form a large condylar fragment. This fracture, described also by Duparc and Filipe,[41] has been called a "spinotuberosity" fracture. It is frequently associated with a subluxation of the rest of the tibia relative to the femur. It has also been called spinoglenoid,[55] or fracture with subluxation of the femoral condyle.[103] The term "spinotuberosity" fracture would seem to be a more adequate description. The spinoglenoid fracture is a rare variety wherein the line is almost parallel to the articular surface of the medial plateau. It is usually observed in very young people in whom the fracture line follows the line of the previous growth plate. The precise mechanism is debated and not precisely known. It could be varus-compression[40,41] or valgus-compression.[32,101]

There are three degrees of severity of this injury in the medial plateau.[41] Grade I shows no displacement. Grade II shows lateral subluxation of the tibia relative to the spinotuberosity fragment, which maintains normal relationship to the femur because of the intact medial and cruciate ligaments. Grade III has lateral tibial dislocation with lateral plateau compression. There are frequently associated lesions of the lateral collateral ligament or avulsion fractures of the fibular styloid. The intercondylar eminence can be avulsed. Lesions of the lateral meniscus are frequently associated.

This type of fracture can also occur laterally. The mechanism is valgus-compression. The fracture is usually associated with a high fracture of the fibula, which may allow a lateral displacement of the plateau and the fibular fragment. There is an abnormal space between fibula and tibia and a superomedial subluxation of the rest of the tibia. These cases often show avulsion fractures of the anterior spine or intraligamentous lesions of the medial collateral ligament and/or medial meniscal lesions.

In type II fracture-dislocation, the incidence of in-traligamentous injuries is 22 percent and is 12 percent for neurovascular injuries.

Type III: Rim-Avulsion Fracture-Dislocation. This fracture occurs laterally more often than medially. The rim fragments are displaced upward and sometimes rotated. They usually come from the rim of the lateral plateau, Gerdy's tuberosity, or fibular styloid. The mechanism for the lateral type is varus force. In addition to ligament avulsion, there can be intraligamentous ruptures of the anterior or posterior cruciate, lateral collateral structures, or iliotibial band. The incidence of intraligamentous injuries in type III is 63 percent and 30 percent have neurovascular injuries.

Type IV: Rim-Compression Fracture-Dislocation. This fracture is different from type III in that the fragments are distally displaced, impacted, or crushed. They are compression fractures of the rim of the medial or lateral plateau. When the rim compression is medial, there are associated avulsions of the fibular styloid or of the anterior spine and intraligamentous lesions of the posterior or anterior cruciate ligaments. When the compressed rim is lateral, there are associated avulsions of the anterior spine and high fractures of the fibula (or tibiofibular dislocation) and often intraligamentous lesions of the medial collateral ligament. The intraligamentous injury rate for type IV is 66 percent with an unexpected low incidence of peroneal nerve and popliteal artery lesions.

Type V: Four-Part Fracture-Dislocation. This fracture is similar to the type VI (comminuted) of Hohl, but in this type there is a bicondylar comminuted fracture; in addition, the intercondylar eminence is fractured and separated from both the shaft and the plateaus. Avulsion fractures of the fibular styloid or fractures of the fibular neck or head are associated frequently. No intraligamentous lesions[86] were observed but the neurovascular injury rate was 50 percent. In conclusion, it is useful to know different classifications, particularly to understand the fracture anatomy and the indications for treatment.

For *practical purposes*, we suggest that the classification of Rasmussen be followed as a guide, with particular attention to certain fracture types well described by others, such as the split (particularly the posteromedial split) (Fig. 15III.5), the spinotuberosity fractures (Figs. 15III.6 and 15III.7), the bicondylar (Fig. 15III.8), and the more severe fracture-dislocations (Fig. 15III.9).

(Text continues on page 463.)

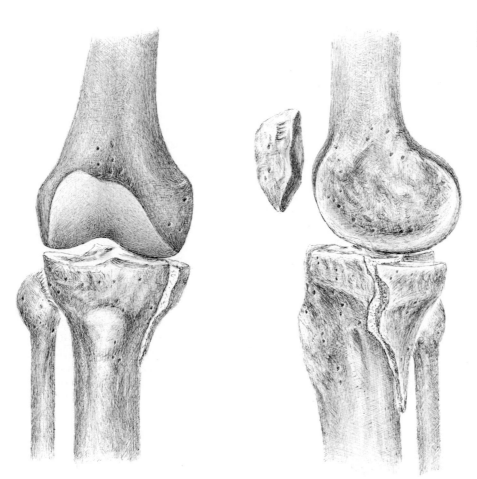

Fig.   15III.5. Posteromedial
frontal split fracture.

Fig. 15III.6. Spinotuberosity medial fracture.

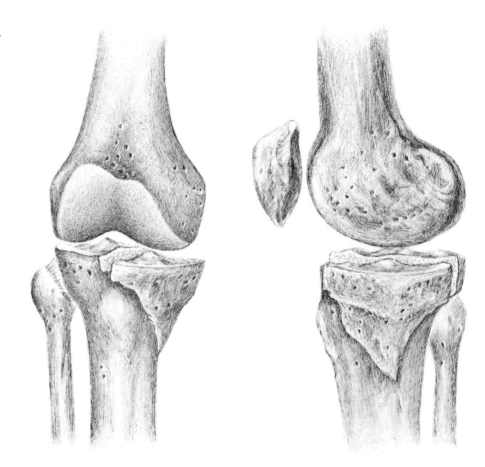

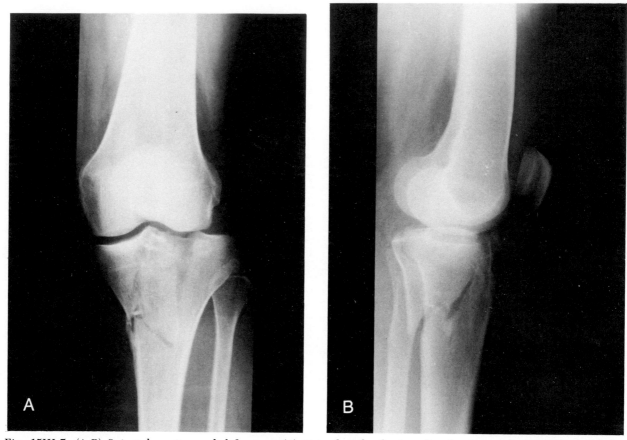

Fig. 15III.7. (A,B) Spinotuberosity medial fracture. (A) Note that the fracture line begins on the lateral side of the intercondylar eminence and that (B) the medial plateau surface is normal. There is often instability because of lateral ligament complex associated injuries.

Fig. 15III.8. Bicondylar fracture.

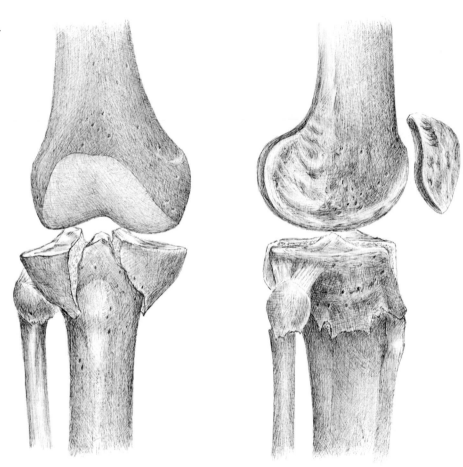

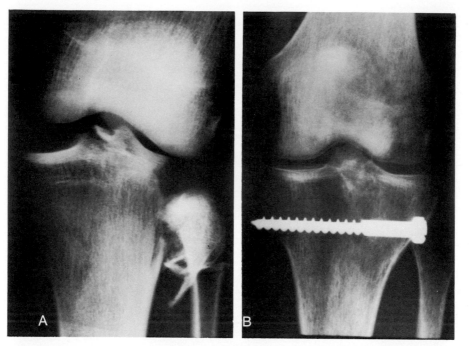

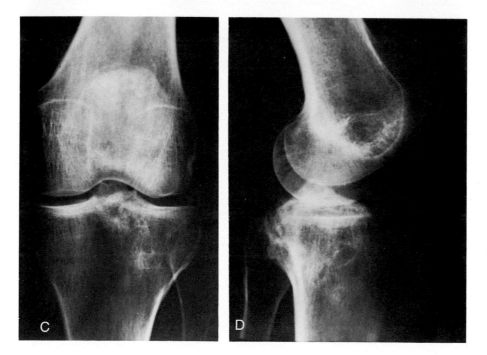

Fig. 15III.9. (A) Fracture-dislocation of the knee. Example of depression of the peripheral part of the lateral plateau with associated medial compartment ligament and anterior intercondylar eminence lesions. (B) Surgical treatment with cancellous screw and repair of the peripheral ligament lesions. (C,D) Show good results at 3 years after removal of the screw.

CLINICAL FINDINGS

An effusion is often present, but if there is an associated tear of the capsule, the blood might have diffused into the periarticular tissues. There is tenderness over the fractured plateau, but this may also be present on the opposite side over the ligament complexes or ligament attachments to bone. Palpation of the knee should be done in flexion, but this may be difficult because of pain and contracture. The patients are sometimes able to do straight leg raising, but this too can be very painful.

Ligament and stability testing should be done as a rule after evacuation of the hemarthrosis. The angular instability is predominantly caused by bone depression and displacement, but it may be also ligamentous. Testing should be done in extension, not in hyperextension, as well as in mild (20 to 25 degrees) flexion. More importance is attributed to the test in extension. If the blood evacuation has not relieved pain sufficiently to allow hamstring relaxation and full extension, the laxity tests should be done under general or spinal anesthesia, particularly in cases for which the surgical indication is in doubt. The instability should be compared with the opposite normal side; the tests for sagittal instability, in flexion and near extension should be checked as well as the abduction and adduction tests.

The extremity should be examined for associated injuries or fractures and for neurovascular complications. Peroneal nerve palsy is comparatively rare but is more frequent in association with fracture dislocations of the knee.

Vascular complications are even more rare but again more frequent in fracture-dislocations. Rasmussen[102] cites an incidence of 2.3 percent of peroneal nerve palsies and 0.3 percent vascular complications in 260 fractures. In Moore's study of fracture-dislocations,[86] 15 percent of patients overall had neurovascular injuries.

Open fractures are infrequent: from 0 percent in Rasmussen's series to 1.6 percent[28] and 3.7 percent.[40] They are more frequent in bicondylar and comminuted fractures.

RADIOLOGIC FINDINGS

Routine frontal and lateral views of the knee will show most of the fractures. However, certain fractures can be seen only in oblique or tunnel views of the knee, which should be obtained at least when there is a diagnostic doubt.[92] Certain depressed areas of the plateaus can be obscured either by the intact portion of the same plateau or by the contralateral unaffected plateau. The horizontal beam lateral view can be useful in trauma patients with knee effusion before knee aspiration to demonstrate a fat–fluid level indicating an intra-articular fracture.

The normal posterior slope of the tibial plateaus (10 to 15 degrees) may be a cause of error in the measurement of the amount of depression in the anteroposterior view of the knee. This measurement is important for the indications for appropriate treatment. The depth of depression can be measured from a reference line parallel to the intact remnants of the lateral plateau. In other cases the depth can be measured from the level of the contralateral plateau. Measuring depressions is difficult in bicondylar fractures because of the lack of a reference line. An error of 2 to 3 mm can occur even when the radiographs are of good quality and the distance from tube to film constant.[99] But owing to the posterior inclination of the plateaus, there could be a larger error.[87] Experimentally obtained depression of 10 mm can measure from 6 to 14 mm by changing the inclination of the central beam over the tibial crest. The position of the depression, anterior or posterior is also important. For posterior depressions, the error would be greater. Therefore, the anteroposterior view should be taken with a 15-degree craniocaudal inclination relative to the vertical plane.

Measurement of condylar widening caused by the separation and lateral displacement of a marginal split fragment is also difficult. We measured the total width of the two tibial plateaus just below the joint line in the anteroposterior view and compared it to the width of the femoral condyles just above the joint.[104] It has been shown[83] that these two measurements are normally equal. Condylar widening can therefore be measured as the difference between the two measurements.

The routine anteroposterior, lateral, oblique, and tunnel views of the knee should be carefully studied with particular reference to the areas of ligament attachments for possible avulsion fragments. The intercondylar eminences, the medial and lateral epicondyles of the femur, the fibular head, the tibiofibular joint, and the lateral or medial margins of the tibial plateaus should be scrutinzed. The osseous landmarks of the normal knee should be kept in mind.

A lateral view of the tibia shows[25] the medial tibial spine which projects more superiorly than the lateral one. In some patients a bony spicule can be identified anterior to the medial tibial spine (Parson's knob) and it shows precisely the site of insertion of the anterior cruciate ligament. Usually the lateral spine proceeds to an even curve in a posterior direction until reaching the posterior contour of the lateral tibial plateau. The medial tibial condyle can be identified in the lateral view by its posterior squared-off appearance and by its posterosuperior position relative to the smaller lateral tibial condyle. The lateral tibial plateau can be identified following the posterior descending portion of the lateral spine, it is smaller and does not have a squared-off appearance. Following the lateral spine more posteriorly and inferiorly along the posterior aspect of the tibia, a radiodensity can be found in the lateral view which normally intersects the fibular head. This represents the posterior tibial groove, which is helpful to diagnose dislocations or subluxations of the tibiofibular articulation. This joint can also be readily seen in the oblique (45 to 60 degrees internal rotation) views of the knee.

Varus and valgus stress films are recommended to show the association of ligament injuries.[51,62–64] The angular stresses are applied to the knee in extension and in mild flexion, preferably with the patient under anesthesia, to eliminate pain. According to Martin,[80] despite experimental resection of the lateral plateau, an abduction force, although able to create a valgus deformity, is unable to open the medial joint space if the medial collateral ligament is intact. The medial "clear space" should be measured at a distance of 5 mm from the tibial edge and averages 6.5 mm (range 5 to 10 mm) in the normal knee. In 22 clinical cases of lateral plateau fracture, some with ligament tears, there was a difference of 5.3 mm between normal and abnormal ligaments. A medial opening of more than 1 mm greater than the normal side would tend to indicate[80] a lesion of the medial collateral ligament.

On the other hand, stress films were thought by others[101] to be of academic interest, time consuming, and of little or no therapeutic consequences. Concomitant collateral ligament injury may contribute to instability but is of minor importance compared with the bone damage and may be ignored in most cases. General fibrosis of torn capsular structures will produce stability if there is good functional contact between the the femur and tibia. Moore et al.[88] did

bilateral stress films in varus and valgus in 208 patients with unilateral tibial plateau fractures after a follow-up of more than 10 years. There was no significant difference between fractured and healthy sides.

We believe that stress films are of interest in those fracture types known to have a higher incidence of severe ligamentous lesions like the fracture-dislocations,[86] the spinotuberosity fracture,[38,41] the posteromedial split type,[111] and the marginal types.[120] Stress films are also important to show the presence of fragments due to ligament avulsions. Those fragments are often revealed only by the stress films, when the joint opens.

Fracture anatomy is most accurately delineated by tomography.[92,112] The classification of the fracture types, so important to the therapeutic decision, can be undertaken only knowing precisely the location, the extent, and the displacement of the fracture or depressed fragments. Plateau depression, which can be overlooked on standard films, is best demonstrated by tomography. This was emphasized by many.[40,45,46,50,130] Classification based solely on standard films is unreliable. Underdiagnosis of depressed osteochondral fragments is the most common mistake.

INDICATIONS FOR TREATMENT

Up to 30 years ago the treatment was mainly conservative, and only a few surgeons used open reduction and internal fixation.[5,96,97,125] Subsequently the number of surgeons in favor of surgical treatment has increased progressively.[1,4,16,22,23,28,33,39,40,54,56,60,69,84,98,102,103,106,111] It is thought that with surgical treatment, the factors that determine the short- and long-term results can be adequately dealt with. This involves joint surface reconstruction with minimum incongruity and irregularity; stable fixation allowing early mobilization for good range of motion and for surface reconstitution and molding; correct treatment of associated ligament and meniscal lesions; and last but not least, stability and correct alignment.

On the other hand, many surgeons favor conservative treatment of various types, including cast immobilization,[19] traction mobilization, and cast braces.[2,3,6,8,11,12,13,21,30–32,37,44,48,49,108,109,114,118,119] Conservative treatment is believed to have a satisfactory percentage of good and excellent short- and long-term results, from the functional point of view, even in treating severely displaced fractures. The anatomic results are less than ideal in many cases, but function is more important than restoration of anatomy.

Attempts to compare the results of nonsurgical and operative treatment are very difficult because of different case groups, ages, type of causative violence, displacement, indications, preferences of the surgeon, and different lengths of follow-up.[24,36,113] In a retrospective study[104] in which similar types of fractures were compared, we showed that surgical treatment gives only a slightly better percentage of satisfactory clinical results and a definitely higher incidence of satisfactory radiographic results.

Recently many investigators have done studies designed to evaluate the indications for surgical versus conservative treatment primarily on the basis of fracture type, amount of displacement, and preoperative instability. We will report their conclusions, bearing in mind that there is not a definitive answer yet.

Roberts[105] has shown that nondisplaced, stable fractures, and local compression, stable fractures, can be successfully treated by conservative methods, particularly traction and early mobilization. Surgery is indicated in many displaced fractures, mostly split-compression types, with instability. Early mobilization is the key to maximum joint function.

Porter[99] has related the degree of depression and the area of depression in "crush" fractures of the lateral tibial plateau (i.e., split-compression or pure compression fractures, excluding the pure split and the bicondylar) to the results of conservative and open treatment. The only factor that appears to influence the results is the extent of the original depression and, if this is severe, the degree of reduction obtained by the treatment. There is nothing to be gained by open reduction if the depression is < 10 mm, as conservative treatment gives good results. If the depression is more severe, a good result can only be achieved if the articular surface is successfully reconstructed. This is possible only by surgical means.

For Hohl,[62–64] the indications change according to type of fracture. In general, undisplaced fractures (≤ 3 to 4 mm) require conservative measures. Local compression or split-compression fractures can be treated conservatively when there is < 8-mm displacement in depression and if the split fragment is large and only minimally displaced outward. Attempts toward closed reduction can be made particularly in split-compression fractures. But if these ef-

forts fail or if stress testing demonstrates more than 5 degrees of valgus instability in near-complete knee extension, open reduction is mandatory. Internal fixation is also necessary for most total condylar depressions and split fractures, particularly the frontal split fracture of the posterior medial condyle. Most comminuted bicondylar fractures are treated nonsurgically, chiefly with traction and manipulative reduction, because of the difficulties in obtaining a stable fixation.

Other workers agree on the indication for this last type of fracture.[1,28,36] Anatomic reduction is difficult and traction with early mobilization is the treatment of choice.

The limit of lateral plateau surface depression beyond which operation is necessary is 5 mm for other investigators.[1,4,56,58,96,98,129] It is essentially the mixed, split-compression fracture that requires, surgical treatment.[18,39]

For Rasmussen,[102] malalignment and instability are far more important than deformity of the joint surfaces. Patients without clinical impairment of stability of the extended knee in the frontal plane, irrespective of the appearance of the surfaces, are treated conservatively mostly by a cast. Instability in flexion (at > 20 degrees) is considered irrelevant. Instability should be examined in extension but not in hyperextension, because this locks the condyles against the plateaus and tightens the ligaments and posterior capsule giving a false impression of stability.[61] A 10-degree increase of lateral instability compared with the normal side is considered an indication for operative treatment. This is mainly attributable to loss of skeletal support and, to a smaller extent, to ligament damage. Fractures of the lateral plateau of the compression type with or without marginal split fragments, with depressions of > 5 mm, but without impairment of stability, have excellent results treated nonsurgically. For this type of fracture many would advocate surgical treatment. Surgical restoration of the surface anatomy should be the goal if the fracture involves the medial plateau.

It is useful to know the percentage distribution of unstable fractures among the different types according to Rasmussen's classification. Of the lateral split-compression fractures, 70 percent are unstable, 24 percent of pure compression fractures are unstable, mainly the anterior and central variants, while only 9 percent of posterior compression fractures are unstable. A fracture with compression and associated split marginal fragment is usually unstable, because the support beneath the femoral condyle is lost, as the marginal fragment is separated and dislocated laterally. Compression fractures without a split fragment are usually stable, as the peripheral margin of the lateral plateau is often sufficient to support the femur with the knee in extension, but instability is found if the intact lateral margin is very narrow. Not all anterior compression fractures are unstable, despite the fact that the knee is tested in extension, because the depression of the surface is usually < 5 mm. As the fracture is produced with the knee in extension, impingement between the femoral intercondylar area and the intercondylar eminence of the tibia soon ensues. A posterior compression fracture, which takes place with the knee in flexion, usually shows much greater depression, because the deep intercondylar notch allows more penetration of the femur into the posterior plateau, but objective instability is infrequent because the knee is tested in extension.

Forty-five percent of the medial plateau fractures are unstable. Usually it is a split fracture, with the medial plateau separated *en bloc* and attached to the femur with the capsule and ligaments. In other instances a compression fracture of the lateral plateau is associated and most of these cases are unstable.

Fifty-two percent of the bicondylar fractures are unstable but instability in this type of fracture can occur at the joint level or at the subcondylar level. When the fracture is purely split, there is usually little displacement and instability. If there is an associated element of compression of the lateral plateau, instability is more frequent. The same applies to the fractures in which there is an additional metaphyseal fracture.

Apley[2] and De Mourgues[30–32] treat most cases with traction-mobilization on the belief that articular defects "fill in" with fibrocartilage which, although not shown on the films, provides good support. These workers believe that surgical treatment should be restricted to young patients, with fractures having a few large fragments that are easy to fix and then only in the best environmental conditions. On the other hand, cast immobilization has several disadvantages, particularly the prolonged rehabilitation needed. Traction-mobilization provides the possibility of early motion, with its beneficial effects.[107] There are two disadvantages: the long period in the hospital and the long protection of weight bearing.

For Schatzker et al.,[111] a "collective" approach to the tibial plateau fractures is misleading. For simple pure cleavage fractures of the lateral plateau, excellent results can be obtained by closed methods only if displacement is minimal. Any degree of condylar spreading which results in widening of the tibial plateau or condylar depression should be operated. Articular defects never "fill in." The combined cleavage and depression fractures, if displaced, always result in knee joint instability which persists, if reduction is not achieved. Therefore, if any degree of instability is present initially, the fracture must be treated surgically. In the pure central depression fracture, many cases are stable and do not require surgical treatment. If any doubt exists as to stability, stress studies are needed in different degrees of flexion, even if this requires general anesthesia; if instability is found, accurate reduction is necessary. Medial plateau fractures carry the worst prognosis, probably because of associated lateral ligament lesions, and require surgical operation. In pure bicondylar fractures, although good results can be obtained by cast bracing, a good reduction has to be maintained; if this fails, open reduction and internal fixation should be carried out. Fracture with dissociation of diaphysis and metaphysis is unsuitable for any type of traction; it is often grossly displaced, but results are surprisingly good with surgical treatment.

For Burri et al.[16] and the Association for the Study of Internal Fixation (ASIF) school, optimal results can be obtained only with reconstruction, as anatomically accurate as possible, of the joint surfaces. For fractures with displacement and depression and for combined types or for comminuted fractures, this can only be obtained surgically. Strong internal fixation is necessary to maintain reduction and to allow early mobilization without a cast. The prognosis improves according to the experience of the surgeon and the accuracy of reduction and rigid internal fixation.

Sarmiento et al.[109] have wide experience with functional bracing and have applied this method to plateau fractures. Early motion is essential; capsular contractures favor the development of arthritis. Often patients function well with minimal or no symptoms despite residual incongruity if there is no limitation of motion. The condition of the fibula seems to determine the angular stability of these fractures under weight-bearing functional conditions. Fractures of the medial plateau, with or without associated fibular fractures, and particularly those with significant obliquity, readily collapse into varus: internal fixation and early motion is the treatment of choice. Isolated fractures of the lateral plateau with an intact fibula do not significantly collapse because of the support provided by the fibula. Such fractures with minimal depression or incongruity can be treated with early bracing of the extremity and partial graduated weight-bearing. Fractures of the lateral condyle with associated fibular fractures tend to collapse into valgus probably because of the loss of support of the fibula. Those fractures should not be braced and subjected to early mobilization and weight-bearing. The greater the displacement and obliquity of the fibular fracture, the greater the mechanical inability to provide support of the lateral condyle. Fractures of both plateaus usually do not show further collapse or angular deformity after bracing if the proximal fibula is fractured and displaced. The load-bearing stresses can be equally distributed through both plateaus. If the fibula is intact the medial condyle usually collapses creating a varus deformity. Therefore, fractures of both condyles with an intact fibula should be operated on.

Scotland and Wardlaw[114] use cast-bracing as the only treatment of compression lateral plateau fractures and bicondylar fractures, after a short period of traction-mobilization. These workers also use cast-braces after screw fixation in wedge fractures. Varus and valgus deformity does not change in the brace. Patients are allowed to bear weight freely. Cast-bracing eliminates the two disadvantages of the traction-mobilization method, namely, prolonged bed rest and protected weight-bearing, while retaining the advantages of early motion.

The problem of associated meniscal lesions has relevance to the indications for treatment. Different investigators have found different incidences of meniscal tears, ranging from a low 17 percent[88] to a high 85 percent.[33] Some of the statistics may show an abnormally high incidence of meniscal tears because meniscectomy was done very frequently, if not routinely, for exposure of the depressed segment, apparently with no ill effects.[99,101] Several workers report incidences above 50 percent.[28,84,85,122] Bakalim and Wilppula[4] found an incidence of 48 percent of true meniscal tears but tried to resuture the peripheral detachments. Burri et al.[16] removed the menisci in 18 percent and resutured them in 9 percent of cases. Moore[86] did not find meniscectomy necessary for exposure. Several investigators—and we agree with them—have suggested preserving the meniscus and

removing it only if torn in its substance; every effort should be made to resuture meniscal tears.[64,88, 105,111,120,125] Peripheral lesions can heal spontaneously with some form of immobilization, or perhaps without it. The absence of symptoms, attributable to lesions of the menisci, at follow-up, both in conservatively treated cases as well as in surgically treated ones, has been noted by many.[2,11,21,32,97,99,118]

The question of associated soft-tissues and ligament injuries is important for surgical indications. There is no unanimity of opinion. On the basis of theoretical considerations, and on the law of Bistolfi-Hulten of the inverse proportion between bone and soft tissue injuries, ligament lesions have been believed rare by many investigators. In contrast, Martin[80] showed that medial joint space opening on valgus stress films can only occur if there is medial ligament injury associated with the lateral plateau defect. Experimentally produced lateral tibial plateau fractures had a very low incidence of associated medial collateral ligament or cruciate ligament lesions.[72]

Clinical studies have shown different incidences of ligament injuries. For some the instability attributable to soft tissue injury was only transient.[8,102] Forster et al.[51] found 22 percent of knees with angular instability on the basis of stress-film studies. Roberts[105] found a 12 percent incidence of ligament lesions; he considered stress films important in leading to surgical repair of the damaged ligament. Porter[99] found a low incidence of 1 percent medial collateral ligament lesions on initial clinical examination and another 4 percent anterior cruciate ligament instability at follow-up. Wilppula and Bakalim[127] repaired the ligaments in 25 percent of their surgical cases, a very high incidence. Rasmussen[102] based his figures on the following criteria: evidence of avulsed fragments on radiographs at the critical sites, surgical demonstration of tears, and Pellegrini–Stieda lesions at follow-up. He found an incidence of approximately 10 percent of ligament lesions (5.4 percent anterior cruciate, 3.8 percent medial collateral, 0.4 percent posterior cruciate). Such injuries do not usually require surgery, and stress films may be of academic interest. Hohl[62] believed stress films to be important and that ligament ruptures should be surgically repaired. Schatzker et al.[111] have found an incidence of 7 percent, the anterior cruciate lesions being the most common. Burri et al.[16] have repaired the ligaments in 7 percent of their surgical cases.

Dejour et al.[27] have found an incidence of approximately 15 to 20 percent. They distinguished two groups of cases: (1) fractures of one plateau with ligament lesions on the opposite side; and (2) fractures of one plateau associated with avulsion fractures of the intercondylar eminence. Stress films are fundamental to show the instability and to disclose the avulsed fragments. The treatment of ligamentous lesions is surgical.

Moore[86] described a separate group of fracture-dislocations of the knee associated with a high incidence of ligament problems requiring surgical treatment as opposed to the regular plateau fractures which do not show significant soft tissue damage.[86,88]

We believe that severe ligament lesions in the most common plateau fractures occur infrequently. There can be intraligamentous stretching, but this can be treated conservatively.

On the other hand, certain fracture types—the spinotuberosity, the marginal, the posteromedial split, and the fracture-dislocations—are more frequently associated with ligament lesions or avulsions. Stress films in case of doubt are useful.

Surgical repair of the torn ligaments, particularly in the fracture-dislocations, in which most of the instability is in the soft tissues, is indicated. It is, we believe, rarely indicated in the common lateral plateau fractures, because instability is predominantly attributable to bony lesions. The instability is greatly reduced after reduction and fixation of the fracture fragments. Only in cases of persistent instability caused by severe associated ligament damage should a ligament repair be attempted. This is particularly true for the cruciate lesions.

In conclusion, we believe that the most important single parameter upon which our surgical indications are based is instability in extension. Other factors are important as well, including the fracture type and displacement, age of the patient, the violence of injury, and associated lesions or fractures. Certain fractures involving the medial condyle (the split and the spinotuberosity) more often require operation. Bicondylar fractures have the worst prognosis with any form of treatment.

CONSERVATIVE TREATMENT

Conservative treatment of tibial plateau fractures includes simple early active exercises and mobilization, cast immobilization, traction-mobilization, and cast-bracing. Closed reduction in association with the above-mentioned forms of conservative treatment can be obtained by the manipulative method and by the traction-compression method.

Early Active Exercises or Mobilization.   This form of therapy, in bed without weight-bearing, has been used particularly in minimally displaced and stable fractures or in cases with minimal depression and crushing, and primarily in patients for whom age or general condition preclude other forms of treatment. This treatment implies avoidance of weight-bearing for a period that can vary from 2–8 weeks, according to the evolution of the fracture and its consolidation. An alternative method in similar situations is a Robert-Jones dressing for 2 to 3 weeks to diminish pain, followed by exercises without weight-bearing. Undisplaced fractures generally tend not to displace further, but follow-up radiographs are necessary. Weight-bearing should be delayed until fracture healing is evident. This is difficult to see in fractures with minimal central compression of the lateral condyle, but depressed cancellous bone heals rapidly.

Cast Immobilization.   The cast is applied from groin to ankle or groin to foot, with the knee near full extension (5 degrees of flexion). A spica cast has been used by some.[37]

Cast treatment has been used mostly for undisplaced or minimally displaced fractures of the various types. It has also been used for compression, split-compression, and split fractures up to 10 mm of local depression, 5 mm of lateral separation, and up to 10 degrees of instability. We tend to use it only in selected cases, particularly for the compression type without instability.

The cast is worn for an average of 3 to 6 weeks, after which a period of rehabilitation of at least 2 to 4 weeks without weight-bearing is instituted. Partial weight-bearing is resumed at 9 to 12 weeks according to the severity of the fracture, and complete weight-bearing at 12 to 16 weeks. There are variations according to different types of fractures, follow-up radiographs in individual cases, and different surgeons' experience. Cast treatment generally maintains correct alignment and fragment position, but displacement in the cast can occur particularly in unstable fractures.

Traction and Mobilization.   This therapy has been widely used.[2,30–32] It has the characteristic of producing and maintaining reduction and correct alignment. At the same time it allows early active and passive mobilization. It has been used for a wide range of indications from undisplaced or minimally displaced fractures of various types, to split, and split-compression displaced fractures, wherein the traction can reduce the marginal split fragments attached to the intact ligament and capsule. Traction has also been used for local compression fractures with intact peripheral rims, bicondylar and comminuted fractures.

The preservation of the lateral meniscus, which covers most of the load-bearing area of the plateau, might explain the good results after traction-mobilization in spite of insufficient reduction. The articular defects uncovered by the lateral meniscus are filled with some fibrocartilaginous tissue stimulated by avoidance of weight-bearing and by the molding effect of motion, as has been shown experimentally,[64] at arthrotomy,[5,77,102] and with arthrography.[36] Movement promotes cartilage repair.[107]

Traction has been used alone, for a duration of 3 to 8 weeks, or followed by cast or cast-braces. Return to weight-bearing follows the same rules as after plaster cast immobilization. Rules vary from author to author and according to type of fracture and individual selection. Traction treatment has also been found useful for open fractures with contaminated wounds.

Traction is applied with a Steinmann pin or Kirschner wire through the os calcis and the extremity is elevated with a thigh support. It is important to bring the knee into full extension periodically and to avoid rotation of the traction pin in the bone during range of motion exercises, which are carried out routinely during the day. The traction bow has to rotate freely around the pin. Traction of approximately 3 to 4 kg is applied and exercises begun after a few days. An Unna-boot bandage is used for the forefoot, with light traction to keep the foot in a vertical position. The bandage is removed during the exercises. Traction is continued for 4 weeks (split fractures), 4 to 6 weeks (split-compression), and 8 to 12 weeks (bicondylar or complex fractures). Weight-bearing is delayed for 3 months overall. The patients can usually get up after 6 weeks. A relatively long hospitalization stay is needed.

The Apley system has been reported to have the virtue of making the patient feel more comfortable, hence early motion can begin. No closed reduction is attempted. Skeletal traction is applied with a Denham pin, threaded for part of its length, and inserted at right angles to the tibia at least 10 cm below the fracture. Hooks are attached to each end of the pin and from each hook a loop of cord runs over a pulley at the foot of the bed each with a 2.5-kg weight. The foot of the bed is elevated 25 cm. The leg lies on a pillow. A split mattress at the foot of the bed facilitates bending. The patient can sit up in the bed.

The os calcis traction apparatus used by Hohl[64] allows full extension in the resting position and 90 degrees of passive flexion. It has been widely used in the United States.

Attempts at closed reduction are sometimes worthwhile with the manipulative method or the traction-compression method. Local compression fractures do not lend themselves to closed reduction maneuvers; however, for split, split-compression fractures of the lateral condyle, medial plateau fractures, bicondylar and comminuted fractures, the system can be used. Naturally redisplacement is always possible and the reduction should be continuously monitored.

Cast-Bracing. This method is a relatively recent form of treatment.[13,108,109,114] It has the advantage of maintaining fragment position or reduction and alignment while allowing motion at the knee and ankle. It also allows progressive weight-bearing.

Experience with this type of treatment is brief, but it has been used for various types of fractures: mono- and bicondylar, compression or split-compression types, as well as comminuted fractures. The stability of the fracture based on the conditions of the fibula and the stability of the knee are important considerations in installing this type of treatment. Patients with split or very unstable fractures are not the best candidates. It can be used for a variable length of time (4 to 12 weeks), alone or after a period of traction. Partial weight-bearing can be resumed with the cast-brace early in the process of healing, but close and frequent supervision is necessary.

SURGICAL TREATMENT

CLOSED OR PERCUTANEOUS INTERNAL FIXATION

This technique[26,84] may be useful, when the skin condition is less than ideal, when the fracture is open and contaminated, and when the age or general condition of the patient does not suggest extensive surgery. It may also save the patient unnecessary meniscectomy, done to achieve a better exposure.

The patient is placed with the knee slightly flexed and in traction on an orthopedic table, with image intensifier. In the case of a split-compression fracture, an elevation of the depressed fragment can be done with a spatula through a small incision. The fractures are fixed by means of cancellous bone screws and washers or bolts. The same technique has been used recently for minimally displaced fractures as a means of fixation in situ.[16] Edeland[42] has suggested a new device for reducing central compression fractures, which involves the introduction of a curved probe through a cortical window in the uninjured condyle under image intensifier control. A tube and plunger are needed for deposition of bone grafts.

Rasmussen[102] has popularized a method of closed reduction and internal fixation with limited exposure using a wire loop. The method[59,69] is simple, avoids the implantation of a lot of metal, and at the same time may provide a more secure fixation than screws or bolts in cancellous porotic bone.

The patient is placed on a fracture table in heavy traction, which usually causes reduction of the joint surfaces. Condylar widening can be reduced manually. Through a small lateral incision two Kirschner wires are introduced with perforated pointed ends from lateral to medial, one anterior, and one posterior, in front of the fibula, and parallel to the joint. The skin is incised medially between the two wires. A stainless steel wire (1 mm) is introduced into the perforated end of one K wire and the other end of the steel wire is passed close to the surface of the tibial bone so as not to constrict the soft tissues and is then introduced into the second K wire. By pulling the K pins laterally, the stainless steel wires are brought laterally and are tightened and twisted. The knot is buried in the cortex.

This method alone has been used successfully in about 30 percent of Rasmussen's surgical cases. The same method of fixation, after open reduction and reconstruction of the joint surface by means of bone grafting, was used in the remaining cases.

OPEN REDUCTION AND INTERNAL FIXATION

Incisions. One of the most widely used skin incisions is the lazy S incision done with the knee in flexion.[34,93,99,101] The upper arm is longitudinal and parallel to the biceps; the incision then swings gently anteriorly at the level of the joint line and the lower arm is placed on the lateral side of the tibial tubercle and can be extended inferiorly. Another widely used skin incision, performed again with the knee in flexion, is an arcuate or gently curved incision across the injured condyle.[16,63,105] The incision usually begins at the level of the lateral femoral epicondyle proceeding distally and anteriorly, crossing the joint line lateral to the patellar tendon, at the level of the tubercle of Gerdy, then proceeding more distally lateral to the tibial crest. The lazy S incision usually gives a larger exposure and permits easier visualization of the peroneal nerve, when needed. Other skin incisions are the straight lateral parapatellar incision,[28] the inverted L incision,[84] and the oblique incision.[18,28] The champagne-cup Y incision of the ASIF school is used rarely in bicondylar fractures, for fear of vascular problems in the flap.[90]

The subcutaneous tissues must be dissected minimally, and the fascia (the fibers of the iliotibial band) must be split in line with the skin incision near the joint line and reflected distally and posteriorly. Exposure of the lateral tibial plateau is facilitated by elevating the meniscus with the femur, doing a submeniscal arthrotomy, severing the meniscotibial coronary ligaments anterolaterally and laterally. The meniscus is frequently found undamaged in its substance, or sometimes detached peripherally at the level of the coronary ligaments and therefore should be saved and its peripheral attachments resutured at the end of the procedure. A meniscectomy for better lateral exposure has been found necessary by some[28,99,102] with no ill effects, but the trend today is to save the meniscus whenever possible for its important functions and for prevention of osteoarthritis.[4,16,63,88,105,111] When the fracture is located posteriorly, its visualization is more difficult. In this case the meniscus can be freed posterolaterally along with the lateral collateral ligament, which at times can be severed, and subsequently resutured.[64] Gossling and Peterson[57] have described a surgical approach that uses the incision of Gariépy, with detachment of the lateral collateral mechanism and the biceps from the fibula. The meniscus can be released from the coronary ligaments and elevated but, if intact, is subsequently repaired and the collateral ligament complex resutured. The conjoined collateral structures, consisting of collateral and arcuate ligament, biceps tendon, and posterior edge of fascia lata, are reattached with a heavy nonabsorbable suture through a drill hole in the resected proximal end of the fibula. In our opinion this approach is generally unnecessary.

None of the described incisions is ideal should a knee anthroplasty become necessary. The two exposures are incompatible and it is inevitable that a skin bridge will be left between incisions. We believe that the lazy **S** incision provides the best compromise; the incision for knee anthroplasty can re-use the lower part and diverge superiorly. We have done this uneventfully on a number of occasions.

When an approach to the medial side is required for medial plateau fractures or for ligament repair, a medial parapatellar incision is performed alone or in association with the lateral incision. The latter must be placed more posteriorly and laterally to avoid skin problems. Once again the possible need for future anthroplasty must be considered in planning the incisions.

Particularly for bicondylar fractures, an osteotomy of the tibial tuberosity can be used for an extensive anterior approach, fixing it back with a staple at the end of the procedure.[95] More often, surgery for bicondylar fractures is done through two incisions or, if possible, using only lateral incisions.

Compression Fractures. The treatment of compression fractures of the lateral condyle involves careful elevation of the depressed fragment(s) to the original level of the articular surface. This can be done through a window in the condyle below the surface, followed by the use of elevators or spatulae. There is wide agreement that the elevated fragments should be supported by a bone graft inserted in the space created below the articular surface.[16,99,105,111] Cancellous grafts or bone blocks from the iliac crest to support or reconstruct the surface have been used extensively.[74] The inverted patella has been used occasionally to provide a new articular surface.[66,124,128] On other occasions, the grafts can be removed from the adjacent femoral condyle or the lateral tibial surface through a linear extension of the same incision. In this latter case, a cortical graft is used which is thought by some to give better support. It is inserted from the window in the plateau, horizontally[91] toward the intact medial cancellous bone. Wires,[52] bolts, wire loops, or Knowles pins[58,105] can be inserted just below the graft. The fibula can be also used as a vertical cortical supporting structure.[67,105]

Heterologous bank bone has been used occasion-

ally in addition to autologous bone.[4] Other materials have been used for support, but there is no adequate documentation for their use. Porous ceramics (tricalcium phosphate) have been suggested.[7,17] Bone cement (methylmethacrylate) has been used sporadically.[93]

Mixed Split-Compression Fractures. In the case of mixed split-compression fractures, the split fragment can be opened like a book, elevation of the fragments is done through the fracture, and sometimes excising some of the depressed loose and potentially necrotic fragments. After this, the split fragment is repositioned at an adequate level and is impacted. Bone grafts must be added in cases of subchondral defects.[16,93,111] Internal fixation is obtained by the usual means: simple wire loops, multiple pins, cancellous screws and washers, bolts, and Knowles pins. If there is a question of stability of the lateral cortex, or if there is a metaphyseal element to the fracture, as in bicondylar fractures, contoured support **T** or **L** buttress plates must be used.[16,90,106,111]

The use of buttress plates is also helpful in cases of severe depression fractures that have required bone grafting.

Split Fractures. For these fractures internal fixation is usually accomplished with simple screws and washers, but again, if there is serious doubt as to the stability of the lateral cortex, a support buttress plate has to be used. A modified technique has been suggested for the treatment of rim fractures, including an osteotomy of the condyle, elevation and grafting with a wedge of bone, and fixation with a staple.[43]

Bicondylar Fractures. The surgical problem can be difficult owing to the need for extensive exposure. A single lateral support plate can suffice at times. Stabilization of the medial fragment is achieved by compression of the screws. On other occasions, two plates placed on both sides will be required.

Complete, severe intraligamentous lesions or avulsions require repair. Bony avulsion of a cruciate ligament can be reinserted with a wire suture through bone. Because a wire may cut out it is sometimes possible to fix an anterior cruciate avulsed with a fragment of bone from the tibia with a screw placed distally using the lag screw principle (*en rappel*). Avulsion of the other ligaments requires different fixation means according to the circumstances (e.g., nonabsorbable sutures, wire sutures through bone, screws,

(Text continues on page 478.)

Table 15III.4. Results of Treatment for Tibial Plateau Fractures

Investigators	No. of Cases	Fracture Types	Treatment	Follow-up (years)	Evaluation Method	Results	Osteoarthritis	Remarks
Hohl and Luck[64]	227	All types	Conservative 81% (cast, traction) Surgical 19% (screws, bolts)	2–13	Hohl and Luck functional method[64]	Excellent, good, 72%, local depressions, treated conservatively 75–87% excellent or good	Correlation between residual depression and valgus deformity and valgus deformity and osteoarthritis	Open reduction makes anatomical results better, but no great difference in functional results, particularly for local depressions; depth of residual depression in cases treated conservatively had relation to functional results; immobilization for more than one month had negative effect on function
Duparc and Ficat[40]	159	All types	Conservative 46% (cast) Surgical 54% (screws, bolts)	Short term	Similar to Hohl and Luck[64]	Excellent or good: Conservative treatment, 62%; surgical treatment, 84%	Mostly due to mechanical factors like articular surface residual step-offs or angular deformity; frequent radiologically; but often silent clinically	Symptomatic osteoarthritis should lead the clinician to look for malalignment or instability
Merle d'Aubigné and Mazas[84]	76	All types	Conservative 63% Surgical 37%	Short term	Similar to Hohl and Luck	Excellent or good, 83%		Bicondylar and lateral split-compression gave the worst results; cast was used at least for one month in both groups (longer in the conservative group); 12% had < 90 degree range of motion
Roberts[105]	100	Undisplaced, 39% Local compression, 26% Split-compression, 35%	Conservative two-thirds (traction, cast) Surgical one-third (mostly split-compression)	1–12	Hohl and Luck method[64]	Excellent, good Overall, 72% Undisplaced (mostly conservatively), 80% Local compression (mostly traction), 81% Split-compression (mostly surgically), 76%	Often no relationship between clinical and radiologic results	Main reason for unacceptable results was residual ligament instability not always recognized upon initial examination and not repaired; the best results obtained with traction-mobilization; meniscus should be preserved; stress films

472

Author	No.	Type	Treatment	Follow-up	Grading	Results	Comments
Anger et al.[1]	175	All types	Conservative Cast, 40.5% Traction, 34% Surgical 25.5%	1–4	Duparc and Ficat[40] method	Excellent, good Overall, 65% cast, 51% traction, 83% operation, 68%	are useful; torn ligaments should be repaired; early mobilization is important Internal fixation and early mobilization is the suggested treatment when there is more than 5 mm displacement; traction gave the best results but it was not used in the worst cases
Apley[2]	60	All types	Conservative 100% (traction)	1–10	Functional grading (Apley)[2]	Excellent, good 80%	Eight years later the same cases were studied again, and the same results were found with no deterioration clinical nor radiographic Degenerative changes seen on roentgenograms do not imply bad function
DeMourgues and Chaix[31,32]	137	All types	Conservative 100% (traction)	1–14	Duparc and Ficat[40] method	Excellent, good 75%	Range of motion was 90 degrees in 91% of cases. Stability was excellent in 70%; some residual valgus is well tolerated; results were 70% excellent or good with > 5 years follow-up Osteoarthritis was very rare and did not deteriorate with time
Porter[99]	68	Lateral plateau "crush" fracture (compression or split-compression)	Conservative (traction, cast) 70% Surgical 30%	3–13	Hohl and Luck[64] criteria	Excellent, good: A < 10 mm depression, treated closed 96% B > 10 mm depression treated closed 47% treated open 80%	Depth of depression had important bearing on the results; knees with > 14 mm depression had poor prognosis, no matter how treated; no patients had symptoms of instability; ligaments were operated in most of the knees with lesions detected preoperatively by stress films; lateral meniscectomy was done routinely; early motion is essential; knees with > 10 mm depression best treated with surgery

(Continued)

Table 15III.4. (*continued*)

Investigators	No. of Cases	Fracture Types	Treatment	Follow-up (years)	Evaluation Method	Results	Osteoarthritis	Remarks
Bakalim and Wilppula[4]	197	All types	Conservative (cast) 53% Surgical 47% (bone grafting)	2–9 Average 4.5	Hohl and Luck[64] criteria	Excellent, good, 75% Conservative treatment, 86% Surgical treatment, 61.5%	Moderate to severe osteoarthritis present in 32%; it was related to the amount of displacement; good reduction was associated with arthrosis in 28%, poor reduction (widening or depression > 5 mm, angulation > 10 degrees) had arthrosis in 79%	A cast was used for 9 weeks average in both groups with no ill effects; non-weight-bearing period averaged 12 weeks, secondary depression may occur, prolonged period suggested; anatomic restoration of articular surface recommended for it correlates with results and development of arthrosis; the method of treatment of menisci had no effects upon results; acceptable end results obtained with residual depression and/or widening < 5 mm
Rasmussen[102]	204	All types	Conservative, 56% (cast) Surgical, 44% with minimal fixation, and often graft.	4–11 Average 7.3	Quantitative numerical system, for functional and for radiologic results[102]	Acceptable Overall, 87% Closed, 95% Open, 80%	Total lack of correlation between anatomical and functional results; incidence of arthrosis 17–21%; more frequent in bicondylar (42%) than medial (21%) or lateral (16%) fractures; arthrosis incidence was 13% in knees with normal alignment, 31% in those with valgus, 79% with varus; arthrosis incidence was 18% when there was no instability, 14% when instability was present only in flexion, 46% if present in extension; no correlation with residual depression, some with condylar widening; arthrosis correlated with functional results	Forty lateral depressions with/without split, treated conservatively because without instability > 10 degrees obtained 96% acceptable results; knee motion better if cast kept < 6 weeks in both groups; instability in extension is the main factor indicating surgical treatment, not the appearance of the articular surface

Rinonapoli and Aglietti[104]	128	All types	Undisplaced 42 (conservative, cast) Displaced: A. Conservative 35 B. Surgical 51 (open reduction, screws fixation, cast immobilization)	2–16 8–18 2–9	Modified Hospital for Special Surgery rating system: excellent, 95-100; good, 85-94; fair, 75-84; poor, < 75	Excellent, good undisplaced, 93% displaced: A conservative, 63% B surgical, 72%	A and B: Arthrosis present in 20% of knees without deformity, 22% valgus, 40% with varus; arthrosis present in 10% of stable knees, 35% unstable in extension; radiographic results much better in operated cases, 90% versus 66% satisfactory, but arthrosis more frequent (31%) in operated cases than in conservatively treated (17.5%); arthrosis more frequent in bicondylar fractures	Two comparable groups, A, B, treated conservatively or surgically; range of motion was inferior in B (17% < 100 degrees) than in A (8% < 100 degrees); age of patient is a negative factor; bicondylar fractures have the worst prognosis; time in the cast, up to 45 days, did not influence results or range of motion in A; in B the use of the cast for more than 1 month had a positive bearing on the overall results, but a negative one on range of motion
Masse and Mazas[81]	56	All types	Mostly surgical	Min 10	Functional and radiologic grading (not specified)	Excellent, good, 82%	Irregularities of the articular surface are well tolerated if knee is stable and well aligned	A previous study had shown only 62.5 satisfactory results, there was a late improvement, two factors associated with unsatisfactory results: laxity and axial malalignment
Burri et al.[16]	278	All types	100% surgical (ASIF) A Inexperienced surgeons, 127 B Experienced surgeons, 151	Average, 32 months	Functional subjective evaluation	Subjective, good to acceptable 89% 97%	Arthrosis present in A 53–82%, depending on severity of displacement; in B it was present in 37–50%, again according to displacement	Prognosis improves with experience of the surgeons; accurate reconstruction of the articular surface, rigid internal fixation to allow early mobilization are essential: group A had less meniscal reinsertions, more meniscectomies, fewer ligament reconstructions than B; this might explain difference in the results. There were more complications in group A

(Continued)

Table 15III.4. (*continued*)

Investigators	No. of Cases	Fracture Types	Treatment	Follow-up (*years*)	Evaluation Method	Results	Osteoarthritis	Remarks
Schatzker[111]	70	All types See classification[111]	Conservative, 56% Surgical, 44%	9–74 months Average, 28 months	Functional evaluation[110]	Acceptable overall, two-thirds closed, 58% open, 78%		Type I fractures obtained 100% acceptable results, type II 66%, type III 80%, type IV 50%, type V 50%, type VI 64%; results deteriorate if the knee is immobilized for more than four weeks. Osteoporosis negatively affects the results; the knees treated by open reduction, bone grafting, fixation with cancellous screws and buttress plating of the lateral cortex obtained 88% acceptable results; a bad reduction never leads to a good result
Drennan et al.[37]	53	Central depression Split compression Bicondylar Comminuted	Conservative 100% (closed reduction and spica cast for 5 to 6 weeks)	Average, 3.8	Modified Hohl and Luck method, good result requires 5 to 100 degrees range of motion	Excellent, good, 85%		Split-compression fractures gave inferior results than pure central compressions; it is important to separate the articular surfaces to obtain good bone and fibrocartilaginous healing; initial displacement correlates with quality of results

Moore[86]	132	Fracture-dislocations of various types, see classification (Moore)
		
		I
		II
		III
		
		IV
		
		V
			Conservative, 35%
			Surgical, 65%
			
			47% ⎫
			61% ⎪ %
			95% ⎬ surgi-
			         ⎪ cally
			44% ⎪ treat-
			         ⎭ ed
			64%
				n.ot given			Fracture-dislocations studied in five groups with increasing incidence of neurovascular impairment; type V rarely obtain a normal knee; they are much more serious injuries than pure fractures of the plateaus; patients with intraligamentous injuries do not do as well as the rest of the group; there is a 50% incidence of neurovascular impairment; almost all group III, IV, and V knees are unstable

Scotland and Wardlaw[114]	29 Split, 7 Compression or bicondylar 22		Operation and cast-brace Cast-brace alone (3 to 12 weeks)	2.5 years period	Rasmussen criteria	Excellent, good, 96%	The varus or valgus deformity remained the same before and after treatment with the cast-brace; the patients could bear weight early

477

or staples). The principles of acute ligament repairs do not differ from those without fractures. In this context, the surgeon must anticipate loss of motion because of the more prolonged immobilization. Cast-braces can be used successfully in the management of such cases.

POSTOPERATIVE REGIMEN

The postoperative regimen is very important. In general, there is a trend toward earlier mobilization,[62–64,96,105,106,120] particularly after surgery. There is no doubt that early postoperative mobilization is a major factor in producing a successful result. If the internal fixation is absolutely stable, active motion can start as early as the first postoperative week. Certainly mobilization should not be done at the expense of loss of reduction or wound healing. Mobilization after surgery can start in traction or in a cast-brace.

In a comparative series[104] of conservatively and surgically treated cases we showed that the range of motion was slightly better in the conservatively treated patients. However, this finding was probably attributable to the trauma of the operation itself, because both groups were casted. Range of motion was better in conservatively treated cases that were not immobilized compared with operatively treated cases in which no cast was used.

It seems therefore that early mobilization or limited use of cast immobilization is particularly important for operated cases. Schatzker et al.[111] have shown that far more acceptable results have been obtained in both nonsurgical and surgical cases if immobilization for fewer than 4 weeks was used.

Although there is a reasonable trend toward earlier postoperative mobilization, the meaning is different from one investigator to another. A relatively long period of immobilization was suggested by Chuinard.[19] Bakalim and Wilppula,[4] with an average immobilization postoperatively of 9.4 weeks, showed very good results. Rasmussen,[102] using plaster after surgery in 95 percent of cases for 2 to 12 weeks, concluded that immobilization of up to 6 weeks is no obstacle to the restoration of a normal range of motion. With immobilization for more than 6 weeks there are increasing risks of joint stiffness. Naturally if additional surgery to the ligaments has been done, the issue is more complicated. In those cases the knee should not be immobilized for the usual 5 to 6 weeks,

which is the custom in ligamentous repairs. We believe that for the sake of early mobilization one should be prepared to sacrifice an anterior cruciate repair particularly in older patients. Moore,[86] on the other hand, has no fear of immobilizing a knee with a fracture-dislocation, in which ligament work has been done, for 6 weeks, but the ligament lesions are far more important in a fracture-dislocation. In summary, the review of the literature and our own experience would suggest that if cast immobilization is needed, 4 weeks can be used safely. This would give the bone and the associated soft tissue lesions, if any, a good chance to heal without important problems of knee stiffness. This is also in keeping with experimental studies: the knees of monkeys with osteocartilaginous defects formed adhesions after 1 month of immobilization.[64]

In terms of delay in weight-bearing there is a consensus of opinion that the period of non-weight-bearing, both after conservative and surgical treatment, should be long enough to achieve secure stability of the fracture. Usually this depends on the type of fracture. The non-weight-bearing period is longer for fractures that have required bone-grafting procedures. The same applies to bicondylar or comminuted fractures or to cases in which a ligament reconstruction was done. Usually partial weight-bearing is begun at 9 to 12 weeks and full weight-bearing at 12 to 16 weeks. The application of a cast-brace reduces the time off weight-bearing in experienced hands.

COMPLICATIONS

The incidence of postoperative complications varies widely. Roberts[106] reported 10 percent of infections and 6 percent of peroneal nerve palsies, Rasmussen[102] reported a 6 percent infection rate, 3 percent of peroneal nerve palsies, and 3 percent of deep vein thrombosis. Bakalim and Wilppula[4] had a similar incidence of 3 percent infections and 5 percent deep vein thrombosis.

Burri et al.[16] found an interesting difference in the complication rate according to the experience of the surgeon. The cases treated by the less experienced surgeons had 14 percent incidence of hematoma (as compared with 6 percent) and a 15 percent incidence of deep and superficial infection (as compared with 0.7 percent).

(Text continues on page 486.)

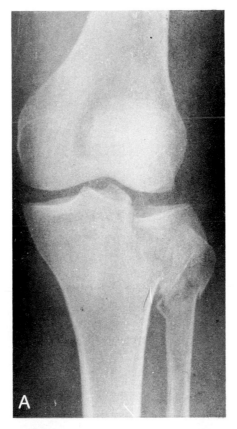

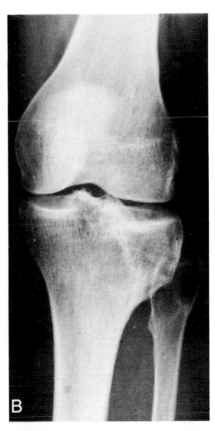

Fig. 15III.10. Female age 47. (A) Lateral plateau fracture with split fragment, treated with cast immobilization for fifteen days. (B) Ten-year follow-up roentgenograms. Excellent clinical and good radiographic result. (From Rinonapoli, E., and Aglietti, P.: Comparison of treatment by open and closed reduction of comparable cases of articular fractures of the proximal tibia. Ital. J. Orthop. Traumatol. [Suppl.], *I*: 105, 1977, with permission.)

Fig. 15III.11. Female age 38. (A) Lateral plateau open fracture treated with cast for 30 days. (B) Good clinical and radiographic results. (From Rinonapoli, E., and Aglietti, P.: Comparison of treatment by open and closed reduction of comparable cases of articular fractures of the proximal tibia. Ital. J. Orthop. Traumatol. [Suppl.], *I*: 105, 1977, with permission.)

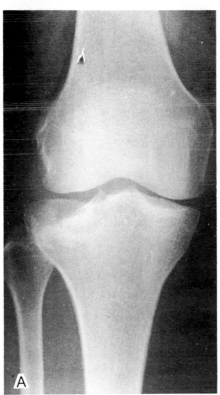

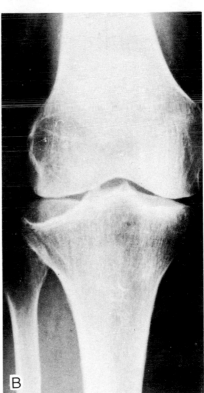

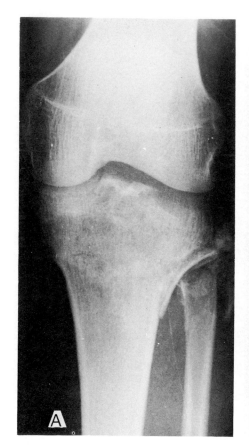

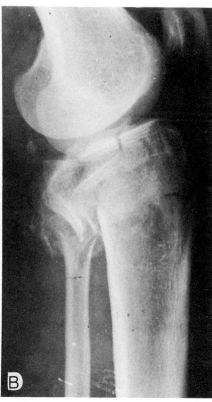

Fig. 15III.12. Male age 59. (A,B) Mixed lateral plateau fracture with predominantly posterior depression, treated with traction for 3 weeks.

(C,D) At 9 years follow-up, good clinical and fair radiographic results.

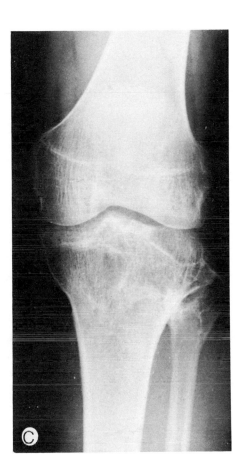

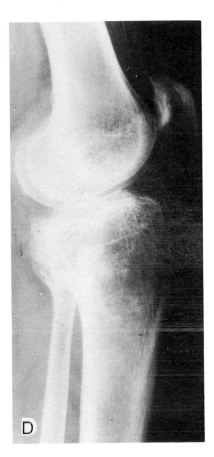

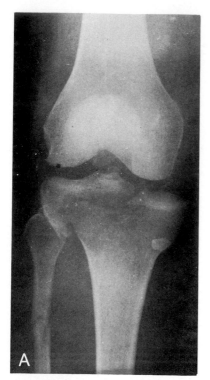
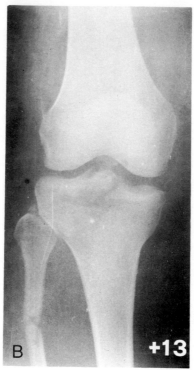
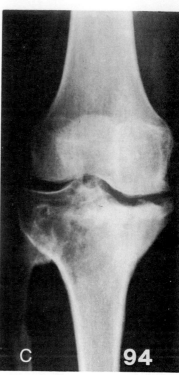

Fig. 15III.13. Female age 34. (A) Lateral plateau fracture of the "spinoglenoid" type, (B) treated with 45 days' traction. (C) The 13-year follow-up showed a clinically excellent result but a poor radiographic outcome, with sclerosis and possible necrosis of the medial tibial plateau. (From Rinonapoli, B., and Aglietti, P.: Comparison of treatment by open and closed reduction of comparable cases of articular fractures of the proximal tibia. Ital. J. Orthop. Traumatol. [suppl.], I:105, 1977, with permission.)

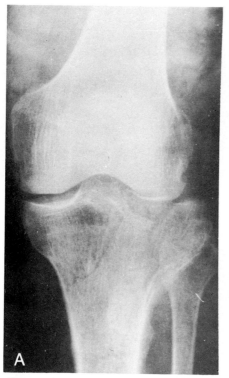
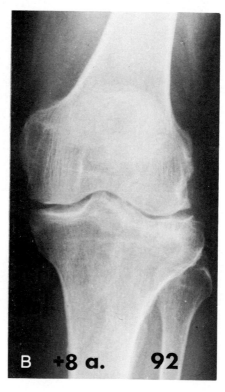

Fig. 15III.14. Female age 45. (A) Lateral plateau fracture with depression and split. Treated conservatively with traction for thirty days. (B) At 8 years follow-up, excellent clinical result with some lateral compartment arthritis.

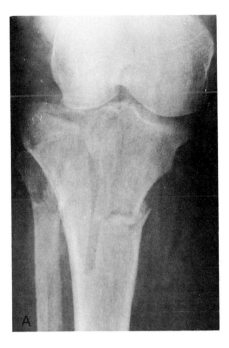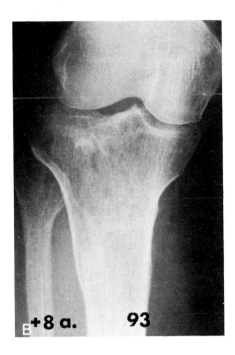

Fig. 15III.15. Male age 50. (A) Medial spinotuberosity fracture with severe comminution of the lateral articular surface, treated with cast for 45 days. (B) At 8 years follow-up, excellent clinical result despite some varus malalignment.

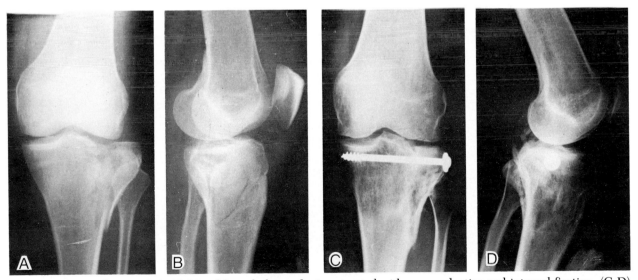

Fig. 15III.16. Male age 45. (A,B) Mixed lateral plateau fracture treated with open reduction and internal fixation. (C,D) At 3 years follow-up, clinically excellent result and good radiographic result. (From Rinonapoli, E., and Aglietti, P.: Comparison of treatment by open and closed reduction of comparable cases of articular fractures of the proximal tibia. Ital. J. Orthop. Traumatol. [Suppl.], *I*: 105, 1977, with permission.)

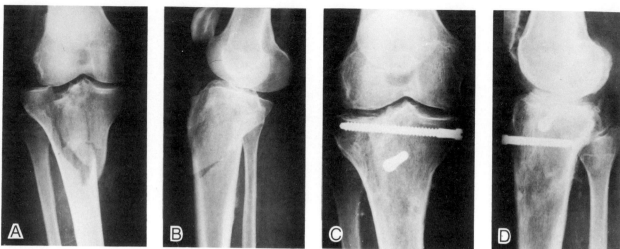

Fig. 15III.17. Male age 73. (A,B) Medial plateau fracture of the spinotuberosity type, with lateral plateau involvement treated with internal fixation with two screws. (C,D) At 6 years follow-up, clinically excellent and good radiographic results with some lateral osteoarthritis. (From Rinonapoli, E., and Aglietti, P.: Comparison of treatment by open and closed reduction of comparable cases of articular fractures of the proximal tibia. Ital. J. Orthop. Traumatol. [Suppl.], *I*: 105, 1977, with permission.)

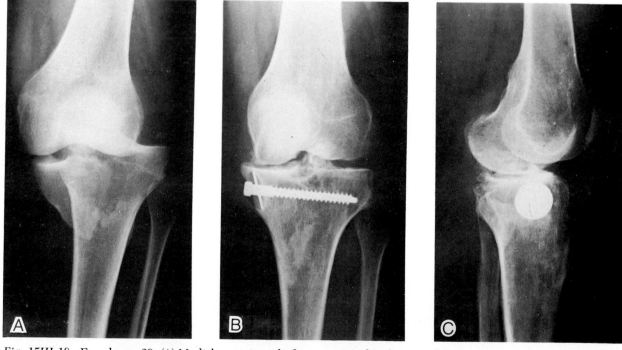

Fig. 15III.18. Female age 39. (A) Medial posterior split fracture treated with internal fixation of the split fragment. (B,C) At 6 years follow-up, good clinical result with fair radiographic result. Note medial arthritis and resorption around washers. (From Rinonapoli, E., and Aglietti, P.: Comparison of treatment by open and closed reduction of comparable cases of articular fractures of the proximal tibia. Ital. J. Orthop. Traumatol. [Suppl.], *I*: 105, 1977, with permission.)

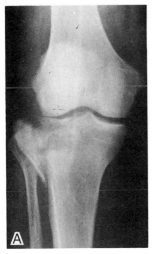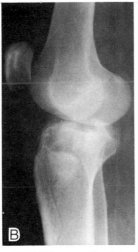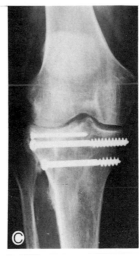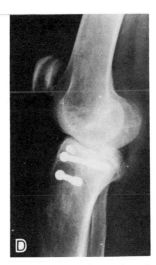

Fig. 15III.19. Male age 50. (A,B) Mixed lateral plateau fracture treated with internal fixation and bone grafting. (C,D) At 5 years, excellent clinical result, with good to fair radiographic result. Note some lateral compartment osteoarthritis. (From Rinonapoli, E., and Aglietti, P.: Comparison of treatment by open and closed reduction of comparable cases of articular fractures of the proximal tibia. Ital. J. Orthop. Traumatol. [Suppl.], *I*: 105, 1977, with permission.)

Fig. 15III.20. Male age 46. (A) Bicondylar fracture treated with cast for 45 days. (B) At 5 years follow-up, good clinical and radiographic results. (From Rinonapoli, E., and Aglietti, P.: Comparison of treatment by open and closed reduction of comparable cases of articular fractures of the proximal tibia. Ital. J. Orthop. Traumatol. [Suppl.], *I*: 105, 1977, with permission.)

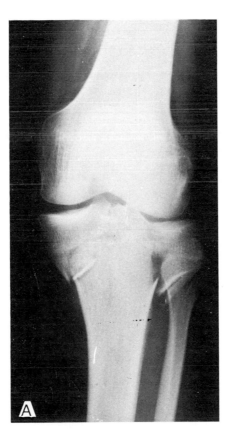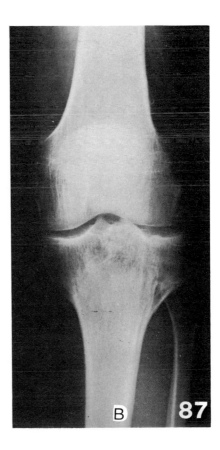

Schatzker and Schulak[110] found a 27 percent incidence of postoperative complications. Peroneal nerve palsy was the most frequent, but it could not be stated for sure whether it was caused by the operation or was present from the beginning. Infection accounted for 7 percent of complications.

Pseudoarthrosis of tibial plateau fractures is very rare. Two cases have been described in the literature.[76,110]

RESULTS AND CONCLUSIONS

The results of some of the most important series of cases treated conservatively or surgically are reported in Table 15III.4.

A comparison of the results is almost impossible. There are differences in fracture types, age of patients, velocity of injury, methods of treatment, selection of indications, and evaluation methods.

To help the reader, mention has been made of the most important variables and the principal conclusions with particular reference to prevention of osteoarthritis.

In conclusion, tibial plateau fractures are difficult lesions. It is most important to correct the presence of instability and the malalignment as well as the articular surface disruption. There are clearly many options whereby a satisfactory result can be attained after a tibial plateau fracture. Conservative (Figs. 15III.10–15) and surgical (Figs. 15III.16–20) treatments have achieved similar results. Selection is therefore difficult. We believe that surgical treatment offers the possibility of better results, but one should remember that it is necessary to have the correct equipment and environment and the personal skills and experience to perform these often difficult surgical procedures. The results of poor open reduction and internal fixation are far worse than the results of conservative treatment.

Ultimate salvage of a poor result often tibial plateau fractures is either tibial osteotomy (Chapter 19) or total knee replacement (Chapter 20).

REFERENCES

1. Anger, R., Naett, R., Wolfe, F., et al.: Étude critique du traitement des fractures articulaires de l'extrémité supérieure du tibia. Rev. Chir. Orthop. *54*: 259, 1968.

2. Apley, A.G.: Fractures of the tibial plateau. Orthop. Clin. North Am., *10*: 61, 1979.
3. Badgley, C.E., and O'Connor, S.J.: Conservative treatment of fractures of the tibial plateau. Arch. Surg., *64*: 506, 1952.
4. Bakalim, G., and Wilppula, E.: Fractures of the tibial condyles. Acta Orthop. Scand., *44*: 311, 1973.
5. Barr, J.S.: The treatment of fracture of the external tibial condyle (bumper fracture). J.A.M.A., *115*: 1683, 1940.
6. Barrington, T.W., and Dewar, F.P.: Tibial plateau fractures. Can. J. Surg., *8*: 146, 1965.
7. Benum, P., Lyng, S., Bø, O., et al.: Porous ceramics as a bone substitute in the medial condyle of the tibia. Acta Orthop. Scand., *47(2)*: 158, 1976.
8. Bick, E.M.: Fractures of the tibial condyles. J. Bone Joint Surg., *23*: 102, 1941.
9. Bistolfi, S.: Contributo allo studio del meccanisomo delle fratture monocondiloidee della tibia da causa indiretta. Chir. Organi Mov., *16*: 451, 1931.
10. Bohler, L.: The Treatment of Fractures, 5th Ed. New York, Grune & Stratton, 1958.
11. Bradford, C.H., Kilfoyle, R.M., Kelleher, J.J., et al.: Fractures of the lateral tibial condyle. J. Bone Joint Surg. [Am.], *32*: 39, 1950.
12. Branciforti, S., and Zappoli, S.: Contributo alla terapia delle fratture del piatto tibiale. Chir. Organi Mov., *37*: 275, 1952.
13. Brown, G.A., and Sprague, B.L.: Cast brace treatment of plateau and bicondylar fractures of the proximal tibia. Clin. Orthop., *119*: 184, 1976.
14. Bruckner, H.T.: Bumper fractures of the tibia. Northwest Med., *37*: 102, 1938.
15. Burke, D.L., Ahmed, A.M., Miller, J., et al.: Pressure distribution on tibial plateaus. Load transmission role of the meniscus. Proc. Orthop. Res. Soc., *23*: 105, 1977.
16. Burri, C., Bartzke, G., Coldewey, J., et al.: Fractures of the tibial plateau. Clin. Orthop., *138*: 84, 1979.
17. Cameron, H.U., McNab, I., and Pilliar, R.M.: Evaluation of a bio-degradable ceramic. In Program of Meeting of the American Society of Biomaterials, 1976. (Abst.)
18. Cauchoix, J., and Deburge, A.: Fractures de l'extrémité supérieure du tibia. Encyclopédie Médico-chirurgicale. Appareil Locomoteur, Vol. II. Paris, Editions Techniques, 1970.
19. Chuinard, E.G.: Fractures of the condyles of the tibia. Clin. Orthop., *37*: 115, 1964.
20. Cornacchia, M., Marrè, F., and Raffelini, R.: Rilievi comparativi fra trattamento cruento e incruento nelle fratture del piatto tibiale. Minerva Ortop., *18*: 346, 1967.

21. Cotton, F.J.: Fender fractures. Surg. Gynecol. Obstet., *62*: 442, 1936.

22. Courvoisier, E.: Les fractures intraarticulaires de l'extrémité supérieure du tibia. Helv. Chir. Acta., *32*: 257, 1965.

23. Courvoisier, E.: Les fractures des plateaux tibiaux. AO Bull., 1973.

24. Courvoisier, E.: Fractures des plateaux tibiaux. Traitement opératoire ou traitement conservateur? Rev. Chir. Orthop., *61*(Suppl. 2): 280, 1975.

25. Danzig, L.A., Newell, J.D., Guerra, J., Jr., et al.: Osseous landmarks of the normal knee. Clin. Orthop., *156*: 201, 1981.

26. Decoulx, J., and Capron, J.C.: Traitement chirurgical à foyer fermé de certaines fractures de l'extrémité supérieure du tibia. Rev. Chir. Orthop., *60*(Suppl. 2): 324 1974.

27. Dejour, H., Chambat, P., Caton, J., et al.: Les fractures des plateau tibiaux avec lesions ligamentaires. Rev. Chir. Orthop., *67*: 593, 1981.

28. Del Torto, V.: Il trattamento delle fratture articolari dell' estremo possimale della tibia. G. Ital. Ortop. Traumatol., *3*(Suppl. I): 81, 1977.

29. Delvecchio, E., and Antongiovanni, G.: Fratture del piatto tibiale: Considerazioni eziopatogenetiche e terapeutiche. Minerva ortop., *28*: 657, 1977.

30. De Mourgues, G.: Traitement non opératoire des fractures des plateaux tibiaux. In Duparc, J. et al. (eds.): Les fractures du genou. 107–116. Paris, Expansion Scientifique Française, 1975. (Cahiers d'enseignement de la SOFCOT:I).

31. De Mourgues, G., and Chaix, D.: Traitement des fractures des plateaux tibiaux. Rev. Chir. Orthop., *50*: 103, 1961.

32. De Mourgues, G., and Chaix, D.: Traitement des fractures des plateaux tibiaux. Rev. Chir. Orthop., *55*: 575, 1969.

33. Denicolai, F., Crova, M., and Gallinaro, P.: Considerazioni sul trattamento chirurgico delle fratture del piatto tibiale. Chir. Organi Mov., *64*(2): 153, 1978.

34. DePalma, A.F.: Diseases of the Knee. Philadelphia, J.B. Lippincott, 1954.

35. DiStefano, V.J.: Function, post-traumatic sequelae and current concepts of management of knee meniscus injuries. Clin. Orthop., *151*: 143, 1980.

36. Dovey, H., and Heerfordt, J.: Tibial condyle fractures. A follow-up of 200 cases. Acta Chir. Scand., *137*: 521, 1971.

37. Drennan, D.B., Locher, F.G., and Maylahn, D.J.: Fractures of the tibial plateau. Treatment by closed reduction and spica cast. J. Bone Joint Surg. [Am.], *61*: 989, 1979.

38. Duparc, J.: Les fractures articulaires de l'extrémité supérieure du tibia. In Duparc, J. et al. (eds.): Les fractures du genou. 93–106. Paris, Expansion Scientifique Française, 1975. (Cahiers d'enseignement de la SOFCOT:I)

39. Duparc, J.: Traitement opératoire des fractures articulaires de l'extrémité supérieure du tibia. In Duparc, J. et al. (eds.): Les fractures du genou. 117–129. Paris, Expansion Scientifique Française, 1975. (Cahiers d'enseignement de la SOFCOT:I).

40. Duparc, J., and Ficat, P.: Fractures articulaires de l'extrémité supérieure du tibia. Rev. Chir. Orthop., *46*: 399, 1960.

41. Duparc, J., and Filipe, G.: Fractures spino-tubérositaries ou fractures avec subluxation de l'extrémité supérieure du tibia. Rev. Chir. Orthop., *61*(8): 705, 1975.

42. Edeland, H.G.: Open reduction of central compression fractures of the tibial plateau. Preliminary report of a new method and device arrangement. Acta Orthop. Scand., *47*(6): 686, 1976.

43. Edeland, H.G.: A method for the treatment of rim fractures of the tibial condyle. Description of a new surgical technique and a new fracture fixation device. Acta Orthop. Belg., *44*: 293, 1978.

44. Eliason, E.L., and Ebeling, W.W.: Nonoperative treatment of fractures of the tibia and femur involving the knee joint. Surg. Gynecol. Obstet., *57*: 658, 1933.

45. Elstrom, J., Pankovich, A.M., Sassoon, H., et al.: The use of tomography in the assessment of fractures of the tibial plateau. J. Bone Joint Surg. [Am.], *58*: 551, 1976.

46. Fagerberg, S.: Tomographic analysis of depressed fractures within the knee joint, and of injuries to the cruciate ligaments. Acta. Orthop. Scand., *27*: 219, 1958.

47. Fairbank, T.J.: Knee joint changes after meniscectomy. J. Bone Joint Surg. [Br.], *30*: 664, 1948.

48. Fairbank, T.J.: Condylar fractures of the knee joint. Proc. R. Soc. Med., *48*: 95, 1955.

49. Fernandez-Esteve, F.: Resultados clinicos-radiograficos finales del tratamiento de las fracturas del tercio distal del femur y del tercio proximal de la tibia mediante los yesos funcionales conformados. Rev. Esp. Cir. Osteoartic., *13*: 29, 1978.

50. Flamand, J.P., and Danis, A.: Reflexions à propos de 60 cas de fracture des plateaux tibiaux. Acta Chir. Belg., *66*:673, 1967.

51. Forster, E., Mole, L., and Coblentz, J.: Etude des lesions ligamentaires dans les fractures du plateau tibial. Ned. Tijdschr. Geneeskd., *105*: 2173, 1961.

52. Fryjordet, A., Jr.: Operative treatment of tibial condyle fractures. Acta Chir. Scand., *133*: 17, 1967.

53. Gallinaro, P., and Crova, M.: Eziopatogenesi e classificasione delle fratture del ginocchio. G. Ital. Ortop. Traumatol., *3*(Suppl. I): 23, 1977.

54. Garcia Suarez, G., Garcia Garcia, F.J., Martinez Zubieta, P., et al.: Tratamiento quirurgico de las fracturas intraarticulares de la meseta tibial. Rev. Esp. Cir. Osteoartic., *13*: 97, 1978.

55. Gérard-Marchant, P.: Fractures des plateaux tibiaux. Rev. Chir. Orthop., *26*: 499, 1939.

56. Godoli, N., Guerra, A., Lanfranchi, R., et al.: La terapia delle fratture del piatto tibiale. Chir. Organi Mov., *62(3)*: 235, 1975.

57. Gossling, H.R., and Peterson, C.A.: A new surgical approach in the treatment of depressed lateral condylar fractures of the tibia. Clin. Orthop., *140*: 96, 1979.

58. Gylling, U., and Lindholm, R.: Fracture of the tibial condyle. Ann. Chir. Gynaec. Finniae., *42*: 229, 1953.

59. Gottfries, A., Hagert, C.G., and Sörensen, S.E.: T and Y fractures of the tibial condyles. A follow-up study of cases treated by closed reduction and surgical fixation with a wire loop. Injury, *3*: 56, 1971.

60. Gui, L.: Fratture e lassazioni. Bologna, Aulo Gaggi Editore, 1973.

61. Hallén, L.G., and Lindahl, O.: The lateral stability of the knee joint. Acta Orthop. Scand., *36*: 179, 1965.

62. Hohl, M.: Tibial condylar fractures. J. Bone Joint Surg. [Am.], *49*: 1455, 1967.

63. Hohl, M. and Larsan, R.L.: Fractures and dislocations of the knee. p. 1131. In Rockwood C.A., and Greene, D.P., eds.: Fractures, Vol. 2. Philadelphia, J.B. Lippincott, 1975.

64. Hohl, M., and Luck, J.V.: Fractures of the tibial condyle. A clinical and experimental study. J. Bone Joint Surg. [Am.], *38*: 1001, 1956.

65. Hulten, O.: Uber die indirekten Brüche des tibiakopfes nebst beiträgen zur Röntgenologie des Kniegelenks. Acta Chir. Scand., Suppl 15, *66*:1, 1929.

66. Jacobs, J.E.: Patellar graft for severely depressed comminuted fractures of the lateral tibial condyle. J. Bone Joint Surg. [Am.], *47*: 842, 1965.

67. Jackson, D.W.: The use of autologous fibula for a prop graft in depressed lateral tibial plateau fractures. Clin. Orthop., *87*: 110, 1972.

68. Jackson, J.P.: Degenerative changes in the knee after meniscectomy. Br. Med. J., *2*: 525, 1968.

69. Jakobsen, A.: Operative treatment of lateral tibial condyle fractures. A follow-up study of 68 cases. Acta Orthop. Scand., *23*: 34, 1953.

70. Johnson, F., Leitl, S., and Waugh, W.: The distribution of load across the knee. A comparison of static and dynamic measurements. J. Bone Joint Surg. [Br.], *62*: 346, 1980.

71. Johnson, R.J, Kettelkamp, D.B., Clark, W., et al.: Factors affecting late results after meniscectomy. J. Bone Joint Surg. [Am.], *56*: 719, 1974.

72. Kennedy, J.C., and Bailey, W.H.: Experimental tibial-plateau fractures. Studies of the mechanism and a classification. J. Bone Joint Surg. [Am.], *50*: 1522, 1968.

73. Krause, W.R., Pope, M.H., Johnson, R.J., et al.: Mechanical changes in the knee after meniscectomy. J. Bone Joint Surg., [Am.], *58*: 599, 1976.

74. Lee, H.G.: Osteoplastic reconstruction in severe fractures of the tibial condyles. Utilization of the anterior superior iliac spine. Am. J. Surg., *94*: 940, 1957.

75. Lotke, P.A., Lefkoe, R.T., and Ecker, M.L.: Late results following medial meniscectomy in an older population. J. Bone Joint Surg. [Am.], *63*: 115, 1981.

76. Lucht, U., and Pilgaard, S.: Fractures of the tibial condyles. Acta Orthop. Scand., *42*: 366, 1971.

77. Maisel, B., and Cornell, N.W.: Conservative treatment of fractures of the tibial condyles. Surgery, *23*: 591, 1948.

78. Maquet, P., Simonet, J., and deMarchin, P.: Biomécanique du genou et gonarthrose. Rev. Chir. Orthop., *53*: 111, 1967.

79. Maquet, P.G., Van De Berg, A.J., and Simonet, J.C.: Femorotibial weight-bearing areas. J. Bone Joint Surg. [Am.], *57*: 766, 1975.

80. Martin, A.F.: The pathomechanics of the knee joint. I. The medial collateral ligament and lateral tibial plateau fracture. J. Bone Joint Surg. [Am.], *42*: 13, 1960.

81. Masse, Y., and Mazas, F.: Devenir à long terme des fractures des plateaux tibiaux. Rev. Chir. Orthop., *63(2)*: 203, 1977.

82. Medlar, R.C., Mandiberg, J.J., and Lyne, E.D.: Meniscectomies in children. Report of long-term results (mean 8.3 years) of 26 children. Am. J. Sports Med., *8*: 87, 1980.

83. Mensch, J.S., and Amstutz, H.C.: Knee morphology as a guide to knee replacement. Clin. Orthop., *112*: 231, 1975.

84. Merle d'Aubigné, R., and Mazas, F.: Formes anatomiques et traitement des fractures de l'extrémité supérieure du tibia. Rev. Chir. Orthop., *46*: 289, 1960.

85. Monticelli, G., and Pizzetti, M.: Sulle lesioni meniscali e legamentose nelle fratture del piatto tibiale. Atti S. O.T.I.M.I., *3*: 326, 1958.

86. Moore, T.M.: Fracture-dislocation of the knee. Clin. Orthop., *156*: 128, 1981.

87. Moore, T.M., and Harvey, J.P., Jr.: Roentgenographic measurement of tibial plateau depression due to fracture. J. Bone Joint Surg. [Am.], *56*: 155, 1974.

88. Moore, T.M., Meyers, M.H., and Harvey, J.P.: Collateral ligament laxity of the knee. Long term com-

parison between plateau fractures and normal. J. Bone Joint Surg. [Am.], *58*: 594, 1976.

89. Morrison, J.B.: The mechanics of the knee joint in relation to normal walking. J. Biomech., *3*: 51, 1970.

90. Müller, M.E., Allgöwer, M., Schneider, R., and Willenegger, H.: Manual of Internal Fixation. Technique recommended by the AO Group. New York, Springer-Verlag, 1979.

91. Neviaser, J.S., and Eisenberg, S.H.: Diagnostic and therapeutic obstacles encountered in tibial plateau fractures. Bull. Hosp. Joint Dis., *17*: 48, 1956.

92. Newberg, A.H., and Greenstein, R.: Radiographic evaluation of tibial plateau fractures. Radiology, *126*: 319, 1978.

93. Nixon, J.E., and DiStefano, V.J.: Injuries of the knee. p 709. In Heppenstall, R.B., ed.: Fracture Treatment and Healing. Philadelphia, W.B. Saunders, 1980.

94. Noyes, F.R., and Grood, E.S.: The strength of the anterior cruciate ligament in humans and rhesus monkeys. J. Bone Joint Surg. [Am.], *58*: 1074, 1976.

95. Olerud, S.: Osteotomy on the tibial tuberosity in fractures of the tibial condyle. Acta Orthop. Scand., *42*: 432, 1971.

96. Palmer, I.: Compression fractures of the lateral tibial condyle and their treatment. J. Bone Joint Surg. [Am.], *21*: 674, 1939.

97. Palmer, I.: Fractures of the upper end of the tibia. J. Bone Joint Surg. [Br.], *33*: 160, 1951.

98. Perey, O.: Depression fractures of the lateral tibial condyle. Acta Chir. Scand., *103*: 154, 1952.

99. Porter, B.B.: Crush fractures of the lateral tibial table. Factors influencing the prognosis. J. Bone Joint Surg. [Br.], *52*: 676, 1970.

100. Postel, M., Mazas, F., and De La Caffinière, J.Y.: Fracture-separation posterieure des plateaux tibiaux. Rev. Chir. Orthop., *60*(Suppl. II): 317, 1974.

101. Rasmussen, P.S.: Tibial condylar fractures as a cause of degenerative arthritis. Acta Orthop. Scand., *43*: 566, 1972.

102. Rasmussen, P.S.: Tibial condylar fractures: Impairment of knee joint stability as an indication for surgical treatment. J. Bone Joint Surg. [Am.], *55*: 1331, 1973.

103. Rieunau, G., Ficat, P., Utheza, G., et al.: Le traitement des fractures articulaires de l'extrémité superieure du tibia. Rev. Chir. Orthop., *57*(Suppl. I): 209, 1971.

104. Rinonapoli, E., and Aglietti, P.: Comparison of treatment by open and closed reduction of comparable cases of articular fractures of the proximal tibia. Ital. J. Orthop. Traumatol., *3*(Suppl. I): 99, 1977.

105. Roberts, J.M.: Fractures of the condyles of the tibia. An anatomical and clinical end-result study of 100 cases. J. Bone Joint Surg. [Am.], *50*: 1505, 1968.

106. Rombold, C.: Depressed fractures of the tibial plateau. J. Bone Joint Surg. [Am.], *42*: 783, 1960.

107. Salter, R.B., Simmonds, D.F., Malcolm, B.W., et al.: The biological effect of continuous passive motion on the healing of full thickness defects in articular cartilage. An experimental investigation in the rabbit. J. Bone Joint Surg. [Am.], *62*: 1232, 1980.

108. Sarmiento, A., Kinman, P.B., and Latta, L.L.: Closed functional treatment of fractures. New York, Springer-Verlag, 1981.

109. Sarmiento, A., Kinman, P.B., and Latta, L.L.: Fractures of the proximal tibia and tibial condyles: A clinical and laboratory comparative study. Clin. Orthop., *145*: 136, 1979.

110. Schatzker, J., and Schulak, D.J.: Pseudoarthrosis of a tibial plateau fracture. Report of a case. Clin. Orthop., *145*: 146, 1979.

111. Schatzker, J., McBroom, R., and Bruce, D.: The tibial plateau fracture: The Toronto experience 1968–1975. Clin. Orthop., *138*: 94, 1979.

112. Schioler, G.: Tibial condylar fractures with a particular view to the value of tomography. Acta Orthop. Scand., *42*: 462, 1971.

113. Schulak, D.J., and Gunn, D.R.: Fractures of the tibial plateaus. Clin. Orthop., *109*: 166, 1975.

114. Scotland, T., and Wardlaw, D.: The use of cast bracing as treatment for fractures of the tibial plateau. J. Bone Joint Surg., [Br.], *63*: 575, 1981.

115. Seedhom, B.B., Downson, D., and Wright, V.: Functions of the menisci—A preliminary study. J. Bone Joint Surg. In proceedings [Br.], *56*: 381, 1974.

116. Shires, P.R.: Tibial condylar fractures. Postgrad. Med. J., *40*: 543, 1964.

117. Shrive, N.: The weight-bearing role of the menisci of the knee. In proceedings J. Bone Joint Surg. [Br.], *56*: 381, 1974.

118. Slee, G.C.: Fractures of the tibial condyles. J. Bone Joint Surg. [Br.], *37*: 427, 1955.

119. Soderberg, L.: End results in conservatively treated compression fractures of the lateral tibial condyle. Acta Orthop. Scand., *29*: 49, 1960.

120. Solonen, K.A.: Fractures of the tibial condyles. Acta Orthop. Scand., *63*(Suppl.): 1, 1963.

121. Tapper, E.M., and Hoover, N.W.: Late results after meniscectomy. J. Bone Joint Surg. [Am.], *51*: 517, 1969.

122. Tessari, L., and Spina, G.M.: Le lesioni meniscali e legamentose quali complicanze di fratture del piatto tibiale. Clin. Ortop., *13*: 573, 1961.

123. Ulin, R.: Unusual etiology of "fender fractures." N. Engl. J. Med., *210*: 480, 1934.

124. Vives, P., Massy, E., and Fichelle, G.: Reimplacement du plateau tibial par la rotule pédiculisée. Rev. Chir. Orthop., *61(6)*: 543, 1975.

125. vonBahr, V.: Depressed and comminuted fractures of lateral tibial tuberosity. Acta Chir. Scand., *92*: 139, 1945.

126. Walker, P.S., and Erkman, M.J.: The role of the menisci in force transmission across the knee. Clin. Orthop., *109*: 184, 1975.

127. Wilppula, E., and Bakalim, G.: Ligamentous tear concomitant with tibial condylar fracture. Acta Orthop. Scand., *43*: 292, 1972.

128. Wilson, W.J., and Jacobs, J.E.: Patellar graft for severely depressed comminuted fractures of the lateral tibial condyle. J. Bone Joint Surg. [Am.], *34*: 436, 1952.

129. Wolf, M.D., and White, E.H.: Depressed fractures of the tibial plateau. Surg. Gynecol. Obstet., *116*: 457, 1963.

130. Zalcman, R., and DeGeeter, L.: Intérêt de la tomographie pour l'étude du bilan lésionnel des fractures des plateaux tibiaux. Acta Orthop. Belg., *39*: 556, 1973.

16 Knee Synovitis

Charles L. Christian

SYNOVIAL PHYSIOLOGY

Because of the large capacity of the knee joint bursa and its accessibility to arthroscopy, biopsy, and physiologic measurements, much of current knowledge of the biology of human synovial tissue derives from the study of this articulation. The tissue lining the synovial spaces is sometimes referred to as a membrane, but there are no membranous structures that separate the loosely arranged and discontinuous lining cells from highly vascularized subsynovial tissue. Except for hyaluronate, the dominant glycosaminoglycan of the synovial fluid, which is synthesized by specialized synovial lining cells, the composition of normal synovial fluid is essentially a dialysate of plasma. It contains water, electrolytes, freely diffusible solutes, and a small amount (no more than 2 g/dl) of low-molecular-weight protein, mainly albumin. The selective permeability of synovial tissue for various-size solutes, and its alteration in inflammatory states, is monitored by the endothelial barrier in a complex network of microvessels deep to the lining cells.

The normal human knee contains 1 to 4 ml of synovial fluid, usually too little to be sampled for study. Because of a difference in oncotic pressure between joint fluid and surrounding tissues, there is a net negative intra-articular pressure in the resting state (averages: 4 mm Hg); hence the cavity is a potential space that is maintained in a collapsed state by its subatmospheric pressure.[3] With certain maneuvers, such as isometric flexion of the lower extremity, the intracavitary pressure drops to as low as -100 mm Hg, a change that probably contributes significantly to joint stability. The pressure dynamics of the knee are dramatically altered by effusions.[4] Isometric flexion of the lower extremity produces positive pressure (range 200 mm Hg) when the knee is distended with 100 ml of saline, and pressure changes approximately double that are observed in comparably effused knees of patients with rheumatoid arthritis. Passive flexion of knees with 100 ml effusions can generate pressures as high as 800 mm Hg—the setting for bursal rupture syndromes.

As noted above, diffusion of most molecules into the joint space is controlled by vascular permeability and, for water-soluble solutes, entry into the joint space is determined by molecular size.[9] By a process that has not been characterized, glucose, the primary energy source for metabolism of articular cartilage, enters the synovial space more rapidly than it leaves. This phenomenon, which results in synovial fluid glucose levels in excess of blood glucose, is dramatically reversed in some patients with rheumatoid arthritis, in which synovial fluid glucose may be undetectable. The basis for this pathologic condition, whether altered diffusion or accelerated consumption of glucose, is unknown.

BIOLOGY OF INFLAMMATION

Few biologic processes rival the complexity of those mediating inflammation: heat, erythema, swelling, and pain. The tissue responses that result in inflammation are (1) changes in vascular tone and permeability, (2) activation of enzymes that attack lipid membranes of cells, and (3) an increase in the number of cells. The events that mediate such changes involve numerous complex biochemical processes, including (1) release of vasoactive amines; (2) generation of several enzymes from plasma substrates or from cells that affect the tone and permeability of blood vessels and promote blood coagulation or fibrinolysis; (3) activation of complement, yielding chemotactic, anaphylactic, and cytotoxic principles; (4) production of prostaglandins via action of multiple enzymes on arachidonic acid; (5) formation of oxygen derived products; and (6) release of lysosomal enzymes from inflammatory cells.

Evidence suggests that the complex processes we call inflammation are important elements in normal homeostastis and that they help defend the host against a variety of noxious stimuli and promote healing. In a sense, the tissue injury associated with inflammation, the unwanted clinical problem, is a by-product of such host responses initiated by infectious, immunologic, chemical, or traumatic stimuli. Much of the injury to articular cartilage, bone, and other periarticular structures in patients with synovitis can be attributed to the same enzymatic and cytotoxic principles discussed under chemical mediation above. In addition, the hyperplastic synovial tissue forming pannus in rheumatoid arthritis and certain other chronic forms of synovitis is a source of collagenase which, in conjunction with other enzymes or by itself, can cleave collagen substrate in cartilage, bone, and other articular and periarticular structures.

Until recent years the development of anti-inflammatory drugs derived from studies of in vivo models of inflammation in experimental species, but recent knowledge that virtually all anti-rheumatic agents inhibit one or more pathways of enzymatic degradation of arachidonic acid, has led to move rapid in vitro screening of compounds and development of a new generation of nonsteroidal anti-inflammatory agents. The clinical employment of these and other agents is described later in this chapter.

DIFFERENTIAL DIAGNOSIS OF KNEE SYNOVITIS

At the outset of inquiry, the physician's mind should be open to the full range of considerations that can be manifested as knee synovitis, being aware of the temptation to concentrate prematurely on limited diagnostic categories. Is the problem restricted to that articulation, or is the knee involvement only part of a more generalized joint disease or a systemic illness? Reliance on the laboratory and differential diagnosis, before exploiting the discriminating power of the medical history and physical examination to focus diagnostic considerations, is wasteful and results in errors; more often, it results in the failure to order the right test.

CLUES FROM THE MEDICAL HISTORY AND PHYSICAL EXAMINATION

ANATOMIC DISTRIBUTION AND PATTERN OF INVOLVEMENT

Monarticular synovitis of the knee, although it can be a manifestation of any rheumatic syndrome, is more likely to result from mechanical derangement, trauma, infection, gout, calcium pyrophosphate deposition disease (CPPD), and hemarthrosis.

Polyarticular patterns of disease may result from infection, gout, and CPPD, but the more common diagnostic categories are rheumatoid arthritis, osteoarthritis, systemic lupus erythematosus (SLE), and psoriatic arthropathy. Involvement of the knees and more distal articulations of the lower extremities is a frequent feature of Reiter syndrome, ankylosing spondylitis, sarcoidosis, and the arthropathy associated with inflammatory bowel diseases. Asymmetric polyarthritis can be an early feature of many syndromes, but it is more common with gout, CPPD, and psoriatic arthropathy. When the more distal extremity joints are affected, patterns of involvement of interphalangeal, metacarpophalangeal, and carpal–metacarpal joints can be virtually diagnostic of rheumatoid arthritis, psoriatic arthropathy, or osteoarthritis. Diffuse dactylitis (sausage digits) can be an early sign of psoriatic arthropathy or Reiter syndrome.

CONSTITUTIONAL SYMPTOMS

Fever in excess of 38°C should focus attention on infectious etiologies of synovitis, as well as SLE, juvenile rheumatoid arthritis, and other connective tissue syndromes. Shaking chills is a particularly important symptom in considering infectious arthritis. Morning stiffness and fatigue are common features of rheumatoid arthritis and other systemic inflammatory arthropathies.

SKIN LESIONS

In any patient with synovitis there should be a careful search for characteristic skin and nail manifestations of psoriasis. Nodules of the skin or subcutaneous tissue and tophi should suggest rheumatoid arthritis and gout respectively. Multiform cutaneous lesions, particularly in sun-exposed areas, are significant features of SLE. A common form of sarcoidosis (Löfgren syndrome) consists of lower extremity arthritis (particularly ankles and feet) in association with erythema nodosum. Of special significance in considering infectious arthritis (e.g., disseminated gonococcemia) are vesicular, necrotic, and purpuric skin lesions.

OCULAR INVOLVEMENT

The following ocular patterns of disease are noteworthy: conjunctivitis/Reiter syndrome, iridocyclitis/juvenile rheumatoid arthritis, ankylosing spondylitis and Reiter syndrome, keratoconjunctivitis/Sjögren's syndrome and rheumatoid arthritis, scleritis or scleromalacia/rheumatoid arthritis.

GENITOURINARY INVOLVEMENT

The following associations have diagnostic significance in consideration of knee arthritis: urethritis and cervicitis/gonococcal disease and Reiter syndrome, glomerulonephritis/SLE and Henoch-Schönlein purpura, urolithiasis/gout and hyperparathyroidism and mucocutaneous lesions/Reiter syndrome and Behçet syndrome.

GASTROINTESTINAL ASSOCIATIONS

Gastrointestinal associations include diarrhea/arthropathy of inflammatory bowel disease, Reiter syndrome and Whipple disease, stomatitis/Reiter syndrome, Behçet syndrome and SLE, xerostomia and sialadenitis/Sjögren's syndrome, rheumatoid arthritis, SLE and other connective tissue syndromes, and proctitis/gonococcal disease.

RESPIRATORY AND CARDIAC INVOLVEMENT

Pleuritis, pericarditis, and interstitial pneumonitis can be manifestations of any of the systemic connective tissue syndromes, particularly SLE, rheumatoid arthritis, and progressive systemic sclerosis. Involvement of cardiac valves should suggest bacterial endocarditis, acute rheumatic fever, ankylosing spondylitis, SLE, and Reiter syndrome.

NEUROLOGIC ASSOCIATIONS

Neurologic associations include peripheral neuropathy/vasculitis syndromes, SLE, and rheumatoid arthritis, seizures or organic central nervous system (CNS) disease/vasculitis, SLE and Lyme disease, radiculopathy/osteoarthritis, Lyme disease and ankylosing spondylitis, myelopathy/rheumatoid arthritis, osteoarthritis and neuropathic joint disease, entrapment neuropathy/rheumatoid arthritis, and other inflammatory arthropathies.

MISCELLANEOUS

Myalgia and weakness are common manifestations of all the systemic connective tissue syndromes. Raynaud symptoms have their highest frequency in progressive systemic sclerosis, also significantly associated with SLE. Clubbing of fingers and toes should suggest pulmonary osteoarthropathy, bacterial endocarditis, and inflammatory bowel disease.

DEMOGRAPHIC CHARACTERISTICS

Family History

Gout, ankylosing spondylitis, and osteoarthritis can be pertinent to diagnostic considerations. Syndromes with male predominance include gout, ankylosing spondylitis, and Reiter syndrome; the frequency of SLE, rheumatoid arthritis, and progressive systemic sclerosis is higher in women.

Promiscuous Sexual Orientation

Promiscuity is pertinent in consideration of gonococcal disease and Reiter syndrome. The frequency of disseminated gonococcemia is increased in homosexual males.

ASSOCIATED DRUG THERAPY

The following associations are noteworthy: penicillin and many other drugs/serum sickness syndromes, adrenocortical steroids/osteonecrosis, osteoporosis, fracture, procaineamide and hydralazine/drug-induced SLE, diuretics/gout, and anticoagulants/hemarthrosis.

OTHER ASPECTS OF CLINICAL ASSESSMENT

The discussion of differential diagnosis noted above is not intended as a specific or restricted guide to diagnosis; it is presented to emphasize the diversity of clinical information that can be collected from the doctor/patient dialogue and the power that such data can have in directing subsequent evaluation. Oversimplification is inherent in any arbitrary diagnostic guide. Some examples relative to the above discussion include the following:

1. Although gout and CPPD are typically monarticular and acute, chronic and polyarticular forms occur.
2. Rheumatoid and psoriatic arthropathy, although usually polyarticular, can affect single articulations.
3. Syndromes ordinarily manifested as joint synovitis (e.g., rheumatoid arthritis, gout infections) can be expressed as synovitis of bursae or tendons.

4. In contrast to the traditional classification of arthropathies, some clinical forms of osteoarthritis are characterized by variable, sometimes marked, inflammation.
5. The demographic characteristics cited are of importance only in a statistical sense; diseases such as gout, Reiter syndrome, gonococcal arthritis, and juvenile rheumatoid arthritis occur in both sexes and at any age.
6. Constitutional symptoms such as stiffness and fatigue are most characteristic of rheumatoid arthritis but occur with any systemic disease.

Some historic items not discussed above deserve emphasis.

Mode of Onset. Was the beginning of symptomatology abrupt or gradual? Was there associated trauma or participation in unusual physical activities?

Chronology. Diagnostic considerations for acute rheumatic syndromes are different and generally broader than those for chronic disease. Recent onset synovitis, particularly if associated with fever or other evidence of sepsis, deserves prompt consideration of infectious etiologies. Episodic and remittent patterns of disease can occur with most rheumatic syndromes, but are more common with gout, CPPD, and traumatic syndromes. The clinical picture of acute rheumatoid arthritis may be identical to remittent forms of synovitis associated with suspected or proven viral syndromes, such as rubella, hepatitis, and mononucleosis.

Functional Alterations. Severity of disease and the extent of disability can often be better quantified in the medical history than from the physical examination. To what extent have activities of daily living, maintenance of vocation, participation in sports, and so forth been affected by the illness?

FORMULATION AFTER COMPLETION OF MEDICAL HISTORY AND PHYSICAL EXAMINATION

At the completion of the clinical evaluation, the diagnosis may be known, and limited laboratory tests may be indicated in order to confirm the diagnosis. If a definite diagnosis is lacking, a strategy should have evolved regarding the most likely diagnosis and some important questions should be addressed: How serious is the illness? Are the rheumatic symptoms part of a more generalized disease? Can subsequent diagnostic evaluation be staged or is there a sense of urgency in obtaining a diagnosis? Does the patient require immediate hospitalization? How can the laboratory most efficiently and economically be employed in clarifying the problem?

LABORATORY STUDIES

The number of rheumatic syndromes that can be confirmed by laboratory examination is small; in the great majority of cases, diagnosis derives from an integration of clinical information with laboratory data that is supportive or confirmatory but not definitive.

Examples of laboratory procedures with high specificity include (1) identification of urate and calcium pyrophosphate crystals in synovial fluids of patients with gout and CPPD, respectively; (2) isolation of bacterial forms in patients with pyarthrosis; (3) early recognition of osteomyelitis and avascular osteonecrosis by radionuclide bone scan; (4) documentation of vasculitis and myositis in biopsy specimens from patients with relevant syndromes; (5) demonstration of arterial aneurysms by arteriography in patients with vasculitis syndromes; and (6) verification of mechanical derangements by arthrography.

With the exceptions noted above, biochemical, pathologic, immunologic, and radiographic studies have statistical, not definitive, relevance to the diagnosis of rheumatic disease (e.g., rheumatoid factors in rheumatoid arthritis; antinuclear antibodies and hypocomplementemia in SLE, hyperuricemia, and gout; HLA-B27 typing in the spondyloarthropathies; increased serum enzymes in myositis syndromes). These and other laboratory procedures, although lacking absolute specificity, may be decisive when interpreted in the light of clinical information. The presence of hypocomplementemia and antinuclear antibodies (particularly anti-dsDNA antibodies) can discriminate between SLE and polyarteritis in patients with arthritis and renal disease. The radiographic demonstration of hilar adenopathy in a patient with lower extremity arthritis and erythema nodosum helps identify patients with a generally benign form of sarcoidosis (Löfgren syndrome).

The discussion that follows is organized according to the different categories of laboratory tests, summarized in Table 16.1.

BASIC LABORATORY STUDIES

The simplicity and low cost of the routine studies noted in Table 16.1 warrant their performance in most patients presenting with undiagnosed rheumatic symptoms. (One can cite some exceptions: persons otherwise in good health, presenting with painful Heberden nodes, shoulder bursitis, tenosynovitis or an obvious traumatic synovitis.) The erythrocyte sedimentation rate (ESR) tends to separate cases into the two broad categories: inflammatory and noninflammatory rheumatism; the routine blood studies, urinalysis, and chemical profile can provide clues for further study regarding the presence of systemic disease. The inclusion of uric acid methods and tests of liver dysfunction in automated analyses permit detection of hyperuricemia and can help identify a relatively common clinical syndrome, HB hepatitis arthropathy. (Concomitant salicylate therapy can spuriously elevate uric acid levels and liver enzymes.)

SYNOVIAL FLUID ANALYSES

As noted in the introduction to this discussion, cytologic, bacteriologic, and polarized light microscopic analysis of joint fluid provide more discriminating and diagnostic information than any other category of tests. Table 16.2 summarizes synovial fluid findings in various types of synovitis. Leukocyte counts in excess of $50,000/mm^3$ suggest sepsis, but levels in that range can be seen in multiple forms of inflammatory arthropathy. The importance and the specificity of polarized light microscopy and bacteriologic studies are self-evident. Two comments regarding arthrocentesis deserve mention: (1) If a joint effusion is demonstrable in an undiagnosed patient with acute synovitis, tap it, as the opportunity might pass; and (2) for bacteriologic studies, the physician should not trust routine routing of samples to the laboratory.

IMMUNOLOGIC STUDIES

The list of serologic procedures in Table 16.1 is not comprehensive, but it includes most tests that are relatively standardized and available in most clinical settings. The presence of anti-dsDNA antibodies is the most specific serologic feature of SLE and should

Table 16.1.   Laboratory Tests for Knee Synovitis

Laboratory Procedures	*Relevance/Usefulness in Diagnosis*
Basic studies	
Complete blood count	Simple and inexpensive tests that have nonspecific relevance to inflammatory and/or systemic disease and that are appropriate for general health assessment
Erythrocyte sedimentation rate	
Urinalysis	
Stool guaiac	
Chemical profile (automated)	Myositis/enzyme elevation, gout/hyperuricemia, liver dysfunction/hepatitis arthropathy or vasculitis, metabolic bone disease/alkaline phosphatase, and serum calcium
Synovial fluid studies	
Complete blood count	Differentiation of noninflammatory from inflammatory and septic disease
Polarized light microscopy	High relevance and specificity for gout and pseudogout (CPPD)
Gram stain	High relevance and specificity for bacterial synovitis (other biologic specimens should be cultured)
Culture	
Immunologic studies	
Rheumatoid factor tests	80% positive in RA but positive in other rheumatic and nonrheumatic illnesses
Antinuclear antibodies (ANA)	90% positive in SLE but positive in other rheumatic and nonrheumatic illnesses
Anti-dsDNA antibodies	70% positive in Active SLE; most specific serologic test for SLE, but occasionally positive in other rheumatic syndromes
Serum complement (or components)	70% abnormal (reduced) in active SLE, also reduced in other syndromes
STS (serologic test for syphilis)	20% positive in SLE (biologic false-positive Wassermann)
FTA (fluorescent treponemal antibody)	Positive in syphilis; negative in SLE
ASLO	80% positive in ARF and in uncomplicated β-hemolytic streptococcal infection
HB$_s$ antigen	Positive, indicates recent infection or carrier state, relevant to preicteric hepatitis arthropathy and to HB, associated with vasculitis
Serum or urine immunoelectrophoresis	Detection of monoclonal immunoglobulins, relevant to amyloid, cryoglobinemia, lymphoma, and detection of immunodeficiency states
HLA-B$_{27}$ antigen	HLA antigen associated with increased risk of spondyloarthropathies, important epidemiologic tool, not a diagnostic test
Immunoglobulin quantification	Detection of monoclonal immunoglobulins, relevant to amyloid, cryoglobulinemia, lymphoma, and detection of immunodeficiency states
Cryoglobulins	Positive in "essential cryoglobulinemia," RA, SLE, vasculitis syndromes, lymphoproliferative diseases
Microbiologic studies	
Culture for bacterial, fungal, mycobacterial species of relevant biologic fluids and/or tissues	High relevance and specificity for infectious arthritis (gonococcal and others), bacterial endocarditis
Pathologic studies	
Muscle/skin/nerve biopsies	High degree of specificity for histopathological diagnoses (myositis, vasculitis, panniculitis), sarcoidosis
Temporal artery biopsy	High degree of specificity for temporal arteritis, if positive; does not exclude diagnosis, if negative
Synovial biopsy	Rarely diagnostic but important in ruling in or out infection when that is suspect
Other biopsies	Renal (glomerulonephritis), rectal (amyloidosis), lip (Sjögren), lymph node (lymphoma, sarcoidosis)
Radiographic studies	
Chest radiograph	Relevant to Löfgren syndrome (hilar adenopathy), Wegener granulomatosus, pulmonary osteoarthropathy, interstitial pneumonitis, pleural disease
Joint(s) radiograph	Infrequently diagnostic except in chronic forms of arthritis and CPPD
Gastrointestinal (barium) studies	Demonstration of esophageal and pharyngeal dysmotility (myositis and PSS), ulcerative colitis, and Crohn's disease (enteropathic arthropathy)
Radionuclide bone scan	Permits early diagnosis of osteomyelitis, avascular osteonecrosis, and osteoid osteoma
Arthrography	Demonstration of mechanical disorders, ruptured bursa
Arteriography	Documentation of vasculitis syndromes via demonstration of aneurysms

Continued

Table 16.1. (*continued*)

Laboratory Procedures	Relevance/Usefulness in Diagnosis
Other studies	
Hematologic	
Bone marrow	Important in considering rheumatic manifestations of leukemia, lymphoma, metastatic cancer, plasma cell dyscrasias, and disseminated tuberculosis, and in exploring bases for cytopenias
Coombs/haptoglobin/retics	Consideration of hemolytic complications of rheumatic syndrome
Serum iron and TIBC	Consideration of hemochromatosis arthropathy, differentiation of iron deficiency from anemia of chronic disease
Coagulation profile	Identification of intravascular coagulation in SLE and vasculitis and the presence of circulating anticoagulants
	Aid in diagnosis of neuropathic and myopathic syndromes
EMG and nerve conduction studies	
Chemistries	
Thyroid chemistries	Diagnosis of hypothyroid arthralgia syndrome or myopathy
Lipid studies	Recognition of rheumatic complications of hyperlipidemia
24-hour uric acid excretion	Differentiation of overproduction versus underexcretion as bases for hyperuricemia
24-hour urine protein	Indicators of activity/severity of renal disease in patients with SLE, vasculitis,
Creatinine clearance	amyloidosis

Abbreviations: ARF, acute rheumatic fever; CPPD, calcium pyrophosphate deposition disease; EMG, electromyogram; HB$_s$, hepatitis B viral surface antigen; HLA, human leukocyte antigen; PSS, progressive systemic sclerosis; SLE, systemic lupus erythematosus.

be performed in patients with clinical features compatible with SLE who are ANA positive. (The same rule applies to serum complement measurement, although hypocomplementemia has a lower order of specificity for the disease.) Several partially characterized antinuclear reactivities have been identified by immunologic techniques: anti-Sm antigen, antiribonucleoprotein (RNP), and others, but the tests for their detection are not routine. (Anti-Sm is relatively specific for SLE and anti-RNP titers are highest in a "mixed connective tissue disease" that most closely resembles progressive systemic sclerosis.) Rheumatoid factors, usually detected by the latex agglutination test, have the highest association with rheumatoid arthritis but the results of this test rarely alter clinical impressions.

Table 16.2. Synovial Fluid Analysis

Classification	Conditions	Appearance	Viscosity (Mucin Clot)	WBC/mm³ (Mean)	% PMN	Crystals
Normal	—	Yellow, clear	Good	<200	<25	—
Noninflammatory	Osteoarthritis, trauma, mechanical derangements, (also early, mild, or subsiding "inflammatory" arthropathies)	Yellow, clear to slightly turbid (red or xanthochromic with hemarthrosis)	Good	200–2,000	<25	Gout/sodium urate/needle-shaped, negative birefringence; pseudogout/calcium pyrophosphate dihydrate/rhomboidal or punctate, weakly positive birefringence
Inflammatory	Rheumatoid arthritis, gout, pseudogout, psoriatic arthropathy, others, and some infectious syndromes	Yellow, slightly turbid to turbid	Fair to poor	2,000–50,000 (20,000)	25–90	Gout, pseudogout. Same as above
Septic	Bacterial, fungal, or tuberculous infection	Yellow to white, turbid to purulent	Poor	20,000–300,000 (80,000)	50→ > 90	— —

MICROBIOLOGIC STUDIES

As noted in Table 16.1 and in the discussion of synovial fluid analysis above, bacteriologic studies play critical roles; they are diagnostic and they lead to specific and curative therapy.

PATHOLOGIC STUDIES

The relevance of histopathologic study of biopsy tissue to diagnosis is summarized in Table 16.1. The pathologic specificity of such analyses is explicit, but multiple clinical syndromes can be associated with myositis, necrotizing vasculitis, or glomerulonephritis. The characteristic lesions of temporal (or cranial) arteritis have clear diagnostic and therapeutic implications.

RADIOGRAPHIC STUDIES

Conventional radiographic studies have significant but limited bearing on rheumatologic diagnosis, but the newer angiographic, radionuclide, and arthrographic techniques have high degrees of specificity for certain conditions (Table 16.1).

OTHER STUDIES

The roles of procedures in this category for diagnosis, grading of severity, and recognition of complications of rheumatic syndromes are summarized in Table 16.1. Additional procedures could be added, including pulmonary function tests, electrocardiogram (ECG), electroencephalogram (EEG), and cerebrospinal fluid (CSF) analysis, serum amylase, urine homogentisic acid, and others.

MEDICAL MANAGEMENT OF SYNOVITIS

Only management principles are summarized here; for more detailed description of the treatment of various rheumatic syndromes, the reader is referred to the standard textbooks of rheumatology listed in the bibliography.[11] The treatment of certain problems referable to knee synovitis is summarized elsewhere in this text, including mechanical derangements (see Chapters 9–15), osteonecrosis (both idiopathic and secondary to adrenocortical steroid therapy) (see Chapter 18), and severe knee joint deformities for which osteotomy (see Chapter 19) or joint replacement (see Chapters 20, 21, 24) are appropriate.

NONSTEROIDAL ANTI-INFLAMMATORY DRUGS

For nearly all forms of knee synovitis, sustained or intermittent use of a nonsteroidal anti-inflammatory drug (NSAID) is usually appropriate. Included in this class of drugs are salicylate preparations, indomethacin, phenylbutazone, and several newer agents, which are listed along with recommended dosages in Table 16.3. All these compounds inhibit prostaglandin biosynthesis, but there may be other actions that mediate, in part, anti-inflammatory effects. All the drugs have levels of anti-inflammatory activity not far removed from that of aspirin. Relative to aspirin there appear to be variable but probably lower levels of gastrointestinal toxicity associated with the newer drugs. In any form of chronic synovitis, such as rheumatoid arthritis, benefits from NSAID therapy require sustained and systematic use of the drugs. A common error is to conclude that a given medication brought no benefit, when in fact such therapy was not given a fair trial. Salicylate preparations have two important advantages relative to other NSAID: (1) low

Table 16.3. Nonsteroidal Anti-inflammatory Drugs

Generic Name	Proprietary Name	Dose Range (mg)
Aspirin		600–1200 QID
Fenoprofen calcium	Nalfon	300–600 QID
Ibuprofen	Motrin	300–800 TID
Indomethacin	Indocin	25–50 TID
Meclofenamate sodium	Meclomen	50–100 QID
Naproxen	Naprosyn	250–500 BID
Phenylbutazone (oxyphenylbutazone)	Butazolidin (Tandearil)	100–200 TID
Sulindac	Clinoril	150–200 BID
Tolmetin	Tolectin	400 TID
Piroxican	Feldene	20 QD

cost, and (2) questions of absorption or toxicity can be easily checked by obtaining salicylate levels.

PHYSICAL MEDICINE MEASURES

The goals of physical therapy for patients with knee synovitis are (1) to combat or reverse muscle weakness, (2) to preserve, to the extent possible, normal alignment of the lower extremity, and (3) to maintain joint motion. Achievement of these objectives rests with the institution of an exercise program that the patient can maintain; adjuvant measures are heat (hot packs, hydrotherapy, diathermy, or ultrasound), rest, and splints. Physical therapy programs need to be individualized. If synovitis is very acute, nothing more than rest, isometric exercises, and gentle passive motion may be appropriate. Rest (avoidance of loaded or weight-bearing exercises) for patients with active knee synovitis is not inconsistent with the goals of maintaining muscle power and motion.

MANAGEMENT OF SPECIFIC FORMS OF SYNOVITIS

RHEUMATOID ARTHRITIS

Basic Management

The basic management relevant to all patients with rheumatoid arthritis includes aspirin, or equivalent NSAID, and a physical medicine program tailored to the pattern of disease and disability. Most patients experience periods of improvement sufficient for the maintenance of vocational activities.

Table 16.4 lists medications applicable to the treatment of rheumatoid arthritis and generally reserved for patients who have not responded to the basic regimen noted above.[1] These agents are quite different chemically, but share three features: (1) their mode of action is unknown but seems to be independent of anti-inflammatory effect, (2) they are slow acting (i.e., require several weeks or more of therapy before improvement ensues), and (3) efficacy is not predictable. Some patients fail to experience remissions with such therapy. Of the therapeutic agents listed in Table 16.4, gold compounds are most widely employed, but penicillamine therapy is gaining in acceptance and has

the advantage over gold in that it can be administered orally. Cytotoxic drugs are reserved for patients with very high risk patterns of disease that are not responsive to other modes of therapy.

Adrenocortical Steroid Therapy

Although these drugs are the most potent of the anti-inflammatory agents, the high incidence of toxicity associated with their systemic administration precludes such therapy, except in special circumstances. Patients with very high levels of disability that do not respond to more conservative regimens may be candidates for systemic corticosteroid therapy; in such cases, accepting the risk of drug toxicity may be preferable to that of chronic invalidism. The dose should be restricted to the lowest level, preferably 10 mg of prednisone or less daily.

When major levels of disability are attributable to one or few joints, intra-articular preparation such as methylprednisolone acetate (20 to 40 mg) may induce periods of improvement that last for several weeks or more. Injections in individual joints should not be repeated more frequently than every two or three months because of the risk of accelerated cartilage destruction.

Surgical Rehabilitation

Discussions elsewhere in this text deal with the indications for various surgical procedures that contribute to the management of chronic rheumatoid synovitis of the knee (see Chapter 21). Improvements in the techniques of total knee replacement over the past decade has made this the treatment of choice for patients with major joint destruction (see Chapter 20). Because of the availability of this salvage procedure, early (prophylactic) synovectomy is performed less frequently, but it is still an appropriate technique for patients with sustained chronic knee synovitis that are demonstrating early signs of bone or cartilage erosion.

PSORIATIC ARTHROPATHY

Patterns of arthritis associated with psoriasis are varied. In the main, the spectra of disease manifestations and the management are the same as for rheumatoid arthritis, with the exception that there is no

Table 16.4.   Remittive* Agents Employed in the Treatment of Rheumatoid Arthritis

Generic Name	Proprietary Name	Initial Dose	Maintenance Dose	Toxicity
Gold compounds Aurothioglucose Aurothiomalate	Solgonal Myochrysine	Weekly injections (IM) beginning 10 mg, increasing to 50 mg, continuing until total dose of 1,000 mg or remission ensues	50 mg at 2–4-week intervals	Skin rash Myelosuppression Nephritis
Antimalarial drugs Hydroxychloroquine	Plaquenil	400 to 600 mg/day for several weeks, or until remission ensues	200–400 mg/day	Skin rash Corneal deposits Retinitis (careful ophthalmologic examination recommended at 3–6-month intervals) Gastrointestinal intolerance
Penicillamine	Cuprimine	125–250 mg/day increasing by 125–250 mg increments every 2–3 months until remission ensues or toxicity develops (maximum daily dose 1,000 mg)	Maintain level of therapy associated with remission, gradually decreasing dose if remission continues	Skin rash Myelosuppression Nephritis Loss of taste
Cytotoxic drugs Cyclophosphamide Azathioprine	Cytoxan Imuran	100–200 mg/day in single AM dose	Maintain level of therapy associated with remission, gradually decreasing dose if remission continues	Myelosuppression (additional toxicity associated with cyclophosphamide includes hair loss, gonadal failure, hemorrhagic cystitis and bladder tumors; large volume of water ingestion and frequent emptying of bladder recommended)

*Colloquialism for disease modifying agents.

demonstrated role for penicillamine as a remittive agent.

SPONDYLOARTHROPATHIES

This term encompasses a group of inflammatory arthropathies affecting primarily, but not exclusively, the spine and axial skeleton.[7] It includes ankylosing spondylitis, Reiter syndrome, and the spondylitis associated with psoriasis, with inflammatory bowel disease, and with juvenile polyarthritis. There are many bases for separating this group of disorders from rheumatoid arthritis, including the high incidence of the transplantation antigen HLA-B27, but to the extent that knee synovitis may be a prominent, sometimes initial manifestation of the syndromes, management is similar to that described for rheumatoid arthritis. (There is no demonstrated role for the remittive agents such as gold compounds and penicillamine in the management of the spondyloarthropathies.)

GOUT

During the past two decades there has been dramatic improvement in the characterization, diagnosis, and management of gout.[10] Recognition that synovitis is induced by deposition of sodium urate crystals has led to the most definitive basis for recognition of the problem: demonstration of characteristic crystals in joint fluid by compensated polarized microscopy.

The long-term management of gout has been greatly simplified by the availability of allopurinol, an inhibitor of xanthine oxidase that decreases biosynthesis of uric acid. It should be emphasized, however, that allopurinol has no role in the treatment of acute gout; such therapy may initiate or perpetuate an attack of synovitis. The goal of allopurinol therapy is to prevent attacks by chronically lowering serum uric acid levels.

The treatment of choice for acute gouty synovitis is indomethacin (100 to 200 mg/day for several days) or comparable doses of other NSAID. These agents are generally prompt and predictable in their effect and less toxic than colchicine, but the latter drug administered intravenously (2 mg) is the treatment of choice for patients with concurrent peptic ulcer disease or in patients with congestive heart failure (salt-retaining effect of NSAID may aggravate congestive failure).

CALCIUM PYROPHOSPHATE DEPOSITION SYNDROMES

The concept of CPPD syndromes has evolved over the past two decades, since McCarty[6] defined the relationship between chondrocalcinosis and intrasynovial calcium pyrophosphate crystal deposition to a variety of rheumatic syndromes. Acute CPPD synovitis (pseudogout) most commonly affects the knee. Chronic patterns of disease include those that clinically resemble degenerative joint disease and others with a chronic inflammatory arthropathy which, when polyarticular, can mimic rheumatoid arthritis. The incidence of chondrocalcinosis increases with age; most elderly subjects with this radiographic finding do not have symptoms attributable to CPPD.

The diagnosis of CPPD syndromes depends on the demonstration of characteristic crystals in synovial fluid by compensated polarized microscopy.

Management of the chronic forms of disease is aspirin or other NSAID. Acute CPPD synovitis may respond to joint aspiration alone; alternatively, intra-articular corticosteroid therapy or the use of NSAID similar to that employed for acute gout can be used.

OSTEOARTHROSIS (DEGENERATIVE JOINT DISEASE)

Osteoarthrosis represents degenerative changes in joints in response to (1) unknown factors that predispose to cartilage wear, (2) mechanical stresses, or (3) alterations in joints resulting from any type of inflammatory arthropathy.[5] (See Chapters 9, 10, 15, 17–20). It is primarily noninflammatory in nature, but in a few subjects, joint synovitis (either primary to the condition or a response to degenerative changes) is prominent.

Medical management consists of (1) patient education in avoidance of mechanical stress and in the performance of a relevant exercise program, (2) aspirin or other NSAID therapy, and (3) intra-articular corticosteroid therapy at infrequent intervals in selected situations.

The role of surgical rehabilitation of patients with knee osteoarthrosis is discussed elsewhere in this text.

INFECTIOUS SYNOVITIS

As discussed elsewhere in this chapter, the highest order of priority in early evaluation of patients with knee synovitis is the consideration of infectious etiologies.

The recognition of rheumatic expressions of defined viral syndromes, such as rubella, HB hepatitis, and mononucleosis, supports the contention that acute self-limited synovitis, usually symmetric polyarthritis resembling early rheumatoid arthritis, may result from infection with a variety of viral agents. Lyme arthritis is a less predictably remittent illness (some patients have sustained synovitis for months), which is caused by a tick-borne infectious agent.[2] The response of some patients with early Lyme disease to antibiotic therapy has been noted. A spirochetal organism isolated from ticks and from affected patients appears to be the etiological agent. The disease occurs primarily in the Northeast seaboard area during the summer months and is frequently preceded or accompanied by an unusual skin lesion at the site of the tickbite.

To the extent that most instances of pyarthrosis derive from hematogenous implantation of microorganisms, any bacterial form capable of gaining access to the circulation may be seeded in joints.[8] In most clin-

Table 16.5.   Intravenous Antibiotic Therapy Based on Culture Identification of Organism

Organism	Antibiotic	Alternate Drug
Staphylococcus	Nafcillin 100–150 mg/kg/24 hr in four doses	Cephalothin 100 mg/kg/24 hr
Streptococcus	Penicillin G 15–20 million units/24 hr in four doses	Cephalothin 100 mg/kg/24 hr
Neisseria gonorrhoeae	Penicillin G 6–10 million units/24 hr in four doses	Erythromycin 2 gm/24 hr
Hemophilus influenzae	Ampicillin 50 mg/kg/24 hr in four doses	Chloramphenicol 50 mg/kg/24 hr
Gram-negative organisms including *Escherichia coli, Enterobacter* spp., *Klebsiella, Proteus,* and *Salmonella*	Gentamicin 5 mg/kg/24 hr in three doses	Amikacin 15 mg/kg/24 hr
Pseudomonas	Tobramycin 5 mg/kg/24 hr in three doses	Amikacin 15 mg/kg/24 hr

ical settings, *Neisseria gonorrhoeae* and *staphylococcal* species account for the great majority of pyarthroses. *Streptococcus pyogenes, S. pneumoniae, S. viridans,* and gram-negative bacteria are significant causes in a few subjects. *Hemophilus influenzae* arthritis, rare in adults, is a basis for septic synovitis in approximately 10 percent of children with pyarthroses. Successful therapy in pyarthrosis is dependent on early diagnosis and prompt institution of appropriate therapy. All the common antibiotics gain access into the synovial bursa from systemic administration. Surgical incision and drainage is not required unless gross suppuration is present, and exudate is inaccessible to periodic aspiration. Table 16.5 summarizes recommended antibiotic regimens for various bacterial species. The duration of therapy is individualized, but for gonococcal arthritis it is usual practice to continue therapy for one week after subsidence of synovitis and for staphylococcal and gram-negative microorganisms, parenteral therapy is recommended for 3 to 4 weeks, followed by 2 to 4 weeks of appropriate oral therapy.

Tuberculous synovitis, typically a chronic monarthritis, is now a relative rarity in Western countries; its highest incidence is in elderly subjects with reactivated disease. When the problem is suspected on the basis of pattern of synovitis and positive purified protein derivative (PPD) of tuberculin skin reaction, obtaining synovial tissue via arthrotomy or arthroscopy for culture is warranted.

OTHER FORMS OF SYNOVITIS

The rheumatic syndromes described above, as well as trauma (see Chapters 11–15) constitute the most common bases for knee synovitis. Other considerations enter into the differential diagnosis of the problem as well, such as synovial tumors (see Chapter 26), pigmented villonodular synovitis, hemarthrosis (complicating coagulation dyscrasias (see Chapter 24), trauma or anticoagulant therapy), and synovitis provoked by entry of foreign material into the knee joint. In addition to primary synovial tumors, pulmonary osteoarthropathy associated with lung neoplasia and leukemias may result in synovitis.

REFERENCES

1. Bunch, T.W., and O'Duffy, J.D.: Disease-modifying drugs for progressive rheumatoid arthritis. Mayo Clin. Proc., *55(3)*: 161, 1980.
2. Hardin, J.A., Steere, A.C., and Malawista, S.E.: Immune complexes and the evolution of Lyme Arthritis: Dissemination and localization of abnormal Clq binding activity. N. Engl. J. Med., *301*: 1358, 1979.
3. Jayson, M.I.V., and Dixon, A.St.J.: Intra-articular pressure in rheumatoid arthritis of the knee. I. Pressure changes during passive joint distension. Ann. Rheum. Dis., *29*: 261, 1970.
4. Jayson, M.I.V., and Dixon, A.St.J.: Intra-articular pressure in rheumatoid arthritis of the knee. III. Pressure changes during joint use. Ann. Rheum. Dis., *29*: 401, 1970.
5. Lee, P., Rooney, P.J., Sturrock, R.D., et al.: The etiology and pathogenesis of osteoarthrosis: A review. Semin. Arthritis Rheum., *3*: 189, 1974.
6. McCarty, D.J., ed.: Conference on pseudogout and pyrophosphate metabolism. Arthritis Rheum., *19*: 275, 1976.
7. Moll, J.M.H., Haslock, I., Macrae, I.F., et al.: Asso-

ciations between ankylosing spondylitis, psoriatic arthritis, Reiter's disease, intestinal arthropathies and Behcet's syndrome. *Medicine, 53:* 343, 1974.

8. Schmid, F.R.: Bacterial arthritis. In McCarty, D.J., ed.: Arthritis and Allied Conditions (9th Ed.). Philadelphia, Lea & Febiger, p. 1363, 1979.
9. Simkin, P.A., and Pizzorno, J.E.: Transynovial exchange of small molecules in normal human subjects. J. Appl. Physiol., *36:* 381, 1974.
10. Wyngaarden, J.B., and Kelley, W.N.: Gout and Hyperuricemia. New York, Grune & Stratton, 1976.

BIBLIOGRAPHY

Katz, W.A., ed.: Rheumatic Diseases: Diagnosis and Management. J.B. Lippincott, Philadelphia, 1977.

Kelley, W.N., Harris, E.D., Jr., Ruddy, S., and Sledge, C.B., eds.: Textbook of Rheumatology, W.B. Saunders, Philadelphia, 1981.

McCarty, D.J., ed.: Arthritis and Allied Conditions, 9th Ed. Lea and Febiger, Philadelphia, 1979.

Scott, J.T., ed.: Copeman's Textbook of the Rheumatic Diseases, 5th Ed. Churchill Livingstone, Edinburgh, 1978.

17 Surgical Pathology of Arthritis

M.A.R. Freeman

The view of the surgical pathology in osteoarthritis (OA) and rheumatoid arthritis (RA) set out in this chapter is based on the author's clinical and operative observations. Although this presentation stands mostly on common ground, it is somewhat controversial, to be viewed as a working hypothesis requiring confirmation or refutation. This discussion is limited to my personal view for clarity of exposition, without reference to those generally accepted observations that can be found readily in the literature. I make no claim to originality.

INITIATION OF OA AND RA OF THE KNEE

Osteoarthritis of the knee as of other joints, is almost certainly attributable fundamentally to mechanical events. For example, a rise in the contact pressures applied to articular cartilage produced by meniscectomy or the malunion of tibial or femoral fractures (Fig. 17.1) may give rise to OA in the presumably overloaded compartment, but not initially elsewhere in the knee. The initial changes affect the cartilage, and it is at least probable that fragmentation of the collagen fiber network, caused by fatigue failure in the face of raised contact stresses, is the fundamental event.[5]

Changes in the bone subjacent to the cartilage are negligible until the cartilage is lost. They then appear to be caused by bone-to-bone contact and by the resultant mechanical disturbances (including abrasive wear and a rise in contact stresses) in the bone; certainly most changes in the bone can be explained on this basis,[4] and pain is not significant until bone is exposed in the articular surface. One bone alteration, osteophyte formation, represents an exception to this generalization, since osteophytes can form at the margin of intact surfaces (in knees displaying degenerative changes in other parts of the joint).

This view of the genesis of OA would suggest that abnormalities in the knee might be focal initially, affecting only those areas in which the contact stresses are increased. This expectation is confirmed on the gross scale by the frequent finding of macroscopically unicompartmental degenerative changes (Fig. 17.2); it has now been further shown that the unfibrillated cartilage in knees such as that shown in Figure 17.2 is for practical purposes, normal histologically and thus functionally.[1]

Thus in summary, OA may be viewed as a focal mechanical disorder that ends up destroying first the articular cartilage and thereafter the bone. Because the bone starts out in a normal state, its destruction begins slowly and is further retarded by reactive new bone formation.

Adult human articular chondrocytes do not appear to be capable of undergoing mitosis[14] (Chondrocyte cluster formation has been interpreted as evidence of chondrocyte mitosis, but in my view, clusters prob-

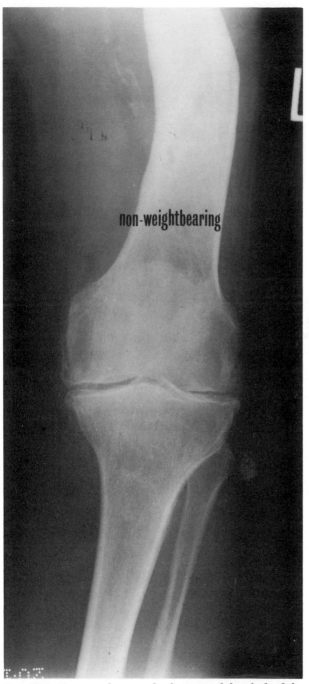

non-weightbearing

Fig. 17.1. Varus malunion of a fracture of the shaft of the femur with medial osteoarthrosis in the ipsilateral knee. It is tempting to suggest that the degenerative changes in this knee were produced by the medial shift in the resultant of the forces acting on the joint after the malunion.

ably arise from the loss of matrix between previously separated cells rather than from cell division.) Thus true healing of an articular cartilage defect cannot occur. Even an effective reactive cellular response to incipient destruction of the matrix seems unlikely, in view of the extreme slowness of collagen turnover in cartilage and the complexity of the organization of the fibers in this tissue.[9,11] Thus true healing of cartilage ulcers and the regression of fibrillation do not appear to be realistic therapeutic possibilities.

Although true healing cannot (and in my view, does not) occur, healing by scar formation is a possibility. As a consequence, exposed bone surfaces can be recovered by functionally useful fibrocartilage. This tissue, derived from granulation tissue reaching the exposed bone surface from the marrow spaces, first becomes loosely fibrous and then fibrocartilaginous in response to compression. This sequence implies that gaps in the bone surface are a prerequisite for this process and hence that a dense, sclerotic surface is unlikely to acquire soft tissue coverage. Equally, soft tissue coverage cannot be expected if the bone in question is constantly subjected to abrasive wear by the opposing condyle, since this must result in the destruction of any granulation tissue that reaches the surface. These facts imply that in order to achieve healing by fibrocartilage (i.e., by scar formation), two conditions must exist: (1) bone sclerosis must not be far advanced or, if it is, gaps in sclerotic surfaces must be made surgically; and (2) the high contact pressures originally responsible for cartilage destruction must be eliminated to preserve any granulation tissue reaching the surface. The first of these implications provides the rationale for surgical drilling of sclerotic surfaces and the second for osteotomy.

In contrast to OA, RA appears to be caused by the generalized destruction of cartilage by lysozymal enzymes, perhaps particularly collagenase derived from leukocytes. Because the cartilage is destroyed as part of a generalized enzymatic attack (much as it is in septic arthritis), its loss is also generalized. Cartilage that has been mechanically weakened by enzymatic attack will of course be more than usually susceptible to mechanical destruction. Thus the cartilage lesions in RA may be worse in some places than in others, although the cartilage is nowhere normal, that is, the lesions are both general (enzymatic) and focal (mechanical). This contrasts with the essentially focal nature of the lesions of OA.

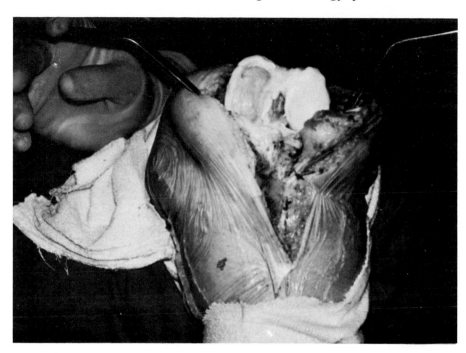

Fig. 17.2. Unicompartmental osteoarthrosis of the tibiofemoral joint. Recent work (see text) has demonstrated that if the cartilage in the intact compartment is not fibrillated, it is functionally normal.

Two other surgically relevant considerations follow from the generalized inflammatory nature of the cartilage destruction in RA: (1) destruction of cartilage, leading to bone exposure, might be expected to occur more rapidly in RA; and (2) cartilage healing by scar formation, which might conceivably be induced in OA, seems inconceivable in RA. Finally, the hyperemia in the joint, disuse, and even medicinal therapy produce osteoporosis; thus bone destruction, like cartilage destruction, is more rapid in RA.

The initial cause of the synovitis in RA is unknown, but it seems clear that its bad prognosis for the joint can be traced to the resultant enzymatic attack on the cartilage; a synovitis without this enzymatic attack, such as that which occurs in rheumatic fever, leaves the joint unscathed. Thus the prognosis for the joint in RA is similar to that in septic arthritis and unlike that in rheumatic fever because in both RA and septic arthritis, but not in rheumatic fever, leukocytes reach the joint cavity to produce generalized enzymatic destruction of the cartilage. Enzymatic attack might conceivably be prevented by synovectomy, but clinical experience shows that this procedure is at best unpredictably beneficial. In contrast to the uncertain effect that removal of the synovium has on the cartilage, the removal of the cartilage (by arthrodesis or total knee replacement) predictably aborts, indeed effectively cures the synovitis. This clinical observation suggests that the synovitis may be in some way attributable to the presence of cartilage in the joint, a speculation now strongly supported by experimental work, as reviewed by Cooke.[2]

In summary, RA appears to be caused by a generalized enzymatic attack on cartilage to which focal mechanical factors may be added. The destruction of both cartilage and bone is not only more generalized than in OA, but is also usually more rapid. Because any cartilage that remains in the joint is mechanically very abnormal, osteotomy is unlikely to be useful. Perhaps because residual cartilage is actually responsible for the synovitis in the first place,[2] the only surgical treatments that might, a priori, be expected to be successful are those involving the ablation of cartilage (i.e., arthrodesis and total joint replacement).

If this general view of the surgical pathology in OA and RA is correct, it should be possible to demonstrate the presence of bone and cartilage loss in the knee and to explain the various misalignments (e.g., varus and valgus) seen in the clinical setting on this basis. This description would constitute a rational, anatomic basis for such surgical procedures as osteotomy and knee replacement. Before considering the knee in this way, however, it is helpful to review briefly the presumably similar surgical pathology in

OA and RA of the hip, since this joint has been available for study for many years and the findings are now not a matter of controversy.

RELEVANT CHANGES IN THE HIP

Bone and Cartilage Loss.   In OA this change usually occurs superolaterally at the zenith of the femoral head and acetabulum, but it may occur medially. In the former situation, it accounts for the wandering acetabulum, for lateral subluxation, for a break in Shenton's line, and for true shortening of the leg. Measured by the latter, a loss of 2 cm of bone is not uncommon. Medial bone and cartilage loss leads to protrusio acetabulae, a change that occurs more commonly in RA than in OA. Just as in the hip, where bone loss may be predominantly lateral or medial, at the knee it will be shown that bone loss may also be predominantly medial or lateral. In this connection there is an interesting but ill-defined similarity between lateral bone loss at the hip (producing lateral subluxation of the femur) and medial bone loss at the knee (producing varus and lateral subluxation of the tibia). Both are common osteoarthrotic patterns in contrast to their opposites (protrusio at the hip and valgus at the knee), which occur mainly in RA. If the former is the result of some shared mechanical feature of the hip and knee, it may be speculated that the obliquity of the femoral shaft may have some bearing on the matter. Thus if the lower limb is thought of as a vertical pelvis, an oblique femur, and a vertical tibia, axial compression would tend to "squeeze" the upper end of the femur laterally and the lower end of the femur medially, thereby producing lateral tibial subluxation.

Soft Tissue Contracture.   This change affects particularly the muscles on the anterior and medial aspects of the hip, accounting for fixed flexion and fixed adduction. Of these, the most dramatic, well-known example is a contracture of the adductor muscles (especially of adductor longus), accounting for the persistence of an adduction deformity after hip replacement unless corrected by adductor tenotomy. Adhesions around ligaments may also maintain deformities.

Osteophyte Formation.   Osteophytes grow by endochondral ossification.[4] Thus osteophytosis occurs particularly in OA, where peripheral cartilage persists. In RA, the generalized loss of cartilage tends to prevent osteophyte formation. Osteophytes grow only in soft tissue spaces, the best example being the space created in the cavity of the hip inferomedial to the femoral head by bone loss at the zenith and lateral migration of the head. Although osteophytes may limit movement mechanically (and thus help to maintain deformity) it is difficult to conceive that their growth could actually produce deformity by pushing the bones into an abnormal position.

Ligamentous Elongation.   This alteration appears never to occur to any significant extent in the arthritic hip, even in RA. Hypermobility and dislocation, which would be expected if gross elongation did occur, are never seen.

Ligamentous Rupture.   This bone change affects only the intracapsular ligament in the hip (the ligamentum teres). Whether the ligament is destroyed by enzymatic digestion or by mechanical attrition is unclear. In RA both seem possible, whereas in OA the latter is more likely.

SUMMARY

At the hip, the processes responsible for the development and maintenance of deformity appear to be the loss of cartilage and bone occurring either laterally or medially and soft tissue adhesions and contractures (affecting ligaments and muscles, respectively). Ligamentous elongation either does not occur or does so only to a slight extent. Ligament rupture affects only intracapsular ligaments (the ligamentum teres) which can be exposed to mechanical attrition. Osteophytes grow by endochondral ossification into soft tissue spaces. They thus only appear where cartilage persists.

If bone loss and soft tissue contracture are the cause of deformity at the hip, and if significant ligamentous elongation does not occur at this joint, it would not be unreasonable to expect that the same would be true of the knee. This view is, however, controversial; valgus and varus instabilities in the arthritic knee have been attributed (presumably by analogy with similar instability after ligamentous injury) to elongated or defective medial and lateral collateral ligaments, respectively. However, although instability in the arthritic knee might theoretically be attributed to elongation, it is equally possible that instability might be caused by bone loss on the concave side of the joint, a view that would be consistent with the morbid anatomy of the arthritic hip. On this view, valgus or varus instability at the arthritic knee could be accounted for by postulating the presence of bone loss, and fixed valgus or varus deformity by postulating a combination of bone loss and soft tissue contracture.

The existence of these alternative pathologic explanations for valgus and varus is not simply of academic interest, since if these and other misalignments are to be reversed rationally, the nature of the underlying structural abnormalities must first be understood.

NATURE OF MORBID ANATOMIC CHANGES RESPONSIBLE FOR DEFORMITY OF THE KNEE IN OA AND RA

This topic is dealt with by considering first instability in a varus and valgus direction and then the same two malalignments, but with the addition of fixed deformity. Other abnormalities of alignment seen in the arthritic knee are then considered.

VARUS INSTABILITY

Theoretically, varus instability might be caused by (1) rupture and/or elongation of the lateral soft tissues (as after soft tissue trauma), or (2) a loss of bone medially, or both. Both pathologic processes would produce the same physical sign on the examination couch, that is, it would be possible to displace the tibia from neutral to varus alignment and back again. In contrast, if the knee were to be compressed axially (as on bearing weight or during muscular contraction), a knee with normal bones would tend to be stabilized in normal alignment, whereas a knee with bone loss would tend to be driven into the position of deformity (Fig. 17.3). It is a commonplace radiologic observation in the arthritic knee (1) that bone loss is present (Fig. 17.4), and (2) that the affected knee falls into a position of deformity on bearing weight (Fig. 17.5), hence the near-irrelevance of taking non-weight bearing x-ray films in the arthritic knee. It may be concluded—even without visual inspection of the articular surfaces of the knee—that bony defects are

responsible, at least in part if not wholly, for varus instability.

The possibility remains that lateral collateral ligament elongation or rupture may also play a part in the genesis of varus instability. I have never observed a frank rupture of the lateral collateral ligament and capsule at operation in uninjured knees. Although this finding does not exclude the possibility that this lesion occurs, it must mean that if it does occur, it is indeed rare.

Elongation of a collateral ligament (as against rupture) seems to be a more likely possibility, indeed, its existence is strongly suggested by radiographic appearances such as those shown in Figure 17.6. The question has to be asked, however, "What mechanism might be responsible for elongation (especially in OA, where damage to the ligament secondary to a prolonged synovitis or by collagenase—both conceivable in RA—seem very unlikely)?" A probable answer is that as the deformity on bearing weight increases, a point is reached at which the line of action of the resultant forces acting on the knee passes medial to the most medial point of bony contact in the joint. At or a little before this stage, the knee will tend to hinge open laterally, thus subjecting the lateral and midline soft tissues to persistent tension. Since it seems most unlikely that the collateral and cruciate ligaments are persistently subjected to tensile forces in the normal knee, the result may well be that the collateral ligament is overstressed. According to this analysis, ligamentous elongation might be expected to increase the malalignment in a knee that is already significantly malaligned as a consequence of bone loss, but not to initiate the malalignment.

That this is indeed the case may be demonstrated at operation by using a special surgical instrument known as a Tenser (Chapter 20). This instrument and its mode of action are illustrated in Figures 17.7 and 17.8. It will be seen that if a Tenser were to be used to tighten the two collateral ligaments in a varus knee that before operation had been unstable (i.e., fully correctable to neutral alignment passively), three possibilities would theoretically arise. First, if the lateral collateral ligament had elongated but not ruptured, the collateral ligaments would tighten to leave the knee in persistent varus (Fig. 17.8A). Second, if only a medial bone defect were present, the medial blade of the Tenser would open more than the lateral, but the two collateral ligaments would then tighten with

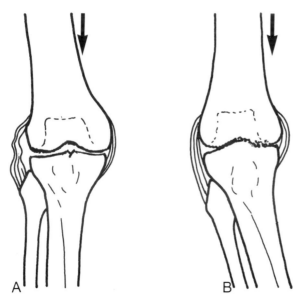

Fig. 17.3. (A) Diagram showing a knee without bone defects but with laxity of the lateral collateral ligament loaded in compression, as during one-leg stance. Because the line of action of the load on the knee passes through the area of contact between the femoral and tibial condyles, there is no tendency for the joint to open laterally; thus normal alignment is maintained. (B) Diagram showing a knee with a medial bone defect during one-leg stance. The load now acts to close the defect, causing the knee to buckle into varus malalignment. (From Freeman, M.A.R., ed.: Arthritis of the Knee. Springer-Verlag, Berlin-New York, 1980, with permission.)

the knee in anatomic alignment (Fig. 17.8B). Finally, if the lateral collateral ligament had ruptured, it would not be possible to tense it, so that the lateral compartment of the knee could be opened infinitely, turning the knee into ever-increasing varus (Fig. 17.8C). I have never observed the last of these possibilities. The first possible outcome has occurred suggesting elongation of the ligament on the convex side of the deformity. This happens mainly in OA and in RA. The usual outcome is the second.

It may be concluded that material elongation of the lateral collateral ligament is a late event and that rupture is rare or nonexistent. Thus varus instability in OA (and when it occurs, in RA) is initiated by medial bone loss. Simple trigonometry shows that, roughly speaking, 1 cm of medial bone and cartilage loss will result in 10 degrees of varus malalignment. Since 2 cm of tissue loss is commonplace at the hip, 13 degrees of varus (i.e., 20 degrees of deformity relative

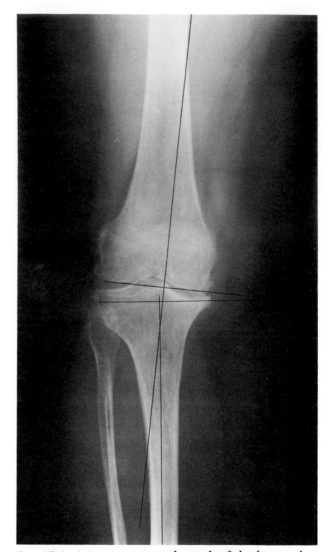

Fig. 17.4. Anteroposterior radiograph of the knee, taken with the patient supine. The vertical line over the tibia represents the tibial axis, that is, this line passes from the center of the knee to the center of the ankle. A horizontal line has been drawn perpendicular to this axis. Medially this line passes through the floor of the medial tibial defect. Laterally it passes approximately 1 cm below the lateral tibial condyle. Thus about 1 cm of bone has been lost medially. A second vertical line has been drawn to show the femoral axis. A line drawn perpendicular to this axis passes across the surface of both femoral condyles. Thus no bone has been lost from the femur. Note that the femoral and tibial axes are not parallel, that is, the knee is in varus. Since the knee is unloaded, this implies the presence of a medial soft tissue contracture.

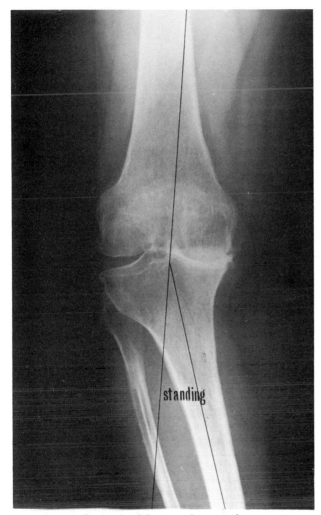

Fig. 17.5. Radiograph of the same knee as shown in Figure 17.4, now taken with the patient standing. Note that the femoral condyle has fallen into the tibial defect to increase the malalignment. Compare this x-ray film with the diagram shown in Figure 17.3B. (From Freeman, M.A.R., ed.: Arthritis of the Knee. Springer-Verlag. Berlin-New York, 1980, with permission.)

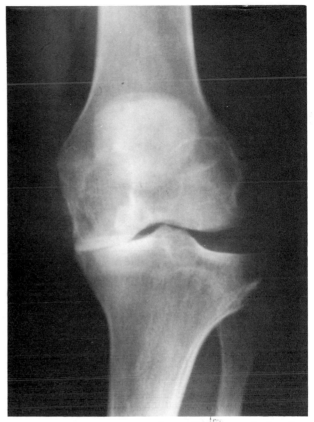

Fig. 17.6. Anteroposterior radiograph of a weight-bearing varus knee, showing the appearance of opening of the lateral compartment of the joint. This appearance suggests that the lateral collateral ligament has been elongated, perhaps as a consequence of tensile stresses developing in it secondary to the varus malalignment. Although the lateral compartment appears to have opened, the radiologic space between the lateral femoral and tibial condyles is in fact partly occupied by articular cartilage and meniscus. The actual elongation of the lateral collateral ligament is therefore less than it appears on this x-ray film. (From Freeman, M.A.R., ed.: Arthritis of the Knee. Springer-Verlag, Berlin-New York, 1980, with permission.)

to an initial 7 degrees valgus) might be a frequent finding at the knee.

The appearances produced by such bone loss in the tibial and femoral condyles of an OA varus knee are shown in Figure 17.9. In contrast to the usual femoral defect in a valgus knee, the femoral defect in the varus knee is typically small. This may perhaps be attributed to the fact that the bone of the distal femur is stronger than that of the tibia, and hence less likely to be crushed, whereas medial patellar subluxation,

leading to damage to the medial femoral condyle by the patella, occurs only rarely, if at all.

As bone is lost from the medial side of the joint, the intercondylar eminence of the tibia (1) moves upward relative to the femur, and (2) tilts (as the tibia as a whole tilts), so that its apex moves laterally (Fig. 17.10). The combined effect of these two displacements is to produce impingement within the knee between the normally nonarticular central parts of the femur and tibia. By analogy with such abnormal bony

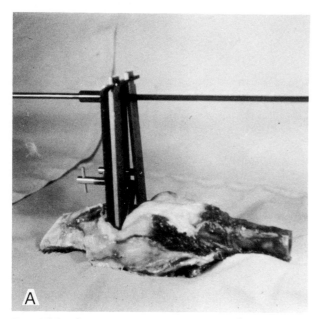

Fig. 17.7. The Tenser, an instrument used in ICLH arthroplasty of the knee, with which the presence or absence of soft tissue contractures can be demonstrated at operation. Before insertion of this instrument, the cruciate ligaments are divided, and the tibial plateau is sectioned at right angles to the anatomic axis of the bone. The instrument is used in the extended knee (A) to separate first one and then the other femoral condyle from the tibia, thereby tensing the medial and lateral soft tissues in turn. A bar passes through the tibial plate at right angles to the latter. The distal end of this bar must lie over the center of the ankle. The proximal end of the bar will lie over the hip when the soft tissues are tensed only when there is neither contracture nor elongation of these tissues on either side of the joint (B). Thus by tensing the tissues and noting the relationship of the proximal end of the bar to the hip, the surgeon can judge the presence and magnitude of soft tissue contracture or elongation.

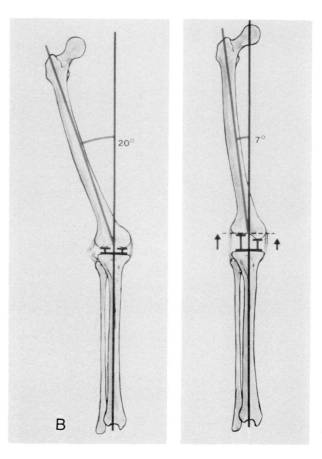

contact elsewhere (e.g., between the fibula and os calcis), this process might be expected to be painful and to lead gradually to the formation of a false midline joint in the knee. The latter does indeed occur, so that the knee comes to transmit load medially and centrally, but not laterally (Fig. 17.10).

The formation of a false midline joint in OA is encouraged by the formation of osteophytes at the margins of the femoral intercondylar notch. Such osteophytes are possibly formed by a crushing of the articular margins of the notch, rather than by endochondral ossification, the process by which osteophytes nor-

mally grow (see above). Whatever their origin, the osteophytes on the medial and lateral edges of the notch eventually fuse to bury the cruciate ligaments and produce a continuous, false, central articular surface. Progressive destruction of the weight-bearing medial and central areas of the knee may eventually reestablish weight-bearing contact between the lateral condyles so that finally the lateral surface also become eburnated to produce a "switch-back knee."

VALGUS INSTABILITY

All the arguments and observations applied above to varus instability apply to valgus instability as well, save that the bony defects are now lateral and the soft tissue defects are medial. Such bony defects are illustrated in a RA knee in Figure 17.11. It should be noted that the tibial defect involves particularly the posterior three-quarters of the condyle, the anterior margin being relatively spared (Fig. 17.11C). This

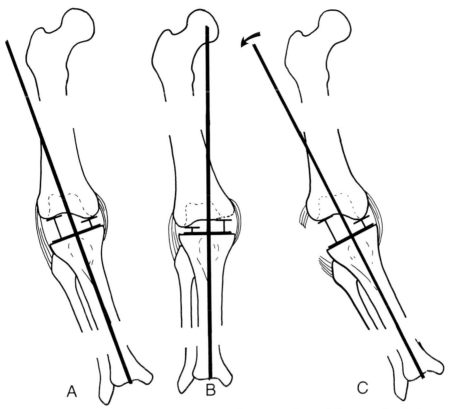

Fig. 17.8. Diagrams illustrating the detection of soft tissue elongation, bone defects, and soft tissue rupture. (A) The Tenser in place, with its blades opened, in a knee having no bone defect, but an elongated lateral collateral ligament (such as that shown in Figure 17.3A). The blades of the Tenser could be opened more widely in the lateral compartment than in the medial compartment of the knee, turning the joint into varus. (B) The Tenser in place, with its blades opened, in a joint having preoperatively a medial tibial and femoral defect (such as that shown in Figure 17.3B), but no soft tissue contracture. The blades can now be opened more widely on the medial than on the lateral side of the joint. When the medial and lateral soft tissues are equally tense, this knee will lie in normal alignment. (C) The Tenser in place, with its blades opened, in a knee having preoperatively a ruptured lateral collateral ligament. In such a knee the lateral blade could theoretically be opened infinitely, turning the knee into progressively increasing varus.

may be attributed to the fact that the femur does not articulate with, and thus will not mechanically damage, the anterior part of the tibial condyle. The lateral femoral condyle is often more grossly destroyed than the lateral tibial plateau (Fig. 17.11B) an observation that may be attributed to the fact that it is exposed to damage, not only from the tibia, but from the laterally subluxated patella as well. Lateral patellar subluxation is often present in such knees; its cause and consequences are discussed under lateral patellar subluxation below.

As with varus instability, it may be concluded that valgus instability is initially caused by bone loss laterally and that this loss can be explained mainly on

simple mechanical grounds. Using the Tenser, my experience has been the same as in knees displaying varus instability. This suggests that elongation of the medial collateral ligament is a late secondary event.

FIXED VARUS DEFORMITY

Theoretically, a fixed varus deformity could be attributable only to one of two possible events: (1) ligamentous elongation laterally combined with growth of the lateral condyles, or (2) collapse of the bone medially combined with contracture of the medial soft tissues (Fig. 17.12). The former seems inconceivable:

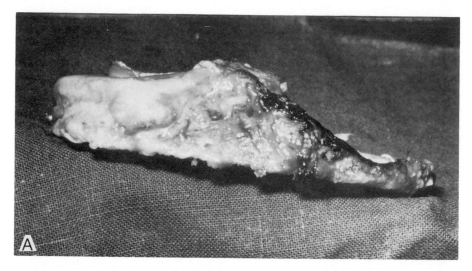

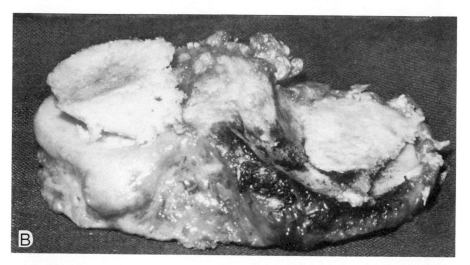

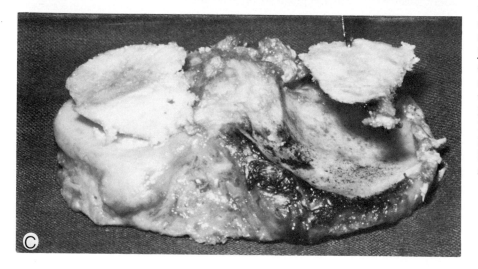

Fig. 17.9. Surgical specimens taken from the knee shown in Figures 17.4 and 17.5. (A) Frontal appearance of the bone removed from the tibia. Note that more bone has been removed laterally than medially, because of the pathologic loss of bone from the medial tibial condyle. The anterior edge of the tibia has been stained with methylene blue. (B) The fragments of bone resected from the distal aspects of the femoral condyles have now been added to the tibial specimen shown in A. The distal femoral condyles have been sectioned at right angles to the mechanical (hip, knee, ankle) axis of the femoral shaft. Here the medial femoral and tibial condyles are in contact, that is, the pathologic specimen is in the position shown in Figure 17.5. (C) Same specimen shown in B. The medial femoral bone fragment has now been lifted to place it on the same horizontal level as the lateral femoral fragment, that is, the specimen is now in an anatomic position, creating a space on the medial side of the joint due to the loss of about 1 cm of bone and cartilage. Closure of this defect creates the varus malalignment shown in Figure 17.5. (From Freeman, M.A.R., ed.: Arthritis of the Knee. Springer-Verlag, Berlin-New York, 1980, with permission.)

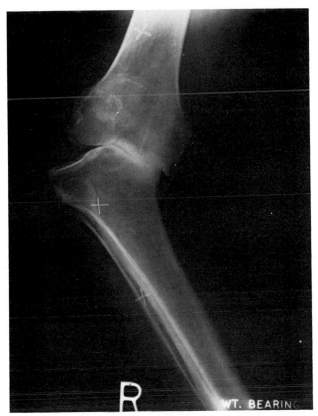

Fig. 17.10. Anteroposterior radiograph of a weight-bearing knee in varus showing contact between the intercondylar eminence of the tibia and the midline of the femur, resulting in load-carriage medially and centrally but not laterally. Note that the areas of bone-carrying load are relatively sclerotic and that the tibial intercondylar eminence has tilted laterally so as to contact the lateral femoral condyle (see also Figure 17.6). Both this knee and that shown in Figure 17.6 appear to display lateral tibial subluxation, but in the latter the medial side of the medial femoral and tibial condyles are in line, whereas here they are not, partly because the medial flare of the tibial condyle has been destroyed. On the lateral side of the joint, the lateral tibial condyle projects beyond the lateral femoral condyle and the lateral collateral ligament and capsule are elongated.

growth (as distinct from marginal and intracartilaginous surface osteophytosis) of the condyles is seen neither in RA nor in OA. In contrast, contractures (e.g., at the hip causing fixed adduction, and at the knee causing fixed flexion), are a common finding. It may be concluded that contracture formation, not growth, is at work, a conclusion that reinforces the view put forward earlier that instability is caused as much by bone loss as by soft tissue elongation.

It remains to consider the nature of the contractures that may be responsible. Surgeons will be familiar with the concept of a contracture at the hip, as already discussed. Although such lesions are clinically commonplace, the precise nature of the pathologic events responsible for them is unclear; presumably they arise from a mixture of shortening and fibrosis in muscles and adhesion formation around muscles and ligaments. Whatever their precise pathologic nature, it is now suggested that similar contractures occur in the arthritic knee (and indeed in all arthritic joints) and that they are responsible for the maintenance of fixed tibiofemoral deformities in varus, valgus, flexion, and external rotation, for fixed lateral tibial and patellar subluxation, and in part for an inability to flex the knee fully.

In fixed varus deformity, the presence of such contractures can easily be demonstrated at operation. With the Tenser in place and the condyles fully separated in such a knee, a varus deformity persists and the contracted tissues can be felt and seen to be tight. These tissues include the medial collateral ligament, the medial half of the posterior capsule, and the muscles crossing the medial side of the knee (the cruciate ligaments may also be involved, but they have been resected by the time the Tenser is inserted). In addition, medial osteophytes may tent the medial collateral ligament and hence contribute to the maintenance of deformity by effectively shortening this ligament. The contracted structures are more easily displayed on the lateral side.

FIXED VALGUS DEFORMITY

This deformity is maintained by lateral contractures that affect most obviously the muscles inserted into the iliotibial tract and the biceps. If the tract and the tendinous part of the biceps are divided, their cut ends spring apart (Fig. 17.13) to permit separation of the lateral femoral and tibial condyles with consequent correction of the valgus deformity. In addition to the contractures mentioned above, a fixed valgus deformity may be maintained by adhesions (contractures) between the lateral femoral condyle on the one hand and the posterior capsule and lateral ligament on the other. Contracture of, or adhesions around,

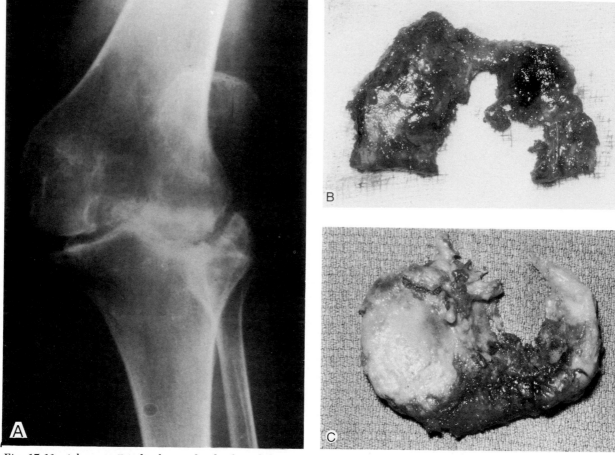

Fig. 17.11. A knee in RA displaying fixed valgus deformity. (A) An anteroposterior radiograph of the non-weight-bearing knee. The valgus deformity is caused by femoral and tibial defects. It persists in the non-weight-bearing knee because it is held, whether the knee is weight-bearing or not, by the presence of a lateral soft tissue contracture. Note the lateral subluxation of the patella. (B) Surgical specimen removed from the distal femur shown in A by resection of the bone at 83 degrees to the long axis of the femoral shaft (i.e., at 90 degrees to the mechanical axis of the femur). On the lateral side (right), little or no bone has been removed because of the preexisting defect. (C) Specimen removed from the tibia by transecting it at right angles to the axis of the shaft. Note that once again little or no bone has been removed from the lateral side. Note that the tibial and the femoral defects are mainly posterior. (Parts B and C from Freeman, M.A.R., ed.: Arthritis of the Knee. Springer-Verlag, Berlin-New York, 1980, with permission.)

the cruciate ligaments may also prevent full correction of the deformity. It should be appreciated that both in valgus and in varus, the extent of the contracture may be less than that of the bone loss: such a knee will display some degree of instability superimposed on an element of fixed deformity. Only the latter is caused by contracture, whereas the bone defect underlies both the instability and the fixed deformity.

FIXED FLEXION

The position of comfort in the knee (i.e., the position of maximum intrasynovial volume) is one of about 15 degrees of flexion. If pain prevents the knee from being voluntarily extended beyond this point, contractures (in this case probably caused chiefly by adhesion formation) involving the posterior capsule (becoming adherent both to itself and to the posterior

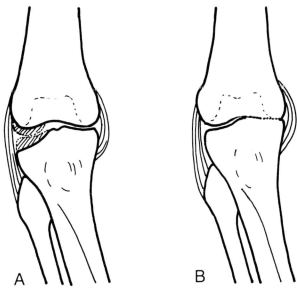

Fig. 17.12. Diagrams showing two mechanisms that might theoretically produce a fixed varus deformity. (A) The varus deformity has been produced by growth of the lateral femoral and tibial condyles combined with elongation of the lateral collateral ligament, which would seem impossible. (B) The fixed deformity has been produced by a medial tibial defect similar to that shown in Figures 17.3, 17.4, 17.5, and 17.9, combined with a medial soft tissue contracture. This seems likely in reality.

femoral condyles), the hamstring muscles, and to a lesser extent the cruciate ligaments may develop and physically prevent full extension. Weight-bearing on the flexed knee then loads the distal and posterior femoral condyles, where they articulate with the posterior half of the tibial condyles at loads significantly greater than those borne by the weight-bearing extended knee.[13] If, as commonly happens in RA, the loaded bone collapses, the femur in effect sinks downward into the posterior part of the tibial condyles until the tibial intercondylar eminence comes to abut against the roof of the femoral intercondylar notch (Fig. 17.10). Eventually a groove is formed running across the anterodistal aspect of the femoral condyles into which the anterior margin of the tibia locks as the knee is extended (Fig. 17.14). Both bony impingements prevent extension. Midline impingement may cause an attrition rupture of the anterior cruciate ligament—especially in RA when the ligament may be weakened enzymatically and is rarely protected by osteophytes.

Such ruptures might be considered analogous to ruptures of the ligamentum teres at the hip.

LOSS OF FLEXION

This abnormality is simply the reverse of a flexion deformity, although it is not usually thought of as such. Viewed in this light, however, it may be regarded as being caused by (1) a contracture of the quadriceps muscle and cruciate ligaments, and (2) adhesions between the collateral ligaments and the sides of the femoral condyles, and perhaps by (3) posterior osteophytosis.

LATERAL SUBLUXATION OF THE PATELLA

This problem is seen particularly in valgus externally rotated RA knees and is presumably caused by the action of the quadriceps muscle, which must have a tendency to pull the patella laterally if the knee is in valgus with external rotation of the tibia (Fig. 17.15). It is permitted by bone loss (as are valgus and varus tibiofemoral deformities), in this case bone being lost from the anterolateral femoral condyle and from the patella (Fig. 17.16). In my experience, the deformity is usually fixed, as the lateral patellar retinaculum becomes contracted.

EXTERNAL ROTATION OF THE TIBIA

This deformity is usually seen in RA valgus knees in women and is most obvious in the flexed, rather than the extended, joint. There appear to be three possible sources for a deforming external rotation force; the laterally subluxed extensor mechanism, tensor fasciae lata and gluteus maximus acting via the iliotibial tract, and the biceps muscle. It seems possible that this external rotation thrust is exacerbated by a loss of the internal rotator power of the popliteus muscle, since (in my experience) the intra-articular tendon of this muscle is usually absent from the rheumatoid (but not from the osteoarthrotic) knee. The tendon is presumably ruptured by being ground between the collapsing lateral femoral and tibial condyles. (So-called posterior ruptures of the knee are probably in fact caused

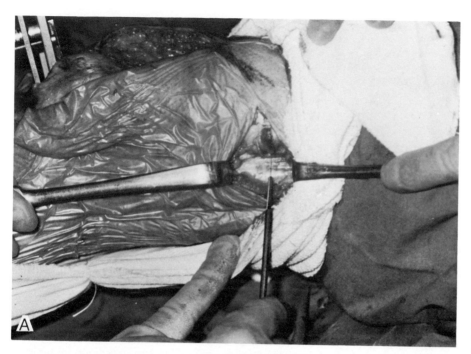

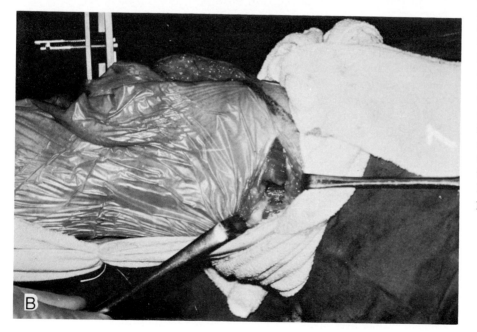

Fig. 17.13. (A) Lateral view of a knee with fixed valgus deformity during operation. The iliotibial tract is about to be divided. At this stage of the operation, the medial and lateral soft tissues had been tensed, but even so the knee lay in valgus. This implies the presence of a lateral soft tissue contracture. (B) The iliotibial tract has now been incised, and the lateral blades of the Tenser (top left) have been opened further, separating the lateral tibial and femoral condyles and correcting the valgus deformity. This has caused the cut edges of the iliotibial tract to separate (the proximal edge not seen here). A contracture of the iliotibial tract (perhaps involving particularly the tensor fascia lata muscle) was mainly responsible for the fixed valgus malalignment in this knee. (From Freeman, M.A.R., ed.: Arthritis of the Knee. Springer-Verlag, Berlin-New York, 1980, with permission.)

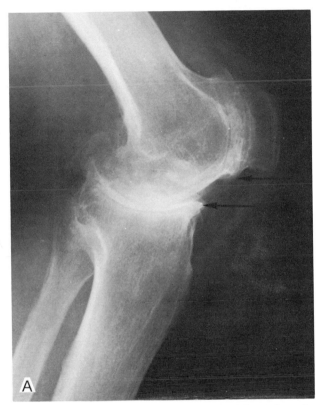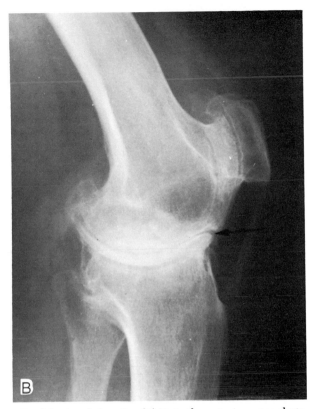

Fig. 17.14. Lateral radiographs of an osteoarthritic knee having a fixed flexion deformity. (A) Note the anterior osteophyte on the tibia (arrow). (B) A groove is seen on the distal end of the femur (arrow) in the slightly flexed knee; the tibial osteophyte and the femoral groove contact each other (arrow) to limit extension.

by the discharge of synovial contents through the hole in the posterior capsule left by the retraction of this tendon from the joint rather than by a rupture of the capsule. The capsule itself is very strong and is never found to be ruptured at operation. Arthrographically, the synovial leak in posterior ruptures is lateral, that is, it corresponds in position to the point of exit of the popliteus tendon.)

Such unbalanced external rotation forces would themselves be capable of rotating the tibia only to its normal extreme, but not beyond. In my view, the hyperexternal rotation that occurs in these knees is permitted by the lateral tibial and femoral bone loss that occurs in the valgus knee, since this will effectively relax posterior cruciate control over the lateral, but not over the medial compartment of the knee. As a consequence, the equivalent of a posterior drawer sign can occur laterally but not medially; that is, the lateral, but not the medial, tibial condyle is free to

sublux posteriorly. Thus the tibia rotates externally. Once rotated, the same contractures that maintain fixed valgus in the extended knee (i.e., contractures of the iliotibial tract and of the biceps) will maintain fixed external rotation in the flexed knee. Finally, the whole circumference of the tibia may become adherent to the capsule in its new position of external rotation.

HYPEREXTENSION

This condition is usually seen in knees displaying fixed valgus deformities (i.e., in knees with contractures of the iliotibial tract) (Fig. 17.17). For the first 5 to 10 degrees of flexion, the iliotibial tract passes in front of the axis of rotation of the knee, acting as an extensor. Its contracture in the absence of a fixed flexion deformity may therefore lead to hyperexten-

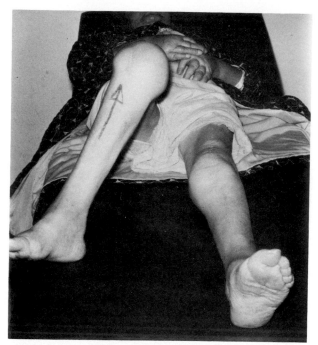

Fig. 17.15. Right knee (arrow) in RA, showing valgus, external rotation, and lateral subluxation of the patella in the flexed knee. (From Freeman, M.A.R., ed.: Arthritis of the Knee. Springer-Verlag, Berlin-New York, 1980, with permission.)

sion. The tendency for this deformity to develop should theoretically be exacerbated by bone loss from both sides of the knee, since this would loosen all those ligaments lying behind the axis of tibiofemoral rotation, normally preventing hyperextension. If, as is frequently the case in the rheumatoid knee, the anterior cruciate ligament has been ruptured, its contribution to the limitation of extension will be also lost.

THE STABLE NEUTRAL KNEE

From what has been said above, it can be seen that a stable arthritic knee in neutral alignment might be attributable either to the absence of both bone loss and soft tissue abnormality or paradoxically to the presence of symmetrical bone loss (medially and laterally) and soft tissue contracture (medially and laterally).

THE LOOSE KNEE

In such knees, which are rare, there is both medial and lateral bone loss without soft tissue contracture. Alternatively, and theoretically, both collateral liga-

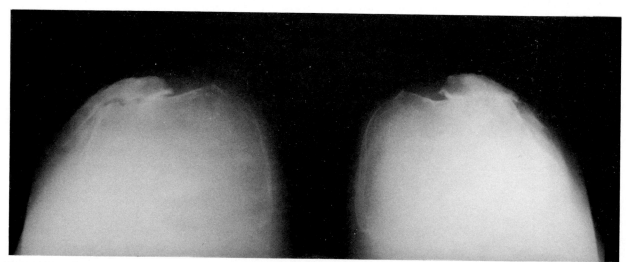

Fig. 17.16. Skyline radiograph of the knee shown in Figure 17.15. Note the lateral subluxation of the patella permitted by destruction of the patella itself and of the lateral femoral condyle (see also Fig. 17.11A). It will be recalled that the anterior prominence of the lateral femoral condyle is normally greater than that of the medial femoral condyle, the reverse of the situation seen in this knee. (From Freeman, M.A.R., ed.: Arthritis of the Knee. Springer-Verlag, Berlin-New York, 1980, with permission.)

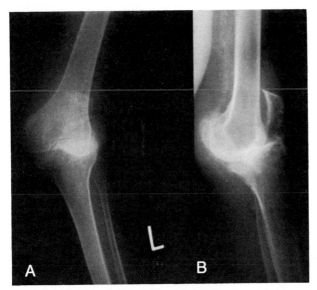

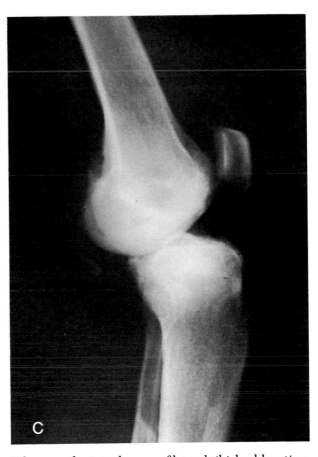

Fig. 17.17. (A,B) Knee in RA, showing hyperextension and valgus malalignment, the latter being fixed. (C) Similar anterior subluxation in OA. In both knees, the anterior cruciate ligament was found to be ruptured at operation. Hyperextension appears to be caused by a contracture of the iliotibial tract in the absence of fixed flexion (see text). Such a contracture must have been present in the knee illustrated in (B) because of (1) the presence of a fixed valgus deformity, and (2) at operation the use of the Tensor demonstrated the contracture. (From Freeman, M.A.R., ed.: Arthritis of the Knee. Springer-Verlag, Berlin-New York, 1980, with permission.)

ments might elongate. They are, however, never absent; all knees of this kind that I have treated could be stabilized in neutral alignment with the Tensor.

LATERAL SUBLUXATION OF THE TIBIA

Although lateral subluxation of the tibia, usually combined with varus, is a well-recognized clinical entity (see Figs 17.6 and 17.10), it is not clear why in some, but not in all, knees the tibia tends to shift laterally on the femur as the loss of medial cartilage and bone turns the knee into varus. Indeed to some extent the appearance of lateral subluxation may be illusory (Fig. 17.10). Perhaps in such knees, before the onset of degenerative changes, the long axis of the tibia intersects that of the femur not in the plane of the knee but further proximally, that is, perhaps the tibia is congenitally somewhat laterally placed in these knees.

Whatever the initial cause of lateral tibial subluxation, it is permitted (as are all other abnormalities of alignment) by bone and cartilage loss—in this case from the tibial intercondylar eminence or the medial side of the lateral femoral condyle, or both. A contracture of the popliteus muscle, running from the tibia medially to the femur laterally, then holds the tibia laterally. In support of the view that a popliteus contracture is responsible, division of the popliteus tendon in knees displaying lateral tibial subluxation eliminates the tendency, otherwise seen after replacement of the surfaces with an unconstrained prosthesis, for the tibia to move laterally relative to the femur as the knee nears full extension.

A connection exists between subluxation of the patella and of the tibia. Both occur in a lateral direction, and they might be causally connected since the extensor mechanism must be carried laterally with the tibia. Thus, at least in theory, a vicious regress may be initiated in the following manner. The tibia subluxes laterally carrying the patella with it. The resulting increased lateral thrust in the patellofemoral joint promotes the destruction of the anterior aspect of the lateral femoral condyle and of the patella, thereby allowing the patella to sublux even further laterally. Once the patella has moved laterally, quadriceps activity must tend to pull the tibia laterally. If such a knee already has a medial tibiofemoral defect (as a consequence of which it is in varus), this lateral patellar pull would displace the proximal tibia bodily laterally, rather than turning the bone into valgus, that is, there would be increasing lateral subluxation of the tibia in a varus knee.

It is perhaps significant in this context that the tibia, for practical purposes, always subluxes laterally, not medially, and that both the commonly occurring bone defects (a medial defect in the tibia and a lateral defect in the femur) produce a joint line that slopes upward and laterally, an abnormality that might lead to lateral tibial subluxation.

CONCLUSIONS

The fundamental pathologic event, on the gross scale, in the knee in OA and RA is the destruction first of cartilage and then of bone. If, as is usual, this happens asymmetrically, it manifests itself as malalignment, with lateral tibiofemoral defects causing valgus, medial tibiofemoral defects causing varus, and lateral patellofemoral defects causing lateral patellar subluxation.

When the tibiofemoral or patellofemoral joints become malaligned, the lines of action of the forces acting on both joints are altered—unfortunately in such a way as to increase the forces acting on the destroyed area of the knee. As a consequence, bone destruction tends to be progressive.

The most important pathologic process in muscle–tendon units is contracture formation; in ligaments it is adhesion formation. Such contractures and adhesions hold the bones in a position of deformity. They also limit movement.

The ligaments of the knee are rarely, if ever, destroyed in arthritis, the only exception to this being the anterior cruciate ligament, which is sometimes destroyed by attrition between the tibia and femur in RA. The collateral ligament on the convex side of a valgus or varus deformity may stretch if the deformity

is sufficient to generate tensile forces on its convex side. Such elongation is late and secondary to the bone defect.

PROGRESSION OF THE PATHOLOGY

In OA the mechanism by which the pathology becomes progressively worse seems clear; that is, the forces that initiated the cartilage and bone damage in the first place continue to act and thus accentuate the defect. Indeed a vicious circle is established because not only does the force accentuate the defect, but the defect accentuates the force. Thus, for example, a varus position produced by a medial defect has the effect of moving the resultant of the forces acting on the knee medially, thereby increasing the force acting on the defect. Similarly, a flexion deformity in excess of 10 degrees increases the magnitude of the tibiofemoral compressive forces.[13]

Since this force always acts in the flexed knee, the more posterior parts of the tibial condyles are affected (since the femur articulates posteriorly with the tibia in flexion), whereas the anterior tibia is spared. As a result, the femur sinks into the posterior two-thirds of the tibial condyles leaving the anterior margin of the tibia as an upwardly projecting ridge that strikes the femur as the knee extends. Thus, by a vicious circle similar to that affecting the varus knee, the forces perpetuate and accentuate fixed flexion deformity.

Although precisely similar considerations as those applying to the varus knee might be thought to apply to the valgus knee, gait analysis suggests that contrary to theoretical expectations, the resultant is not always shifted laterally.[6] Possibly, this is because patients can compensate better for a valgus deformity (by altering the placement of their feet as they walk) than they can for a varus deformity.

Misalignment of the patella must of course affect the tibiofemoral joint force. Thus lateral patellar subluxation, which often accompanies tibiofemoral valgus, can be expected to shift the line of action of the quadriceps muscle (and thus the resultant of the tibiofemoral forces) laterally in extension. In flexion, the same lateral patellar subluxation will lead to tibial external rotation to produce the complex deformity of valgus, lateral patellar subluxation, external rotation in flexion, and often fixed flexion.

In RA, all the same mechanical considerations apply, but in addition it is widely thought that an active synovitis, attributable to some fundamental but unknown causative agent, is at work. In my own (admittedly speculative) view, such a primary synovitis continues only as long as cartilage remains in the joint, since it seems to be this tissue that provokes the synovial reaction.[13] This perhaps explains the fact that, once the cartilage is entirely lost, the rheumatoid synovitis may burn itself out. It may also explain the clinical observation that a synovitis may recur after a synovectomy (because cartilage persists), but rarely after a total replacement (because cartilage is then absent from the joint). There is, however, another possible cause for an active synovitis in RA, and indeed to a lesser extent in OA. This is the continuous release of bone and cartilaginous debris into the synovial cavity. According to this argument, the synovitis in RA would merely be viewed as a more violent variety of that occurring, for example, in the presence of a torn meniscus and might be thought to be more florid in RA than in OA because enzymatic attack and osteoporosis (and hence the rate of bone and cartilage destruction) is greater in the former. This synovitis, like the disturbance of joint forces, could be seen as being secondary to the bone defects, not the cause of them.

There is another feature of the arthritic knee that may appropriately be considered here. This feature concerns the magnitude and duration of action of major forces in the joint as contrasted with those in the hip. As regards the magnitude of such forces, gait analysis studies and static analysis suggest (but do not prove, since no direct measurements are available) that peak forces in everyday activities, such as walking, are greater in the hip than in the tibiofemoral joint. For example, in the hip, Paul[12] finds the maximum force to be about five times the body weight during level walking, and Morrison in the same laboratory finds the peak tibiofemoral force to be about three times body weight.[10]

The patellofemoral force may equal or even exceed that in the tibiofemoral joint but only on activities such as unsupported squatting; generally, it is lower.

Not only are the peak forces on activity lower in the knee, there is also evidence that true off-loading is possible in this joint. Thus at the tibiofemoral joint it is well known that the damaged surfaces of the tibia and femur can be seen to separate on an x-ray film when the patient lies down, hence the need to take radiographs of this joint during weight-bearing if it is to be fully assessed clinically. At the hip no such separation occurs. This radiologic fact probably accounts for the well-known clinical observation that night pain is an important clinical feature in arthritis of the hip, but not of the knee, since in the latter the structures responsible for the pain (i.e., the exposed bone surfaces) can be off-loaded at night.

That the forces in the knee are probably smaller in magnitude and more intermittent in action than in the hip may account for the generally slower evolution and relatively less severe pain in OA of the knee than of the hip. That the tibiofemoral joint can be unloaded when the patient lies down probably accounts for the rarity of significant night pain in OA of the knee as compared with its frequency at the hip. In RA, the much greater area of cartilage in the knee and the fact that because the joint is more peripheral its cartilage is more permeable,[8] probably account for the increased incidence of rheumatoid synovitis in the knee as compared with the hip.

IMPLICATIONS FOR TREATMENT

From what has been said above it seems unlikely that a conservative form of treatment for OA will ever be found. Other than instructing the patient to reduce body weight, moderate activities, and use a stick, nothing can be done to alter the forces acting on the knee. Once cartilage has been damaged, the inability of the chondrocyte to undergo mitosis makes it as unlikely that new cartilage can be induced pharmacologically as it is that new brain tissue (i.e., new neurons) can be induced after a cerebrovascular accident (CVA). Analgesics can, of course, relieve pain, and I believe there is no convincing evidence that the so-called anti-inflammatory agents have any action whatsoever except insofar as they have analgesic properties. There remains the possibility of surgery.

Osteotomies could be expected to move the line of action of the resultant of the forces acting on the tibiofemoral joint, but not to alter its magnitude. From what has been said above, it would seem reasonable to expect that to off-load a defect, say in the medial tibial condyle, in this way might enable fibrocartilage to form on the exposed bone surface (provided that this is not too densely sclerotic, when additional drilling might be helpful). Such an osteotomy might be expected to be more predictably beneficial for a medial defect causing varus than for a valgus knee since recent gait analysis studies[6] (referred to above) show that in the former the resultant force is always displaced medially when the patient walks, whereas in the latter its line of action is not always displaced laterally. This theoretical expectation conforms with clinical experience.

Theoretically, however, and indeed in practice, osteotomy would seem to have limitations. First, it will do nothing for lateral tibial subluxation nor for instability unless, in the case of the latter, contractures happen to form postoperatively to stabilize the joint. Second, overcorrection might induce degenerative changes in the opposite compartment, whereas undercorrection will fail to solve the problem in the damaged compartment. A priori it seems impossible to guarantee the achievement of the perfect alignment (whatever that may be), especially when it is borne in mind that some collapse may occur at any loaded fracture site, that is, at the osteotomy as it unites, thereby altering the alignment produced at operation. The symptomatic unpredictability of this procedure may be attributable to the fact that pain relief probably depends on off-loading the damaged compartment enough to permit formation of fibrocartilage, while taking care not to overload the opposite side, a difficult compromise to achieve.

At the patellofemoral joint, the theory behind the Maquet procedure[7] is sound, but in practice the cosmetic and wound-healing problems associated with this operation may represent unacceptable disadvantages.

Thus, in theory, as in practice, osteotomy might be expected to be most useful for the early varus knee, for which it is the tibia that should be angulated, since the defect is tibial. Such an operation might theoretically be expected to produce healing by the formation of functionally useful fibrocartilaginous scars on the surfaces of the exposed bones, provided these are not too sclerotic; indeed, there is now arthroscopic evidence that this does happen.[3]

Apart from fibrocartilage formation, the only way in which exposed bone surfaces can be recovered with insensitive material so as to relieve pain is by the use of implants. If such an implant and the subjacent bone on which it rests are not to be destroyed by the same forces as those originally producing the defect, the height of the implants must be adjusted so as to re-

align the limb perfectly. In a knee with a contracture, the requisite space for the implant cannot be obtained until the contractures have been surgically reversed. Since these objectives can now be achieved technically, there is, theoretically at least, a prospect that properly executed replacement—either total or unicompartmental—can restore the function of an osteoarthrotic knee in the same way that properly executed dentistry can restore the function of a carious tooth.

In RA it seems unlikely that anything useful would be gained from transferring load from one compartment to another, since the loss of cartilage is generalized. Thus osteotomy seems unlikely to be helpful in RA. In contrast, synovectomy might at first sight have something to offer. But in practice, synovectomy has not proved reliably beneficial. This outcome would be expected on the basis of the views set out above, which imply that the synovitis in RA is secondary—either, early in the disease, to an immune mechanism involving cartilage, or later to detritus. Neither of these primary events will be affected by synovectomy. Indeed, according to this analysis, this operation appears to be directed against a consequence of the fundamental pathology, not against the fundamental pathology itself.

Therefore, as in OA, replacement seems to offer the only serious prospect of surgical relief—and for the same reasons, namely, exposed bone surfaces are covered and the joint realigned. Two points are of special relevance to RA, however. First, unicompartmental replacement, which might, at least theoretically, be useful in those cases of OA in which the cartilage in the apparently uninvolved tibiofemoral compartment is now known to be essentially normal, can have no place in RA in which none of the cartilage is normal. Second, if the synovitis in RA represented a primary pathologic process, it should continue after the joint surfaces have been replaced so as eventually to loosen the prosthesis and once again destroy the joint. Replacement in these circumstances would be futile. In practice, the synovitis in RA remits after resurfacing, and I have not thus far seen a recurrent rheumatoid flare in a satisfactorily replaced joint. This observation is easy to understand, indeed it is predictable, if it is accepted that the two causes of synovitis in RA are an autoimmune response to cartilage and the release of detritus, since total resurfacing removes both cartilage and debris from the joint. Thus not only does total replacement control the local symptoms of RA, it "cures" the disease in that joint. Since conservative measures for RA are today (1983) at best only marginally effective in the present state of the art, I believe that surgery represents the only fundamentally effective treatment available for this disease of the knee.

REFERENCES

1. Brocklehurst, R., Hill, M.V., Bayliss, M., et al.: Biochemical studies of femoral condyle cartilage removed at operation for total knee replacement. In preparation.
2. Cooke, T.D.V.: How does the mechanism of cartilage destruction influence surgical management of the rheumatoid joint? J. Rheumatol. 7: 119, 1980.
3. Fujisawa, Y., Masuhara, K., Matsumoto, N., et al.: The effect of high tibial osteotomy on osteoarthritis of the knee. An arthroscopic study. Clin. Orthop. Surg. *11*: 576, 1976.
4. Freeman, M.A.R.: The pathogenesis of primary osteoarthrosis: An hypothesis. p. 40. In Apley, A.G. (Ed.): Modern Trends in Orthopaedics, Vol. 6. London, Butterworths, 1972.
5. Freeman, M.A.R., and Meachim, G.: Aging and degeneration. In Freeman, M.A.R. ed.: Adult Articular Cartilage, 2nd Ed. Tunbridge Wells, England, Pitman Medical, 1979, p. 487.
6. Johnson, F., Leitl, S., and Waugh, W.: The distribution of load across the knee. A comparison of static and dynamic measurements. J. Bone Joint Surg. [Br.], 62: 346, 1980.
7. Maquet, P.: Considérations biomécaniques sur l'arthrose du genou. Un traitement biomécanique de l'arthrose femoropatellaire. L'avancement du tendon rotulieu. Rev. Rhum., *30*: 779, 1963.
8. Maroudas, A.: Biophysical chemistry of cartilaginous tissues with special reference to solute and fluid transport. Biorheology, *12*: 233, 1975.
9. Meachim, G., and Stockwell, R.A.: The Matrix. p. 10. In Freeman, M.A.R., ed.: Adult Articular Cartilage, 2nd Ed. Tunbridge Wells, England, Pitman Medical, 1979.
10. Morrison, J.B.: Biomechanics of the knee joint in relation to normal walking. J. Biomech. 3: 51, 1970.
11. Muir, I.H.M.: Biochemistry. p. 187. In Freeman, M.A.R., ed.: Adult Articular Cartilage, 2nd Ed. Tunbridge Wells, England, Pitman Medical, 1979.
12. Paul, J.P.: Bio-engineering studies of the forces transmitted by joints. Part II. Engineering analysis. p. 369. In Kenedi, R.M., ed.: Biomechanics and Related Bio-Engineering Topics. Oxford, Pergamon Press, 1964.
13. Perry, J., Antonelli, D., and Ford, W.: Analysis of knee-joint forces during flexed-knee stance. J. Bone Joint Surg. [Am.], *57*: 961, 1975.
14. Stockwell, R.A., and Meachim, G.: The chondrocytes. p. 113. In Freeman, M.A.R., ed.: Adult Articular Cartilage. 2nd Ed. Tunbridge Wells, England, Pitman Medical, 1979.

18 Osteonecrosis

John N. Insall
Paolo Aglietti
and
Peter G. Bullough

Spontaneous osteonecrosis of the knee was first described as a distinct nosologic entity by Ahlbäck, et al.[2] in 1968.

Previously the typical or similar lesions had been studied by various investigators in Italy[10,17,62] and in France[21,61] and interpreted as chondritis or osteochondritis of the elderly.

Several papers have since been devoted to this peculiar condition. Some have studied the clinical and diagnostic problems,[8,15,18,28,44,47,65] others the prognosis,[49] the pathology,[3] the pathophysiology,[23] the radiology,[73] and the treatment.[1,38,45,60]

THE TYPICAL PRESENTATION

In the typical case the patient, who is usually over 60, presents with a precise and dramatic description of severe pain with sudden onset, well localized to the medial side of the knee. Often the patient recalls exactly the activity he or she was doing at the onset of symptoms. In the acute phase the pain can be so severe that it does not disappear at night.

On clinical examination in the acute phase the knee appears locked, that is, the patient cannot fully bend or fully extend the knee because of pain, effusion, and muscle contracture. The examiner can find an area of precise and severe tenderness over the medial femoral condyle above the joint line in the flexed knee.

Roentgenograms show no abnormal findings at first. This sometimes leads to an incorrect diagnosis, such as torn meniscus, and often to a delay in diagnosis, hence adequate treatment. The patient may not be x-rayed again for several months, when arthritis and deformity might already be present.

When the roentgenograms are normal, the bone scintigraphy is already markedly abnormal, with elevated counts over the knee, particularly over the medial femoral condyle (Fig. 18.1). Seldom does a case of osteonecrosis of the knee show normal scintigraphy in this phase.

After 2 or 3 months, roentgenograms show abnormal findings, with flattening and radiolucency of the subchondral bone of the medial femoral condyle (Fig. 18.2). A few months later, they show degenerative changes in addition to the necrotic lesion (Fig. 18.3).

PATHOLOGY

Osteonecrosis indicates death of a segment of the weight-bearing portion of the condyle with associated subchondral fracture and collapse.

The advent of total knee replacement has enabled

527

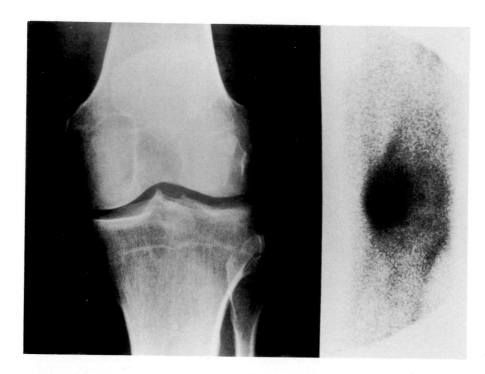

Fig. 18.1. In the early stages of acute osteonecrosis of the knee the radiographs are normal, but bone scintigraphy shows markedly abnormal findings.

Fig. 18.2. A few months after the onset of symptoms radiographs show flattening and a radiolucency.

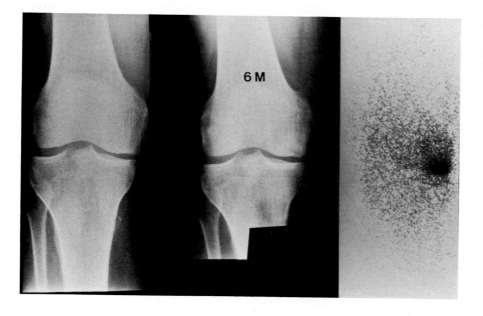

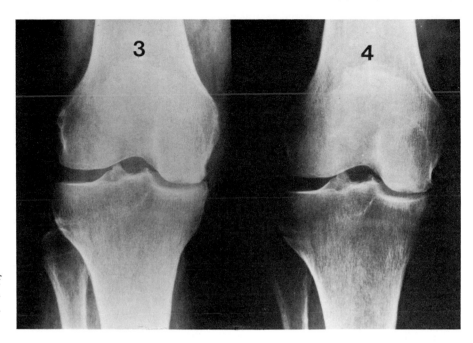

Fig. 18.3. With the passage of time, degenerative changes occur in the medial compartment.

the pathologist to document precisely what happens both macroscopically and histologically. Sagittal sections of the femoral condyle are of particular value, as they clearly show all the layers of the lesion (Figs. 18.4 and 18.5).[3]

The lesion can be observed in different pathologic stages. Upon opening a knee with osteonecrosis in an early stage, one finds only an area of slight flattening or discoloration of the articular cartilage.

Probing with an instrument usually shows an area of variable size in the condyle depressible like a ping-pong ball. At the edges of the lesion one might find an irregular line of demarcation on the surface, with a ridge of cartilage of altered color.

In a later stage of the disease, the demarcation can become more pronounced (Fig. 18.6); gradually a flap becomes manifest (Fig. 18.7). The fragment of cartilage, with a thin layer of dead subchondral bone, can easily be freed from its base with a forceps. It is usually hinged anteriorly. The shape of the lesion is oval, with a longer sagittal diameter.

More advanced cases show only remnants of the fragment as evidence of a degenerative process involving the entire compartment. A crater can be found covered by material which varies from dead detritus to regrown fibrocartilage.

In the sagittal sections of the distal femur, removed at the total knee replacement operation, one can see

in the typical case a cartilage layer of normal thickness and color, without any gross fibrillation or fissuring. Just below it is a thin layer of whitish-yellowish necrotic subchondral bone, sometimes in a fragmented state.

Proceeding toward the depth of the condyle one encounters a clear, empty space, corresponding to the subchondral fracture which has begun at the margin and propagated parallel to the surface as part of a biomechanical process through necrotic bone. In the bed of the crater, above the fracture cleft, one can see necrotic detritus and necrotic trabeculae. The bone around the necrotic area gradually acquires normal gross characteristics, with signs of intense perifocal reparative reaction and sometimes sclerosis.

In a more advanced case, in which degenerative changes have already begun, it might be difficult to find in the pathology section the typical necrotic lesion. Sometimes only after close scrutiny can the pathologist find the remnants of a worn-down crater and fragment. We believe that osteonecrosis of the knee, as in the hip, is an important and underestimated cause of osteoarthritis.

Histologically, the articular cartilage is not only viable but normal or almost normal, at least in a relatively early stage. The chondrocytes are grouped normally with normal-staining matrix around them.

Later, if the process has been going on for awhile,

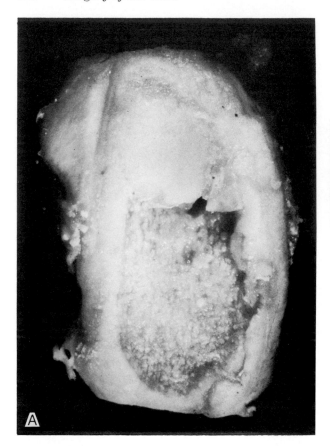

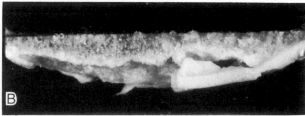

Fig. 18.4. (A) Most of the necrotic fragment in this specimen has fallen out of its bed, revealing the necrotic base of the lesion. (B) Sagittal section shows a small portion of the cartilage and attached necrotic bone remaining. This case demonstrates how, in the late stages, it may no longer be appreciated that the destructive joint disease with which the patient presents had begun as a focus of osteonecrosis.

there might be cloning of the chondrocytes, early fibrillation or erosion, and the gray layer of the tidemark might become wavy and thicker. The subchondral bone shows all the typical characteristics of necrosis; that is, the marrow exhibits cell lysis, disruption of fat cells, blood vessels, and stroma, and the osteocytic lacunae in the trabeculae are empty or have pyknotic nuclei. The marrow in a more advanced case shows a typical dusky or smokey appearance. There are no signs of reaction here.

In the more superficial layers of the base of the crater one can find again some necrotic trabeculae and an intense fibrovascular granulation tissue with histiocytes and osteoclasts reabsorbing the necrotic tissues. Here and there can be seen islands of fibrocartilage. The appearance is very much similar to that of a fracture callus.

Proceeding toward the depth of the condyle, the perifocal reaction gradually shifts toward new bone formation, and one can observe deposition of new immature bone around dead trabeculae or thickening of trabeculae and sclerosis. This type of reparative reaction can be very deep in the condyle.

ETIOLOGY

While the term "spontaneous" relates to the clinical presentation of the typical case, "idiopathic" indicates that the etiology of this condition is still unknown. Two main theories of the etiology of osteonecrosis can be identified: the vascular and the traumatic theories.

Osteonecrosis of the knee has yet to be experimentally reproduced. The etiologic hypotheses are therefore generally borrowed by analogy from osteonecrosis of the hip, because the two diseases are pathologically similar.[3,26]

The vascular theory is the most widely accepted theory for etiology of this condition in the hip and has been applied to the knee, but in a rather arbitrary and undocumented fashion.

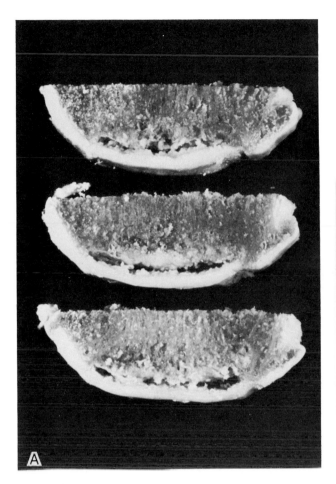

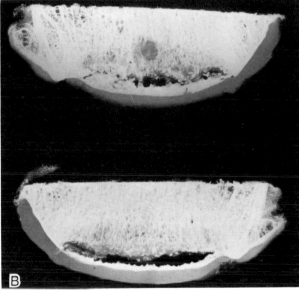

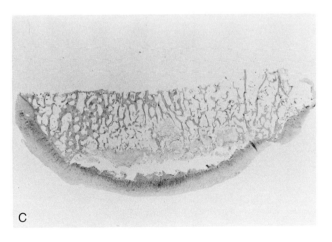

Fig. 18.5. (A) Gross inspection of the medial femoral condyle reveals smooth cartilage, but with a focally depressed area demarcated by a well-defined circumferential groove. In frontal sections a transarticular fracture can be seen. These changes give rise to the typical radiographic findings already illustrated. (B) Radiograph of the same specimen illustrated in A, showing the subchondral bone plate still attached to the cartilage. The radiolucent crescent is similar to that seen in the hip in early osteonecrosis. (C) Histologic preparation of the same specimens.

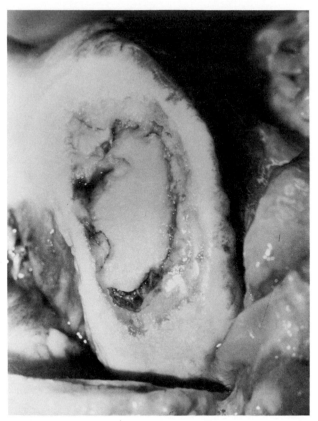

Fig. 18.6. Demarcation of a large area of osteonecrosis of the medial femoral condyle.

The blood supply to the femoral condyles has been studied in the clinical setting mainly with injection techniques.[13,59,63] Most of the blood supply comes from the superior genicular arteries and from the middle genicular artery with several intraosseous "radiate" arteries with rich and free anastomoses between them. It therefore seems difficult to conceive of a vascular arterial insult as the cause of a bone infarct.[7]

Fat embolism has been suggested as a possible mechanism in several cases of osteonecrosis of the hip, particularly when secondary to steroid treatment.[14,24,25,34,35] This mechanism has been denied by other workers.[27] Fat globules can be also found post mortem in the femoral heads of normal or osteoarthritic patients.

The vascular theory has recently acquired new strength from the studies on bone microcirculation. Every vascular insult on the arterial or venous side or directly on the bony and marrow sinusoids may lead to bone ischemia. Bone microcirculation is contained within an unexpandable compartment; an increase in bone marrow pressure can cause bone ischemia. An elevation in bone marrow pressure has been found in both the hip and the knee in osteonecrosis of idiopathic and steroid-associated types,[22,23,31,66,70,74] although this has also been found in osteoarthritis of the knee.[6]

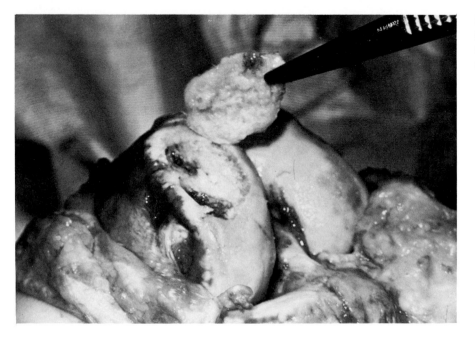

Fig. 18.7. A flap of largely intact articular cartilage is common; when raised, the area of necrosis is revealed.

The most recent hypothesis[66,68,69,71] as a cause of increased bone pressure and decreased blood flow relates to the size of the individual marrow fat cells, which has been found to be increased after cortisone treatment. A similar mechanism can be suggested for necrosis secondary to alcoholism.

That osteonecrosis of the knee is secondary to some form of trauma has been implied by some.[44,45,51] A fracture in the subchondral bone could occur first, followed by surrounding necrosis. A particular mechanism with expression of synovial fluid through the cartilage and subchondral bone into the marrow space has been postulated by Lotke et al.[44] The subchondral plate of an elderly person could be weakened by bone porosis, but this has not been documented for patients with idiopathic osteonecrosis.

CLINICAL ASPECTS

Idiopathic osteonecrosis of the knee is more frequent in women (3:1) and is most often seen in patients over age 60 (4:1). The disease is bilateral in fewer than one-fifth of cases.

The typical sudden onset of the disease is found in most cases, although the occasional case has a gradual beginning and poorly localized pain. A history of traumatic origin is true for a few patients (about 10 percent).

Of the symptoms and signs, an effusion is present frequently at the beginning. Locking or pseudolocking is common, and a flexion contracture often develops in more severe cases. In almost all cases, the lesions are localized in the weight-bearing area of the medial femoral condyle. Only a few are localized in the medial condyle, toward either the periphery or the intercondylar notch. Lateral condylar necrosis is very rare.

Recently osteonecrosis of the medial tibial plateau has been described as a cause of pain on the medial side of the knee, particularly in elderly women.[43] Histologic proof of such an entity has not been fully documented so far, but we are convinced of the existence of such a possibility (Fig. 18.8). It must be differentiated from stress fractures;[20,55,72] also, stress fractures demonstrate an increased scintigraphic uptake.

RADIOGRAPHIC ASPECTS

Radiographically, five stages of osteonecrosis can be described in an effort to follow the pathologic sequence (Fig. 18.9).

Stage I. Roentgenograms are entirely normal. It is well known that at the beginning of the disease and for the first 2 to 3 months the roentgenograms can be normal. Usually a lesion develops. Recently a series of cases with "spontaneous resolution" and roentgenograms that remain normal has been described[44] with histologic proof. The diagnosis is therefore based mainly on scintigraphy. We believe that such a condition indeed exists, but to be absolutely sure of the diagnosis can be difficult. If no roentgenographic changes are apparent 6 months from the onset of symptoms, the patient will remain in stage I.

Stage II. By carefully reviewing the roentgenograms in an early phase one can detect an area of slight flattening on the convexity of the condyle (Fig. 18.10), usually for a brief period. This finding implies an impending subchondral fracture.

Stage III. The typical stage III case shows an area of radiolucency with a distal sclerosis and a faint halo of bony reaction. Pathologically this finding corresponds to necrosis without obvious flap formation and sequestration (Fig. 18.11).

Stage IV. The typical stage IV case shows a calcified plate (*sequestrum,* or "flap fragment") with a radiolucency surrounded by a definite sclerotic halo (Fig. 18.12).

Stage V. Finally, stage V of the disease represents narrowing of the joint space, as well as subchondral (both tibial and femoral) sclerosis and osteophyte formation typical of osteoarthritis (moderate to severe) (Fig. 18.13).

Most frequently encountered are stages III and IV. There is a relationship between stage of disease and time from onset, as stages III and IV are usually diagnosed within 1 year, and it takes more than 2 years to develop the changes typical of secondary osteoarthritic stage V.

A periosteal reaction on the medial femoral me-

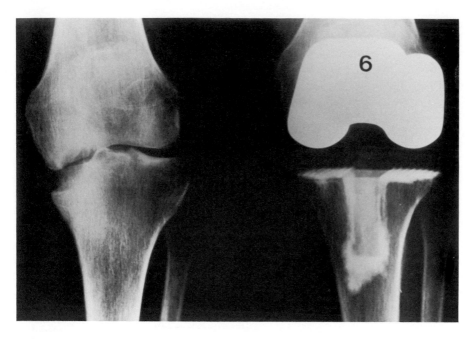

Fig. 18.8. This case shows an area of osteonecrosis in the medial femoral condyle. In addition, a large defect is found in the medial tibial plateau. This tibial lesion probably also represents an area of osteonecrosis, but to date histologic proof for this entity is lacking.

taphysis is often noted, while loose body formation is rare.

It is very important to measure two quantifiable parameters. The first is the area of the lesion,[49] obtained by multiplying the greatest diameters in the frontal and sagittal planes (Fig. 18.14AB). This area can vary from a few square millimeters to more than 10 cm^2.

The second critical parameter is the ratio in the anteroposterior view between the necrosis and the width of the condyle,[45] which can reach more than 80 percent (Fig. 18.15).

SCINTIGRAPHIC ASPECTS

The disease was first documented using ^{85}Sr by Bauer and co-workers.[2] Subsequently ^{18}F was used as well, but during the past few years preference has been given to technetium-99m phosphate compounds. Of the ^{99m}Tc phosphate compounds used (P-P, PyP, EHDP, MDP), we believe that the most suitable is now ^{99m}Tc-MDP (methylenediphosphonate) because of the characteristics of the isotope and the combined substance.[30,67]

The isotope is easily prepared and obtained, has a

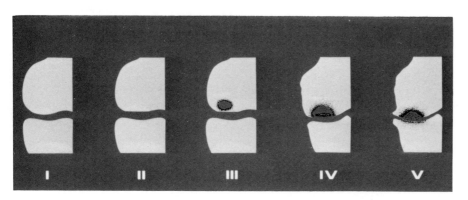

Fig. 18.9. Five stages of osteonecrosis (see text).

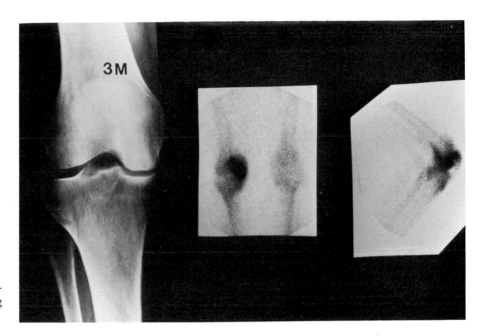

Fig. 18.10. Stage II osteonecrosis, showing slight flattening of the medial femoral condyle.

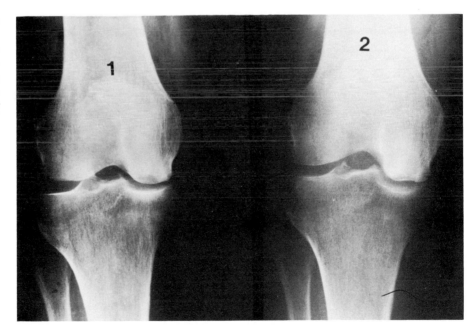

Fig. 18.11. Stage III osteonecrosis shown radiographically. (Left) Obvious radiolucency without flap formation 1 year after symptoms began. (Right) Early stage IV lesion 1 year later, showing the beginning of flap formation

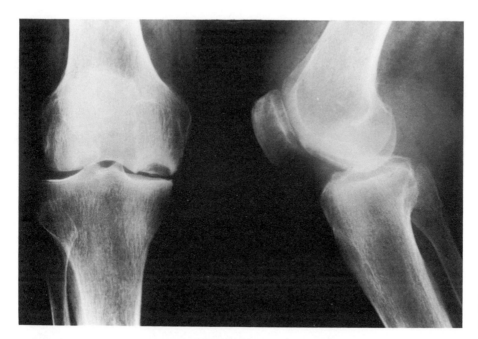

Fig. 18.12. Late stage IV osteonecrosis showing an obvious calcified flap on radiography.

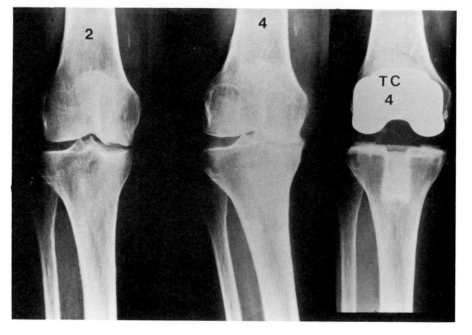

Fig. 18.13. Stage V osteonecrosis with advanced osteoarthritis, shown radiographically in sequence. (Left) Stage IV lesion 2 years after onset of symptoms. (Middle) By 4 years, the lesion has progressed to a medial compartment osteoarthritis, in which it may be difficult or impossible to identify the original cause. (Right) Same knee 4 years after total knee replacement.

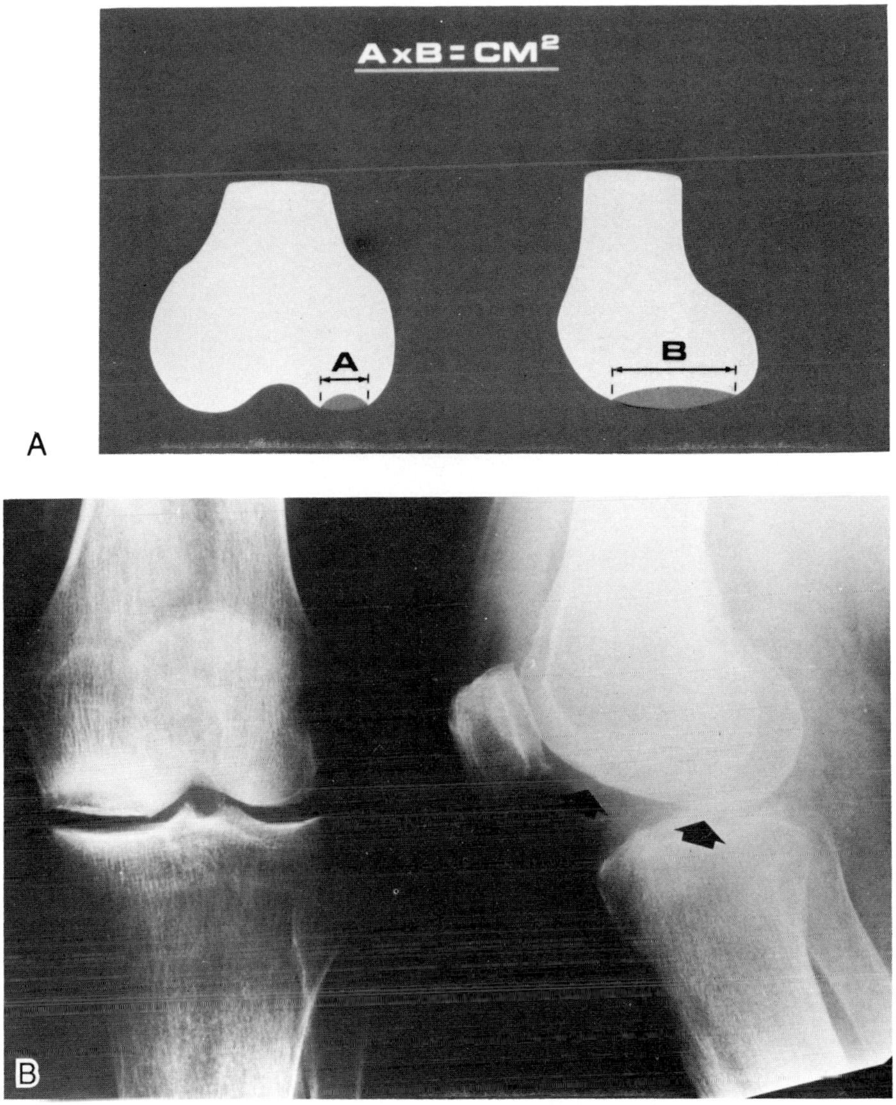

Fig. 18.14. (A) The area of the lesion is expressed in square centimeters by multiplying A × B. (B) In practice, this may be difficult because although the size of the lesion may be readily apparent in the anteroposterior view, it is often difficult to measure in the lateral view.

short half-life (6 hours), and has a pure gamma emission. The MDP has a rapid blood clearance and a very useful ratio of bone: soft tissues, with better bone imaging.

As far as mechanisms of fine localization are concerned, there are several hypotheses,[12] namely, absorption on hydroxyapatite crystals, immature collagen binding, alkaline phosphatase, and calcium phosphate targeting.

As far as the mechanisms of distribution of ^{99m}Tc-MDP are concerned, it is well established that there is increased perifocal blood flow as well as increased osteogenic activity.[12,57] The mechanisms of distribution are therefore rather aspecific. Blood-flow images, blood-pool images, and delayed bone-scan images can be obtained.[29]

In the acute phase of osteonecrosis, bone scintigraphy is very helpful and the only way to confirm the diagnosis before changes show up roentgenographically.

There is a very high uptake of ^{99m}Tc-MDP in the knee, particularly localized in the medial upper quadrant. As there is some diffusion of images in the anteroposterior view, the femoral or tibial localization of the increased uptake must be detected in the lateral view (Fig. 18.16).

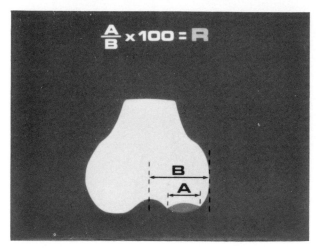

Fig. 18.15. A second method of expressing the size of the lesion is the ratio of A (size of necrosis) to B (width of the condyle).

As the healing proceeds there is a gradual loss of the uptake in the medial upper quadrant, although one can still detect a focal spot for a long period of time. If there is a significant arthritic evolution, the scintigraphy remains positive with increased uptake on the medial compartment both in the femur and tibia.

Osteonecrosis of the knee has never been shown to undergo a phase with a scintigraphically detectable defect, as is true of the hip.

OTHER STUDIES

Although in a certain number of patients with "idiopathic" osteonecrosis of the knee certain blood tests (e.g., cholesterol, triglycerides, SGOT, uric acid, and lipoproteins) have been found abnormal, we do not know the real etiologic and statistical significance of this.

Obesity seems to play a role, as it has been found in more than 60 percent of cases.[1]

An association with such factors as varus alignment[18] or medical diseases has not been documented.

Steroid-induced or -associated osteonecrosis of the knee is well known and documented, particularly in lupus erythematosus and after renal transplantations.[19] Although we believe that steroid treatment (particularly with high doses or for long periods) can be associated with necrosis of the knee and other bones, the characteristics of these types of necroses are different.[74] Apart from age and sex, which are related to the primary disease, the necrosis is often bilateral and can be localized anywhere in the knee, particularly in the lateral femoral condyle; it is often asymp-

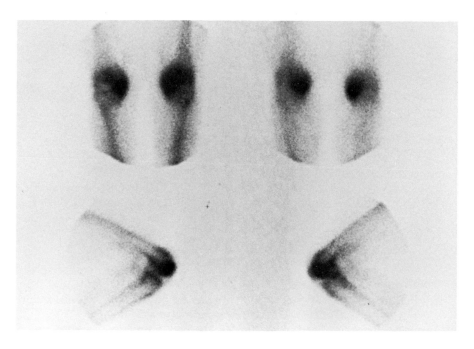

Fig. 18.16. The localization of the scintigraphic uptake is best seen in the lateral view.

tomatic, and bone scintigraphy itself can be misleading. The lesions can be very large and occupy a large section of the condyle, sometimes more than one condyle. They can be associated with necrosis in other bones (e.g., humeral head, hip, lateral humeral condyle, talus). The typical subchondral fracture through necrotic bone may be present, or there may be a lesion more similar to a bone infarct, with near-normal condylar surfaces.

DIFFERENTIAL DIAGNOSIS

OSTEOCHONDRITIS DISSECANS

The etiology of osteochondritis dissecans (OCD) remains obscure.[53] Some favor a "constitutional" theory[48,53,56] (hereditary predisposition, endocrinologic dysfunction, abnormalities of collagen and epiphyseal development), particularly in the juvenile forms. For the adult forms, a traumatic (exogenous and also endogenous trauma) origin is favored.[4,5,54] An interesting theory has been well documented in domesticated animals,[52] with anomalies of ossification a primary factor. The relevance of such findings to osteochondritis dissecans in humans remains unknown.

The localization in OCD is different from that in osteonecrosis (ON). In most cases the OCD lesion is located in the lateral aspect of the medial femoral condyle, toward the intercondylar notch (Fig. 18.17). Sometimes the area extends toward the weight-bearing portion of the condyle, but two-thirds to three-fourths of cases are located near the notch.[5,40,58]

Predilection of age and sex is also different. OCD occurs in the juvenile or in the young adult; it may present between ages 10 to 50 years, but the peak incidence occurs between ages 15 to 20.[5,40,58] Males are involved two or three times more frequently than are females.[5,40,58]

A history of trauma[5,40] is given by approximately one-half of patients with OCD, but this is rare in ON. The typical case of OCD has an insidious or gradual onset[40] of symptoms; acute onset is rare (apart from cases with sudden detachment of the fragment and locking, which usually occurs in an already symptomatic knee).

Radiologically, apart from the already described differences in location, there is often collapse of the ON lesion, subjected to weight-bearing forces, while the OCD lesion rarely collapses, being subjected because of its location, mainly to tangential forces. The triad of deformity, joint narrowing, and osteoarthritis is a very frequent and often rapid consequence of ON,[2,49,60] while it is a rare complication in juvenile OCD and a very slow and progressive one in the adult forms of OCD;[41] loose body formation is frequent in OCD and rare in ON.

Scintigraphic studies[42] have been performed in OCD, showing a low level of activity (Fig. 18.18). Bone marrow pressure studies in the condyles of OCD are infrequently altered, presenting some proof of a more localized nature of OCD, as compared with ON.[23]

Histologically[11] in OCD the fragment of bone being separated does not show signs of necrosis, unless it has been completely detached. There is a clear-cut fibrocartilage layer between the fragment and the underlying base of the crater, with signs of attempts at repair and endochondral ossification toward the ossific nucleus. The perifocal sclerotic reaction is narrow and does not deepen in the condyle. One sees neither the typical subchondral necrosis and fracture (with a cleft) nor fibrovascular granulation tissue in the base of the crater which is found in ON.

OSTEOARTHRITIS

Osteoarthritis (OA) usually has a gradual onset. Radiologically there is narrowing of the joint space without areas of necrosis or subchondral fractures. Scintigraphically there is increased uptake on both sides of the joint, and usually more so in the tibia.[60] The uptake increase never reaches the values produced in osteonecrosis.

Typical ON has been found to occur as well in knees already showing symptoms and signs of osteoarthritis. By contrast, OA is a very frequent later consequence of osteonecrosis of the condyle.

MENISCAL TEARS

When no radiolucency is seen on roentgenograms, scintigraphic studies are a useful means of differentiating ON from torn menisci, which occur also in the older population with some frequency.

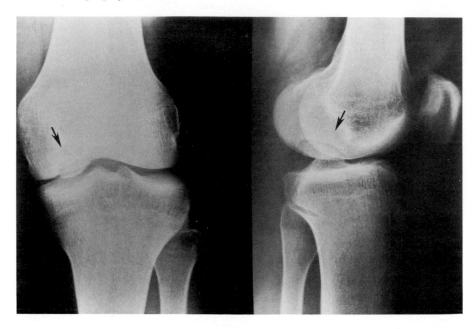

Fig. 18.17. A typical lesion of osteochondritis dissecans shown radiographically in the lateral aspect of the medial femoral condyle. This location is different from the typical location of osteonecrosis.

Torn menisci usually have no uptake increase. One can use an arthrogram or arthroscopy to reveal a meniscal lesion, but one must be careful to interpret a degenerative meniscal tear as the cause of symptoms, since degenerative tears of the medial meniscus are found with great frequency in the age groups under discussion.[50] Most tears must be asymptomatic.

The results of medial meniscectomy in the older population are controversial,[36,46] although perhaps not as bad as originally thought, particularly if there is no associated arthritis and if done arthroscopically,[33] but removing a meniscus in a patient with incipient osteonecrosis may only result in severe deterioration of the involved compartment.

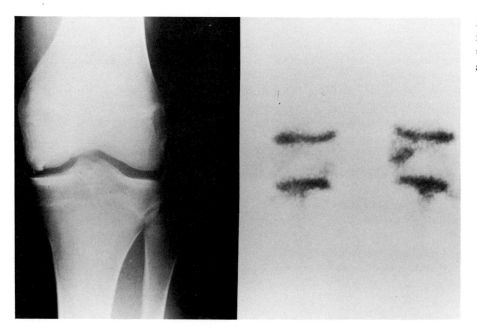

Fig. 18.18. Scintigraphic studies in osteochondritis dissecans usually display a low level of activity.

PES ANSERINUS BURSITIS

Pes anserinus bursitis is another source of severe pain in the medial aspect of the knee. Roentgenograms and scintigrams are normal; the pain is located in the medial tibia well below the joint line.

NATURAL HISTORY AND PROGNOSIS

Several parameters may be considered in assessing the clinical and functional future as well as the chances of developing osteoarthritis in a knee with osteonecrosis.

We believe that the main prognostic parameters are the area of the lesion,[49] the ratio of the lesion to the size of the condyle,[45] and the stage of the lesion.[38]

That the area of the lesion is important in predicting which knee will go on to develop severe osteoarthritis was first shown more than 10 years ago.[49] The group with favorable evolution had an average lesion size of 2.4 cm^2 (Fig. 18.19), while the group with severe evolution had an average size of 10.4 cm^2. Conservative treatment was therefore proposed for lesions of < 3.5 cm^2 and surgery for lesions of > 5 cm^2.

That this is true has been also found more recently.[60] In knees treated conservatively, those without osteoarthritis were shown to have average lesion size of 2.3 cm^2, those with osteoarthritis of 3.7 cm^2.

We believe that the area of the lesion is important not only in predicting osteoarthritic changes, but in determining the clinical and functional grade of the knee as well. While knees with lesions of > 5 cm^2 have a poor clinical and radiographic prognosis, with rapid development of severe osteoarthritis (Fig. 18.20), knees with lesions of < 5 cm^2 have a better clinical and radiographic prognosis (OA slow and slight).

There might be a "gray" zone in the 3.5- to 5-cm^2 range, but these lesions usually behave as do all lesions of < 5 cm^2.

The ratio of width of lesion to width of condyle in the anteroposterior view has also been recently proposed as a guide to prognosis[45] from a clinical and radiographic standpoint. The average ratio in the knee with favorable prognosis was 32 percent, and in the knees with poor prognosis, 57 percent. We think that this type of measurement, deprived of the possibility

of errors attributable to magnification, is very important. Knees with less than 40 percent lesions have a better clinical and roentgenographic prognosis (development of OA, severity, and time evolution) than do knees with more than 40 percent. Lotke et al.[45] found 50 percent to be the borderline between good and poor prognosis (Fig. 18.21).

The stage of the lesion is also thought to be important.[38] The earlier the stage of the lesion at the time of diagnosis or surgery, the better the prognosis. One problem with staging is that if it is done only radiologically there might be mistakes in interpreting the lesion, particularly stage III.

At surgery some stage III lesions may prove to be stage IV. The reverse is more rare. Nevertheless, we have found that radiographic staging is important to the prognosis, at least from a radiographic point of view (development of OA). More precise staging can be achieved at arthrotomy or by arthroscopy.[39]

Overall it should be noted that in due time most knees with osteonecrosis develop osteoarthritis. We have found that at 2 years almost all patients have at least grade I OA (narrowing of joint space) (Fig. 18.22), but more severe grades after the same period of time are present in one-third of patients.

TREATMENT

There are several options regarding treatment:
1. Conservative treatment.
2. Arthrotomy to remove the fragment and drill the base of the crater, for a stage IV lesion, or to drill through the cartilage in a stage III lesion. (In a stage III lesion, which is closed, a bone-grafting procedure can be done through a window in the medial side of the medial femoral condyle, as advocated by Koshino.[38] Autologous osteocartilaginous transplant from the back of the condyle has been also suggested for severe lesions.[16] If the lesion is in a stage of degeneration and secondary osteoarthritis, one can clean the crater and drill its base.)
3. High tibial osteotomy, which can be associated with an arthrotomy, in order to decrease the load in the medial (or rarely lateral) compartment.
4. Total knee replacement of the monocompartmental or of the more complete types.

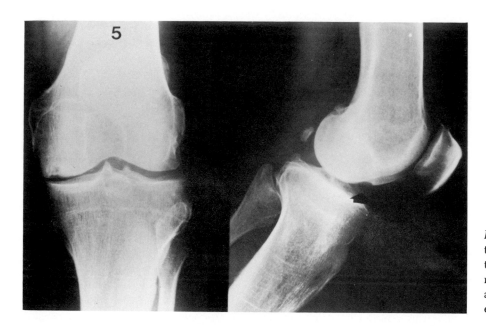

Fig. 18.19. When the area of the osteonecrotic lesion is small, the prognosis is favorable. This radiograph of a knee 5 years after onset shows only minor evidence of osteoarthritis.

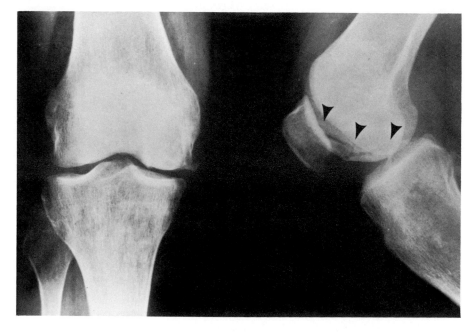

Fig. 18.20. Osteonecrotic lesion measuring 5 cm². The prognosis is poor.

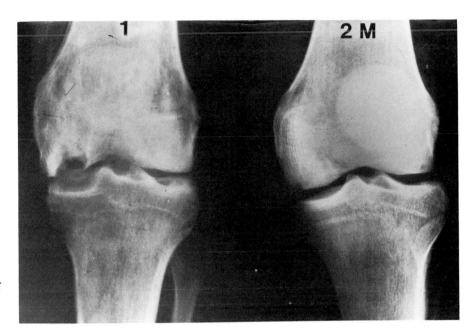

Fig. 18.21. This large osteonecrotic lesion occupies more than 50 percent of the width of the medial femoral condyle. The prognosis is poor.

Fig. 18.22. Even with small lesions, most knees with osteonecrosis show some evidence of osteoarthritis after 2 years.

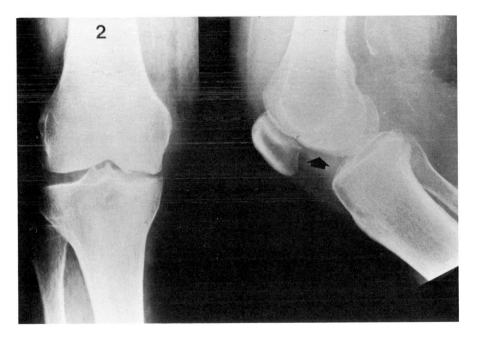

There are only a few papers dealing specifically with the results of treatment. Rozing et al.[60] described 90 knees followed for at least 2 years, 42 of which were treated conservatively and 48 surgically (arthrotomy, osteotomy with and without arthrotomy, total knee replacement mostly of the total condylar type). Koshino[38] presents the results of 37 knees treated with tibial osteotomy alone, tibial osteotomy and bone grafting, osteotomy and drilling, with a follow-up from 2 to 8 years. Lotke et al.[45] reported on 17 knees treated conservatively and 28 treated with total knee replacements of various types followed for variable but relatively short periods. Finally, our most recent paper[1] reported the results of 101 knees followed for 2 to 16 years (5 years average), 22 treated conservatively, 11 with arthrotomy (curettage and drilling after removal of the fragment, or drilling alone), 31 with osteotomy of the tibia (20 with arthrotomy), and 37 with total knee replacement (32 total condylar).

CONSERVATIVE TREATMENT

Conservative treatment consists of weight bearing relief, analgesics, and straight leg raising exercises.

Excellent or good results in this group of knees with a relatively small lesion are obtained in approximately 71 percent,[60] 81 percent,[1] or 90 percent[45] of cases, according to various investigators. The knee score increases, but not to a significant level. On the other hand, the necrotic lesion remains unchanged, improves, or gets worse in about equal proportions. Degenerative changes are present in the end stages, in almost all cases, but often are not severe. The varus deformity also increases with time. This group of patients therefore continues to function relatively well, with limited symptoms and with slow progression of arthritis.

ARTHROTOMY

When an arthrotomy is done as the only surgical procedure (with drilling or with fragment removal, or with curettage and drilling), the results are excellent or good in 77 percent,[60] or 55[1] percent of cases, according to various investigators. The knee score does not improve significantly, and roentgenographic deterioration of arthritis is present in most knees at the end stages. The limb axis remains about the same,

while the necrotic lesion is usually unchanged. Therefore, the apparently good results achieved with arthrotomy alone might well have occurred without surgical intervention, because the results were similar to those obtained in patients not operated on.

HIGH TIBIAL OSTEOTOMY

High tibial osteotomy can be performed alone or in association with various intra-articular procedures (usually at the same surgical intervention). Most of the osteotomies described in the literature[1,60] are of the closed-wedge type above the tibial tuberosity, without internal fixation and with early weight-bearing in a cylinder cast. Osteotomies can also be done with internal fixation or with compression clamps.[38]

Excellent or good results can be obtained in a high proportion of cases ranging from 86 percent,[38] 87 percent,[1] and 96 percent.[60] Koshino[38] used a slightly more rigorous classification of the postoperative knee scores than did the other two series. The knee scores significantly improved at follow-up in all quoted series.

According to both Rozing et al.[60] and Koshino,[38] intra-articular procedures are frequently indicated in addition to the high tibial osteotomy (Fig. 18.23). It is believed that the cartilage flap that may overlie the necrotic lesion is unable to reunite spontaneously and acts as an obstacle to the healing of the cartilage.

The average postoperative score in the knees with tibial osteotomy and bone grafting (all stage III) was significantly better in the Koshino series than reported in knees treated with tibial osteotomy and drilling alone. However, in our recent and more comprehensive study,[1] we did not find a significant difference in the results when arthrotomy procedures (such as drilling or curettage and drilling) were associated with the osteotomy.

The necrotic lesion improves after osteotomy in most cases, and our series[1] demonstrates no difference whether an arthrotomy is associated or not.

In the Koshino series,[38] knees treated with bone grafting or drilling together with osteotomy showed significantly greater roentgenographic improvement. As far as osteoarthritis is concerned, osteotomy seems to slow down or stop the evolution of the degenerative process. Again we did not find, as did Koshino, that this is significantly better when arthrotomy is also done.

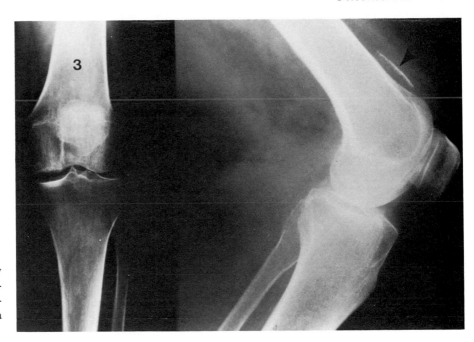

Fig. 18.23. Although loose body formation is rare in osteonecrosis, arthrotomy is occasionally needed for removal of a calcified and detached flap.

Adequate correction with osteotomy should be achieved. The average femorotibial angle (standing films) in the knees with excellent results in Koshino's cases and our series is 170 degrees (10 degrees valgus) (Fig. 18.24). The ideal range seems to be 6 to 15 degrees of valgus. For the rare case of a knee with lateral condyle osteonecrosis, the ideal correction seems to be 4 degrees valgus.[38]

We have used osteotomies in knees with varus deformities secondary to the collapse of the medial femoral condyle and degenerative changes of the medial compartment.

Fig. 18.24. After high tibial osteotomy, the femorotibial angle should be 170 degrees (10 degrees of valgus). It seems to make little difference to the result whether the area of osteonecrosis is debrided or not. In this case a good result after osteotomy was maintained for 13 years.

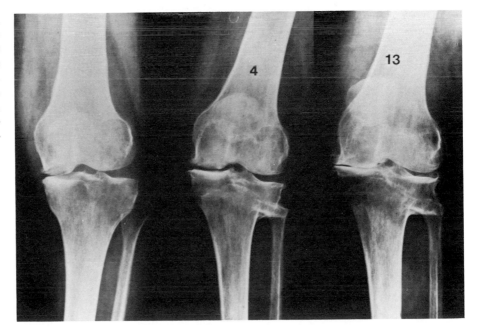

We do not think an osteotomy is indicated if the alignment of the knee is normal, but we have performed it in cases showing reduction of the normal valgus (in the 1 to 5 degrees valgus category).

The quality and longevity of results after a high tibial osteotomy for osteonecrosis are similar to results with primary osteoarthritis. Pain relief is very satisfactory, as is walking capacity and range of motion. Associated arthrotomies do not negatively influence range of motion even after cast immobilization if no internal fixation is used. Fair or poor results have been attributed mainly to residual pain, sometimes due to insufficient correction. A particular problem has been flexion contracture, which is often present preoperatively and tends to remain as such postoperatively.

TOTAL KNEE REPLACEMENT

We believe that total knee replacement has an important role in the treatment of osteonecrosis of the knee. The selection between osteotomy and replacement should be made on the basis of the same guidelines used in osteoarthritis.

Such factors as advanced age, low level of activity, severity of the lesion and of deformity, and presence of instability, flexion contracture, or synovitis, tend to influence the decision toward replacement.

Unicompartmental arthroplasty, because of the nature of the disease, would seem particularly suitable for osteonecrosis. Unfortunately our experience with this type of prosthesis[32] has not been positive. Fixation of the femoral and tibial components, residual pain from the patellofemoral joint, progression of arthritis, and deterioration of the results with the passage of time are the main problems encountered. Our experience has not been shared by others,[9,37,64] however, and unicondylar prostheses are still used for osteonecrosis.

Our preference favors a more complete form of replacement, such as the total condylar (Fig. 18.25). For this model we have used both types I and II and the more recent posterior stabilized version. In a group of 37 total knee replacements (32 total condylar, two unicondylar, and three duocondylar), excellent or good results have been obtained, with an average 5-year follow-up, in 90 percent of cases. There have been only two revisions (one unicondylar and one duocondylar). The postoperative scores are significantly increased over the preoperative ones, and the quality of the results, including pain relief, is similar to that for total knee replacement performed for osteoarthritis.

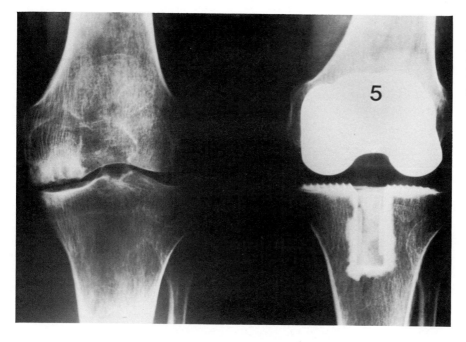

Fig. 18.25. When a replacement is chosen, a total condylar arthroplasty produces more predictable results than does unicompartmental replacement.

We do not agree with the statement[45] that proximal tibial osteotomy has been unsuccessful for severe osteonecrosis of the knee, but we consider the results of knee replacement superior to those obtained by tibial osteotomy, although statistically to a low level of significance. The follow-up period is now sufficient for us to make the above judgment as to the merits of this procedure and is almost reaching the length of follow-up for osteotomies.

CONCLUSIONS

1. Osteonecrosis is a frequent cause of acute knee pain in the elderly.
2. Etiology is unknown and probably none of the current theories even closely approaches reality.
3. Scintigraphy is a useful diagnostic means, particularly in cases demonstrating normal roentgenograms.
4. The real incidence is as yet undefined. There are self-resolving cases, mistakes can be made because the initial roentgenograms are negative, and probably several cases of osteoarthritis of the knee are secondary to osteonecrosis, which is recognized with difficulty in an advanced case.
5. Conservative treatment is sufficient in a significant proportion of cases.
6. A period of observation of about 6 months is useful.
7. Small lesions with slowly progressing osteoarthritis can be treated conservatively for long periods of time.
8. Surgical treatment may be reserved for cases with lesions of > 5 cm^2 and a ratio of more than 40 percent.
9. Arthrotomy alone does not significantly alter the evolution of the disease.
10. High tibial osteotomy, alone or in combination with arthrotomy, is a highly successful operation.
11. When osteotomy is done, the results in our hands have not been significantly different whether arthrotomy was done or not.
12. Total knee replacements, particularly of the total condylar type, give a very high success rate, and the quality of the results is probably slightly superior to that produced with osteotomy.
13. We believe that knee replacement should be reserved for the older age group with fewer activity expectations, in cases with severe necrosis, severe arthritis, and deformity.

REFERENCES

1. Aglietti, P., Insall, J., Deschamps, G., et al.: The results of treatment of idiopathic osteonecrosis of the knee. In press J. Bone Joint Surg. [Br.], 1983.
2. Ahlbäck, S., Bauer, G.C.H., and Bohne, W.H.: Spontaneous osteonecrosis of the knee. Arthritis Rheum., *11*: 705, 1968.
3. Ahuja, S.C., and Bullough, P.G.: Osteonecrosis of the knee. J. Bone Joint Surg. [Am.], *60*: 191, 1978.
4. Aichroth, P.: Osteochondral fractures and their relationship to osteochondritis dissecans of the knee. J. Bone Joint Surg. [Br.], *53*: 448, 1971.
5. Aichroth, P.: Osteochondritis dissecans of the knee. A clinical survey. J. Bone Joint Surg. [Br.], *53*: 440, 1971.
6. Arnoldi, C.C., Lemperg, K.R., and Linderholm, H.: Intraosseous hypertension and pain in the knee. J. Bone Joint Surg. [Br.], *57*: 360, 1975.
7. Arnowsky, S.: Personal communication, 1982.
8. Bauer, G.C.H.: Osteonecrosis of the knee. Clin. Orthop., *130*: 210, 1978.
9. Bauer, G.C.H.: Personal communication, 1982.
10. Bortolotti, E.: La osteocondrite dissecante del ginocchio nell'età senile. Minerva Ortop., *13*: 742, 1962.
11. Chiroff, R.T., and Cooke, C.P.: Osteochondritis dissecans: A histologic and microradiographic analysis of surgically excised lesions. J. Trauma, *15*: 689, 1975.
12. Christensen, S.B., and Arnoldi, C.C.: Distribution of ^{99m}Tc phosphate compounds in osteoarthritic femoral heads. J. Bone Joint Surg. [Am.], *62*: 90, 1980.
13. Crock, H.V.: The blood supply of the lower limb bones in man. Baltimore, Williams and Wilkins, 1967.
14. Cruess, R.L.: Cortisone induced avascular necrosis of the femoral head. J. Bone Joint Surg. [Br.], *59*: 308, 1977.
15. Daumont, A., Deplante, J.P., Bouvier, M., et al.: L'osteonecrose des condyles fémoraux chez l'adulte. A propos de 30 cas personnels. Rev. Rhum. Mal. Osteoartic., *43*: 27, 1976.
16. De La Caffinière, J.Y.: La translocation ostéocartilagineuse autogène dans les nécroses condyliennes du genou chez le vieillard. Rev. Chir. Orthop., *64*: 653, 1980.
17. Delfino, C., and Turrini, P.: Contributo allo studio della condrite dissecante dell'età senile. Arch. Ist. Osp. Santa Corona, *31*: 516, 1966.

18. Duparc, J., and Alnot, J.Y.: Osteonecrose primitive du condyle fémoral interne du sujet agé. Rev. Chir. Orthop., *55*: 615, 1969.

19. Elmstedt, E.: Avascular bone necrosis in the renal transplant patient: A discriminant analysis of 144 cases. Clin. Orthop., *158*: 149, 1981.

20. Engber, W.D.: Stress fractures of the medial tibial plateau. J. Bone Joint Surg. [Am.], *59*: 767, 1977.

21. Fages, A.: De l'osteonecrose aseptique de l'epiphise fémorale inférieure. A propos de 30 observations. Thèse Méd Paris, *25*: 1965,

22. Ficat, P., Arlet, J., Vidal, R., et al.: Resultats therapeutiques du forage-biopsie dans les osteonecroses femorocapitales primitives. Rev. Rhum. Mal. Osteoartic., *38*: 269, 1971.

23. Ficat, P., Arlet, J., and Mazières, B.: Ostéochondrite disséquante et ostéonécrose de l'extrémité inférieure du fémur. Sem. Hôp. Paris, *51*: 1907, 1975.

24. Fisher, D.E.: The role of fat embolism in the etiology of corticosteroid-induced avascular necrosis. Clin. Orthop., *130*: 68, 1978.

25. Fisher, D.E., and Bickel, W.H.: Corticosteroid induced avascular necrosis. J. Bone Joint Surg. [Am.], *53*: 859, 1971.

26. Glimcher, M.J., and Kenzora, J.E.: The biology of osteonecrosis of the human femoral head and its clinical implications. II The pathological changes in the femoral head as an organ and in the hip joint. Clin. Orthop., *139*: 283, 1979.

27. Glimcher, M.J., and Kenzora, J.E.: The biology of osteonecrosis of the human femoral head and its clinical implications. III Discussion of the etiology and genesis of the pathological sequelae: Comments on treatment. Clin. Orthop., *140*: 273, 1979.

28. Glimet, T., Fages, A., Welfling, J., et al.: L'ostéonécrose primitive du genou chez le sujet agé. Sem. Hop. Paris, *48*: 879, 1972.

29. Greyson, N.D., Lotem, M.M., Gross, A.E., et al: Radionuclide evaluation of spontaneous femoral osteonecrosis. Radiology. *142*: 729, 1982.

30. Hughes, S.: Radionuclides in orthopaedic surgery. J. Bone Joint Surg. [Br.], *62*: 141, 1980.

31. Hungerford, D.S.: Pathogenetic considerations in ischemic necrosis of bone. Can. J. Surg., *24*: 583, 1981.

32. Insall, J., and Aglietti, P.: A five to seven-year followup of unicondylar arthroplasty. J. Bone Joint Surg. [Am.], *62*: 1329, 1980.

33. Jackson, R.W., and Rouse, D.W.: Results of partial arthroscopic meniscectomy in patients over forty years of age. J. Bone Joint Surg. [Br.], *64*: 481, 1982.

34. Jones, J.P.: Alcoholism, hypercortisonism, fat embolism and osseous avascular necrosis. In Zinn, W.M.

(ed.): Idiopathic Ischemic Necrosis of Femoral Head in Adults. Stuttgart, Georg Thieme, 1971, p. 113.

35. Jones, J.P., and Sakovich, L.: A technique for staining bone fat. Arthritis Rheum., *8*: 448, 1965.

36. Jones, R.E., Smith, E.C., and Reisch, J.S.: Effects of medial meniscectomy in patients older than forty years. J. Bone Joint Surg. [Am.], *60*: 783, 1978.

37. Jones, W.T., Bryan, R.S., Peterson, L.F.A., et al.: Unicompartmental knee arthroplasty using polycentric and geometric hemicomponents. J. Bone Joint Surg. [Am.], *63*: 946, 1981.

38. Koshino, T.: The treatment of spontaneous osteonecrosis of the knee by high tibial osteotomy with and without bone-grafting or drilling of the lesion. J. Bone Joint Surg. [Am.], *64*: 47, 1982.

39. Koshino, T., Okamoto, R., Takamura, K., et al.: Arthroscopy in spontaneous osteonecrosis of the knee. Orthop. Clin. North Am., *10*: 609, 1979.

40. Linden, B.: The incidence of osteochondritis dissecans in the condyles of the femur. Acta Orthop. Scand., *47*: 664, 1976.

41. Linden, B.: Osteochondritis dissecans of the femoral condyles. A long term follow up study. J. Bone Joint Surg. [Am.], *59*: 769, 1977.

42. Linden, B., and Nilsson, B.E.: Strontium-85 uptake in knee joints with osteochondritis dissecans. Acta Orthop. Scand., *47*: 668, 1976.

43. Lotke, P.A., and Ecker, M.L.: Osteonecrosis of the medial tibial plateau. Orthop. Trans. *5*: 485, 1981.

44. Lotke, P.A., Ecker, M.L., and Alavi, A.: Painful knees in older patients. J. Bone Joint Surg. [Am.], *59*: 617, 1977.

45. Lotke, P.A., Abend, J.A., and Ecker, M.L.: The treatment of osteonecrosis of the knee. Presented at the Annual Meeting of the American Academy of Orthopedic Surgeons, Atlanta, Georgia, February 11, 1980.

46. Lotke, P.A., Lefkoe, R.T., and Ecker, M.L.: Late results following medial meniscectomy in an older population. J. Bone Joint Surg. [Am.], *63*: 115, 1981.

47. Magard, M., Maitrepierre, J., and Durant, J.: L'osteonécrose primitive du genou des sujets ages. Rev. Rhum. Mal. Osteoartic., *36*: 697, 1969.

48. Mubarak, S.J., and Carroll, N.C.: Juvenile osteochondritis dissecans of the knee: Etiology. Clin. Orthop., *157*: 200, 1981.

49. Muheim, G., and Bohne, W.H.: Prognosis in spontaneous osteonecrosis of the knee. J. Bone Joint Surg. [Br.], *52*: 605, 1970.

50. Noble, J., and Hamblen, D.L.: The pathology of the degenerate meniscus lesions. J. Bone Joint Surg. [Br.], *57*: 180, 1975.

51. Norman, A., and Baker, N.D.: Spontaneous osteone-

crosis of the knee and medial meniscal tears. Radiology, *129*: 653, 1978.

52. Olsson, S.E.: Osteochondrosis in domestic animals. Acta Radiol. [Suppl.] (Stockh.), *358*: 1978.

53. Pappas, A.M.: Osteochondrosis dissecans. Clin. Orthop., *158*: 59, 1981.

54. Petrie, P.W.R.: Aetiology of osteochondritis dissecans. Failure to establish a familial background. J. Bone Joint Surg. [Br.], *59*: 366, 1977.

55. Prather, J.L., Nusynowitz, M.L., Snowdy, H.A., et al.: Scintigraphic findings in stress fractures. J. Bone Joint Surg. [Am.], *59*: 869, 1977.

56. Ribbing, S.: The hereditary multiple epiphyseal disturbance and its consequences for aetiogenesis of local malacias, particularly the osteochondrosis dissecans. Acta Orthop., *24*: 286, 1955.

57. Riggs, S.A., Wood, M.B., and Kelly, P.J.: The relationship between blood flow and Tc^{99m} labeled methylenediphosphonate uptake in bone scanning. Transactions of the 28th Annual Meeting O.R.S., New Orleans, 1982.

58. Roberts, J.M.: Osteochondritis dissecans. In Kennedy, J.C. (ed.): The Injured Adolescent Knee, Baltimore, Williams & Wilkins, 1979, pp. 121–140.

59. Rogers, W.M., and Gladstone, H.: Vascular foramina and arterial supply of the distal end of the femur. J. Bone Joint Surg. [Am.], *32*: 867, 1950.

60. Rozing, P.M., Insall, J., and Bohne, W.H.: Spontaneous osteonecrosis of the knee. J. Bone Joint Surg. [Am.], *62*: 2, 1980.

61. Rubens-Duval, A., Villiaumey, J., Lubetzdi, D., et al.: L'ostéochondrite du genou du sujet agé: Intérêt de la biopsie synoviale. Rev. Rhum. Mal. Ostéoartic., *33*: 709, 1964.

62. Scaglietti, O., and Fineschi, G.: La condrite dissecante dell'età senile. Arch. Putti, *20*: 1, 1965. *20*: 1, 1965.

63. Scapinelli, R.: Studies on the vasculature of the human knee joint. Acta Anat., *70*: 305, 1968.

64. Scott, R.D., and Santore, R.F.: Unicondylar unicompartmental replacement for osteoarthritis of the knee. J. Bone Joint Surg. [Am.], *63*: 536, 1981.

65. Serre, H., Simon, L., Sony, J., et al.: L'osténécrose primitive du genou chez le sujet agé. Presse Med., *78*: 2119, 1970.

66. Solomon, L.: Idiopathic necrosis of the femoral head: Pathogenesis and treatment. Can. J. Surg., *24*: 573, 1981.

67. Sy, W.M.: Gamma images in benign and metabolic bone diseases. Boca Raton, Florida, C.R.C. Press.

68. Wang, G.J., Sweet, D.E., Reger, S.I., et al.: Fat cell changes as a mechanism of avascular necrosis of the femoral head in cortisone treated rabbits. J. Bone Joint Surg. [Am.], *59*: 729, 1977.

69. Wang, G.J., Moga, D.B., Richemer, W.G., et al.: Cortisone induced bone changes and its response to lipid clearing agents. Clin. Orthop., *130*: 81, 1978.

70. Wang, G.J., Lennox, D.W., Reger, S.I., et al.: Cortisone-induced intrafemoral head pressure change and its response to a drilling decompression method. Clin. Orthop., *159*: 274, 1981.

71. Wang, G.J., Hubbard, S.L., Roger, S.I., et al.: Femoral head blood flow in long term steroid treatment (study of rabbit model). Transactions of the 28th Annual Meeting of the O.R.S., New Orleans, 1982, p. 188.

72. Wilcox, J.R., Moniot, A.L., and Green, J.P.: Bone scanning in the evolution of exercise-related stress injuries. Radiology, *123*: 699, 1977.

73. Williams, J.L., Cliff, M.M., and Bonakdarpont, A.: Spontaneous osteonecrosis of the knee. Radiology, *107*: 15, 1973.

74. Zizic, T.M., and Moore, R.: Steroid associated ischemic necrosis of the knee. Presented at the 47th Annual Meeting of the American Association of Orthopedic Surgeons, Atlanta, 1980.

19 Osteotomy

John N. Insall

Osteotomy for correction of limb deformities must be among the oldest of orthopedic procedures. The first known report on osteotomy performed on the tibia was written in 1875 by Volkmann,[42] who performed the operation to correct a deformity of the knee joint. Jones and Lowett,[23] in their textbook on orthopedic surgery, described tibial osteotomy as a form of treatment for deformities of the knee joint. Steindler[39] suggested tibial osteotomy as a treatment for osteoarthritis of the knee. Lange[29] recommended osteotomy in rickets and for post-traumatic conditions to correct abnormal angulations and thereby prevent the occurrence of degenerative arthritis. The operation was slow in gaining acceptance, as the procedure was widely regarded as dangerous, largely because it was known that fractures of the proximal tibia were sometimes associated with arterial injuries. Jackson[18] is generally given credit for describing tibial osteotomy as a safe, effective procedure performed specifically for degenerative arthritis.

Debeyre and Patte[8] were the first to present a detailed report on corrective osteotomy in osteoarthritis of the knee. From a series of 54 osteotomies performed over a 10-year period, they presented the results of 18 operations in 14 patients. Because an excellent result was obtained in five knees with imperfect correction of deformity, Debeyre and Patte concluded that the effect of osteotomy not only redistributed the load passing across the knee joint, but in some way modified the blood circulation as well. The concept of altered circulation has subsequently received support from Helal[16] and Arnoldi et al.,[1] who ascribed the beneficial effect to a lowering of the intraosseous venous pressure.

The venous pressure theory notwithstanding, most investigators believe that the effects of osteotomy are purely mechanical.[31] Jackson and Waugh[19] reported good results in 10 patients for whom the expressed purpose of the operation was to "make the leg look straight." Coventry[4] reported the early results of tibial osteotomy at the Mayo Clinic, and the same author has subsequently published the results of his own series of cases, which began in 1960.[5,6] Coventry recommends a technique performed through a lateral approach, as originally suggested by Gariepy.[12] A portion of the fibular head is excised and the osteotomy performed above the tibial tubercle. A staple is used for fixation.

Coventry stresses the mechanical aspects of the operation, the object being to obtain a knee in balance with symmetric loading both medially and laterally. The importance of correct postoperative alignment has been recognized by many investigators, although the most desirable position remains debatable. Although all agree that varus deformities must be corrected into valgus.

SELECTION

In the past, tibial osteotomy was used to correct both varus and valgus deformities of any degree; even today in parts of the world where for various reasons total knee replacement is not widely performed, the operation is still performed to correct severe deformities. It has become apparent, however, that there are certain relevant contraindications to tibial osteotomy.

VALGUS DEFORMITIES

It was noted by Wardle[43] that correction of valgus produced an obliquity or tilting of the knee joint axis in the coronal plane, which he did not believe to be of consequence (Fig. 19.1). Bauer et al.[2] found a similar obliquity and were also of the opinion that apart from producing an inelegant appearance in the radiograph it did not matter. Subsequent studies[5,37,38] have provided a different viewpoint. While it may be true that minor degrees of joint obliquity are compatible with a good clinical result, when the tilting exceeds 10 to 15 degrees, the mechanical effect is to shift the loading of the joint from the lateral compartment only as far medially as the tibial spine and not as intended to the more normal medial compartment. With time, pronounced obliquity also tends to cause the femur to sublux medially on the tibia; ultimately, a late varus angulation may develop. This joint obliquity after osteotomy for valgus is caused by greater loss of substance from the lateral femoral condyle than from the lateral tibial plateau (the reverse of what is seen in medial compartment gonarthrosis). Exactly why the pattern of articular degeneration should be this way has not been fully explained, unless it be that the underlying cause for idiopathic gonarthrosis is structural, having its origin in an anatomic variation. In this regard it is interesting that post-traumatic lateral osteoarthritis caused by a depressed fracture of the lateral tibial plateau responds much better to tibial osteotomy, and in this instance one can assume that before the injury the structure of the knee joint was normal.

Apart from the undesirable joint obliquity, there is another disadvantage to wedge osteotomy for valgus. When the base of the wedge is medial, bone is removed from between the origin and insertion of the

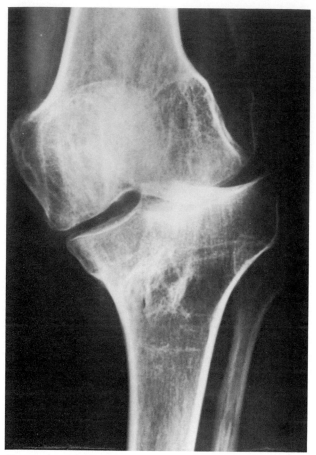

Fig. 19.1. Tibial osteotomy for valgus deformity produces an obliquity of the joint axis, which leads to weight transfer only as far as the lateral aspect of the tibial spine.

superficial medial ligament (the most important medial stabilizer of the knee), and the relative lengthening of the ligament will therefore predispose to joint instability (Fig. 19.2). This problem cannot be avoided by making a dome osteotomy; it can only be solved by an opening wedge osteotomy and a bone graft. Unfortunately, osteotomies of this type are often slow in healing.

SEVERE VARUS DEFORMITY

Not only is a deformed limb awkward to walk on, but progression of medial gonarthrosis occurs because of the biomechanical alteration caused by angulation. Abnormal stress on the medial articulation causes progressive loss of cartilage and bone, in turn increas-

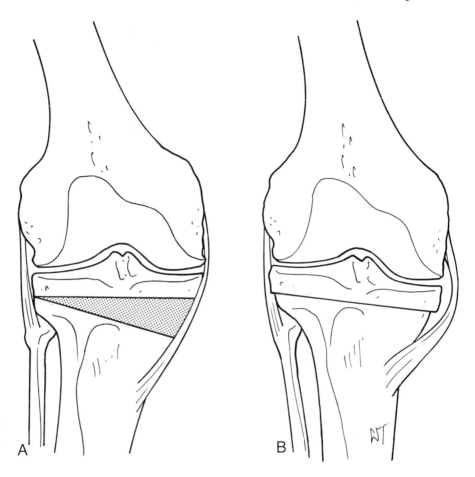

Fig. 19.2. Removing a wedge with the base medial effectively lengthens the superficial medial collateral ligament.

ing the deformity. This vicious circle is exacerbated by stretching of the lateral ligament and capsular structures causing more instability and more deformity (Fig. 19.3A,B). The instability and loss of substance produce what Kettelkamp et al.[25] call the "teeter" effect. Loss of substance makes it difficult or impossible to obtain two-plateau loading, and the laxity makes prediction of the weight-bearing alignment after osteotomy equally difficult. The amount of instability that contraindicates osteotomy does not lend itself to precise definition, but fortunately there is a close correlation between deformity and instability. Knees with < 10 degrees of deformity when standing are nearly always stable, but when the deformity exceeds 10 degrees instability is found more often. When the deformity is ≥ 15 degrees, the instability attributable to a combination of loss of substance and soft tissue stretching can be expected to prejudice the result of osteotomy. Coventry,[5] although generally in

agreement that 10 degrees of varus should be the upper limit of deformity in a knee being considered for osteotomy, also recommends that laxity be corrected by soft tissue reefing on the lateral aspect after the bone wedge has been removed.

Maquet,[31,32] however, disputes the belief that the degree of deformity influences the outcome of osteotomy. He has reported on 41 patients who had either a varus deformity > 15 degrees or subluxation evident on weight-bearing radiographs. In 32 knees, an excellent result was obtained after osteotomy. Maquet describes a barrel vault osteotomy for correction in these patients (Fig. 19.4). He does not consider a closing wedge osteotomy above the tibial tubercle satisfactory, as there is not enough room to remove a wedge of sufficient size. He does not believe that soft tissue laxity requires reefing and states that tightening occurs spontaneously if slight overcorrection is obtained.

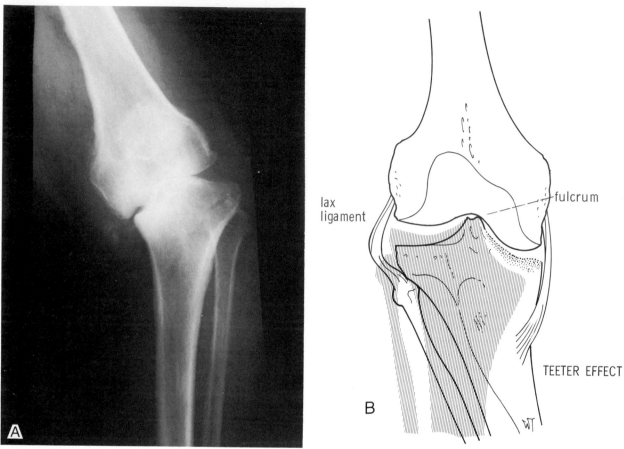

Fig. 19.3. (A) Severe varus deformity is caused by medial bone erosion of the tibia; stretching of the lateral ligaments occurs later because of the stresses of walking on a deformed limb. (B) A combination of bone loss and ligament instability makes the knee difficult to balance (see teeter effect).

PATELLOFEMORAL ARTHRITIS

Patellofemoral symptoms after osteotomy are not generally held responsible for failure in a significant number of cases although Kettelkamp et al.[25] have suggested that this may be partly attributable to lack of specific inquiry into patellofemoral function. Stair climbing and other activities that stress the patello-femoral joint are often not included in the evaluation of results. However, radiographically severe patello-femoral arthritis definitely does not contraindicate osteotomy, which may improve patellofemoral function by a subtle alteration in patellar tracking or by anterior advancement of the tibial tubercle (Fig. 19.5). Tibial tubercle advancement is sought as part of the technique described by Maquet but often occurs inadvertently when such displacement is not deliberately intended. There is certainly general agreement that patellofemoral arthritis is not a major cause of failure after osteotomy; nonetheless, when patellar symptoms are suspected preoperatively on clinical grounds, the patient should be warned that these symptoms may continue afterward. Such symptoms include difficulty in stair climbing, arising from a low chair, and pain at rest or at night. Signs of patellar dysfunction include pain and crepitus on active extension, patellofemoral tenderness, and a persistent effusion.

These symptoms and signs may raise suspicion of significant patellofemoral arthritis but are not diag-

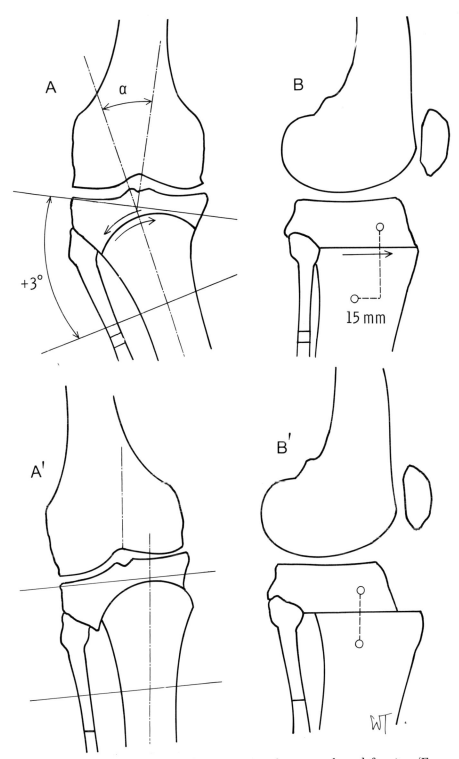

Fig. 19.4. Barrel vault osteotomy for correction of severe valgus deformity. (From Maquet, P.: Valgus osteotomy for osteoarthritis of the knee. Clin. Orthop., *120*: 143, 1976, with permission.)

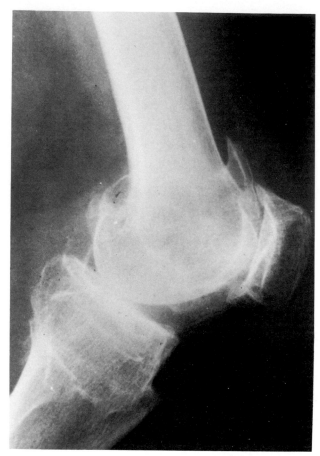

Fig. 19.5. Patellofemoral arthritis is not usually a contraindication to osteotomy. Sometimes a small advancement of the tibial tubercle occurs even though, as in this case, it was not specifically intended.

nostic. However, suspicion in a borderline case may tip the selection of procedure toward total knee arthroplasty.

FLEXION CONTRACTURE

Minor degrees of fixed flexion can be corrected at the osteotomy site, but when the contracture exceeds 20 degrees, an excessive and undesirable anterior tilt of the tibial plateau will result. Thus a flexion contracture of ≥ 20 degrees is a contraindication to tibial osteotomy unless the deformity can be corrected by a posterior capsulotomy. Generally, though, this is not possible because the block to further extension is caused by intra-articular osteophytes and bony proliferation.

DIMINISHED MOTION

Osteotomy cannot improve the range of motion present in the knee, and there may be some slight loss afterward. A range of motion of < 70 degrees is therefore a contraindication to osteotomy particularly when, as is often the case, restricted motion is associated with a fixed flexion contracture. Loss of motion may be associated with severe patellofemoral arthritis, and large intercondylar osteophytes (Fig. 19.6), in addition to the drawback of restricted motion, articular damage is usually widespread, and the joint is too far gone to benefit much from osteotomy.

PATIENT AGE

Now that total knee replacement has become an established and reliable operation, it must be considered as an alternative to osteotomy. In addition to

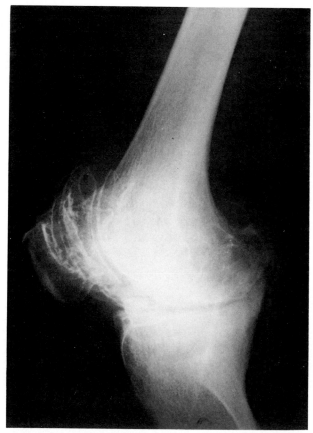

Fig. 19.6. Diminished motion is associated with advanced patellofemoral arthritis and proliferative osteophytes.

any of the factors considered above possibly turning the decision in favor of replacement, there is the question of age. Current prosthetic designs have proved decently durable, offer a higher proportion of excellent results, and give a more rapid recovery than osteotomy, particularly in bilateral cases. On these grounds alone, replacement seems preferable to osteotomy in most patients over the age of 60, with exceptions being made for those who perform heavy manual labor and those who continue to be active in vigorous sports. However, there is another, more important reason for preferring replacement in older patients. In a recent study of the results of osteotomy,[24] we found that patients who were over the age of 60 at the time of their surgery did less well than patients who were under this age. The difference could not be attributed to any other factors, such as more severe preoperative deformity or length of follow-up. The effect of age on the result has not been previously reported; perhaps it indicates either that cartilage damage is more widespread or that previously unloaded cartilage is less resilient in older patients when subjected to weight-bearing after osteotomy than is the case in younger subjects.

GOAL OF OSTEOTOMY: POSTOPERATIVE ALIGNMENT

Although one of the beneficial effects of osteotomy may be alteration in the vascularity or venous pressure within the bone, the major effect is mechanical.[27] Many studies have shown a relationship between clinical improvement and postoperative alignment, but there is no absolute agreement concerning the optimal position of the leg after osteotomy. Several different methods of assessing deformity and its subsequent correction are available.

FEMOROTIBIAL ANGLE (Bauer et al.[2])

The femorotibial (FT) angle is the simplest and perhaps most widely used method (Fig. 19.7). The long axes of the femur and tibia are represented by appropriate lines drawn on the radiograph and the angle formed by their intersection at the knee joint make up the femorotibial angle. The normal according to Kettelkamp and others is 175 degrees or 5 degrees of valgus.[26] The femorotibial angle is only meaningful

when measured on radiographs showing weight-bearing, as x-ray films of supine or unstressed subjects will not demonstrate loss of substance or ligament laxity. The diagnostic importance of this standing investigation cannot be overemphasized; in fact, the diagnosis of gonarthrosis may not be made at all if this investigation is omitted (Fig. 19.8A,B). The examination should be made with the loaded knee in single-leg stance, but without the patient maintaining balance by leaning to the affected side.

The normal femorotibial angle will vary according to body type and will not be the same for those of short and wide stature as for tall and thin persons. FT measurement is therefore an approximation that will also be influenced by a flexion contracture, which can alter the apparent degree of angulation. However, because of its simplicity it is widely used. Many workers have reported their results with reference to this measurement, although there has not been agreement over the desired postoperative position. Bauer et al. recommend a postoperative FT angle of between 177 and 164 degrees (three to 16 degrees of valgus). Coventry considers the normal FT angle to be a valgus deviation of 5 to 8 degrees (175 to 172 degrees) and recommends an overcorrection of 5 degrees, with the ultimate objective of osteotomy to achieve a valgus deviation of 10 to 13 degrees (170 to 167 degrees). Kettelkamp et al. recommend 5 degrees of valgus[26] (175 degrees) as the objective of osteotomy, and MacIntosh and Welsh[30] consider 5 to 7 degrees of valgus correct (175 to 173 degrees). We are in agreement with Coventry and we recommend correction to at least 170 degrees. Excessive valgus, although perhaps cosmetically unacceptable, does not prejudice function; we have cases placed in excessive valgus who continue to function well many years after osteotomy. Kettelkamp et al. cite one patient with 23 degrees of valgus and a good functional result.

DETERMINATION OF MECHANICAL AXIS USING STANDING RADIOGRAPHS INCLUDING HIP, KNEE, AND ANKLE

This method has many advocates including Harris and Kostuik,[15] Maquet,[32] Johnson et al.,[22] Hagstedt,[13] and Koshino and Tsuchiya.[28] Standing radiographs in single-leg stance are measured on the hypothesis that the weight-bearing axis will normally pass from the center of the hip through the center of

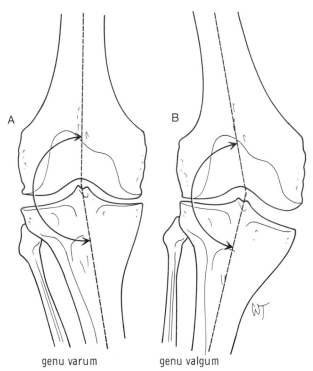

genu varum   genu valgum

Fig. 19.7. The femoral tibial angle is the simplest method of expressing varus and valgus alignment.

the knee to the center of the ankle. Deviations from this axis therefore imply that either the medial or the lateral compartment is excessively loaded. Harris and Kostuik use the deviation from the mechanical axis to determine the wedge size required (Fig. 19.9). Maquet recommends 2 to 4 degrees of overcorrection in excess of that required to restore a normal mechanical axis.[32]

The relevance of this method of static measurement is debatable. Morrison[33] has shown that in the normal knee loading is predominantly medial. Johnson et al.[22] have paired the information obtained from static full-length films including the hip and ankle with the results obtained from dynamic gait analysis. They conclude that the assumption of knee balance inherent in the concept of the mechanical axis is false. The results of gait analysis after tibial osteotomy further showed that even when corrected by osteotomy into more valgus than the mechanical axis, nearly one-half the patients still loaded the medial compartment more than the lateral. Johnson et al. concluded that while determination of the mechanical axis may be useful in predicting wedge size, it does not in itself ensure

that the desired weight transfer to the lateral compartment will be achieved. The explanation for the lack of correlation between the mechanical axis and actual weight-bearing in the knee is in the difference between the static and dynamic situations. In a static normal knee the vertical reaction from the floor passes through the center of the knee; there are no horizontal forces. The load is then shared equally between the lateral and medial compartments. Force platform measurements in a normal knee at the center of the stance phase have indicated that there will now be an additional horizontal component to the floor reaction causing the vector to be directed medially to the knee. The effect will be to increase the load in the medial plateau. The results from gait analysis have indicated that the division of load between the lateral and medial compartments of the knee will usually be more medial than might be predicted from a static analysis, except when there is a varus deformity of more than 5 degrees when both methods will predict the same result.

THREE-POINT MEASUREMENT
(Edholm et al.[10,11])

The three-point technique measures both angulation and instability (Fig. 19.10). The examination is performed supine with the knee stressed first into varus and then into valgus by means of a special jig. In each position, views of hip, knee, and ankle are obtained using a reference grid. On each of the two films of the knee three lines are drawn: the hip–ankle line from the center of the femoral head to the center of the ankle; the hip–knee line from the center of the femoral head to the center of the tibial eminence, and the knee–ankle line from the center of the eminence to the center of the ankle. The medial–lateral instability is measured as the angle through which the knee–ankle line has moved in relationship to the hip–knee line between the two measurements. The varus or valgus deviation of the knee is defined as the angle between the hip–knee line and the middle position of the knee–ankle line, that is, the bisector of the instability angle. If this bisector makes a medial deviation, it is regarded as a varus deviation; if it makes a lateral deviation, it is a valgus deviation. As the varus or valgus deviation of healthy subjects was found to be near zero, the wedge size at osteotomy

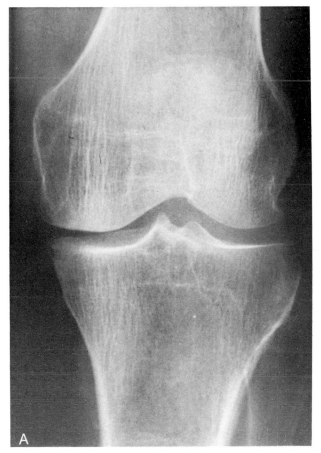 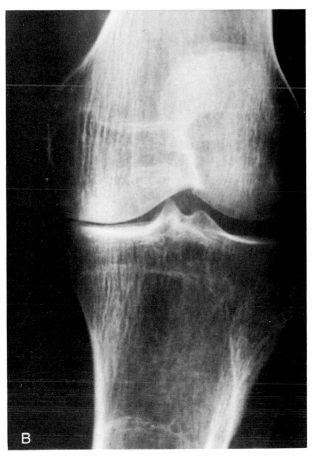

Fig. 19.8. Importance of weight-bearing radiographs. (A) Supine view. (B) Same knee shown weight-bearing.

is estimated so that the deviation after operation would be zero. Thus the size of the wedge should be the same as the deviation determined by the three-point measurement technique.

This method was applied to 21 patients undergoing tibial osteotomy; it was found that on average the knees were slightly undercorrected.[35]

The three methods all have their advantages. The FT angle measurement is simple, the mechanical axis predicts the correct static alignment for a particular individual, and the three-point measurement assesses instability. However, none is entirely accurate, and the complexity of the three-point measurement would seem to preclude it from general use. Gait analysis, although interesting, cannot predict the amount of correction required and is also of limited application because of the equipment needed. Until a more foolproof method is available, the best way to assess an arthritic knee may be to obtain a single full-length standing film to assess the mechanical axis and, when the other knee is uninvolved, the normal femorotibial angle for that particular individual. Thereafter, the femorotibial angle alone can be used for calculating the wedge size that results in 5 degrees of overcorrection and also for future follow-up examinations.

SITE OF OSTEOTOMY

In their original report, Jackson and Waugh recommended an osteotomy below the tibial tubercle and, in a more recent publication, a dome osteotomy at the level of the tubercle.[21] Maquet uses either a wedge osteotomy or for large corrections a barrel vault osteotomy above the level of the tubercle for the reason that not enough bone exists in the proximal tibia to remove a very large wedge. Generally the preferred method is the Gariépy method of wedge osteotomy done through the cancellous bone of the upper tibia proximal to the tibial tubercle. Osteotomies in this site have a broad area of contact and are therefore intrinsically stable and able to heal rapidly (Fig. 19.11) compared with the more unstable and slower healing osteotomies performed at a more distal level (Fig. 19.12). The inability to remove a really large wedge of bone from this site has become unimportant, at least in the United States, because patients with severe deformity are usually treated by total knee replacement. As total knee arthroplasty becomes more generally accepted, this will also be the case in many other parts of the world, except perhaps in those countries in which the expense of a prosthesis continues to be prohibitive. Large corrections can be obtained by Maquet's technique or by the combination of closing and opening wedge osteotomy using an iliac graft to maintain the open wedge. The opening wedge technique also has the advantage of tightening medial collateral ligament laxity (Fig. 19.13).

WEDGE SIZE

If patients selected for osteotomy have a femorotibial angle of ≤ 190 degrees (10 degrees varus) and the desired postoperative alignment is 170 degrees, a wedge of up to 20 degrees must be removed from the upper tibia. After assessment by the means discussed above the wedge size can be calculated and appropriately drawn on a radiograph of the upper tibia. However, when this calculation is translated to the actual osteotomy, further difficulties will be encountered. There is always some magnification in the radiograph, especially when a flexion contracture of the knee is present. Although a number of jigs have been devised for removing a wedge of proper size,[34] none has achieved any kind of general recognition. For most surgeons the wedge is removed by eye and confirmed by a visual and perhaps radiographic check of alignment after the osteotomy is completed.

Unfortunately, the alignment of the leg on the operating table may not be the alignment that eventually results when the patient is standing and walking. It is in the execution of wedge removal that most errors are likely to occur, and because of a natural reluctance to place the leg in excessive valgus, the error is nearly always on the side of undercorrection. Bauer et al.[2] and Coventry[5] have stated that 1 mm of

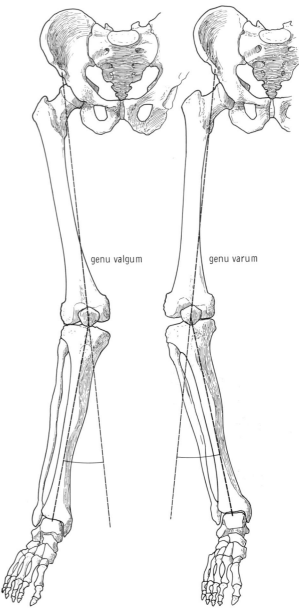

genu valgum   genu varum

Fig. 19.9. The mechanical axis (see text). (From Myrnerts, R., ed.: High tibial osteotomy in medial osteoarthritis of the knee. Linkoping University Medical Dissertations, No. 77. Linkoping 1979, Vimmerby, VTT-Grafiska, 1979, with permission.)

wedge measured at the base gives 1 degree of correction. This has to be an approximation, but one that is fairly accurate when the patient is female. For men, who generally have a larger bone size, the calculation is likely to lead to undercorrection. For men of av-

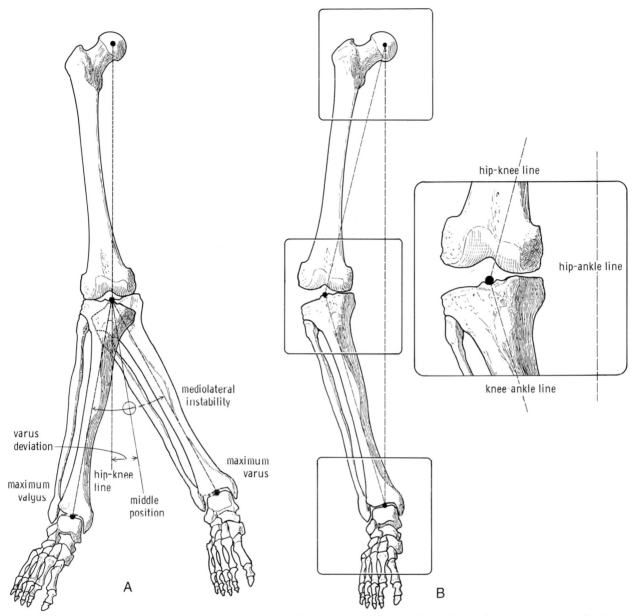

Fig. 19.10. (A,B) Three-point measurement (see text). (From Myrnerts, R., ed.: High tibial osteotomy in medical osteoarthritis of the knee. Linkoping University Medical Dissertations, No. 77. Linkoping 1979, Vimmerby, VTT-Grafiska, 1979, with permission.)

erage size, a wedge of 10 mm base size gives about 8 degrees of correction.

Sharp osteotomes are preferred for the osteotomy itself, for while an oscillating saw is more precise than an osteotome, the rate of bony union is likely to be slower because of thermal necrosis (in the single case of nonunion at The Hospital for Special Surgery, a power saw was used to do the osteotomy).

Considering the importance given to accurate correction, it seems curious that no one has yet devised a simple yet accurate method of actually performing the osteotomy.

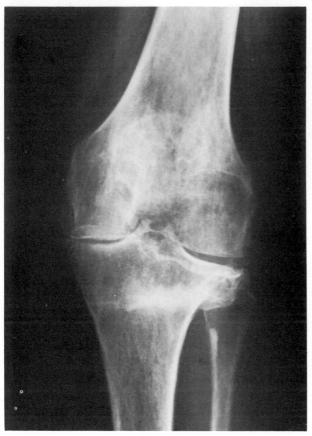

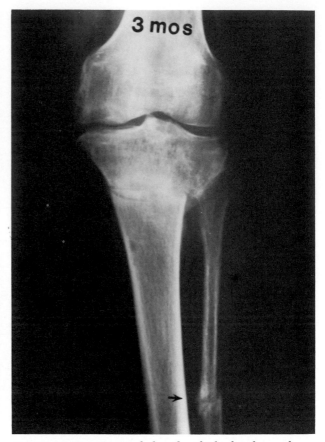

Fig. 19.11. Preferred site for high tibial osteotomy is through the cancellous bone of the upper tibia above the tibial tubercle. Union is usually rapid.

Fig. 19.12. Osteotomies below the tibial tubercle are slower and less predictable in uniting.

THE FIBULA

Unless the base of the wedge is entirely above the fibular head, the fibula will exert a tethering effect and prevent closure of the osteotomy. This can be dealt with in a number of ways (Fig. 19.14).

Osteotomy of the Fibular Shaft (Wardle,[43] Jackson and Waugh[19])

Through a short incision over the middle third of the fibula an oblique osteotomy is performed. The need for a separate incision is a minor disadvantage. More importantly, the tethering effect is not fully relieved because the proximal fragment of the fibula remains attached to the distal fragment of the tibia through the fibers of the interosseous membrane.

These fibers will often cause a medial shift of the distal tibial fragment that, although not critically important, does reduce the area of bony contact and may cause the wedge to spring open laterally, particularly when internal fixation is not used.

Fibular Head Excision (Gariépy,[12] Coventry[5])

The lateral ligament and insertion of biceps femoris are detached from the fibular styloid and a portion of the fibular head is excised to provide access to the lateral part of the upper tibia. After the osteotomy a repair of the lateral soft tissues is possible. The only disadvantage is the risk of peroneal nerve injury. Coventry did not have a peroneal palsy in his series, but Harris and Kostuik, using a similar technique, reported two in 44 osteotomies.

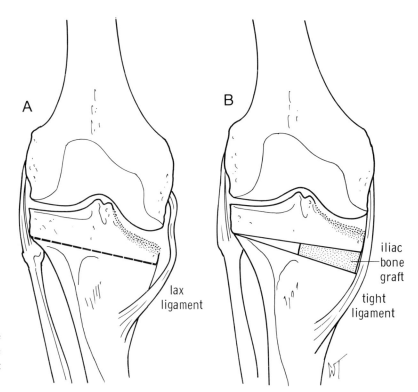

Fig. 19.13. An opening wedge osteotomy with an iliac bone graft can be used to correct unstable varus knees.

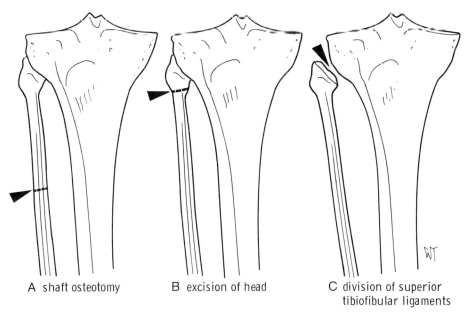

A shaft osteotomy B excision of head C division of superior tibiofibular ligaments

Fig. 19.14. Methods of relieving the tethering effect of the fibula. (A) Osteotomy of the fibular shaft. (B) Excision of the fibular head. (C) Division of the superior tibiofibular joint. (From Bauer, G.C.H., Insall, J., and Koshino, T: Tibial osteotomy in gonarthrosis [osteoarthritis of the knee]. J. Bone Joint Surg. [Am.], *51*: 1545, 1969, with permission.)

Division of the Superior Tibiofibular Joint

A transverse incision is used extending from the level of the tibial tubercle posteriorly to the fibular head. Once the muscles from the upper tibia are stripped, the superior tibiofibular joint is exposed and divided either with an osteotome or a periosteal elevator. When the fibular head is free, the posterior aspect of the tibia is accessible; after the osteotomy, the fibular head slides proximally on the proximal tibial fragment. The peroneal nerve is protected throughout by the fibular head itself; no peroneal nerve palsies have occurred with this method. A possible disadvantage is that the lateral ligament is made lax because it is attached to the fibular styloid. However, the iliotibial tract, which is a much more important lateral stabilizer in extension, remains unaltered in its attachment to the proximal tibia, and the biceps femoris readily adapts to a small change in its resting length. In any event, an increase in lateral instability has not been observed with this technique, although as performed by us until recently, a cast has been used. Currently internal fixation is being performed after this type of exposure, also without any discernible decrease in lateral stability.

Of the three methods of dealing with the fibula, shaft osteotomy seems unnecessary. Either fibular head excision or division of the superior tibiofibular joint provide excellent exposure of the upper tibia and relief of the tethering effect of the fibula at the same time. One method carries possible risk of peroneal nerve injury and the other of increasing lateral instability. Neither complication has occurred in the hands of the originators, and the choice between the two methods therefore seems a matter of personal preference.

FIXATION

Cast (Fig. 19.15)

The simplest method of fixation is to use a well-padded and molded cylinder cast extending from the upper thigh to the ankle. The cast must be molded above the medial malleolus, above the lateral aspect of the knee and in the upper medial thigh, to obtain three-point fixation. As cylinder casts inevitably slip, a thick layer of felt is placed around the ankle to minimize discomfort from the weight of the cast settling on the foot. Even so, a cast is cumbersome and universally disliked in elderly patients, however well applied. The operative cast should preferably remain in place until osteotomy healing has occurred. There is

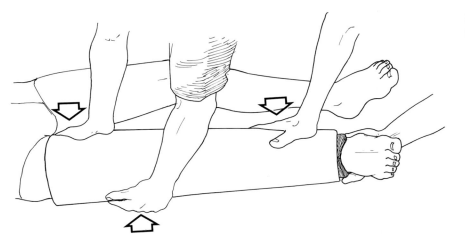

Fig. 19.15. Three-point fixation in a cast after osteotomy.

a real danger of loss of position if the cast needs changing in the first few weeks after surgery because adequate molding is often prevented because of pain. To apply a postsurgical cast that will remain for 2 months requires some practice and skill. The cast must be applied as tightly as possible in order to minimize slippage. With a tight cast, the circulation must be closely observed and the cast split, if need be, although this has never proved necessary at The Hospital for Special Surgery.

Staples

Coventry has for many years advocated the use of a stepped staple which has proved most satisfactory. In his entire series he has not noted loss of position after an initially satisfactory correction, which he attributes to the fixation provided by the staples. Coventry, however, does use a cast in addition to the staples, while Harris and Kostuik[15] consider the cast unnecessary and use only a compression dressing postoperatively. To some extent the fixation afforded by staples depends on the quality of the cancellous bone of the upper tibia; when there is osteoporosis, the staples may fail to hold and back out from the bone. The staples may actually hold the osteotomy apart if the osteotomy is not fully closed and compressed at the time of their insertion.

Plate and Screw (Fig. 19.16)

A method of internal fixation is attributed to Weber. A semitubular plate containing five to seven holes (depending on bone size) is bent to a right angle through the second hole with bending irons. The long arm of the plate is driven into the proximal fragment until flush with the lateral cortex. A long cortical bone screw is then inserted through the hole in the short arm so that it passes medially and distally at approximately 45 degrees in order to engage the medial cortex. The screw is inserted with the osteotomy fully closed; compression is obtained by tightening the screw further. The plate and screw act, in fact, as an enormous staple, but with the advantage that compression can be applied: the apparatus also cannot back out. The plate and screw method is simple, does not require extensive stripping of the upper tibia, and can be used for an osteoporotic bone.

Fixation by Blade or Y Plates (Fig. 19.17)

Fixation of the osteotomy with blade plates or Y plates of Arbeitsgemeinschaft für Osteosythesefragen (AO) design is practiced in Europe, but not widely in the United States. Very secure fixation is obtained at the expense of a wider exposure with greater soft tissue stripping from the lateral aspect of the tibia. The method has not become popular in the United States probably because of a relative unfamiliarity with the necessary equipment and techniques.

External Fixation with Transfixion Pins and Frame (Fig. 19.18)

Single or double Steinmann pins are passed through proximal and distal fragments and held with Charnley clamps or a similar external frame. This method has been advocated by numerous workers who emphasize that firm fixation allows early motion, which is particularly important if routine arthrotomy is practiced at the time of osteotomy. Complications are pin tract infections and peroneal nerve palsy. MacIntosh and Welsh[30] report nine pin tract infections and 14 peroneal nerve palsies in 116 knees; Jackson et al.[21] 13 pin tract infections and eight palsies; Maquet[32] no infections but three palsies; and Beltrami et al.[3] nine infections and 12 nerve palsies. Pin and frame fixation is appealing because of its relative simplicity, but clearly these complications must be considered before choosing the method.

COMPLICATIONS OF OSTEOTOMY[20]

Notwithstanding early misgivings, high tibial osteotomy has generally proved a relatively simple and complication-free procedure even in elderly patients. However, significant and serious complications can occur that in some instances seem related to a particular technique. The complications noted in 10 clinical series[3,5,13,15,17,21,30,32,35,43] totaling 804 osteotomies were analyzed. Sixty infections were reported, of which 55 were superficial and five were deep. Thirty-seven of the infections occurred in association with transfixion pins and an external frame. Fifty-six peroneal nerve palsies were reported, 37 associated with transfixion pins. Eight intra-articular fractures occurred, most of

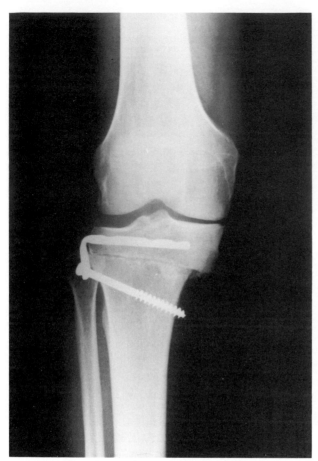

Fig. 19.16. Plate and screw fixation.

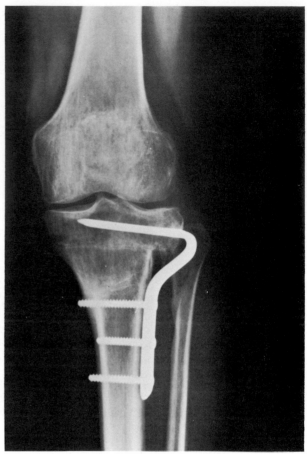

Fig. 19.17. Blade-plate fixation.

which were caused by a proximal tibial fragment that was made too thin.

In regard to general complications, one vascular injury was reported to what was thought to be the anterior tibial artery; the operative procedure was aborted, but when no sequelae occurred, the osteotomy was successfully completed at a later date. Most probably the artery involved was the peroneal rather than anterior tibial. There were no cases reported of injury to the popliteal artery. Coventry had one patient in whom gangrene developed after osteotomy and who required an above-knee amputation. This patient had preexisting arterial insufficiency, and the gangrene was not in any way caused by arterial injury at the time of surgery.

Twenty-nine cases of clinically diagnosed deep vein

thrombosis and 13 cases of pulmonary embolism were recorded. Two patients died after pulmonary embolism. Most authorities have not considered either deep vein thrombosis or pulmonary embolism a particular problem after osteotomy, but perhaps a 0.25 percent death rate from pulmonary embolism requires second thoughts. Curiously, both of the reported deaths occurred with the pin and frame fixation method, and presumably early motion was practiced.

TECHNIQUE OF OSTEOTOMY

Three methods are described in detail, two of which can be combined with transfixion pins, staples, or plate and screw fixation.

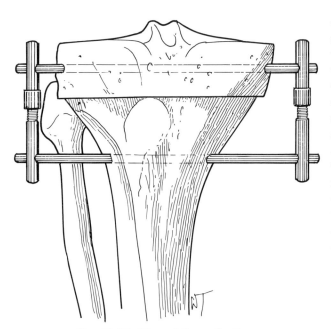

Fig. 19.18. Pin and frame fixation.

OSTEOTOMY WITH DIVISION OF SUPERIOR TIBIOFIBULAR JOINT (Fig. 19.19A–G)

This method has been used for the past 10 years at The Hospital for Special Surgery. The patient is placed supine with a small sandbag placed beneath the left buttock in order to prevent external rotation of the leg. The knee is flexed about 45 degrees over folded sheets. A tourniquet is used routinely.

A transverse skin incision is made extending from the tibial tubercle to the fibular head. Skin flaps are raised proximally and distally. A vertical incision is made in the knee capsule lateral to the patellar tendon and extended distally along the lateral aspect of the tibial tubercle and the crest of the tibia. A transverse incision is made through the fascia at the upper limit of the anterolateral musculature at right angles to the first incision and extending posteriorly to the superior tibiofibular joint. The muscles are stripped from the anterior crest and lateral surface. The lateral condyle is exposed by reflecting the fascial attachments proximally. The anterior surface of the superior tibiofibular joint is thereby exposed, and using an osteotome or a periosteal elevator, the fibers of the capsule of this joint are divided completely so that the fibular head can move freely on the tibia. The pos-

terior surface of the tibia is then exposed by driving a periosteal elevator across to the medial border. Anterior exposure can be increased by removing a portion of the patellar ligament insertion from the tibial tuberosity. A retractor is placed posteriorly and another anteriorly beneath the patellar ligament. A wedge of the appropriate size is marked with methylene blue on the lateral condyle of the tibia. The proximal cut should be at least 1.5 cm distal to the joint surface, which can be located either with a needle or by direct inspection. The osteotomy is inclined medially and distally to allow for the normal medial slope of the upper tibia and for bone erosion that may have occurred in the medial tibial condyle; otherwise, if the osteotomy is made too transverse, the joint may be entered medially. Using a sharp osteotome, the osteotomy is completed about three-quarters of the way across the tibia, and the wedge of bone is removed so that the remainder of the osteotomy can be completed under direct vision. The medial bone at the apex of the wedge is weakened by placing several drill holes through it; the medial cortex is divided last without damaging the medial soft tissue attachments and the superficial medial ligament. The osteotomy should then close without resistance; when any degree of force is needed, the reason must be sought. Usually the fibular head remains attached to the tibia, or the medial cortex has not been fully divided. Forcible correction may fracture the proximal fragment[20] and must therefore be avoided. When the wedge closes, the fibular head slides proximally on the upper tibia; correction can be maintained by gentle pressure. A long alignment rod, such as that used for total knee arthroplasty, assesses the degree of correction, so that when aligned with the center of the ankle and tibial tubercle, the proximal end of the rod passes at least 2.5 cm (1 inch) medial to the hip joint. If the position is satisfactory, the wound is closed and the position maintained with a well-fitting plaster cylinder.

Partial weight-bearing is permitted 2 days after surgery, and the patient is progressed to walking with a cane as soon as pain allows, normally within 2 weeks of surgery. Unless the postoperative cast becomes uncomfortable or very loose, it is not changed. A radiologic assessment of the osteotomy is made 4 weeks after surgery, mainly to confirm that position has not been lost. The cast is removed 8 weeks after surgery,

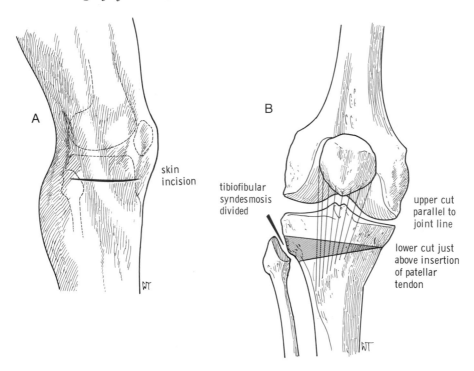

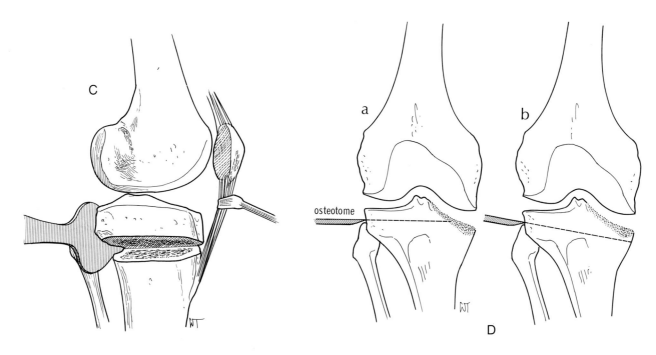

Fig. 19.19. Hospital for Special Surgery technique of osteotomy. (A) Skin incision. (B) Division of superior tibiofibular joint and outline of osteotomy. (C) Lateral view of required exposure with a retractor placed posteriorly. (D) The osteotomy must not enter the medial side of the joint, hence must be inclined distally as well as medially. (Figure continues)

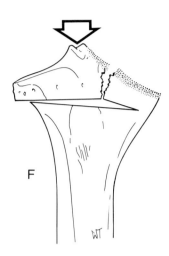

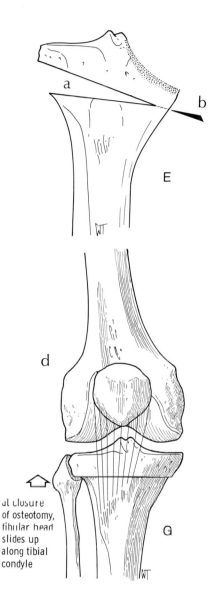

Fig. 19.19 (Continued). (E) The apex of the wedge is slightly medial to the medial cortex, permitting removal of this bone before the osteotomy is completed. (F) If force is used to close the osteotomy, a fracture of the proximal fragment may result. (G) Completed osteotomy.

al closure of osteotomy, fibular head slides up along tibial condyle

and a clinical and radiologic assessment of union is made. In most patients, the osteotomy is solid and knee flexion can then begin. If there is doubt about the degree of bony union, a further cylinder cast is applied for another month, as loss of correction can still occur at this stage (Fig. 19.20A,B).

Quadriceps exercises and straight leg raising are done throughout the convalescent period and are continued after cast removal. Lifting of weights is generally not recommended for fear of overstressing the arthritic knee.

TECHNIQUE OF INTERNAL FIXATION BY BLADE-PLATE FIXATION (FIG. 19.21A–D) (HOSPITAL COCHIN, PARIS)

A most satisfactory method of internal fixation has been developed by surgeons at the Hospital Cochin.[7] A vertical incision is made beginning midway between the patella and fibular head and extending distally for about 12 cm to the crest of the tibia. The upper tibia is exposed by making a fascial incision along the crest of the tibia extending proximally to

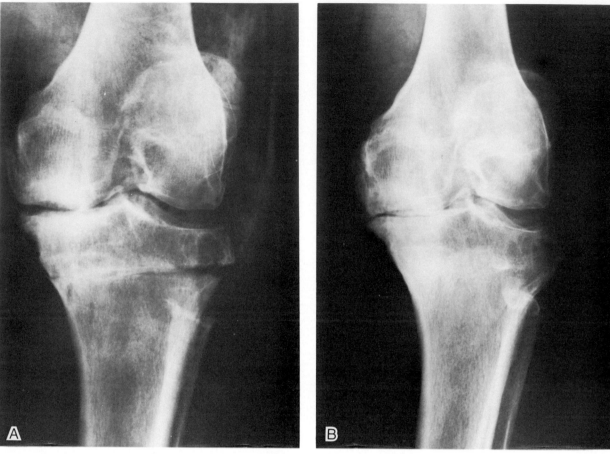

Fig. 19.20. Loss of correction. (A) Position was lost during a cast change; the base of the wedge has opened. (B) The result is undercorrection with union of the osteotomy in slight varus.

the fibular head. The patellar ligament and tibial tubercle are exposed by a vertical incision along the lateral border of the patellar ligament, which may be continued proximally through the lateral patellar retinaculum as far as the vastus lateralis, if a lateral patellar release is indicated. The tethering effect of the fibula is removed either by fibular shaft osteotomy or by separation of the superior tibiofibular joint. The lateral joint line is identified with a needle, and a point is selected midway between the tibial tubercle and fibular head 12 mm distal to the surface of the lateral tibial plateau. By means of a special jig, a guide wire is driven transversely across the upper tibia. The jig can be set for a predetermined amount of correction to overcorrect the mechanical axis by 3 to 5 degrees. The jig is normally set for use with a 90-degree

blade plate, but when greater correction is required, it can be used with an alternative 100-degree blade plate. The track for the blade plate is cut in the proximal fragment with a cannulated cutting tool, which is passed over the guide wire and aligned with the jig. The tool is driven into the tibia for a distance of 6 to 7 cm. The osteotomy is marked with methylene blue; the proximal limb is parallel with the guide wire and situated 12 mm distal to it. The wedge-size calculation is made. After wedge removal, the osteotomy is completed, the previously selected blade plate is driven over the guide wire and fixed to the tibial cortex with three screws. Radiographic checks are made at two stages, the first after insertion of the guide wire and the second after insertion of the plate. The method by virtue of the plate and the special jig provides

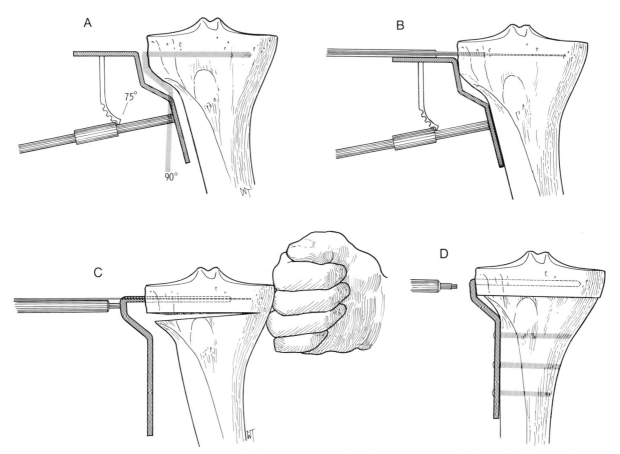

Fig. 19.21. Blade-plate fixation. (A) The guide instrument is set for the correction angle desired. (B) A guide wire is drilled into the proximal tibia. (C) After completion of the osteotomy, the blade plate is driven into the proximal tibia over the guide wire. (D) The blade is screwed to the tibia. (From d'Aubigné, A.M.: Joint realignment in the management of osteoarthritis. In Straub, L.R., and Wilson, P.D., Jr., eds.; Clinical Trends in Orthopaedics. New York, Thieme-Stratton, p. 246, 1982, with permission.)

automatic correction. The fascia is closed over a suction drain. Because anterior compartment syndromes have been reported by the originators of this technique, care must be taken to avoid traumatizing the muscles during the operation and to avoid a postoperative hematoma.

Aftercare

A compression dressing is applied that is removed after 1 week, at which time knee rehabilitation exercises are begun. Walking is permitted with crutches, but weight-bearing is delayed until union of the osteotomy has occurred.

OSTEOTOMY WITH EXCISION OF FIBULAR HEAD (Coventry[5]) (Fig. 19.22A–F)

With tourniquet applied to the thigh, the knee is flexed to 90 degrees (a position that relaxes the neurovascular structures and allows them to fall posteriorly); a lateral incision is made through the distal part of the iliotibial band parallel and anterior to the fibular collateral ligament and extending proximally as far as the level of the joint space. The tendon of the biceps femoris and fibular collateral ligament are removed by sharp dissection from the head of the fibula as a wide-conjoined tendon, and the fibular head is excised with an osteotome. During this procedure,

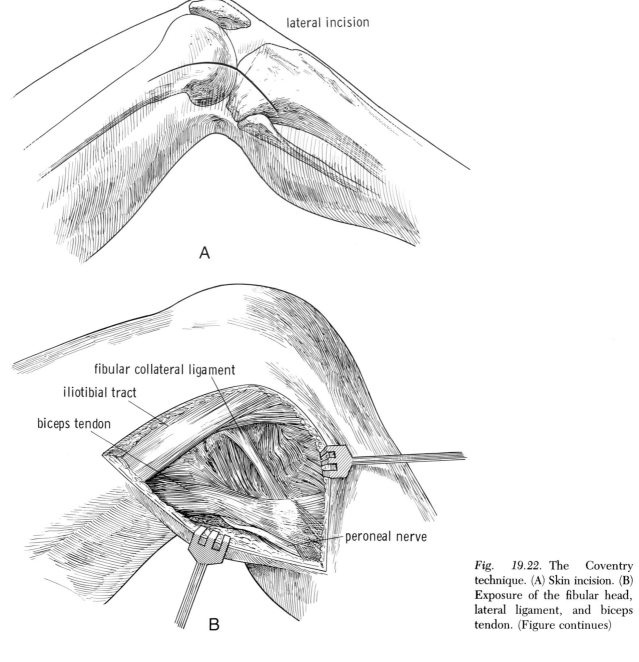

Fig. 19.22. The Coventry technique. (A) Skin incision. (B) Exposure of the fibular head, lateral ligament, and biceps tendon. (Figure continues)

a finger is placed on the peroneal nerve to identify and protect it. It is best not to dissect it out and isolate it, but rather to keep it covered by its envelope of fatty tissue. A small incision through the capsule of the knee will then permit visualization of the lateral lip of the tibia for purposes of orientation. The soft tissues are stripped from the front of the tibia ante-riorly as far as the patellar tendon and posteriorly for the full width of the posterior surface of the tibia so that both the anterior and the posterior tibial cortex can be seen. An osteotomy is then carried out under direct vision using a wide osteotome. The upper limb of the wedge is first marked out along a plane 2 cm below and parallel to the articular surface, so that the

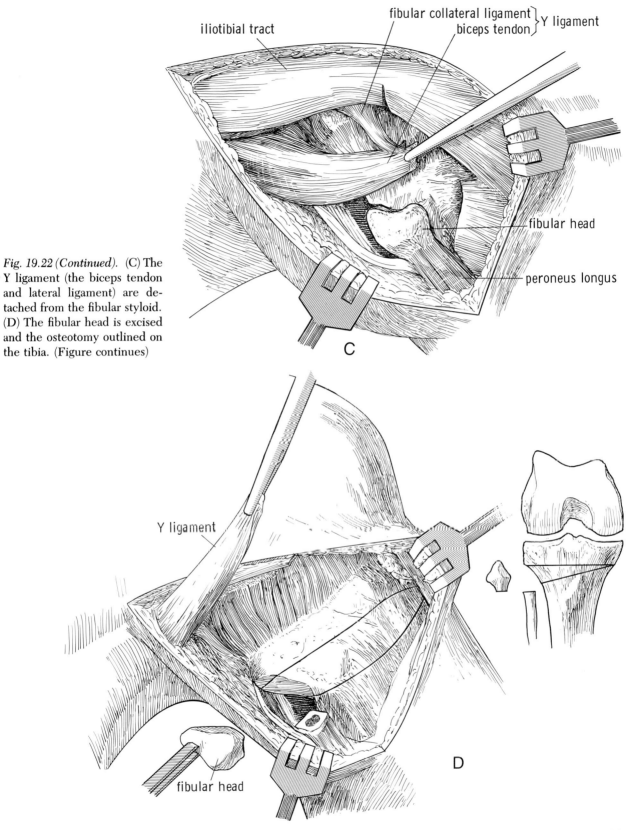

iliotibial tract

fibular collateral ligament
biceps tendon

Y ligament

fibular head

peroneus longus

Fig. 19.22 (Continued). (C) The Y ligament (the biceps tendon and lateral ligament) are detached from the fibular styloid. (D) The fibular head is excised and the osteotomy outlined on the tibia. (Figure continues)

C

Y ligament

fibular head

D

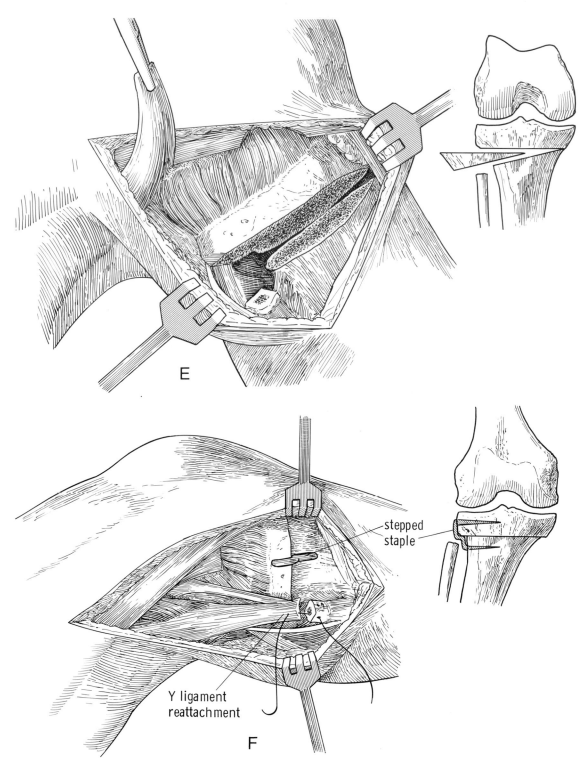

E

F

stepped
staple

Y ligament
reattachment

Fig. 19.22 (Continued). (E) Completed osteotomy. (F) The osteotomy is closed and
held with a staple; the Y ligament is reattached to the fibula. (From Coventry, M.B.:
Osteotomy about the knee for degenerative and rheumatoid arthritis. Indications, operative technique, and results. J. Bone Joint Surg. [Am.], 55: 23, 1973, with permission.)

proximal fragment will be large enough to accommodate the staple and provide fixation. The appropriate wedge is then marked out below the previously established line and the wedge is removed. After it has been removed, the opposite (medial) cortex of the tibia is perforated with a 6.4 mm osteotome in a few places, so that the cortical bone can be easily fractured. The knee is then extended, and cut ends of the bone are brought together and held securely with a stepped staple. The tourniquet is released, blood vessels are coagulated, and the knee is placed in 45 degrees of flexion while the operation is completed. The biceps tendon and fibular collateral ligament which are in the form of a Y ligament are reattached by a suture through a drill hole in the neck of the fibula; this attachment is then reinforced by sutures through the iliotibial band and the anterior coronal fascia. The incision in the fascia lata is then approximated with horizontal mattress sutures. One suction drain is inserted posteriorly before the wound is closed. A modified Robert Jones dressing (cotton cast with posterior plaster splint) is used for 8 days after operation. A cylinder cast is then applied for about 5 weeks, and weight-bearing with crutches is allowed. Union has usually occurred by this time. After cast removal, active exercises are commenced. Manipulation to gain motion is almost never indicated. The patient continues to use crutches usually for about 4 weeks after the cast has been removed until he or she can walk well, without pain or swelling. The patient then uses a cane, which can gradually be discarded with improving gait.

RESULTS

Numerous reports in the literature attest to the effectiveness of high tibial osteotomy in relieving pain and improving function.[36,40]

Jackson et al.,[21] to whom the operation is most often attributed, reported on 70 osteotomies. Forty-six had a varus deformity and the follow-up ranged from 1 to 8 years. The osteotomy was at the level of the tuberosity by a curved osteotomy convex upward. The fibula was divided through a separate incision. Fixation was by a cast in one group and by transfixion pins and frame in the second group. In the 46 varus knees, complete relief of pain was achieved in 31, partial relief in 13, and no relief in two. In the plaster fixation group, delayed union occurred in three patients and bone grafting was done (Fig. 19.23). In the transfixion pin group dorsiflexion weakness of the foot was noticed in eight patients. There were also four superficial wound infections and 13 pin tract infections in the pin group.

Devas[9] reported on 28 knees of which 21 were preceded by, or combined with, excision of the patella. Fixation was by transfixion pins and compression clamps. The follow-up was a minimum of 6 months. The results were classified as good in 22, fair in three, and bad in two. Two patients had a peroneal nerve palsy.

Bauer et al.[2] emphasized the importance of obtaining correct alignment. In a group of 63 arthritic knees, most of which had a varus deformity, high tibial osteotomy resulted in a stable, mobile, painless knee in

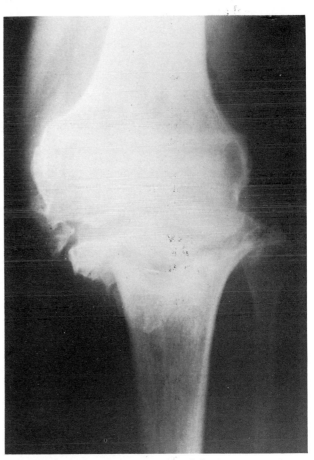

Fig. 19.23. Delayed or nonunion of the osteotomy is rare but does occur occasionally, especially when the proximal fragment is thin, perhaps because of avascular necrosis.

43 patients. Harris and Kostuik[15] based their results on the patient's subjective evaluation. Their results were as follows: 26 good, five fair, and five poor results. No patient suffered a decrease in range of motion.

Coventry[5] described his personal results with tibial osteotomy over an 11-year period. His series included 86 knees in which the osteotomy was done for degenerative arthritis. A good result, defined as relief of all or most of the pain, 90 degrees or more of motion, and with functional activity equal to the status before onset of symptoms, was obtained in 76 knees. A fair result was obtained in seven knees. These patients had bothersome pain, limited motion, mild instability, or a combination of these symptoms, but were able to work; also, the pain was less severe than it had been before operation. Three knees had a poor result, one of which was attributable to a postoperative femoral artery thrombosis, resulting in a below-the-knee amputation. One other knee had a good result for 8 years, after which pain and deformity occurred. The third poor result was in a patient with previous extensive osteochondritis dissecans for whom pain was unrelieved.

In a later report, Coventry[6] gave his results with a longer follow-up, with 61.8 percent of patients rating themselves as having less pain than before osteotomy, even 10 years after surgery. Functionally, 64.7 percent of patients felt better. Coventry concluded that the major complication is recurrence of deformity and stated that this can be minimized by achieving at least 7 degrees of valgus axial alignment (up to 10 degrees is allowable) and by excluding from operation knees with bicompartmental involvement. None of the seven knees corrected to > 10 degrees of valgus was unsatisfactory.

Insall et al.[17] followed 51 osteoarthritic knees treated by high tibial osteotomy for at least 5 years. From the viewpoint of patient satisfaction, and in terms of pain relief, stability, motion, and walking ability, the overall result was satisfactory in 33 of the 51 knees (three with valgus and 30 with varus deformity) and unsatisfactory in 18 knees (three with valgus and 15 with varus deformity). All 18 unsatisfactory results became apparent within 3 years. Of these 18, 13 were unsatisfactory within 1 year, most of them immediately after operation. Two knees deteriorated in the second postoperative year and three in the third postoperative year. From this observation it seems that an unsatisfactory clinical result tends to be apparent

relatively early. The eventual result seemed to be influenced by the amount of preoperative deformity. When this was between 180 and 190 degrees 23 of 26 knees (88 percent) were stable, mobile, and painless after osteotomy. Of three failures, two were overcorrected and one was undercorrected. In contrast, when a preoperative deformity exceeded 190 degrees, a satisfactory result was obtained in only 7 of 19 knees (Fig. 19.24). Of the 12 failures, 11 were associated with undercorrection and one with overcorrection. However, Maquet[32] states that a properly planned osteotomy can succeed even when the preoperative angular deformity exceeds 195 degrees. He

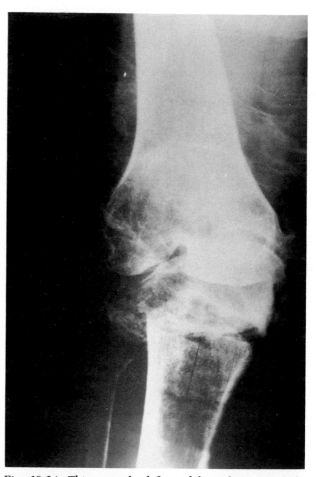

Fig. 19.24. This severely deformed knee has apparently been corrected after osteotomy with cast immobilization. However, note that much of the correction has occurred in the knee joint itself and the medial joint space has opened widely. When the cast is removed the knee will relapse to a varus position.

recommends preoperative evaluation with full-length standing radiographs from which a precise preoperative drawing can be made showing the amount of correction required. A very precise osteotomy giving some overcorrection must then be performed above the tibial tubercle. As the amount of bone available may not be sufficient to remove a large wedge, he recommends a curved barrel vault osteotomy. Fixation is by Steinmann pins and an external frame. Maquet records excellent results in 32 of 41 patients. Good results were obtained in five patients and fair and poor results in four patients. There were three peroneal nerve palsies.

MacIntosh has practiced a combined tibial osteotomy and open joint debridement since 1961. The osteotomy is fixed with Steinmann pins and external Charnley-type clamps. MacIntosh and Welch[30] report on 116 procedures followed for an average of 5.4 years. At this time, 81.9 percent of the knees were rated good or satisfactory (64 good, 31 satisfactory, and 21 failed). Ten knees required a manipulation and there were 9 pin tract infections and 14 peroneal nerve palsies. Four osteotomies required bone grafting for nonunion.

Vainionpää et al.[41] report on 103 knees followed for an average of 6.9 years. The result was good or fair in 86 knees (83.5 percent). An average of 3.4 years after osteotomy, deterioration was demonstrable in 26 knees in which the initial result had been good; this is a higher incidence of deterioration than in previously published series. In 16 of the 103 knees, a total arthroplasty was subsequently performed because of a poor result an average of 7.6 years after the osteotomy. These workers recommended an optimal postoperative alignment of 170 to 173 degrees.

The most recent review at The Hospital for Special Surgery has been in general agreement with the above study and has differed in some important aspects from our previous reports.[24] Ninety-five knees with an average follow-up of 8.5 years (range 5 to 14 years) were examined. All had osteonecrosis or medial compartment osteoarthritis with a femorotibial angle of < 190 degrees in 87 knees and > 190 degrees in eight knees. The average age at osteotomy was 60 years, with 47 being younger and 48 being older than the average. The results were assessed using the rating system that for many years has formed the basis of our studies on total knee arthroplasty and which is described elsewhere. At follow-up, 63 percent were in excellent or good categories and 37 percent fair or

poor. Twenty-four knees were subsequently revised to a total knee replacement.

This group of cases overlapped but by no means coincided with the cases reported in 1974. Thus, in this group there were no valgus knees; only 8 percent had a varus deformity exceeding 190 degrees compared with 42 percent with this degree of deformity in the earlier series. Six of the eventual fair and poor results were apparent within the first 3 years and in the remainder, deterioration occurred after that time; even at 5 years 80 knees or 83 percent still had either an excellent or good rating.

We have previously recommended a correction aimed at achieving a femorotibial angle of 170 degrees ± 5 degrees. Using this criterion, 75 knees were properly corrected, of which 64 percent still had a satisfactory result at the time of follow-up (Fig. 19.25). Fourteen knees were undercorrected and 50 percent

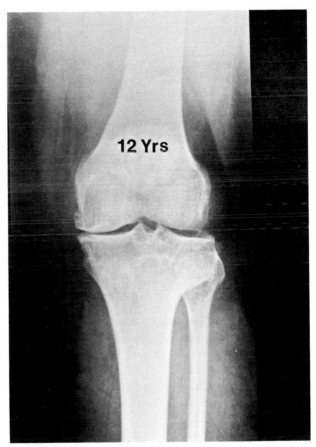

Fig. 19.25. This varus knee was corrected to a femorotibial angle of 170 degrees (10 degrees of valgus). The result remains excellent after 12 years.

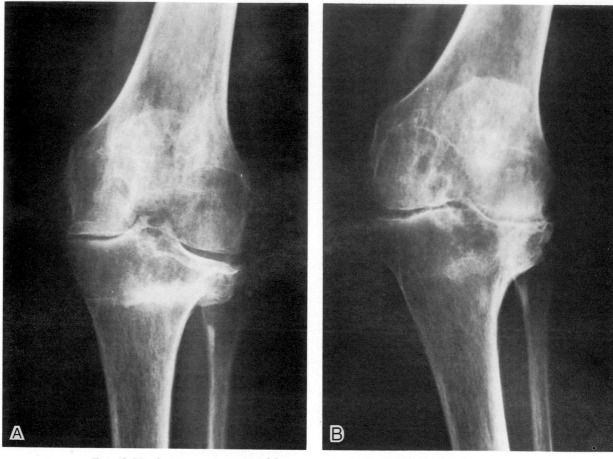

Fig. 19.26. Overcorrection caused by progressive arthritis. (A) Postoperative film one year after osteotomy showing a femorotibial angle of 170 degrees. (B) At 7 years after osteotomy, the femorotibial angle was 160 degrees, resulting from progressive loss of lateral articular space.

had a satisfactory result. Six knees were overcorrected, 83.5 of which still had a satisfactory result when examined.

If 170 degrees is taken as the minimum acceptable correction, and no limit is placed on overcorrection, there were 59 knees with a postoperative alignment of >170 degrees and 33 (56 percent) had an excellent or good result. In contrast, when the femorotibial angle was 170 degrees or less 27 of 37 knees (73 percent) were in the excellent or good categories (Fig. 19.26).

One other factor emerged from this study that to my knowledge has not been mentioned before. Patients who were under the age of 60 at the time of osteotomy did much better than did patients who were older. Thus, in the under-60 group 76 percent had a

satisfactory result compared with 51 percent of the 48 osteotomies done in patients over the age of 60. Other possible variables, such as extent of deformity and adequacy of correction, were examined and found to be equally distributed in both groups.

In summary, the results confirm that high tibial osteotomy is a useful and reliable operation for varus gonarthrosis. The ideal correction would seem to be between 170 and 165 degrees, and the utmost precision in planning, performing, and fixing the osteotomy is important. Full-length standing radiographs are most useful in this regard, but are probably no more valid than the femorotibial angle in predicting the load transfer to the lateral compartment. Staples or cast fixation seem preferable to pin and frame tech-

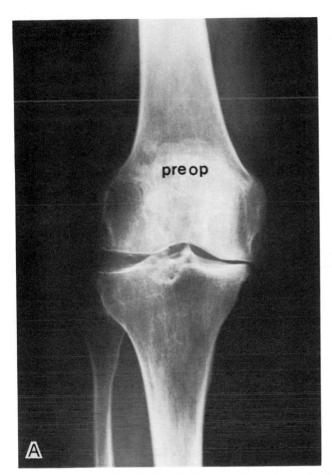
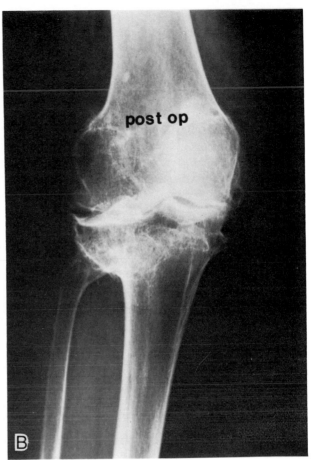

Fig. 19.27. (A) Preoperative radiograph of a varus knee suitable for high tibial osteotomy. (B) Although properly corrected to a femorotibial angle of 170 degrees, 10 years after osteotomy progressive arthritis involving both lateral and medial compartments is noted.

niques in that the latter have a high incidence of infection and nerve palsy. Adequacy of selection and technique notwithstanding, there is evidence of deterioration in the results with time because of progressive arthritis in previously unaffected areas of the joint (Fig. 19.27A,B). Finally, there is also some evidence that the best results of osteotomy are in younger patients, providing a further reason for preferring total knee arthroplasty in the elderly.

FEMORAL OSTEOTOMY

The preceding discussion of high tibial osteotomy has alluded to the undesirability of using this technique for the treatment of lateral compartment osteoarthritis with valgus deformity. Although in early series on osteotomy no distinction was made between varus and valgus, in recent years it has become apparent that valgus knees do not respond as well to tibial osteotomy.[14] There are a number of reasons for this.

HIP DEFORMITIES

When valgus angulation and arthritis are secondary to long-standing adduction contracture of the ipsilateral hip joint, correction of the knee deformity by osteotomy will not be successful. In these cases the hip deformity must be corrected first either by osteotomy or arthroplasty, depending on circumstances.

Valgus deformity is sometimes associated with a long-standing arthrodesis of the hip in correct position without adduction. This situation may be an exception in that correction of the knee deformity alone will suffice. Likewise, a valgus knee is sometimes found associated with congenital dysplasia of the hip; it may be the product of manipulation and the prolonged immobilization of the knee in early life incurred as a result of treatment of the hip condition. Again, when there is no fixed adduction of the hip, osteotomy of the knee is sufficient, although each case requires careful evaluation. The patient is asked to stand with the feet spread apart as far as is possible; when the femur on the affected side becomes vertical in this position, correction of the knee deformity alone is indicated, whereas when the femur remains adducted, the hip deformity must be corrected first.

OBLIQUITY OF THE TIBIAL PLATEAU

When valgus deformity is corrected in the tibia, tilting of the joint axis in the frontal plane will be found. This is because (with the exception of post-traumatic arthritis secondary to a tibial plateau fracture) lateral compartment arthritis is associated with a deficiency of the lateral femoral condyle. The obliquity was first noted by Wardle, who considered it unimportant, a viewpoint supported by Bauer et al., who described the tilting as inelegant but inconsequential. Further studies showed these opinions to be incorrect. While minor degrees of tilting may be compatible with a good result, when the obliquity exceeds 12 to 15 degrees it becomes significant; instead of transferring weight from the lateral to the medial compartment, marked tilting causes the weight

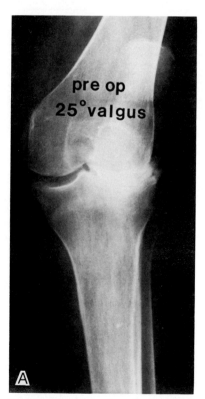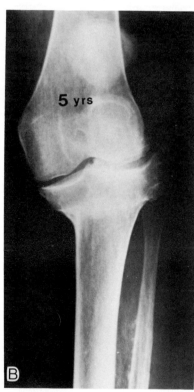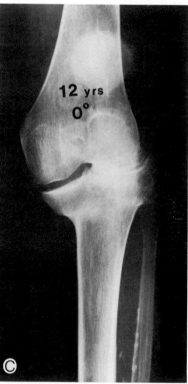

Fig. 19.28. Correction of valgus deformity by tibial osteotomy. (A) Preoperative radiograph. (B) After 5 years the result is excellent; the obliquity of the joint axis is 15 degrees. (C) At 12 years, medial subluxation of the tibia has occurred, but the result still remains good. This case is unusual, and tibial osteotomy for valgus does not usually give such a satisfactory result.

transfer to shift only to the lateral part of the inter-condylar eminence and with time a medial subluxation of femur on tibia is likely.

INSTABILITY

As with the corresponding varus deformities, long-standing valgus angulation leads to stretching of the medial collateral ligament. However, unlike the case of varus angulation, wedge osteotomy for valgus accentuates the medial collateral laxity because the medial base of the osteotomy lies between origin and insertion of the ligament. This can of course be partially solved by a reconstruction of the medial collateral ligament by distal advancement. This solution was attempted in some of our cases without success because the staples used for fixation backed out, resulting in marked instability.

OVERCORRECTION INTO VARUS

The ideal postoperative position after correction of valgus deformity is 175 degrees but, because of the teeter effect, it is very difficult to obtain this correction when there is medial laxity. To avoid recurrence of valgus, a position closer to 180 degrees is needed. We have also found a tendency to overestimate the necessary wedge size, which again leads to overcorrection.

Overcorrection may also occur during the healing phase in spite of accurate postoperative correction. Most likely, this is caused by allowing weight-bearing in a cylinder cast. Morrison and others have shown that in the normal knee weight bearing during the stance phase of gait is predominantly medial so that presumably the same will be true after osteotomy leading to a tendency for the osteotomy to deform into varus. It is difficult to prevent this tendency by providing an adequate degree of immobilization in the cast especially when the patient is obese. The same mechanism exists after correction of varus deformity and may contribute to undercorrection.

Shoji and Insall[37] reviewed the experience at The Hospital for Special Surgery. Forty-nine knees were examined with an average follow-up of 31 months (range 13 to 69 months). Pain relief was complete in

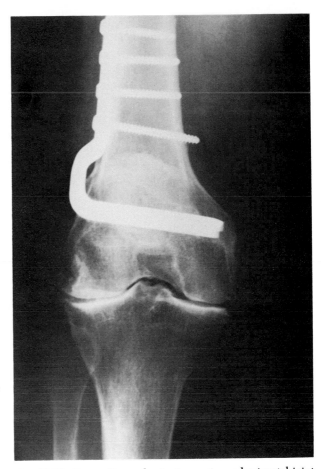

Fig. 19.29. Lower femoral osteotomy gives a horizontal joint line.

53 percent, partial in 14 percent, and not obtained in 33 percent. Only 17 of the 49 knees were stable, mobile, and painless, in contrast to 42 of 63 knees in an earlier series from the Knee Service assessed by Bauer et al.

We agree with Coventry that a satisfactory result can be obtained when the postoperative alignment is correct and when the plateau tilt does not exceed about 12 degrees (Fig. 19.28A–C). In practice, however, the technical difficulties in obtaining the required position have led us to correct valgus deformities by low femoral osteotomy. We also believe that while some degree of joint tilting is acceptable, it surely must be better for the plane of the joint to be parallel with the ground which can only be achieved by femoral osteotomy (Fig. 19.29).

In selecting cases for femoral osteotomy, the alternative of total knee replacement must be considered. Because femoral osteotomy requires a lengthy period of partial weight-bearing on crutches, it is less suitable than high tibial osteotomy for elderly patients; hence the age and expected activity level of the patient are of paramount importance. Severe instability (usually associated with severe deformity) is also a contraindication to osteotomy, because instability will persist even when the alignment is correct. Panarthritis, severe patellofemoral arthritis, a flexion contracture exceeding 30 degrees, and an arc of motion of < 80 degrees are also contraindications.

As with high tibial osteotomy, there will be borderline cases in which making the correct choice is difficult and in which both osteotomy and replacement seem equally appropriate. Under these circumstances the surgeon must turn to personal experience and familiarity with the two procedures. Within this context, it must be noted that for severe deformity and instability, both relative contraindications to osteotomy, the technical difficulties in performing total knee replacement are greatest. For this reason, surgeons relatively inexperienced in total replacement may prefer to stretch the indications for osteotomy somewhat.

TECHNIQUE OF LOW FEMORAL OSTEOTOMY (FIG. 19.30)

The incision preferred on the Knee Service is similar to that used for total knee replacement but because the exposure required is of the lower femur, the distal portion of the incision does not need to be fully developed. This approach is preferred because of the complete accessibility to both sides of the lower femoral metaphysis, which is not obtained by the alternative of separate medial and lateral incisions. The wedge is removed with the base medial and the osteotomy is fixed with a four-hole 90-degree hip plate applied to the lateral aspect of the bone. The available blade plates do not fit well on the medial side of the lower femur and there is little room proximally for applying a compression device because of femoral vessels in the adductor canal.

The exposure gives excellent access to the lower 20 cm of the femur. The periosteum is stripped from the lateral and posterior aspects and from a small area

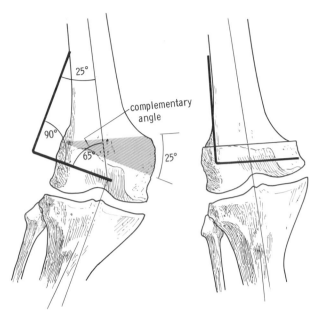

Fig. 19.30. Technique of lower femoral osteotomy (see text).

medially, so that Bennett retractors can be passed around the femur at the site of osteotomy immediately proximal to the femoral groove. The osteotomy wedge size is calculated from preoperative standing radiographs, preferably full length, including the hip and ankle joints. Cut-out drawings are made on the radiograph to predict accurately the amount of correction; from this the wedge size is calculated, remembering that there will be a magnification factor of about 15 percent, although the predetermined angle will remain the same when translated to the bone. The osteotomy is marked on the lower femur with methylene blue and placed in such a manner that after removal of the wedge, the osteotomy line will be as transverse as possible. This is best achieved by inclining the distal arm of the wedge obliquely so that it lies parallel to the articular surfaces. The proximal arm of the osteotomy is made transversely across the bone. If correctly done, such an osteotomy would produce an alignment of 180 degrees, whereas the desired postoperative alignment is between 175 and 180 degrees. Therefore, a slight adjustment is made in the inclination of the distal arm of the wedge. When there is a coexistent flexion contracture, this can usually be corrected by impacting the anterior cortex of the proximal fragment into the distal fragment.

When the osteotomy is marked the guide for the blade plate is driven into the lateral femoral condyle at an angle to the femoral shaft that is complimentary to the osteotomy angle. The positioning of the guide should also allow for correction of flexion contracture. A 90-degree blade plate is driven in part way until the plate impinges proximally against the lateral femoral shaft. The osteotomy is then performed with a power saw. The knee should be flexed to make the soft tissues more easily retractable and to ensure that the posterior vessels fall away from the bone. (The vessels, in any event, are protected by posteriorly placed retractors.) When the osteotomy is complete, the bone wedge is removed and the osteotomy closed, allowing the blade plate to be driven in fully. The plate is clamped to the femoral shaft and a compression device affixed proximally. When the osteotomy has been compressed, three screws are inserted and the compression device removed. The fourth most proximal screw is inserted, and finally a cancellous bone screw is passed through the neck of the blade plate into the distal fragment. The knee should now be aligned in full extension with 2 to 3 degrees of valgus position.

Generally a debridement of the knee is not recommended in the belief that this contributes little to the success of the procedure and may increase postoperative adhesions. However, in valgus knees, the patella often tracks laterally; in this event, patellar osteophytes are removed and the lateral retinaculum and lower fibers of vastus lateralis are divided. The tourniquet is released and major bleeding points coagulated. The leg is rewrapped with an Esmarch bandage and the tourniquet reinflated. A routine wound closure over one or two suction drains is performed and if a patellar realignment is needed the incision in the quadriceps tendon is overlapped so that the vastus medialis is sutured more laterally. When sutured, the closure should be tested by flexing the knee to a right angle.

When the wound is closed a Robert Jones compression dressing reinforced with two plaster splints is applied. The drains are removed in 24 to 36 hours.

Aftercare

When the wound is healed the dressing is removed and flexion exercises are begun. Normally flexion is regained quite easily, but if this is not so at 6 weeks,

a gentle manipulation under anesthesia is performed. Partial weight-bearing with crutches is allowed beginning 2 weeks from surgery, but full weight-bearing without support is not permitted until there is clinical and radiologic evidence of bone healing, which is normally about 3 months from surgery. During this period, weight-bearing is not generally well tolerated because of pain. The necessary prolonged use of crutches makes the technique rather unsuitable for elderly patients.

Complications

The only complication of note that has occurred at The Hospital for Special Surgery was an arterial hemorrhage from the lowest perforating artery, necessitating a return to the operating room. In this same patient a wound infection subsequently developed after the second procedure; later the blade plate was removed because of recurrent infection. This patient has a follow-up of 10 years and the result is rated as good in spite of intermittent episodes of recurrent infection.

Results

From the paucity of information concerning the results of low femoral osteotomy I conclude that the operation is seldom performed. Wardle graphically demonstrated loss of flexion in a small number of cases, but as these were done without internal fixation and therefore required lengthy cast immobilization, this result might have been expected. We reviewed a small series of 15 cases with a follow-up of 1 to 10 years. The results at follow-up were satisfactory (excellent or good) in all in spite of recurrent infection in one case (already described). Range of motion exceeded 90 degrees in all cases. The recovery period was often very slow, and it was usually 6 months before patients were able to appreciate any benefit from the procedure. This reservation aside, femoral osteotomy was a satisfactory procedure.

OSTEOTOMY FOR GENU RECURVATUM (FIG. 19.31)

A recurvatum deformity of the knee presents a particular difficulty because (1) it is difficult to control the proximal fragment of the tibia, and (2) cast im-

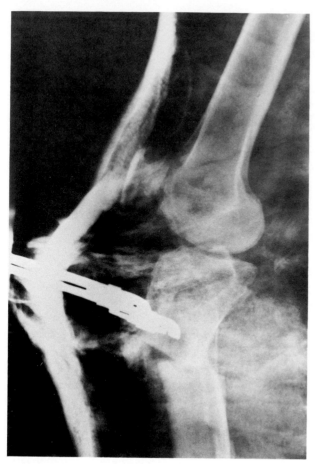

Fig. 19.31. Osteotomy for genu recurvatum (see text). A pin with traction bow attached is incorporated in the cast to prevent flexion of the small proximal fragment.

mobilization is inadequate. The osteotomy can be done in one of two ways. One method involves removing a wedge of appropriate size above the level of the tibial tubercle based posteriorly and fixing the fragments with a blade plate (as described for correction of varus).

Because there is sometimes difficulty in obtaining good apposition of the fragments, I prefer the following method, in which a midshaft fibular osteotomy is performed through a separate incision, and the tibial osteotomy is done immediately distal to the tibial tubercle through a transverse incision. The osteotomy may be wedge shaped but simple transverse division of the bone will suffice. The proximal fragment is controlled by a Steinmann pin connected to a traction bow by means of which it can be held extended while

the distal part of the tibia is flexed the required amount. A long leg plaster cast is applied incorporating the Steinmann pin and traction bow. The Steinmann pin is maintained for 6 weeks, by which time the osteotomy is sufficiently consolidated for a plaster cast alone to be adequate for the remainder of the healing time.

REFERENCES

1. Arnoldi, C.C., Lemperg, R.K., and Linderholm, H.: Intraosseous hypertension and pain in the knee. J. Bone Joint Surg. [Br.], *57*: 360, 1975.
2. Bauer, G.C.H., Insall, J., and Koshino, T.: Tibial osteotomy in gonarthrosis (osteo-arthritis of the knee). J. Bone Joint Surg. [Am.], *51*: 1545, 1969.
3. Beltrami, P., Calandriello, B., and Coli, G.: Axial deviations of the knee with secondary arthrosis. Correction by high osteotomy of the tibia and fibula. Ital. J. Orthop. Traumatol., *2*: 163, 1976.
4. Coventry, M.B.: Osteotomy of the upper portion of the tibia for degenerative arthritis of the knee. A preliminary report. J. Bone Joint Surg. [Am.], *47*: 984, 1965.
5. Coventry, M.B.: Osteotomy about the knee for degenerative and rheumatoid arthritis. Indications, operative technique, and results. J. Bone Joint Surg. [Am.], *55*: 23, 1973.
6. Coventry, M.B.: Upper tibial osteotomy for gonarthrosis. Orthop. Clin. North Am., *10(1)*: 191, 1979.
7. d'Aubigné, R.M.: Joint realignment in the management of osteoarthritis. In Straub, L.R., and Wilson, P.D. Jr., eds.: Clinical Trends in Orthopaedics. New York, Thieme-Stratton, p. 246, 1982.
8. Debeyre, J., and Patte, D.: Place des osteotomies de correction dans le traitement de la gonarthrose. Acta Orthop. Belg., *27*: 374, 1961.
9. Devas, M.B.: High tibial osteotomy for arthritis of the knee. A method specially suitable for the elderly. J. Bone Joint Surg. [Br.], *51*: 95, 1969.
10. Edholm, P., Lindahl, O., Lindholm, B., et al.: Knee instability. Acta Orthop. Scand., *47*: 658, 1976.
11. Edholm, P., Lindahl, O., Lindholm, B., et al.: Knee instability and tibial osteotomy. Acta Orthop. Scand. *48*: 95, 1977.
12. Gariépy, R.: Genu varum treated by high tibial osteotomy. In Proceedings of the Joint Meeting of the Orthopaedic Associations of the English-Speaking World. J. Bone Joint Surg. [Br.], *46*: 783, 1964.
13. Hagstedt, B.: High tibial osteotomy for gonarthrosis. ISBN 91-7222-069-4 Lund, 1974.

14. Harding, M.L.: A fresh appraisal of tibial osteotomy for osteoarthritis of the knee. Clin. Orthop., *114*: 223, 1976.

15. Harris, W.R., and Kostuik, J.P.: High tibial osteotomy for osteo-arthritis of the knee. J. Bone Joint Surg. [Am.], *52*: 330, 1970.

16. Helal, B.: The pain in primary osteoarthritis of the knee. Postgrad. Med. J., *41*: 172, 1965.

17. Insall, J., Shoji, H., and Mayer, V.: High tibial osteotomy. A 5-year evaluation. J. Bone Joint Surg. [Am.], *56*: 1397, 1974.

18. Jackson, J.P.: Osteotomy for osteoarthritis of the knee. In Proceedings of the Sheffield Regional Orthopaedic Club. J. Bone Joint Surg. [Br.], *40*: 826, 1958.

19. Jackson, J.P., and Waugh, W.: Tibial osteotomy for osteoarthritis of the knee. J. Bone Joint Surg. [Br.], *43*: 746, 1961.

20. Jackson, J.P., and Waugh, W.: The technique and complications of upper tibial osteotomy. J. Bone Joint Surg. [Br.], *56*: 236, 1974.

21. Jackson, J.P., Waugh, W., and Green, J.P.: High tibial osteotomy for osteoarthritis of the knee. J. Bone Joint Surg. [Br.], *51*: 88, 1969.

22. Johnson, F., Leitl, S., and Waugh, W.: The distribution of load across the knee. J. Bone Joint Surg. [Br.], *62*: 346, 1980.

23. Jones, R., and Lowett, R.W.: Orthopaedic surgery. New York, William Wood, 1924. Cited by Ahlberg, A., Scham, S., and Unander-Sclarin, L.: Osteostomy in degenerative and rheumatoid arthritis of the knee joint. Acta Orthop. Scand., *39*: 379, 1968.

24. Joseph, D., Insall, J., and Msika, C.: High tibial osteotomy: A long term clinical review. Presented at The American Academy of Orthopaedic Surgeons Annual Meeting, Anaheim, California, 1983.

25. Kettelkamp, D.B., Leach, R.E., and Nasca, R.: Pitfalls of proximal tibial osteotomy. Clin. Orthop., *106*: 232, 1975.

26. Kettelkamp, D.B., Wenger, D.R., Chao, E.Y.S., et al: Results of proximal tibial osteotomy. The effects of tibiofemoral angle, stance-phase flexion-extension, and medial-plateau force. J. Bone Joint Surg. [Am.], *58*: 952, 1976.

27. Koshino, T., and Ranawat, N.S.: Healing process of osteoarthritis in the knee after high tibial osteotomy through observation of strontium-85 scintimetry. Clin. Orthop., *82*: 149, 1972.

28. Koshino, T., and Tsuchiya, K.: The effect of high tibial osteotomy on osteoarthritis of the knee. Int. Orthop., *3*: 37, 1979.

29. Lange, M.: Orthopädisch-Chirurgische Operationslehre, Munich, Bergman, p. 660, 1951.

30. MacIntosh, D.L., and Welsh, R.P.: Joint debridement—A complement to high tibial osteotomy in the treatment of degenerative arthritis of the knee. J. Bone Joint Surg. [Am.], *59*: 1094, 1977.

31. Maquet, P.G.J.: Biomechanics of the Knee. New York, Springer-Verlag, 1976.

32. Maquet, P.: Valgus osteotomy for osteoarthritis of the knee. Clin. Orthop., *120*: 143, 1976.

33. Morrison, J.B.: Bioengineering analysis of force actions transmitted by the knee joint. Biomed. Eng., *3*: 164, 1968.

34. Myrnerts, R.: The SAAB jig: An aid in high tibial osteotomy. Acta Orthop. Scand., *49*: 85, 1978.

35. Myrnerts, R., ed.: High tibial osteotomy in medial osteoarthritis of the knee. Linkoping University Medical Dissertations, No. 77. Linkoping 1979, Vimmerby, VTT-Grafiska, 1979.

36. Seal, P.V., and Chan, R.N.W.: Tibial osteotomy for osteoarthrosis of the knee. Acta Orthop. Scand., *46*: 141, 1975.

37. Shoji, H., and Insall, J.: High tibial osteotomy for osteoarthritis of the knee with valgus deformity. J. Bone Joint Surg. [Am.], *55*: 963, 1973.

38. Shoji, H., and Insall, J.: High tibial osteotomy for osteoarthritis of the knee. Int. Surg., *61*: 11, 1976.

39. Steindler, A.: Orthopedic Operations. Indications, Technique and End Results. Springfield, Ill. Charles C. Thomas, 1940.

40. Torgerson, W.R., Jr., Kettelkamp, D.B., Igou, R.A., Jr., et al.: Tibial osteotomy for the treatment of degenerative arthritis of the knee. Clin. Orthop., *101*: 46, 1974.

41. Vainionpää, S., Läike, E., Kirves, P., et al.: Tibial osteotomy for osteoarthritis of the knee. A five to ten year follow-up study. J. Bone Joint Surg. [Am.], *63*: 938, 1981.

42. Volkmann, R.: Osteotomy for knee joint deformity. Edinburgh. Med. J., translated from Berl. Klin. Wochenschr., 794, 1875.

43. Wardle, E.N.: Osteotomy of the tibia and fibula. Surg. Gynecol. Obstet., *115*: 61, 1962.

20 Total Knee Replacement

John N. Insall

HISTORY[124]

The concept of improving knee joint function by modifying the articular surfaces has received attention since the nineteenth century. In 1860 Verneuil[142] suggested the interposition of soft tissues to reconstruct the articular surface of a joint. Subsequently pig bladder, nylon, fascia lata, prepatellar bursa, and cellophane were some of the materials used. The results were disappointing. In 1861 Ferguson[34] resected the entire knee joint and began motion on the newly created subchondral surfaces (Fig. 20.1). When more bone was removed, the patients developed good motion but lacked the necessary stability, whereas with less bone resection, spontaneous fusions often resulted. These early attempts were usually performed on knees damaged by tuberculosis or other infectious processes with resulting ankylosis and deformity. The results were sufficiently poor to discourage anything more than occasional attempts in severe cases.

Encouraged by the relative success of hip cup arthroplasty, Campbell[15] reported the successful use of the metallic interposition femoral mold in 1940. A similar type of arthroplasty was developed and used at the Massachusetts General Hospital. The results published by Speed and Trout[134] in 1949 and by Miller and Friedman[104] in 1952 were not very good, and this type of knee arthroplasty never achieved wide recognition.

In 1958 MacIntosh[94] described a different type of hemiarthroplasty he had used in treating painful varus or valgus deformities of the knee. An acrylic tibial plateau prosthesis was inserted into the affected side to correct deformity, restore stability, and relieve pain. Later versions of this prosthesis[95] were made of metal (Fig. 20.2) and the somewhat similar McKeever prosthesis[93] showed considerably more success and were extensively used, particularly in rheumatoid arthritis. Gunston[49,50] carried MacIntosh's ideas a step further and, instead of using a simple metal disk interposed within the joint, substituted metallic runners embedded in the femoral condyles, articulating against polyethylene troughs attached to the tibial plateau. To make a four-part system of this kind feasible, it is necessary to find a means of fixing the components rigidly to the bone. The solution was provided by acrylic cement.

Although the Gunston polycentric prosthesis was the first cemented surface replacement of the knee joint, the work of Freeman and Swanson has had an even greater influence on the direction of both prosthetic design and surgical technique. The design objectives for a prosthesis (Fig. 20.3A,B) were outlined

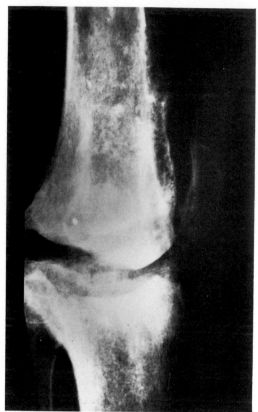

Fig. 20.1. Resection arthroplasty creates a mobile but usually unstable joint.

by Freeman et al.[41] in 1973. The most important of these objectives are the following:

1. A salvage procedure should be readily available. The implantation of the prosthesis should require the removal of no more bone than for primary arthrodesis and should leave large, flat surfaces of cancellous bone.
2. The chances of loosening should be minimized.
   a. The femoral and tibial components should be incompletely constrained relative to each other so that twisting, varus, or valgus moments cannot be transmitted to the bonds between prosthesis and skeleton.
   b. The friction between the components should be minimized.
   c. Any hyperextension-limiting arrangement should be progressive and not sudden in action.
   d. The prosthetic component should be fitted to the bone by means which spread the loads over the largest possible areas of the bone prosthesis interface.
3. The rate of production of wear debris should be minimized and the debris produced should be as innocuous as possible. This leads to a preference for metal-on-plastic-bearing surfaces, which should be as large as possible to keep the surface stresses low.
4. The probability of infection should be minimized by having compact prosthetic components with few dead spaces.
5. The consequences of infection should also be minimized by avoiding long intramedullary stems and intramedullary cement.
6. A standard insertion procedure should be available.
7. The prosthesis should give motion from 5 degrees of hyperextension to at least 90 degrees of flexion.
8. Some freedom of rotation should be provided.
9. Excessive movements in any direction should be resisted by the soft tissues, particularly the collateral ligaments.

All these objectives remain valid today, although two additional points cited in this article remain issues for debate. These are (1) the place of the cruciate ligaments in total knee arthroplasty, and (2) the need to replace the patellofemoral joint and the desirability of patellar resurfacing.

Other early examples of resurfacing prostheses (Figs. 20.4A,B and 20.5A,B) were the geometric,[22,23] the duocondylar,[113,132] the UCI,[31,147] and the Marmor.[87,99–101]

CONSTRAINED PROSTHESES

A second line of development in knee arthroplasty occurred in parallel to the concepts of interposition and later surface designs. In 1951, Walldius[146] developed the hinged prosthesis that bears his name. The device was initially made of acrylic and later of metal.

Shortly thereafter, Shiers[127] described a similar device with even simpler mechanical characteristics (Fig. 20.6). A hinged prosthesis has a considerable appeal. Technically it is easy to use as the intramedullary stems make the prosthesis largely self-aligning, and all the ligaments and other soft tissue constraints can be sacrificed because the prosthesis is self-stabilizing. The extent of damage to the knee is therefore of no

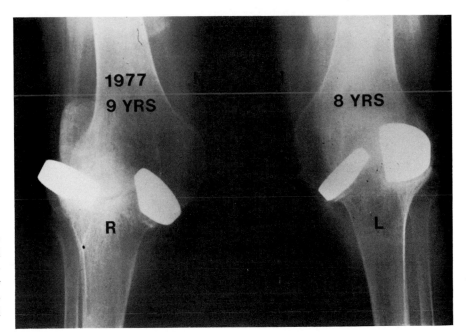

Fig. 20.2. MacIntosh hemiarthroplasty used in rheumatoid arthritis often restores alignment and stability for a few years. However as in this bilateral case, late dislocation and sinkage are common.

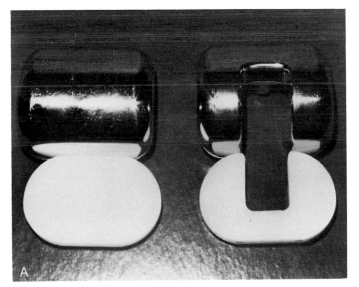

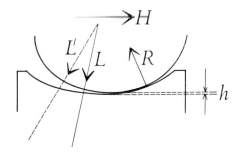

H = horizontal force
R = reaction at condyles
L = collateral force
L' = force from oblique fibers
h = increase in height

Fig. 20.3. (A) The original Freeman-Swanson prosthesis used two one-piece components. (B) Stability is obtained by the roller-in-trough concept; dislocation can occur only if one component runs uphill on the other. Distraction is resisted by capsular and collateral ligament tension.

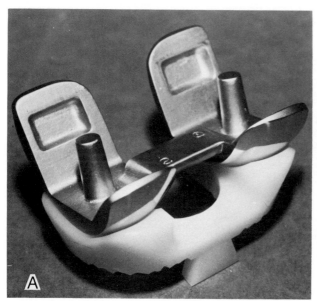

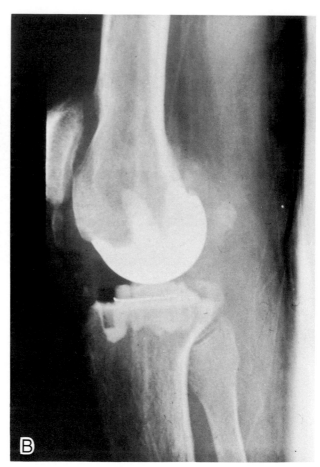

Fig. 20.4. (A,B) An early and widely used surface replacement was the geometric prosthesis.

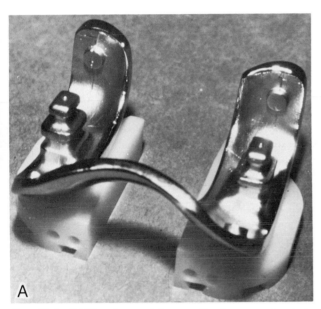
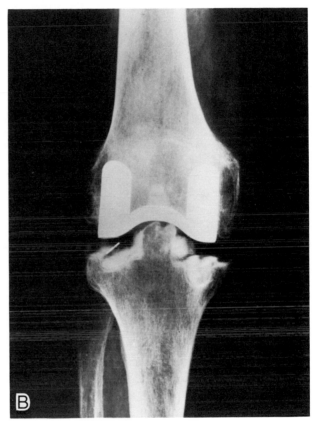

Fig. 20.5. (A) The duocondylar prosthesis was anatomic in concept, retained both cruciate ligaments when these were present, but did not resurface the patellofemoral joint. Sinkage and loosening of the tibial components were an eventual problem with this design. (B) An anteroposterior radiograph with the duocondylar prosthesis inserted. Radiolucent lines around both tibial components are visible.

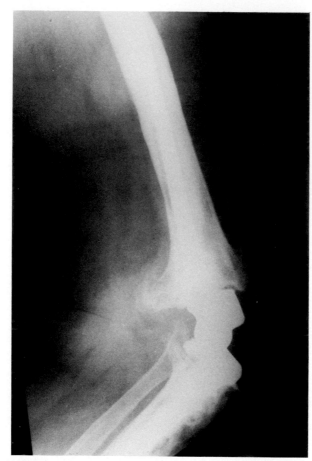

Fig. 20.6. The Shiers prosthesis was a simple uniaxial metallic hinge.

consequence, and even the most extreme deformities can be corrected by dividing the soft tissues and resecting sufficient bone. Of course, the early hinged designs were uncemented, although later developments such as the Guepar were designed from the outset to be used with methylmethacrylate cement.

EVOLUTION OF PROSTHETIC DESIGN

The prostheses discussed up to this point are now more or less obsolete. Although the early results were quite encouraging, further follow-up demonstrated various problems that have to this day given total knee replacement a bad reputation.

A review of the literature of the last several years,

relevant to total knee arthroplasty, reveals many articles giving follow-up on designs no longer in common use.[1,13,19,31,64,81,82,103,110,112,113,115,130,132,148,149] These published reports on results using early models are somewhat difficult to compare because of different rating methods. A review conducted at The Hospital for Special Surgery between 1971 and 1973 is probably representative. This paper[72] compared four different models: the unicondylar (Fig. 20.7), the duocondylar, geometric, and Guepar (Fig. 20.8) designs. The results were expressed using a knee-rating scale (HSS) that totaled 100 points.

The knees were divided into four groups. Those that rated excellent scored 85 or more points. These knees approached the normal, and the knee was obviously much improved in the opinion of both the patient and the examiner. Knees with ratings between 70 and 84 were considered to have a good result. Such knees had been obviously improved by the arthroplasty, but the result was not as good as in the previous group. Knees designated as fair had a point range of 60 to 69. This group mostly comprised knees in which the result of the arthroplasty was deficient in some way (persistent pain, moderate instability, or unsatisfactory range of motion), but also included some in which the rating of the arthroplasty was downgraded by the patient's general condition (e.g., multiple joint involvement in rheumatoid arthritis or because of systemic disease). Rated as failures were those knees that had a postoperative score of less than 60. These knees were evidently unsatisfactory and below the rating achieved by knee fusion (which scores a 60 on the HSS knee-rating scale). This classification included knees in which the prosthesis had been removed or replaced and knees in which the improvement if any did not seem to justify the risk of arthroplasty.

Considering the entire group of 178 arthroplasties studied in the four different models (23 unicondylar, 60 duocondylar, 50 geometric, and 45 Guepar), the results were considered excellent in 47 (26 percent), good in 66 (37 percent), fair in 37 (21 percent), and poor in 28 (16 percent) (Fig. 20.9). There was no statistically significant difference between the results obtained with each of the four prostheses studied. However, because it is easier to improve a bad knee than a relatively good one, the percentage of improvement was much greater with the Guepar than with the unicondylar (120 percent versus 45 percent).

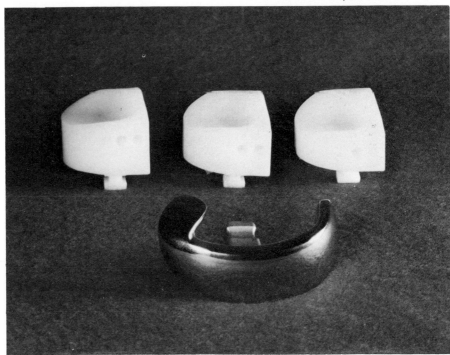

Fig. 20.7. The unicondylar prosthesis was designed to resurface only the affected femorotibial compartment. The shape and curvature of the component were similar to the duocondylar design.

Fig. 20.8. The Guepar hinge was like the Shiers uniaxial metallic hinge, but with the axis placed more posteriorly and femoral resurfacing for the patellar articulation.

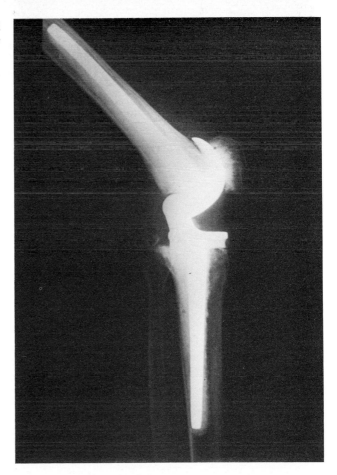

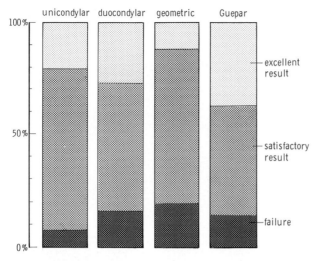

Fig. 20.9. Graph showing comparative results of 4 early prosthetic models.

Three specific problems are identified from this study: patellar pain, component loosening, and surgical technique. However, because the Guepar hinge was inserted into the worst knees originally, it gave the greatest percentage of improvement in the knee rating scale. At the time of the study, the conclusion reached was that the Guepar prosthesis appeared superior in a number of ways. It had been selected for use in the most severely involved knees and yet equalled any of the other prostheses in the quality of results both in rheumatoid arthritis and in osteoarthritis. It also gave the lowest proportion of failures and was the only model to improve range of motion postoperatively. However, the potential problems of loosening and mechanical failure with the Guepar prosthesis were noted. Most Guepar prostheses at The Hospital for Special Surgery were inserted from 9 to 12 years ago, and these expected problems have

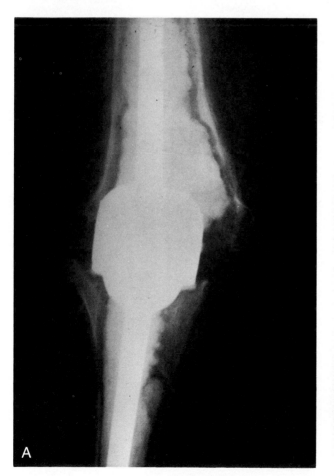

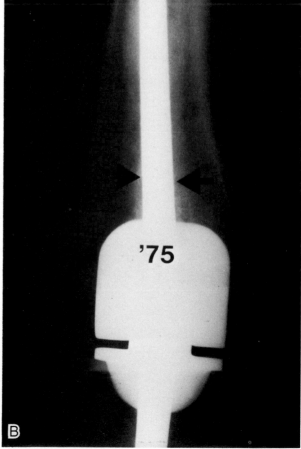

Fig. 20.10. (A) Radiograph of a grossly loose Guepar prosthesis 5 years after the initial insertion. (B) Stem breakage occurred with the Guepar prosthesis, usually at the site shown here in the radiograph 5 cm proximal to the joint.

now to some extent materialized.[80] Approximately 80 percent of the prostheses are loose both clinically and radiographically, but are not necessarily symptomatic (Fig. 20.10A). There have also been seven cases of stem breakage (four femoral and three tibial) (Fig. 20.10B).

PATELLAR PAIN

None of the four early prosthetic models studied made any provision for patellofemoral function. Patellectomy did not seem to offer a solution to the problem of patellofemoral arthritis (Fig. 20.11). Thirty-eight patellectomies were performed in the group as a whole, three of which were done at a later date than the arthroplasty because of persistent patellar pain. A complaint of pain after patellectomy was as frequent in those patients as in patients in whom patellectomy had not been performed. In addition, patients with a patellectomy suffered from inadequacy of the extensor mechanism. In the Guepar group of 45 knees, pain on patellar compression was found in 22 on follow-up and patellar erosion was observed in five patients. Patellar subluxation frequently occurred with the Guepar prosthesis in spite of a wide lateral release of the patellar retinaculum at the time of arthroplasty (Fig. 20.12). However, this was often not apparent to

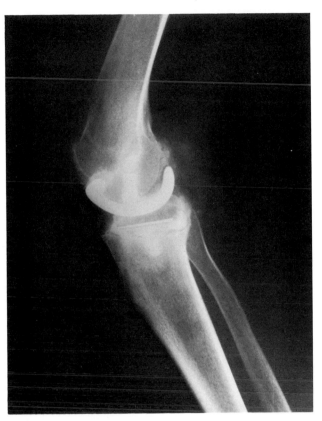

Fig. 20.11. Patellectomy is not a satisfactory solution to patellofemoral pain. Patellectomy was done in conjunction with a unicondylar prosthesis.

Fig. 20.12. Patellar subluxation and dislocation often occurred with the Guepar prosthesis. It was not always symptomatic.

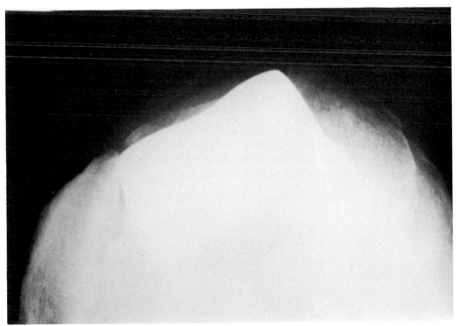

the patient and may be considered an incidental finding. Subluxation of the patella did not necessarily correlate with complaints of postoperative pain. However, with the geometric prosthesis, 29 of 50 knees had pain on patellofemoral compression. Patellar subluxation was found in nine knees, and all were painful.

LOOSENING

A radiolucent line surrounding the prosthetic components was seen with great frequency. With the condylar replacements the radiolucency was usually observed around the tibial component. It was present in 70 percent of knees with the unicondylar, 50 percent with the duocondylar, and 80 percent with the geometric prosthesis. A radiolucent line was observed around the femoral component in 45 percent of the patients with a Guepar prosthesis. The radiolucent line was slightly more frequent in osteoarthritic than in rheumatoid patients; it was observed in all knees with osteoarthritis in which the geometric prosthesis was used. Radiolucent lines are by no means always symptomatic, but when complete, progressive, and associated with pain on weight-bearing, they generally indicate failure of fixation. Our subsequent experience has shown that the incidence of radiolucency for a particular prosthesis correlates well with the eventual amount of component loosening.

On the basis of early analysis of these data, it was clear that tibial loosening represented a failure in prosthetic design. The flat, cancellous surface of the upper tibia is not a suitable bed for a flat prosthetic component because of poor resistance to shear stress. Moreover, this bone is not of sufficient strength to resist subsidence of the tibial component even if excavations are made to accommodate fixation fins on the bottom of the tibial prosthesis (Fig. 20.13). It was concluded that some form of cortical fixation would be essential for a successful series of total knee arthroplasties.

PROSTHESIS SELECTION AND SURGICAL TECHNIQUE

Like many others, we initially believed in the concept of a graduated system[143] in which selection of a prosthesis depended upon the severity of damage found

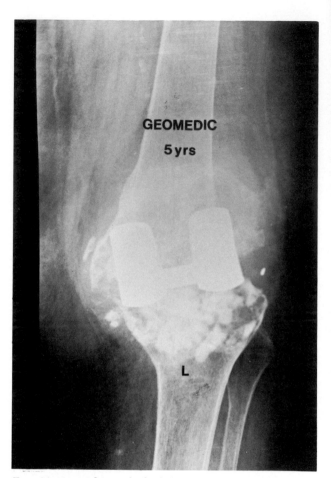

Fig. 20.13. Failure of tibial fixation was a too frequent problem with many early prosthetic designs. The problem was primarily attributable to collapse of the cancellous bone of the upper tibia, with sinkage of the component.

in the arthritic knee (Fig. 20.14). For example, knees with cartilage erosion restricted to one femorotibial compartment were replaced with a unicondylar prosthesis, whereas in the most severely damaged and deformed knees, a hinged prosthesis was used. The bicondylar prosthesis occupied an intermediate position with respect to the severity of arthritis. While the use of a hinged prosthesis is not technically demanding, the early condylar designs were difficult to insert and align and there was very little margin for error. Obviously the advantage of even the most sophisticated prosthetic design is lost if the surgical placement is incorrect. Furthermore, an inherent drawback in a graduated system of prostheses is that a model may be used for degrees of deformity ex-

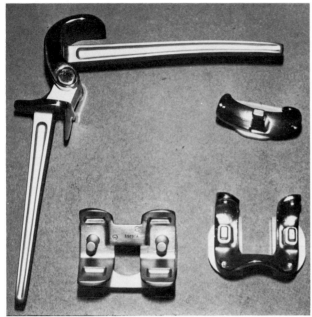

Fig. 20.14. The graduated system concept selected the prosthesis according to the degree and extent of damage. The prostheses shown here in a clockwise direction are: the unicondylar, duocondylar, geometric, and Guepar prostheses.

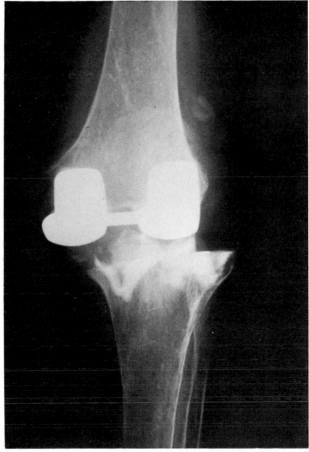

Fig. 20.15. This geometric prosthesis translocated and dislocated. This was the condition of the knee before the prosthesis was inserted and represents an error of selection of prosthesis.

ceeding the limits for which the prosthesis was designed. This error can of itself be a cause for failure (e.g., dislocation) (Fig. 20.15). Clearly, there is no purpose in selecting one prosthetic design over another unless some advantage can be shown. For example, in this particular comparative study we did not find that the unicondylar prosthesis offered any advantage over bicondylar models.

INFECTION

Although deep periprosthetic infection was not a frequent cause of failure for the condylar designs, it has subsequently proved a major problem with the Guepar prosthesis. With further follow-up 12 of 108 prostheses became infected (four early and eight late). This incidence of 11 percent is likely to rise as late infection occurs even many years after the arthroplasty. The most recent example was an 85-year-old woman who had a Guepar prosthesis inserted in 1972. She did very well for 8 years until the onset of acute deep sepsis. There was no obvious focus elsewhere to suggest a metastatic infection. Because of her age

and the extreme toxicity caused by virulent infection, a midthigh amputation had to be performed. Although this is the only example of an amputation following an infected prosthesis at The Hospital for Special Surgery, there have been reports of other, similar occurrences in the literature.[3] It seems likely that the Guepar prosthesis will fare little better than other hinged designs. Young[154] found that in a series of hinged prostheses all had failed by the end of 10 years. Hui and Fitzgerald[61] reported an 11.7 percent infection rate in 77 Guepar arthroplasties followed for two or more years. They comment on the difficulty of obtaining arthrodesis if the prosthesis has to be removed. DeBurge[28] had a failure rate of 34 percent with the Guepar prosthesis attributable to major complications. Bargar et al.[8] also counseled against the use of constrained prostheses, although their complication rate was somewhat less than that reported by other workers. Only Wilson et al.[153] have reported favorable results over a long period of time using an uncemented Walldius prosthesis. The overall infection rate was 3.2 percent and clinical evidence of loosening occurred infrequently. The 20 knees followed for an average of ten years showed little evidence of progressive deterioration. They attribute this to the absence of cement. Walldius himself[147] has recently written on 27 years' experience with his prosthesis and states that good results are obtained in 80 percent of patients with a high degree of preoperative disability. No details are given.

No hinged prostheses have been used on the Knee

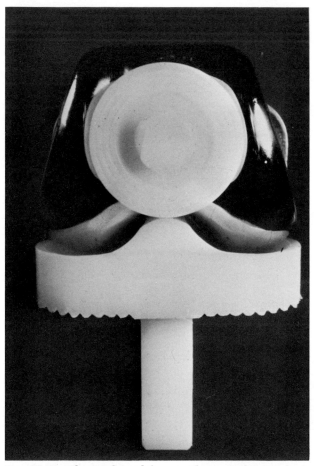

Fig. 20.16. The total condylar prosthesis is the standard surface replacement used in the Hospital for Special Surgery.

Service at The Hospital for Special Surgery since 1976 despite a large referral practice of difficult revision arthroplasty problems.

The experience quoted above has led to a convergence of prosthetic designs, particularly in the United States.

At The Hospital for Special Surgery dissatisfaction with the early prostheses led to the design of the total condylar and duopatellar prostheses.

CLASSIFICATION OF PROSTHESES

It seems unnecessary to advocate a complicated system of classification. It is recommended that prostheses be divided into two categories, each subdivided as follows:
Surface replacements
    Unicondylar
    Bicondylar
        Cruciate retaining
        Cruciate excising
        Cruciate substituting
Constrained prostheses
    Loose with some degree of rotation and varus–valgus rock permitted; bearing surface usually metal or polyethylene
    Rigid: fixed-axis metal hinges

SURFACE REPLACEMENTS

TOTAL CONDYLAR PROSTHESIS
(Fig. 20.16)

Although coined as the name of a specific prosthesis, the total condylar has more recently been given a generic meaning to describe a whole range of surface prostheses that share general characteristics with the original: some of these later models differ in design details that may prove important in the long run.

The total condylar[71,73,74] prosthesis designed in 1973, was a true total replacement of the knee in that the patellofemoral joint was replaced as well as the femorotibial compartment. It is still widely used in its original form and is therefore probably the oldest prosthesis of which this can be said. The salient features of the design are the following:
1. *Femoral component:* Made of cobalt chromium al-

loy. Contains a symmetrically grooved anterior flange separating posteriorly into two symmetric condyles, each of decreasing radius posteriorly and having a symmetric convex curvature in the coronal plane.

2. *Tibial component:* Made of high-density polyethylene in one piece with two separate biconcave tibial plateaus that mate (articulate) precisely with the femoral condyles in extension, thus permitting no rotation in this position. In flexion the fit ceases to be exact and rotation and gliding motions are possible. The symmetric tibial plateaus are separated by an intercondylar eminence designed to prevent translocation or sideways sliding movements. The peripheral margin of the articular concavities is of an even height both anteriorly and posteriorly. The deep or bony surface of the component has a central fixation peg 35 mm in length and 12.5 mm in width. The anterior margin of the peg is vertical, but the posterior margin is oblique, conforming with the posterior cortex of the tibia.

3. *Patellar component:* Made of high-density polyethylene. It is dome-shaped on its articular surface, conforming closely to the curvature of the femoral flange. A dome was selected because this shape does not require rotary alignment as would an anatomic prosthesis. The bony surface of the prosthesis has a central, rectangular fixation lug.

DUOPATELLAR PROSTHESIS

The total condylar prosthesis was designed for cruciate excision. In contrast, the duopatella,[33] a sister prosthesis designed later than the total condylar as a replacement for the duocondylar model, was intended to preserve existing cruciate ligaments, particularly the posterior cruciate. The general shape of the tibial runners is anatomic in the sagittal plane. Coronally, the condyles are flat with a median curvature.

The anterior connecting bar of the duocondylar was extended into a femoral flange. The initial version of the duopatella had two separate tibial plateaus identical to the duocondylar, being flat in the sagittal plane, but with a median curvature coronally to prevent translocation. The deep surface was dovetailed for cement fixation. Later the two components were joined, and a central fixation peg similar to that of the total condylar was added. A posterior cruciate cut-out was provided.

The patellar component of the duopatella is identical to that of the total condylar.[75]

CRUCIATE RETENTION VERSUS EXCISION

One of the functions of the cruciate ligaments, in addition to providing static stability, is to impose certain movements on the joint surfaces relative to one another. The anterior cruciate ligament is not of much consequence in the arthroplasty and in fact is often absent in arthritic knees. The posterior cruciate, on the other hand, although it may be attenuated is usually present. The posterior cruciate causes the femoral condyles to glide posteriorly on the tibial articular surface as the knee is flexed.[84] In the normal knee the shape of the tibial plateau does not restrain this rolling motion, and the laxity of the meniscal attachments permits the menisci to move posteriorly with the femur. This anatomic function is crucial in prosthetic designs; if the cruciate ligaments are retained the tibial component must be flat or even posteriorly sloped[42] (Fig. 20.17). Posterior impingement occurs if a cruciate-retaining prosthesis has a dished tibial component (Fig. 20.18). These considerations are reflected in the design of the total condylar and duopatellar prostheses. It is incorrect to preserve the posterior cruciate using a total condylar design unless the articular shape of the tibial component is suitably modified to resemble that of the duopatella. Likewise, cruciate excision with the duopatella may lead to subluxation.

ARGUMENTS FOR CRUCIATE EXCISION

Advantages

1. *Fixation.* Optimal fixation of the tibial component can be obtained by resting the component on all aspects of the upper tibial cortex or by using a short intramedullary peg. This is easier to arrange when the cruciate ligaments are excised.

2. *Correction of deformity.* Removal of the cruciate ligaments is an essential element in the soft tissue release of a fixed varus or valgus deformity. Clear-

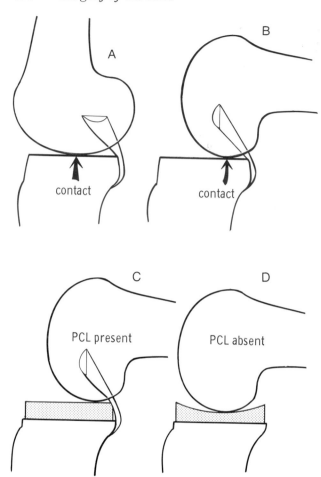

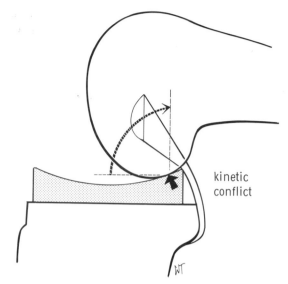

Fig. 20.18. Kinematic conflict occurs if concepts are mismatched. In this case the posterior cruciate ligament is preserved using a dished tibial component. Impingement occurs posteriorly with flexion.

Fig. 20.17. The effect of posterior cruciate retention on prosthetic design. Because of the rollback enforced by the PCL, (A, B) the prosthetic tibial surface must be flat to allow this movement. (C) When the PCL is absent a dished tibial plateau is used.

ance of the intercondylar area of the knee also provides full exposure of the posterior capsule, facilitating its release for correction of fixed flexion deformity.

3. *Technique.* It is technically easier to cut straight across the top of the tibia than to cut around the intercondylar eminence: therefore accurate placement of the prosthetic components is more likely. In addition, it is unlikely that the size and geometry of the prosthetic components can exactly reduplicate the original shape of the knee. Thus the cruciate ligaments that originally interacted with that shape may be in conflict with the new prosthetic surfaces. This will be accentuated by any

surgical error in placement, and in particular components that are inserted too tight. If the components are too loose, however, the cruciates will be rendered nonfunctional and might well be excised in the first place. It is our experience that it requires considerable skill to insert a cruciate retaining prosthesis correctly.

4. *Cement removal.* Excision of the intercondylar structures enables cement to be removed posteriorly because of access through the empty intercondylar space.

5. *Intercondylar impingement.* There can be no intercondylar impingement after the arthroplasty, and this area as a source of postoperative pain is eliminated.

6. *Mobility.* In preoperatively stiff knees the range of flexion frequently cannot be increased until the cruciate ligaments are released.

Disadvantages

1. *Posterior subluxation* (Fig. 20.19). If the components are inserted too loose, either unavoidably because of the pathology in the knee or because of technical error, posterior subluxation or dislocation in flexion may occur.

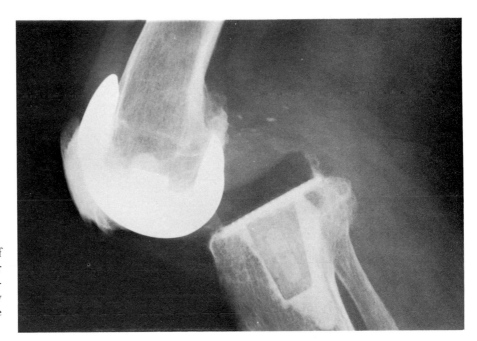

Fig. 20.19. A disadvantage of PCL excision is that posterior subluxation can occur in flexion. Usually this is caused by faulty technique, but in some knees it may be unavoidable.

2. *Increased stress on the bone–cement interface.* A cup-shaped articulation such as possessed by the total condylar or ICLH prostheses provides stability through the shape of the components. In the sagittal plane, the femoral component has a smaller radius of curvature than that of the tibial component, providing partial conformity. If a horizontal force is applied horizontal displacement occurs until the femoral component begins to ride out of the trough. A vertical distraction is then produced that tightens one or both collateral ligaments giving a force and corresponding reaction of the metal–plastic contact point. Ultimately this force is transmitted to the bone–cement interface. When the cruciates are retained the tibial surface is flat, the horizontal forces are absorbed by the ligaments and not transmitted to the tibial component. The additional forces generated by cruciate excision may therefore predispose to tibial loosening.
3. *Roller-in-trough design.* This design is not compatible with normal flexion. In fact it is difficult to obtain more than 90 degrees of flexion with designs of this kind. Some increase in flexion can be obtained by sloping the articular surface posteriorly so that the trough is tilted backward.

ARGUMENTS FOR CRUCIATE RETENTION

Advantages

1. Preservation of the cruciate ligaments means that the normal rolling and gliding movements of the femur on the tibia occur to some degree. It is therefore possible to design a prosthesis that has a greater range of flexion because posterior impingement is less likely.
2. Posterior stability is ensured by the presence of intact ligaments.
3. Horizontal forces are dissipated by the ligaments rather than transmitted to the prosthesis and thence to the bone–cement interface.

Disadvantages

1. *Technique.* Discussed above.
2. *See-saw effect* (Fig. 20.20). The rolling movement of the femur changes the metal–plastic contact point from anterior in extension to posterior in flexion. Thus, in extension the anterior part of the tibia is compressed, there is a tendency for the compo-

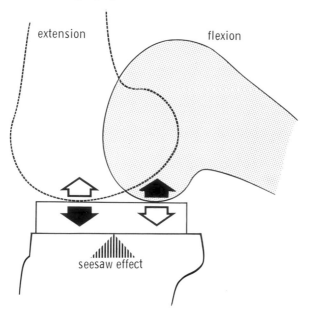

Fig. 20.20. The see-saw effect. The back-and-forth movement on the tibial component caused by PCL retention creates a rocking motion that may cause loosening.

nent to tilt anteriorly, and a distraction force exists posteriorly at the bone–cement interface. In flexion the situation is reversed. This alternating compression–distraction may ultimately affect fixation.

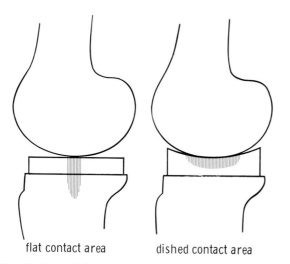

Fig. 20.21. A dished component permits greater conformity, hence a larger contact area. The smaller contact area with a flat tibial component increases the stresses on the polyethylene.

3. *Subluxation.* Because the prosthesis provides no inherent stability, ligament deficiency may result in subluxation.
4. *Increased wear.*[13] The consequent reduction in contact area due to a curved surface (the femoral component) articulating against a flat surface (the tibial plateau) results in a higher contact stress on the polyethylene (Fig. 20.21). This can lead to increased surface failure of the polyethylene and a higher rate of wear.

SUMMARY OF COMPARATIVE DESIGNS

Whether cruciate-retaining prosthetic designs are better than cruciate-sacrificing designs has not yet been determined. Both concepts have theoretical advantages and disadvantages, but whether these are important in practical terms is not certain. It will require several more years of follow-up study before any clear superiority is defined for either design. There are some instances where cruciate retention is impossible and in these cases a cruciate sacrificing design must be used. In knees with a lesser degree of deformity either design can be used according to the surgeon's preference and particular expertise.

It must be emphasized that the concepts and designs are separate and cannot be mixed. Unfortunately some current total knee models do just this. An extreme example is the geometric prosthesis, which retains the cruciate ligaments and yet has a totally conforming articulation. A tight posterior cruciate ligament in these circumstances makes the knee "open like a book" because of posterior impingement. The amount of plastic distortion, cold flow, and the high rate of tibial loosening reported with the geometric are likely due to this conflict between prosthetic surfaces and ligament restraint. It is incumbent upon the surgeon to examine carefully an unfamiliar design that retains the cruciates to be certain that the geometry of the prosthesis is correct for its intended purpose.

CURRENT DESIGNS OF SURFACE REPLACEMENT

The Freeman-Swanson, or ICLH, prosthesis was designed in England at the London Hospital and Imperial College, but most other prostheses of this type have originated in the United States; currently this category accounts for most implants in general use. Examples are the total condylar, the duopatella, and the Townley; more recent derivatives include the posterior stabilized condylar,[76] the geopatellar, the anametric,[37,140] the kinematic, the porous-coated anatomic,[62] the multiradius, and the Cloutier.[18] In many respects these prostheses are closely related, suggesting that there is a developing consensus on how and with what the knee joint should be replaced. While it is true that differences do exist between these designs, most seem of trivial consequences (e.g., some prostheses are asymmetric, requiring left and right versions). An important distinguishing feature is the question of cruciate retention (see above). Although the evidence available at present suggests that both types when correctly selected and implanted will give equally good short term clinical results, there is evidence from gait analysis that differences do exist between various models that may be of long-term consequence. Andriacchi and Galante[2] compared various parameters of gait using a variety of prostheses (total condylar, geomedic, duopatella, Gunston, and Cloutier). An age-matched group of 14 elderly normal subjects was also studied. It was found that the gait of patients after total knee replacement was different than normal. The patients all had a shorter than normal stride length, reduced knee flexion during midstance and an abnormal pattern of flexion–extension moments at the knee. This abnormality was found to be independent of the design of the device. The major difference between prostheses was observed in climbing up or downstairs. The normal subjects used on average about 85 degrees of knee flexion climbing up stairs and about 90 degrees descending stairs. The only prosthesis that equaled this range of motion was the Cloutier, a design that preserves both cruciate ligaments and is almost unconstrained. Patients with the total condylar prosthesis used the least knee motion (about 70 degrees) both going up and down the stairs (this was the only cruciate excising prosthesis tested). Patients with other prostheses occupied an intermediate position between these two (all preserved at least the posterior cruciate ligament). It remains to be seen whether this information has any clinical significance, although clearly other things being equal, it is desirable for the gait to approach the normal.

Another important difference between prostheses is the method of tibial fixation. The total condylar, duopatella, and posterior stabilized condylar employ central peg fixation, whereas others (ICLH, multiradius, porous-coated anatomic, and anametric) have two or more short studs. Although the subject of chapter 22, it is pertinent to mention this aspect of fixation because it relates to prosthetic design. Long-term studies using central peg fixation are available (total condylar and duopatella), and tibial loosening has been rare with both types (Fig. 20.22). With longer intramedullary stems on the tibial component (variable axis), no loosening at all has been reported.[107] There is thus clinical evidence that a central peg or stem added to the tibial component virtually eliminates tibial loosening even using conventional cementing techniques. The optimal length of the stem remains debatable. Too long a stem is difficult to remove and results in stress transfer from the cancellous bone of the upper tibia to the cortical bone of the diaphysis. Too short a stem, on the other hand, will be insecure.

There is also good evidence from early experience with knee arthroplasty that separate tibial components are susceptible to fixation failure.[97,113,128] Neither an anterior bar (with cruciate cut-out) nor the use of fixation studs is helpful. Walker et al.[145] tested a variety of tibial components by applying compressive load with anteroposterior force, rotational torque or varus–vulgus moment (Fig. 20.23). The relative deflections, both compressive and distractive, were measured between the component and the bone. The fewest deflections occurred with one-piece metal components. Whether a central peg or two lateral studs was used did not seem to make much difference. Thick plastic components behaved much like metal-backed ones, except when a cruciate cut-out was made. Metal backing thus seems particularly desirable for cruciate retaining implants.

Clinical data on more recent implants using metal tray and two stud fixation is not available. However, Freeman has used an all-plastic component with "magic pegs"[11] (in effect, two lateral studs) and peripheral cortical contact (the plastic is trimmed to fit the upper tibia) since 1977. The incidence of tibial loosening up to this time is about 4 percent,[39] suggesting that for polyethylene components the central peg may be better than two lateral studs: whether this also applies to metal tray designs is uncertain. However, laterally

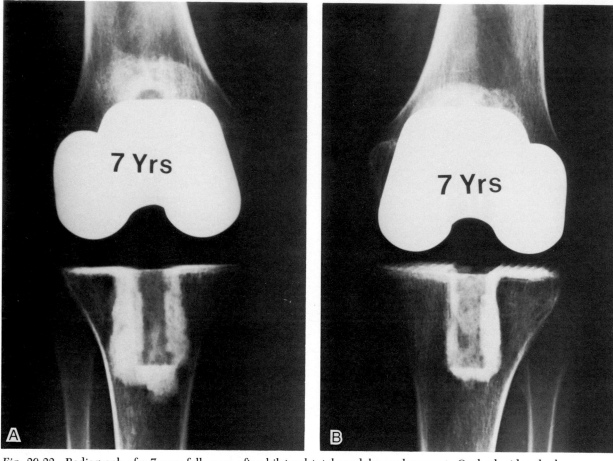

Fig. 20.22. Radiograph of a 7-year follow-up after bilateral total condylar replacement. On both sides the bone cement interface appears secure, although the central cement fill is larger than ideal.

placed studs or posts require the destruction of supporting cancellous bone, whereas a central peg removes bone where it is already weakest and also provides fixation to the posterior cortex of the upper tibia (the strongest bone in the region).

Support of the plastic by means of a metal tray or endoskeleton (Fig. 20.24A,B) is desirable when the bone of the upper tibia is deficient (severe erosive arthritis or revision operations), but when the bone is of good quality, metal backing may not offer an advantage. One-piece plastic components with a central peg have a low rate of loosening but in 30 to 40 percent of cases a partial radiolucency develops. For the most part these radiolucencies appear within the first year, are nonprogressive and are of dubious clinical significance. The addition of a metal tray reduces the incidence of radiolucency, but with a central peg design bone reabsorption because of stress shielding may occur beneath the metal tray and the weakening of cancellous bone support may eventually increase the incidence of late subsidence. Thus, laboratory data must be accepted with caution and the application of metal-backed tibial components for all cases cannot yet be unequivocally recommended.

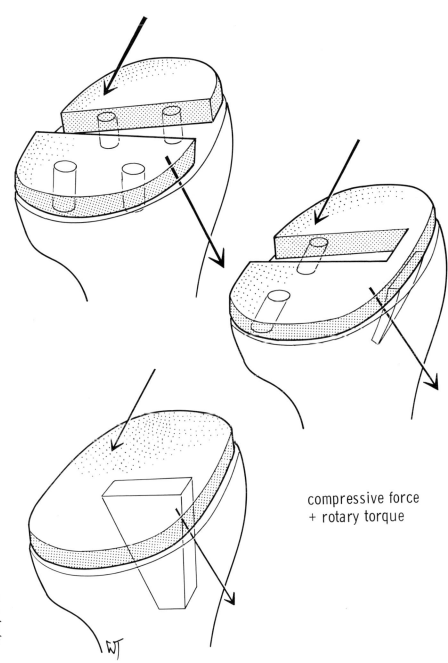

compressive force
+ rotary torque

Fig. 20.23. Deflections at the bone–cement interface showing different configurations of tibial component. (Courtesy of Dr. Peter Walker.)

606 Surgery of the Knee

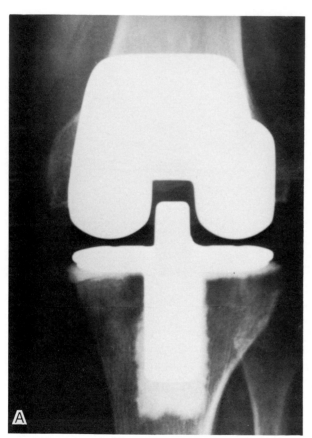
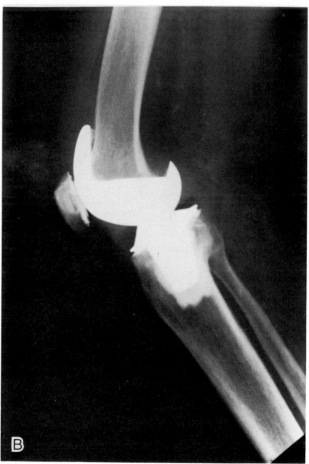

Fig. 20.24. (A,B) Anteroposterior and lateral radiographs of a tibial component with an endoskeleton. Metal backing of this type may in the long run enhance fixation.

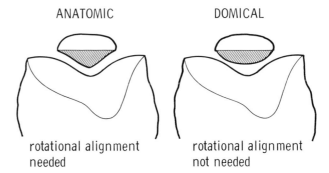

ANATOMIC   DOMICAL

rotational alignment   rotational alignment
needed   not needed

Fig. 20.25. Rotational alignment is needed with a patellar replacement of anatomic shape.

Until recently most patellar components were dome shaped. This configuration is not ideal because the convex contour might be expected to wear poorly on the basis of engineering experience (in an articulation, the softer material should be concave). A component that is a semirectangle (e.g., the ICLH) or anatomic (porous-coated anatomic) has a more desirable configuration in this respect, but requires careful rotary alignment to prevent binding against the femur (Fig. 20.25). In addition, correct static alignment, even if achieved at operation, may not predict the functional pull of the quadriceps in active use and the more desirable wear characteristics can be offset by increased torque on the component caused by malalignment. In any event, wear with a dome-shaped component has not proved a problem (Fig. 20.26), and the clinical experience has been most satisfactory.

While a femoral flange is now an almost universal attribute, the need to resurface the patella itself is not fully accepted. At The Hospital for Special Surgery it is done routinely both in rheumatoid arthritis and in osteoarthritis, in every case in which the patella will accept an implant, irrespective of the condition of the patellar articular cartilage. This policy arose from the early experience with selective replacement when relatively normal patellae were not resurfaced (Fig. 20.27A,B). Although most of these patients did well, a proportion required reoperation to insert a patellar button, and this number exceeded those in whom a complication developed from the implant itself[123] (Fig. 20.28). Patellar fractures caused by weakening of the patellar bone have occurred, but for the most part have not required reoperation and have not significantly influenced the quality of the

Fig. 20.26. The appearance of a dome shaped patella at reoperation for suspected sepsis after 5 years. All the components were rigidly fixed, and the patellar component was virtually unmarked.

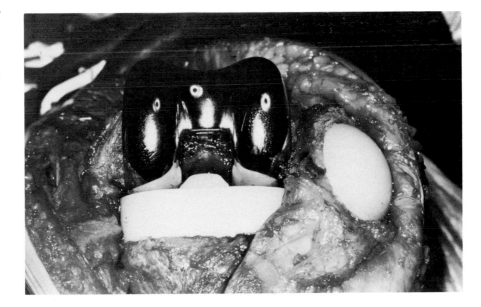

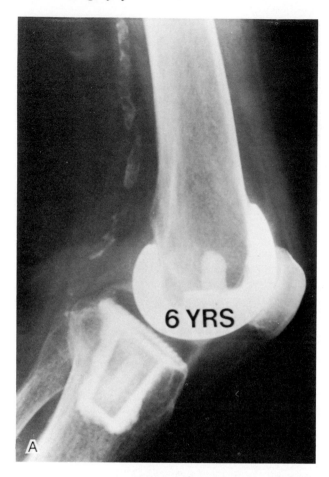

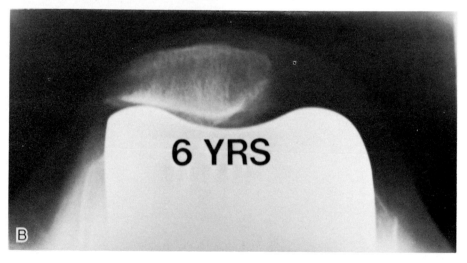

Fig. 20.27. (A,B) Lateral and skyline patellar views of a knee replacement without patellar resurfacing.

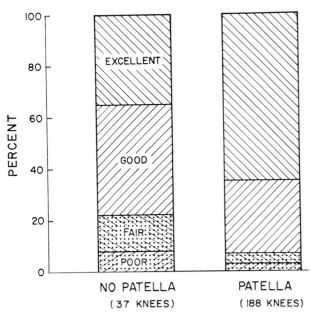

OVERALL GROUP

Fig. 20.28. The clinical results are slightly better when a patellar component is used.

arthroplasty.[137] Loosening and wear have not to date caused clinical difficulties. While there does seem a trend toward this viewpoint, Sledge and Ewald[131] recommend a selective approach in osteoarthritis replacing only damaged patellae. They believe that in rheumatoid arthritis the patella should be replaced in every case so as to remove all articular cartilage from the joint.

THE POSTERIOR STABILIZED CONDYLAR KNEE[76] (Fig. 20.29)

This is a development of the total condylar design. Because the TCP, like the ICLH, provides anteroposterior stability in part by the dished shape of the tibial articulation (acting together with tension in the collateral ligaments), it was logical to carry the concept a step further by providing more active and concrete posterior cruciate substitution. This function was assumed by a central spine which articulates against a transverse cam on the femoral component. In the first version of the prosthesis (TCP II) the cam mechanism provided a purely passive restraint against pos-

terior displacement and, incidently, an anterior stop preventing hyperextension (Fig. 20.30). This latter function proved both unnecessary and undesirable.[69] The TCP II was used in 1976 and 1977 and was superseded in 1978 by the current design, the posterior stabilized (PS) knee. In the PS knee, the central spine was much reduced in size, reshaped, and repositioned so that with flexion, the spine engages with the femur at 75 degrees. Thereafter, with further flexion, the cam imposes a progressive rollback of the femoral condyles to prevent posterior impingement (Fig. 20.31). The standard version is designed to reach 120 degrees, but a version designed to fulfill local custom needs in Asia allows 140 degrees of flexion. In extension the spine does not engage the femur anteriorly until the knee is in 20 degrees of hyperextension (a position that should never be reached). The cam mechanism permits an increasing amount of rotation as the knee is flexed, up to a maximum of 20 degrees at right angle flexion. No varus–valgus stability is provided, and the two components disengage freely if stressed in these directions (Fig. 20.32). In order to provide the capacity for greater flexion, some minor modifications were made in the curvatures of the femoral component, and the tibial articulation was inclined posteriorly at an angle of 10 degrees, so that the anterior lip of the articulation is approximately 5 mm higher than the posterior lip (Fig. 20.33). As the intercondylar recess now dovetails into the femur, the fixation lugs were removed from the medial and lateral condyles, which is an advantage because important bone stock is preserved in these areas. The fixation peg on the tibial component remains the same, and the patellar button is unchanged. As will be discussed later, the PS knee has behaved in vivo in the same manner as the TCP except for significant gains in the range of flexion and the associated functional activities that go with greater motion.

THE ICLH PROSTHESIS[38,40,42–44,106]

The ICLH implant was originally known as the Freeman-Swanson (Fig. 20.34); the first prosthesis was inserted at the London Hospital in 1970. The general principle was that of a roller-in-trough. The trough was formed by the top surface of a thin polyethylene tibial component, and the roller by a femoral component consisting of a roughly U-shaped shell that

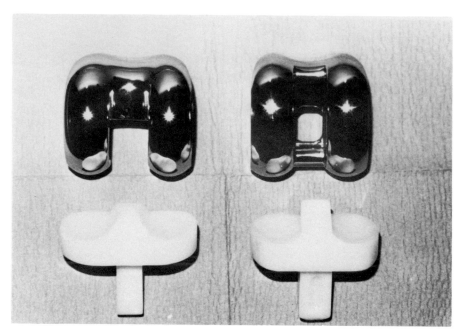

Fig. 20.29. (Left) Total condylar prosthesis. (Right) posterior stabilized condylar knee, a newer derivative providing posterior cruciate substitution by means of a central cam mechanism. (From Insall, J.N., Lachiewicz, P.F., and Burstein, A.H.: The posterior stablized condylar prosthesis. A modification of the total condylar design. Two to four year clinical experience. J. Bone Joint Surg. [Am.], *64:* 1317, 1982, with permission.)

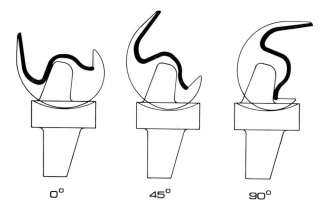

0°   45°   90°

Fig. 20.30. The TCP II was a precursor of the posterior stabilized knee that provided a passive stop against posterior displacement in flexion, as well as a hyperextension stop in extension. (From Insall, J.N., Tria, A.J., and Scott, W.N.: The total condylar knee prosthesis: The first five years. Clin. Orthop. *145:* 68, 1979, with permission.)

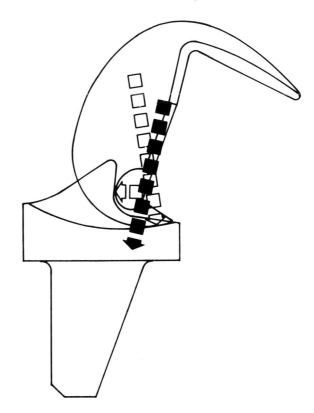

Fig. 20.31. The cam mechanism of the posterior stabilized knee simulates the function of the posterior cruciate ligament and causes a rollback of the femur on the tibia with flexion. The resulting vector of forces passes distally through the fixation peg. (From Insall, J.N., Lachiewicz, P.F., and Burstein, A.H.: The posterior stabilized condylar prosthesis. A modification of the total condylar design. Two to four year clinical experience. J. Bone Surg. [Am.], *64:* 1317, 1982, with permission.)

Fig. 20.32. Neither the TCP II nor the posterior stabilized knee provides varus or valgus restraint. (From Insall, J.N., Trio, A.J., and Scott, W.N.: The total condylar knee prosthesis: The first five years. Clin. Orthop., *145:* 68, 1979, with permission.)

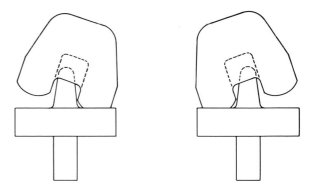

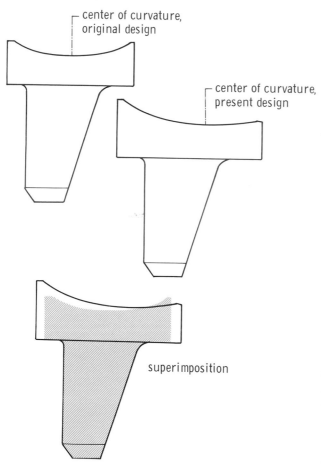

superimposition

Fig. 20.33. The articular surface of the tibial component of the posterior stabilized knee is inclined posteriorly 10 degrees.

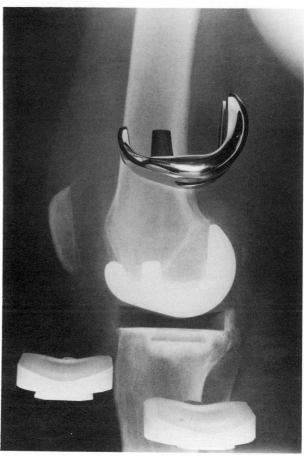

Fig. 20.34. The original version of the Freeman-Swanson prosthesis (courtesy of M.A.R. Freeman).

fitted onto rectangularly trimmed femoral condyles. The geometry of a cylindrical roller in a reciprocally shaped trough was somewhat modified. The femoral component on its articular surface had successively a posterior cylindrical portion that engaged with the correspondingly curved part of the trough, an inclined distal flat that formed part of the hyperextension-limiting mechanism, and an anterior cylindrical portion that provided a bearing surface for the patella or patellar tendon.

The prosthesis has been successively modified by Freeman (Fig. 20.35); the problems and their solutions were as follows.[40,44]

Loosening and Sinkage of the Tibial Component (Fig. 20.36). The first version of the tibial component was made small enough to be implanted into all

knees; as a consequence, in most knees the prosthesis rested on a part of the cross section of the tibia. In 1975 a large-area tibial component was introduced together with a specially designed power-driven instrument to trim excess polyethylene at operation. Finally, in 1977 a fixation change was made by the addition of two "magic pegs"—medial- and lateral-finned UHMWP studs about 2 cm in length. The pegs are driven into slightly undersized circular holes causing the fins to fold upward; in position, the fins either penetrate into the cancellous bone or remain compressed against the pegs. The intention is not bone ingrowth but immediate mechanical fixation.[11] The tibial component can be implanted with or without cement.

Patellar Pain. Ten early patients had a concomi-

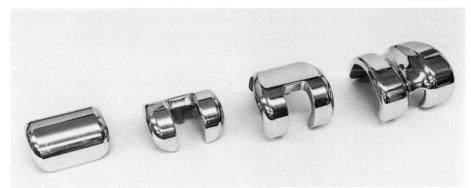

Fig. 20.35. Successive modifications have been made to the original femoral component of the Freeman-Swanson prosthesis (courtesy of M.A.R. Freeman).

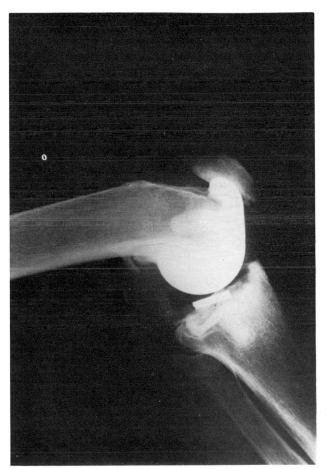

Fig. 20.36. Tibial component loosening and sinkage and patellar pain and impingement were problems with the early version of the Freeman-Swanson prosthesis.

tant patellectomy with a number of disastrous failures in wound healing; subsequently, the patella was retained. In 1975 the posterior surface of the patella was resected and in 1977 a high anterior flange femoral component was added; patellar resection (without replacement) continued until 1978, when resurfacing of the patella with polyethylene begin routinely. The polyethylene component was concave to fit against the convex femoral component and thus required correct alignment during insertion into the patella.

Posterior Cementophytes. With the original monocondylar femoral prosthesis it was difficult to clear cement from the posterior part of the joint. In 1975 a bicondylar femoral component was made, and the tibial component was inserted first. When the bicondylar femoral component was subsequently cemented, excess cement extruded into the empty intercondylar notch, from which it could be removed.

RECENT DEVELOPMENTS

The ICLH prosthesis is now known as the Freeman-Samuelson (Fig. 20.37), the latest modifications include the following:

1. A groove on the anterior flange of the femoral component to restrain the patella and prevent lateral subluxation
2. A raised anterior lip to the tibial component and division of the trough into separate articulations by

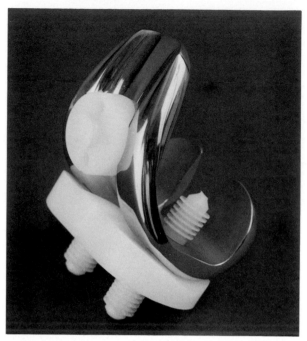

Fig. 20.37. The current version of the Freeman-Samuelson prosthesis (courtesy of M.A.R. Freeman).

an intercondylar eminence to prevent translocation

3. The addition of "magic peg" fixation to the femoral and patellar components

As this section proposes to deal mainly with cruciate-removing prostheses, which I consider most suitable for replacement in osteoarthritis, the cruciate-retaining types will not be further discussed here. The rationale and use of the duopatellar prosthesis[35] (a typical cruciate-preserving design) are described in Chapter 21.

It is appropriate, however, to mention an interesting and ingenious design developed in Oxford by Goodfellow and O'Connor.[48] The prosthesis uses polyethylene "menisci" inserted between the femoral and tibial condyles: the designers recognizing that intact cruciates impose a rollback on flexion, designed the prosthesis to accommodate this movement. The femoral and tibial condyles are resurfaced with metal, and stability and alignment are restored to the knee by blocking open the joint medially and laterally with polyethylene disks of varying thicknesses (in a similar manner to the MacIntosh prosthesis). The polyeth-

ylene menisci are retained only by their shape and ligament tension and move with the femur on flexion and extension of the knee. Dislocation of the polyethylene disks is an obvious possibility, but the designers have stated that this is a rare occurence provided the prosthesis is correctly inserted. Early clinical data show that varus and valgus deformities are correctable, provided that some postoperative flexion contracture is accepted: the flexion contracture tends to decrease with time.

UNICOMPARTMENTAL REPLACEMENT

Unicompartmental replacement of the osteoarthritic knee is widely used both in the United States and in Europe.[68,73,83,96,101,122,129] The concept has been recommended because only the abnormal joint surfaces are removed, and the total amount of bone excised is minimal. The amount of foreign material used (metal, polyethylene, and cement) quantitatively is also minimal. Finally, it has been claimed that the operative time and complications are less.

Unicompartmental designs include the polycentric, unicondylar, the modular (Fig. 20.38), the St. Georg, the Manchester, and the most recent version of the Freeman. All are similar in concept and are intended to replace osteoarthritic knees in which one compartment alone is involved. The ligaments, including the cruciates, must all be present and relatively normal. Therefore, the prosthesis cannot be used in severely involved arthritic knees with large deformity, severe instability, or a significant flexion contracture. Likewise, the procedure has no place in the treatment of rheumatoid panarthritis. Therefore the indications for unicompartmental replacement in varus gonarthrosis are essentially the same as for high tibial osteotomy. For lateral compartment arthritis, another alternative choice is lower femoral osteotomy.

The unicondylar prosthesis[70] (Fig. 20.7) consists of a metallic femoral replacement of approximate anatomic design: the sagittal curvature increases posteriorly and in the frontal plane the curvature mimics the median half of the femoral condyles. Therefore two mirror image femoral components are required with a central peg and anterior flange for fixation and

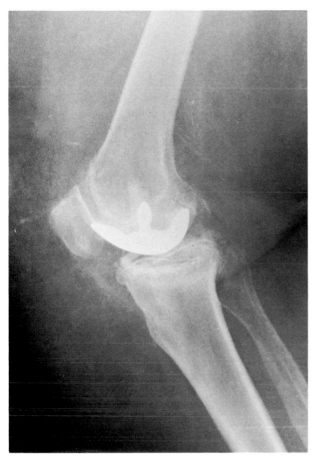

Fig. 20.38. Lateral radiograph of unicompartmental Marmor modular prosthesis.

alignment. They are available in either small or large sizes. The polyethylene tibial component is flat in the sagittal plane and curved in the frontal plane to conform with the femoral component. The deep surface is dovetailed for cement fixation, and the component is available in several thicknesses. Fixation lugs have been added to the tibial component at the Robert B. Brigham Hospital in Boston.

The modular, St. Georg, and Freeman prostheses differ in that the components in the coronal plane are flat.

Unicompartmental replacements are tricky to insert and require much precision. The surgical technique may therefore play a big part in the ultimate success of the device.

CONSTRAINED PROSTHESES

These implants provide all the required stability for the knee joint, and therefore both cruciate and collateral ligaments may be excised or absent. Most experience has been with the metal-to-metal hinges (Walldius, Shiers, and Guepar). There is a considerable amount of literature devoted to these specific prosthetic designs. Infection and loosening have been major problems. Arden[3] reported 26 infections in 209 Shiers prostheses (12 percent), Bain[7] had 10 infections in 100 Walldius prostheses. Watson et al.[148] found 35 of 38 Shiers prostheses to show signs of loosening. Considerable bone resection is required for implantation and much of the remaining cancellous bone is lost during the removal of the implant. The femur and tibia resemble hollow cones of cortical bone after such removals. In one series of Guepar hinges only three of 14 attempts at fusion resulted in a bony arthrodesis.[80] The long-term results of hinged prosthetic total knee designs have been discouraging and their continued use cannot be recommended. Several newer designs with metal-on-polyethylene articulations have attempted to solve these problems by allowing rotary and gliding movements while continuing to provide the necessary stability. Examples include the TCP III, the stabilocondylar,[112] spherocentric,[133] Attenborough,[5,6] Deane,[27] and Sheehan[126] prostheses.

While the mainstream of prosthetic replacement undoubtedly lies with surface replacement, full constraint is occasionally required for revision surgery and for a few primary cases. As far as the latter group is concerned, it is estimated that between 90 and 99 percent are replaceable using a surface prosthesis the exact proportion being dependent on the experience and technical skill of the surgeon. The data on the newer constrained prostheses are too recent and incomplete to judge whether they will fare better than the older metal-on-metal designs, although it is probable that they will. In any event, it is preferable for the patient to leave the operating table with a stable arthroplasty, even if this means the use of a constrained design rather than an unsatisfactory and unstable surface replacement that is doomed to failure from the outset. A constrained prosthesis such as listed above should therefore be kept as a backup "in the cupboard;" moreover, the presence of this security encourages a neophyte surgeon to perform boldly the necessary soft tissue releases, which are the key to successful surface replacement arthroplasty.

TCP III (Fig. 20.39)

The total condylar prosthesis III (TCP III) evolved from the total condylar and stabilocondylar designs. The stabilocondylar[112] was developed at The Hospital for Special Surgery in 1974 and possesses an articulation very similar to the TCP. Stability is provided by a rectangular tibial post that fits snugly within a reciprocal recess in the femoral component. The two are linked together by a transverse pin passing through a loose slot in the tibial post. Insertion of this prosthesis is rather complicated, as the linkage makes it necessary to insert the femoral and tibial components together. This is made possible by inserting a separate tibial intramedullary stem that is passed through the tibial component once in place.

It soon became apparent that the actual linkage was seldom needed and thus the unlinked TCP III evolved. The rectangular post and recess mechanism remain the same, but the tibial component is now made in one piece with an attached intramedullary stem, 7 cm in length. The tibial component is available in UHMWP or reinforced with metal backing. The femoral component is available with and without intramedullary stems. The patellar component is the TCP dome.

The TCP III is mainly a backup prosthesis available as an intraoperative choice for revisions or in cases of technical error. It is also occasionally used as a primary prosthesis for knees with severe valgus or flexion deformities in which it is judged that a postoperative peroneal palsy is probable from stretching of the nerve.

THE SPHEROCENTRIC PROSTHESIS[85,133] (Fig. 20.40A,B)

The spherocentric knee is a nonhinged intrinsically stable knee joint prosthesis that permits controlled triaxial rotation and is designed specifically for use in severely deformed or unstable knees. There are three metal-on-high-density polyethylene-bearing surfaces: a ball-in-socket joint located within the femoral component and two runner and track joints between the femoral and tibial condyles. The ball-and-socket joint is composed of a central metal sphere on top of a column rising from the tibial component, which in the articulated prosthesis is contained within a polyethylene socket within the femoral component. The ball-and-socket joint formed permits triaxial rotation, but dislocation is not possible in any direction. The center of the sphere lies above the joint surfaces and posterior to the long axis of the femur, thus approximating the location of the average flexion axis of the normal knee. The location, dimensions, and contour of the metal femoral runners and their mated tibial polyethylene tracks serve to guide and control flexion, varus–valgus movement, and torsion and to increase the total bearing surface of the joint. The con-

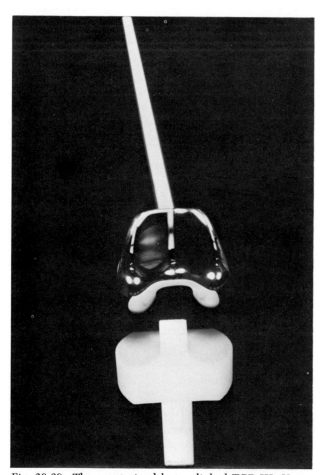

Fig. 20.39. The constrained but unlinked TCP III. Varus and valgus constraint is provided by the rectangular central peg on the tibial component.

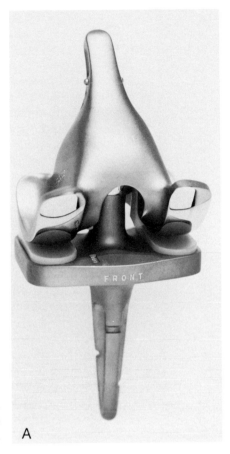
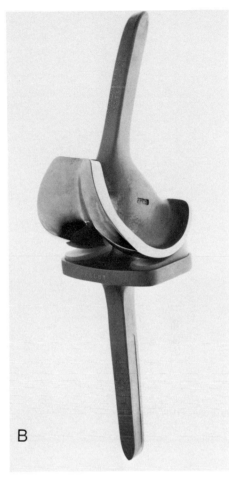

Fig. 20.40. Spherocentric prosthesis. (A) Standard version. (B) Long-stemmed variant with patellar flange (courtesy of Drs. Kaufer and Matthews).

tours of the femoral condylar surfaces in the sagittal plane include an anterior part with a larger radius of curvature that is not concentric with the surface of the sphere and a posterior part with a smaller radius of curvature that is concentric with the surface of the sphere. As the knee approaches full extension, the anterior surfaces of the femoral condylar runners with their larger radius of curvature bear increasingly on the plastic tibial tracks, thereby unloading the top of the sphere and resisting hyperextension by gradual deceleration. Impact loading during extension is thereby minimized, and at full extension the prosthesis is fixed and completely stable in all directions except flexion. As the prosthesis flexes the femoral condylar surfaces slowly lift off the plastic tibial track gradually transferring all of the load to the dome of the sphere. At a maximum flexion of 120 degrees, the prosthesis permits up to 30 degrees of tibial rotation and up to 5 degrees of varus–valgus motion. All ar-

ticulating surfaces are metal on plastic. The prosthesis possesses short intramedullary stems for both femur and tibia. The prosthesis can be used for either the right or the left side.

THE ATTENBOROUGH PROSTHESIS[5,6] (Fig. 20.41)

The stabilized gliding knee prosthesis represents a compromise between a constrained hinge and an unconnected surface prosthesis. It is a two-piece prosthesis with normal gliding movement for flexion and extension. A stabilizing rod between the femoral and tibial components permits some lateral and rotational laxity while acting in place of the cruciate ligaments and in place of, or in addition to, the collateral ligaments. Excessive rotational and lateral movements tighten the soft tissues and produce a gradual decel-

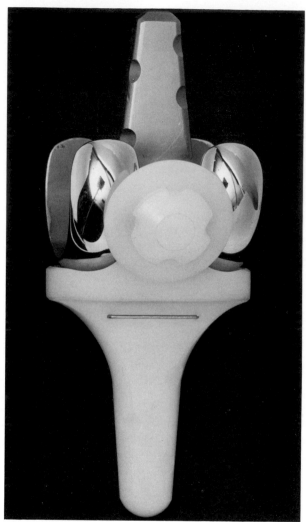

Fig. 20.41. Attenborough prosthesis.

THE SHEEHAN PROSTHESIS[126]
(Fig. 20.42)

Both components have intramedullary stems, that on the femoral component is inclined so that left and right prostheses are required.

The femoral component has separate bearing surfaces with a gap for the stabilizing stud of the tibial component that interlocks between the femoral-bearing surfaces and engages an inner radius, ensuring stability of the joint. Cruciate stability is simulated by preventing anterior–posterior movement, but sliding and rolling movements are permitted. Collateral ligament stability is achieved by the same mechanism, allowing 2 to 3 degrees of movement in the extended position and 6 to 7 degrees when the knee is flexed. The external surface of the femoral component has a curvature simulating that of the normal knee, permitting a constantly changing instant center of rotation. The intercondylar notch of the femoral component widens posteriorly to allow approximately 20 degrees of rotation at a right angle.

The tibial component is made of polyethylene; it has two bearing surfaces and an expanded intercondylar stud. The polyethylene portion is attached to a metal base and intramedullary stem.

INDICATIONS FOR TOTAL KNEE REPLACEMENT[66]

It goes without saying that to warrant knee joint replacement symptoms and disability must be severe. Patients who have had an unsatisfactory arthroplasty naturally gravitate to surgeons whose expertise lies in that area, and I have seen cases in which the selection of the original operation was questionable. While it is no longer true that a patient should consent to an arthrodesis before undergoing an arthroplasty a frank discussion with the patient concerning the consequences of failure is essential. Medical management should be continued as long as possible and alternative techniques such as tibial osteotomy selected when feasible.

In the presence of severe and unremitting symptomatology, total knee arthroplasty is indicated in the following circumstances:

1. *Rheumatoid panarthritis.* Here, it is indicated regardless of age.

eration of movements. The stabilizing rod possesses a sphere at its proximal end contained within a recess in the femoral component and is held in place by a polyethylene circlip. Once in place, it cannot be removed except by destruction. The distal end of the stabilizing rod passes down a vertical channel within the tibial component and with movements of the knee it is free to move up and down within the tibial channel like a plunger. The articular surface possesses moderate cupping and an intercondylar eminence. Both components have short stems.

There is a dome-shaped polyethylene tibial component. The implant can be used in patients with severe deformity and instability. For revision cases a "high tibial" component is available to fill the gap between the bone ends.

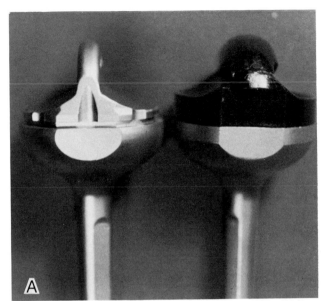

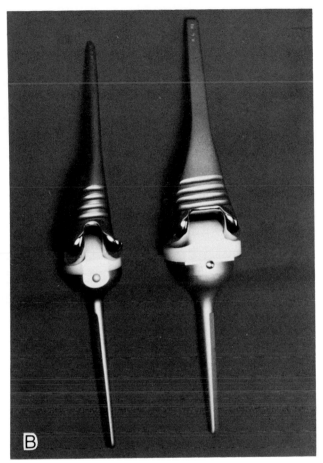

Fig. 20.42. The Sheehan prosthesis. (A) The tibial polyethylene stud. (B) Assembled prosthesis (courtesy of Dr. Sheehan).

2. *Gonarthrosis.* Here the age of the patient, occupation, level of activity, sex, and weight are all factors that must be considered. In general terms, arthroplasty should be avoided in patients under 60 years of age, manual laborers, athletes, and those grossly overweight. Men will tend to abuse the arthroplasty more than women, so that the sex of the patient is also important. The surgeon must review these factors in his own mind and discuss them with the patient before arriving at a recommendation.

3. *Post-traumatic osteoarthritis.* There may rarely be an indication for knee replacement in the younger patient following intra-articular fracture or other traumatic injuries to the joint. This is discussed further in the section on Arthrodesis, Chapter 23.

4. *Failure of high tibial osteotomy.* When high tibial osteotomy has failed to relieve symptoms or when symptoms recur after an interval due to progressive arthritis total knee replacement can be done without difficulty. No adverse effects due to the osteotomy have been observed with regard to tibial fixation.

5. *Patellofemoral osteoarthritis.* In most cases, patellofemoral osteoarthritis is not an indication for total replacement of the joint, and the condition is better managed by another technique. Femorotibial narrowing on a weight bearing radiograph is therefore usually a prerequisite for joint replacement, but occasionally an elderly patient will present with very severe patellofemoral arthrosis without significant femorotibial narrowing despite patchy articular degeneration found throughout the joint at arthrotomy. This type of case, although rare, does better with total joint replacement than with any other method.

6. *The neuropathic joint.* Joint replacement in neuropathic states is controversial and represents a technical challenge as instability and deformity are often extreme. I believe that knee replacement is feasible provided that a surface replacement can be used, the joint is thoroughly debrided, and correct alignment and stability achieved. Metal-backed components with longer than usual stem fixation are desirable.

CONTRAINDICATIONS TO KNEE REPLACEMENT

1. A sound painless arthrodesis in good position should not be converted to a knee arthroplasty. Prospects of a successful arthroplasty are not good, and a constrained prosthesis is usually required. Should the arthroplasty fail, re-arthrodesing the knee may not succeed.
2. Genu recurvatum associated with muscular weakness and paralysis is likely to recur after a surface replacement, and the stresses imposed on a constrained prosthesis will probably loosen it.
3. Gross quadriceps weakness.
4. Active sepsis. When infection is caused by a susceptible organism thorough debridement and appropriate antibiotic therapy may be followed by a later replacement after eradication of infection (see section on management of the infected arthroplasty). Tuberculous joints can be managed in a similar manner. When the infecting organism cannot be adequately treated because, for example, of the potential toxicity of the necessary antibiotic therapy, arthrodesis is the better choice.

SURGICAL TECHNIQUE

The success of any total knee replacement depends on four factors: patient selection, prosthetic design, prosthetic materials, and surgical technique.

Prosthetic design has evolved to the point where little further toward improvement in the results can be expected from continued refinement in design. Current prostheses possess many basic similarities and, if correctly inserted, most will give satisfactory results. However, whereas total hip arthroplasty is relatively forgiving of surgical error, total knee replacement is not. Component malposition of 5, 10, or even 20 degrees, may not affect the outcome in arthroplasty of the hip. In knee replacement an error of 5 degrees is significant and 10 degrees often catastrophic (Fig. 20.43). Furthermore, even when the components themselves are correctly positioned, the adjustment of tension in the soft tissues must also be exactly right for the arthroplasty to function. In the hip, for instance, a loose fit between the components is not in itself of great consequence. Shifting the greater trochanter downward will often compensate and, pro-

vided the hip is prevented from dislocating during the early postoperative phase, the soft tissues aided by the muscles acting across the joint will adjust and contract, ending with a stable arthroplasty and, at worst, slight shortening of the leg. In contrast, the knee surgeon must consider not only the overall soft tissue tension, but the relative tightness, both medially and laterally (Fig. 20.44), and in the positions of flexion (Fig. 20.45) and extension. All must be correct at the end of the operation. Prolonged immobilization does not usually improve inadequate soft tissue balance, and muscle development will not prevent subluxation or dislocation of the components. Therefore unlike the hip, the component placement and overall alignment must be correct within narrow tolerance limits, and the soft tissues must be adjusted while in the operating theater. When these requirements are not met, the arthroplasty will at best be suboptimal, and often a total failure.

PRINCIPLES OF SURGICAL TECHNIQUE[67,68]

Regardless of the type of prosthesis, there are some common surgical principles that apply to the use of surface replacements of the knee whether or not the cruciate ligaments are to be excised. As will be discussed later, the instrument systems available for different designs of prostheses vary considerably and in some instances the sequence recommended for making the bone cuts is not the same as the following description. Most prostheses have femoral components of various sizes, and tibial components of various thicknesses, so that component size can be roughly adjusted to the dimensions of the knee. Attempting to replace the knee with components that are grossly mismatched in size is likely to be difficult and unsatisfactory, so that an adequate inventory of component parts is essential.

The simplest knee to replace is one in which only the articular cartilage is damaged, so that normal alignment is retained, the ligaments are unaltered, and there are no bone defects. The following description applies to a knee of this kind and it is assumed that the tibial component is in one piece and that the femoral component has the deep surface shaped to fit right-angle bone cuts.

The bone ends must be reshaped so that they may

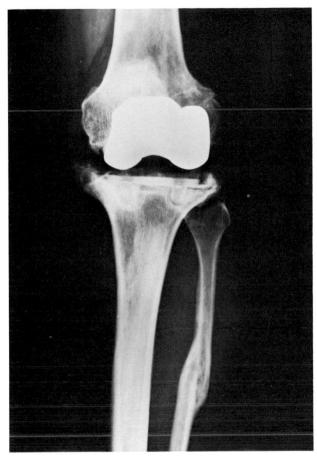

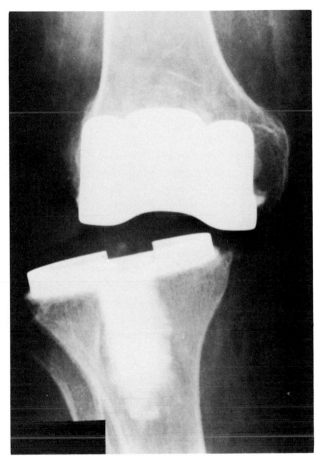

Fig. 20.43. Component malposition even of minor degree is likely to have long-term significance. This knee, which is in slight varus, is likely to fail. A pronounced lateral radiolucency is present.

Fig. 20.44. Instability in extension caused by improper mediolateral ligament balance.

Fig. 20.45. Instability in flexion. (Left) Posterior subluxation with a Freeman-Swanson prosthesis. (Middle) Revised to a total condylar prosthesis with subluxation. (Right) Instability solved by the use of a TCP II.

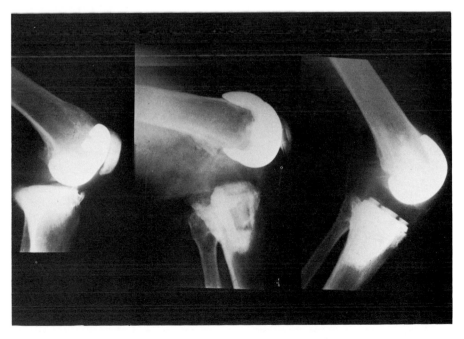

be capped by the components, which must fit so that the new prosthetic geometry will be compatible with existing ligament lengths throughout the range of motion. Although instruments are desirable to aid in precision, a "cookbook" approach to knee arthroplasty is deplorable. In order to be consistently successful the surgeon must understand clearly the basic principles of arthroplasty and be able to work by eye when necessary. Given this degree of skill, comprehensive instrumentation helps attain the desired level of precision.

The basic operation is carried out in the following manner using a sequence of steps that are easy to follow and that experience has shown are not fundamentally altered by the myriad of pathologic variations encountered in knees with complex deformities.

CREATION OF THE FLEXION GAP

The femoral condyles are measured using dummy components or templates and a prosthesis is selected which roughly approximates the original size of the femur, particularly in its anteroposterior dimensions.

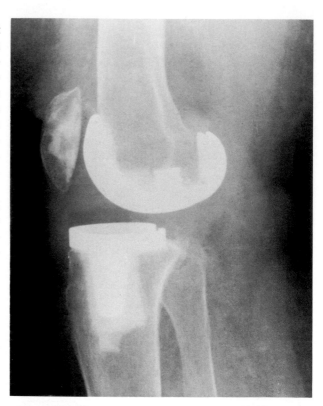

Fig. 20.47. Excessive posterior cruciate tightness causes the tibia to sublux forward.

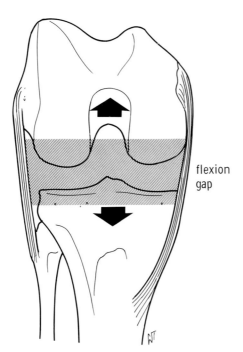

Fig. 20.46. The flexion gap is created first removing bone from the tibial plateaus and posterior femoral condyles.

The flexion gap (Fig. 20.46) is created by removing the posterior femoral condyles and the surface of the tibial plateau so that the resulting space can be filled by the combined bulk of the femoral and tibial components. The space must not be too small to accept the thinnest available tibial component nor too large to be filled by the thickest standard component. In the former instance the prosthesis cannot be inserted, and in the latter the fit will be undesirably loose so that the components may dislocate. When the cruciates are retained subluxation in flexion is less likely but extra care must be taken to prevent the fit being excessively tight. It is not enough for the flexion space to accept the components: they must fit without anterior displacement of the tibia; this will happen when excessive tension forces the posterior cruciate ligament to assume a more vertical orientation (Fig. 20.47).

Because it is desirable for the anterior femoral flange to fit flush with the anterior femoral shaft, the best point of reference for beginning the bone cuts is the anterior femoral cortex (Fig. 20.48). The first jig should

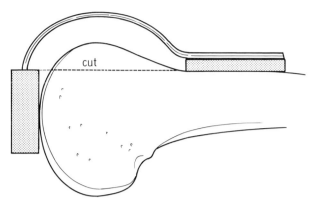

Fig. 20.48. First femoral jig is aligned with the anterior cortex of the femur.

various blocks for femurs of different size

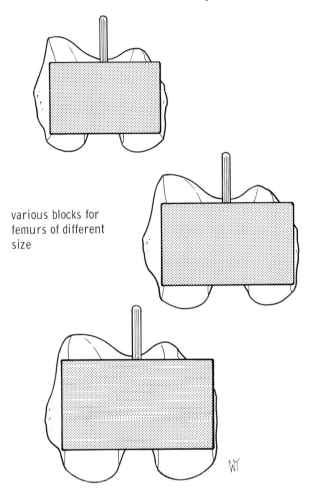

Fig. 20.49. Sizing the femoral condyle.

therefore indicate the level of anterior and posterior femoral resection and the amount of bone to be removed from the upper tibia. The properly selected size of the femoral component should result in roughly equal amounts of bone being removed anteriorly and posteriorly from the femur (Fig. 20.49). When the tibial bone is also removed the resulting space should snugly accommodate the components. The selection of the tibial component thickness may need some fine tuning to get the best fit; this is most conveniently done by using a series of appropriate spacers.

Rotation and Alignment in Flexion

Two anatomic features often accentuated in arthritic states must now be considered: (1) the medial slope of the tibial plateau, which is normally inclined at an angle of 3 to 5 degrees from the horizontal; and (2) lateral ligament laxity in flexion, which normally occurs to provide for the greater mobility of the lateral femoral condyle in the flexed position.

Prosthetic components inserted anatomically would therefore (1) have a medial slope to the tibia, and (2) permit excessive lateral rotational laxity when the knee is flexed (Fig. 20.50).

Imitating the normal anatomy in knee replacement thus does not seem desirable. Designing prosthetic components to allow greater lateral excursion seems unnecessarily complex, and when rotation is to be shared equally by the medial and lateral articulations, the adjacent soft tissues must therefore be of symmetric length. Also, since the normal knee is loaded to a greater extent medially than laterally,[79] and the

prosthetic components are designed for equal distribution of weight, a second adjustment is required.

Because of the inequality of ligament length in flexion, when bone is resected symmetrically from the tibia and the posterior femoral condyles, the resulting space between the bone ends upon distraction of the joint will be trapezoidal rather than rectangular (Fig. 20.51).

If soft tissue balance is to be given priority the slack in the lateral ligament can be taken up by increasing the medial slope of the tibial cut. However, equal loading on the two sides of the tibial component is more likely when the component is positioned at right angles to the long axis of the bone.

Relating these considerations to technique, the preferred compromise is to (1) cut the tibia at right angles to the long axis of the bone, and (2) after dis-

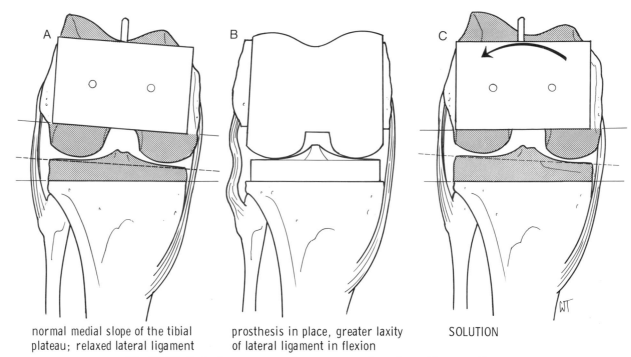

normal medial slope of the tibial   prosthesis in place, greater laxity   SOLUTION
plateau; relaxed lateral ligament   of lateral ligament in flexion

Fig. 20.50. Imitating tne normal anatomy results in lateral laxity in flexion.

tracting the ligaments, rotate the position of the femoral component relative to the femoral condyles until it becomes parallel with the tibial cut (Fig. 20.52).

If the position of the hip is fixed this maneuver would result in external rotation of the knee, ankle and foot during gait. However, when the hip is mobile the result is merely a small compensatory internal rotation movement at the hip joint.

THE EXTENSION GAP

The cuts already performed have produced a rectangular space between the bones in flexion which is snugly filled by the femoral component and a selected thickness of tibial component. The precise dimension of this gap has been assessed with a spacer. An amount of bone must now be removed from the distal femur to create a second rectangular gap of exactly similar size with the knee extended (Fig. 20.53). This is done by distracting the knee and marking the femur at an appropriate level, once again parallel to the tibial cut. (In this given instance, it has been assumed that the overall alignment was correct to begin with so that provided both collateral ligaments are symmetrically

tensioned in this step, the overall postoperative alignment will automatically be correct.) After bone removal, the resulting gap should therefore accept the same spacer used in flexion.

Note that the flexion gap determines the extension gap and not vice versa. The tibia is always cut at the same level to preserve the strongest cancellous bone immediately beneath the articular surface. A component approximately the size of the femur is chosen and a precise fit obtained by using the thickest tibial component that will fit in flexion. The level of distal femoral resection is adjusted to correspond. This principle holds true for structurally intact knees but becomes even more important when there is contracture, deformity, and instability.

Component Position and Alignment

In our opinion it is undesirable to mimic the normal medial slope of the tibial plateau during knee replacement. It is also not necessarily correct to restore the original anatomical alignment of the knee and in a unilateral case the replaced knee will not always have the same alignment as the other uninvolved knee. Whereas the average physiological valgus is estimated

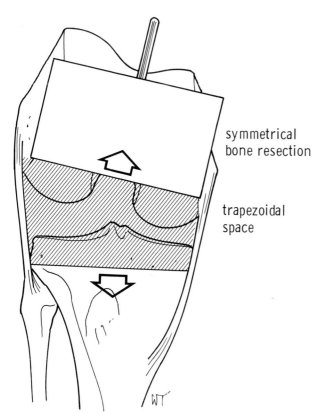

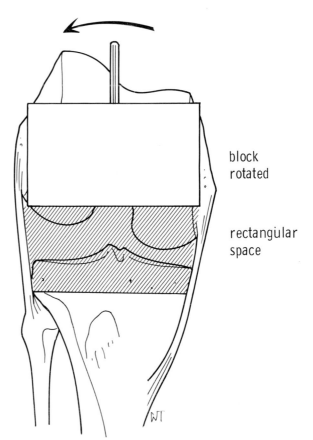

symmetrical
bone resection

trapezoidal
space

block
rotated

rectangular
space

Fig. 20.51. In the osteoarthritic knee, lateral laxity is accentuated; when symmetric bone is excised from the posterior femoral condyles, the resulting space upon distraction is trapezoidal.

Fig. 20.52. By externally rotating the femoral component and removing an asymmetric amount of bone from the posterior femoral condyles, soft tissue length is equalized and the resulting space is rectangular.

at 5 to 7 degrees, the range is considerable particularly in men, and the preexisting femorotibial angle may have been zero or even a few degrees of varus. In as far as is possible, equal loading across the prosthetic joint is the objective; this may mean positioning in more valgus than is "normal" for a particular individual.

In the early days of knee replacement, subtleties of component position and alignment were not fully appreciated, and it was generally considered sufficient to make the leg look straight. Today, restoration of the mechanical axis (i.e., a line drawn through the hip, knee, and ankle) is considered ideal (Fig. 20.54). To achieve this, a long alignment rod is essential.

Lotke and Ecker[91] studied the effect of alignment on the results using the geometric prosthesis. They defined perfect position as a knee aligned in 3 to 7 degrees of valgus, the tibial component in a perfectly horizontal position in both planes, the femoral com-

ponent in 4 to 6 degrees of valgus, and both femoral and tibial components centered in the midline of the joint; 100 points were allotted to a knee filling these radiographic criteria. Deviations from the ideal position resulted in subtractions from the total score. Fewer than 10 percent of their patients achieved a perfect score; Lotke and Ecker found a statistically significant correlation between good clinical results and good radiographic scores.

Our current recommendation for perfect positioning is similar to that proposed by Lotke and Ecker, except that we prefer a slightly more valgus position. Thus the positioning of the tibial component is horizontal in all planes, the femoral component is in 6 to 9 degrees of valgus in the anteroposterior view, and horizontal in the lateral view. The overall alignment is in 6 to 9 degrees of valgus, a position that corre-

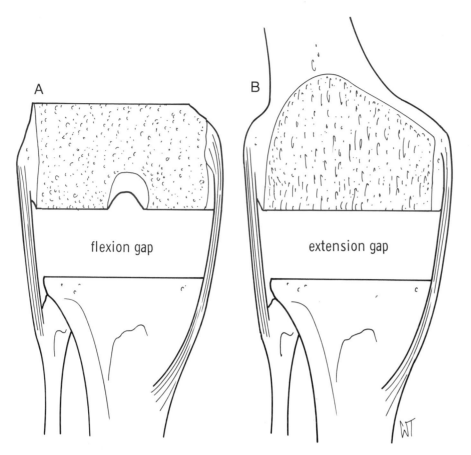

Fig. 20.53. The extension gap must exactly equal the flexion gap.

sponds very closely to the so-called mechanical axis regardless of the patient's body build.

BONE TRIMMING

The final stage of the operation consists of shaping the bone ends to receive the components. Thus anterior and posterior chamfering of the femur and trimming of the intercondylar notch are usually required. A fixation hole or holes must also be excavated from the tibia.

INSTRUMENTATION

Whereas the skilled surgeon may be able to replace the knee consistently by eye, most will need the aid of instruments. Unfortunately, varying size of components from different manufacturers precludes the use of general instruments for all prostheses. However, a set of instruments to perform the basic steps of the operation outlined above have been developed for use with the total condylar and Freeman-Samuelson prostheses, which by chance have components of almost exactly similar dimensions. In the interests of standardization, it is hoped that eventually all knee prostheses will share basically similar sizing, thus making some instruments interchangeable. Certainly idiosyncracies in such matters as beveling and the size and shape of fixation studs or stems will always require specific instrumentation for individual prostheses to perform the trimming stage of the operation.

FREEMAN-INSALL INSTRUMENTS

These are basic instruments for the fundamental steps of knee replacement. Further separate instruments are required for cutting fixation holes and be-

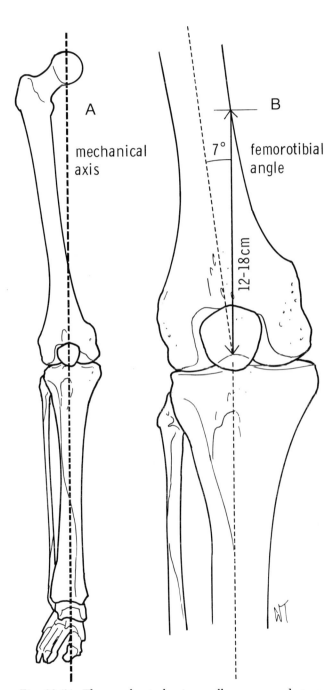

Fig. 20.54. The mechanical axis usually corresponds to a femorotibial angle of about 7 degrees and the mechanical axis intersects the medial femoral cortex 12–18 cm proximal to the knee.

veling the lower femur. Freeman also uses a polyethylene trimmer to shape the tibial component.

The Flexion Cuts. There is an expanding block (template) (Fig. 20.55) for assessing the anteroposterior dimension of the femur, and thus the appropriate femoral prosthetic size. Upon selection of the appropriate size the block is fitted with a hoop that locates it in relationship to the anterior femoral shaft. A vertical bar is attached to a tibial cutting block that is free to slide up and down (Fig. 20.56). With the knee flexed 90 degrees, the assembled instrument is positioned so that the vertical bar is aligned proximally over the tibial tubercle and distally through the center of the ankle joint. The sliding tibial cutting block is adjusted to a position that removes the smallest amount of tibial bone yet provides an adequate anchoring surface for the prosthesis. The tibial block is pinned to the bone.

The rotation of the femoral block is adjusted so that (1) it is parallel to the tibial block (Insall) or (2) it is symmetrically placed across the femoral condyles (Freeman).

After both blocks have been pinned to their appropriate bones, the anterior hoop and the vertical bar are removed. The blocks are left in place indicating the bone to be resected from the anterior and posterior femoral condyles and from the tibial plateau. The blocks also serve as a saw guide (Fig. 20.57).

The Extension Gap. The tenser is an instrument devised by Freeman (Fig. 20.58) to tense the ligaments and align the knee. The instrument is inserted upon the cut surface of the upper tibia and allows distraction of the medial and lateral compartments separately. Correct alignment is confirmed by a straight bar running through the instrument and extending proximally to the hip and distally to the ankle (Fig. 20.59). The tenser is used to fine-tune the alignment and has attached proximally a cutting block for the distal femur. The position of this block may be adjusted according to the thickness of the tibial component preselected for the flexion gap (Fig. 20.60). When the extension, alignment, and stability are considered satisfactory, the femoral cutting block is pinned to the anterior face of the femur and the tenser is removed. The distal femur is resected using the cutting block as a saw guide. Assessment of the extension gap is completed by inserting the appropriate spacer already used for the flexion gap.

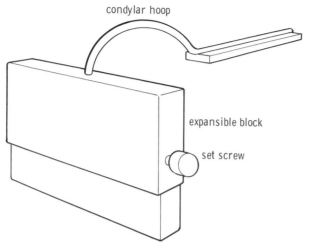

Fig. 20.55. Instead of separate templates, the first femoral cutting jig of the Freeman-Insall instrumentation uses an expanding block.

PITFALLS IN TECHNIQUE

OVERALL ALIGNMENT AND FAILURE TO LOCATE THE HIP JOINT

The external landmarks that are easiest to find on most patients are the anterior superior iliac spine, the center of the knee joint, and the center of the ankle joint. The foot and ankle should be draped in such a manner as not to obscure the malleoli. A two-piece 90-cm (36-inch) alignment rod (the two-piece design facilitates autoclaving) that extends from the hip to the ankle joint is recommended. The position of the hip joint is the most difficult landmark to find and may be approximated by several methods:

1. The hip joint lies at a point midway between the anterior superior iliac spine and the middle of the symphysis pubis.

2. It may be estimated by measuring one, two, or three fingerbreadths medially from the anterior-superior iliac spine depending on whether the patient is tall and thin, of average build, or short and fat, respectively.

3. In obese patients the surgeon's ability to locate the anterior-superior iliac spine is impaired by the panniculus that may overlie the area. The femoral head is located using radiographic control and marked with an ECG electrode taped to the skin

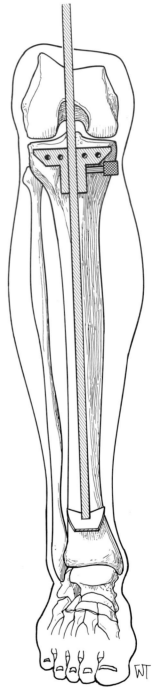

Fig. 20.56. The tibial cutting block is attached to a vertical alignment bar that permits adjustment to the position of the tibial cutting block.

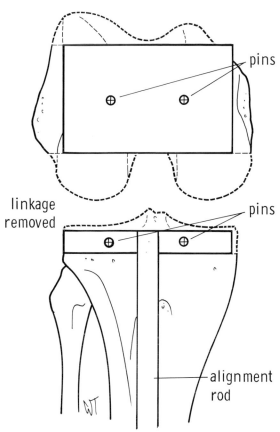

Fig. 20.57. After positioning, the blocks are pinned to their respective bones and the anterior hoop and vertical bar are removed.

or other suitable device. This method, although time consuming, is the most accurate of all, but obtaining radiographs in the operating theater may be difficult when a clean air enclosure is used.

4. As the mechanical axis corresponds to approximately a 7 degree femoral-tibial angle, the femoral cutting block is positioned at 7 degrees of valgus in relationship to the distal femoral shaft.

5. In an average-size limb, the mechanical axis intersects the medial cortex of the femur 12 to 18 cm proximal to the knee joint (the exact distance can be calculated for each individual case). The femoral cutting block is provided with a proximal extension rod positioned appropriately with reference to the medial femoral cortex.

CUTTING THE TIBIA WITH A MEDIAL SLOPE

This error occurs as a result of several factors:

1. There is a natural inclination to follow the original articular surface of the tibia, which is often exaggerated by medial erosion in osteoarthritis.

2. The fat pad obscures the lateral part of the tibia, and the patellar tendon also intrudes on this region.

3. The tibial alignment rod may be positioned proximally medial to the tibial tubercle with its distal end inclined toward the ankle.

All encourage a resection of the tibia that inclines medially. If not recognized and corrected, the medial

Fig. 20.58. The Freeman tenser (courtesy of M.A.R. Freeman).

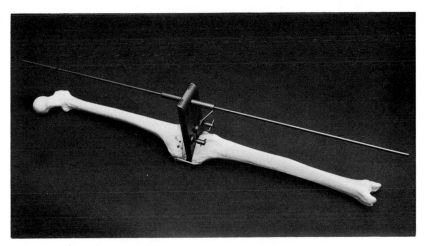

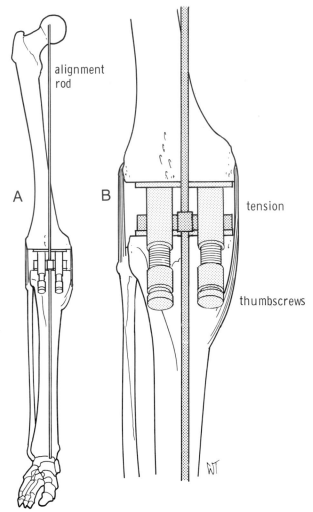

Fig. 20.59. By adjusting the medial and lateral thumbscrews, the alignment rod is brought into the mechanical axis.

slope will affect the overall alignment of the leg. When recognized, an excessive valgus placement of the femoral component may be made, although the exact amount is difficult to judge because the alignment rod must now lie medial to the hip joint. This obliquity of the joint axis caused by miscutting of the tibia is one of the commonest errors in knee replacement; even if not associated with an overall malalignment, it is likely to cause uneven loading and uneven wear of the prosthesis. Also more of the medial corticocancellous bone is removed weakening the medial support of the tibial component.

MISJUDGING THE SOFT TISSUE TENSIONS

Unequal gap size in flexion and extension results in (1) anteroposterior instability in flexion, or a flexion contracture in extension, and (2) mediolateral instability in extension.

These soft tissue errors should not occur if the basic steps are followed as outlined or, if they do, should be recognized by instrument checks before cementing the components. The remedy for both errors is to adjust the position of the femoral component. Error 1 is corrected by the removal of more bone from the distal femur until the extension gap equals the flexion gap (Fig. 20.61). Error 2 is caused by removal of excessive bone from the distal femur. Here adjustment of gap size is not possible by the trimming of further bone from the tibia nor by inserting a thicker tibial component, which is prohibited because the component will not fit in flexion. The solution is to "build up" the position of the femoral component until the knee becomes stable (Fig. 20.62). A stemmed component is useful, as are screws or wire mesh protruding from the distal end of the femur.

ROTATIONAL MALALIGNMENT OF THE TIBIAL COMPONENT

A rotational error in the placement of the tibial component can result in uneven femorotibial tracking (Fig. 20.63A, B) (or, when extreme, rotary subluxation and dislocation). More likely, rotary malposition will affect the patellofemoral joint. Patellar tracking is determined largely by the position of the tibial component and internal rotation, with respect to the bone, can lead to patellar dislocation (Fig. 20.64). The difficulty with rotary positioning of the tibial component is that the tibial tubercle is often eccentrically placed toward the lateral side of the knee so that a component placed in the center of the tibia will not necessarily lie directly behind the tubercle. For correct positioning the tibia must be rotated so that the tubercle lies anterior (albeit laterally placed). A marking line (real or imaginary) is drawn on the tibial surface running through the tubercle in an anteroposterior direction. The tibial component should be positioned at right angles to this line. Thus, the component should face in the same direction as the tubercle, but not necessarily directly toward it.

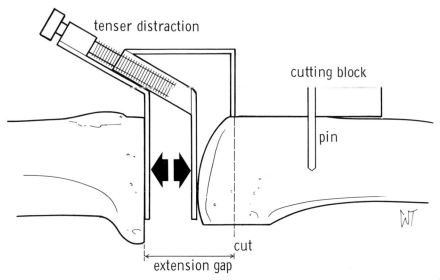

Fig. 20.60. The distal femoral cutting guide is controlled by the tenser and positioned to create an extension gap of the correct dimensions.

Finally, a peculiar form of malrotation may be noticed after inserting the components, even though both appear correctly positioned. As the knee is flexed, the lateral tibial plateau fails to glide smoothly on the femoral condyle, and is seen to sublux forward although at the same time the tracking of the medial condyle appears normal. This internal rotation with flexion is caused by excessive tightness of the popliteus tendon and, as the popliteus muscle seems to serve no useful function after knee replacement, it should be excised. A tight popliteus is analogous to a tight PCL in cruciate-sparing designs but is limited in effect to the lateral compartment.

MANAGEMENT OF INSTABILITY, DEFORMITY, AND CONTRACTURE

The technique just described applies only to knees with normal anatomy, and of course such joints rarely require replacement. In most cases some degree of instability, deformity, contracture or a combination of these elements will be found. Moreover, even in knees without initial deformity some change in alignment may be required (for example, in the patient who is habitually bow-legged). While some minor degree of postoperative ligament asymmetry or laxity may be tolerated, it is better to obtain near-perfect stability through surgical technique.

Some workers use a constrained prosthesis for unstable or deformed knees. Kaufer and Matthews[85] have stated that optimal results are not achieved with a resurfacing knee prosthesis when there is $\geq$ 20 degrees of fixed varus or valgus deformity, $\geq$ 30 degrees of fixed flexion deformity, or gross preoperative instability with incompetence of two or more of the major knee ligaments. For this group of patients, they recommend a constrained prosthesis (the spherocentric).

It has been our experience that such prostheses are very rarely required for a primary knee arthroplasty, although they may be needed in occasional revision cases. Such almost universal use of a resurfacing knee prosthesis is only possible when the nature of the underlying pathology is recognized, and when the surgeon is versed in the soft tissue techniques necessary for correction.

INSTABILITY, ANGULAR DEFORMITY, AND CONTRACTURE

In most arthritic knees, instability initially develops because of loss of cartilage and bone; this is more or less symmetrical in rheumatoid arthritis and usually

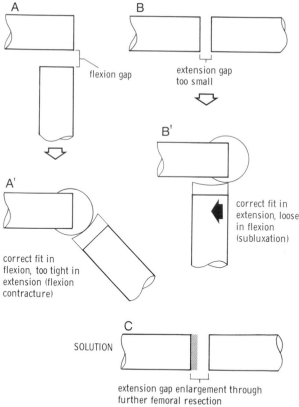

Fig. 20.61. Unequal gap size is a frequent technical error. When the extension gap is too small, the knee will not fully extend; if a thinner tibial component is used, the prosthesis will be too loose in flexion. The solution is to excise more bone from the distal femur.

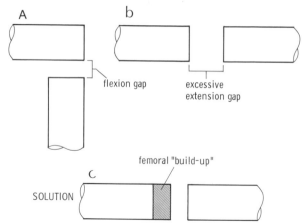

Fig. 20.62. When the extension gap is too large equalization cannot be obtained by further bone resection. The prosthesis must be built up on the femoral side.

asymmetrical in osteoarthritic knees. Instability by itself (i.e., without any accompanying adaptive changes in the ligaments) can be managed by applying the standard surgical technique and principles. All that is needed to provide a stable arthroplasty is to remove relatively less bone when inserting the prosthesis so that the bulk of the prosthetic components themselves (the spacing effect) restores ligament length to normal. Instability that can be corrected by these means is known as symmetric instability (Fig. 20.65).

However, in advanced arthritis there are nearly always adaptive changes that take place in the ligaments. For example, in the usual varus deformity of osteoarthritis, the medial collateral ligament becomes shortened in part due to osteoarthritic overgrowth on the medial side of the knee and in part to actual contracture of the ligament because its physiologic length

is not maintained (because of loss of medial bone). The process is akin to the contracture of the posterior capsule associated with a longstanding flexion deformity. The effect of contracture of the medial ligament is a varus deformity that is fixed and cannot be passively corrected.

In addition, in the same example, adaptive changes occur in the lateral ligament and capsule which become stretched by the stresses of walking on a knee which is in a fixed varus position (Fig. 20.66). Thus an "asymmetric instability" is now present, the elements of which are asymmetric loss of bone medially, contracture of the medial ligament, and stretching of the lateral ligament. It is obvious that this type of instability cannot be corrected simply by the spacing effect of the prosthesis because the collateral ligaments have now become permanently altered, with one being shorter and the other longer than normal.

In valgus deformity there is the reverse occurrence with contracture of the lateral ligamentous capsule and iliotibial band and stretching of the medial collateral ligament (Fig. 20.67). In fixed valgus deformity, particularly in rheumatoid arthritis, there may also be a fixed external rotation deformity of the tibia presumably caused by contracture of the iliotibial band (a situation analogous to a similar contracture seen in poliomyelitis).

In addition to angular deformities and contractures, there may be flexion contracture, flexion instability, and restricted motion of the knee (this latter may be thought of as an extension contracture).

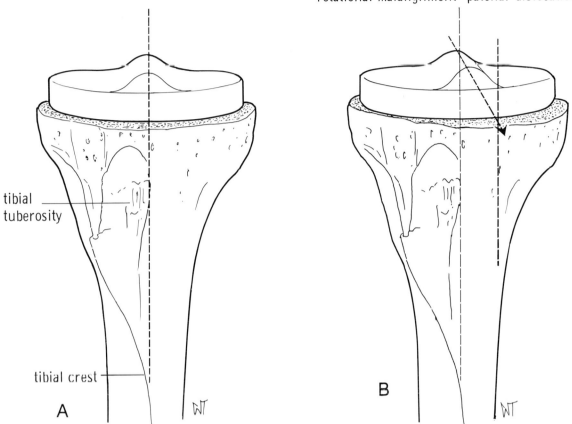

Fig. 20.63. The tibial component should be aligned with the tibial tubercle. (A) Correct position. (B) The tibial component internally rotated on the tibia.

Fig. 20.64. Gross rotary malposition of the tibial component leads to patellar dislocation.

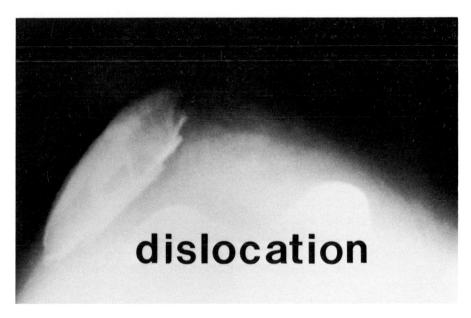

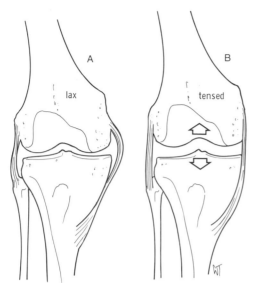

Fig. 20.65. Symmetric instability. The ligaments, although lax, are of equal length. Both alignment and stability are restored by tensioning the ligaments.

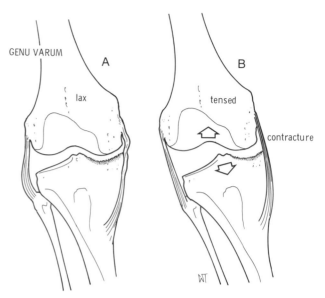

Fig. 20.66. Asymmetric instability in varus. The medial ligament is shorter than the lateral.

FLEXION CONTRACTURE

Flexion contracture is not usually very pronounced in osteoarthritis and seldom presents much of a technical problem (Fig. 20.68). The more extreme degrees are seen in rheumatoid arthritis. In patients who have been unable to walk for years and who have spent most of their time sitting in a wheelchair, fixed flexion deformities of ≥ 90 degrees can occur. The contracture is caused by shortening of the posterior capsule.

FLEXION INSTABILITY

Flexion instability caused by primary pathology is seen only in rheumatoid arthritis, but may be caused secondarily during the course of surgery by ligament release or an inaccurate cut on the tibia that removes too much bone.

In rheumatoid arthritis, more bone is sometimes lost from the posterior femoral condyles than from their distal aspect, so that when viewed laterally, the lower femur looks like a drumstick or chicken leg (Fig. 20.69A). This condition, therefore, may be suspected from the roentgenographic appearance (Fig. 20.69B) and confirmed at surgery, when distraction of the knee in flexion produces excessive separation

of the joint surfaces. Paradoxically, flexion instability often coexists with flexion contracture, compounding the technical problem to be solved. Extra thick components are needed to fill the flexion gap and to make the knee stable in flexion, while at the same time thinner components than usual are required in extension to overcome the flexion contracture.

Flexion instability resulting from excessive tibial resection is a technical mistake and should not occur. Except in most unusual circumstances, the level of tibial resection is always immediately below the subchondral end plate. The surgeon may choose to make an excessively large tibial resection when there is considerable asymmetric loss of bone from the tibia so as to obtain a flat tibial surface (Fig. 20.70). This also is an error not only producing a wide flexion space but also placing the component on relatively weak cancellous bone (the density of cancellous bone decreases with distance from the end plate). Compensation for asymmetric loss of bone should be made with protruding screws, titanium mesh or best of all an asymmetric tibial component (Fig. 20.71A,B). The use of metal enclosed plastic and an intramedullary prosthetic stem may also be helpful in obtaining adequate component anchorage.

The creation of an enlarged flexion space by ligament release for the purpose of correcting angular deformity may require some amplification. As previ-

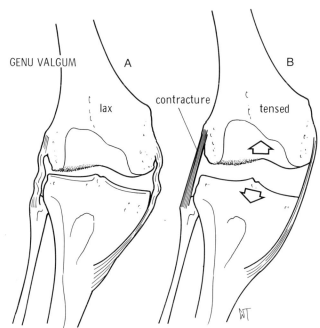

Fig. 20.67. Asymmetric instability in valgus.

ment release is done after sizing the flexion gap but before cutting the distal femur an enlarged flexion gap will result.

It is of critical importance that ligament asymmetry be assessed and corrected before any of the bone cuts are made. The extent of ligament contracture or stretching must be assessed also in two positions: as near to full extension as the knee will go and at 90 degrees of flexion. Once the knee is exposed, the joint must be levered apart until the ligaments become fully tight in both of these positions, which can be done most simply by inserting a periosteal elevator into the sides of the joint and prying the joint surfaces apart. Distraction instruments such as a ratchet-handle laminar spreader are also extremely helpful but sometimes cannot be used for the initial assessment because when one side of the knee is extremely tight, there may not be sufficient room to permit insertion. Thus a laminar spreader can be inserted to distract the loose side of a joint while the joint surfaces on the tight side are pried apart by a manually held instrument. By these means, ligament asymmetry is identified and must now be overcome.[59]

ously stated, the abnormal anatomy found in angular deformity is ligament asymmetry (one ligament contracted and the other stretched). The presence of a stretched ligament is normally readily perceived when the knee is examined in extension, but may not be at all obvious once the knee is flexed because of the tethering effect of the contracted ligament. However, once the contracted ligament has been released, the joint is now free to open until the previously elongated opposite ligament becomes tight. When liga-

TECHNIQUE FOR
SOFT TISSUE RELEASE

A standard midline approach is used unless otherwise indicated (e.g., a previous scar). The skin incision should be of adequate length so that retraction is not required during the procedure. The capsule

Fig. 20.68. In a flexion contracture the posterior capsule is shortened and adherent.

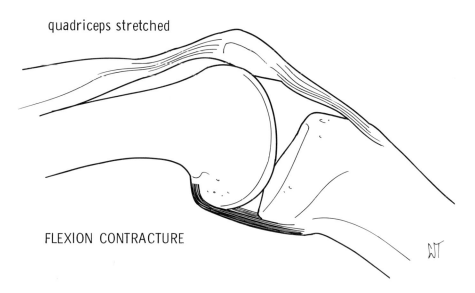

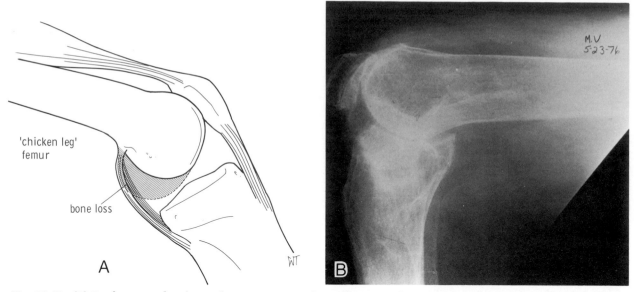

Fig. 20.69. (A) In rheumatoid arthritis there is excessive loss of bone on the posterior aspect of the femoral condyles. (B) Lateral radiograph showing this condition. Unless the technique recognizes and adjusts for it, flexion instability will result.

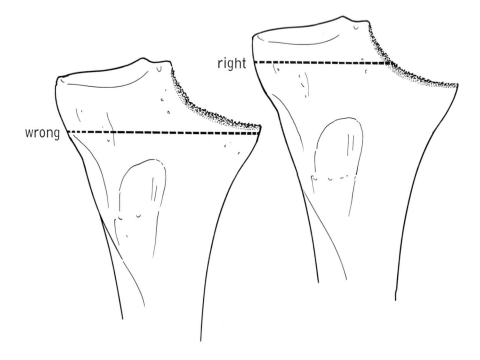

Fig. 20.70. When there is asymmetric bone loss from the upper tibia, the tibial resection must not be too distal but rather at the usual level.

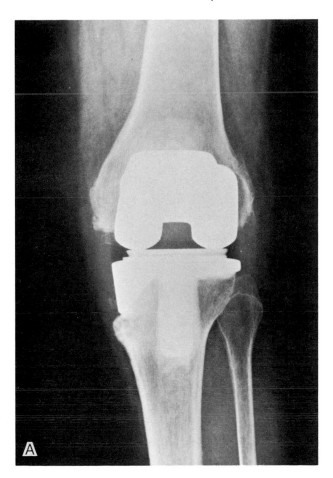

Fig. 20.71. (A,B) Asymmetric bone loss should be compensated for by an asymmetric tibial component.

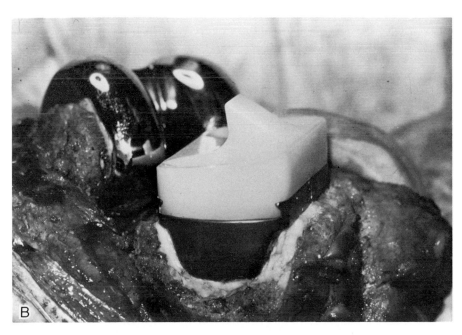

incision into the extensor mechanism passes over the medial third of the patella and runs distally medial to the patellar ligament and tibial tubercle. This incision is also virtually straight and permits a secure closure that will allow early motion without risk of disruption. By making an overlapping closure, proximal realignment can also be done if it is required to correct patellar tracking. The incision is extensile and can be continued both proximally and distally as needed for further exposure. In all cases the exposure must permit complete displacement of the tibia in front of the femur by freeing the collateral and capsular attachments to the tibia sufficiently to allow the tibia to be "button holed" forward. While the attachment of the patellar ligament to the tibial tubercle can be partially freed, avulsion must not be allowed, and the maintenance of continuity between the patellar ligament and distal periosteum is essential.

VARUS DEFORMITY (Fig. 20.72A–F)

Ligament balance is achieved by progressively releasing the medial soft tissues until they reach the length of the lateral ligamentous structures. The extent of the release can be monitored by periodically inserting the laminar spreaders and judging alignment with an aligning rod. The end point of the release is a position in which the rod passes in a line from the center of the ankle over the tibial tubercle to the hip joint (a location that will be from one to three fingerbreadths medial to the anterior-superior iliac spine, depending on individual stature). The cruciate ligaments must be completely excised *before* starting the release because their presence will often inhibit correction. Because the lateral ligament is stretched and elongated, the end point of a medial release is a lengthening of the medial structures beyond their original length. Cruciate ligaments, being in the center of the knee, usually retain approximately normal length regardless of alterations that occur in the collateral ligaments and thus will not permit the stretching that is the objective of the release procedure.

The medial release is done by removing medial osteophytes from the femur and the tibia (including the protruding flare of the tibial plateau) and raising a sleeve of soft tissue from the upper medial tibia that

is allowed to slide proximally. The sleeve consists of periosteum, deep medial ligament, superficial medial ligament, and the insertion of the pes anserinus tendons. More posteriorly at the joint surface the sleeve is continuous with the semimembranosus insertion and posterior capsule.

Distally, the release may include the deep fascia investing soleus and popliteus muscles. The sleeve is made by continuing the standard approach distally on the anteromedial surface of the tibia for 8 to 10 cm and stripping the periosteum medially from the tibia. The knee is flexed, and the leg is progressively externally rotated to gain posterior access. The distal attachment of the superficial medial ligament can be initially left intact; in moderate deformities, this will be the extent of the release needed. When this is not the case, the release is continued posteriorly and distally by further subperiosteal stripping. Correction of deformity occurs gradually and is aided by the intermittent stretching action of the medial laminar spreader. With a progressive release, there is no discontinuity between the medial soft tissue structures; the result is balance with some overall lengthening of the limb (the amount of lengthening is dependent upon the degree of preoperative stretching of the lateral structures).

As stated earlier, the ideal postoperative alignment with regard to prosthetic placement and function is independent of the original anatomy. This is to say that in a patient who has always been bowlegged and has later developed unilateral osteoarthritis, it is not sufficient to match the alignment of the replaced knee with that of the opposite "normal" (which in this case means varus). Whatever the original appearance may have been, the relationship of hip, knee, and ankle must be correct after prosthetic replacement (a femorotibial alignment of 6 to 9 degrees of valgus). Otherwise, the prosthetic components will be unequally loaded and will be subjected to excessive varus stress.

At the completion of varus release, the limb is already aligned in the proper position, no further correction is needed, and the bone cuts can be made in a standard manner to place the components in position. After insertion of components of the correct size, the knee should be fully stable and not require immobilization because of the release. Motion can be started at the usual time (when wound healing has progressed enough to allow it) and walking with full weight-bearing is allowed within a few days of surgery.

VALGUS DEFORMITY (Fig. 20.73A–C)

The principles for the correction of fixed valgus are the same as for fixed varus; however, there are certain differences in performing the release because of the anatomy. The popliteal nerve passes on the lateral side of the knee and along with other structures is stretched beyond its original length. (There is no corresponding structure on the medial side of the knee.) The ligamentous, capsular, and fascial attachments are also different, hence the release must be done from the femur rather than the tibia.

The harmful effects of the inevitable stretching of the peroneal nerve can be partially mitigated by dissection of the nerve, especially that portion that passes around the fibular neck extending to and including the position where the deep portion of the nerve passes beneath a fibrous raphe into the anterior compartment of the leg (Fig. 20.74). The rationale for this dissection is that interference of nerve function is due not only to stretching but to fascial compression, especially at the sites mentioned. The iliotibial band also has no counterpart on the medial side and when contracted not only maintains fixed valgus but also (because it remains tight even with flexion of the knee) a fixed external rotation of the tibia. The iliotibial band cannot be stripped and progressively lengthened as with the medial sleeve, and often complete transection is required. Fixed valgus deformity may also be associated with lateral patellar subluxation. This can of course be corrected by dividing the lateral patellar retinaculum at the patellar border, but if this is done, there is considerable interference with the blood supply. (There is evidence that fatigue fracture of the patella may be caused by avascular necrosis.) The patella should be repositioned by a release that has the least effect on patellar vascularity; by dissection in the interval between the iliotibial band and the biceps femoris, the patella can be reduced preserving all the vessels that arise from the inferior lateral genicular artery and perhaps some of those derived from the superior genicular artery.

These considerations dictate a modification of the surgical approach in two alternative ways. First, the skin incision may be placed more laterally reaching the peroneal nerve by subcutaneous dissection and, by similar undermining of the other flap, making the usual medial arthrotomy incision into the knee. The other method is to use two incisions, one anteriorly, and another posterolaterally over the peroneal nerve. Division of the iliotibial tract and release of the patellar retinaculum is then done subcutaneously using both incisions to obtain exposure.

Whichever approach is chosen, the capsular incision is made in the usual manner and the patella dislocated laterally. The lateral capsule is cut from the femoral condyle, together with the lateral ligament and popliteus tendon. At the level of the lateral femoral condyle, the posterior capsule and sometimes the lateral head of gastrocnemius require division. As is the case on the medial side, the amount of correction obtained at each stage is determined by an alignment check after insertion of laminar spreaders. Usually the amount of dissection so far described is sufficient to provide balance and correction. In severe cases, particularly those with associated external rotation deformity, the iliotibial band must also be divided. After lateral release there is no permanent laxity in extension and no instability when walking. However, there may be a functional instability in flexion because of the need to excise the cruciate ligaments. Thus, even when using the thickest components there is a tendency toward posterolateral rotatory subluxation. Normally, in the process of healing, the processes of scar formation and readherence of the lateral capsule prevent this from becoming a clinical problem. However, there is some unpredictability in the healing process, and it is safer after lateral release to use components that assume posterior stability (posterior stabilized condylar prosthesis).

Needless to say, the full lateral dissection as described will divide all the elements that contribute to associated external rotation contracture, with the exception of the biceps femoris. Very rarely partial or complete division of this muscle may also be required.

FLEXION CONTRACTURE

Unlike angular deformity, lesser degrees of flexion contracture can be overcome by removing relatively more bone from the femur and tibia, but there are disadvantages to this approach. The amount of bone

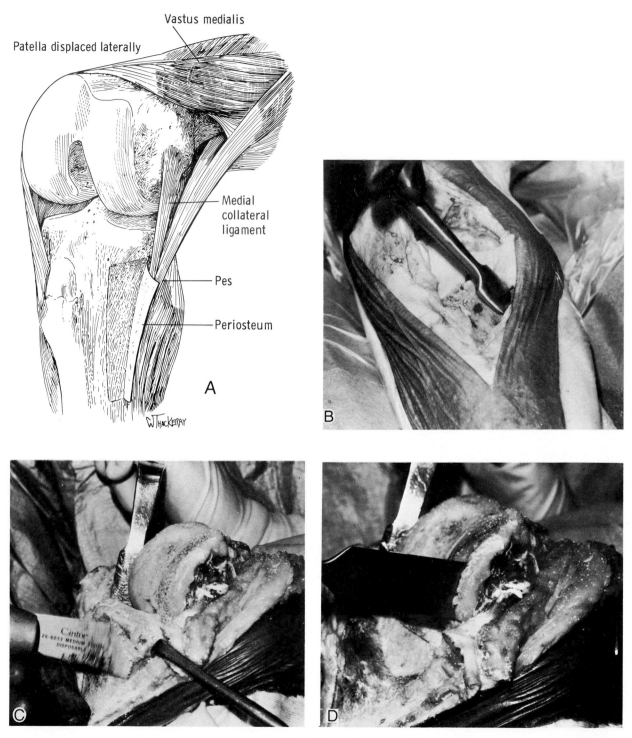

Fig. 20.72. Varus release. (A) The structures to be reflected from the upper tibia. (B) The exposure is begun by sub-periosteal stripping beneath the superficial medial collateral ligament. (C) The protruding medial flair of the tibia is removed with a saw. (D) Osteophytes are removed from around the margin of the femoral condyle. (E) Completed release. Only the superficial medial collateral ligament remains intact but (F) this too can be detached if necessary.

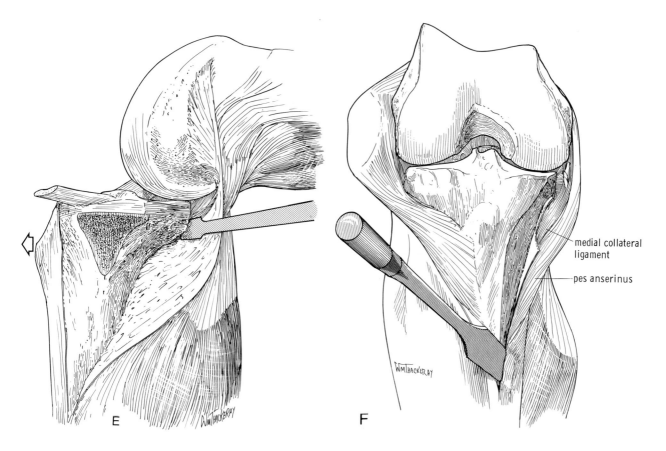

medial collateral
ligament

pes anserinus

E

F

that can be removed from the femur is limited by the attachment of the collateral ligaments and excessive resection of the tibia produces a large gap between the bone ends in flexion which is likely to produce flexion instability. Also, excessive bone removal, be it from femur or tibia, results in shortening of the leg, hence lengthening of the quadriceps and extensor mechanism (which may very well already be stretched), resulting in a permanent extension lag. Beyond this point further correction can only be obtained by posterior capsulotomy. In a longstanding contracture, the normal posterior recess is obliterated, and the capsule is adherent to the femoral condyles. The recess must first be recreated by stripping adherent capsule, although this maneuver alone seldom results in much correction. Cruciate ligament excision removes the central portion of the posterior capsule, leaving the medial and lateral segments lying anterior to the respective heads of gastrocnemius. These segments must be separated from contiguous collateral capsule by vertical incisions made at the medial and lateral posterior corners. (Because there are no important structures posterior to the capsule in these areas, the vertical incisions can be made blindly with confidence and safety.) The medial and lateral segments of the posterior capsule can now be divided sharply under direct vision (Fig. 20.75). Often in rheumatoid arthritis the capsule is greatly thickened and intimately adherent to the gastrocnemius muscle, which must also be divided. The objective of the capsulotomy is to cut all fibrous structures from one side of the knee to the other, exposing the popliteal layer of fat. Because the thickest capsule is in the medial and lateral recesses, there is little likelihood of injury to a vital structure. However, needless to say, the division of the posterior capsule requires care and a light touch. The necessary exposure can be made easier by prior removal of bone from the upper tibia and posterior femoral condyles (an exception to the rule that soft tissue release must precede all the bone cuts). When flexion deformity is associated with fixed valgus, the approach is considerably simplified because the lat-

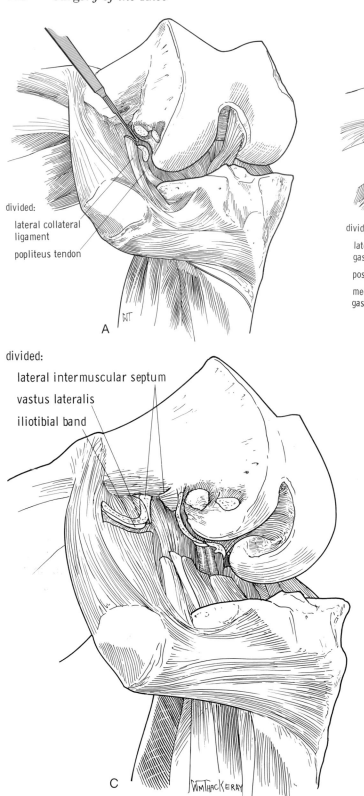

divided:

lateral collateral
ligament

popliteus tendon

A

divided:

lateral intermuscular septum

vastus lateralis

iliotibial band

C

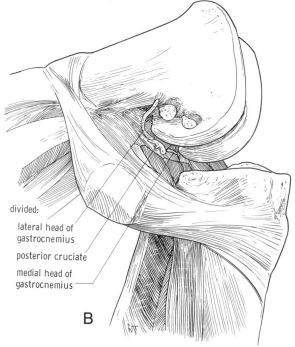

divided:

lateral head of
gastrocnemius

posterior cruciate

medial head of
gastrocnemius

B

Fig. 20.73. (A–C) Valgus release is done on the femur releasing completely the soft tissues from the lateral femoral
condyle and, if necessary,
transversely dividing the iliotibial band.

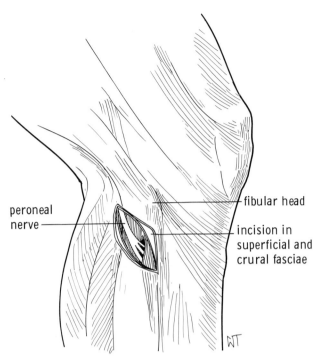

Fig. 20.74. For severe valgus deformities in which there is anticipated stretching of the lateral soft tissues, release of the fascia overlying the lateral popliteal nerve is recommended.

eral release can be done first, and the posterior capsule approached from the lateral side, allowing retraction of the popliteal vessels.

Correction of severe flexion contracture may also stretch and compress the peroneal nerve. Decompression of the nerve through a separate posterolateral incision is recommended to prevent foot drop. After correction of flexion deformities the knee may be springy; and to prevent recurrence of contracture during the postoperative period, the knee is splinted in extension from one to three weeks.

FLEXION INSTABILITY

When the condition is primary (rheumatoid arthritis), it should be recognized by the initial ligamentous assessment and appropriate allowance made in deciding the level of tibial resection (sometimes less than usual).

When caused by the effect of ligament release or by the error of excessive tibial resection, flexion instability may not be recognized until the time comes to fit the trial components, when excessive anteroposterior motion in flexion will be apparent.

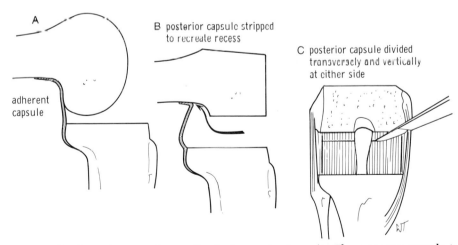

Fig. 20.75. Posterior capsulotomy for flexion contracture. (A) The posterior capsule is adherent. (B) The original recess is reestablished. (C) The cruciate ligaments have already been excised; only the medial and lateral parts of the posterior capsule need division. Often the underlying gastrocnemii are adherent and must be divided as well. At the margin of the collateral ligaments, vertical incisions in the capsule must be made.

There are two remedies. One is to restore flexion stability by using a thicker tibial component, thereby filling the flexion gap and restoring collateral ligament tension. This means an appropriate adjustment to the extension gap or the knee will not fully extend with the thicker component in place. Extra bone must be removed from the distal femur equal to the difference between the tibial component originally selected and the thickness needed to give stability. Another alternative to respacing the knee is to use components that in themselves provide posterior stability. In some cases this may be the preferred solution.

THE STIFF KNEE

Long-standing stiffness at or near full extension, even though caused primarily by intra-articular adhesions, inevitably leads to secondary quadriceps contracture.

QUADRICEPS CONTRACTURE
(Fig. 20.76)

The use of the standard midline approach may have disadvantages because excessive tightness in the rectus femoris can lead to avulsion of the tibial tubercle during knee flexion. This is difficult to repair satisfactorily and is best avoided by early recognition that such a problem is likely. The inverted V incision of Coonse and Adams[21] is recommended and completely avoids the risk of distal avulsion. The quadriceps tendon and the patella are turned distally leaving a broad-based attachment to the tibia. Immediate and extensive exposure is obtained.

The V incision may be closed as a Y thus lengthening the rectus femoris or by selective reattachment of the vasti according to their degree of tightness. Usually very little V–Y lengthening is required, and sufficient quadriceps mobilization is obtained by reattaching the vastus lateralis at a higher level. The result of the inverted V incision is satisfactory motion at the expense of a mild extension lag (which usually diminishes with time).

INTRA-ARTICULAR ADHESIONS

Posterior adhesions and contracture of the posterior cruciate ligament will cause the knee to "open like a book" (Fig. 20.77). Instead of the normal rolling and gliding motions, a posterior hinge is formed so that increased flexion is accompanied by a progressive anterior displacement of the tibia on the femur. To prevent the same pattern of motion after replacement, the posterior cruciate must be excised and the normal posterior recess reestablished by capsular stripping. Vertical incisions medially and laterally are often needed to separate the posterior capsule from the collateral capsule.

Of all the techniques described, the release of extension contracture is perhaps the least satisfactory, and it is the uncommon case in which the result will be as good following other kinds of release because

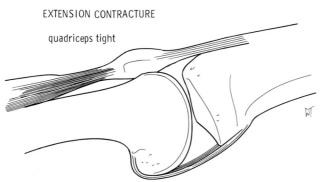

EXTENSION CONTRACTURE

quadriceps tight

Fig. 20.76. In an extension contracture not only are there intra-articular adhesions, but the quadriceps muscle itself is shortened and tight.

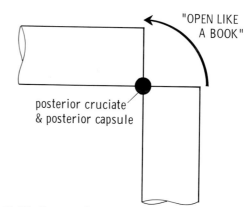

"OPEN LIKE A BOOK"

posterior cruciate & posterior capsule

Fig. 20.77. In some knees contracture of the posterior cruciate ligament causes the knee to "open like a book." Normal motion cannot be reestablished until the ligament is divided.

of the failure to restore both normal motion and quadriceps strength.

SUMMARY

Soft tissue release techniques are designed to restore normal alignment and motion with the preservation of sufficient ligamentous integrity to enable the use of a surface knee joint replacement. The techniques require cruciate ligament excision, so that anteroposterior stability after the arthroplasty is dependent in part on collateral ligament tension and in part on the surface geometry of the prosthesis which must possess some degree of cupping. Additional anteroposterior stability can be obtained, when necessary, by using a prosthesis that possesses an intercondylar cam with a cruciate substituting function.

The alternative to soft tissue release techniques is to obtain correction of deformity by additional bone resection; a constrained prosthesis that assumes ligament function is then required. However, constrained prostheses have higher rates of loosening, breakage, and infection, so that their use should be limited to as few cases as possible. With experience soft tissue release techniques make it possible to correct most deformities and to permit the use of a surface replacement prosthesis.[75]

THE PATELLA

Routine resurfacing is recommended whenever this is practical (the patella must be of sufficient size and thickness to accept a prosthesis). Resection of the articular surfaces is done by eye, holding the patella fully everted. The line of resection runs from the margin of the medial articular surface to the margin of the lateral articular surface (Fig. 20.78), landmarks that are not always clearly seen, especially when the

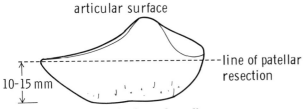

Fig. 20.78. The line of patellar resection.

articular surface

line of patellar resection

10-15 mm

---

anatomy is distorted by arthritis. A common error is to resect only the lateral facet which results in oblique placement of the patellar component. An even thickness can be judged by palpation leaving 1 to 1.5 cm of patella to provide adequate anchorage. Most patellar components require a fixation hole which is made with a drill or gouge. The hole should be no bigger than necessary and should be undercut slightly. A domed patellar component does not require rotary alignment, but with faceted components the positioning must be judged by observing patellar tracking with the trial components. When a congruent position is obtained marking is made on the patella for reference during cementing. Some bone, usually on the lateral side, will normally overhang the component and should not be trimmed away to avoid weakening the remaining patellar bone. Finally, with the component in place, patellar tracking should be tested observing the rule of "no thumb." The patella should remain in place throughout the range of motion without being held. If subluxation or tilting is observed, a lateral retinacular release is indicated, which can be done obliquely from the inside of the knee (Fig. 20.79). The lateral retinacular release is continued proximally into the lower fibers of vastus lateralis and distally as far as necessary to provide smooth patellar tracking. Some of the lateral retinacular arteries are of necessity divided, but by being careful it may be possible to preserve some of the lateral arterial supply to the patella (Fig. 20.80).

FIXATION

Methods of fixation and cementing techniques are the subject of Chapter 22. Some generalities are in order here. Tourniquet release before final insertion of the components is recommended for control of bleeding from larger vessels, particularly those that lie posteriorly and that are inaccessible after the components are in place. This means that the bone surfaces become covered with blood, and so before cementing, the tourniquet is reinflated and a pulsatile water lavage system is used to clean the exposed cancellous bone thoroughly of blood, marrow, and fat. The bone should then be dried before applying cement to the exposed cancellous surfaces.

Using standard cementing techniques, penetration of 2 to 3 mm into the cancellous bone can be ob-

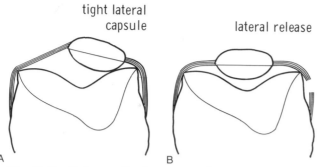

tight lateral
capsule

lateral release

A   B

Fig. 20.79. If the patella does not track smoothly without a tendency to displace, a lateral release is done.

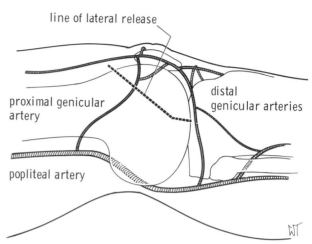

line of lateral release

proximal genicular
artery

distal
genicular arteries

popliteal artery

Fig. 20.80. The lateral release is done obliquely to preserve the distal genicular arteries.

tained. With low viscosity cement and pressurization, penetration may be excessive even if fixation is superior. The revision of components for infection, malposition or subluxation is most difficult and considerable bone must be sacrificed. Whatever technique is used, once the components are cemented it is essential that all excess cement be trimmed from around the components to prevent cement particles from breaking loose. The presence of entrapped cement between the articular surfaces leads to three body wear and rapid destruction of the polyethylene. The most likely places for cement to remain are behind and above the posterior femoral condyles and at the posterior and lateral aspects of the tibial plateau. Good exposure during the operation and while cementing provides for more complete cement removal. Insertion of the components one at a time is also recommended for the same reason.

AFTERCARE OF TOTAL KNEE ARTHROPLASTY PATIENTS

Intravenous antibiotics (usually oxacillin or cephalosporin) are administered immediately preoperative and for 48 hours postoperatively. No further antibiotic prophylaxis is recommended. All patients receiving a total joint implant are given a card upon discharge regarding the administration of prophylactic antibiotics to prevent possible metastatic infections. We recommend that antibiotic coverage be given when there is a known infection elsewhere in the body or for dental manipulations, genitourinary tract instrumentations, or other major surgery in which there is a possibility of bacteremia. We recommend a ceph-

alosporin four times a day for 24 hours preceding and 48 hours after the invasive procedure. This information is printed on a card to allow another treating physician to contact us should there be any question regarding the use of antibiotics for prophylactic coverage during any procedure. We have found the other medical disciplines to be most cooperative in this program.

The prevention of thrombophlebitis and pulmonary embolism[19,32] should be a major goal of every orthopedic surgeon who performs total knee arthroplasty. In a recent study of 643 patients undergoing total knee arthroplasty at The Hospital for Special Surgery,[136A] 64 percent were found to have evidence of thrombophlebitis, as indicated by a positive venogram on postoperative day 5. This result occurred despite all types of prophylactic anticoagulation including aspirin,[78] reomacrodex, and mini-heparin. All the patients also had a preoperative lung scan and a postoperative lung scan on day 6. There was an 11 percent incidence of postoperative lung scan changes consistent with small pulmonary emboli, although only a few of these patients had clinical symptoms or signs of pulmonary embolism. As with other investigators, we found the clinical diagnosis of deep venous thrombosis to be totally unreliable, with numerous examples of both false-negative and false-positive findings.[53] All patients with clinical or scintographic evidence of pulmonary embolism also had positive venography, suggesting that the positive venogram, although not itself associated with local symptoms, is of clinical significance. Patients with a positive venogram or lung scan are therefore anticoagulated for 2 to 3 months unless there are also correlating clinical symptoms and signs of pulmonary embolism in which case the anticoagulation is continued for 6 months. Anticoagulation is accomplished using coumadin. We do not recommend the use of heparin in therapeutic doses except in life-saving situations because of the considerable risk of a hemarthrosis in the knee.

In an effort to reduce the incidence of deep venous thrombosis following total knee surgery, we have used intermittent compression stockings on the lower extremity, applied immediately postoperatively in the operating room under the usual dressing. An early review of the first 50 patients so treated indicated a reduction in positive venography from 64 to 11 percent.[36]

The total knee patients are allowed to walk on the third or fourth postoperative day using a walker or crutches with weight-bearing as tolerated. The patients are disconnected from the pulsatile stockings while walking, but otherwise remain connected during the first 5 postoperative days. The compressive Robert Jones dressing is removed after the venogram on the fifth postoperative day, and active assisted flexion exercises are begun if the condition of the wound is satisfactory. Quadriceps-strengthening exercises are not stressed during this phase of rehabilitation because of the risk of damaging the capsular closure. We have encountered patients who have suffered a patellar dislocation during the course of physiotherapy, particularly when lifting weights. We therefore prefer to delay muscle strengthening exercises for 2 weeks and then begin only with straight leg raising exercises.

The patients remain in hospital until they (1) walk independently with a cane, (2) can climb stairs, and (3) have 90 degrees of flexion. The use of a static bicycle is a great aid in gaining flexion. The patients begin with the seat raised to its maximum height with progressive lowering of the seat as the range of motion improves. A gentle manipulation under anesthesia is indicated during the third postoperative week when flexion is not satisfactory. We have found that the manipulation rate is greatly reduced in patients having a lateral retinacular release during surgery. In a recent study we found that in one group of patients who did not have a lateral release the incidence of postoperative manipulation was 66 percent.[76] In another group using the same prosthesis, surgical technique and postoperative program, except for the addition of the lateral retinacular release, the incidence of manipulation fell to less than 20 percent. While manipulation of itself is usually an uncomplicated and uneventful process, it does involve a second anesthetic and is undesirable when the patient is receiving anticoagulation therapy. Also, patients undergoing a lateral release seem to have a much easier time with their postoperative physiotherapy, with much less pain and discomfort. For these reasons, we are now advocating a more routine use of lateral release.

COMPLICATIONS OF KNEE REPLACEMENT[86,151]

GENERAL COMPLICATIONS

Despite the advanced age of most patients and the frequency of associated medical conditions such as arteriosclerotic heart disease, hypertension, diabetes and chronic pulmonary disorders, the general complications of knee replacement are relatively few. At The Hospital for Special Surgery in a consecutive series of 1,500 arthroplasties there were no intraoperative deaths, although one patient undergoing bilateral sequential Guepar prostheses died of fat embolism[10] in the recovery room. Six patients suffered a cerebral vascular accident within 2 days of surgery, one of which was fatal. Three patients died of pulmonary embolism in the third postoperative week (in the first group of 400 arthroplasties performed before any form of thromboembolic prophylaxis was used). Two patients died of myocardial infarction during the postoperative period. Two of the early cases died from septicemia secondary to an infected prosthesis approximately one year after operation. All other deaths were unrelated to the operative procedure.

Urinary retention and urinary tract infections occurred with some frequency, especially in bilateral cases (21 percent). Postoperative catheterization was often required. The organism most frequently recovered was *Escherichia coli*. All cases eventually responded to conservative measures and appropriate antibiotic therapy. In none of these was the postoperative urinary tract infection related to the development of a deep wound infection in the operated knee.

LOCAL COMPLICATIONS

WOUND DRAINAGE AND DELAYED WOUND HEALING

In a series of 220 total condylar arthroplasties[73] studied some years ago, 49 knees did not have primary wound healing or had some wound drainage. Forty-one had cultures taken of which 35 were negative. The most frequently isolated organism was Staphylococcus epidermidis. One case with skin necrosis became secondarily infected (mixed organisms) and eventually developed a deep wound infection. With this exception, early wound drainage was not related to periprosthetic infection (although this was not true in another study of the Guepar prosthesis).[80] Most cases of delayed wound healing were attributed to beginning physical therapy and motion too soon in the postoperative course. In the early part of the series therapy was begun on the second postoperative day. We now recommend delaying the onset of knee flexion until the fifth postoperative day or until the wound is completely sealed and dry. Walking, however, can begin as soon as tolerated by the patient. Delaying physical therapy in this manner has resulted in a reduction in the frequency of wound drainage and in the most recent group of patients studied using the posterior stabilized condylar knee, the incidence of wound complications was 15 percent. It is also advisable to release the tourniquet before closing the wound in order to ligate or coagulate the major bleeding points, reinflating the tourniquet before wound closure. Suction drainage should be used for 24 hours.

In the total condylar series of 220 knees, seven had skin necrosis or wound separation. Three required secondary closure and two, skin grafts. Skin necrosis is particularly likely in previously operated knees, especially when midmedial or midlateral incisions (such as were once used for synovectomy) are already present. In such cases, it may be necessary to use a midline anterior incision for the arthroplasty, and breakdown of a skin bridge (usually laterally) may occur. Medial parapatellar skin incisions are particularly prone to skin necrosis, whereas lateral parapatellar skin incisions, although presenting no particular healing difficulties, may be objected to because when lateral retinacular release is also needed, the skin incision comes to lie directly over the prosthetic components. A straight midline incision therefore seems better than either type of parapatellar incision.

THROMBOEMBOLIC AND VASCULAR COMPLICATIONS

Anticoagulation therapy may occasionally result in a hemarthrosis particularly when heparin is used. With coumadin therapy the risk is small provided the prothrombin time is kept at a level about 1.5 times above the control. Prolonged swelling of the operated leg, not necessarily related to deep vein thrombosis, is a common complaint and may persist for several months after the arthroplasty. Supporting stockings and active exercise together with an increased activity level eventually resolve swelling.

Vascular or arterial complications have fortunately been rare, and the absence preoperatively of peripheral pulses has not been regarded as a contraindication to surgery provided that the capillary circulation was adequate. Vascular complications have occurred in only three patients in more than 3,000 arthroplasties.

In one elderly patient with osteoarthritis, extensive lateral soft tissue release was done to correct a valgus deformity. The release apparently interfered with the collateral circulation to the distal leg by dividing the lateral genicular artery and its branches. Postoperatively the foot was cold and pulseless and an arteriogram showed a blockage of the popliteal artery above the knee with no collateral runoff whatsoever. Nevertheless, by the time the arteriogram had been completed, warmth and a capillary circulation had returned to the foot, so the patient was treated conservatively. Thereafter recovery was uneventful and the patient has now been followed for 2 years without further evidence of vascular insufficiency. This case indicates however, the need for careful assessment when an extensive soft tissue dissection is contemplated because of the risk of interrupting a supportive collateral circulation system (Fig. 20.81).

The second case was a rheumatoid patient with vasculitis in whom postoperative gangrene developed in the toes, which later led to an above-knee amputation.

A third patient, with post-traumatic arthritis, had a vascular insufficiency before surgery confirmed by arteriography; the vascular consultant believed that a knee replacement was not contraindicated, and the patient's disability seemed to warrant the risk. At surgery some purulent fluid was encountered, so that after taking cultures the procedure was aborted and the wound was closed. Postoperatively an area of skin necrosis developed over the wound that took several months to heal. By this time the knee had become so stiff that all thoughts of an arthroplasty were abandoned and the knee eventually ankylosed. Gangrene subsequently developed in the toes, later requiring an above-the-knee amputation. In this instance the amputation was not directly related to the patient's surgery.

NERVE PALSY

While we have encountered one case of transient paralysis of the popliteal nerve after correction of a severe flexion contracture, most nerve palsies involve the peroneal nerve. This is composed of fibers from the dorsal portion of the 4th and 5th lumbar and 1st and 2nd sacral nerves. As the nerve courses down from the thigh it curves laterally behind the head of the fibula to reach the two heads of the peroneus longus. The nerve flattens as it passes between these two heads, as a result the bundles become separated exposing unprotected nutrient vessels. It then curves around the neck of the fibula and divides into deep and superficial branches.

The deep peroneal nerve continues under the extensor digitorum longus along the anterior aspect of

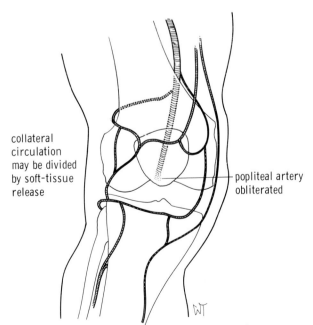

collateral circulation may be divided by soft-tissue release

popliteal artery obliterated

Fig. 20.81. In elderly patients, extensive soft tissue releases may interrupt a vital collateral circulation.

the intraosseous membrane. It sends motor branches to the tibialis anterior, extensor digitorum longus, extensor hallucis longus, and the peroneus tertius. The nerve continues distally, ending in the medial and lateral terminal branches, which among other functions supply sensation to the first web space of the foot.

The superficial peroneal nerve passes distally between the peronei and extensor digitorum longus. Motor branches are given off to both the peroneus longus and brevis. In the lower one third of the leg the nerve branches into the medial and intermediate dorsal cutaneus nerves. These terminal branches complete the sensory enervation of the foot.

A total of 2,626 total knee arthroplasties were performed at The Hospital for Special Surgery from January 1974 to December 1980. During that time there were 23 peroneal nerve palsies in 22 patients.[116] One patient developed a peroneal palsy after both total knee arthroplasties, which were done 5 months apart. The preoperative deformity was varus in five knees, neutral alignment in seven knees, and valgus in 11 knees. In addition, some degree of flexion contracture was found in 14 patients, being severe in nine patients. Five patients underwent exploration and release of the peroneal nerve and a nerve palsy developed despite this precaution. These explorations were done in knees with severe flexion contractures (30 degrees and 80 degrees) and in severe valgus deformities (27 degrees, 35 degrees, and 40 degrees).

The time of appearance of the problem was variable and ranged from discovery in the recovery room to the sixth postoperative day. Most cases were noted early, with eight found in the recovery room and another eight discovered during the first postoperative day. Three were noted on postoperative day 2, two on postoperative day 3, and two on postoperative day 6. The motor fibers of the tibialis anterior and extensor hallucis longus muscles were affected in all cases; a sensory deficit was noticed in 20 cases (87 percent). The peroneus longus muscle was affected in nine cases (39 percent). Six patients underwent electromyographic evaluation during the early postoperative period; the findings were those of a diffuse motor neuropathy in the mild cases and of denervation potentials in muscles supplied by the deep branch of the common peroneal nerve in the more severely involved cases.

The treatment rendered on discovery of these findings varied according to the discretion of the surgeon involved. The most frequent therapeutic measure was to loosen the Robert Jones dressing and place the knee in a more flexed position. In two cases this maneuver brought immediate improvement of both motor and sensory deficits.

The time interval between discovery and the beginning of the return of function ranged from immediately in the two cases mentioned to 6 months. Motor improvement occurred first, with sensory return lagging behind.

In 13 cases, traction[29,54,55,92] secondary to correction of a valgus or flexion deformity, or both, was the cause of the palsy. In three cases the use of medial and lateral splints to hold the knee with "tight" components in full extension with consequent traction on the nerve by this stretching mechanism was implicated as the etiology. In four cases the dressing containing medial and lateral plaster splints was considered too tight or improperly padded, causing direct pressure on the peroneal nerve. In three cases no explanation could be determined.

Seventeen of the peroneal palsies were extensive enough to require a drop-foot brace. The other six were mild and did not need any dorsiflexion assist.

At follow-up examination a residual deficit was found in all 18 patients in whom a sensory deficit had been present. Motor power was clinically normal in six of the patients (28 percent), the remaining 15 patients had motor power clinically assessed in the poor to good range. Full clinical recovery occurred in only two patients, neither of whom had a sensory deficit initially. This recovery occurred within 6 months in both cases. Four additional patients had complete motor recovery but still had a residual sensory deficit.

The following factors contribute to the development of peroneal nerve palsy: (1) stretching of the nerve in valgus and flexion contractures, (2) fascial compression of the nerve and its vascular supply, (3) direct pressure from the dressing, and (4) rare idiopathic cases in which none of the above mechanisms seem to apply.

It is apparent that patients with excessive total deformities are candidates for developing peroneal nerve palsies. The large soft tissue dissections required to balance the more severe deformities may be responsible for increased traction or vascular compromise in this area. The alternative method of bone sacrifice to correct large deformities, although appealing because of the elimination of the need for obtaining soft tissue balance, does not eliminate peroneal nerve palsy although it may be less likely.[85] The bone-sacrificing method also leaves a residual leg length discrepancy that is permanent and frequently of more consequence than a peroneal nerve palsy. Contrained prostheses have a higher loosening rate in the long run.

Recovery of paralysis of the peroneal nerve is usually partial with sensory deficits that may be permanent. Residual motor deficits are not usually of clinical significance despite occasional marked weaknesses, especially of the great toe extensors. Immediate knee flexion upon recognition of the palsy is recommended.

FRACTURES

Fractures around the prosthesis[56] are of three kinds: (1) intraoperative, (2) caused by stress or fatigue, and (3) caused by a fall or other injury.

INTRAOPERATIVE FRACTURES

These fractures can occur in either the tibial plateau or the femoral condyles (Fig. 20.82). They are most likely when bone is brittle and can occur when the prosthesis is driven hard onto the bone. Tibial fractures are seldom of consequence and require no special treatment. Femoral condyle fractures may displace and then require internal fixation with screws. When the bone is very soft (rheumatoid arthritis) the femoral component in particular may be driven into the bone more than intended, resulting in a malposition of the components. This can only be avoided by taking great care in such patients.

Intraoperative fractures seldom require any special postoperative management except perhaps a longer than usual period on crutches. Motion does not need to be delayed.

STRESS OR FATIGUE FRACTURES[114]

Stress fractures adjoining the components occur in the patella, femur (Fig. 20.83), and tibia and may result in recurrent deformity and component loos-

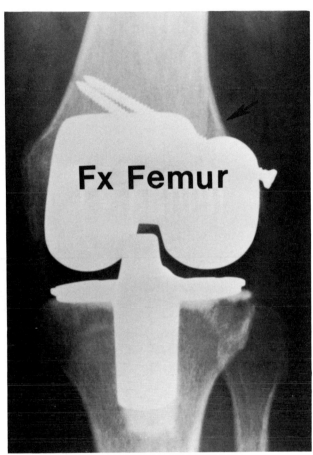

Fig. 20.82. An intra-operative fracture of the lateral femoral condyle occurred in this case. After fixation with two screws, the aftercare was uneventful and weight-bearing as usual was permitted.

ening. When the femoral or tibial components are involved revision is usually required.

FRACTURES CAUSED BY
A FALL OR OTHER INJURY

Most fractures occur in the lower femur adjoining the prosthesis. They may be comminuted and displaced. Fractures seem more likely to occur in this region if the femur was breached at operation by notching of the anterior femoral cortex (Fig. 20.84). This was likely to happen before a complete range of femoral sizes became available because of the need to fit a relatively small prosthesis onto a large bone. Femoral fractures may at times need internal fixation,

but usually can be managed by applying skeletal traction through the tibia or the os calcis. Six weeks traction allowing early motion is usually sufficient for adequate healing with retention of motion. Even though the radiological appearance shows residual displacement of the fragments after healing the final functional result is often excellent. Internal fixation with a blade plate is often complicated by the presence of the femoral component or cement and should in general be avoided.

TIBIAL TUBERCLE AVULSION

Avulsion of the tibial tubercle (Fig. 20.85) is most often an intraoperative complication that is best avoided rather than treated. Exposure can be difficult in knees that are tight or stiff, and with the patella dislocated laterally, considerable traction is exerted upon the insertion of the patellar ligament. Avulsion of the tubercle during intraoperative maneuvers can easily happen, and if the periosteum tears across, an adequate reconstruction is very difficult if not impossible. Two preventive measures are possible:

1. Make the vertical capsular incision onto the tibia 1 cm medial to the tibial tubercle, so that a cuff of periosteum is reflected in continuity with the ligamentum patellae. If the insertion then begins to peel away from the tibial tubercle, the periosteal cuff is taken with the patellar ligament and preserves soft tissue integrity distally.
2. When the knee is very tight and avulsion appears likely, the exposure is converted to a quadriceps turndown by cutting obliquely across the quadriceps tendon from its apex into the vastus lateralis until the quadriceps tendon, and the patella can be turned distally and laterally to provide adequate exposure. Quadriceps turndown is particularly useful for revision operations. It requires three weeks of immobilization before beginning flexion, and although a slight extension lag may occur, the result is infinitely better than after a tibial tubercle avulsion.

Avulsion can also occur as a result of a manipulation or a fall. It has also been reported spontaneously during postoperative physical therapy, but probably this is more in the nature of a spontaneous detachment of an insertion already weakened by the operative exposure. A manipulative avulsion is avoidable pro-

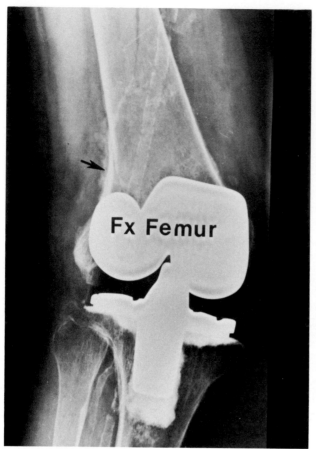

Fig. 20.83. In this rheumatoid patient a lateral soft tissue release was done to correct a severe valgus deformity. Two months after operation, pain and a recurrent valgus deformity developed. A stress fracture of the lateral femoral condyle was observed that healed in a position of deformity. The femoral component in this case is apparently not loose, and the knee is painless.

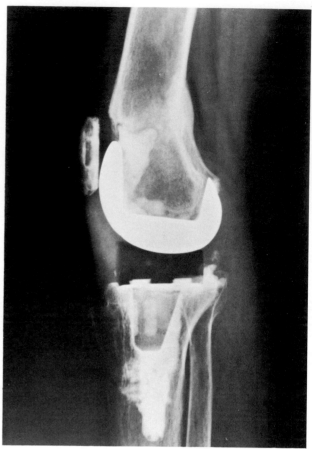

Fig. 20.84. The saw has violated the anterior cortex of the femur. The weakened bone makes it susceptible to fracture.

vided that the quadriceps muscle is paralyzed by a muscle relaxant before the manipulation is done.

Once established, the author knows of no satisfactory method of repairing an avulsed tibial tubercle. Avulsion is most likely when the tibial bone is osteoporotic and this factor complicates the repair. Open repair by suture, screw or staple should be done but all too often rerupture occurs even after six to eight weeks of immobilization.

Rupture of the patellar ligament or quadriceps mechanism can also happen, and although repair is more satisfactory than after tibial avulsion, late stretching is likely.

PATELLAR COMPLICATIONS

SUBLUXATION AND DISLOCATION

Two factors are involved in causing a postoperative patellar subluxation or dislocation:

1. The rotation of the tibial component. Malposition of the tibial component results in excessive lateral placement of the tibial tubercle. The correct placement has been discussed, and in extreme cases revision of this component is necessary. However, proximal realignment is often sufficient to restore patellar stability but distal realignment should not be done because of the difficulty in obtaining satisfactory reattachment of the patellar ligament, especially when a tibial component stem is present.

2. Incorrect patellar tracking due to a tight lateral

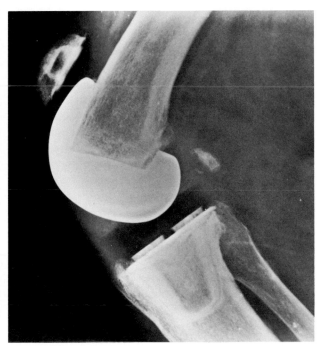

Fig. 20.85. The patellar ligament has been avulsed from the tibial tubercle, and the patella is very high riding. There is a 40 degree extension lag.

retinaculum or quadriceps malalignment. The patella must track smoothly at the conclusion of the operation without the need for digital pressure to hold it in place. A lateral retinacular release is done when needed.

When a patellar dislocation occurs in spite of these precautions, a proximal realignment is nearly always sufficient to control it. The technique used will be found in the section on patellar disorders (see Chapter 11).

SOFT TISSUE IMPINGEMENT[76]

Occasionally cases will be found in which there is postoperative grating and catching upon active extension of the knee. The radiographs appear entirely normal. No evidence of patellar subluxation is found. The cause is soft tissue entrapment between the peripatellar synovium and capsule and the femoral component. Most often this involves a portion of the suprapatellar synovium which becomes irritated, inflamed and swollen. Occasionally a sizable mass can result which can be caught against the anterior lip of the

intercondylar recess of the femoral component. As a rule symptoms from this type of soft tissue impingement are relatively mild, but we have on occasion performed an arthrotomy to remove the soft tissue mass. Excision results in a cure.

PATELLAR FRACTURES[137]

Patellar fractures after total knee arthroplasty can occur with and without patellar resurfacing, although they are more common when a patellar implant has been used. Fractures are of two types:

1. *Traumatic fractures.* These occur as a result of fairly major trauma, such as a fall downstairs. This type of fracture is usually displaced (Fig. 20.86) and requires open operation to reapproximate the fragments because there is usually a tear through the extensor mechanism as well as a fracture through the patella. Operative repair is somewhat complicated by the presence of the patellar button and often rather soft patellar bone, so it may be difficult to reduce the fragments accurately and fix them satisfactorily. The retinacular tears should also be carefully repaired.

2. *Fatigue fractures.* These occur spontaneously without significant trauma and often are asymptomatic, being noticed only on routine radiography. There are three types:

    a. *Horizontal fractures* (Fig. 20.87). In this type the patella separates horizontally, one portion usually containing the patellar implant remaining in its normal position, with the other fragment subluxing laterally. Thus the mechanism of fracture is due to improper patellar tracking and is akin to a patellar dislocation. The extensor mechanism is usually weakened particularly when the displaced fragment is a major one which carries with it the attachments of the quadriceps tendon and patellar ligament. Operative repair to reposition the major fragment with or without excision of the button and smaller fragment is sometimes required, being dictated by the amount of extensor mechanism inadequacy.

    b. *Vertical fractures* (Fig. 20.88). The fracture occurs in a vertical plane, often with separation of the fragments. The fracture almost invariably passes through the patellar fixation

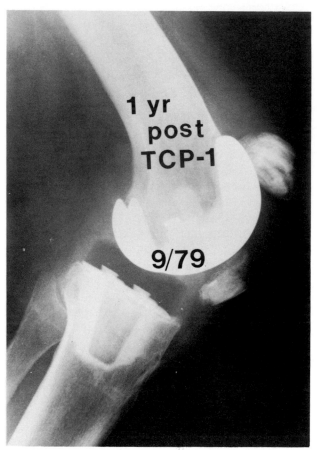

1 yr post TCP-1

9/79

Fig. 20.86. Post-traumatic vertical fracture of the patella, requiring open reduction.

hole. Often in spite of wide separation of the fragments, the extensor mechanism is remarkably normal presumably because at least partial continuity remains and the medial and lateral retinaculae are intact. The presentation may be one of transient mild pain and swelling, but at times the fracture seems entirely asymptomatic. Usually no specific treatment is required. Patients are told not to climb stairs with the affected leg until all pain and swelling have gone, but otherwise they may use the leg normally. The fracture may unite with bone or fibrous tissue.

c. *Comminuted and displaced fractures.* This is the most common type and appears to be a combination of types 1 and 2. The presentation is nearly always asymptomatic, no extensor weakness is demonstrable, and as these are often discovered on routine follow-up, the exact timing of the fracture may be difficult to pinpoint. No treatment is required unless the patellar implant is loose when removal of the button is indicated.

A number of factors seem to be implicated in the development of fatigue fractures.

1. Improper patellar tracking seems the major factor in the horizontal and perhaps some of the comminuted displaced fractures. This should be preventable by careful attention to patellar tracking at the time of surgery, performing a lateral release when the patella does not track without digital pressure.

2. Weakening of the patella because of resection of its articular surfaces and the making of a central fixation hole for the patellar implant. Usually cortical bone will protrude laterally beyond the surface of the implant due to the elliptical shape of the patella, and if this bone is trimmed to prevent possible lateral impingement, the patella is further weakened. Trimming is therefore not recommended.

3. Avascularity due to the large medial retinacular incision and sometimes a lateral release that will also divide the lateral retinacular vessels. There is in a sense a dilemma: a lateral release is necessary to prevent patellar dislocation and horizontal fractures, but the performance of the release further

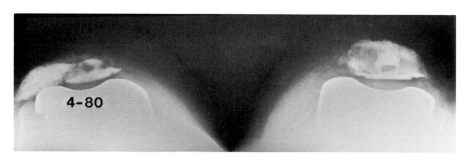

4-80

Fig. 20.87. Horizontal fatigue fracture of the patella.

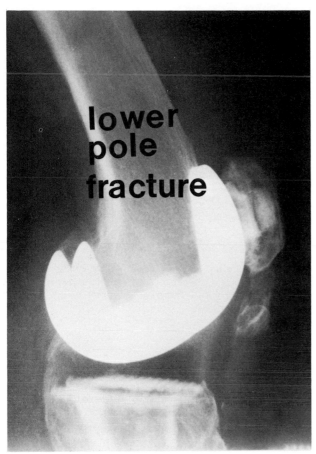

Fig. 20.88. Vertical fatigue fracture of the patella. In contradistinction to the traumatic fractures, this type usually heals spontaneously, as occurred in this case.

compromises the patellar blood supply and increases the chance of vertical fractures. We believe that patellar tracking receives priority and that a lateral release should be performed whenever necessary. It has been suggested by some workers that excision of the fat pad will impair the patellar arterial supply. This concept is probably erroneous because the main vessels lie more superficially in the retinacular layer and thus are not affected by excision of the fat pad. However, much of the venous drainage from the patella occurs through the fat pad,[24] and thus by causing back pressure due to venous insufficiency, fat pad excision may indirectly compromise the arterial supply.

4. Patient activity. In a sense patellar fractures are a complication of success as they are seen in the most active patients with the greatest range of motion

(Fig. 20.89) and who therefore tend to use the knee arthroplasty in a normal manner for stair climbing, arising from a chair and other stressful activities. Patellar fractures have been seen more frequently with the posterior stabilized condylar prosthesis. Patients with this prosthesis have an average range of flexion 25 degrees greater than most other implants, and most use the knee normally for climbing up and down stairs.

In a recent retrospective study[137] at The Hospital for Special Surgery, 18 patellar fractures occurring after total condylar arthroplasty were studied. Two open reductions were performed for traumatic fractures, one closed reduction and cast immobilization for a separated vertical fracture, and one patellectomy was performed in conjunction with a revision procedure. The results in this group were rated as good in three and fair in one due to persistent quadriceps weakness and an extension lag.

The remaining fourteen knees were either not treated at all or managed conservatively by simple measures. The results were excellent in 10 and good in four. None of this group had demonstrable quadriceps weakness or an extension lag (Fig. 20.90). In one however, the patellar button worked itself loose and presented under the skin, whence it was removed through a small incision.

BREAKAGE AND WEAR

Breakage of components is rare and usually restricted to hinges and linked designs. For example, with the Guepar prosthesis breakage may occur in the femoral stem about 3 cm proximal to the joint (Fig. 20.91). Fracture of the tibial stem in a corresponding position is a more rare occurrence. Breakage is manifest by instability, pain and deformity, but does not necessarily call for immediate revision. One of our patients had a fracture of the femoral stem associated with an episode of transient pain three years after the arthroplasty. Although some instability was present, she functioned at a high level with little or no pain for another 5 years before revision became necessary for an increasing varus deformity.

Breakage has also been reported with other linked components. The Herbert prosthesis, using a ball-and-socket linkage, had such a high incidence of mechanical failure[108] that the prosthesis was withdrawn

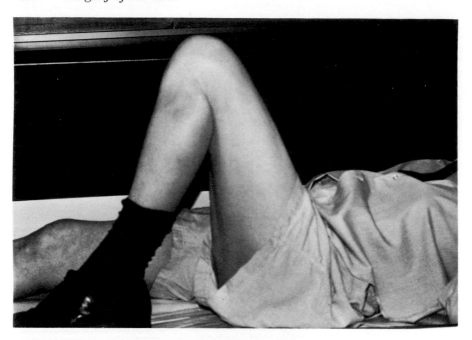

Fig. 20.89. Patients with flexion well beyond 90 degrees are susceptible to fatigue fractures of the patella because of the greater stresses imposed on the bone.

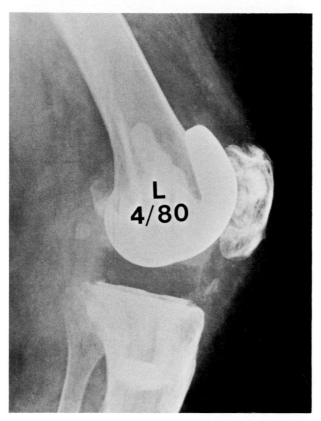

Fig. 20.90. A healed fractured of the lower pole of the patella. This patient has an excellent result and no quadriceps weakness.

from use. The spherocentric knee replacement, on the other hand, using a similar ball-and-socket linkage, has not so far been reported to suffer from mechanical failure. Sheehan[126] has encountered five cases in which the polyethylene tibial stud fractured, one the result of a fall on a polished floor. The stabilizing post of the stabilocondylar prosthesis has also suffered from distortion and fatigue failure in two of our patients. No mechanical failures have been reported with Attenborough or TCP III prostheses.

Mechanical failure in surface replacement is very rare. We have encountered three fractured femoral components in the early version of the uni- and duocondylar prostheses. In these the femoral runner was made of considerably thinner metal than used on subsequent designs, and it is not expected that a similar fatigue failure will be seen in current models.

WEAR

Retrieval analysis of removed total joint implants has consistently revealed polyethylene particles in the synovium.[15] In addition, acryllic debris and occasionally metallic debris particles have also been seen. Inspection of the removed components often reveals embedded cement particles in the polyethylene component with scratching, pitting, and burnishing of the

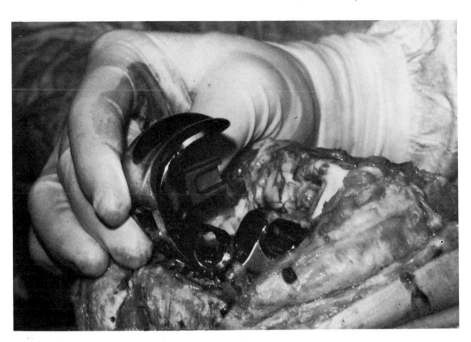

Fig. 20.91. A broken Guepar prosthesis.

articular surface (Fig. 20.92). Distortion of the polyethylene and gross deformation of the component due to cold flow (Fig. 20.93) may also occur and is particularly likely when the tibial component is thin. Some of the earlier designs possessed a component that was deliberately made thin in order to minimize bone removal, and in addition, often had a cruciate cut-out. This combination led in some instances to gross distortion and deformation, which contributed to loosening of the component. (The early UCI design was prone to this mode of failure.) It is now considered that unless reinforced with a metal tray, a minimum thickness of 8 mm is desirable. Also, as mentioned previously, a one-piece component (that is without a cruciate cut-out) contributes greatly to rigidity.

Metal femoral components may be observed to have scratches in the highly polished articular surface in more than one-half the retrieved specimens.

It is believed that most of the debris is generated from free cement particles that have become entrapped between the articular surfaces. Careful surgical technique can lessen cement entrapment, however, even in the absence of evidence of cement or three body wear, polyethylene failure at the articular surface may be observed. This is manifested by pitting, scratching, burnishing, and abrasion of the surface. The amount of surface failure is highly correlated with the level of patient activity, body weight,

and length of implantation and seems to be of a greater degree than noted in retrieval analysis of total hip implants.[58]

The durability of a spherically convex polyethylene patellar implant may be questioned in that this shape theoretically causes more wear. Retrieval analysis at The Hospital for Special Surgery of 35 patellar buttons[60] did not indicate that the rate of wear is greater than that of the tibial plateau. There is however, some deformation of the polyethylene, usually with elongation in the long axis and some flattening of the convex shape where it articulates with the femoral component.

Several things have been done to improve the wear characteristics of ultrahigh-molecular-weight polyethylene in total joint arthroplasties. The manufacturers have voluntarily increased the molecular weight of the polyethylene, which theoretically gives it better-wear characteristics. Another solution currently being evaluated is the addition of carbon fragments to the polyethylene. Yet a third attempt to correct this problem has been the addition of metal backing to provide a better support and allow less deformation (Fig. 20.94). These latter solutions have the effect of increasing the stiffness of the polyethylene which for a corresponding body weight will result in a decreased surface area for transmission of the load applied. This increased force per unit area, however, will certainly result in

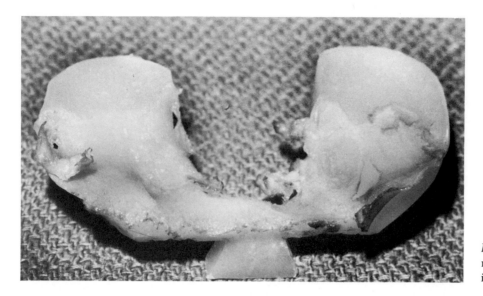

Fig. 20.92. A retrieved geometric tibial component showing severe wear.

a higher rate of wear which may cancel the advantage gained by a harder surface. A number of clinical trials are currently in progress to determine the outcome of such attempts at improving wear characteristics.

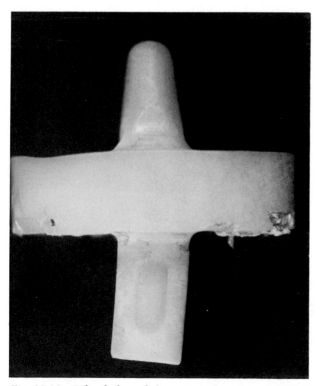

Fig. 20.93. Polyethylene deformation of a removed TCP II tibial component.

INADEQUATE MOTION

The range of motion obtained after arthroplasty is dependent on several factors, including body habitus, patient motivation, adequacy of physical therapy, and prosthetic design. However, probably the most important determinant is the range of motion that existed before the arthroplasty. A knee that is very stiff to begin with is difficult to mobilize satisfactorily because of quadriceps contracture and capsular fibrosis. Even if an adequate range of motion is achieved in the operating theater, this may not be realized postoperatively. For this reason very stiff or ankylosed knees should be approached with caution and with the expectation that 45 to 60 degrees of flexion is the likely end result. Arthrodesed knees in which more extensive damage to the extensor mechanism might be expected, and in which the ligaments were probably divided should not be considered for arthroplasty at all. A linked design is more successful in improving motion than a surface replacement because the ligaments and capsule not being required for stability can be excised. The difficulty in exposing a very stiff knee has been alluded to and a quadriceps turn-down incision is recommended. A partial quadricepsplasty can be achieved if only the vastus medialis and rectus femoris components of the quadriceps are resutured, leaving the vastus intermedius and vastus lateralis completely or partially unattached.

It has been our policy to manipulate knees postoperatively if motion is not rapidly regained, and usu-

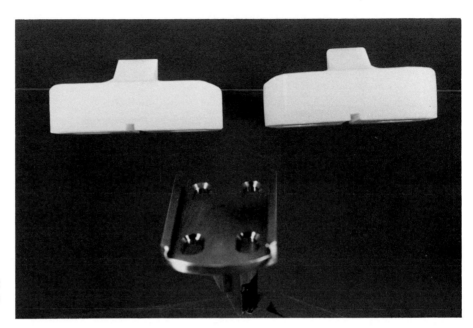

Fig. 20.94. Metal tray support of the polyethylene prevents deformation.

ally this is done during the third postoperative week when flexion is not 75 degrees or more by this time. A general anesthetic with full muscular relaxation is needed because if tone remains in the quadriceps muscle the increased resistance may damage the patellar ligament or its insertion and possibly cause a fracture adjoining the prosthesis. The purpose of the manipulation is to overcome intraarticular adhesions and this can be done with less force when quadriceps resistance is eliminated. We have manipulated between one third and one-half of all our arthroplastics in this manner so that the total number of manipulations is now more than 1,000. Only two complications have been recorded: one was a supracondylar femoral fracture in a knee that was ankylosed before the arthroplasty, and the other a patellar ligament avulsion also occurring in a previously stiff knee. Both these complications were early in our experience when the value of muscle-relaxing agents was not appreciated and might have been avoided had the quadriceps been paralyzed.

Some of our patients may not have needed a manipulation and might have regained motion if left alone to continue physical therapy. Fox and Poss[37] studied 343 total knee replacements performed in a twelve month period in which 81 (23 percent) were manipulated, the indication being the failure to achieve 90 degrees of comfortable, active flexion by the end of the second postoperative week. Manipulation did not increase the ultimate flexion of the knee when compared with the larger group of knees that were not manipulated at all. However, their study did not address the critical question of whether the knees chosen for manipulation would have done just as well without. Some patients do not easily regain flexion of the knee after arthroplasty, and in some restriction of motion may be permanent. We have seen examples of this in patients who were not manipulated either because a second anesthetic was prevented by a medical problem, or because the surgeon involved did not consider manipulation desirable. A selective manipulation is done for the following reasons: (1) it improves the immediate course by allowing more normal function and by making the continued physical therapy easier and less painful. It also facilitates earlier discharge from the hospital; and (2) to prevent permanent restriction of motion in certain patients who are not easily identified until it is too late for manipulation to be effective.

We believe that prediction of the postoperative range of motion is more certain for cruciate-removing designs. Accurate tensioning is required with cruciate retention to prevent the posterior cruciate ligament from acting as a check rein; this happens when the geometry of the prosthesis is of different curvature than the preexisting anatomic surfaces, causing the posterior cruciate to tighten with flexion.

Other intraarticular causes of loss of flexion are excess posterior cement and adhesive capsulitis. The latter is likely to follow a hematoma or other wound healing problem which results in a long delay in physical therapy. Even so most patients gradually regain motion given sufficient time. When a lateral retinacular release has not been done, tightening of the lateral capsule makes flexion difficult; in particularly resistant cases, a lateral retinacular release followed by a manipulation will sometimes successfully regain motion.

Sympathetic dystrophy is an extreme example of adhesive capsulitis in which the whole joint is chronically swollen and the capsule greatly increased in thickness. Usually the other signs associated with a sympathetic dystrophy are present and the patient invariably complains of excessive pain.

A persistent flexion contracture is usually the result of incorrect bone cuts at surgery or failure to strip and divide the posterior capsule. The latter maneuver is necessary when there is a severe (>40 degrees) preoperative flexion contracture and is in practice limited to rheumatoid knees. Very rarely does this degree of contracture develop in gonarthrosis. With this exception, a postoperative flexion contracture is due to removal of an inadequate amount of bone from the distal femur, and normally, this should be noticed when inserting the appropriate spacer in extension. If the components have already been fitted, it is tempting to overcome the flexion contracture by excising more bone from the upper tibia; to recut the distal femur requires more reshaping and is a more complicated and troublesome process. However, if the flexion contracture is relieved by removing extra tibial bone, the flexion gap will also be enlarged and, as a result, the tibia may dislocate posteriorly. Therefore, it is the femur that must be reshaped; only then will the correct flexion balance be retained.

All prosthetic designs allow at least 90 degrees of flexion; hinges and some other linked designs may give more than this. With regard to surface replacement, the total condylar and Freeman-Samuelson models are designed to reach 90 degrees. Cruciate retention combined with flat tibial plateaus in theory allows more motion, and in practice about 100 degrees of flexion is obtained with these models (e.g., duopatella). The posterior stabilized knee provides for cruciate substitution by a cam mechanism and has provided the best range of motion of any prosthesis that we have used so far (an average of 115 degrees in a recent clinical study).[76]

INSTABILITY, SUBLUXATION, AND DISLOCATION

Instability after knee arthroplasty can be subdivided into five types: extension instability, flexion instability, rotary instability, translocation, and genu recurvatum.

EXTENSION INSTABILITY

Instability in extension can be either symmetric or asymmetric. Either type is accentuated when there is malposition of the components or overall malalignment of the extremity. Conversely the effects of extension instability are lessened, and sometimes masked altogether when position and alignment are correct.

Symmetric instability is caused whenever the thickness of the components is less than the extension gap between the bone ends. It can be caused by removal of excessive bone from the distal femur either because of miscalculation or because the collateral ligaments were not tensioned properly when making the point of resection. The patient's state of muscular relaxation can be a contributing cause when using manual force to tension the ligaments, and although deep anesthesia is not necessary for the rest of the operation, proper relaxation is required for this stage. Alternatively mechanical distraction with laminar spreaders or a tenser device make the mistake less likely.

Sometimes extension instability due to excessive bone resection can be solved by the use of thicker components. However, if the flexion gap has already been cut correctly, it may not be possible to insert a thicker tibial component (because it will not be accommodated in flexion). A thicker femoral component must therefore be used which, although available on a custom basis, is not routinely part of most total knee systems. Therefore, the femoral component must be built up, which can be accomplished to a limited degree by omitting the chamfer cuts causing the prosthetic component to sit proud of the distal femur. Alternatively, the build-up can be done with screws or titanium mesh; a stemmed femoral component is desirable when a considerable build-up is necessary.

Extension instability can also be caused when a ligament release to correct fixed varus or valgus deformity is done inappropriately after the bone cuts have been made, for the effect then is not only to

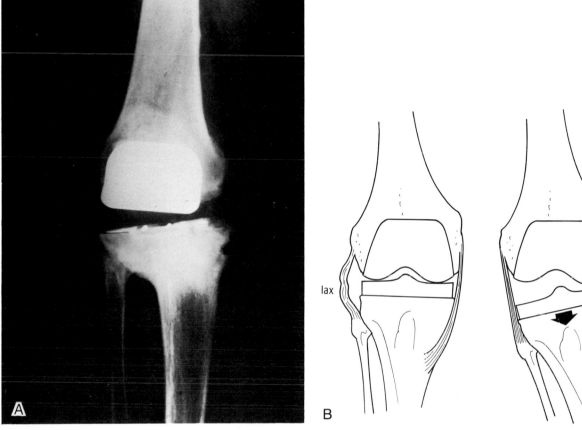

Fig. 20.95. (A) This arthroplasty is unstable, but not because of a ligament deficiency. (B) The medial ligament was not released, hence an asymmetric instability remains.

balance the ligaments but also to increase the extension gap. In varus release both gaps are increased (although not always to the same degree), and it is often possible to solve the problem by the use of thicker components as the concomitant increase in the flexion gap permits a greater range of tibial components to be tried. After valgus release, only the extension gap is increased, eliminating this option. When the ligament releases are completed first this particular problem will not arise, but sometimes, particularly in valgus knees, the amount of release can be underestimated until the components have been actually fitted.

ASYMMETRIC INSTABILITY

This is perhaps the most frequently encountered variant of instability. Most arthritic knees possess some degree of ligament asymmetry, and if the bone cuts are made without regard to this fundamental anomaly the arthroplasty will be unstable on one side (Fig. 20.95A,B). The most usual mistake in technique is to inadequately release a tight ligament due to a natural fear of causing instability. In practice, this apprehension is not justified for, whereas I have seen many knees that remained unstable because of insufficient release, I have seen none that subluxed because of the opposite condition. This is not to say that ligament balancing should be done carelessly, particularly when the deformity is mild. Postoperative instability can follow inadvertent division of a medial ligament in a correctly aligned knee for which no release at all was required.

Apart from such iatrogenic causes asymmetrical instability is very rarely due to complete absence of ligaments. This situation might be expected in some post-traumatic cases, but even then the torn ligaments normally heal so that the end result is stretching rather than absence. It is often believed that the ligaments in rheumatoid knees are incompetent or sometimes destroyed by synovitis, but if so, it must be most unusual. It is true that in some loose rheumatoid knees, some degree of postoperative stretching can occur, so that a tight fit is desirable. Sometimes the stretching present before surgery is so extreme that balancing becomes impractical because of the amount of overall leg lengthening required to equalize the ligaments (Fig. 20.96). This is a very rare but occasional indication for a constrained prosthesis.

Bone loss accompanying severe instability and deformity is not in itself an indication for a constrained prosthesis. It is a technical mistake to cut back excessively on either the tibia or the femur to produce a flat bone surface. On the tibial side large asymmetric defects, usually medial, are often found. Resection at the bottom level of the defect removes a large amount of tibial bone; the remaining cancellous bone is weak and often the cross-sectional area of the tibia is reduced. It is preferable to resect the tibia at the usual level as if no defect existed and then build up the uneven surface on one side with protruding screws, wire mesh or a bone graft. Best of all, the defect can be filled using an asymmetric tibial component (Fig. 20.97). Suitable wedge-shaped components are offered as custom components by several manufacturers and may soon become part of regular inventory.

Femoral defects are usually lateral and it may be that the indicated level of resection removes bone

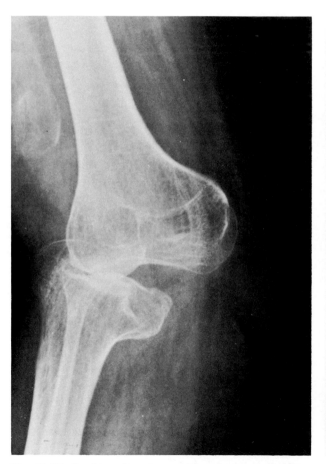

Fig. 20.96. In this valgus knee, although the medial ligament is not absent, it is so elongated that soft tissue balancing by lateral release is impractical. This is an indication for a constrained prosthesis.

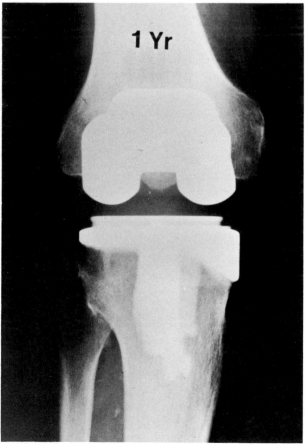

Fig. 20.97. A large medial tibial bone deficiency has been compensated by the use of a medial wedge tibial component. The articular surface of the prosthesis is standard total condylar and is not constrained.

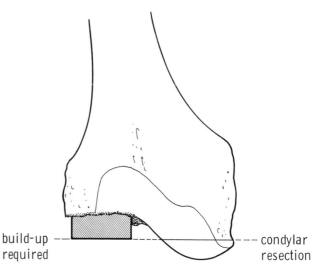

build-up — required

condylar — resection

Fig. 20.98. In some valgus knees, the level of femoral resection may pass distal to the lateral femoral condyle. Lateral augmentation of the femoral component is required.

from the medial femoral condyle but passes distal to the lateral (Fig. 20.98). The same solutions apply. Screws or mesh are satisfactory solutions, but augmented components are preferred.

While stems are a means of gaining extra fixation to the bone, use of a stem should not be confused with constraint in the prosthetic joint itself, although most constrained or hinged prostheses also have long intramedullary stems. Particularly in revision operations constrained prostheses are often used unnecessarily not because the instability cannot be managed by other means, but because the stabilizing prostheses has a stem.

FLEXION INSTABILITY

Whereas extension instability is due to excessive femoral bone excision, flexion instability is usually caused by removing too much tibial bone. One of the reasons relates to the surgeon's desire for a flat tibial surface when a defect is present (see above). Another cause is when too little femoral bone has been removed so that with the components inserted the knee does not fully extend. At this point it is tempting to use a thinner tibial component. The knee now extends fully but when flexed becomes unstable so that the tibia dislocates backward. A similar end result is reached when the components are made to fit in extension by removing more tibial bone: once again,

the components will be too loose in flexion. The correct, although more troublesome solution, is to recut the distal femur so that the originally chosen components now fit properly not only in extension but in flexion as well.

In arthritic knees with mild deformity and good initial stability flexion instability will not occur if the flexion gap is assessed properly before cutting the distal femur to ensure that adequately thick components can be used. The flexion gap must be assessed first and thus the order of the bone cuts is important. Instrumentation that begins with distal femoral resection can be dangerous in this respect because it does not allow fine tuning of the flexion and extension gaps and thus must be used only with cruciate retaining prosthetic designs.

In arthritic knees that are deformed and unstable, there may be difficulty obtaining flexion stability even with correct technique, the reason being that ligament release does not affect the flexion and extension gaps equally. The ligament release is intended to equalize length and provide symmetry in extension. Considerable asymmetry may persist in flexion. For example, in varus knees, after ligament balancing in extension the lateral soft tissues often remain lax in flexion, which is only an exaggeration of the normal condition. Cutting the femur anatomically (removing symmetrical amounts of bone from both condyles) will leave a flexion gap that is not rectangular but which is narrower medially than laterally and this asymmetry may result in rotary subluxation with the lateral tibia dropping posteriorly. The remedy is to distract the knee and cut the end of the lower femur obliquely but parallel to the upper tibial cut (thereby externally rotating the femoral component).

In the valgus knee, a lateral release involves stripping the soft tissue from the lateral femoral condyle, and therefore there is always a lateral laxity in flexion at the end of surgery (Fig. 20.99). Normally, readherance to the lateral femur and scar formation make this temporary, but dependence on scarring for stability is unpredictable and the potential for late lateral rotary subluxation exists.

An alternative solution to asymmetric instability in flexion after correction of both varus and valgus deformities is to use a cruciate substituting prosthesis.

Rotary instability can occur for the reasons just discussed but a more usual cause is malposition of the tibial component, which may cause a conflict between the movement of the articulation and the tension in the soft tissues. This is usually apparent at the time of a trial fit and thus can be corrected before cementing. Otherwise removal and repositioning of the tibial component is essential, because in time the polyethylene will distort and allow a progressive instability. Apparent malrotation of the tibial component is observed when the popliteus tendon is too tight and flexing the knee causes the lateral part of the tibial component to sublux forward (the tibia internally rotates). This movement is often hidden by the patellar ligament and fat pad when the patella is in place. It should always be looked for because the remedy is simple: division of the popliteus tendon allows the lateral tibial plateau to drop back in flexion and immediately congruent tracking is restored.

Translocation.   This is possible in some designs that do not possess an intercondylar eminence. Usually the tibia moves laterally on the femur. The dis-

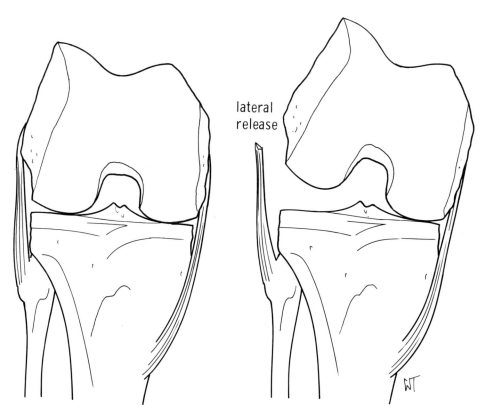

lateral release

Fig. 20.99. After lateral release for the correction of valgus, the knee is always inherently unstable in flexion. A lateral rotary instability may develop that will be exacerbated if there is any malrotation of the tibial component.

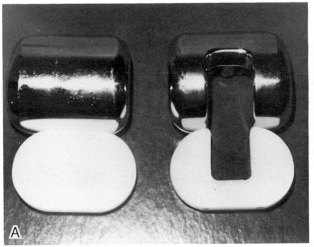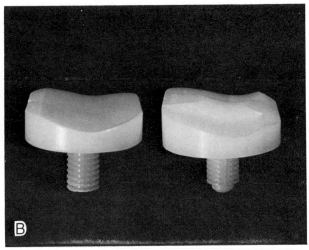

Fig. 20.100. (A) In the original Freeman-Swanson prosthesis, translocation is not resisted and, in the cruciate cut-out version of the prosthesis, may result in dislocation. (B) The latest version of this model has an intercondylar eminence on the tibial component (right) to prevent sideways sliding motion.

placement is likely when the popliteus tendon is tight and when there is a medial slope to the tibial cut. When the design has separate tibial components or a large cruciate cutout, translocation results in subluxation or dislocation of the articular surfaces. In the Freeman-Swanson design (Fig. 20.100), the consequences are less serious because, although the femoral component separates into individual runners, the tibial component is a one piece trough. Models with flat tibial components are most prone to translocation: dishing reduces the tendency and a raised intercondylar eminence virtually eliminates it.

Genu Recurvatum. The condition of genu recurvatum occurs almost exclusively in rheumatoid arthritis and patients with muscle paralysis. Recurvatum and anterior subluxation of the tibia have been reported after polycentric arthroplasty in rheumatoid arthritis. Although it is generally true that a knee that does not hyperextend at the conclusion of surgery will not develop recurvatum later, an exception is those patients who have lack of muscle control. Patients with long-standing weakness from poliomyelitis may develop osteoarthritis and often also have recurvatum. A replacement should not be undertaken unless there is good power in the quadriceps muscle, but sometimes a functioning quadriceps is present in an otherwise almost flail extremity. These knees should be approached with great caution because in the ab-

sence of hamstring and calf musculature a slowly developing recurvatum is likely using any kind of surface replacement. Probably if these knees are to be replaced at all there is an indication for a constrained prosthesis with an extension stop, but of course the increased risk of loosening with such a device must be carefully weighed before making a decision.

LOOSENING

Component loosening, usually of the tibial component,[30] was the most frequent cause of failure with hinged prostheses and early surface replacements. The results of hinges often appear deceptively good when the follow-up time is short because loosening is a time-related phenomenon and usually heralded by the development of a complete radiolucency at the bone-cement interface (Fig. 20.101). On the other hand, with the surface replacements, most component loosening occurs within the first two years, although the incidence of loosening does increase slowly thereafter (Fig. 20.102). Therefore, a 2-year follow-up examination of a surface replacement model serves as a good indication of the security of fixation while similar data for a constrained prosthesis may be misleading. For example, Deburge et al.[28] report with the Guepar prosthesis a 2 percent loosening rate before 2

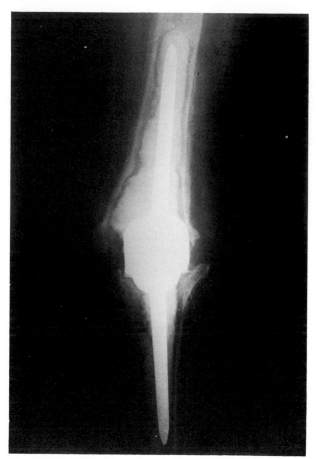

Fig. 20.101. With hinge designs, loosening is time related.

rigidity of polyethylene can be compromised by excessively thin components and generous cruciate cutouts. Modifications to the tibial components have been made in subsequent designs. The total condylar prosthesis, for example, has a one-piece tibial component and a central fixation peg and no component loosening was seen in 220 knees followed from 3 to 5 years. Because loosening is more frequent in osteoarthritis,[152] we have studied 100 osteoarthritic knees after total condylar replacement followed from 5 to 9 years. Two components have loosened, one of which was associated with malposition and malalignment. In both cases a complete radiolucent line developed around the tibial component before loosening became symptomatic. One was aligned postoperatively in a slight varus and developed a medial radiolucency after 1 year. Subsequent radiographs showed a progressive medial sinkage of the tibial component with bending of the polyethylene, although the component did not become clinically loose until 5 years had past.

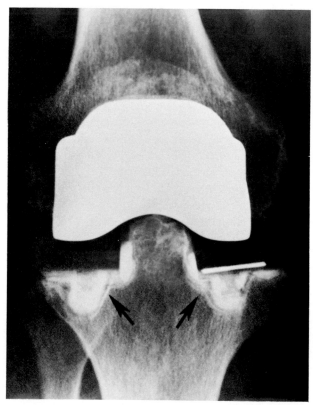

Fig. 20.102. Complete radiolucent lines are frequently seen around two-piece polyethylene tibial components.

years: at five years a total of 15 percent of the prostheses had aseptic loosening. More sophisticated constrained designs also seem to share this characteristic, albeit to a lesser degree. Kaufer and Matthews[85] using the spherocentric prosthesis report a 7.7 percent loosening after an average follow-up of 34 months. In addition 10 percent of the femoral and 14 percent of the tibial components showed a progressive radiolucency, indicating further incipient loosening.

There is reason to believe that the high failure rate due to tibial component loosening (Fig. 20.103) represents a design problem[144] that is now on the way to solution (Fig. 20.104). High rates of loosening have been reported with polycentric, geometric and early Freeman-Swanson designs.[47] In addition to loosening, plastic deformation and cold flow were reported with the original UCI prosthesis[149] indicating that the

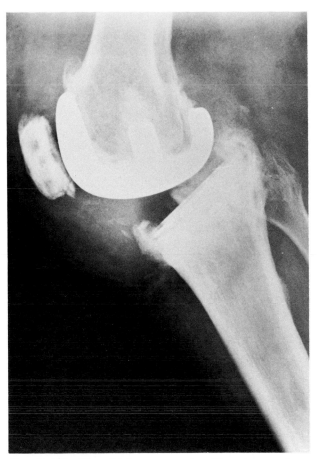

Fig. 20.103. Flat tibial components, although one-piece, are inadequately supported by the cancellous bone of the upper tibia and are susceptible to sinkage usually in anterior or medial directions.

The other case of tibial loosening was in a correctly aligned knee which developed a complete and progressive tibial radiolucency by the third postoperative year. Thereafter progressive pain was felt and a revision was performed at 5 years. This case was unique in the series of 100 knees and made more curious because the opposite knee done on the same day with similar technique and showing similar postoperative positioning did not have a radiolucency at all. Complete radiolucent lines of this type are rare and are considered attributable to infection until proved otherwise (Fig. 20.105). In this particular case, however, all the cultures were negative.

This series of cases represented early experience with the total condylar prosthesis and the technique of fixation was suboptimal by today's standards. No

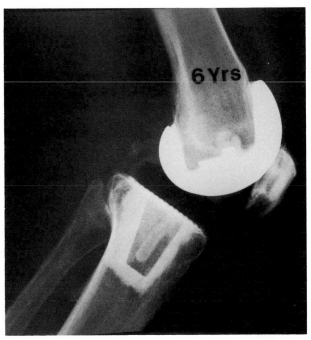

Fig. 20.104. The addition of a central fixation peg to the tibial component virtually eliminates tibial component loosening.

attempt was made to clean the bone ends other than by simple irrigation, and the cement was not injected or forcibly packed to penetrate the bone. Notwithstanding, only the two cases described loosened and a further radiographic analysis showed that no other complete radiolucent lines were present. However, a partial radiolucency was present in 31 percent of the knees at 1 year and 39 percent of the knees at 5 years. In some of the knees a radiolucency appeared where none was present before and in others an existing radiolucent line became slightly more prominent. Any reading of radiolucent lines is somewhat subjective and can be affected by positioning and radiographic technique. Thus, while there seemed to be a general tendency toward a slight increase in radiolucency with time, in some other knees regression of radiolucent lines appeared to be taking place. Both occurrences may be the result of artifact as shown by fluoroscopy in a few patients; by this method we have shown that even a prominent radiolucency can be made to disappear by just a small change in positioning. Our conclusion from this study was that there was no evidence of significant fixation problems with the polyethylene tibial component using single peg

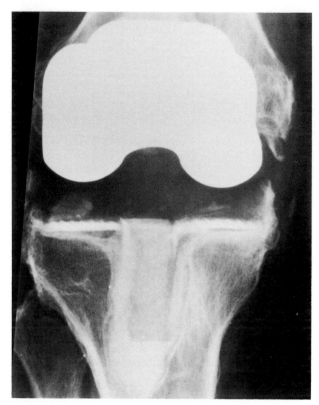

Fig. 20.105. With the total condylar prosthesis, a complete radiolucency is attributed to low-grade infection until proved otherwise.

fixation at the end of 5 years minimum follow-up time.

The addition of metal reinforcement to support the polyethylene may further enhance fixation. Murray and Webster[107] report their results with the variable-axis prosthesis, which has metal reinforcement as well as intramedullary stems on both components, in a study of 55 prostheses with a minimum 2-year follow-up, there was no clinical or radiographic evidence of loosening. However, 37 patients had a lucent line measuring 0.5 to 1.5 mm at the bone–cement interface at some location around the prosthetic components. This was most common beneath the tibial plateau.

Improved cementing techniques[105] using bone lavage, pressure injection, and low-viscosity cement might be expected to reduce radiolucent lines further and improve fixation (Chapter 22). No discussion of component loosening is complete without reference to component positioning. Lotke and Ecker[91] noted a statistically significant positive correlation between a good clinical result and a well-positioned geometric prosthesis. They devised for the purpose clinical and radiographic scores, both with a total of 100 points. They were not able to correlate mechanical failure with the radiographic score because the series was relatively small. However, four of the five failures had the tibial component positioned in varus. With a device such as the total condylar prosthesis possessing secure fixation characteristics it is even harder to correlate loosening with positioning. However, one of our two cases of tibial loosening was positioned in varus and clearly demonstrated progressive sinkage and bending of the polyethylene. We believe strongly that longer follow-up will eventually demonstrate definite connection between positioning and longevity of fixation (Fig. 20.106).

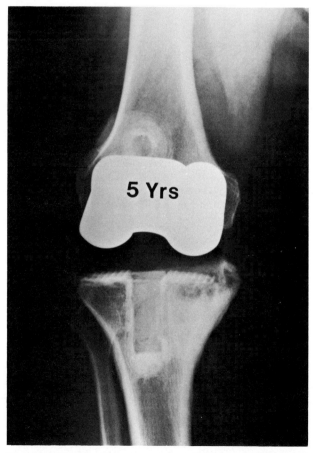

Fig. 20.106. The importance of axial alignment. This total condylar knee prosthesis was positioned at surgery in slight varus, which gradually increased over a 5-year period. Collapse of the medial bone support with distortion of the polyethylene can be seen.

INFECTION[63,109,118]

Persistent symptoms following total knee replacement in the absence of a clear mechanical explanation should alert the surgeon about the possibility of infection. Although diagnosing acute severe infection with local and general symptoms poses no particular problem, occasionally latent infections can manifest themselves mainly by knee pain with mild or no general symptomatology. The wound can be benign and the usual laboratory tests and radiologic findings may prove negative.

Metastatic or hematogenous infections[4,25,26,52,135] can produce an acute and severe symptomatology resembling early deep infections in their manifestation despite their late onset. In some cases there is an apparent association with preceding infection at sites remote from the knee, such as teeth,[117] ulcers, lungs, gastrointestinal tract, and genito-urinary tract. In these cases seeding onto the prosthetic knee occurs most likely through transient bacteremia.

INCIDENCE OF INFECTION

It is well known that joint infection occurs more frequently in patients with rheumatoid arthritis,[45,65] who often are immunologically deficient. In addition, frequently these patients have had previous operations and sometimes the placement of previous incisions may predispose to skin necrosis which can lead by extension to a deep prosthetic infection. For these reasons the infection rate for rheumatoid arthritis at The Hospital for Special Surgery is about 3 percent compared with 0.5 percent for osteoarthritic knees.

The surgeon can influence the ultimate infection rate not only by his technique but also by his selection of prostheses. For example, using surface replacements such as the duocondylar, duopatellar, or total condylar prostheses, the overall infection rate is less than 1 percent. On the other hand, for metal-on-metal constrained hinge prostheses such as the Guepar, the infection rate may approach 15 percent with many of these infections occurring late, sometimes several years after implantation. The reason for this very high incidence of infection is not altogether clear but is probably related to the amount of metallic debris,[111,120] which in turn causes a sac containing fluid and debris to form around the prosthesis. Impregnation of the bone and soft tissues with metallic fragments and the extent of the bone–cement interface may be other factors, particularly when the prosthesis becomes loose. Disturbingly, constrained prostheses with metal-on-plastic-bearing surfaces also seem to share a higher infection rate. For example, the stabilocondylar prosthesis also had an infection rate of 8.3 percent in a small series of 36 cases. Although because the numbers are small this may represent a meaningless statistical fluctuation, we have concluded that both constraint and intramedullary stems should be avoided in prosthetic designs whenever possible.

Skin necrosis (Fig. 20.107) with secondary deep extension has already been alluded to. Incisions placed at the side of the knee, such as were at one time used for synovectomy, are not suitable for total knee replacement and their presence may sometimes cause

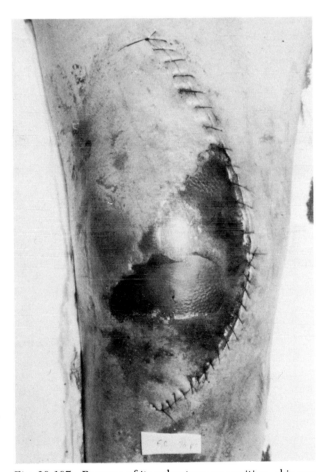

Fig. 20.107. Because of its subcutaneous position, skin necrosis is a particular hazard in knee joint replacement. Overaggressive debridement can lead to deep infection. When necrosis occurs, the knee should be immobilized until the eschar separates.

unavoidable skin necrosis. If this complication occurs it is recommended that the knee be immobilized for as long as is necessary until spontaneous separation of the eschar occurs. Early and aggressive attempts at debridement have in our experience led to deep contamination that might have been avoidable.

Wound drainage defined as leakage from the incision sufficient to draw comment in the progress notes is a frequent occurrence and often requires no modification of the postoperative regiment. When profuse wound drainage occurs the knee should be immobilized until it stops, but on no account should antibiotics be given for fear of masking latent deep infection. Some degree of wound drainage occurs in about 25 percent of our cases and may be further subdivided as culture negative and culture positive. There seems no relationship between culture positive wound drainage and subsequent deep infection, so we prefer to avoid the term "superficial" infection.

DEEP INFECTION

Deep or periprosthetic infection may be either *early*, defined as within three months of surgery, or *late* occurring after this time.

EARLY INFECTION

An early infection, provided that its course is not modified by injudicious use of antibiotics, is usually not difficult to recognize. The clinical course is abnormal with prolonged pain, swelling, inflammation and fever. The white cell count and sedimentation rate remain elevated.

The recommended procedure to establish the presence of infection is a knee aspiration performed under strict aseptic precautions. The fluid aspirated is sent immediately to the bacteriologic laboratory for direct smear, Gram stain, anaerobic, microbacterial and fungal cultures and sensitivities. Occasionally the infecting organism can be an indolent type of bacteria. In order to increase the chances of bacterial growth, the aspirate should be inoculated as soon as possible in the appropriate broth and culture medium. A transport system with a culture medium to support the bacteria during the time of transport is recommended.

If enough fluid is aspirated from the knee a complete cell count and differential may also give valuable information. If the complete count shows more than 25,000 polymorphonuclear leukocytes per milliliter and the differential count more than 75 percent of these white cells, infection should be suspected. Obviously the higher number of polymorphonuclear leukocytes, the greater the possibility of infection. Fluid should also be sent for glucose and protein levels. In the normal synovial fluid, protein levels are about one-third serum levels, whereas in infection they approach serum levels. Glucose values in synovial fluid are similar to those of plasma. In the presence of infection synovial glucose values are lowered due to the presence of organisms which utilize sugar in their metabolism. Thus, a low glucose and a high protein are compatible with infection. If the diagnosis is still unclear once all this information is gathered, and if the clinical suspicion of infection is strong, an open biopsy is indicated. At surgery a thorough debridement is done; frozen tissue sections, complete Gram stains, cultures of the tissue, and the macroscopic appearance of the wound should also provide diagnostic information. In early infections of this type the prosthetic components should be left in situ and after debridement the wound should be closed over widebore suction drains. These drains are removed at 36 hours, and we do not favor closed suction irrigation due to the risk of exogenous super infection.

Intravenous antibiotic therapy is begun under the supervision of an infectious disease specialist subsequently modified if necessary according to the sensitivities of the organism. Antibiotic blood levels are monitored against cultures of the infecting organism with the objective of maintaining peak bacteriocidal concentrations at a minimum eightfold dilution.

The wound is inspected after 2 weeks, and the wound is reaspirated under strict aseptic conditions. When the wound is benign and the cultures are negative, antibiotic therapy is continued for a further 4 weeks. When this is not the case, reoperation with removal of the prosthetic components and all cement is performed.

We do not believe that infections complicating total knee replacement should be treated with antibiotic therapy alone.[120] This treatment might suppress the symptoms of infection transiently and may be indicated only as a temporary measure if surgery is contraindicated due to medical reasons or if the patient does not accept it. Antibiotic therapy alone[102] is unlikely to cure the infectious process. Furthermore, its use can complicate the problem by selecting resistant strains. For various reasons, in five of our early cases antibiotic therapy only was given. Two of these patients eventually died of septicemia related to their infectious process, two developed draining sinuses which later required removal of the prosthesis, and in only one, after a follow-up of 2 years, was the infection apparently dormant.

We also condemn procrastination and the prolonged use of oral antibiotics, particularly when infection is only suspected and not confirmed by bacteriological evidence. The end result of this course is likely to be an indolent, subclinical infection and a painful prosthesis. In addition, it may make subsequent culture of the organism very difficult even after the components have been removed so that proper and appropriate antibiotic therapy is impossible and ultimate salvage of the arthroplasty by reimplantation of another prosthesis becomes much less likely.

LATE INFECTION

Late infection is much more common than an early one and the diagnosis is usually straightforward unless antibiotics have previously been given. The usual presentation is of acute pain and swelling in the knee of a patient with a previously satisfactory arthroplasty. Aspiration as described above will usually provide the diagnosis. However, in cases that have received antibiotics the diagnosis may be much more difficult. We believe that any painful prosthesis for which a cause is not readily apparent, should be assumed infected until proven otherwise.

The treatment for proven or suspected late deep infection is incision, drainage, thorough debridement of the involved tissues and removal of the prosthetic components along with the acrylic cement (Fig. 20.108). This course should be followed even in suspected cases because only cultures obtained from the bone-cement interface may be positive. Even when preoperative cultures have been obtained, antibiotic therapy is not given until the components are out and multiple cultures obtained, because sometimes more than one infecting organism may be present. Once adequate specimens have been obtained, antibiotic therapy is commenced and later modified if necessary according to the sensitivities.

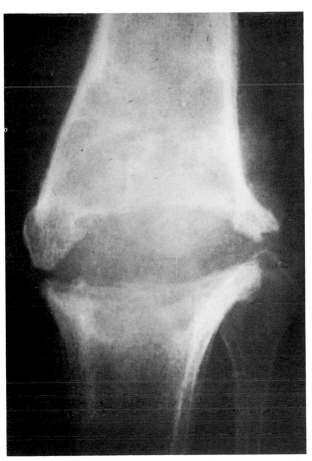

Fig. 20.108. For proven or suspected deep infection, the treatment is complete removal of the prosthetic components and all acrylic cement.

Adequate preoperative planning is necessary and the availability of special instruments is recommended. Removal of the prosthetic components and acrylic cement can prove a difficult task, particularly if the septic process is of recent onset. In this case the prosthetic components most likely will not be loose, and removal of the tight interdigitation between bone and cement demands a laborious, patient, meticulous technique in order to prevent unnecessary loss of bone stock. The removal of hinged total knee replacements with intramedullary stems into the femur and tibia can also prove rather difficult. For these, special cement osteotomes and a high-speed cement drill are helpful. A custom-made sliding hammer (Fig. 109A,B) with a special attachment to lock on to the prosthesis is also available.

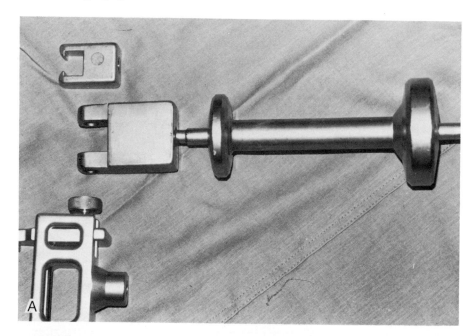

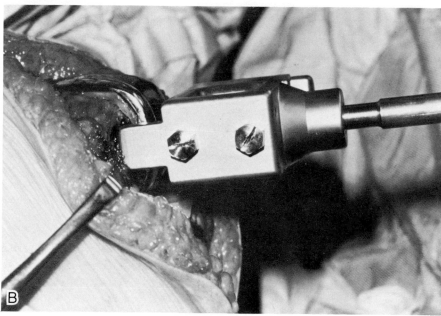

Fig. 20.109. (A,B) A sliding hammer with special attachments is very helpful for removing prosthetic components, especially those with stems.

All scarred, inflamed, and devitalized tissues should be thoroughly excised leaving viable, healthy, well-irrigated tissues.

Primary wound closure can usually be performed over closed suction tubes, which are removed after 24 to 48 hours. The knee is immobilized in a bulky Robert Jones dressing with plaster splints. Unless there are clinical signs that suggest problems we prefer to leave this dressing untouched for a few weeks. We do not advise skeletal traction and prefer to leave the bone ends in contact to reduce dead space.

When the cultures and sensitivities are finally available the subsequent course is planned. When the diagnosis of infection is erroneous and all cultures are negative, a new prosthesis can be reimplanted as soon as primary wound healing has occurred (generally about

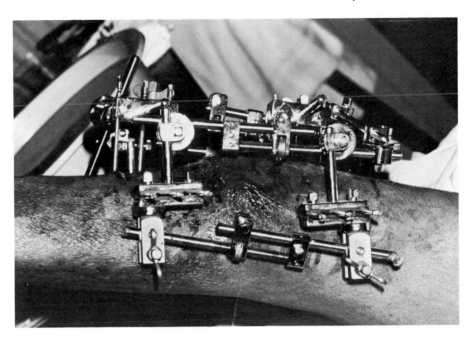

Fig. 20.110. When secondary arthrodesis is indicated after removing prosthetic components, transfixation pins can be inserted without reopening the wound.

2 weeks from the first operation). When the infecting organism is resistant to antibiotic therapy or when adequate blood levels cannot be obtained without undue risk of toxicity to the patient, secondary arthrodesis is performed by inserting multiple transfixation pins and applying an external compression apparatus. Usually this can be done without reopening or otherwise disturbing the wound (Fig. 20.110). Arthrodesis is most likely needed when the infecting organism is gram negative.

When the organism is susceptible, the wound is inspected after 6 weeks of intravenous therapy with the appropriate antibiotic having been completed. If the wound is completely benign and the patient has had an uneventful postoperative period, we would consider reinsertion of another total knee prosthesis.[72A] If at this time the wound still shows signs of inflammation, a long cylinder cast is applied and the patient is started on ambulation and discharged home as soon as he is independent. Further inspection of the wound is made a month later and if now benign, reinsertion of another total knee prosthesis is reconsidered. On the other hand, if the wound is not benign the knee is placed in a Prenyl brace until it becomes stable enough to discontinue the orthosis. If the knee persists to be unstable a formal fusion might be indicated although in most instances the fibrous

ankylosis of the knee provides a painless lower extremity allowing the patient to be brace free (Fig. 20.111). Obtaining a successful bony arthrodesis in the knee with considerable loss of the bony surfaces may be a difficult task.[12,51]

In suitable cases, provided the patient accepts and understands the increased risk of recurrence of infection, a new total knee prosthesis can be inserted at this time. Frozen tissue sections are obtained at the time of surgery to assess tissue inflammation as well as Gram stain cultures of the tissues. The macroscopic appearance of the wound should be completely benign; all scarred and devitalized tissue is now excised leaving only viable, well-irrigated, healthy tissues. Exposure can sometimes be difficult after prolonged immobilization, and there is danger of causing an avulsion of the tibial tubercle while attempting to mobilize the patella and flex the knee. If this event seems likely, a modification of the Coonse and Adams quadriceps turndown exposure is used by making an oblique incision across the tip of the quadriceps tendon into the vastus lateralis muscle.

Again, preoperative planning is essential in order to have available adequate prosthetic components to facilitate a satisfactory biomechanical reconstruction. When there is bone stock deficit, a special custom design prosthesis might be necessary. In lieu of this

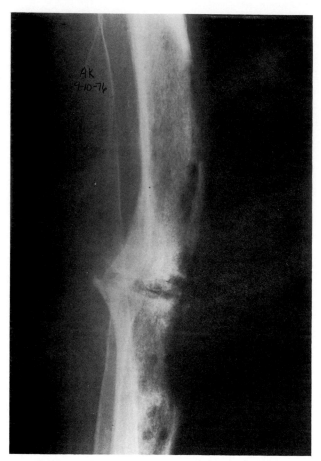

Fig. 20.111. A fibrous anklyosis sometimes provides a satisfactory result after removal of an infected prosthesis.

we have found titanium mesh useful in building up significant bony defects (Fig. 20.112A,B). In most cases, proper alignment can be reestablished with adequate tissue tension. Excision of the patella has proved helpful in cases where the skin closure was too tight. Normally reconstruction can be achieved using standard total condylar components or variants thereof, even when the removed prosthesis was a hinge or other more constrained design. The soft tissue capsule that forms around the knee provides an excellent substitute for the collateral ligaments and, after adequate spacing with the prosthetic components, both alignment and stability can be restored. At the time of surgery it is important to avoid any further bone resection.

Sometimes the use of constrained components is unavoidable. When this is so we select the TCP III, which has intramedullary stems on both components and restricts varus/valgus, anteroposterior, and rotary motions by means of a centrally positioned peg. However, stemmed components should be avoided whenever possible because of the risk of recurrent infection. It should also be remembered that while a stemmed component in the tibia, femur or both is required because of bone deficiency, constraint at the prosthetic surfaces is not automatically required unless in addition there is uncontrollable ligamentous instability. We have found this to be seldom the case so that by mixing and matching components bony deficiency can be compensated where needed while avoiding constraint in the arthroplasty itself.

The use of antibiotic impregnated cement has been recommended for reimplantation after infection;[16,98] we have not done this in any of our cases and thus cannot comment.

POSTOPERATIVE MANAGEMENT AFTER REIMPLANTATION

Postoperative management after reimplantation is the same as for a primary arthroplasty unless a quadriceps turn down was done to facilitate exposure. In this event the knee is immobilized with plaster splints for 3 weeks before beginning motion. On the assumption that the knee was sterile at the time of reimplantation, we do not believe there is a need for prolonged antibiotic therapy. In fact the antibiotic prophylaxis given to cover reimplantation is the same as we use for primary arthroplasty (oxicillin or cephalosporin) and the antibiotic may well be different from that used to cure the infection itself. Postoperative antibiotics are given for 2 days intravenously after reimplantation and then totally discontinued. No further oral therapy is given subsequently.

RESULTS OF TREATMENT[119]

Since 1976 it has been the policy of the Knee Service to reimplant a new prosthesis whenever possible. During this period 24 cases of septic failure have been managed and in 18 a reimplantation was done.[77] Reimplantation was not done in some cases for a variety of reasons. In two cases the infection was caused by mixed organisms making antibiotic therapy diffi-

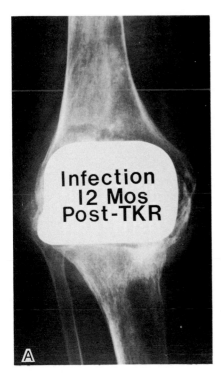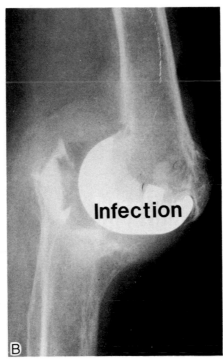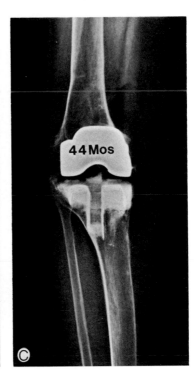

Fig. 20.112. (A,B) In this infected Freeman-Swanson prosthesis, the tibial component had sunk and rotated 90 degrees, creating a large, bony deficiency in the tibia. (C) During implantation of a duopatellar prosthesis, the tibial defect was filled with titanium wire mesh and cement. Follow-up on this case is nearly 4 years.

cult, and in three cases the age and general condition of the patient made removal and reimplantation unfeasible. In one case the patient refused surgery. Four of these cases were treated by incision and drainage and prolonged antibiotic therapy. The result was suppression of the infection in two, a draining sinus in one, and in the fourth case, the patient died of an unrelated cause, but with persistent infection in the knee. The two patients with a mixed infection had the prosthesis removed and a fusion attempted. Arthrodesis was obtained in one and a pseudarthrosis in the other.

The remaining 18 patients had a removal of the prosthesis followed by reimplantation 6 weeks to 3 months later according to the protocol described. The infecting organism was gram positive (*Staphylococcus aureus, Staphylococcus epidermidis,* and *Streptococcus*) in 16 and gram negative in two knees. These latter infections occurred in a bilateral case but one year apart. The infecting organism was an encapsulated pseudomonas, a variant that proved unusually sensitive to therapy so that reimplantation was considered possible.

The follow-up after reimplantation ranges from 3 months to 5 years, and at the time of writing all have remained infection free. Ten of the cases have been followed for more than 2 years after reimplantation. The quality of the arthroplasty has been generally good, approaching that of the primary operation. All have a satisfactory range of motion and good stability. Three have extensor mechanism weakness and an extension lag. In two this preexisted the infection and in the third a patellectomy was done to obtain wound closure. One case we reexplored 1 year after reimplantation because of persistent pain and stiffness. No evidence of infection was found and all cultures proved negative. Components were left undisturbed and the wound was closed after dividing adhesions. The result in this patient remains unsatisfactory due to a suspected sympathetic dystrophy.

ILLUSTRATIVE CASE

A 65-year-old woman underwent bilateral total knee replacement in 1972. The prosthesis was a duocondylar on the left and a Guepar on the right. Both knees did very well for four years and had an excellent rating. In 1976 she was admitted to another hospital with a fever and chills and swelling of the right leg was noted. She was transferred to The Hospital for Special Surgery in an extremely toxic condition with massive swelling and inflammation of the right leg extending proximally to the upper thigh. A large quantity of grossly purulent fluid was aspirated from the right knee joint, many gram-positive organisms were seen on a smear and cultures later grew *Staphylococcus aureus*. Immediate removal of the prosthesis was not done because her general condition was so poor, but after 2 days of intravenous fluids and large doses of oxacillin, there had been no improvement and the cellulitis of the right thigh was undiminished. As a life-saving measure, the prosthesis and acrylic cement were removed in an operation lasting about 3 hours. The wound was closed primarily over two suction drains, which were removed after 36 hours. She made a remarkable improvement, and within a week her temperature was normal and all signs of toxicity had disappeared. At 6 weeks the wound was inspected but slight redness still remained. Because of this she was sent home in a cylinder cast and allowed partial weight-bearing with crutches. At 3 months after removal of the infected prosthesis, the wound was completely benign and the sedimentation rate normal. A second operation was performed to reimplant a new prosthesis. In spite of the nature of the previous prosthesis, an adequate capsule remained and the bone stock was relatively good. It was found that a standard total condylar prosthesis could be fitted after a minor build-up of the medial tibia with titanium wire mesh (Fig. 20.113). Postoperatively some skin necrosis developed anteriorly, which delayed physical therapy for another 6 weeks. Once knee flexion was started, she regained motion easily, and 5 years later her knee has an excellent rating. The range of motion is from 0 to 95 degrees, alignment and stability are excellent, and there is normal muscle strength without an extension lag. She has received no further antibiotic therapy since reimplantation, and there has been no evidence of recurrent infection. The radiographs have remained unchanged without radiolucency at the bone–cement interface.

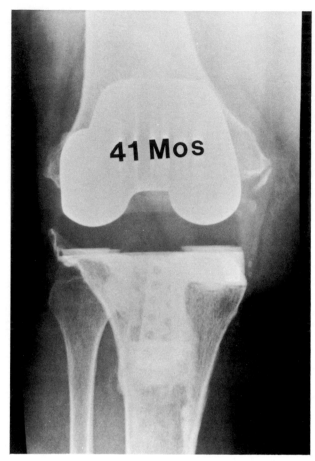

Fig. 20.113. After a Guepar prosthesis had been removed for infection, a standard total condylar prosthesis was reimplanted with a medial build-up using titanium mesh.

REVISION OF TOTAL KNEE ARTHROPLASTY

Revision of total knee arthroplasty is a surgical procedure new to the last decade. The earlier models of total knee prostheses were basically hemiarthroplasties and gave good service for several years. The early metal and plastic prostheses for knee replacement tended to be unicompartmental and then bicompartmental in design and, with the passage of time, the unresurfaced compartments usually developed progressive arthritis and recurrence of pain. Hinge-type prostheses were also susceptible to loosening because of the excessive restraint; either failure occurred at the bone–cement interface or the component broke.

While component loosening was by far the major cause of failure (and therefore revision) with early

Table 20.1. Other Prostheses

Defect	N	%
Loosening	29	60
Progressive osteoarthritis	10	21
Infection	6	13
Subluxation	1	2
Breakage	1	2
Stiffness	1	2
	48	100

prosthetic designs (Table 20.1) this is not the case with later models such as the total condylar prosthesis (Table 20.2). In a recent study of both our own patients and those referred to us, failure was caused by malposition, loosening, infection, and subluxation in about equal numbers. Malposition usually resulted in patellar dislocation that could not be controlled without correction of the tibial component. Both malposition and subluxation are mostly attributable to errors in surgical technique, hence avoidable.

However, in the past revision surgery has been undertaken for four reasons: pain, loosening, sepsis, and instability. These are, however, not mutually exclusive categories as a loose component can also become infected or vice versa, and all have some component of pain. Likewise, instability can result from a failure to balance the soft tissues, poor choice of prosthesis, or progressive loosening.

We have evolved several useful techniques that have been helpful in such revision arthroplasty.[57] Quadriceps mechanism turndown in the fashion of Coonse and Adams has been extremely useful in increasing exposure without avulsing the patellar tendon from the tibial tubercle and can easily be converted from the standard midline approach which we recommend for knee exposure. Skeletonization of the ends of the bones by subperiosteal dissection of both tibia and femur is also recommended as a means of gaining exposure. To some degree the medial tibia is always dissected to permit anterior displacement and dislocation of the components prior to their removal. Skel-

Table 20.2. Total Condylar Prosthesis

Defect	N	%
Malposition	7	29
Loosening	6	25
Infection	6	25
Subluxation	4	17
Stiffness	1	4
	24	100

etonization of the distal femur can be done in addition if exposure is still inadequate or if there is difficulty removing articulated components. Femoral skeletonization is, however, most useful for reinserting a knee prosthesis after the treatment of infection.

We have also found the need for special devices to remove the components and cement. A large sliding hammer with various gripping devices is invaluable for extraction especially of hinge-type prostheses. A high-speed low-torque pneumatic drill is useful for cement removal. A fiber optic headlamp facilitates removal of cement from the intramedullary canal.

As a general principle revision surgery should be performed as soon as failure is diagnosed. This is to prevent excessive bone loss which is often the major problem in revision surgery. For example, once components are loose and have shifted in position, failure is inevitable and procrastination only results in progressive bone destruction and the creation of large defects. A more satisfactory revision operation is obtained by early intervention.

All cases must be reviewed carefully preoperatively giving thought to the type of prosthesis that will be required for the revision. Any special components that may be needed must be ordered. It is important to remember that radiographic defects usually prove larger than imagined once all cement, necrotic bone, and granulation tissue have been removed. Small cancellous bony defects of the tibial plateaus may be managed with titanium mesh to contain and reinforce the cement; cancellous bone screws help position the components. Larger defects should be managed with custom designed metal trays to fill the bony defects with metal and not cement (Fig. 20.114A,B). This principle can be applied to the femoral component as well. The femoral components are modified with posterior, anterior or distal augmentation to accommodate bone loss on the posterior, anterior or distal portions of the femoral condyle (Fig. 20.115).

The tibial metal trays designed to fill bony defects are topped by interchangeable heights of polyethylene to allow for proper ligament balancing. These tibial components are sometimes attached to intramedullary rods for further fixation and for the management of adjoining fractures in the proximal or middle tibial shaft (Fig. 20.116). Femoral components can be similarly modified with an intramedullary rod for supracondylar fractures.

It is seldom possible to retain the cruciate ligaments in revision surgery, and it is difficult to secure

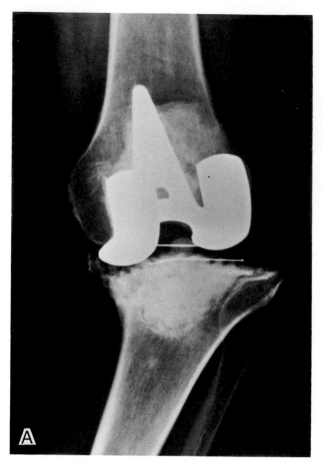
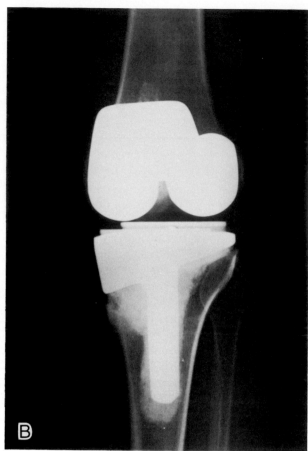

Fig. 20.114. (A,B) In the revision of this prosthesis with severe collapse of the medial tibia, a custom-made prosthesis with a full wedge was used. The articular surfaces of the revision prosthesis are standard posterior stabilized condylar design.

satisfactory ligament balancing in both flexion and extension. We therefore recommend the posterior stabilized condylar prosthesis as most suitable for revision operations and this is our most frequent choice. It is necessary to have available at all times a total condylar III or similarly constrained design to allow for collateral ligament substitution when ligament stability has been lost. The total condylar III compensates for lack of medial and lateral collateral ligaments in addition to the anteroposterior stability provided by the posterior stabilized knee.

The revision of hinged knees can be a particular challenge (Fig. 20.117). The removal of the components can be a formidable task particularly when there has been stem breakage. However, the major difficulty again lies in the bony defects because collateral ligaments or a functional substitution by a fibrous cap-

sule is often found. The hinge can therefore be usually revised with a modified posterior stabilized design.

When the revision is done as a staged procedure (in, for example, cases of suspected or confirmed sepsis) there is the opportunity to obtain a mold of the bone ends after prosthetic removal. This allows an accurate revision prosthesis to be constructed. This procedure should be followed whenever the gross appearance suggests possible sepsis or when frozen sections show evidence of acute inflammation. The two-stage procedure is also useful when available components do not provide a satisfactory reconstruction. It is then better to take molds as suggested and complete the reconstruction at a later date when more satisfactory components have been fabricated.

The results of revision surgery are nearly as good

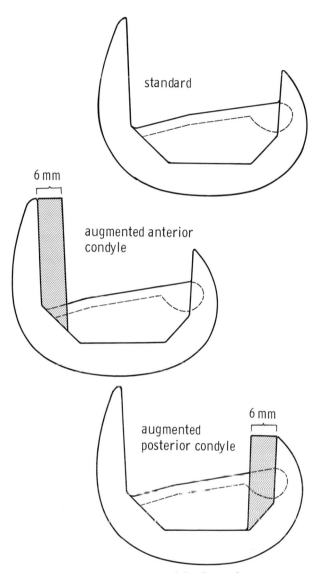

Fig. 20.115. Augmentation of the femoral component.

standard

6 mm

augmented anterior
condyle

augmented
posterior condyle

6 mm

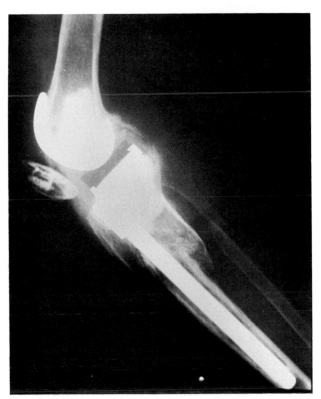

Fig. 20.116. The tibial component of this posterior stabilized prosthesis had a fluted intramedullary rod for the management of an ununited upper tibial fracture.

as with the primary operation.[138] In a recent study the proportion of good and excellent results was 85 percent. However, there were fewer excellent and more good results than in a comparable group of primary operations. As a group, the revision cases did not have quite the complete pain relief normally found after knee replacement. Extensor mechanism problems, such as patellar subluxation, quadriceps weakness, and extension lag were relatively more common, and a few knees did not regain a full range of motion. However, in most cases restricted motion was

not a difficulty. The average range of motion post revision is almost the same as the primary operation.

Radiographic evaluation revealed that radiolucent lines were much more frequent in the revision cases and were often complete (Fig. 20.118) These lines were often visible soon after surgery and in some cases reflect the difficulty of cleaning the bone ends after removing the previous component. Often, thick fibrous membranes have a tenacious hold on the bone so that complete removal is not possible without removing the bone itself. In addition, a cortical shell often forms around a loose component beneath which is found very weak cancellous bone. Removal of this cortical shell seems quite undesirable as bone strength is further compromised. Radiolucencies after revision do not have the same implication as for primary cases and even complete radiolucencies usually appear quite stable. A radiolucency after revision therefore does not herald another episode of loosening but may account for the less complete pain relief that is sometimes observed.

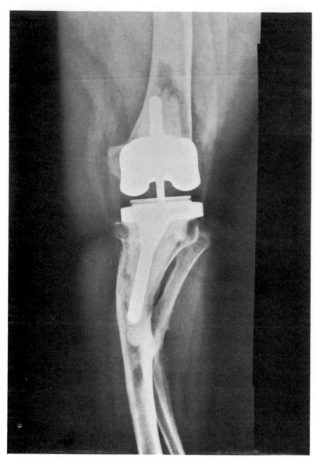

Fig. 20.117. This bizarre prosthesis is a posterior stabilized design used for the revision of a hinged prosthesis. An angulated tibial stem was used because of bone deformity of the upper tibia.

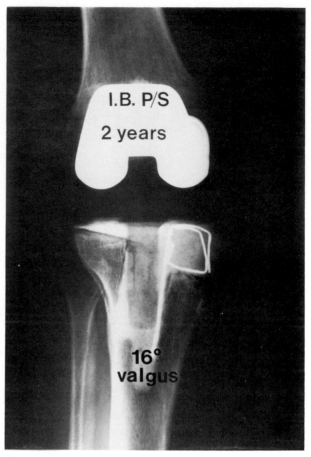

Fig. 20.118. Prominent radiolucent lines are usual after revision surgery; they do not have the same significance that they would in primary cases. Note that this case has been placed in excessive valgus because of the marked medial bone deficit.

RESULTS OF TOTAL KNEE ARTHROPLASTY

ASSESSMENT OF RESULTS[150]

There is no uniform method of assessing the results of a knee arthroplasty, which makes comparison of different prostheses difficult, if not impossible. Numerical rating systems are most often used in the United States. This method gives points to various aspects from the history and examination with a total most often coming to 100 points. However, the allotment of points for pain, function, motion, and so on varies from one scheme to another. For example, one

system may give 30 points to freedom from pain, another 40 points, and a third 50 points.

The Hospital for Special Surgery knee arthroplasty score sheet is reproduced (Fig. 20.119). Out of a total of 100 points, the method allots 30 points for absence of pain, 22 points for function, 18 points for range of motion, and 10 points each for muscle strength, stability, and absence of flexion contracture. From this total, subtractions are made for walking aids, varus or valgus alignment, and extension lag. An excellent result exceeds 85 points, a good result is from 70 to 84 points, a fair result from 60 to 69 points, and a poor result under 60 points. As a successful knee fusion achieves 60 points, this was chosen as the cut-off between fair and poor results.

THE HOSPITAL FOR SPECIAL SURGERY
KNEE SERVICE
Knee Rating Sheet

Name_____ HSS #_____ Preoperative date_____

		LEFT						RIGHT					
	Score	pre	6mo	1yr	2yr	3yr	4yr	pre	6mo	1yr	2yr	3yr	4yr
PAIN (30 points)													
Walking: none	15												
mild	10												
moderate	5												
severe	0												
At rest: none	15												
mild	10												
moderate	5												
severe	0												
FUNCTION (22 points)													
Walk:													
walking & standing unlimited	12												
5-10 blocks, standing >30 min	10												
1-5 blocks, standing 15-30 min	8												
walk <1 block	4												
cannot walk	0												
Stairs: normal	5												
with support	2												
Transfer: normal	5												
with support	2												
ROM (18 points) each 8° = 1 point													
MUSCLE STRENGTH (10 points)													
cannot break quadriceps	10												
can break quadriceps	8												
can move through arc of motion	4												
cannot move through arc of motion	0												
FLEXION DEFORMITY (10 points)													
none	10												
5°-10°	8												
10°-20°	5												
>20°	0												
INSTABILITY (10 points)													
none	10												
0°-5°	8												
6°-15°	5												
>15°	0												
TOTAL													
SUBTRACTIONS:													
one cane	1												
one crutch	2												
two crutches	3												
extension lag of 5°	2												
10°	3												
15°	5												
Deformity (5°=1 point) varus													
valgus													
TOTAL SUBTRACTIONS													
KNEE SCORE													

Fig. 20.119. H.S.S. knee arthroplasty rating system.

The HSS rating system has been in use for 10 years. We support a point-rating system because by combining subjective and objective information it provides a complete picture of the arthroplasty. When the parameters are expressed separately it is more difficult to comprehend the true nature of the results. For example, consider two patients, the first having a painless arthroplasty with very restricted motion and the second a painful arthroplasty with good motion. Using the point system, neither arthroplasty will be satisfactory. However, if the parameters are expressed separately this information will be recorded as one knee painless, one knee painful, one knee stiff, and one knee with good motion. There is no means of knowing whether this represents one very good painless knee with good motion and one very bad result that is both painful and stiff or two mediocre results. Given the number of different parameters involved in assessing a knee arthroplasty, it becomes impossible to know if the results are mostly excellent with a few very poor cases having multiple deficiencies or consist of a larger number of mediocre cases with each knee having a single deficiency.

One drawback to any scoring system is the point loading allocated to each of the various parameters. Does one ascribe one-third or one-half of the total number of points to relief of pain? What is the relative importance of range of motion and walking ability? The other disadvantage is converting the total point score into the conventional excellent, good, fair and poor categories. While it is easy to recognize excellent and poor results, there is a gray area between the fair and good result. For this reason we advocate paying the most attention to excellent and poor ratings in assessing results.

The function assessment chart proposed by the British Orthopaedic Association does not attempt to produce a final score but collects all the essential information necessary to rate the results of an arthroplasty (Fig. 20.120). However, without making the conversion to an overall rating, results are difficult to understand. This is illustrated by a recent symposium which presented the results of the prostheses most frequently used in Great Britain.[6,17,44,89,125,126] From the mass of information available this reader found it impossible to make comparisons between the various prostheses described. Whether or not unanimity on how to express results is ever reached, at the time of writing the differences in rating systems remain.

A second difficulty is that in order to be meaningful, the follow-up time must be sufficient. Most studies have reported patients followed from 2 to 4 years, which is not long enough to uncover all possible problems. Longer follow-up information is available for some prostheses, but these models have either been discontinued or modified to such an extent (e.g., the ICLH prosthesis) that the information is no longer relevant.

Bryan and Peterson[14] have stated that a 2-year follow-up was of little value in predicting the long term results of non-constrained surface replacements (polycentric arthroplasty). They reported 86 percent good results at two years but the results subsequently deteriorated so that after seven years good results were noted in only 64 percent. Causes of failure noted were loosening of tibial components, settling, unexplained pain, lax ligaments, dislocation, and patellar problems.

There is reason to believe that current resurfacing designs will not deteriorate in the same manner. The total condylar prosthesis is probably the oldest resurfacing model which is still widely used in its original form. (The Townley prosthesis, a cruciate-retaining design, has existed for a similar period, but a change has been made to the tibial component and a polyethylene patellar replacement has been added to the design.)

A total condylar prosthesis was first implanted at The Hospital for Special Surgery in January 1974. The first 100 consecutive patients to have the total condylar prosthesis implanted for gonarthrosis on the Knee Service were recently studied. The diagnosis in all patients was osteoarthritis because they are generally the most active patients and will give the best assessment of problems related to long-term prosthetic viability. The minimum follow-up period was 6 years and the maximum was 9 years (average: 6.6 years). At the end of this time there had been 13 deaths (17 knees) and eight patients (eight knees) were lost to follow-up. Thus, there were 100 arthroplasties in 79 patients available for review. The average age was 68.2 years and the average weight 76.6 kg. A patellar replacement was used in all but nine knees.

At follow-up, 70 knees (70 percent) were rated excellent, 23 knees (23 percent) good, two knees (2 percent) fair, and five knees (5 percent) poor. The average postoperative range of motion was 96 degrees (range: 75 to 120 degrees).

KNEE FUNCTION ASSESSMENT CHART

(BRITISH ORTHOPAEDIC ASSOCIATION RESEARCH SUB-COMMITTEE)

NAME

Hospital number   Age

Occupation   Sex

DIAGNOSIS

DURATION OF DISEASE   General   (years)
                             Knee   (years)

SIDE

PREVIOUS KNEE OPERATIONS

OTHER JOINTS (See Appendix)

STATE OF OTHER KNEE   Normal
                              Slightly affected
                              Moderately affected
                              Severely affected
                              Replaced

STATE OF HIPS   RIGHT   LEFT
                              Normal
                              Slightly affected
                              Moderately affected
                              Severely affected
                              Replaced

STATE OF FEET/   RIGHT   LEFT
ANKLES   Normal
                              Slightly affected
                              Moderately affected
                              Severely affected
                              Replaced

FOLLOW UP (MONTHS)

1. ASSESSMENT BY THE PATIENT

   A. After treatment the patient is:

       (4) Enthusiastic
       (3) Satisfied
       (2) Non-committal
       (1) Disappointed

   B. Is the patient's present disabiity due to the affected knee?

       (4) Entirely
       (3) Mainly
       (2) Partially
       (1) Scarcely at all

2. PAIN

   (4) None
   (3) Mild pain, not interfering with activities or sleep
   (2) Moderate pain, either reducing activities or disturbing sleep
   (1) Severe pain

3. ABILITY TO WALK

           Distance Or Time

   (5) > 1 kilometre (unlimited)   >60 minutes
   (4) Up to 1 kilometre   30–60 minutes
   (3) Up to 50 metres   10–30 minutes
   (2) 50–100 metres (outdoors)   5–10 minutes
   (1) Indoors only   Indoors only
   (0) Unable   Unable

4. WALKING AID

   (4) None
   (3) Stick outside
   (2) Stick always
   (1) Two sticks/crutches/frame
   (0) Unable to walk

5. GAIT

   (4) Normal free swing
   (3) Slight limitation of swing
   (2) Minimal movement
   (1) Stiff knee

6. FLEXION DEFORMITY   7. MAXIMUM FLEXION

   (5) 0 degrees
   (4) <10 degrees   (4) >100 degrees
   (3) 11–20 degrees   (3) 81–100 degrees
   (2) 21–30 degrees   (2) 61-80 degrees
   (1) >30 degrees   (1) <60 degrees

8. EXTENSION LAG
   Additonal to flexion contracture if present

   (4) 0 degrees
   (3) <10 degrees
   (2) <20 degrees
   (1) >20 degrees

9. VALGUS ANGLE   10. VARUS ANGLE
   When the tibia is   When the tibia is
   stressed laterally   stressed medially

                           (5) 0 degrees
   (4) 0–10 degrees   (4) <10 degrees
   (3) <20 degrees   (3) <20 degrees
   (2) <30 degrees   (2) <30 degrees
   (1) >30 degrees   (1) >30 degrees

11. ABILITY TO GET OUT OF CHAIR

   (4) With ease
   (3) With difficulty
   (2) Only by using arms
   (1) Unable

12. ABILITY TO CLIMB STAIRS
   (4) Normal
   (3) One step at a time
   (2) Only with a bannister, stick or both
   (1) Unable or only by bizarre method

APPENDIX

STATE OF OTHER JOINTS

SLIGHTLY AFFECTED

   Infrequent pain
   Minor stiffness—no functional deficit
   Walking minimally affected. No support required

MODERATELY AFFECTED

   Moderate pain
   Joint stiffness producing some function deficit
   Walking interrupted and support required

SEVERELY AFFECTED

   Severe pain
   Stiffness with marked functional disability
   Unable to walk or walking with difficulty using a major support

Fig. 20.120. BOA knee function assessment chart.

Good and excellent results had no pain and were not limited functionally in their everyday activities by the knee itself (although in some cases there was limitation due to age, general medical condition, or involvement of other joints).

The two fair results were attributable to unexplained pain in one case and a patellar tendon avulsion with consequent quadriceps weakness in the other.

The five poor ratings were due to loosening in two knees, posterior subluxation in one knee, component malposition in one knee, and sepsis in one knee.

In the two cases with tibial loosening, the result was rated after 2 years as good in one knee and fair in the other. The initially good result was correctly positioned but 3 years after operation, developed a complete and progressive radiolucency around the tibial component. Thereafter increasing pain was felt and a revision was performed because of pain at 5 years. The component was loose as the radiograph suggested. The other patient that initially had a fair rating was positioned in varus at the time of surgery, and the knee was always painful on the medial side. Over the years the varus deformity increased and subsidence of the medial tibial component was noticed associated with bending of the polyethylene. At reoperation after 5 years, the component was found

to be loose with considerable bone necrosis of the medial tibia. The case of malposition was somewhat similar in that the knee was positioned in varus at the time of surgery. This patient also complained of pain from the beginning, but no change in the position of the tibial component was observed. The knee was explored because of persistent complaints after 3 years. There was no obvious cause for the pain found at operation and all the components were rigidly fixed. However, because of the malposition and residual deformity, the tibial component was removed and a new component inserted correcting the knee to 7 degrees of valgus. This patient has subsequently been pain free.

It seems therefore that malposition can by itself be a cause of pain, perhaps due to bone overload which in time can lead to loosening. In the entire series only one case that was correctly positioned and aligned at surgery subsequently loosened. The appearance of a complete radiolucency around the tibial component was unique to this case and is so unusual that we have considered the finding due to an infection until proven otherwise.

The radiolucent lines at the bone–cement interface were studied on serial radiographs. Thirty-one percent of the knees had a radiolucency present on some

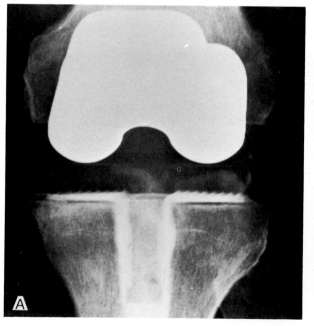 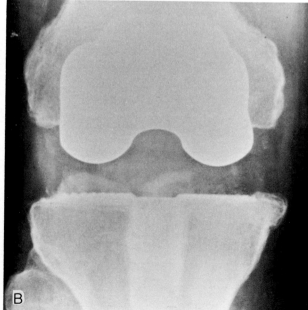

Fig. 20.121. (A) Radiograph taken 1 year after implantation shows a pronounced radiolucent line beneath medial and lateral tibial plateaus. (B) Radiograph of the same knee taken at 5 years shows a barely visible radiolucency.

prosthetic surface at 1 year. Thirty-nine percent had a radiolucency after 5 years, and thus eight knees that initially had no radiolucencies subsequently developed them. The most common locations for radiolucency were the medial and lateral plateaus of the tibial component. With the one exception noted, no knee prosthesis had a complete circumferential radiolucency, and in a few knees an initially prominent radiolucency became less pronounced with time although it did not completely disappear (Fig. 20.121A,B). In order to determine whether any measurable wear was taking place in the polyethylene, the thickness of the tibial component was measured in serial radiographs. Although apparent thinning of the polyethylene was seen in some knees, an equal number had a thicker measurement after 5 years than at 1 year. We concluded that these differences could be accounted for by positioning and projection, and in no case were we able to demonstrate unequivocal evidence of polyethylene wear.

It seems from this clinical and radiographic study that modern designs of knee surface replacement are acceptably durable and in fact compare well with total hip replacement. There is no evidence that either component loosening or polyethylene wear are likely to prove major problems, and projecting from our results we believe that for patients over age 60, a knee prosthesis will last for the remainder of life in most

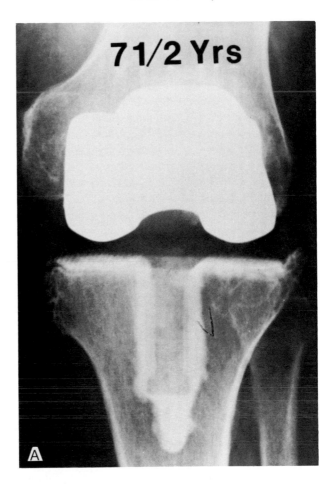

Fig. 20.122. (A,B) Anteroposterior and patellar views of a total condylar prosthesis $7\frac{1}{2}$ years after implantation. No detectable change in the appearance of the implants had taken place since the 1-year radiographs.

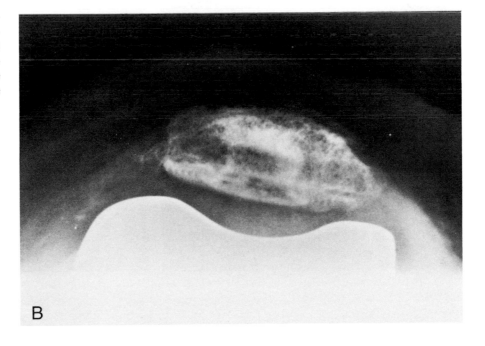

cases (Fig. 20.122A,B). For younger patients who are also likely to be more active, current data are inadequate to form an opinion concerning the durability of the implants.

The use of unicompartmental replacement (Fig. 20.123A,B) is controversial and the published results of these prostheses are conflicting. Insall and Aglietti[68] reported on 22 unicondylar knee replacements with a 5- to 7-year follow-up. Although the results of the unicondylar arthroplasties were initially considered good, they subsequently showed a marked deterioration. At the time of review one knee was rated excellent, seven knees good, four knees fair, and 10 knees poor. Seven knees (28 percent) were revised to a total condylar prosthesis. The lateral replacements did much better than the medial ones. To some extent the poor showing of this prosthesis could be attributed to incorrect selection of patients and deficiencies in surgical technique. Only patients with unicompartmental osteoarthritis are suitable for the procedure, and if there is extensive degeneration in other parts of the joint the operation will be a failure from the beginning. Because patellofemoral arthritis is associated with femoro-tibial arthritis in most knees, more than one-half of this series had a concomitant patellectomy on the assumption that pain relief would be more complete if the patella were removed. In retrospect the decision to remove the patella seems unwise. In both the medial and lateral replacements knees with a patellectomy did worse, although admittedly these tended to be the worst cases to begin with. Incorrect placement of the prosthesis can result in binding of the components during motion due to the rotary movements of the knee that are imposed

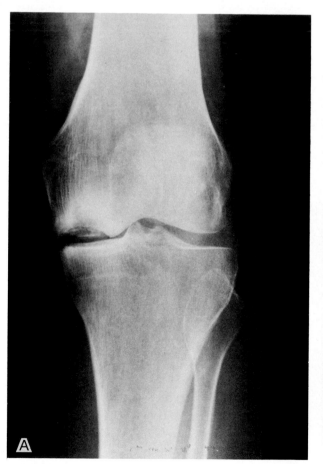
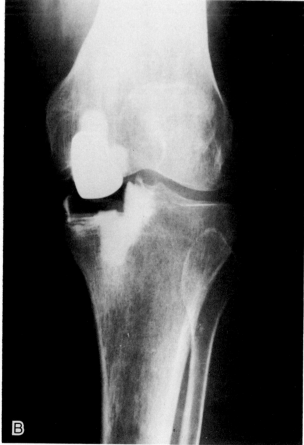

Fig. 20.123. (A,B) Unicondylar replacement for osteonecrosis of the medial femoral condyle. This result remained good at 5 years.

by the intact surfaces and ligaments. It is also difficult in the case of medial replacements to obtain adequate support for the medial tibial component, particularly when bone erosion is present. Three cases of sinkage and a stress fracture of the medial tibia may have resulted from this lack of support. It was also difficult to obtain full correction of varus in the knees with medial compartment replacement and perhaps the results would have been better had a medial ligament release been done in more of the knees. However, Marmor[101] has cautioned against overcorrection; the major reason for failure in our cases was progression of arthritis in the contralateral compartment (Fig. 20.124A,B). This progressive degeneration could be due to mechanical causes and altered joint function after the arthroplasty or to reactive synovitis and embedded particles of bone or methylmethacrylate. Acrylic cement and polyethylene debris were observed in all of the revised knees and a metallic synovitis was also present in two. Debris particles are largely generated by entrapped cement that escapes from beneath the components, particularly when they become loose. This can be reduced by accurate cement trimming, which is difficult with a design such as the unicondylar prosthesis because of the shape of the components and retention of the cruciate ligaments. Cement particles contributed to the severe polyeth-

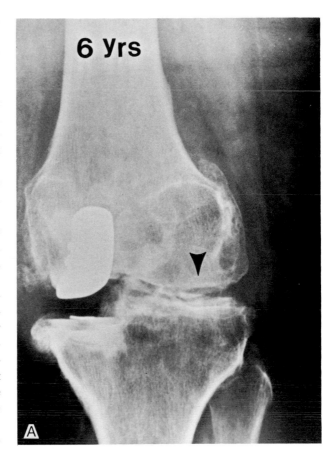

Fig. 20.124. (A,B) The most common reason for failure of unicondylar replacement was progressive arthritis of the unreplaced compartments of the knee. Free or embedded particles of acrylic cement were frequently found.

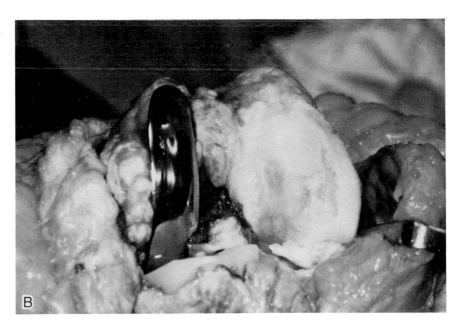

ylene wear that was observed in all knees that underwent revision. The loss of correction that was frequently seen was due to a combination of component loosening, settling and wear.

Laskin,[88] reporting on 37 Marmor modular prostheses, also found results inferior to bicompartmental replacement, particularly for medial osteoarthritis. Recurrent pain, degeneration of the other compartments, and tibial component sinkage were the major problems.

Marmor has reported better results with a minimum follow-up of 4 years on 59 knees with unicompartmental replacement (54 medial and five lateral). The results were good to excellent in 75 percent of the patients with no difference between those with medial and those with lateral disease. Poor results usually were associated with the use of a thin tibial component (6 mm) that was prone to bend and loosen. Scott and Santore[121] reported on 100 knees in 86 patients with osteoarthritis followed for 2 to 6 years. Fifteen of these knees were followed for more than 5 years. Eighty-eight knees had medial and 12 had lateral replacement. The ages of the patients at the time of operation ranged from 46 to 85 years with an average of 71 years. These workers used the same unicondylar prosthesis as that used by Insall and Aglietti, but their clinical results were much better. Pain relief was satisfactory in 92 of the 100 knees. The average range of motion was 114 degrees and 49 percent of the knees had at least 120 degrees of flexion. Seventy-three percent of the 86 patients could walk an unlimited distance without support, and 65 percent could go up and downstairs normally. Eight percent of the knees had radiolucent lines at the bone–cement interface on the femoral side, and 27 percent showed radiolucent lines about the tibial component. Four of these lines extended the full length of the interface, were more than 1 mm wide, and were increasing in size. Three patients had a revision, one because of ligament instability, and two because of femoral component subsidence. All three patients were obese. On the basis of their findings, Scott and Santore continue to recommend unicompartmental replacement for elderly patients with unicompartmental osteoarthritis as confirmed by thorough exploration of the knee at arthrotomy. They estimate that approximately one third of the osteoarthritic knees in which knee replacement is performed fulfill these criteria. Why their results are so much better than those obtained at Special

Surgery using the same prosthesis is unclear. However, as these authors did not note progressive arthritis in any of their patients it seems probable that the shorter follow-up may be the single most important factor in the discrepancy. The ultimate place of unicompartmental replacement in knee arthroplasty must await the results on more patients followed from five to ten years.

Using a modified Walldius prosthesis Young[154] reported that in his experience no prosthesis survived ten years. However, more recently Wilson[153] et al. have reported on a series of uncemented Walldius prostheses which included a group of twelve patients with 20 knee prostheses followed for an average of ten years. Using their own scoring system, the average rating was 80 points and although a zone of radiolucency was observed at the bone-prosthesis junction in most patients, this finding was not associated with either clinical loosening or pain, a finding that the authors attribute to the lack of cement in their cases.

Using a cemented Guepar prosthesis, Deburge et al.[28] report that 15 percent of the prostheses had aseptic loosening at 5 years. However, only one-half the loose prostheses were symptomatic and needed re-operation. The deep infection rate was relatively high (6.6 percent), and the Guepar group report a 1 percent incidence of sudden death occurring during or immediately after surgery. Whether this is caused by fat embolism associated with pressurization of cement is not certain. Hui and Fitzgerald[61] report a 23 percent incidence of major complications with hinged total knee arthroplasty. The incidence of infection rate was 11.7 percent. It seems to be the consensus of opinion that with hinged prostheses (1) there is a higher incidence of complications; (2) the procedure is technically easy and, by virtue of the stems, the prosthesis is largely self-aligning; (3) the short-term results are often good; but (4) results deteriorate with time largely due to late infection and loosening.

A number of prosthetic designs such as the Sheehan, Attenborough and spherocentric, have attempted to provide constraint but overcome the drawbacks of fixed axis hinges. The published information on the first two models indicates that the early results are good,[6,141] but there is as yet no information about the 5-year results.

Kaufer and Matthews[85] have provided more information on the spherocentric prosthesis. Reviewing 82 consecutive spherocentric arthroplasties with an average follow-up of four years, they report an infection rate of 4 percent and 10 percent incidence of aseptic loosening. All patients had either severe preoperative instability or deformity, or both. Deformity was corrected whenever possible by resection of bone rather than soft tissue release, but in spite of this, knees that were initially in valgus were more likely to develop peroneal nerve palsy. Knees that were initially in varus were much more susceptible to aseptic loosening. A prosthetic component was considered to be loose if (1) radiologic change in position was demonstrated, (2) stress radiograms revealed motion between prosthesis and bone, or (3) motion was detected at secondary operation. Loosening was diagnosed between 4 and 30 months after the initial arthroplasty, and all of the knees with loose components had a prior complete and progressive radiolucency. Convery et al.[20] report eight cases of confirmed or suspected loosening in 36 spherocentric arthroplasties followed for an average of 3 years. Because of this loosening they proposed a long stem modification of the prosthesis and believe that the short stem of the original version may have been a factor in the "unacceptable rate of revision" (22 percent). Kaufer and Matthews, while recognizing the need for long stem components in certain special circumstances, continue to recommend the short stem version for routine use because of a concern that long stems may relieve the metaphyseal bone of stress promoting bone atrophy and possibly leading to an increased failure rate. They also prefer the flexibility in placement that short stems allow. In summary, modified constrained prostheses such as the spherocentric seem to occupy an intermediate position between fixed axis hinges and surface replacements, in that infection and loosening are reduced but not to the level achieved with surface replacements.

FUTURE DEVELOPMENTS

It seems clear that the future of knee arthroplasty lies with surface replacement, although the need for a modified constrained prosthesis will continue in special circumstances and for occasional cases. Advances in surgical technique should greatly reduce the need for the latter type.

SURGICAL TECHNIQUE AND INSTRUMENTATION

Most unsatisfactory results after knee arthroplasty using one of the latest resurfacing models are due more to inaccurate insertion and poor surgical technique than to implant deficiencies. Whereas total hip replacement is a relatively forgiving operation, even minor errors in the insertion of a knee prosthesis are clinically evident and may cause complete failure of the arthroplasty. Not only must the overall alignment be correct within a tolerance of less than 5 degrees, but also each component must be placed with similar accuracy, the ligament tension in both extension and flexion must be right, and the patella and quadriceps mechanism must track smoothly in the midline. An error in any one of these areas will not self-correct, but will rather become magnified with time. It is not easy to achieve the necessary precision in a thin patient without significant deformity, and when the patient is obese and the deformity severe the task becomes much more difficult. The unavoidable technical difficulties probably make the operation unsuitable for those surgeons who perform it infrequently. A measure of continuing experience is necessary, and although it is hard to define exactly what this should be, the operation should probably be performed not less than once or twice a month to maintain competence. Otherwise, the patient should be referred to a more experienced surgeon or an alternative operation such as osteotomy should be done. More comprehensive instrumentation is also needed to increase the precision of the bone cuts which cannot be done entirely by eye, even by the most gifted and experienced surgeons. However, instruments are only an aid and cannot substitute for a thorough understanding of the basic principles of the technique. In fact, some of the best results have been published by surgeons who use relatively simple guides, although Freeman, in particular, has always stressed the need for better instrumentation.

PROSTHETIC DESIGN

The major appeal of constrained implants is that the surgical technique is greatly simplified,[46] making the results more reproducible by inexperienced surgeons. For this reason alone, further developments seem justified so that the disadvantages of loosening and infection can be reduced or overcome. At the moment, such examples as the spherocentric, Sheehan, and Attenborough prostheses seem partially successful in this respect.

Less change is forseen in the design of surface replacements, and future development will most likely be one of refining existing concepts. Right and left components, multiple sizes and thicknesses, metal containment of polyethylene, and changes in the articular geometry designed to produce greater motion are the most expected alterations.

Although cement fixation seems perfectly adequate for older patients, it is probably unsuitable for those who are younger and more vigorous. Although the latter group is limited in number, there are some patients with post-traumatic arthritis who fit in this category, and of course rheumatoid patients may require replacement even as teenagers. Alternative methods of fixation are being sought either by the use of porous materials that permit bone ingrowth[139] or by methods that provide immediate interdigitation of components and bone. Most of the information has come from Freeman who has used cementless fixation for more than 4 years; so far the clinical results are indistinguishable from those with cemented prostheses.[11] There is no worthwhile information on the use of porous ingrowth materials at the time of writing. Newer fixation methods must prove themselves at least as good as conventional cement techniques before widespread adoption can be justified and this is certainly not the situation at present.

Metal containment of the polyethylene has been widely adopted mainly on theoretical arguments.[9,90] Early clinical experience appears to show that there is a decreased incidence of radiolucent lines, but the long term effects on fixation cannot yet be judged.

High-density polyethylene is not the most suitable material for a knee arthroplasty. In all designs the polyethylene is loaded close to fatigue failure. While permanent deformation of polyethylene as reported for the UCI prosthesis is not common with more recent designs, Ducheyne et al.[31] have calculated that for a patient weighing 75 kg, permanent deformation can occur at a peak knee joint reaction force of between five and eight times body weight. For a patient weighing 100 kg, the joint reaction force is approximately four to six times body weight. These joint reaction forces are probably only reached with sudden vigorous activities, so that it is the overweight and the younger patients who are at greatest risk. Prudence dictates that running sports and other strenuous activities should be avoided by all patients with a knee arthroplasty. For the time being at least it is the wear characteristics of the polyethylene and not fixation failure that seems the major limiting factor in knee arthroplasty. However, at the moment no newer materials to supersede polyethylene are available.

REFERENCES

1. Andersen, J.L.: Knee arthroplasty in rheumatoid arthritis: An analysis of 240 cases of hemi-, hinge and resurfacing arthroplasties. Acta. Orthop. Scand., Suppl. *180:* 1, 1979.
2. Andriacchi, T.P., and Galante, J.O.: Influence of total knee replacement design on walking and stair climbing. J. Bone Joint Surg. [Am], *64:* 1328, 1982.
3. Arden, G.P.: Total replacement of the knee. J. Bone Joint Surg. [Br.], *57:* 119, 1975.
4. Artz, T.D., Macys, J., Salvati, E.A., et al: Hematogenous infection of total hip replacements: A report of four cases. In proceedings J. Bone Joint Surg. [Am.], *57:* 1024, 1975.
5. Attenborough, C.G.: Total knee replacement using the stabilized gliding prosthesis. Ann. R. Coll. Surg. Engl., *58:* 4, 1976.
6. Attenborough, C.G.: The Attenborough total knee replacement. J. Bone Joint Surg. [Br.], *60:* 320, 1978.
7. Bain, A.M.: Replacement of the knee joint with the Walldius prosthesis using cement fixation. Clin. Orthop., *94:* 65, 1973.
8. Bargar, W.L., Cracchiolo, A. III, and Amstutz, H.C.: Results with the constrained total knee prosthesis in treating severely disabled patients and patients with failed total knee replacements. J. Bone Joint Surg. [Am.], *62:* 504, 1980.
9. Bartel, D.L., Burstein, A.H., Santavicca, E.A., et al: Performance of the tibial component in total knee replacement—Conventional and revision designs. J. Bone Joint Surg. [Am.], *64:* 1026, 1982.
10. Bisla, R.S., Inglis, A.E., and Lewis, R.J.: Fat embolism following bilateral total knee replacement with the Guepar prosthesis. A case report. Clin. Orthop., *115:* 195, 1976.
11. Blaha, J.D., Insler, H.P., and Freeman, M.A.R., et al: The fixation of a proximal tibial polyethylene prosthesis without cement. J. Bone Joint Surg. [Br.], *64:* 326, 1982.

12. Brodersen, M.P., Fitzgerald, R.H., Jr., Peterson, L.F.A., et al: Arthrodesis of the knee following failed total knee arthroplasty. J. Bone Joint Surg. [Am.], *61:* 181, 1979.

13. Bryan, R.S., and Peterson, L.F.A.: Polycentric total knee arthroplasty: A prognostic assessment. Clin. Orthop., *145:* 23, 1979.

14. Bullough, P.G., Insall, J.N., and Ranawat, C.S., et al: Wear and tissue reaction in failed knee arthroplasty. In proceedings J. Bone Joint Surg. [Br.], *58:* 366, 1976.

15. Campbell, W.C.: Interposition of vitallium plates in arthroplasties of the knee. Preliminary report. Am. J. Surg., *47:* 639, 1940.

16. Carlsson, A.S., Josefsson, G., and Lindberg, L.: Revision with gentamicin-impregnated cement for deep infections in total hip arthroplasties. J. Bone Joint Surg. [Am.], *60:* 1059, 1978.

17. Cavendish, M.E., and Wright, J.T.M.: The Liverpool mark II knee prosthesis. A preliminary report. J. Bone Joint Surg. [Br.], *60:* 315, 1978.

18. Cloutier, J.M., Gauthier, F., and Rizkallah, R.: Arthroplasty of the knee using the Marmor prosthesis. In proceedings J. Bone Joint Surg. [Br.], *58:* 142, 1976.

19. Cohen, S.H., Ehrlich, G.E., Kauffman, M.S., et al: Thrombophlebitis following knee surgery. J. Bone Joint Surg. [Am.], *55:* 106, 1973.

20. Convery, F.R., Minteer-Convery, M., and Malcom, L.L.: The spherocentric knee: A re-evaluation and modification. J. Bone Joint Surg. [Am.], *62:* 320, 1980.

21. Coonse, K., and Adams, J.D.: A new operative approach to the knee joint. Surg. Gynecol. Obstet., *77:* 344, 1943.

22. Coventry, M.B., Finerman, G.A.M., Riley, L.H., et al: A new geometric knee for total knee arthroplasty. Clin. Orthop., *83:* 157, 1972.

23. Coventry, M.B., Upshaw, J.E., Riley, L.H., et al: Geometric total knee arthroplasty. II. Patient data and complications. Clin. Orthop., *94:* 177, 1973.

24. Crock, H.: Personal communication, 1980.

25. Cruess, R.L., Bickel, W.S., and von Kessler, K.L.C.: Infections in total hips secondary to a primary source elsewhere. Clin. Orthop., *106:* 99, 1975.

26. D'Ambrosia, R.D., Shoji, H., and Heater, R.: Secondarily infected total joint replacements by hematogenous spread. J. Bone Joint Surg. [Am.], *58:* 450, 1976.

27. Deane, G.: The evolution and clinical use of the Deane intercondylar knee. In proceedings J. Bone Joint Surg. [Br.], *63:* 476, 1981.

28. Deburge, A., and GUEPAR: GUEPAR hinge prosthesis. Complications and results with two years follow-up. Clin. Orthop., *120:* 47, 1976.

29. Denny-Brown, D., and Doherty, M.M.: Effects of transient stretching of peripheral nerve. Arch. Neurol. Psychiat *54:* 116, 1945.

30. Ducheyne, P., Kagan, A. II, Lacey, J.A.: Failure of total knee arthroplasty due to loosening and deformation of the tibial component. J. Bone Joint Surg. [Am.], *60:* 384, 1978.

31. Evanski, P.M., Waugh, T.R., Orofino, C.F., et al: UCI knee replacement. Clin. Orthop., *120:* 33, 1976.

32. Evarts, C.M.: Thromboembolism. In Rockwood, C.A., Jr., and Green, D.P., eds.: Fractures, Vol. 1: Complications. Philadelphia, J.B. Lippincott, p. 174, 1975.

33. Ewald, F.C., Thomas, W.H., Poss, R., Scott, R.D., et al: Duo-patella total knee arthroplasty in rheumatoid arthritis. Orthop. Trans., *2:* 202, 1978

34. Ferguson, W.: Excision of the knee joint; Recovery with a false joint and a useful limb. Med. Times Gaz., *1:* 601, 1861.

35. Finerman, G.A.M., Coventry, M.B., Riley, L.H., et al: Anametric total knee arthroplasty. Clin. Orthop., *145:* 85, 1979.

36. Flawn, L.B., Hood, R.W., and Insall, J.N.: The use of pulsatile compression stockings in total knee replacement for prevention of venous thromboembolism—a prospective study. Orthop. Trans., *6(3):* 457, 1982.

37. Fox, J.L., and Poss, R.: The role of manipulation following total knee replacement. J. Bone Joint Surg. [Am.], *63:* 357, 1981.

38. Freeman, M.A.R. (ed.): Arthritis of the Knee. Clinical Features and Surgical Management. Berlin, Heidelberg, New York, Springer-Verlag, 1980.

39. Freeman, M.A.R.: Personal communication, 1982.

40. Freeman, M.A.R., and Insall, J.N.: Tibio-femoral replacement using two unlinked components and cruciate resection. (The ICLH and Total Condylar Prostheses.) In Freeman, M.A.R., ed.: Arthritis of the Knee. Clinical Features and Surgical Management. Berlin, Heidelberg, New York, Springer-Verlag, p. 254, 1980.

41. Freeman, M.A.R., Swanson, S.A.V., and Todd, R.C.: Total replacement of the knee using the Freeman-Swanson knee prosthesis. Clin. Orthop., *94:* 153, 1973.

42. Freeman, M.A.R., Insall, J.N., Besser, W., et al: Excision of the cruciate ligaments in total knee replacement. Clin. Orthop., *126:* 209, 1977.

43. Freeman, M.A.R., Sculco, T., and Todd, R.C.: Replacement of the severely damaged arthritic knee by the ICLH (Freeman-Swanson) arthroplasty. J. Bone Joint Surg. [Br.], *59:* 64, 1977.

44. Freeman, M.A.R., Todd, R.C., Bamert, P., et al:

ICLH arthroplasty of the knee: 1968–1977. J. Bone Joint Surg. [Br.], *60:* 339, 1978.

45. Garner, R.W., Mowat, A.G., and Hazleman, B.L.: Wound healing after operations on patients with rheumatoid arthritis. J. Bone Joint Surg. [Br.], *55:* 134, 1973.

46. Gibbs, A.N., Green, G.A., and Taylor, J.G.: A comparison of the Freeman-Swanson (ICLH) and Walldius prostheses in total knee replacement. J. Bone Joint Surg. [Br.], *61:* 358, 1979.

47. Goldberg, V.M., and Henderson, B.T.: The Freeman-Swanson ICLH total knee arthroplasty. Complications and problems. J. Bone Joint Surg. [Am.], *62:* 1338, 1980.

48. Goodfellow, J., and O'Connor, J.: Kinematics of the knee and the prosthetic design. In proceedings J. Bone Joint Surg. [Br.], *59:* 119, 1977.

49. Gunston, F.H.: Polycentric knee arthroplasty. Prosthetic simulation of normal knee movement. J. Bone Joint Surg. [Br.], *53:* 272, 1971.

50. Gunston, F.H., and MacKenzie, R.I.: Complications of polycentric knee arthroplasty. Clin. Orthop., *120:* 11, 1976.

51. Hagemann, W.F., Woods, G.W., and Tullos, H.S.: Arthrodesis in failed total knee replacement. J. Bone Joint Surg. [Am.], *60:* 790, 1978.

52. Hall, A.J.: Late infection about a total knee prosthesis. J. Bone Joint Surg. [Br.], *56:* 144, 1974.

53. Harris, W.H., Salzman, E.W., and DeSanctis, R.W.: The prevention of thromboembolic disease by prophylactic anticoagulation. A controlled study in elective hip surgery. J. Bone Joint Surg. [Am.], *49:* 81, 1967.

54. Highet, W.B., and Holmes, W.: Traction injuries to the lateral popliteal nerve and traction injuries to peripheral nerves after suture. Br. J. Surg., *30:* 212, 1943.

55. Highet, W.B., and Sanders, F.K.: The effects of stretching nerves after suture. Br. J. Surg. *30:* 355, 1943.

56. Hirsh, D.M., Bhalla, S., and Roffman, M.: Supracondylar fracture of the femur following total knee replacement. Report of four cases. J. Bone Joint Surg. [Am.], *63:* 162, 1981.

57. Hood, R.W., and Insall, J.N.: Total knee revision arthroplasty: Indications, surgical techniques and results. Orthop. Trans., *5(3):* 412, 1981.

58. Hood, R.W., Wright, T.M., Burstein, A.H., et al: Retrieval analysis of 70 total condylar knee prostheses. Orthop. Trans., *5(2):* 319, 1981.

59. Hood, R.W., Vanni, M., and Insall, J.N.: The correction of knee alignment in 225 consecutive total condylar knee replacements. Clin. Orthop., *160:* 94, 1981.

60. Hood, R.W., Wright, T.M., Burstein, A.H., et al: Retrieval analysis of twenty polyethylene patellar buttons. Orthop. Trans., *5(2):* 291, 1981.

60a. Hood, R.W., Flawn, L.B., Insall, J.N.: The use of pulsatile compression stockings in total knee replacement for prevention of venous thromboembolism—A prospective study. Trans. ORS, *7:* 297, 1982.

61. Hui, F.C., and Fitzgerald, R.H., Jr.: Hinged total knee arthroplasty. J. Bone Joint Surg. [Am.], *62:* 513, 1980.

62. Hungerford, D.S., Kenna, R.V., and Krackow, K.A.: The porous-coated anatomic total knee. In Scott, W.N., ed.: Symposium on Total Knee Arthroplasty. Orthopedic Clinics of North America. Philadelphia, W.B. Saunders Co., *13(1):* 103, 1982.

63. Hunter, G.A., and Dandy, D.: Diagnosis and natural history of the infected total hip replacement. In The Hip Society: The Hip. Proceedings of the Fifth Open Scientific Meeting of The Hip Society. St. Louis, C.V. Mosby, 1977.

64. Ilstrup, D.M., Coventry, M.B., and Skolnick, M.D.: A statistical evaluation of geometric total knee arthroplasties. Clin. Orthop., *120:* 27, 1976.

65. Infection in rheumatoid disease, editorial. Br. Med. J., *2:* 549, 1972.

66. Insall, J.N.: Reconstructive surgery and rehabilitation of the knee. pp. 1980. In Kelley, W.N., Harris, E.D., Jr., Ruddy, S., and Sledge, C.B., eds.: Textbook of Rheumatology. Philadelphia, W.B. Saunders Co., 1980.

67. Insall, J.N.: Technique of total knee replacement. p. 324. In Instructional Course Lectures, The American Academy of Orthopaedic Surgeons, Vol. 30. St. Louis, C.V. Mosby, 1981.

68. Insall, J.N., and Aglietti, P.: A five to seven year follow-up of unicondylar arthroplasty. J. Bone Joint Surg. [Am.], *62:* 1329, 1980.

69. Insall, J.N., and Tria, A.J.: The total condylar prosthesis type II. Orthop. Trans., *3:* 300, 1979.

70. Insall, J.N., and Walker, P.: Unicondylar knee replacement. Clin. Orthop., *120:* 83, 1976.

71. Insall, J.N., Ranawat, C.S., Scott, W.N., et al: Total condylar knee replacement. Preliminary report. Clin. Orthop., *120:* 149, 1976.

72. Insall, J.N., Ranawat, C.S., Aglietti, P., et al: A comparison of four models of total knee replacement prostheses. J. Bone Joint Surg. [Am.], *58:* 754, 1976.

72a. Insall, J.N.: Infection in Total Knee arthroplasty. Instructional Course Lectures. The American Academy of Orthopaedic Surgeons. The C.V. Mosby Co., *31:* 42, 1982.

73. Insall, J.N., Scott, W.N., and Ranawat, C.S.: The total condylar knee prosthesis. A report of two hundred

and twenty cases. J. Bone Joint Surg. [Am.], *61:* 173, 1979.

74. Insall, J.N., Tria, A.J., and Scott, W.N.: The total condylar knee prosthesis: The first five years. Clin. Orthop., *145:* 68, 1979.

75. Insall, J.N., Freeman, M.A.R., Matthews, L.S., et al: Symposium: Present status of total knee replacement. Contemp. Orthop., *2:* 592, 1980.

76. Insall, J.N., Lachiewicz, P.F., and Burstein, A.H.: The posterior stabilized condylar prosthesis. A modification of the total condylar design. Two to four year clinical experience. J. Bone Joint Surg. [Am.], *64:* 1317, 1982.

77. Insall, J.N., Thompson, F.M., Brause, B.D., et al: Two-stage reimplantation for the salvage of infected total knee arthroplasty. Presented at the Annual Meeting of the American Academy of Orthopaedic Surgons. New Orleans, Louisiana, 1982. Orthop. Trans., *6(3):* 369, 1982.

78. Jennings, J.J., Harris, W.H., and Sarmiento, A.: A clinical evaluation of aspirin prophylaxis of thromboembolic disease after total hip arthroplasty. J. Bone Joint Surg. [Am.], *58:* 926, 1976.

79. Johnson, F., Leitl, S., and Waugh, W.: The distribution of load across the knee. J. Bone Joint Surg. [Br.], *62:* 346, 1980.

80. Jones, E.C., Insall, J.N., Inglis, A.E., et al: GUEPAR knee arthroplasty results and late complications. Clin. Orthop., *140:* 145, 1979.

81. Jones, G.B.: Arthroplasty of the knee by the Walldius prosthesis. J. Bone Joint Surg. [Br.], *50:* 505, 1968.

82. Jones, G.B.: Walldius arthroplasty of the knee. J. Bone Joint Surg. [Br.], *52:* 390, 1970.

83. Jones, W.T., Bryan, R.S., Peterson, L.F.A., et al: Unicompartmental knee arthroplasty using polycentric and geometric hemicomponents. J. Bone Joint Surg. [Am.], *63:* 946, 1981.

84. Kapandji, I.A.: The physiology of the joints. Vol. II, The lower limb, p. 120. London, Edinbrugh. Churchill Livingston, 1970.

85. Kaufer, H., and Matthews, L.S.: Spherocentric arthroplasty of the knee. J. Bone Joint Surg. [Am.], *63:* 545, 1981.

86. Kaushal, S.P., Galante, J.O., McKenna, R., et al: Complications following total knee replacement. Clin. Orthop. *121:* 181, 1976.

87. Laskin, R.S.: Modular total knee replacement arthroplasty. A review of eighty-nine patients. J. Bone Joint Surg. [Am.], *58:* 766, 1976.

88. Laskin, R.S.: Unicompartmental tibiofemoral resurfacing arthroplasty. J. Bone Joint Surg. [Am.], *60:* 182, 1978.

89. Lettin, A.W.F., Deliss, L.J., Blackburne, J.S., et al:

The Stanmore hinged knee arthroplasty. J. Bone Joint Surg. [Br.], *60(3):* 327, 1978.

90. Lewis, J.L., Askew, M.J., and Jaycox, D.P.: A comparative evaluation of tibial component designs of total knee prostheses. J. Bone Joint Surg. [Am.], *64:* 129, 1982.

91. Lotke, P.A., and Ecker, M.L.: Influence of positioning of prosthesis in total knee replacement. J. Bone Joint Surg. [Am.], *59:* 77, 1977.

92. Lundborg, G., and Rydevik, B.: Effects of stretching the tibial nerve of the rabbit. A preliminary study of the intraneural circulation and barrier function of the perineurium. J. Bone Joint Surg. [Br.], *55(2):* 390, 1973.

93. McKeever, D.C.: Tibial plateau prosthesis. Clin. Orthop., *18:* 86, 1960.

94. MacIntosh, D.L.: Hemiarthroplasty of the knee using a space occupying prosthesis for painful varus and valgus deformities. J. Bone Joint Surg. [Am.], *40:* 1431, 1958.

95. MacIntosh, D.L.: Arthroplasty of the knee in rheumatoid arthritis. J. Bone Joint Surg. [Br.], *48:* 179, 1966.

96. Mallory, T.H., and Dolibois, J.M.: Unicompartment total knee replacement. A 2-4 year review. Clin. Orthop., *134:* 139, 1978.

97. Manchester Knee arthroplasty, editorial. J. Bone Joint Surg. [Br.], *61:* 225, 1979.

98. Marks, K.E., Nelson, C.L., and Lautenschlager, E.P.: Antibiotic-impregnated acrylic bone cement. J. Bone Joint Surg. [Am.], *58:* 358, 1976.

99. Marmor, L.: The modular (Marmor) knee. Case report with a minimum follow-up of two years. Clin. Orthop., *120:* 86, 1976.

100. Marmor, L.: Results of single compartment arthroplasty with acrylic cement fixation. A minimum follow-up of two years. Clin. Orthop., *122:* 181, 1977.

101. Marmor, L.: Marmor modular knee in unicompartmental disease. Minimum four-year follow-up. J. Bone Joint Surg. [Am.], *61:* 347, 1979.

102. Marsh, P.K., and Cotler, J.M.: Management of an anaerobic infection in a prosthetic knee with long-term antibiotic alone: A case report. Clin. Orthop., *155:* 133, 1981.

103. Mazas, F.B., and GUEPAR: Guepar total knee prosthesis. Clin. Orthop., *94:* 211, 1973.

104. Miller, A., and Friedman, B.: Fascial arthroplasty of the knee. J. Bone Joint Surg. [Am.], *34:* 55, 1952.

105. Miller, J.: Improved fixation in total hip arthroplasty using L.V.C. Surgical Technique Brochure. Zimmer, Warsaw, Ind., U.S.A., 1980.

106. Moreland, J.R., Thomas, R.J., and Freeman, M.A.R.: ICLH replacement of the knee: 1977 and 1978. Clin. Orthop., *145:* 47, 1979.

107. Murray, D.G., and Webster, D.A.: The variable-axis knee prosthesis: two-year follow-up study. J. Bone Joint Surg. [Am.], *63:* 687, 1981.

108. Murray, D.G., Wilde, A.H., Werner, F., et al: Herbert total knee prosthesis. Combined laboratory and clinical assessment. J. Bone Joint Surg. [Am.], *59:* 1026, 1977.

109. Petty, W., Bryan, R.S., and Coventry, M.: Infection following total knee arthroplasty. J. Bone Joint Surg. [Br.], *57:* 394, 1975.

110. Phillips, H., and Taylor, J.G.: The Walldius hinge arthroplasty. J. Bone Joint Surg. [Br.], *57:* 59, 1975.

111. Rae, T.: A study on the effects of particulate metals of orthopaedic interest on murine macrophages in vitro. J. Bone Joint Surg. [Br.], *57:* 444, 1975.

112. Ranawat, C.S., and Brigham, L.: Preliminary evaluation of stabilo-condylar arthroplasty. Orthop. Trans., *1:* 92, 1977.

113. Ranawat, C.S., Insall, J.N., and Shine, J.: Duo-condylar knee arthroplasty. Hospital for Special Surgery design. Clin. Orthop., *120:* 76, 1976.

114. Rand, J.A., and Coventry, M.B.: Stress fractures after total knee arthroplasty. J. Bone Joint Surg. [Am.], *62:* 226, 1980.

115. Riley, L.H., and Hungerford, D.S.: Geometric total knee replacement for treatment of the rheumatoid knee. J. Bone Joint Surg. [Am.], *60:* 523, 1978.

116. Rose, H.A., Hood, R.W., Otis, J.C., et al.: Peroneal-nerve palsy following total knee arthroplasty. A review of the Hospital for Special Surgery experience. J. Bone Joint Surg. [Am.], *64:* 347, 1982.

117. Rubin, R., and Salvati, E.A.: Infected total hip replacement after dental procedures. Oral Surg., *41:* 18, 1976.

118. Salvati, E.A., and Insall, J.N.: The management of sepsis in total knee replacement. p. 49. In Savastano, A.A., ed.: Total Knee Replacement. New York, Appleton-Century-Crofts, 1980.

119. Salvati, E.A., Brause, B.D., Chekofsky, K.M., et al: Reimplantation in infected total joint arthroplasty. Orthop. Trans., *5:* 449, 1981.

120. Schurman, D.J., Johnson, B.L., Jr., and Amstutz, H.C.: Knee joint infections with Staphylococcus aureus and Micrococcus Species: Influence of antibiotics, metal debris, bacteremia, blood, and steroids, in a rabbit model. J. Bone Joint Surg. [Am.], *57:* 40, 1975.

121. Scott, R.D., and Santore, R.F.: Unicondylar unicompartmental replacement for osteoarthritis of the knee. J. Bone Joint Surg. [Am.], *63:* 536, 1981.

122. Scott, R.D., Welsh, R.P., and Thomas, W.H.: Unicompartment unicondylar total knee replacement in osteoarthritis of the knee. Orthop. Trans., *2:* 203, 1978.

123. Scott, W.N., Rozbruch, J.D., Otis, J.C., et al.: Clin-

ical and biomechanical evaluation of patella replacement in total knee arthroplasty. Orthop. Trans., *2:* 203, 1978.

124. Scott, W.N., Tria, A., and Insall, J.N.: Total knee arthroplasty: Past, present, future. Orthop. Surv., *3:* 135, 1979.

125. Shaw, N.E., and Chatterjee, R.K.: Manchester knee arthroplasty. J. Bone Joint Surg. [Br.], *60:* 310, 1978.

126. Sheehan, J.M.: Arthroplasty of the knee. J. Bone Joint Surg. [Br.], *60:* 333, 1978.

127. Shiers, L.G.P.: Arthroplasty of the knee. Preliminary report of a new method. J. Bone Joint Surg. [Br.], *36:* 553, 1954.

128. Shoji, H., D'Ambrosia, R.D., and Lipscomb, P.R.: Failed polycentric total knee prostheses. J. Bone Joint Surg. [Am.], *58:* 773, 1976.

129. Skolnick, M.D., Bryan, R.S., and Peterson, L.F.A.: Unicompartmental polycentric knee arthroplasty. Description and preliminary results. Clin. Orthop., *112:* 208, 1975.

130. Skolnick, M.D., Bryan, R.S., Peterson, L.F.A., et al: Polycentric total knee arthroplasty. J. Bone Joint Surg. [Am.], *58:* 743, 1976.

131. Sledge, C.B., and Ewald, F.C.: Total knee arthroplasty experience at the Robert Breck Brigham Hospital. Clin. Orthop., *145:* 78, 1979.

132. Sledge, C.B., Stern, P., Thomas, W.H., et al.: Two year follow-up of the duo-condylar total knee replacement. Orthop. Trans., *2:* 193, 1978.

133. Sonstegard, D.A., Kaufer, H., and Matthews, L.S.: The spherocentric knee. Biomechanical testing and clinical trial. J. Bone Joint Surg. [Am.], *59:* 602, 1977.

134. Speed, J.S., and Trout, P.C.: Arthroplasty of the knee. A follow-up study. J. Bone Joint Surg. [Br.], *31:* 53, 1949.

135. Stinchfield, F.E., Bigliani, L.U., Neu, H.C., et al: Late hematogenous infection of total joint replacement. J. Bone Joint Surg. [Am.], *62:* 1345, 1980.

136. Stulberg, B.N., Insall, J.N., Williams, G., et al: Deep vein thrombosis following total knee replacement: An analysis of 643 arthroplasties. Presented at the Annual Meeting of the American Academy of Orthopaedic Surgeons, Anaheim, California, March, 1983.

136a. Stulberg, B., Insall, J.N., Hood, R.W., and Williams, G.: Postoperative thrombosis following total knee arthroplasty. Trans. ORS, *7:* 291, 1982.

137. Thompson, F.M., Hood, R.W., and Insall, J.N.: Patellar fractures in total knee arthroplasty. Orthop. Trans., *5:* 490, 1981.

138. Thornhill, T.S., Hood, R.W., Dalziel, R.E., et al: Knee revision in failed non-infected total knee arthroplasty—The Robert B. Brigham and Hospital for Special Surgery Experience. Orthop. Trans., *6:* 368, 1982.

139. Trent, P.S., Besser, W., Dueland, R., et al: Total knee prosthesis combining porous ingrowth and initial stabilization. Trans. Orthop. Res. Soc., *3:* 164, 1978.

140. Turner, R.H., Matza, R., and Hamati, Y.I.: Geometric and anametric total knee replacements. p. 171. In Savastano, A.A., ed.: Total Knee Replacement. New York, Appleton-Century-Crofts, 1980.

141. Vanhegan, J.A.D., Dabrowski, W., and Arden, G.P.: A review of 100 Attenborough stabilised gliding knee prostheses. J. Bone Joint Surg. [Br.], *61:* 445, 1979.

142. Verneuil, A.: De la création d'une fausse articulation par section ou résection partielle de l'os maxillaire inférieur, comme moyen de rémedier à l'ankylose vraie ou fausse de la machoire inférieure. Arch. Gen. Med., *15*(Ser. 5): 174, 1860.

143. Walker, P.S.: Human Joints and Their Artificial Replacements. Springfield, Ill., Charles C Thomas, 1977.

144. Walker, P.S., Ranawat, C., and Insall, J.N.: Fixation of the tibial components of condylar replacement knee prostheses. J. Biomech., *9:* 269, 1976.

145. Walker, P.S., Greene, D., Reilly, D., et al: Fixation of tibial components of knee prostheses. J. Bone Joint Surg. [Am.], *63:* 258, 1981.

146. Walldius, B.: Arthroplasty of the knee joint using endoprosthesis. Acta Orthop. Scand., *24*(Suppl.): 19, 1957.

147. Walldius, B.: Arthroplasty of the knee—Twenty-seven years' experience. p. 195. In Savastano, A.A., ed.: Total Knee Replacement. New York, Appleton-Century-Crofts, 1980.

148. Watson, J.R., Wood, H., and Hill, R.C.J.: The Shiers arthroplasty of the knee. J. Bone Joint Surg. [Br.], *58:* 300, 1976.

149. Waugh, T.R., and Evanski, P.M.: University of California, Irvine (UCI) Knee replacement—Design, operative technique, and results. p. 217. In Savastano, A.A., ed.: Total Knee Replacement. New York, Appleton-Century-Crofts, 1980.

150. Waugh, W., and Tew, M.: Total replacement of the knee. (Letter to the editor). J. Bone Joint Surg. [Br.], *61:* 225, 1979.

151. Wilde, A.H.: Management of complications after knee replacement. In Ahstrom, J.P., ed.: Current Practice in Orthopaedic Surgery. St. Louis, C.V. Mosby, p. 121, 1979.

152. Williams, E.A., Hargadon, E.J., and Davies, D.R.A.: Late failure of the Manchester prosthesis. Its relationship to the disease process. J. Bone Joint Surg. [Br.], *61:* 451, 1979.

153. Wilson, F.C., Fajgenbaum, D.M., and Venters, G.C.: Results of knee replacement with the Walldius and Geometric prostheses. A comparative study. J. Bone Joint Surg. [Am.], *62:* 497, 1980.

154. Young, H.H.: Use of a hinged vitallium prosthesis (Young type) for arthroplasty of the knee. In proceedings of The American Orthopaedic Association. J. Bone Joint Surg. [Am.], *53:* 1658, 1971.

21 Total Knee Replacement in Rheumatoid Arthritis

Clement B. Sledge
and
Peter S. Walker

Are the differences between patients with inflammatory arthritis and those with degenerative arthritis sufficient to warrant a separate chapter in a textbook such as this? Since the entire joint is usually replaced, does it matter what the underlying pathology might be?

Obviously, we and Dr. Insall believe that the answer to these questions is yes. Since rheumatoid arthritis and its variants are systemic diseases, there are immediate significant differences in the overall approach to such patients. In addition, the functional demands placed on the prosthetic joint by the patient with rheumatoid arthritis (RA) will differ from the demands placed on the joint by the patient with osteoarthritis (OA). Finally, there are differences in the pathologic process itself; these differences are significant in respect to the stability of the bone–cement interface and the longevity of the prosthesis in the patient.

The knee is frequently involved in patients with long-standing rheumatoid arthritis. Although involved at the onset of disease in only 8 percent of patients[15] early in the course of the disease process, one or both knees will be involved in nearly 90 percent of patients.[15] Involvement is unilateral in 30 to 35 percent.[15] By comparison, the hip is involved early in the course of the disease in fewer than 10 percent, and fewer than 40 percent of patients with long-standing RA have hip involvement.[14,15,27]

THE PATIENT WITH RHEUMATOID ARTHRITIS

GENERAL CONSIDERATIONS

The patient with rheumatoid arthritis usually has involvement of multiple joints, each interfering with the function of the other joints. Whereas the patient with osteoarthritis may be well served by a knee arthroplasty that permits only limited flexion (because motion in the hip and ankle may partially compensate), the patient with rheumatoid arthritis must achieve maximal knee flexion. As there is often involvement of the upper extremities as well as the lower, rising from the seated position becomes a strenuous problem in the patient with limited knee flexion. To rise, one must either propel the center of gravity (centered in the second sacral vertebra) over the center of support (the foot placed on the floor) or flex the knee 105 degrees to place the center of support below the center of gravity. The alternative is to use the upper extremities to push the body into the upright position. The patient with rheumatoid ar-

697

thritis will rarely be able to propel the torso forward and use the first mechanism. Frequent involvement of the upper extremities makes the last mechanism both difficult and painful. For these reasons, it is highly desirable to achieve at least 105 degrees of flexion in patients undergoing knee arthroplasty for rheumatoid arthritis. The need for combined hip and knee flexion dictates that special attention be given to the choice of prosthetic design for both the knee and the hip, choosing designs that maximize the range of motion.

The patient will require crutches after knee surgery, so it is essential preoperatively to evaluate the ability of the patient to use some form of crutch support. If there is extensive involvement of the shoulder, elbow, or wrist, axillary crutches may not be appropriate. Forearm crutches will sometimes be a suitable alternative, particularly if involvement of the wrist or elbow makes the use of axillary crutches painful. Occasionally, it will be necessary to carry out arthrodesis of the wrist before surgery on the lower extremities so that the patient will be able to use forearm crutches during the postoperative period.[59]

PREOPERATIVE EVALUATION

The first consideration is whether a painful knee in a patient with rheumatoid arthritis requires surgery. If synovitis is the cause of the patient's pain and disability, continued medical management with drugs and physical modalities is appropriate. If medical management fails and the patient is disabled by synovial inflammation and effusion, synovectomy may be considered. Although surgical synovectomy has recently been challenged as an effective modality, in the eyes of most orthopedic surgeons, it still has a useful, if limited, role.[19] The recent development of radiation synovectomy offers promise that local temporary remission of chronic synovitis may be achieved by intra-articular administration of an appropriate radioactive isotope.[4,21,43]

If it can be determined that structural damage to the joint has occurred, it is unrealistic to expect that medication will be sufficient. A trial of anti-inflammatory medication and physical therapy is appropriate, particularly as the use of crutches may allow the acute disabling symptoms to subside to an acceptable level even in the presence of structural damage. If these measures fail and structural damage can be demonstrated on physical or radiographic examina-

tion, arthroplasty can be considered. In general, it is better to perform surgery on each joint as it becomes structurally destroyed instead of waiting until the patient has multiple destroyed joints requiring prolonged hospitalization, repeated anesthetics, and a series of debilitating surgical procedures.

General surgical risk should be assessed, especially from the point of view of the systemic manifestations of the rheumatic diseases. The patient should be in optimal medical condition and, when on steroids, should be on the lowest possible maintenance dose. Obvious sources of infection should be identified and eradicated to prevent postoperative hematogenous seeding of the surgical site. Carious teeth should be extracted before surgery is performed on the joints, and urinary tract infections should be identified and treated. Many female patients have asymptomatic bacteriuria, making urine culture before surgery mandatory. In male patients, prostatic hypertrophy, if severe, should be treated before surgery to avoid postoperative catheterization with its attendant risk of bacterial seeding and infection. It is useful to determine whether the patient is able to void in the supine position as a predictor of the need for postoperative catheterization. Frequently, preoperative practice at supine voiding will eliminate postoperative catheterization.

Most difficult to evaluate is the patient's motivation and ability to participate in the postoperative program. Patients should be evaluated by physical and occupational therapists, both to assess the patient's ability to participate in the program and to determine what special requirements are likely to present during the postoperative period. If multiple procedures are envisioned, it is often useful to perform a simple procedure first, so that the ability of the patient to follow the postoperative program can be assessed. If both hips and knees require surgery, the hip can be used for this assessment. The relief of pain and improvement in function following hip arthroplasty are essentially independent of the patient's cooperation, and the postoperative period is characterized by minimal pain. If the patient is unable to cooperate with a therapy program after hip replacement, it is unlikely that he or she will be able to participate in the postoperative program after a more painful knee arthroplasty, which requires a patient's full cooperation.

The patient with rheumatoid arthritis or its variants poses certain special problems that bear on the results and risks of surgery. Rheumatoid patients undergoing surgery average 10 years younger than patients with osteoarthritis undergoing similar procedures and are expected to live longer with their prosthetic joint.[50] This means that there will be more time for complications to appear, such as delayed infection, late loosening, and wear of the component parts. Much has been written of the increased susceptibility to infection in patients with rheumatoid arthritis; we have recently documented that the patient undergoing total knee replacement in rheumatoid arthritis does have a significantly increased risk of infection (2.7 times greater than that in the patient with osteoarthritis).[50]

PROBLEMS RELATED TO MEDICATION

Approximately 10 percent of patients coming to surgery at our institution are on maintenance steroids; this form of therapy has been shown in some studies to increase the risk of infection.[18] Aspirin, used by almost all patients, may produce difficulties with intraoperative and postoperative bleeding. Careful assessment of bleeding and clotting times is useful, but platelet transfusions are occasionally required.[16,48] Some patients are on chronic immunosuppressive treatment, and the effect of these drugs on postoperative infection must be considered. Although there is controversy regarding the relationship between penicillamine treatment and wound healing,[7,12,54] it is the opinion of most surgeons with experience in the field that wound healing in patients on penicillamine shows a definite delay. This effect may delay the postoperative rehabilitation program until satisfactory wound healing is achieved. In addition to this possible effect on wound healing, penicillamine shares with gold the possibility of producing renal damage resulting in proteinuria and occasionally producing a nephrotic syndrome.[28]

INTERACTION BETWEEN CARTILAGE AND SYNOVIUM

There is both clinical and laboratory evidence to suggest that the rheumatoid process is perpetuated in a given joint by the presence of articular cartilage.[10,47] Whether this is because of sequestered antigen–antibody complexes, the continued release of cartilage breakdown products producing synovial inflammation, or undiscovered factors is unclear. It has been a frequent observation, however, that patients undergoing total knee replacement in whom the patellar cartilage is retained will have involvement of the prosthetic joint in systemic flareups, whereas patients in whom all cartilage has been removed will not experience involvement of the prosthetic knee in such flares.

The quality of bone in patients with rheumatoid arthritis is frequently poor. This may be because of direct involvement of the subchondral trabecular bone by rheumatoid granulation tissue, related to the catabolic effects of chronic steroid use, the bone resorption resulting from excessive production of prostaglandins by rheumatoid synovium,[53] or an excess of parathyroidlike activity in these patients.[29,30] Regardless of the cause, the quality of bone is of great concern in regard to its ability to sustain the forces from the increased function expected after surgery.[35,36] Many prosthetic devices transfer high shear and rotational forces, in addition to the vertical joint reactive forces, directly to the bone–cement interface, which may be unable to withstand these forces over a long period of time. For this reason, it is desirable to use prosthetic devices that are the least constrained and that transfer forces away from the bone–cement interface into the more compliant and forgiving soft tissues.

SPECIFIC DISEASE-RELATED PROBLEMS

Psoriatic Arthritis.   Patients with psoriatic arthritis sometimes have involvement of the skin in the area of the proposed surgical incision. Several investigators report colonization of psoriatic skin with microorganisms and suggest an increased risk of infection after incision through such skin.[1,33,42] Although we have not observed this complication, it is desirable to clear up the skin at the operative site by appropriate local therapy before surgery.

Inflammatory Bowel Disease.   The arthropathies related to inflammatory bowel disease pose a special threat of postoperative infection because of possible late hematogenous seeding from a focus of infection in the bowel.

Systemic Lupus Erythematosus.   In association with osteonecrosis of the knee, SLE presents a very difficult problem for both the patient and the physician. The patients are often young and on large doses of steroids and may have a near-normal life expectancy when they develop osteonecrosis.[20] To implant a prosthetic joint in a young patient invites the long-term failures related to wear and loosening; to do so in a patient on long-term steroid therapy adds the further risk of infection. The presence of renal involvement in these patients may have implications in regard to their life expectancy. In the young patient with a limited life expectancy, prosthetic replacement may well be justified to relieve pain and improve the quality of life for the remaining years. On the other hand, in the patient with a normal life expectancy, there will almost certainly be late problems following joint replacement in the third and fourth decades. These patients often present with avascular necrosis of a femoral condyle with pain, deformity, and functional loss. It may be better to accept the lesser result produced by a high tibial or femoral osteotomy than to carry out knee replacement surgery with the high probability of eventual complication in these young patients.

Reiter's Syndrome, Ankylosing Spondylitis. Patients with Reiter's syndrome[8] as well as those with ankylosing spondylitis[9] have a significant incidence of cardiac involvement. Careful preoperative cardiac assessment should be carried out in such patients.

Juvenile Rheumatoid Arthritis. The patient with juvenile rheumatoid arthritis presents certain unique features that bear directly on the results to be expected from surgical intervention.[56,58] As in patients with ankylosing spondylitis, there appears to be a much greater involvement of the soft tissues surrounding the joint, with the result that the ultimate range of motion achieved after joint arthroplasty is less than would be predicted from the range achieved at surgery. After arthroplasty, there is a progressive loss of motion in these patients, and the effect of this loss on ultimate functional capacity must be anticipated. The young age at which patients with juvenile rheumatoid arthritis undergo arthroplasty exposes their prosthetic joints both to greater functional demands and to a longer period of exposure to late complications, such as infection and loosening.

On the positive side, it must be stated that patients with inflammatory arthritis do have some relative advantages in respect to joint replacement surgery; the goals are usually more limited and the patient will therefore place less stress on the prosthetic joint and on the bone–cement interface than would the more active patient with monarticular osteoarthritis. In addition, pain is usually the dominant consideration in the patient with rheumatoid arthritis undergoing knee surgery, and pain relief is remarkably predictable after arthroplasty.

THE KNEE

KINETICS OF THE NORMAL KNEE

MOTION

The knee joint achieves both flexion and rotation by low femorotibial conformity, especially in the lateral compartment, and by reduction in the sagittal radius of the femoral condyles from front to back. The ligaments and capsule are relatively inelastic and change their length very little during motion.[37,69] There is thus a preferred path of rotation, as flexion proceeds in synchrony with the resultant force and moment vectors of the muscles.[23,32] The relative conformity of the medial articulation and the nonconformity of the lateral compartment produce rotation about an axis centered toward the medial side of the joint.[32,64] Recent measurements in our laboratory on both specimens and normal subjects with the knee loaded showed that the medial condyle remained relatively stationary while the lateral condyle moved backward by about 17 mm as flexion proceeded from 0 to 120 degrees.[32] This produced a total external rotation of the tibia of some 20 degrees (Fig. 21.1). This combination of external rotation and rollback of the lateral femoral condyle permits flexion approaching 140 degrees. Without this mechanism, impingement of the posterior rim of the tibia and the soft tissues behind the knee would limit flexion to between 90 and 105 degrees.

STABILITY

The unloaded knee joint displays considerable laxity, particularly in rotation and anterior–posterior motion when there is no compressive load acting.[24,41,68] This laxity decreases progressively as compressive load is applied, but even at loads of three times body weight the laxity is still significant. In laboratory tests, the

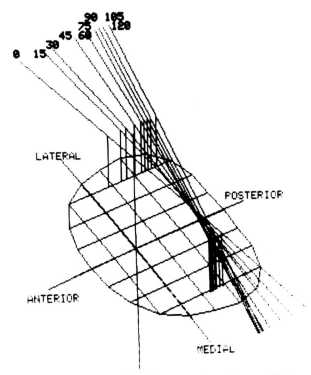

Fig. 21.1. Rotation of the femur on the tibia with flexion. The plane is the upper tibial surface. The transverse angled lines are the femoral axis through the centers of the medial and lateral condyles. The pivot point is close to the medial side.

more the joint is forced to move in a restricted path in one plane, the less are the laxities in other planes.[41,49] It therefore appears that laxity performs the very important function of attenuating the forces on the joint surfaces by permitting additional freedom of motion of the joint, transferring forces to the ligaments and muscles. There are clearly strong reasons for designing replacement joint surfaces that provide laxity characteristics similar to those of the normal knee.

Stability in the normal joint depends on a complex interaction of the muscles, the ligaments, and the joint surfaces. In most situations, force analysis shows that the knee is not stabilized by muscle action alone, but that certain force imbalances are borne by the ligaments and joint surfaces.

In the arthritic knee, the musculature is often weak, but the posterior cruciate ligament and the collateral ligaments are usually intact (although the latter may display a length imbalance). Assuming optimal alignment, it is axiomatic that the external forces and mo-

ments that are not stabilized by muscles are stabilized by the remaining ligaments and by the geometry of the prosthetic surfaces. The aims of joint replacement (other than replacement of the bearing surfaces) are to restore adequate stability and motion to the joint.

The mechanism of stability in a prosthetic joint is essentially an interaction between the geometry of the condylar surfaces and the remaining soft tissue structures. Assume a convex joint surface resting on a flat surface connected by a vertical and an angled ligament (Fig. 21.2A). If a horizontal force is applied, most of the stability is provided by the angled ligament because its elongation is far greater. Consider now partially conforming surfaces without any ligamentous connections (Fig. 21.2B). If a vertical compressive force is acting, and a horizontal force is now applied, stability will be reached when the slope at the point of contact enables the reaction force to balance the resultant of the vertical and horizontal forces. The third case (Fig. 21.2C) is a combination of the two previous cases; stability is produced by a combination of the angled ligament, the joint surfaces, and to a small extent the vertical ligament. It must be realized that ligamentous forces also act to compress the joint surfaces, contributing to stability from the surfaces themselves.

Mediolateral Translation

The femorotibial force in this direction was calculated at 0.2 body weight,[44,45] but Nissan[46] puts it as up to 2.5 times this. In any case, the force will be borne primarily by the intercondylar eminence.[41] The excessive translation that can result from the absence of such an eminence on a prosthesis has been demonstrated.[13] Another function of the eminence is to provide a pivot for varus–valgus angulation.

Anteroposterior Translation

Nissan[46] calculated forces in level walking of up to 200 newtons forward force on the femur relative to the tibia and 100 newtons in the other direction; these forces translated into 400 newtons and 200 newtons in the posterior and anterior cruciates, respectively. However, walking upstairs and up a ramp gave as much as 1,200 newtons and 500 newtons, respectively, in the posterior cruciate.[45] In stooping, the anterior shear force of the femur on the tibia was

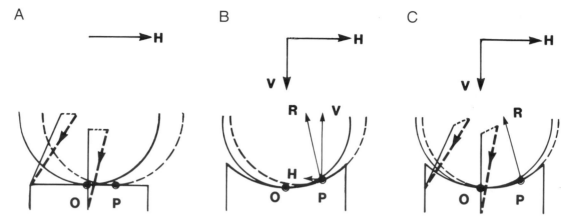

A   **B**   **C**

Fig. 21.2. Mechanisms of stability to a horizontal force. (A) Stability is first from the angled ligament, second from the vertical ligament. The joint surfaces provide no stability. (B) Stability is entirely from the partially conforming surfaces. (C) Stability is from the surfaces, the angled ligaments, and the vertical ligament.

calculated at 1.3 body weight, giving about twice that force in the posterior cruciate.[57] The high shear force was confirmed in another study.[11] Apparently the highest demands are placed on the posterior cruciate, hence in a prosthesis these forces must be stabilized in some way by a retained posterior cruciate, by the conformity of the bearing surfaces, or by both. For a conforming geometry, the surfaces carry all the forces, and stability is unaffected by the presence or absence of the cruciates.[40] In a partially confirming geometry, it is difficult to arrange for a sharing of the force except toward extension (Fig. 21.3). If there is close conformity in extension, most of the force will be carried by the condylar surfaces. As flexion proceeds, however, the smaller radius of the posterior femoral condyles comes into play concurrent with a rollback

of the contact point. The amount of rollback in replacements in which the posterior cruciate has been preserved is generally in the range of 5 to 10 mm. In this situation, the condyles will offer little stability. In the region toward extension, calculations were made of the percentages of the anterior force carried by the cruciate and the condylar surfaces.[65] The governing factor was the difference between the femoral and tibial sagittal radii of curvature. For complete femorotibial conformity, the cruciate carried 0 percent; for a difference in radius of 5 mm, it was 20 percent, while for 10-mm difference in radius, the posterior cruciate carried more than 30 percent. This analysis was broadly confirmed in tests of force transmission in prosthetic components of different curvatures, with and without the posterior cruciate ligament.[62] The

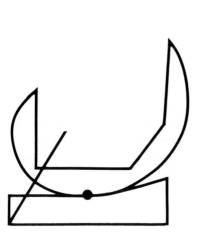
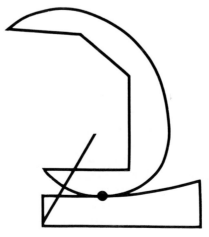

Fig. 21.3. Femoral rollback is mainly caused by the posterior cruciate but relies on a flat tibial surface.

shear force transmitted to the tibial interface was always higher without the posterior cruciate, but the difference decreased with increasing weight-bearing.

Further aspects that would affect the force distribution are stiffness of the ligament, tightness after prosthetic insertion, and variation in tightness in the range of flexion attributable to prosthetic geometry and position. This association was clearly shown by Markolf et al.,[40] in stability tests before and after insertion of knee prostheses, and by Lewis et al.,[37] who showed variations in cruciate ligament tensions with different prosthetic designs. Such considerations explain the practical difficulty in retaining both cruciate ligaments. To achieve effective functioning of both throughout the range would require accuracy of placement and design to within an estimated 2 mm of the optimum.

Varus–Valgus Angulation

During normal activities, such as walking, a few degrees of varus–valgus motion occurs. This will be caused by the general flexibility of the menisci and cartilage surfaces, to the sliding of the femoral condyles on the changing slope of the tibial surfaces, and in extreme cases, to lift off on one side.[41] Since the rheumatoid patient is susceptible to valgus deformity, the greatest resistance to valgus tilting is an advantage. A prosthesis with a broad base of contact and preservation of one or both cruciate ligaments will assist the prime stabilizer, the medial collateral ligament.

Rotation About the Tibial Axis

Several in vivo studies have recorded rotations in the range of 10 to 20 degrees occurring during normal activities. Recent work[32] has shown that this transverse rotation occurs by rolling backward of the lateral femoral condyle, with the medial condyle being stationary or even moving forward (Fig. 21.1). Such a path of rotation occurs during loaded activities, such as walking and stair climbing. However, in vitro studies have shown the considerable laxity that occurs in response to applied torque at all angles of flexion. The rotational laxity in full extension is small, constrained by tense collateral and cruciate ligaments combined with conformity of the joint surfaces and the menisci. However, in flexion, there is consider-

able rotational laxity, primarily because of the loss of conformity of the joint surfaces. This is demonstrated by reduction in laxity of about 25 percent when compressive load is applied.[41] Hence, it appears that laxity in rotation, particularly in flexion, will allow the knee to accommodate readily to different activity patterns by adjusting its rotational path.[3] Prosthetic geometry that prevents laxity and that is even more restrictive in load-bearing will not provide these characteristics and will transfer loads to the bone–cement interface.

POSTERIOR CRUCIATE LIGAMENT

From the above discussion, it is evident that the posterior cruciate ligament is involved in both passive attenuation of knee forces and in actively controlling knee motion.

As the knee flexes, the eccentric position of the posterior cruciate ligament femoral origin produces a tensile force in the ligament. Because of the nonconforming, low-friction articulation, this tensile force is converted into a translatory force, shifting the tibia forward (or forcing the femur to roll back). This rollback produces two major effects, that is, posterior clearance is increased, permitting greater flexion without impingement, and the moment arm of the quadriceps is increased by 20 to 30 percent (Fig. 21.4).

Total knee designs that provide congruent articular surfaces with essentially uniaxial flexion will therefore permit less flexion arc[2,3] and produce a quadriceps force that is demonstrably weaker[50,51] (M. Soudry, P.S. Walker, and C.B. Sledge, unpublished work) (Figs. 21.5 and 21.6). Posterior cruciate function may be built into the prosthesis by an appropriately shaped intercondylar tibial eminence articulating in flexion with the femoral component. This design maximizes flexion and quadriceps power but transfers shear forces normally absorbed by the posterior cruciate ligament to the bone–cement interface.

Is the posterior cruciate ligament involved by rheumatoid inflammatory tissue? If so, it would be common to find the posterior cruciate absent or scarred and shortened from such involvement. Such is not the case. In juvenile rheumatoid arthritis with longstanding flexion deformity of severe degree, the posterior cruciate ligament and posterior capsule are often shortened and must be resected to correct the flexion

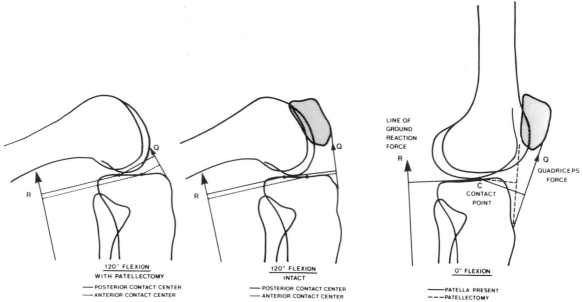

Fig. 21.4. The location of the femoral–tibial contact point in the AP direction has a considerable effect on the force requirements in the quadriceps. Shown are representative positions of the knee in extension and flexion, with the typical direction of the foot-to-ground force R indicated. The quadriceps force Q can then be calculated in terms of R. In extension, the contact points are anterior, whether or not the posterior cruciate is retained. With the patella present, $Q = 1.2R$, and with a patellectomy, $Q = 1.6R$. In this case, the absence of the patella does not drastically increase the demands on the quadriceps. In flexion, the situation is quite different. If the posterior cruciate is present, the contact point is posterior, but if it is absent, the contact point is more anterior. The values of Q are $1.6 \times R$ for the posterior and anterior contact, respectively, a more than twofold difference. In case of a patellectomy, the values are $2.0 \times R$ and $4.9 \times R$. In this case in particular, the posterior contact point is a great advantage, for with anterior contact the quadriceps would have difficulty in generating sufficient force.

deformity. In that situation, it is necessary to use a cruciate-substituting prosthesis. In adult-onset rheumatoid arthritis, however, deformity or absence of the ligament is exceedingly rare. Indeed, in more than 2,000 total knee arthroplasties done in our unit the ligament has been absent or severely attenuated only three times and contracted enough to produce a flexion deformity in three additional patients. Thus, in only six cases out of 2,000 has a cruciate-substituting device been necessary.

STRENGTH OF TRABECULAR BONE AND ITS INFLUENCE ON DESIGN AND TECHNIQUE

The trabecular bone in rheumatoid arthritis is generally weaker and more porous and contains more cystic areas than does normal bone. The compressive strength of trabecular bone in the proximal tibia varies between 11 and 260 percent of normal,[6] the higher values being for sclerotic bone on the lateral plateau in patients with valgus deformity. Lereim et al.[35,36] found that the subchondral bone on the medial plateau demonstrated about one-half the hardness of normal subchondral bone. We have examined cross sections of the proximal tibia in specimens of normal and rheumatoid bone. The area of bony trabeculae cross sections, ranked on a 0 to 100 scale, ranged from 5 to 50 in rheumatoid bone, compared with 20 to 40 in normal bone. The limited data available therefore suggest that some portions of the bone in RA are much weaker than normal. It might be considered that such bone would be inadequate for normal load-bearing, but presumably the limited usage and light weight of most patients with RA prevent excessive failure of the bone.

After prosthetic replacement, it is expected that the activity level will increase significantly. Given the deficiencies in the properties of rheumatoid trabecu-

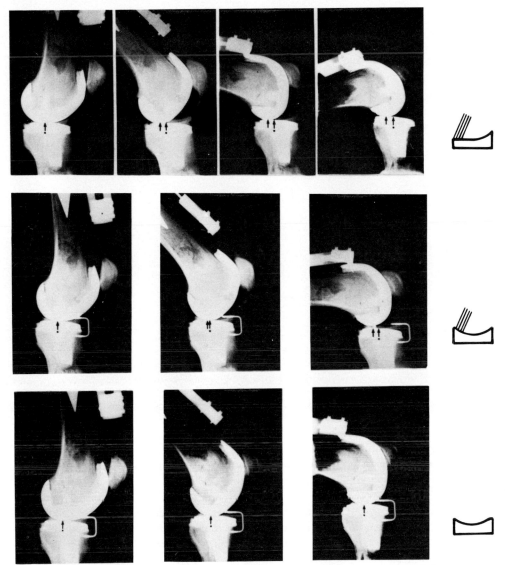

Fig. 21.5. In vitro demonstration of the interaction between tibial geometry and the posterior cruciate ligament. A cadaver specimen was fitted with a total knee prosthesis in which the tibial plastic piece could be changed or the posterior cruciate ligament excised, or both, as diagrammed in the right margin. Radiographs in varying degrees of flexion are illustrated. Arrows locate the contact point between the components. The center of the tibial component is indicated by a dot. (A) The posterior cruciate ligament (PCL) has been retained, and the tibial plastic is flat posteriorily. As flexion progresses to 105 degrees, the contact point rolls back approximately 9 mm. (B) The PCL is again retained, but here the tibial component is conforming. Rollback of the contact point is limited by the upward slope of the tibial component posteriorly. (C) In the absence of the PCL and with conforming geometry, rollback is absent, thereby limiting flexion and quadriceps strength and transferring load to the interfaces. (Experiment conducted by M. Soudry and P.S. Walker.)

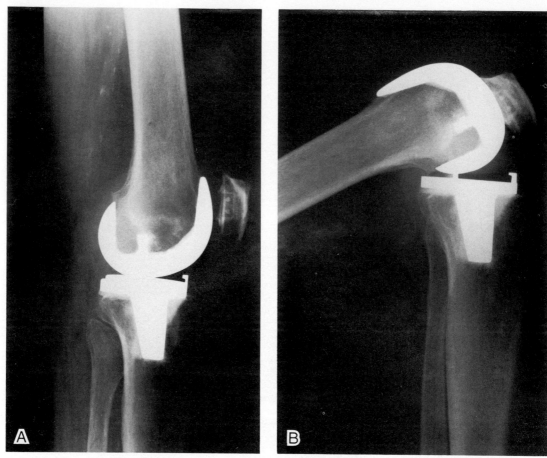

Fig. 21.6. Lateral radiographs of a patient with a flat tibial surface posteriorly and retained postcruciate ligament. (A) In extension, the contact point between the femur and the tibia is about midway back on the tibial surface. (B) In full flexion, the contact point has moved posterially about 10 mm.

lar bone, it is particularly important that the stresses of the implant–bone interface be minimized. The design of the prosthetic components will have a direct effect on the durability of fixation. The excessive loosening rates of the geometric design, with its high conformity and similarly high loosening rates with the thin plastic modular tibial components, is well known.

Various types of tibial components were compared in a laboratory study by subjecting them to a sequence of loads and moments and measuring the component-to-bone movements.[51,66,67] Modular components deflected the most, whereas the best performance overall was demonstrated by one-piece metal-backed components with one or two fixation pegs and with or without a posterior cruciate cut-out. Two finite element studies have generated support of this

view.[5,38] Calculations were made of the interface stresses for different components. Metal trays generally distributed the forces better and reduced the maximum compressive stresses on the underlying cancellous bone compared with the all-plastic components. The only disadvantage of the metal tray was that with extreme eccentric loading, a small tensile interface stress was developed at the side opposite the load.

Plastic pegs carry only a few percentages of the compressive load, but metal pegs carry about 25 percent.[5] This was confirmed experimentally by Reilly et al.,[51] who showed that the bending resistance of metal pegs was substantial, in contrast with plastic pegs, which were ineffective. These features of a metal tray, with reduction in compressive stresses on cancellous bone attributable to better stress distribution and load carrying by the central peg, are seen as advantages in the weak rheumatoid bone which is relatively unstressed before arthroplasty but which will become more stressed as the patient resumes a more active life-style after joint replacement.[66]

Another aspect of tibial fixation that is often overlooked is the percentage of area of the tibial surface that is covered by the component. Clinical failures where an undersized component has gradually subsided into the bone are not uncommon. Complete coverage has been shown to reduce the component–bone movement considerable for a variety of load conditions.[66]

Fixation of the femoral component has been studied relatively little, probably because of a lower incidence of recognized loosening. However, principles similar to those discussed for the tibial side will apply. A metallic component for better stress distribution and maximum area of coverage are two important aspects. The areas that generally give the highest incidence of interface failure are the patellar flange and the posterior condyles. It is important to note that these areas of poor cement intrusion at surgery also have a high shear stress when loaded during walking. Fixation as a whole is preserved by the distal surface, as well as by the fixation pegs. The usefulness of a central fixation stem has not been demonstrated but is often empirically chosen in rheumatoid patients in whom the quality of femoral cancellous bone is found to be particularly poor or during revision in which a large portion of the cancellous bone must be destroyed during the surgical procedure.

CEMENT TECHNIQUE

As was stated earlier, the porosity of rheumatoid trabecular bone is generally greater than that of normal bone, except in cases of lateral sclerosis. The more porous the bone, the easier it will be to clean using the standard techniques of suction and lavage. If the cement is applied under comparable conditions, the cement penetration will be greater in the less dense bone. This will reduce the amount of micromotion between the cement and the bone and will enhance the strength of the bond.

Regarding the interface strength, such factors as compression, shear, and tensile stresses must be con-

sidered, since these occur in physiologic loading conditions. Figure 21.7A shows an example of trabecular bone of average density in which the acrylic cement has barely penetrated the matrix. Many of the trabecular ends are not held at all by the cement, while only the tips of others are encased. When a shear force is applied, cement–bone micromotion will occur at the tips, while the high bending stresses in other trabeculae will lead to resorption or fracture; tensile forces will clearly lead to micromotion at the interface. In the example shown in Figure 21.7B, showing penetration of a few millimeters, the trabecular ends are firmly held, and the stiffness and resistance to compression, shear, and tension will be greatly enhanced.

Measurements of bond strength show the significance of penetration depth. Using trabecular bone from the knee, Krause et al.[31] obtained tensile strengths ranging from 2.5 to 8 mPa, with the higher values for more thorough bone cleaning and greater depth of penetration. Shear strength values increased from 9 to 40 mPa at the original cut surface. However, the interface at the limit of penetration is much weaker, with strength of about one-third of these values.[22] Since failures will occur at the limit of penetration, and the bone is weaker at these lower levels, the bone strength will be lower for excessive penetration. Concurrently, if failure does occur farther into the bone, much more bone has been lost for a revision. The viability of the bone encased in cement must also be questioned, as well as the weakening effect of the trabeculae on the cement mantle. Huiskes and Slooff[25] showed that heat necrosis will almost certainly occur for penetration of $\geq$ 5 mm.

It thus appears, taking all factors into consideration, that the ideal penetration depth is 3 to 5 mm, which would effectively bond to many cross-struts of the bone as well as to the verticals. The aim of the surgical technique should be to meter the correct viscosity of cement and apply sufficient pressure to force it uniformly into the bone to the ideal depth.

SURGICAL TECHNIQUE FOR POSTERIOR CRUCIATE RETENTION

Several aspects of technique assume greater significance in replacement of the rheumatoid knee. There is often a valgus–external rotation deformity requiring

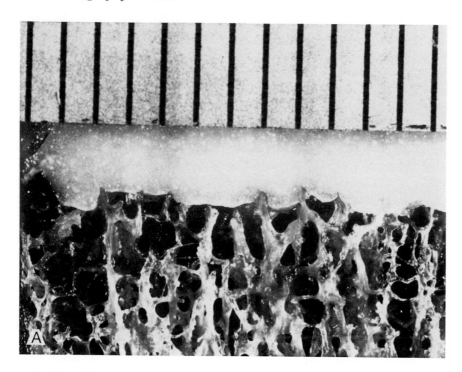

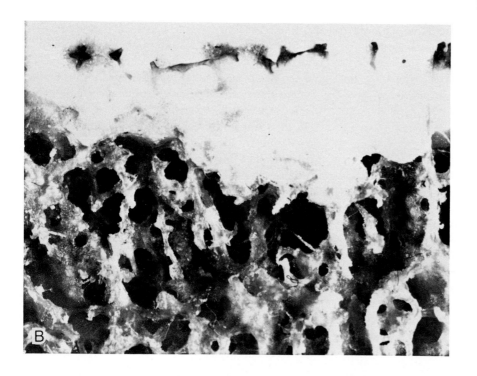

Fig. 21.7. (A) Trabecular bone of average density with little cement penetration. (B) Trabecular bone with ideal penetration after surface cleaning and pressurization of the cement.

release of the popliteus and lateral structures. The cancellous bone is often extremely weak, requiring special precautions to spare the bone–prosthesis interface; these precautions include minimal tibial resection to avoid weaker distal bone, maximum coverage of the exposed cancellous surface of the tibia by the component, filling of the subchondral cysts with bone graft or methylmethacrylate, and the use of stemmed components to distribute forces over the largest available area. The use of minimally constrained prostheses that preserve the posterior cruciate function further protects the interface between the weak bone and the prosthesis.

The tibial surface should be resected first to minimize tibial resection. This cut should be precisely parallel to the long axis of the tibia and just deep enough into the substance of the subchondral bone to provide an appropriate porous interface for interdigitation of cement. The posterior cruciate ligament inserts on the posterior aspect of the tibia behind and distal to the tibial intercondylar spines. It is therefore possible to resect the entire upper tibia without injuring the ligament, but it is usually desirable to leave a small square of posterior intercondylar eminence about 1 cm in width to ensure that the ligament is not damaged by the saw during tibial resection. Once the upper tibia has been resected, ligament balance can be assessed with the knee in extension and in flexion. The access provided by carrying out tibial resection before ligament release facilitates the latter, while failure to perform ligament release before femoral resection leads to excessive bone resection of the femur and the possibility of persistent imbalance. Tension in the collateral ligaments can be assessed by a number of different techniques, but the aim is to restore 7 to 9 degrees of valgus between the long axis of the femur and the long axis of the tibia with both medial and lateral collateral ligaments under equal tension and with the prosthetic components in proper static alignment. The techniques of carrying out this balance have been well described by Insall[26] and by Freeman et al.[17]

It is also important to restore ligamentous balance with the knee flexed to 90 degrees to provide uniform distribution of stress to both collaterals and the posterior cruciate ligament and to avoid rotational deformities in the femoral cut. As the posterior aspect of the femoral articular surface is rarely destroyed

with RA, the gap between the posterior femoral condyle and the resected upper surface of the tibia should be uniform, both medially and laterally. If not, tight structures should be released until the tension in medial, lateral, and posterior cruciate ligaments is equal with the knee flexed to 90 degrees, upward distraction on the femur, and distal traction on the tibia. If this is accomplished, the knee will be stable in flexion and will not have rotary instability in spite of the flattened contours of the posterior aspect of the tibial component. Failure to restore proper tension in the posterior cruciate ligament, on the other hand, will result in rotary instability of the knee with the possibility of rotary subluxation of the femoral component off the back of the tibial component.

Once the ligaments are balanced in both extension and flexion, the posterior femoral cut is made after marking the appropriate amount of resection with the ligaments under tension. The anterior femoral cut is made to accept the largest possible femoral component, taking care to avoid notching the anterior femoral cortex.

In similar fashion, the distal femur is marked for resection with the knee extended, the collateral ligaments manually tensioned, and valgus alignment maintained. Particular attention should be paid to the fit between the posterior femur and the condylar portion of the femoral prosthesis. Since it is difficult to apply cement to this interface, if there is not a close fit posterior forces in flexion will be resisted only by the cement between the distal femur and the prosthesis, which resists shear forces poorly.

The patella is routinely resurfaced in patients with rheumatoid arthritis. There is strong clinical and laboratory evidence that articular cartilage in the rheumatoid joint perpetuates the inflammatory response of the synovium.[10,47] With all cartilage excised, the inflamed synovium becomes quiescent. It is not necessary to perform a synovectomy at the time of knee replacement if all cartilage is removed. Furthermore, with the cartilage removed, the operated joint will not become involved in subsequent flares of rheumatoid activity. Conversely, a knee with the patellar cartilage retained may continue to be mildly inflamed and may participate in flares of inflammatory activity with the possibility of progressive destruction of the remaining patellar cartilage and the possibility of resorption at the bone–cement interface.

Lateral release is often necessary in the rheumatoid knee to correct the valgus and external rotation deformity and to improve patellar tracking. Because of the poor quality of the skin in many of these patients, we prefer to carry out all releases from within the joint, avoiding second incisions and large subcutaneous flaps. With the patella everted, the lateral synovium and capsule are incised vertically about 2 to 3 cm posterior to the lateral patellar border. This exposes the iliotibial band, which can be incised in the same vertical direction. The incision is carried distally to the tibia just behind Gerdy's tubercle, then curved anteriorly to detach the iliotibial band from the tubercle. Proximally the posterior margin of the vastus lateralis is defined and swept anteriorly off the lateral intermuscular septum. The superior lateral geniculate artery is carefully identified and preserved. With the artery retracted out of the way, the incision in the iliotibial band is carried proximally with scissors. If necessary, the vastus lateralis can be elevated from its distal femoral origin along the lateral intermuscular septum. The remaining intact portion of the iliotibial tract is the posterior band behind the vertical incision. If necessary, this remaining portion can be cut transversely proximal to the joint line. If the valgus deformity is still uncorrected, the popliteus muscle and lateral collateral ligament are detached from their femoral origin with a thin sliver of bone. This step is rarely necessary if the iliotibial tract is sectioned as described above, but detachment of the popliteus tendon often facilitates correction of the external rotation deformity of the tibia.

The adequacy of the vertical component of the lateral release is tested by assessment of patellar tracking. The patellar prosthesis should track in the groove of the femoral component easily and smoothly with no tendency to lateral dislocation. Tracking should be assessed before the capsule is closed, and the patella should remain in the groove during flexion without manual force.

In knees with varus deformity, the medial collateral ligament is lengthened in three stages: first, the deep fibers are excised from the tibial insertion; next, the arcuate capsular fibers immediately posterior to the tibial collateral ligament are detached from the medial and posterior rim of the tibia; and finally, if the deformity is not fully corrected, the superficial fibers of the medial collateral ligament are elevated from

their tibial insertion under the pes anserinus using a curved $\frac{1}{2}$-inch osteotome as an elevator. Correction must be tested repeatedly after each step in the release to avoid overcorrection and medial instability.

Although the steps in bony resection and soft tissue release are described separately, the preferred sequence is to resect the proximal tibia first, since that cut is independent of deformity and ligament release and provides access to the capsule and collateral ligaments, improving exposure of the distal femur. Using the flat upper tibial surface of the resected tibia as a benchmark, ligamentous imbalance can be corrected before femoral resections are done.

After completion of bone resection and ligament release, trial components are inserted to test alignment, proper tension of collateral and posterior cruciate ligaments, tracking of the patella, and the range of flexion and femoral rollback. If the components are too tight in flexion, binding may occur or the components may rock. If this happens, a thinner tibial component should be used, or an additional 1 or 2 mm of tibia should be resected. If the sequence of steps outlined above has been followed, this additional tibial resection will not produce excessive laxity in extension. Rather, the slight flexion deformity that usually accompanies excessive tightness in flexion will be corrected. The components should not rock during flexion and extension before cementing. If they do, there is persistent ligamentous imbalance, which should be corrected. The sole purpose of the technique described here is to minimize shear stress at the bone–cement interface. Ligament imbalance demonstrated by the rocking of the uncemented components will produce undesirable forces on the interface and on the weak trabecular bone.

Before cementing the components in place, the tourniquet should be deflated to secure careful hemostasis. This is most easily done before the components fill the resection gap and obscure access to the posterior capsule, lateral gutter, and other bleeding sources. After the tourniquet is reinflated, the cancellous bone surfaces are cleaned with pulsating saline lavage, followed by aspiration of water and fat with suction.

To ensure adequate cement penetration, we prefer to insert both the femoral and tibial components simultaneously, so that the knee can be extended to achieve pressurization of cement. The use of pressure-sensitive film inserted between the components during this maneuver has demonstrated that nearly 1,000 newtons of force are generated on average—far greater than that possible with manual pressure alone. It is not necessary to cement the femoral component at the same time as the tibial to achieve this effect. The femoral component can be inserted without cement, used to pressurize the tibial fixation, then removed to facilitate removal of excess cement behind the tibial component after polymerization. The femur and patella can then be fixed simultaneously with a second mix of methylmethacrylate.

After capsular closure, the knee should be flexed 105 to 110 degrees to ensure adequacy of the closure and proper patellar tracking and to demonstrate that postoperative physical therapy will not compromise the capsular closure. Careful subcutaneous closure with absorbable No. 3-0 sutures is followed by skin closure with continuous No. 4-0 subcuticular nylon. The avoidance of skin sutures prevents the common stitch abscesses that may lead to deep infection.

The extremity is loosely wrapped in a bulky dressing and elastic bandage. Immobilization is provided by a commercial knee immobilizing splint. Prophylactic antibiotics, begun just before induction of anesthesia, are continued for 48 hours. Suction drainage tubes are removed at 24 hours, and at 48 hours the dressing is removed and gentle physical therapy begun. This consists of quadriceps sets, assisted straight leg raising, and side lying active assisted flexion and extension. By day 4 or 5, independent straight leg raising should be achieved. The patient is then allowed to sit on the edge of the bed with the operated knee flexed. Walking with two crutches is begun when the patient obtains 60 degrees of knee flexion and demonstrates muscular control of the extremity. Seventy degrees of flexion should be reached by day 10, and bicycle exercises should be begun at that point. Ninety degrees of flexion should be achieved before discharge on day 14. If 90 degrees is not reached by that time, manipulation under anesthesia is carried out (necessary in fewer than 10 percent of patients). Patients are usually discharged from the hospital by day 14 to 18, walking independently on two crutches. Crutches are continued for 1 month while the patient carries out a formal program of exercises at home, including the use of a stationary bicycle. If these measures are effective in producing adequate motion

and muscular strength at the 6-week follow-up, a single crutch can be used until all support is removed at 3 months.

RESULTS

The goals of surgery are to eliminate pain, provide an adequate range of motion, and restore function with minimal risk. The prosthetic design and surgical technique are chosen to minimize the early risks of infection and delayed wound healing and the late risks of loosening, patellar pain, and component failure.

During the past decade, our group has carried out more than 2,000 metal to plastic knee replacements using these principles. Three careful reviews involving nearly 800 knees having a minimum follow-up of 2 years have been carried out (Table 21.1). Analysis of these series will permit some conclusions about the immediate success of the procedure. An analysis of the radiographs for evidence of progressive loosening will permit some prediction of future problems.

The series of 135 knees reported in 1978[61] involved the duocondylar design in which the patellofemoral joint was ignored. Because of dissatisfaction with that aspect of the design, the duopatellar design was used from 1979 until 1980. With this prosthesis, a flange was provided to resurface the patellar groove of the femur. The option was available to resurface the patella with a polyethylene button, and this option was used approximately 50 percent of the time.[60] An analysis of 747 such replacements was presented in 1979 and published in 1980.[63] At that time, 563 knees were evaluated at a minimum follow-up of 2 years. The duopatellar design used in that series had separate tibial components that were felt to provide less than

Table 21.1. Robert B. Brigham Hospital (RBBH) Total Knee Experience, 1973–1981

	OA (%)	RA (%)	Total
Duocondylar (1978)	28(21)	107(79)	135
Duopatella (1979)[a]	166(29)	397(71)	563
Duopatella (1981)[b]	45(45)	55(55)	100
	239(30)	559(70)	798

Abbreviations: OA, osteoarthritis; RA, rheumatoid arthritis; RBBH,
[a]Two-piece plastic tibia.
[b]One-piece plastic tibia.

Table 21.2. Pain Relief

	No Pain (%)
Duocondylar	83
Duopatella (1979)	94[a]
Duopatella (1981)	95

[a]Ninety-five percent in rheumatoid arthritis, 92 percent in osteoarthritis.

Table 21.3. Range of Motion

	Degrees
Duocondylar	106
Duopatella (1979)	105
Duopatella (1981)	106

ideal tibial fixation.[51] In 1978 we adopted the use of a single plastic tibial component with a short intramedullary stem. This design was the subject of a third series, reported in 1981.[39]

As relief of pain is an important goal of knee replacement, it is gratifying to see that more than 92 percent of patients denied any knee pain at follow-up (Table 21.2).

The importance of achieving 105 degrees of knee flexion in patients with rheumatoid arthritis has been stressed. The average range of motion achieved in these three series was 106, 105, and 106 degrees (Table 21.3); 70 percent of the patients in these series had rheumatoid arthritis.

Function is the result of a complex interaction involving the patient, his or her disease, involvement of other joints, and the operation itself. These interactions are difficult to assess in an objective manner, but numerous tools are available that give an indication of functional result.[52] Table 21.4 shows the overall functional results achieved in all three series of knee replacements at our institution. Only clear successes and clear failures are listed: the ambiguous category of "fair" has been omitted to emphasize the increasing percentage of clearly good results from 67 to 92 percent and the decreasing percentage of clear failures from 14 to 2 percent.

To provide some indication of what the future might bring to these patients in a longer follow-up, a careful analysis of the radiographs has been carried out (Table 21.5). The presence of a radiolucent line at the bone–cement interface was recorded with its thickness and extent. Lines of > 1-mm thickness were

called severe and thought to be of some prognostic significance with respect to future loosening. In all three series, such lines are found in 3 to 4 percent of operated knees. Mild radiolucent lines (< 1 mm and involving only portions of any component interface) have not been progressive and do not appear to predict eventual loosening; they may indeed be more indicative of bone preparation and cement technique. In the most recent series, such lines were seen in 24 percent of knees.[55]

One unequivocal measure of failure is a revision operation. Table 21.6 lists revisions for component loosening, patellar pain, and infection in the three series. Loosening has resulted in revision in 1.3 percent of knees, patellofemoral pain in 1.8 percent, and sepsis in 0.4 percent. The failure rate in all three categories appears to be declining with modifications of design and surgical technique.

It is interesting to compare patients with rheumatoid arthritis with those with osteoarthritis. Table 21.7 examines the categories of pain relief, unsupported stair climbing, and radiographic evidence of severe

Table 21.4. Overall Functional Results

	N	Good–Excellent (%)	Unsatisfactory (%)
Duocondylar	135	67	14
Duopatella	563	85	5
Duopatella	100	92	2

Table 21.5. Radiolucent Lines

	Severe (> 1 mm) (%)	Mild (%)
Duocondylar	4	22
Duopatella (1979)	3	40
Duopatella (1981)	3	24

Table 21.6. Revision

	N	Loosening	Patello-femoral Pain	Sepsis
Duocondylar	135	3	2	0
Duopatella (1979)	563	7	10	3
Duopatella (1981)	100	0	2	0
	798	10 (1.3%)	14 (1.8%)	3 (0.4%)

Table 21.7. Comparison of RA and OA

	OA (%)	RA (%)
Pain-free	92	95
Stairs without support	90	80
Severe radiolucent lines	3.6	2.5

Abbreviations: OA, osteoarthritis; RA, rheumatoid arthritis.

radiolucent lines in these two groups. In all categories, save climbing stairs without support, in which involvement of other joints is probably the major deterrent, the patient with rheumatoid arthritis fares quite well. The infrequency of severe radiolucent lines in these patients with poor bone structure who nonetheless return to active function suggests that the concepts of component design, ligament balance, static alignment of implant placement, cement technique, and preservation of the posterior cruciate ligament are correct principles and provide excellent, durable results in patients with rheumatoid arthritis. Comparison with other series of knee replacement in rheumatoid arthritis in which more constrained or cruciate-sacrificing prostheses have been used suggests that the principles enumerated here are correct, although longer follow-up is necessary to demonstrate this effect unequivocally.[34,55]

REFERENCES

1. Aly, R., Maibach, H.E., and Mandel, A.: Bacterial flora in psoriasis. Br. J. Dermatol., 95: 603, 1976.
2. Andriacchi, T.P., Galante, J.O., and Fermier, R.W.: The influence of total knee replacement design on walking and stairclimbing. J. Bone Joint Surg., [Am.], 64: 1328, 1982.
3. Andriacchi, T.P., Andersson, G.B.J., Fermier, R.W., et al.: A study of lower limb mechanics during stairclimbing. J. Bone Joint Surg. [Am.], 62: 749, 1980.
4. Ansell, B.M., Crook, A., Mallard, J.R., et al.: Evaluation of intra-articular colloidal gold Au 198 in the treatment of persistent knee effusions. Ann. Rheum. Dis., 22: 435, 1963.
5. Bartel, D.L., Burstein, A.H., Santavicca, E.A., et al.: Performance of the tibial component in total knee replacement (conventional and revision designs). J. Bone Joint Surg., [Am.], 64: 1026, 1982.
6. Behrens, J.C., Walker, P.S., and Shoji, H.: Variations in strength and structure of cancellous bone at the knee. J. Biomech., 7: 201, 1974.
7. Burry, H.C.: Penicillamine and wound healing—a potential hazard? Postgrad. Med. J., 50(Suppl.) 2: 75, 1974.
8. Calin, A.: Reiter's syndrome. P. 1033. In Kelley, W.N., Harris, E.D., Jr., Ruddy, S., and Sledge, C.B., Eds.: Textbook of Rheumatology. Vol. II. Philadelphia, W.B. Saunders, 1981.
9. Calin, A.: Ankylosing spondylitis. P. 1017. In Kelley, W.N., Harris, E.D., Jr., Ruddy, S., and Sledge, C.B., Eds.: Textbook of Rheumatology. Vol. II. Philadelphia, W.B. Saunders, 1981.
10. Cooke, T.D., Richer, S., and Hurd, E. et al.: Localization of antigen-antibody complexes in intra-articular collagenous tissues. Ann. N.Y. Acad. Sci., 256: 10, 1975.
11. Dalquist, N.J., Mayo, P., and Seedhorn, B.B.: Forces during squatting and rising from a deep squat. Eng. Med., 11: 69, 1982.
12. Deshmukh, K., and Nimni, M.E.: A defect in the intra- intermolecular cross-linking of collagen caused by penicillamine. J. Biol. Chem., 244: 1787, 1969.
13. Ewald, F.C., Scott, R.D., Thomas, W.H., et al.: The importance of intercondylar stability in knee arthroplasty: Comparison of McKeever, modular and duocondylar types. In proceedings J. Bone Joint Surg. [Am.], 57: 1033, 1975.
14. Fleming, A., Crown, J.M., and Corbett, M.: Early rheumatoid disease. I. Onset. Ann. Rheum. Dis., 35: 357, 1976.
15. Fleming, A., Benn, R.T., Corbett, M., et al.: Early rheumatoid disease. II. Patterns of joint involvement. Ann. Rheum. Dis., 35: 361, 1976.
16. Foker, J.E., Schwartz, R., Smith, D.C., et al.: Surgical problems in immunodeficient and immunosuppressed children. Surg. Clin. North Am., 59(2): 213, 1979.
17. Freeman, M.A.R., and Insall, J.: Tibio-femoral replacement using two un-linked components and cruciate resection. (The ICLH and total condylar prostheses.) p. 254. In Freeman, M.A.R., Ed.: Arthritis of the Knee—Clinical Features and Surgical Management. Berlin, Springer-Verlag, 1980.
18. Garner, R.W., Mowat, A.G., and Hazleman, B.L.: Wound healing after operations on patients with rheumatoid arthritis. J. Bone Joint Surg. [Br.], 55: 134, 1973.
19. Gschwend, N.: Synovectomy. p. 1874. In Kelley, W.N., Harris, E.D., Jr., Ruddy, S., and Sledge, C.B., Eds.: Textbook of Rheumatology. Vol. II. Philadelphia, W.B. Saunders, 1981.
20. Griffiths, I.D., Maini, R.N., and Scott, J.T.: Clinical and radiological features of osteonecrosis in systemic lupus erythematosus. Ann. Rheum. Dis., 38: 413, 1979.
21. Gumpel, J.M., and Roles, N.C.: A controlled trial of

intra-articular radiocolloids versus surgical synovectomy in persistent synovitis. Lancet, *1:* 488, 1975.

22. Halawa, M., Lee, A.J., Ling, R.S., et al.: The shear strength of trabecular bone from the femur and some factors affecting the shear strength of the cement-bone interface. Arch. Orthop. Traumat. Surg., *92:* 19, 1978.

23. Helfet, A.J.: Disorders of the Knee. Philadelphia, J.B. Lippincott, 1974.

24. Hsieh, H.H., and Walker, P.S.: Stabilizing mechanisms of the loaded and unloaded knee joint. J. Bone Joint Surg. [Am.], *58:* 87, 1976.

25. Huiskes, R., and Slooff, T.J.: Thermal injury of cancellous bone, following pressurized penetration of acrylic cement. Trans. Orthop. Res. Soc. *6:* 134, 1981.

26. Insall, J.: Reconstructive surgery and rehabilitation of the knee. p. 1980. In Kelley, W.N., Harris, E.D., Jr., Ruddy, S., and Sledge, C.B., Eds.: Textbook of Rheumatology. Vol. II. Philadelphia, W.B. Saunders, 1981.

27. Jacoby, R.K., Jayson, M.I.B., and Cosh, J.A.: Onset, early stages and prognosis of rheumatoid arthritis: A clinical study of 100 patients with 11 year follow-up. Br. Med. J., *2:* 96, 1973.

28. Jaffe, I.A.: D-Penicillamine. p. 815. In Kelley, W.N., Harris, E.D., Jr., Ruddy, S., and Sledge, C.B., Eds.: Textbook of Rheumatology. Vol. I. Philadelphia, W.B. Saunders, 1981.

29. Kennedy, A.C., Allam, B.F., Boyle, I.T., et al.: Abnormalities in mineral metabolism suggestive of parathyroid over-activity in rheumatoid arthritis. Curr. Med. Res. Opin., *3(6):* 345, 1975.

30. Kennedy, A.C., Allam, B.F., Rooney, P.J., et al.: Hypercalcaemia in rheumatoid arthritis: Investigation of its causes and implications. Ann. Rheum. Dis., *38:* 401, 1979.

31. Krause, W., Krug, W., and Miller, J.E.: Cement bone interface—effect of cement technique and surface preparation. Trans. Orthop. Res. Soc. *5:* 76, 1980.

32. Kurosawa, H., and Walker, P.S.: A new method for describing the motion of the knee. Presented at the Sixth Annual Conference of the American Society of Biomechanics, Seattle, Washington, 1982.

33. Lambert, J.R., and Wright, V.: Surgery in patients with psoriasis and arthritis. Rheumatol. Rehabil., *18:* 35, 1979.

34. Laskin, R.S.: Total condylar knee replacement in rheumatoid arthritis. A review of 117 knees. J. Bone Joint Surg. [Am.], *63:* 29, 1981.

35. Lereim, P., and Goldie, I.: Relationship between morphologic features and hardness of the subchondral bone of the medial tibial condyle in the normal state and in osteoarthritis and rheumatoid arthritis. Arch. Orthop. Unfall-Chir., *81(1):* 1, 1975.

36. Lereim, P., Goldie, I., and Dahlberg, E.: Hardness of the subchondral bone of the tibial condyles in the normal state and in osteoarthritis and rheumatoid arthritis. Acta Orthop. Scand., *45:* 614, 1974.

37. Lew, W.D., and Lewis, J.L.: The effect of knee-prosthesis geometry on cruciate ligament mechanics during flexion. J. Bone Joint Surg. [Am.], *64:* 734, 1982.

38. Lewis, J.L., Askew, M.J., and Jaycox, D.P.: A comparative evaluation of tibial component designs of total knee prostheses. J. Bone Joint Surg. [Am.], *64:* 129, 1982.

39. Liang, M.H., and Jette, A.M.: Measuring functional ability in chronic arthritis. Arthritis Rheum., *24:* 80, 1981.

40. Markolf, K.L., Finerman, G.M., and Amstutz, H.C.: In vitro measurements of knee stability after bicondylar replacement. J. Bone Joint Surg. [Am.], *61:* 547, 1979.

41. Markolf, K.L., Bargar, W.L., Shoemaker, S.C., et al.: The role of joint load in knee stability. J. Bone Joint Surg. [Am.], *63:* 570, 1981.

42. Marples, R.R., Heaton, C.L., and Kligman, A.M.: Staphylococcus aureus in psoriasis. Arch. Dermatol., *107:* 568, 1973.

43. Menkes, C.J., Aignan, M., Galmiche, B., et al.: Le traitement des rhumatismes par les synoviorthèses choix des malades, choix des articulations, modalités pratiques, résultats, indications, contreindications. Rhumatologie, 2(Suppl. 1): 61, 1972.

44. Morrison, J.B.: The mechanics of the knee joint in relation to normal walking. J. Biomech., *3:* 51, 1970.

45. Morrison, J.B.: Function of the knee joint in various activities. Biomed. Eng., *4:* 573, 1969.

46. Nissan, M.: The use of a permutation approach in the solution of joint biomechanics: the knee. Eng. Med., *10:* 39, 1981.

47. Ohno, O., and Cooke, T.D.: Electron microscopic morphology of immunoglobulin aggregates and their interactions in rheumatoid articular collagenous tissues. Arthritis Rheum., *21:* 516, 1978.

48. O'Loughlin, J.M.: Infections in the immunosuppressed patient. Med. Clin. North Am., *59(2):* 495, 1975.

49. Piziali, R.L., Rastegar, J.C., and Nagel, D.: The axis of varus-valgus rotation of the in-vitro human knee joint. Trans. Orthop. Res. Soc. *3:* 239, 1978.

50. Poss, R., Ewald, F.C., Thomas, W.H., et al.: Complications of total hip replacement arthroplasty in patients with rheumatoid arthritis. J. Bone Joint Surg. [Am.], *58:* 1130, 1976.

51. Reilly, D., Walker, P.S., Ben-Dov, M., et al.: Effects of tibial components on load transfer in the upper tibia. Clin. Orthop. *165:* 273, 1982.

52. Riley, L.H., and Hungerford, D.S.: Geometric total knee replacement for treatment of the rheumatoid knee. J. Bone Joint Surg. [Am.], *60:* 523, 1978.

53. Robinson, D.R., Tashjian, A.H., Jr., and Levine, L.: Prostaglandin-stimulated bone resorption by rheumatoid synovia. A possible mechanism for bone destruction in rheumatoid arthritis. J. Clin. Invest., *56(5):* 1181, 1975.

54. Schorn, D., and Mowat, A.G.: Penicillamine in rheumatoid arthritis: wound healing, skin thickness and osteoporosis. Rheumatol. Rehabil., *16:* 223, 1977.

55. Scott, R.D.: Duopatellar total knee replacement—the Brigham experience. Orthop. Clin. North Am., *13(1):* 89, 1982.

56. Scott, R.D., and Sledge, C.B.: The surgery of juvenile rheumatoid arthritis. p. 2014. In Kelley, W.N., Harris, E.D., Jr., Ruddy, S., and Sledge, C.B., Eds.: Textbook of Rheumatology. Vol. II. Philadelphia, W.B. Saunders, 1981.

57. Seireg, A., and Arvikar, R.J.: A mathematical model for the evaluation of forces in lower extremities of the musculoskeletal system. J. Biomech., *6:* 313, 1973.

58. Sledge, C.B.: Joint replacement surgery in juvenile rheumatoid arthritis. Arthritis Rheum., *20:* 567, 1977.

59. Sledge, C.B.: Correction of arthritic deformities in the lower extremity and spine. p. 563. In McCarthy, D.J., Ed.: Arthritis and Allied Conditions. Philadelphia, Lea & Febiger, 1979.

60. Sledge, C.B., and Ewald, F.C.: Total knee arthroplasty experience at the Robert Breck Brigham Hospital. Clin. Orthop., *145:* 78, 1979.

61. Sledge, C.B., Stern, P., Thomas, W.H., et al.: Two year follow-up of the duocondylar total knee replacement. Orthop. Trans., *2:* 193, 1978.

62. Soudry, M., Walker, P.S., Reilly, D., et al.: Interface forces of tibial component: The effect of posterior cruciate sacrifice and conformity. Trans. Orthop. Res. Soc., *8:* 37, 1983.

63. Thomas, W.H., Ewald, F.C., Poss, R., et al.: Duopatella total knee arthroplasty. Orthop. Trans., *4:* 329, 1980.

64. Trent, P.S., Walker, P.S., and Wolf, B.: Ligament length patterns, strength and rotational axes of the knee joint. Clin. Orthop., *117:* 263, 1976.

65. Walker, P.S., and Lawes, P.: The stability and fixation of knee prostheses. In Hastings, G.W., and Williams, D.F., Eds.: Mechanical Properties of Biomaterials. London, John Wiley and Sons, Ltd. 1980.

66. Walker, P.S., Greene, D., Reilly, D., et al.: Fixation of tibial components of knee prostheses. J. Bone Joint Surg. [Am.], *63:* 258, 1981.

67. Walker, P.S., Thatcher, J., and Ewald, F.C.: Variables affecting the fixation of tibial components. Eng. Med., *11:* 83, 1982.

68. Wang, C.J., and Walker, P.S.: Rotatory laxity of the human knee joint. J. Bone Joint Surg. [Am.], *56:* 161, 1974.

69. Wang, C.J., Walker, P.S., and Wolf, B.: The effects of flexion and rotation on the length patterns of the ligaments of the knee. J. Biomech. *6:* 587, 1973.

22 Fixation in Total Knee Arthroplasty

Jo Miller

Replacement arthroplasty of the arthritic knee has evolved, during the last decade, into a highly scientific and orderly procedure. With progressive improvements in implant design and increasing emphasis on the importance of alignment, ligament balancing, and correct orientation of the components, the surgeon can predict success in a large majority of surgical cases.

There continues to be some concern about the problem of fixation of implants to bone. The very high incidence of loosening reported[1] during the early experience with knee replacement was attributed to the use of constrained hinged devices, which placed an unacceptably high load on the interface between implant and bone. The hinges were succeeded, in the early 1970s, by the first resurfacing devices,[4,9] which emphasized conservative resection of bone; even these were constrained, however, because of the relative congruity of the femoral and tibial components, and loosening remained a troublesome problem.

The development of more modern designs, together with a recognition of the importance of alignment and of patient selection, has reduced the problem of gross loosening to a reasonable level.

In spite of numerous reports in the recent literature indicating that revision for loosening is as low as 2 to 3 percent,[22] there is a general dissatisfaction with traditional techniques for implant fixation. Perhaps the published figures from major academic centers are misleading, and surgeons in smaller centers are experiencing a higher incidence of loosening. The appearance of dramatic lucent lines between cement and bone has ominous implications. There can be momentous difficulties encountered in the course of revision surgery necessitated by loosening. Whatever the reason, this dissatisfaction has led to a growing interest in a variety of new techniques, including cementless fixation, fixation by biologic ingrowth, and the use of pressure penetration of low-viscosity cement.

EVALUATION OF FIXATION

In evaluating the success or failure of fixation of implant components, a number of difficulties are found to exist. There is considerable variation among workers in the use of radiologic findings, making the comparison of results from different centers impractical or impossible. Most workers limit loosening statistics to those cases in which a loose component is found at revision surgery. A shift in position of a component,[21] as seen on radiographs, would seem to be indisputable evidence of fixation failure, but such a case may not be included in loosening data if the patient continues to function well. Sinking of the component into the cancellous proximal tibia is a case in point.

Radiolucent lines continue to be a contentious is-

717

sue. In knee implants with opaque cement, the lines are an almost constant finding, but in most cases, their presence does not influence the clinical status of the patient. It has become fashionable to accept these lines as inevitable and to consider them insignificant if they are incomplete, nonprogressive, or less than a specified thickness. Whereas few authorities are willing to accept radiolucencies as an early stage of loosening, almost all would agree that the knee without a hint of lucent lines has superior fixation. There is little uncertainty about the nature of radiolucent lines that develop subsequent to surgery. They represent resorption of bone adjacent to the implant and replacement by a fibrous membrane.[3] There is a loss of contact between implant and bone and thus a loss of rigid mechanical fixation, at the microscopic level at least.

The role of cement as an actual precipitator of bone resorption is a matter of current high interest, and a variety of mechanisms have been postulated. Willert and Semlitsch[25] suggest that wear products accumulating at the bone–cement interface result in granulomatous resorption of bone. Their evidence appears to be indisputable in regard to so-called massive osteolysis in the hip, but is probably not applicable to the simple early lucent line between cement and bone. Freeman et al.[7] have proposed that histiocytes found at the interface between acrylic and bone are responsible for bone resorption, and their presence may be provoked by the cement itself. Goldring et al.[8] found that fibrous membrane recovered from the cement–bone interface has characteristics similar to those of synovial membrane and is capable of generating enzymal products that may contribute to bone resorption.

The single most dominant element in loosening is a mechanical one. There is considerable evidence to suggest that bone resorption results from micromovement between cement and bone[18] and that the size of the radiolucent line is related to the magnitude of the micromovement. The highest incidence of loosening occurs in those situations in which the load imposed on the interface is highest, that is, in hinged or constrained knee designs, in cases in which poor component orientation or leg alignment has been accepted, in very heavy or very active patients, and in cases in which cement technique has been obviously inadequate. Conversely, in situations wherein cement technique has achieved excellent fixation by mi-

crointerlock, the incidence of radiolucent lines has been dramatically low.[15] Thus, the actual performance of the interface will depend on the mechanical integrity of the interface and the demands placed on it. The ability of the interface to resist micromovement appears to be of prime importance.

A radiolucency developing adjacent to a radiolucent implant or radiolucent cement is more difficult to evaluate. A fibrous membrane interposed between a polyethylene implant and bone cannot be seen on a routine radiograph. In such situations, impending loosening will not be detectable, and only the advent of gross displacement or sinkage of a component will confirm loss of fixation.

Radiopaque components inserted without cement are somewhat easier to evaluate. During the weeks following implant surgery, a thin layer of bone joins the ends of the cut cancellous trabeculae,[5,14] and this has been likened to a new subchondral plate.[16] On x-ray film, separation of this plate from the implant by a thin clear zone may indicate that a fibrous membrane is interposed between implant and bone. This sign may be useful in evaluating the presence or absence of ingrowth.

TRADITIONAL CEMENT TECHNIQUES

Most knee arthroplasties performed during the past 12 years have employed traditional cement techniques in which doughy cement is applied by hand to the prepared bone surfaces. Fixation depends on gross interlock between the cement and irregularities, such as drill holes and peg cut-outs, produced on the bone surfaces. Recent reports of nonhinged knee reconstructions[22] indicate a rate of radiolucency of 25 to 45 percent. The incidence appears to be higher in the more constrained designs and may be less in those in which the tibial component incorporates a central peg. The incidence of revision for loosening varies from approximately 2 to 5 percent, depending on the prosthetic model and the length of follow-up. Insall[12] reports, in one of the longest follow-up studies, on 100 total condylar prostheses, 5 to 9 years after surgery, with a 41 percent incidence of radiolucency and only two cases of loosening.

Two small changes have come into use to improve the quality of the interface between cement and bone.

Cleaning of bone surfaces with a pulsating water jet is now widely accepted and serves to open trabecular spaces for cement intrusion. The second advance has been related to the use of cement slightly earlier than the usual dough stage, in order to improve its intrusion characteristics; this advice is followed in some centers.

Two other factors have some influence on fixation of knee implants. Resection of the articular surface of the femur or tibia exposes trabeculae to thermal effects, mechanical trauma, and microvascular damage. These surface trabeculae, of questionable viability, may not be ideal for the establishment of an enduring cement–bone interface.

The second factor is related to the use of a tibial component with a central peg. Cement, poured into the hole cut in the tibia, is constrained, and the rapid introduction of the tibial component in effect pressurizes the cement into bone. It is common in postoperative radiographs to see a cement–bone interface around the peg having a fuzzy appearance, indicating pressurization and microfixation. This well-fixed peg is often accompanied by rather dramatic lucent lines beneath the wings of the tibial component (Fig. 22.1), possibly the result of stress shielding by the well-fixed peg. Riley,[20] who has carefully followed cases done with three different models of the anametric knee, reports that the lucencies beneath the wings of the tibial component are more dramatic in knees in which the implant incorporates a metal base plate and stem. This finding tends to substantiate the stress-shielding concept.

In spite of these theoretical shortcomings to the traditional cement technique, the results of arthroplasties in a large number of reported cases seem satisfactory to date, but a longer follow-up period will be required. The comment by Scott[21] may be prophetic: "It is significant that no revisions have been necessary yet for tibial loosening, but surely this will be required in a certain number of knees with longer follow-up."

FIXATION WITH PRESSURE-PENETRATED CEMENT

Soon after its introduction, fixation with acrylic cement showed evidence of imperfection with the appearance of a radiolucent line between cement and

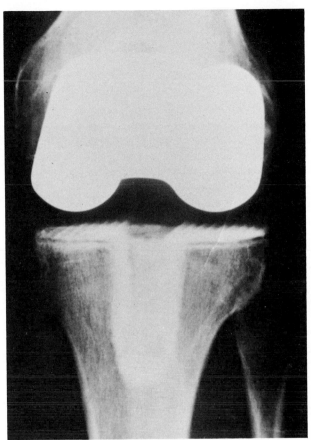

Fig. 22.1. A stemmed tibial component showing excellent fixation of the prosthetic peg and radiolucencies beneath the wings, possibly caused by stress shielding.

bone. As early as 1969, Ling[13] perceived that this might represent the first stage of loosening. In an attempt to improve fixation of cement to bone, he devised a technique for applying pressure to acrylic cement, forcing it to enter the open spaces between the trabeculae in the acetabulum. His data on the prevention of loosening of the acetabular component are dramatic.

In 1976, we began to pursue studies related to improved fixation of acrylic cement. An effort was made to pressurize cement, soon after mixing, forcing it to intrude into cancellous surfaces. The early clinical experiences used a slightly modified ICLH prosthesis and employed a crude cement delivery system with a tip that could be fitted into multiple shallow $\frac{1}{4}$-inch drill holes made on the cut surface of the tibia (Fig.

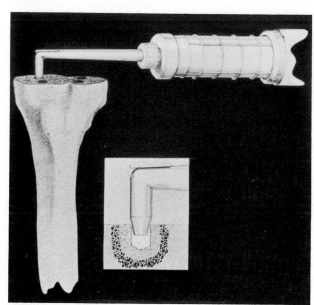

Fig. 22.2. Cement was pressure penetrated into shallow drill holes. This technique, which gave poor control of depth of cement penetration and failed to interlock over the entire surface, is now rarely used.

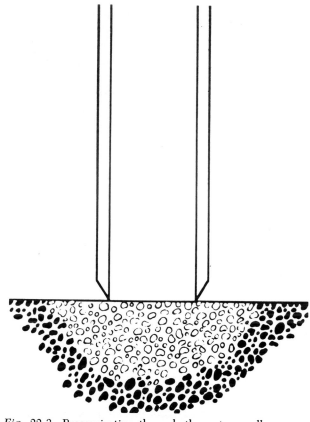

Fig. 22.3. Pressurization through the cut cancellous surface. The cement penetrates to 3 to 6 mm in almost every instance, achieving microinterlock at close intervals.

22.2). The cement flowed into the bone, displacing fat and marrow and interlocking with the trabecular structure. Because penetration was difficult to control, was often excessive, and failed to interlock at every site on the cut cancellous surface, the technique was modified to employ a cement delivery system nozzle that would force the cement through the intact cancellous surface without the need for drill holes (Fig. 22.3). Acrylic cement was used in a very liquid state, soon after mixing. This technique proved superior to the traditional techniques in which doughy acrylic cement was applied to bone by hand. In contrast to the dramatic radiolucent lines frequently developing within 1 year (Fig. 22.4), the interface was characterized by a fuzziness seen immediately after

surgery and that showed no change with the passage of time (Fig. 22.5).

Enough evidence was accumulated by 1978 to justify the establishment of a study of the efficacy of so-called composite structure fixation. The term suggests that the implant will be attached to bone by a system in which all interfaces are secure, so that the entire system functions as a composite structure (Fig. 22.6). A well-established prosthetic design was modified by replacing the tibial stem with four short positioning pegs (Fig. 22.7). The undersurface was made porous by sintering on 250-μm chrome–cobalt spheres in several layers. The device was designed to be used with pressure penetration of cement into cancellous bone.

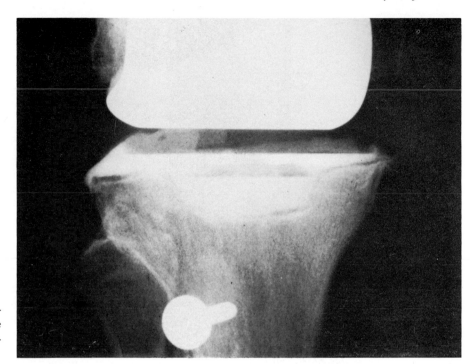

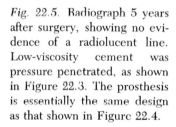

Fig. 22.4. A dramatic radiolucent line developing in a knee implanted with traditional cement techniques.

Fig. 22.5. Radiograph 5 years after surgery, showing no evidence of a radiolucent line. Low-viscosity cement was pressure penetrated, as shown in Figure 22.3. The prosthesis is essentially the same design as that shown in Figure 22.4.

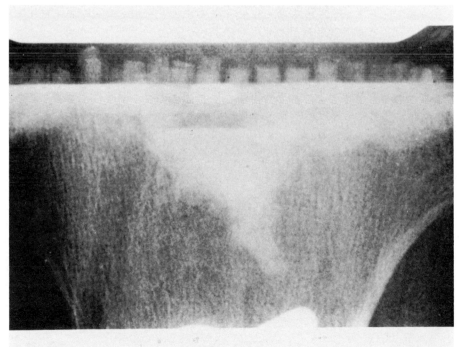

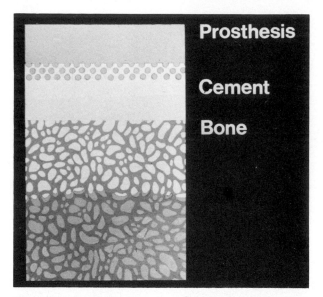

Fig. 22.6. Composite structure fixation suggests a secure interface achieved by the penetration of cement into cancellous interstices of bone and a firm interface by interlock of the cement with the porous undersurface of the prosthesis.

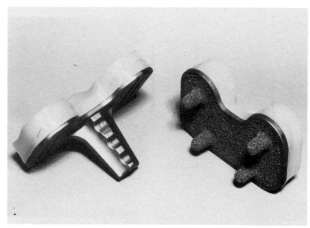

Fig. 22.7. Modifications were made by replacing the tibial stem with four short positioning pegs. The undersurface was made porous by the sintering on of chrome cobalt spheres in several layers.

LOW-VISCOSITY CEMENT

It became apparent that the use of traditional cement in a very liquid phase, within 1 minute of mixing, had a number of disadvantages. Only about 45 seconds of working time was available, and once the cement had passed the 2-minute mark, its ability to intrude into cancellous surfaces was markedly diminished. Even if the cement was successfully employed within this time limit, it then required a further 10 to 12 minutes to polymerize, with the danger of unwanted movements affecting final fixation. The very high level of free monomer soon after mixing also caused some concern. On our advice, a new cement was formulated that became commercially available in early 1979. This product is identical both physically and chemically to traditional doughy cement and owes its low-viscosity characteristics to the nature of the polymer powder; changes in powder bead size and surface characteristics are responsible for the special handling and setting behavior. This cement is designed to have a working time of 3 to 6 minutes and to set at 8 to 10 minutes after mixing (at 71°F; times are dependent on ambient temperature). This prod-

uct has proved somewhat more difficult to use than the traditional cement, but appears to facilitate superior fixation.

SURGICAL TECHNIQUE

Pressure penetration of low-viscosity cement can be used with almost any design of knee, but is most advantageous when employed together with a porous based prosthesis. The cut surfaces of tibia and femur are carefully prepared to receive the implant and are cleaned with a pulsating water jet. The soft tissue is draped to control spill of the cement. The cement is mixed in the usual fashion, introduced into the cement delivery system at about 1½ minutes; at about 2 minutes after mixing, it is applied to the porous undersurface of the prosthesis in a very liquid state.

Pressure penetration of the cement begins at about 3 minutes after mixing (depending on the ambient temperature). The tip of the nozzle is placed firmly against cancellous bone and a single squeeze of the gun trigger introduces about 2 cc of cement into bone. The process is repeated in an orderly fashion over the entire surface. Fat and bone marrow, extruded onto the surface, is suctioned away as it appears. Any cement that spills onto soft tissue is left undisturbed, to be cleaned up at a later time once it has thickened considerably.

At the completion of pressurization, the precoated prosthesis is positioned and seated. Cement penetration is ideally 3 to 6 mm (Fig. 22.8).

Because of the importance of timing in the use of low-viscosity cement, implantation of tibial, femoral, and patellar components must be done sequentially with separate mixes of cement.

CLINICAL RESULTS

A clinical evaluation trial of composite structure fixation was initiated in late 1979 with five centers participating. Approximately 300 knees have been done in these five centers using pressure penetration of low-viscosity cement.

In January 1982, a radiologic survey of all knees with more than 1 year follow-up was carried out with special interest in the appearance of the interfaces. For controls, a similar radiologic evaluation was done on two other types of knees, fixed with traditional

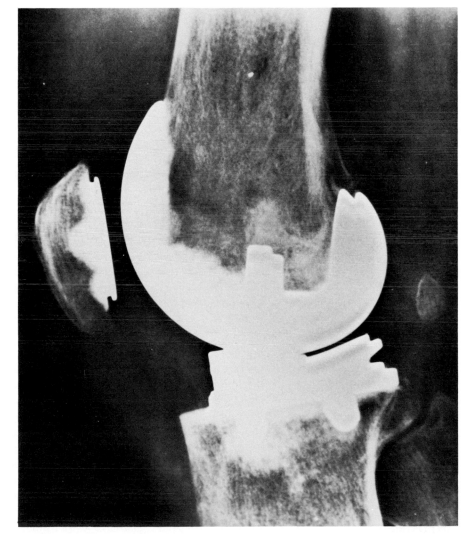

Fig. 22.8. X-ray film of the tibial component 2 years after surgery. The depth of cement penetration is 3 to 6 mm and is considered ideal. No change has occurred at the interface during the course of follow-up.

cement techniques. One design was relatively constrained and the other markedly unconstrained.

In the composite structure knees, the interfaces were judged to be excellent (i.e., no evidence of radiolucent lines of any dimensions at any part of the interface between tibia and implant) in 60 percent of the knees, while in the control series only 4 percent and 13 percent, respectively, had this quality of interface.

An unsatisfactory interface (with a radiolucent line of ≥0.5 mm in width over most of the interface) was found in only 4 percent of the composite structure knees, while the controls showed this finding in 30 percent of cases.

CEMENTLESS FIXATION OF NONPOROUS IMPLANTS

Dissatisfaction with cemented knee implants has stimulated a number of workers to develop designs that depend only on their gross configuration for fixation. The concept is not new. Early replacement arthroplasty designs, developed over 25 years ago, were introduced without cement. Shiers[23] used uncemented hinge devices for at least 10 years, and Walldius[24] continues to advocate the use of implants with a nonrigid type of fixation.

MacIntosh[13A] introduced his metallic tibial resurfacing device more than 20 years ago and has continued to use it without cement. The principles outlined by MacIntosh were adopted more than 10 years ago by Yabsley and his associates,[26] who employed two uncemented polyethylene tibial plateaus together with a cemented geometric femoral component with good results reported (Fig. 22.9). Loosening of the unfixed tibial component has occurred only rarely.

In 1977, Freeman[7] began to use a modification of his original ICLH prosthesis without cement. The tibial component incorporated two polyethylene pegs (Fig. 22.10) with a series of protruding flanges which on insertion into tibial drill holes deformed and interlocked, achieving mechanical fixation of the device (Fig. 22.11). By 1982, Freeman was able to report on more than 50 knees without mechanical loosening. It should be pointed out that Freeman employed a sophisticated instrumentation system so that perfect alignment was always achieved; he also incorporated the principle of full coverage in which the entire cut surface of the tibia is covered by the polyethylene prosthesis, which if necessary, is reshaped in the operating room. He demonstrated evidence of adaptive changes in the bone under the polyethylene plateaus and around the bone pegs without actual ingrowth of bone into the spaces between the flanges.

Histologic studies[6] were carried out on material obtained from patients who had died for unrelated reasons or on tissue obtained at the time of revision (done for reasons other than loosening of the tibial component). These suggest that there is some initial resorption of bone from the cut upper surface of the tibia and replacement with a layer of fibrous tissue, displaying chondroid metaplasia. A thin plate of new bone tends to close off the openings between cut trabeculae. This new bone, surrounding the implant, can be seen radiologically and might be likened to a subchondral plate. Freeman emphasizes that the layer of fibrous tissue between bone and prosthesis is not characterized by the presence of large numbers of histiocytes and cites this as evidence that fixation is more likely to be biologically stable than with cement.

BIOLOGIC FIXATION BY INGROWTH OF BONE INTO POROUS SURFACES

The latent mistrust of traditional techniques for the fixation of arthroplasty components has been most clearly demonstrated by the dramatic interest shown since 1980 in the use of porous implants designed to induce ingrowth of bone and thus biologic fixation. The concept of component fixation by ingrowth, with its implication of long-term endurance, is intuitively attractive to the practicing orthopedic surgeon.

The capacity of bone to grow into a porous implant has been known for at least 15 years,[19] and its potential as a method for fixation of implants was recognized early.[10] Extensive laboratory investigations have been carried out in a number of centers, and the results of animal surgery have been encouraging.

The use of a porous surface implant does not ensure ingrowth unless certain very strict criteria are met. The surface must have porosity characteristics >50 μm and <600 μm with the optimum pore diameter probably lying between 50 and 400 μm.[17] The porous surface must be closely apposed to a viable bone surface and gross immobilization of the implant with re-

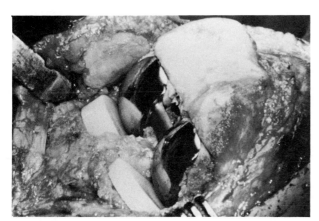

Fig. 22.9. The Dalhousie knee uses a cemented geometric femoral component together with two uncemented polyethylene tibial components similar in configuration to the MacIntosh prosthesis. (Courtesy of Dr. R.H. Yabsley.)

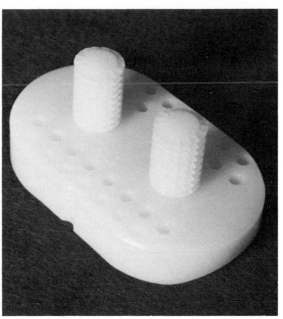

Fig. 22.10. The prosthesis used by Freeman and his associates is polyethylene with two polyethylene pegs incorporating protruding flanges. (Courtesy of M.A.R. Freeman.)

Fig. 22.11. On insertion into drill holes, the flanges deform locking the prosthesis in place. (Courtesy of M.A.R. Freeman.)

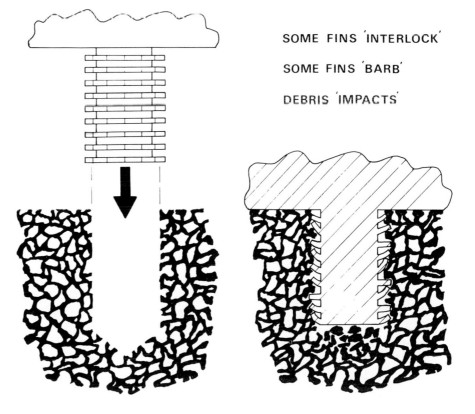

SOME FINS 'INTERLOCK'

SOME FINS 'BARB'

DEBRIS 'IMPACTS'

spect to bone must be maintained for 4 to 6 weeks to allow establishment of ingrowth. Effectiveness of this immobilization is largely dependent on the design configuration of the implant, the accuracy of the fit between implant and bone and, necessarily, the stresses applied to the system by movement of the surgically reconstructed joint as part of the postoperative rehabilitation program.

Failure to meet these requirements will lead to incomplete or abortive ingrowth and the implant will, as a result, interface with bone via a fibrous membrane. Some investigators[2] have suggested that such a result is acceptable or even desirable, comparing the situation with the peridontal membrane of the tooth. The acceptability of fibrous membrane fixation remains unanswered for the moment, but there is reason to believe that such a system will be less enduring than rigid fixation. Clinical experiences with hip arthroplasty, primarily in Europe, seem to indicate a rather high incidence of pain in association with fibrous membrane fixation.

The use of a porous stem implanted in the long axis of a load-bearing system raises the spector of stress shielding of surrounding bone. This complication has not been seen in the clinical series of porous stemmed proximal femoral prostheses, probably because ingrowth has not developed over the entire surface of the implants.

There is little available experimental work with animal models, dealing specifically with problems of knee implant fixation by ingrowth.

In 1980, Hungerford and his associates[11] began to use a knee prosthesis of anatomic configuration, intended for biologic fixation. The design (Fig. 22.12), a semiconstrained resurfacing system, incorporates a relatively coarse porous coat on tibial, femoral, and patellar components. Primary mechanical fixation of the tibial component is achieved with two short-angled pegs and a screw introduced into an expandable plastic sleeve placed in the bone beneath the implant (Fig. 22.13). The femoral component is immobilized by press fit, augmented by two studs. The patella depends entirely on two very short porous pegs for its initial fixation. A sophisticated instrumentation system is used to accomplish the very high level of surgical accuracy necessary if fixation by ingrowth is to be successful.

This knee has been used widely with acrylic cement and in a restricted program without cement.

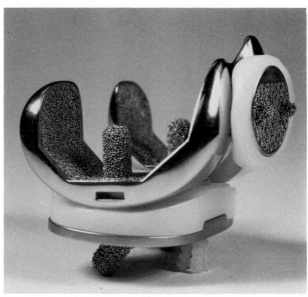

Fig. 22.12. The porous coated anatomic (PCA) prosthesis designed by Hungerford and his associates incorporates a porous undersurface for biologic ingrowth. (Courtesy of D.S. Hungerford.)

Reports are enthusiastic, but data regarding the effectiveness of fixation by ingrowth must be considered preliminary at this time. Hungerford in 1982 published the early results of 16 knees inserted without cement and followed for a minimum of 6 months.[11] There were no cases of loosening and careful radiologic evaluation suggested fixation by ingrowth. A larger series has been presented more recently with similar results.

The Hungerford knee has been used without cement by a number of other groups, and there have been isolated cases of early loosening, perhaps as a result of imperfections in surgical technique. To date, no other models of knee arthroplasty designed for fixation by ingrowth have appeared.

DISCUSSION

Loosening is a persistent problem in total knee arthroplasty and may increase in magnitude in the next decade with a longer follow-up period, as has been the case in hip replacement surgery.

Most knee implants have been done with acrylic cement; it is tempting to blame the cement for the complications. It is evident, however, that in well-

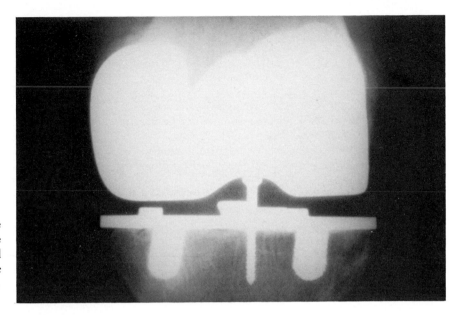

Fig. 22.13. X-ray films of the PCA prosthesis showing the mode of temporary fixation and suggesting fixation by biologic ingrowth. (Courtesy of D.S. Hungerford.)

performed knee surgery, cement carefully used in the traditional fashion will give satisfactory fixation in the vast majority of cases. The concepts that cement has inherent qualities which result in bone destruction are still unconfirmed and are based largely on circumstantial evidence. Secure mechanical microfixation seems to be the most important single factor in the prevention of loosening.

Improved cement techniques appear to offer significant advantages. Pressure penetration of cement into bone achieves an interface mechanically superior to that produced by manual application of cement.

Cementless fixation as proposed by Yabsley and by Freeman has merit and is gathering support, in spite of some concern expressed about the lack of rigid fixation.

Fixation by biologic ingrowth is fundamentally attractive. The concept is not without its dangers and drawbacks. The technique places much greater demands on the skill of the surgeon, and even minor errors may result in failure of fixation. The incidence of early loosening is not yet known. Once established, fixation is likely to be sustained, and late loosening would seem an unlikely event.

What will happen to implants that are not incorporated by bony ingrowth? Will fibrous membrane fixation suffice? A lengthy follow-up period will be required to begin to answer these questions.

Clearly, total knee arthroplasty has so much to offer the patient with knee arthritis, and the alternatives are so few that the operation is here to stay. The problem of fixation must be solved, and the excellent progress made in the last few years promises further improvement in the near future.

REFERENCES

1. Arden, G.P., and Kamdar, B.A.: Complications of arthroplasty of the knee, p. 118. In Total Knee Replacement. London, The Institution of Mechanical Engineers, 1974.
2. Cameron, H.U.: Personal commmunication, 1980.
3. Charnley, J.: Acrylic Cement in Orthopaedic Surgery, p. 24. Baltimore, Williams & Wilkins, 1970.
4. Coventry, M.B.: Tibio-femoral replacement using two components with retention of the cruciate ligaments (the geometric and anametric prosthesis). In Freeman, M.A.R., Ed.: Arthritis of the Knee, p. 191. Berlin, Springer-Verlag, 1980.
5. Freeman, M.A.R.: Personal communication, 1982.
6. Freeman, M.A.R., Bradley, G.W., and Revell, P.A.: Observations upon the interface between bone and polymethylmethacrylate cement. J. Bone Joint Surg. [Br.], *64:* 489, 1982.
7. Freeman, M.A.R., Blaha, J.D., Bradley, G.W., et al.: Cementless fixation of ICLH tibial component. Orthop. Clin. North Am., *13*(1): 141, 1982.
8. Goldring, S.R., Schiller, A.L., Roelke, M.S., et al.: Characterization of the histological lesions associated

with localized bone resorption following total hip replacement. Presented at the Second A.O.A. International Symposium, Boston, May 27–30, 1981.

9. Gunston, F.H.: Polycentric knee arthroplasty. Prosthetic simulation of normal knee movement. J. Bone Joint Surg. [Br.], *53:* 272, 1971.

10. Hahn, H., and Palich, W.: Preliminary evaluation of porous metal surfaced titanium for orthopaedic implants. J. Biomed. Mater. Res., *4:* 571, 1970.

11. Hungerford, D.S., Kenna, R.V., and Krackow, K.A.: The porous-coated anatomic total knee. Orthop. Clin. North Am., *13*(1): 103, 1982.

12. Insall, J.N., Hood, R.W., Flawn, L.B., et al.: The total condylar knee prosthesis in gonarthrosis. J. Bone Joint Surg. [Am.], *65:* 619, 1983.

13. Ling, R.S.M.: Loosening experience at Exeter. Presented at the Second A.O.A. International Symposium, Boston, May 27–30, 1981.

13A. MacIntosh, D.L.: Hemiarthroplasty of the knee using a space occupying prosthesis for painful varus and valgus deformities. J. Bone Joint Surg. [Am.], *40:* 1431, 1958.

14. Miller, J.: Unpublished data, 1978.

15. Miller, J., Krause, W.R., Burke, D.L., et al.: Pressure penetration of low viscosity acrylic cement for improved fixation of arthroplasty components. Orthop. Trans. 6(3): 458, 1982.

16. O'Connor, J., Goodfellow, J., and Perry, N.: Fixation of the tibial components of the Oxford knee. Orthop. Clin. North Am., *13*(1): 65, 1982.

17. Pilliar, R.M.: Experimental basis of bone ingrowth for implant fixation. Presented at the Second A.O.A. International Symposium, Boston, May 27–30, 1981.

18. Reckling, F.W., Asher, M.A., and Dillon, W.L.: A longitudinal study of the radiolucent line at the bone–cement interface following total joint replacement procedures. J. Bone Joint Surg. [Am.], *59:* 355, 1977.

19. Reynolds, J.T.: As quoted by Hahn, H., and Palich, W.: J. Biomed. Mater. Res., *4:* 571, 1970.

20. Riley, L.H.: Personal communication, 1982.

21. Scott, R.D.: Duopatellar total knee replacement: The Brigham experience. Orthop. Clin. North Am., *13*(1): 89, 1982.

22. Scott, W.N., Guest Ed.: Symposium on total knee arthroplasty. Orthop. Clin. North Am., *13*(1): 1982.

23. Shiers, L.G.P.: Arthroplasty of the knee. Preliminary report of a new method. J. Bone Joint Surg. [Br.], *36:* 553, 1954.

24. Walldius, B.: Arthroplasty of the knee using a hinged vitallium prosthesis. Acta. Orthop. Belg., *39:* 245, 1973.

25. Willert, H.G., and Semlitsch, M.: Problems associated with the cement anchorage of artifical joints. In Schaldach, M. and Hohmann, D., Eds.: Advances in Artificial Hip and Knee Joint Technology, p. 325, Berlin, Springer-Verlag, 1976.

26. Yabsley, R.A.: Personal communication, 1982.

23 Miscellaneous Items: Arthrodesis, The Stiff Knee, Synovectomy, and Popliteal Cysts

John N. Insall

ARTHRODESIS

Arthrodesis of the knee is seldom performed nowadays as a primary operation; more usually, it is a salvage procedure. In the latter case bone stock may be grossly deficient, making arthrodesis difficult to achieve.[2,17] Even as a primary procedure under optimal circumstances knee fusion may not always occur. Most series have reported a success rate ranging between 80 and 98 percent, the remainder resulting in a fibrous ankylosis, which can be painful.[6,7,15,31] Therefore, the procedure should not be undertaken lightly; the best possible technique should be used and immobilization made as rigid as can be obtained.

INDICATIONS

Unilateral Post-traumatic Osteoarthritis in a Young Person.[10] An otherwise healthy young man with a severely damaged knee should probably be advised to have an arthrodesis, particularly when his occupation involves manual labor. However, this advice will often be refused by men and rejected out of hand by women who, if at all sophisticated, will demand a knee replacement. This presents a most difficult dilemma for the surgeon, and I confess that I do not know the answer. Certainly, no existing knee replacement is likely to stand up to a lifetime of hard use but, on the other hand, a knee arthrodesis is final and cannot usually be revised to an arthroplasty later on. Fortunately, these cases are rare; when they present, the surgeon must judge each case individually. Sometimes a joint debridement or a realignment by osteotomy will provide a way out, and sometimes counseling will help the patient decide to avoid surgery altogether.

The Multioperated Knee. In these patients the original insult may have been a ligament injury or perhaps a patellar dislocation. Now, 10 or 12 operations later, there is a chronically painful and usually unstable joint, leaving the patient depressed, angry, and hostile. These people represent another therapeutic challenge. Most further surgery of any kind is unwarranted; management should consist of simple conservative management, bracing, attendance at a "pain clinic," and perhaps psychiatric care. For a select few, arthrodesis may be the correct approach.

Painful Ankylosis. In a knee that is already stiff (after sepsis, tuberculosis, or perhaps ancient trauma), an arthroplasty may be either contraindicated or likely to produce a suboptimal result, particularly in terms of motion. When an ankylosis is painful, it is best converted into an arthrodesis. In this situation, the patient is at least aware of the drawbacks of a stiff knee.

729

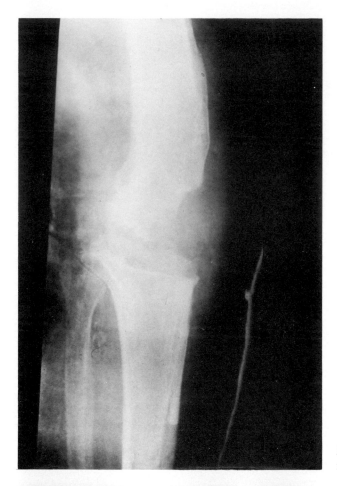

Fig. 23.1. Arthrodesis after removal of a knee prosthesis may be difficult to obtain because of bone deficiency.

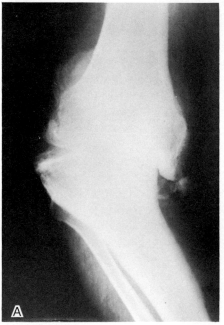

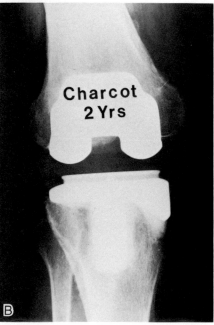

Fig. 23.2. Although arthrodesis can be obtained in a neuropathic joint, total knee replacement is also feasible. (A) Preoperative radiograph of a neuropathic joint. (B) Two years after total replacement with a custom prosthesis. The knee is stable, without swelling and the clinical rating is excellent.

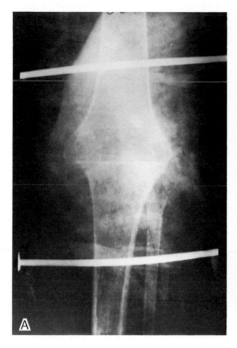
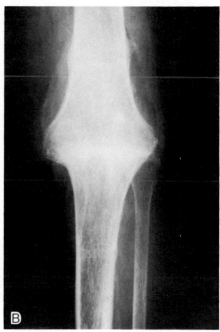

Fig. 23.3. (A, B) Successful compression arthrodesis using a Charnley clamp.

Paralytic Conditions. Muscle weakness caused by poliomyelitis is rare nowadays. It can usually be managed successfully by bracing. However, when associated with genu recurvatum, bracing is difficult and may not be successful.

Failed Knee Arthroplasty. This is currently the major indication for knee fusion, as well as being the most difficult circumstance in which to obtain one (Fig. 23.1). Mechanical failure of an arthroplasty can nearly always be managed by revision. When the failure is caused by sepsis, two-stage reimplantation with another prosthesis may be the best choice (see Chapter 20). Some cases, however, can only be managed by removal of the prosthesis and attempted fusion.

Neuropathic Joint. Arthrodesis of a Charcot joint is difficult to obtain. Success is more likely if preceded by a thorough debridement and synovectomy.[11] Total knee arthroplasty is also feasible in some cases (Fig. 23.2A,B).

TECHNIQUE

Compression Arthrodesis. Compression using a pin and frame technique was popularized by Key[23] and Charnley[4,5] (Fig. 23.3). Today instead of a single pin above and below the knee, multiple transfixation pins are used. Half-pins positioned at right angles to the transfixation pins are sometimes used for added stability. The knee is approached through a midline incision or using previous scars when appropriate. A transverse incision at the level of the knee joint dividing the quadriceps mechanism is also most satisfactory. In primary cases, the joint surfaces are prepared using a saw, preferably with total knee instrumentation to make accurate cuts and obtain the correct alignment. A total of 1.5 to 2 cm of bone must be excised to provide a suitable cancellous surface on both bones. Further bone shortening relaxes the hamstrings and gives greater flexibility at the hip joint, which is desirable if both knees have to be fused.[6] The desired alignment is 0 to 5 degrees of valgus, with the knee flexed 10 to 15 degrees. The patella can be left as it is, or the articular surface can be excised; when this is done the opposing femoral groove should also be removed. When the fusion is done as a salvage technique for failed arthroplasty, further bone should not be removed, but rather the fragments are thoroughly cleaned and the irregular surfaces interdigitated to give the best possible contact. The patella can sometimes be used as a graft to fill large defects. An external fixator is then applied (e.g., the Hoffmann apparatus). Three parallel transfixation pins are passed through the distal femur and three more

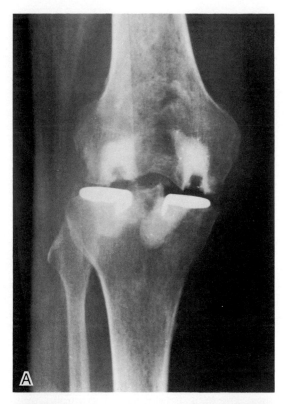

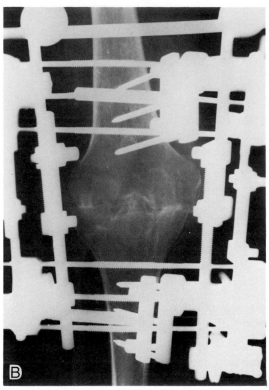

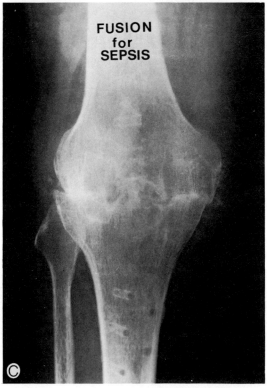

Fig. 23.4. Arthrodesis of the knee with an infected surface inlay prosthesis. (A) Preoperative radiograph. (B) Prosthesis and acrylic cement have been removed and the surfaces opposed to give the best possible bony contact. A Hoffman apparatus has been applied with six transfixation pins and six anterior half-pins. (C) The completed arthrodesis.

through the upper tibia; when the bony surfaces are adequate, this is usually sufficient fixation. When the knee still has a tendency to rock, a further series of six half-pins, three above and three below, are inserted under radiographic control (Fig. 23.4). All the pins are connected by the frame, and compression is applied. Fixation is usually so secure that early weight-bearing is tolerated. The external fixator should remain in place for 3 months.

Intramedullary Rod Fixation (Fig. 23.5). After failure of a hinged arthroplasty, the femur and tibia may resemble hollow cones with little or no cancellous bone remaining; even cortical bone is often irregular, partially devascularized, or impregnated with metallic debris. A great deal of length may have been lost. In these circumstances, Kaufer et al.[22] recommend a period of prolonged immobilization first to clear infection if it were present and second to obtain a fibrous anklyosis. Often the anklyosis will be relatively stable and painless and this situation may be acceptable. When it is not after a suitable length of time (perhaps 1 year after the removal of the components) a long, slightly curved intramedullary nail is inserted. This is passed up the femur from the knee and then in retrograde fashion into the tibia. The nail should be slightly curved to pass easily through the femoral canal and to give some flexion at the arthrodesis and of the maximum diameter that the bones will accept. Kaufer et al.[22] recommend using an overlong nail cut to length with a hacksaw at operation. This method, they maintain, imparts immediate stability and may lead to fusion, even in the most unpromising circumstances. Even if fusion does not occur, the fibrous ankylosis obtained is stable and painless.

COMPLICATIONS OF ARTHRODESIS

Fusion may not occur; when the ankylosis is painful, a repeat procedure with bone grafting is needed. Arthrodesis, even when successful, will not in itself eliminate sepsis, particularly if foreign material such as cement remains. Pin tract infections with the external fixator can be troublesome and may require premature removal of the apparatus. The intramedullary nail may also cause recurrent sepsis. The single bone between hip and ankle is vulnerable; femoral or tibial fractures are not uncommon. Back pain has been reported as an occasional problem. Finally, few patients are fully satisfied even with the best arthrodesis. The leg is awkward and ungainly in modern society. No patient should have an arthrodesis unless he or she has first had an extended trial in a cylinder cast and fully realizes the disadvantages.

THE STIFF KNEE

MANIPULATION

The technique of manipulation under anesthesia is indispensable; many surgeons regard it with apprehension. It is my practice to manipulate knee arthroplasties 2 to 3 weeks after operation when motion is not being regained spontaneously. For other major knee surgery the period is 6 weeks to 3 months. Beyond 3 months, manipulation is likely to be difficult, but I have had success as much as 2 years after surgery. Manipulation is regarded as an aid to physical therapy, and not a substitute for it. Active and passive exercises must be resumed immediately, or the benefit will be lost.

TECHNIQUE

A general anesthetic is given with complete muscle relaxation so that no tension remains in the quadriceps to resist the force applied by the surgeon. To omit relaxation is dangerous and most mishaps occur for this reason. Manipulation is an art that must be acquired individually. My own method is to place the patient's foot and ankle under my arm and, while countertraction from the thigh is provided by an assistant, steady pressure is applied on the lower leg. The exact amount of pressure that can be tolerated without damage can only be learned by experience; it is quite substantial, provided sudden jerky movements are avoided. A few moments of steady pressure are usually rewarded by a palpable and often audible "tearing" in the knee, after which the joint flexes easily. If the knee does not bend readily, pressure of the same degree is continued for 10 to 15 minutes. Persistence usually pays off, but the amount of pressure should not be increased.

Manipulation is most difficult and least likely to succeed when the knee initially is fixed near a position of extension and when the stiffness is long-standing. Manipulation is always worth trying, but for stubborn cases an open procedure is required.

RETINACULAR RELEASE AND QUADRICEPSPLASTY

Retinacular release followed by manipulation is usually successful when limitation of movement is purely intra-articular. A short lateral parapatellar incision is used, the lateral retinaculum is opened, and intra-articular adhesions are divided; occasionally the medial patellar retinaculum will also need division.

When loss of motion has followed a femoral fracture or osteomyelitis of the femur, the cause is usually adhesions between the quadriceps muscle and the

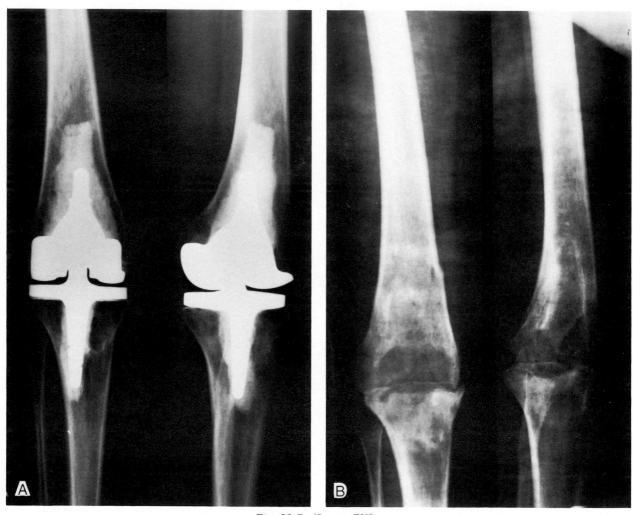

Fig. 23.5. (See p. 735).

Fig. 23.5. Arthrodesis using a long intramedullary rod. (A) Anteroposterior and lateral radiograph of an infected spherocentric prosthesis. (B) Resection arthroplasty approximately nine months after prosthesis removal. Although the limb was free of drainage at this point, the patient requested arthrodesis because of unacceptable instability at the knee. (C) A curved intramedullary rod is in place. A wire fixes the proximal end of the rod to the trochanter to prevent rod migration. (D) Radiograph approximately 1 year postarthrodesis shows a secure fusion. The patient bore weight without any external supports immediately after the operation. (E) Radiograph shows the distal end of the nail within the tibial metaphayis. Note the trabecular bone reaction around the tip of the nail. In those cases in which the tip of the nail is at the diaphyseal metaphyseal junction, or more proximal within the diaphesis, intense periosteal reaction may be noted, which can lead to a displaced fatigue fracture. It is therefore recommended that in all patients the distal tip of the nail should be well within the distal tibial metaphysis. (Courtesy of Dr. Herbert Kaufer.[22])

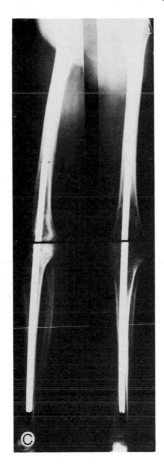

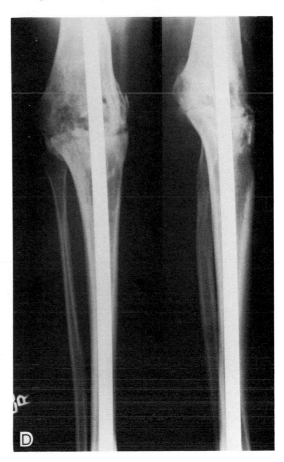

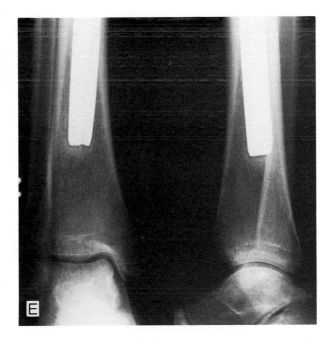

bone. A quadriceps contracture can also follow intra-muscular injections in infancy, leading to fibrosis in the quadriceps and progressive loss of motion. In both types of contracture, it is the vastus intermedius and vastus lateralis that are most affected. The rectus femoris is sometimes shortened in long-standing cases but the vastus medialis is seldom involved. For fibro-sis or adhesions of the quadriceps muscle a quadri-cepsplasty is required.

Thompson Technique

An anterolateral longitudinal skin incision is used in the Thompson technique.[18,32] The lateral patellar retinaculum is incised and intra-articular adhesions divided. When the medial retinaculum is tight, it too is incised. A manipulation is attempted and a few degrees may be gained. The lateral incision is then extended into the vastus lateralis, separating this component of the muscle from the rectus tendon. The tendon of vastus intermedius is located and divided at its point of insertion into the quadriceps tendon; a portion may be excised. A further manipulation is attempted and usually at this point will be successful. When the rectus femoris is tight it can be lengthened in Z fashion, but permanent weakness of extension is likely to result. The vastus lateralis is reattached to the tendon at a higher level or is sometimes left free. The wound is closed over a suction drain. Thompson recommended immobilization of the knee in 90 de-grees of flexion, but this is a hazard to wound healing; I prefer to immobilize the leg in extension until the wound is healed. At 2 to 3 weeks, a second manipu-lation under anesthesia is done followed by intensive physical therapy.

The original Thompson technique sectioned both vasti from the rectus femoris as well as the vastus intermedius (Fig. 23.6). Sectioning the vastus medi-alis is usually unnecessary and may contribute to weak extension and a permanent extension lag. Nicoll[28] found that about one-fifth of cases had a tight rectus, lim-iting flexion.

Judet Technique

Because of the limitations of the Thompson quad-ricepsplasty, Judet described a technique of disinser-tion and distal sliding of the tight quadriceps com-

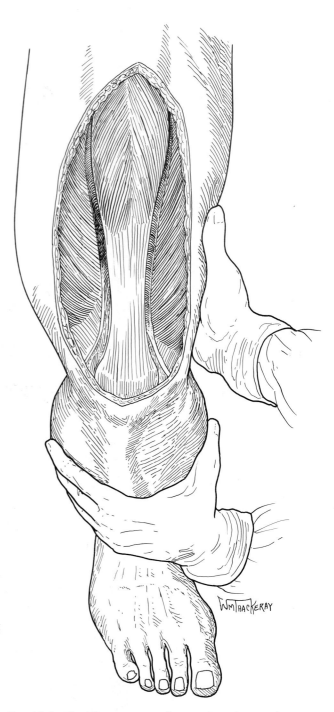

Fig. 23.6. The Thompson quadricepsplasty (see text). Sec-tion of the vastus medialis is seldom necessary.

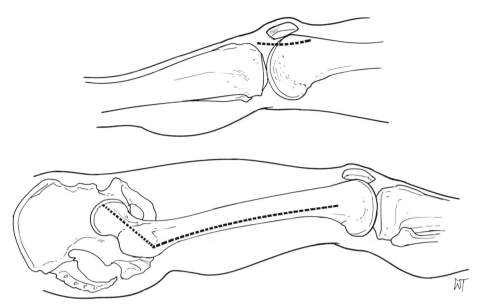

Fig. 23.7. The Judet quadriceps slide with rectus release. (From Daoud, H., O'Farrell, T., and Cruess, R.L.: Quadricepsplasty. The Judet technique and results of six cases. J. Bone Joint Surg. [Br.], *64:* 194, 1982, with permission.)

ponents.[19–21] Daoud et al.[9] recently described a modification of the Judet technique adding a proximal rectus femoris release (Fig. 23.7). Intra-articular adhesions are first divided through a short lateral or short medial parapatellar incision. The knee is manipulated and, if the manipulation is not successful, the lateral incision is extended proximally to the greater trochanter. The vastus lateralis is freed from the linea aspera and from the greater trochanter, and the vastus intermedius is lifted extraperiosteally from the lateral and anterior surfaces of the femur. When the rectus is tight, the incision is extended proximally and the rectus femoris is freed from the ileum and superior acetabulum. The vastus medialis is not disturbed as its origin is solely from the linea aspera. The incisions are closed over a continuous suction drain. After operation the hip and knee joints are flexed to 90 degrees over a box frame and heavy sedation is used. Passive exercises are started at 48 hours. Active assisted exercises are begun at 3 to 5 days. A manipulation under anesthesia is done if the motion obtained at operation is not regained. The aim of surgical treatment should be to achieve flexion of 110 to 120 degrees.

SYNOVECTOMY

The major indication for synovectomy has been rheumatoid arthritis[13,14,25,26,30,33] in the belief that excision of inflamed synovium would (1) relieve swelling and discomfort, and (2) retard progression of arthritis and destruction of articular cartilage (Fig. 23.8). The extent to which synovectomy impedes progression of damage to articular cartilage is controversial, and the prophylactic effect is very difficult to assess because of the unpredictable evolution of the disease.[24] Certainly the synovium that reforms has a more normal cellular lining supported by a dense fibrous stroma.[27] Even in early cases, however, recurrences do occur (about 20 percent in Gariépy's series[12]), and an arthroplasty is more appropriate today for knees showing articular destruction. It has been observed that after total knee replacement, inflammatory changes in remaining synovium subside, leading to the possibility that rheumatoid synovitis may not be a primary factor, but rather caused by degradation products of the articular cartilage itself (see Chapter 17). For these reasons, synovectomy has become much less popular than it was a few years ago. Thus, for

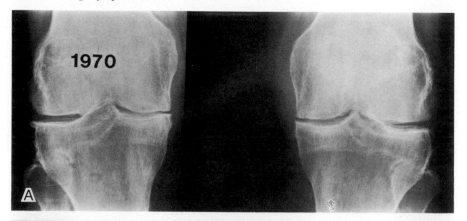

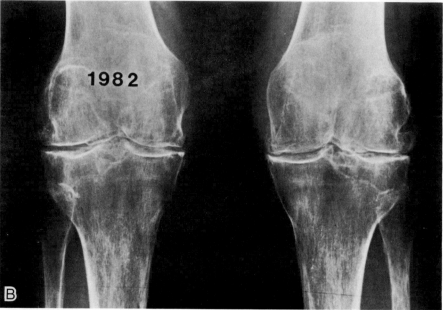

Fig. 23.8. Synovectomy of the knee. (A) Preoperative radiograph of patient with rheumatoid arthritis, showing the presence of a slight joint space narrowing. (B) Twelve years after synovectomy of both knees, little further narrowing has occurred in the interval but periarticular spurring and subchondral sclerosis are now present, suggesting a superimposed osteoarthritis. The patient does not now have a synovitis, but has recently complained of pain when walking.

rheumatoid arthritis synovectomy should be done when the articular surfaces are in good condition and the symptoms from pain and swelling cannot be controlled by medical means and seem in themselves to justify a relatively major operation. Synovectomy is also advised for other synovial diseases, such as pigmented villonodular synovitis and chondrocalcinosis.

TECHNIQUE OF SUBTOTAL SYNOVECTOMY

The purpose of this technique is to remove as much of the abnormal synovium as possible, recognizing that some will always be left behind. In the past it was the custom to perform synovectomy through mid-

medial and midlateral incisions in order to allow the exposure of the anterior and posterior compartments on each side. Although the exposure obtained was very satisfactory for the purpose, this approach should not be used because the placement of the incisions can cause difficulty if a later total knee arthroplasty is required. I prefer a gently curved anteromedial skin incision, which permits access to the anterior and posteromedial compartments. The upper limits of the suprapatellar pouch are defined and the pouch is divided longitudinally in the midline down to the femoral groove. Each side of the pouch is in turn grasped with a rongeur and peeled distally aided by sharp dissection to the level of the joint line. If the synovium can be satisfactorily cleaned from around the menisci, they should be preserved but often this is impossible and the menisci must also be removed. The intercondylar notch is debrided with rongeurs and synovium removed from around the cruciate ligaments together with that covering the fat pad. The medial skin flap is dissected posteriorly to allow a separate capsular incision into the posteromedial compartment, and the synovium is removed piecemeal with rongeurs. When there is an associated popliteal cyst, an extracapsular dissection will usually allow delivery of the cyst into the wound. The posterolateral compartment can be reached in a variety of ways. Sometimes access with rongeurs around the popliteus sleeve is sufficient. Otherwise a separate posterolateral incision can be made, or the compartment can be approached from above through the existing anterior incision. By retracting the patella and vastus lateralis, the lateral aspect of the lower femur is seen. A vertical incision is made through the periosteum coagulating the superior lateral genicular artery. Subperiosteal dissection exposes the posterior surface of the femur and the posterolateral capsule which, with the lateral head of the gastrocnemius, can be separated from the bone to enter the posterolateral compartment.

AFTERCARE

A compression dressing is used 1 week when flexing exercises are begun. A manipulation may be required 3 to 6 weeks after surgery.

POPLITEAL CYSTS[34]

Distention of the semimembranosus bursa gives rise to a popliteal or Baker's cyst[1] (actually, Baker described a tuberculous sac).

In Children. The condition is primary in children. It usually presents as a painless swelling at the back of the knee, which can attain a large size. The reason for the cyst is unknown, although possibly friction of the flexed knee against a school chair or bench may be the cause.[16] The cyst, which may be bilateral, often resolves as the child grows older, so treatment consists of observation and reassurance. Only occasionally is excision indicated.

In Adults. A popliteal cyst in an adult is nearly always secondary to pathologic changes in the knee joint, notably patellofemoral arthrosis, meniscal tears, or any form of chronic synovitis.[3,8] The patient is often made aware of the cyst by aching pain at the back of the knee, a symptom that should be interpreted with caution, as many of the conditions causing the cyst also refer pain to the popliteal fossa. If this is the case, excision will do away with the cyst, but not the pain. The diagnosis of a popliteal cyst is rarely in doubt but can be confirmed readily by aspiration.

RUPTURE OF A POPLITEAL CYST

Occasionally popliteal cysts associated with chronic rheumatoid synovitis can reach a very large size and dissect distally into the calf, at times reaching almost to the ankle.[29] It is usually these rheumatoid cysts that are susceptible to rupture, and the sudden release of synovial fluid into the tissues of the calf musculature can present as a condition resembling acute thrombophlebitis. The leg is swollen and tender, and dorsiflexion of the foot is painful. Arthrography done soon after the rupture will demonstrate dye in the soft tissues, but the synovial leak usually seals rapidly within 1 to 2 days. The condition can be distinguished from thrombophlebitis by venography, and the treatment is rest, elevation, gentle compression, and local heat.

MANAGEMENT OF POPLITEAL CYSTS

Most popliteal cysts require no treatment other than reassurance. When large and tense, the cyst may be aspirated to reduce its size. Very occasionally, excision of the cyst is indicated, although I have not found this necessary in many years.

TECHNIQUE

The patient is placed face down, with the knee slightly flexed. A lazy **S** skin incision crossing the back of the knee is used. The cyst usually lies immediately beneath the deep fascia and is revealed when the fascia is incised longitudinally. The cyst usually presents between the medial head of gastrocnemius and semimembranosus and can be dissected by blunt and sharp maneuvers until its communication with the knee is seen. After excision of the cyst, closure of this isthmus

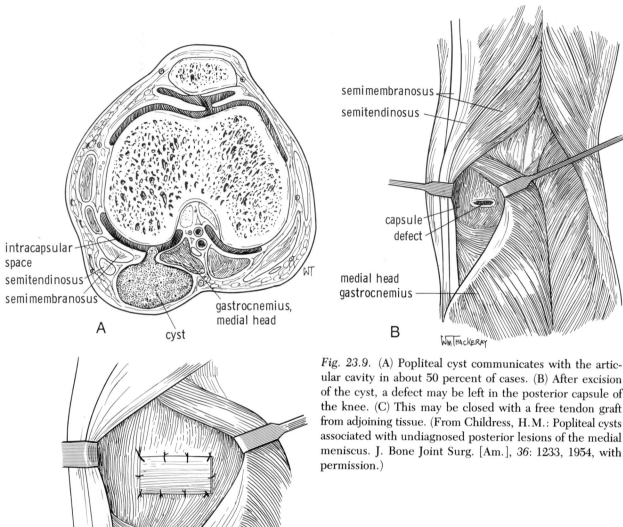

Fig. 23.9. (A) Popliteal cyst communicates with the articular cavity in about 50 percent of cases. (B) After excision of the cyst, a defect may be left in the posterior capsule of the knee. (C) This may be closed with a free tendon graft from adjoining tissue. (From Childress, H.M.: Popliteal cysts associated with undiagnosed posterior lesions of the medial meniscus. J. Bone Joint Surg. [Am.], *36:* 1233, 1954, with permission.)

is generally recommended; Childress recommends suturing a portion of the medial head of the gastrocnemius to the posterior joint capsule (Fig. 23.9).

REFERENCES

1. Baker, W.M.: On the formation of synovial cysts in the leg in connection with disease of the knee joint. St. Bartholomew's Hosp. Rep., *13:* 245, 1877.

2. Brodersen, M.P., Fitzgerald, R.H., Jr., Peterson, L.F.A., et al.: Arthrodesis of the knee following failed total knee arthroplasty. J. Bone Joint Surg. [Am.], *61:* 181, 1979.

3. Burleson, R.J., Bickel, W.H., and Dahlin, D.C.: Popliteal cyst: A clinicopathological survey. J. Bone Joint Surg. [Am.], *38:* 1265, 1956.

4. Charnley, J.C.: Positive pressure in arthrodesis of the knee joint. J. Bone Joint Surg. [Br.], *30:* 478, 1948.

5. Charnley, J.: Arthrodesis of the knee. Clin. Orthop., *18:* 37, 1960.

6. Charnley, J., and Baker, S.L.: Compression arthrodesis of the knee. A clinical and histological study. J. Bone Joint Surg. [Br.], *34:* 187, 1952.

7. Charnley, J., and Lowe, H.G.: A study of the end-results of compression arthrodesis of the knee. J. Bone Joint Surg. [Br.], *40:* 633, 1958.

8. Childress, H.M.: Popliteal cysts associated with undiagnosed posterior lesions of the medial meniscus. J. Bone Joint Surg. [Am.], *36:* 1233, 1954.

9. Daoud, H., O'Farrell, T., and Cruess, R.L.: Quadricepsplasty. The Judet technique and results of six cases. J. Bone Joint Surg. [Br.], *64:* 194, 1982.

10. Dee, R.: The case for arthrodesis of the knee. Orthop. Clin. North Am., *10:*(1) 249, 1979.

11. Drennan, D.B., Fahey, J.J., and Maylahn, D.J.: Important factors in achieving arthrodesis of the Charcot knee. J. Bone Joint Surg. [Am.], *53:* 1180, 1971.

12. Gariépy, R., Demers, R., and Laurin, C.A.: The prophylactic effect of synovectomy of the knee in rheumatoid arthritis. Can. Med. Assoc. J., *94:* 1349, 1966.

13. Geens, S.: Synovectomy and debridement of the knee in rheumatoid arthritis: Part I. Historical review. J. Bone Joint Surg. [Am.], *51:* 617, 1969.

14. Geens, S., Clayton, M.L., Leidholt, J.D., et al.: Synovectomy and debridement of the knee in rheumatoid arthritis: Part II. Clinical and roentgenographic study of thirty-one cases. J. Bone Joint Surg. [Am.], *51:* 626, 1969.

15. Green, D.P., Parkes, J.C. II, and Stinchfield, F.E.: Arthrodesis of the knee. A follow-up study. J. Bone Joint Surg. [Am.], *49:* 1065, 1967.

16. Gristina, A.G., and Wilson, P.D.: Popliteal cysts in adults and children: A review of 90 cases. Arch. Surg., *88:* 357, 1964.

17. Hagemann, W.F., Woods, G.W., and Tullos, H.S.: Arthrodesis in failed total knee replacement. J. Bone Joint Surg. [Am.], *60:* 790, 1978.

18. Hesketh, K.T.: Experiences with the Thompson quadricepsplasty. J. Bone Joint Surg. [Br.], *45:* 491, 1963.

19. Judet, R.: Mobilisation of the stiff knee. In proceedings J. Bone Joint Surg. [Br.], *41:* 856, 1959.

20. Judet, R., Judet, J., and Lagrange, J.: Une technique de libération de l'appareil extenseur dans les raideurs du genou. Mem. Acad. Chir., *82:* 944, 1956.

21. Judet, R., Judet, J., and Lord, G.: Resultats du traitement des raideurs du genou par arthrolyse et desinsertion du quadriceps femoral. Mem. Acad. Chir., *85:* 645, 1959.

22. Kaufer, H., Irvine, G., and Matthews, L.S.: Intramedullary arthrodesis of the knee. Presented at the American Academy of Orthopaedic Surgeons Annual Meeting, Anaheim, California, 1983.

23. Key, J.A.: Positive pressure in arthrodesis for tuberculosis of the knee joint. South. Med. J., *25:* 909, 1932.

24. Laurin, C.A., Desmarchais, J., and Daziano, L., et al.: Long-term results of synovectomy of the knee in rheumatoid patients. J. Bone Joint Surg. [Am.], *56:* 521, 1974.

25. Marmor, L.: Surgery of the rheumatoid knee. Synovectomy and debridement. J. Bone Joint Surg. [Am.], *55:* 535, 1973.

26. Marmor, L.: Synovectomy of the knee joint. Orthop. Clin. North Am., *10*(1): 211, 1979.

27. Mitchell, N., and Shepard, N.: The effect of synovectomy on synovium and cartilage in early rheumatoid arthritis. Clin. Orthop., *89:* 178, 1972.

28. Nicoll, E.A.: Quadricepsplasty. J. Bone Joint Surg. [Br.], *45:* 483, 1963.

29. Perri, J.A., Rodnan, G.P., and Mankin, H.J.: Giant Synovial Cysts of the Calf in Patients with Rheumatoid Arthritis. J. Bone Joint Surg. [Am.], *50:* 709, 1968.

30. Ranawat, C.S., and Desai, K.: Role of early synovectomy of the knee joint in rheumatoid arthritis. Arthritis Rheum., *18:* 117, 1975.

31. Siller, T.N., and Hadjipavlou, A.: Arthrodesis of the knee. p. 161. In the American Academy of Orthopedic Surgeons. Symposium on Reconstructive Surgery of the Knee. St. Louis, C.V. Mosby, 1978.

32. Thompson, T.C.: Quadricepsplasty to improve knee function. J. Bone Joint Surg. *26:* 366, 1944.

33. Verdeck, W.N., and McBeath, A.A.: Knee synovectomy for rheumatoid arthritis. Orthop. Clin., *134:* 168, 1978.

34. Wilson, P.D., Eyre-Brook, A.L., and Francis, J.D.: A clinical and anatomical study of the semimembranosus bursa in relation to popliteal cyst. J. Bone Joint Surg. *20:* 963, 1938.

24 Management of the Hemophilic Knee

John E. Carvell
and
Robert B. Duthie

The hemophilias are a group of genetically transmitted deficiencies of specific clotting factors:

Classic hemophilia (hemophilia A): Caused by insufficient factor VIII

Christmas disease (hemophilia B): Caused by a deficiency of factor IX

von Willebrand's disease: Associated with a prolonged bleeding time and deficiencies of factor VIII, factor VIII-related antigen, and a plasma factor necessary for some platelet reactions.

Classic hemophilia and Christmas disease are transmitted in a sex-linked recessive manner and resemble one another in almost every clinical aspect. The symptomatology and natural history are practically indistinguishable, except that the heterozygous female carrier of Christmas disease has a greater tendency to suffer from abnormal bleeding. In the 30 percent of cases of classic hemophilia patients with no family history, the disorder is probably a spontaneous genetic mutation. von Willebrand's disease is inherited as a simple dominant condition that passes directly from the affected parent to his or her children.

Classic hemophilia in its severe form is a relatively rare disorder, having an incidence of 3–4: 100,000 of the population worldwide. The incidence is doubled when mildly affected cases are taken into account.

Christmas disease is six to eight times less common than the classic hemophilia worldwide; however, it is relatively more common in certain countries, such as Switzerland, which have a localized geographic distribution. von Willebrand's disease is very rare. Table 24.1 shows the relative incidence of the three disorders in admissions to the Nuffield Orthopaedic Centre in the 13-year-period 1966–1979.

Acute hemarthrosis is the most common feature of severe hemophilia and accounts for 85 percent of all bleeding episodes. Because it is a relatively uncommon clinical feature of von Willebrand's disease, other more common causes of swelling in a joint should be considered in the differential diagnosis. An analysis of the distribution of hemarthroses seen in patients treated at the Nuffield Orthopaedic Centre during the past 13 years (Table 24.2), indicates that the knee is the most common site. The high incidence of hemarthrosis in the knee, elbow, and ankle is attributed to the inability of diarthrodial hinge joints to withstand the minor rotatory and angulatory strains imposed on them by either voluntary or involuntary movements. The latter occur during the tossing and turning of sleep and may precipitate many of the bleeding episodes that occur while a child is asleep or confined to bed in hospital as a result of a previous

743

Table 24.1.   Admissions 1966–1979

Disorder	Number of Patients
Hemophilia A	503
Hemophilia B	45
von Willebrand's	7
Total	655

Table 24.3.   Relationship between Blood Levels of Factor VIII and IX and Severity of Bleeding Manifestations

Blood Level of factors VIII and IX (% N)	Bleeding Manifestations
50–100	None
25–50	Tendency to bleed after major injury
5–25	Severe bleeding after surgical operations or minor injury
1–5	Severe bleeding after minor injury; occasional spontaneous bleeding
0	Severe hemophilia with spontaneous bleeding into muscle and joints, possibly crippling

(From Biggs, R., and MacFarlane, R.G., eds.: Treatment of hemophilia and other coagulation disorders. Blackwell Scientific Publications, Oxford, 1966, with permission.)

hemarthrosis. The relatively large amounts of synovium in these joints may be pinched in the articulation and contribute to the bleeding episode.

These observations are made in relationship to the relative sparing of the hip and shoulder ball-and-socket articulations. Although they are subject to considerable load bearing, angulatory, and rotatory forces, they appear to accommodate them more easily.[15]

PATHOLOGY OF HEMOPHILIC ARTHROPATHY

The pathology of joint destruction in hemophilia is not yet clearly defined. Joint involvement is the most important clinical feature of hemophilia in a high percentage of patients. However, because few specimens from patients are available and the changes observed late, any explanation is speculative. We have to rely on more detailed studies of osteoarthrosis, hemochromatosis, and rheumatoid arthritis combined with the results from animal models.

Since the hemophiliac begins life with normal joints,[13,30] chronic hemophilic arthropathy is the result of the exposure of the joint lining tissues to repeated, prolonged intra-articular hemorrhages. It is likely that these will result in damage to the affected joint by a number of mechanisms involving synovial tissue, synovial fluid, and articular cartilage. The advanced articular cartilage breakdown leads to disorganization of joint surfaces, stiffness, and pain.

The severity of the bleeding tendency and the degree of joint destruction in hemophilia A and Christmas disease are directly related to the circulating levels of factors VIII and IX, respectively (Table 24.3).[10,14,23,59]

Several mechanisms, general and local, physical and chemical, may contribute to the aetiology of hemophilic arthropathy.

Table 24.2.   Distribution of Acute Hemarthroses in Patients Treated at the Nuffield Orthopaedic Centre, Oxford, 1966–1979

Site	N
Knee	363
Elbow	198
Ankle	110
Shoulder	28
Wrist	21
Hip	20
Hand	18
Foot	12
Total	770

GENERAL PHYSICAL FACTORS

The number of hemarthroses and the severity of joint destruction clearly relate to the level of the relevant circulating factor. The prolonged intra-articular presence of blood, which may be under high pressure,[39] may contribute to damage to the synovium as well as destruction of articular cartilage.[48] The intra-articular pressure may be further raised by the position of flexion.[39] Consequently, the flexion deformity and fixed flexion contracture commonly seen with hemarthrosis affecting the knee may combine to produce very high intra-articular pressures.

LOCAL PHYSICAL FACTORS

The hematoma may remain fluid and continue to increase in size in the untreated hemophiliac for some time. This results from deficiency of thromboplastin activity in the synovium and fibrous capsule, and its direct communication with the capillaries may exert an intra-articular pressure equivalent to the systemic blood pressure.[30] Prolongation of this raised intra-articular pressure system may contribute to the already high pressure.

The excess clot formed as a result of continued hemarthrosis is unlikely to be removed completely by the fibrinolytic process; organization of the remaining clot will lead to excess dense fibrous tissue formation. Fibrosis has been shown to be a constant feature of subsynovial tissue.[49] The synovial tissue is the primary site of joint hemorrhage[47]; indeed, the hyperemic synovium may be subject to recurrent bleeding after the initial hemarthrosis, one hemarthrosis predisposing to further bleeding. Dense intra-articular and subsynovial fibrosis may lead to capsular fibrosis and joint contracture.

The content of synovial fluid is altered by the presence of fluid blood, clot, plasmin, and lysosomal enzymes released from inflamed synovial tissue. Such an alteration may have a direct effect on the nutrition of articular cartilage in the hemophiliac.

The nutrition of articular cartilage is altered by immobilization,[57] the reaction being defined as chondrofibrosis[36] and has been shown to be independent of direct pressure across the joint line.[56] In the hemophiliac, raised intra-articular pressure and immobilization appear to act in sequence on the affected joint. Any hemarthrosis will induce reflex immobility by pain, which may then become a permanent feature as a result of intra-articular adhesions, joint surface damage, and capsule contracture.

CHEMICAL FACTORS

Biopsies of synovium from hemophiliac patients show a marked thickening and villus proliferation that affects the entire lining layer of younger patients; this proliferation gradually disappears with age, until the synovial lining layer is flat and devoid of villi. Despite this, synovial lining cells retain their ability to de-grade red blood cells and hemoglobin after hemarthrosis.

Small round cell inflammatory infiltrates appear in the perivascular subsynovial tissue and around hemosiderin deposits, accompanied by a nonspecific angiomatoid reaction.[48] The inflammatory reaction stimulates the pleuripotential synovial cells to become actively phagocytic[22] and enables them to ingest iron particles.

The role of iron in the pathophysiology of hemophilic arthropathy is not yet established; however, the work of Stein at Oxford has contributed much to our understanding of this subject.[49] Stein was able to demonstrate that cytoplasmic deposits of iron were to be found in the synovial cells, in subsynovial tissue, and in the chondrocytes of the superficial layer of the articular cartilage. These findings were substantiated by light and electron microscopy, and supplemented by x-ray microprobe analysis. These cytoplasmic deposits have been termed true siderosomes by Stein. They have been variously described as siderosomes[43,44] and residual bodies,[19] but are defined as membrane-bound structures showing a conglomerate of amorphous, electron-dense particles that contain an even denser area on electron microscopy, slightly eccentrically located, which could be called a pseudonucleus. In a review of hemophilic synovial biopsies, Stein demonstrated that all the cells containing siderosomes showed signs of degeneration and disintegration and concluded that iron in the form of cytoplasmic true siderosomes contributed directly to early degeneration and disintegration of these cells.

The alteration in the cell physiology of the chondrocyte brought about by repeated hemarthrosis combined with the alteration in chemical and physical properties of the cartilage matrix may combine to produce the pathologic entity of severe articular cartilage damage in chronic hemophilic arthropathy.[9,46]

The process of degeneration and necrosis seen in chondrocytes containing true siderosomes in the superficial and upper cartilage zones may lead to a disruption of the surface continuity of cells, as well as a loss of matrix, which will result in further fissuring and cracking of the cartilage. The intracellular iron deposits have been associated with the deposition of insoluble calcium pyrophosphate[46] and the deterioration in cartilage matrix.[9] Sokoloff[48] has postulated that a salt might be formed between ionic iron and the sulfated proteoglycans of the ground substance.

Therefore, the addition of polyvalent cations may increase matrix deformability and reduce its capacity to recover from applied stress.

Large areas of cartilage destruction have been noted adjacent to heavily pigmented synovium.[52] It is known that proteolytic enzymes may degrade cartilage and high levels of hydrolytic enzymes, particularly cathepsin-D. Cathepsin-D has been detected in the synovium and synovial fluid of hemophilic joints.[23] The enzyme has a potent chemotactic effect and may play a part in maintaining a chronically inflamed synovium. Cathepsin-D may also degrade the extracellular matrix of articular cartilage participating in further cartilage degeneration.

Plasmin, a proteolytic enzyme resulting from the activation of serum plasminogen, also contributes to articular degeneration in chronic hemophiliac arthropathy. Derived from blood, plasmin can be activated in synovial fluid as a result of trauma to synovium and cartilage. Cartilage is capable of activating plasminogen, which escapes into the joint as a result of the increased vascular permeability of synovium after hemarthrosis. The plasmin formed onto articular cartilage substrate escapes inhibition by the excess inhibitor to plasmin in the blood and synovial fluid. Plasmin then exerts a proteolytic papainlike action on the articular cartilage and permits chondroitin sulfate to leak out into the bloodstream, where some of it will be excreted as glucuronic acid.[33]

Fibrosis of the synovial lining of a hemophilic joint may lead to altered metabolic function of the synovial lining cells, one function of which is the synthesis and

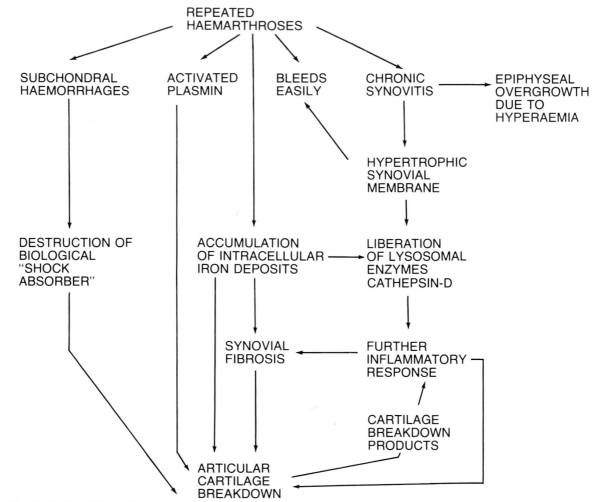

Fig. 24.1. Possible pathogenesis of chronic hemophilic arthropathy. (From Stein, H., and Duthie, R.B.: The pathogenesis of chronic haemophilic arthropathy. J. Bone Joint Surg. [Br.], *63*: 4, 1981, with permission.)

secretion of glycosaminoglycans,[42] particularly chondroitin sulfate. Another function of the synovial membrane is the secretion of hyaluronic acid into the synovial fluid. The surface of normal articular cartilage is covered by a layer of hyaluronic acid with protein, which protects the underlying tissue from mechanical and enzymatic damage by blood cells and fibroblasts in synovial fluid. This layer of hyaluronic acid could not be demonstrated on hemophilic articular cartilage by histochemical or electron microscopic studies[49] and may be absent. It signifies further extensive damage to the articular cartilage and emphasizes the deleterious effect of the impairment of the synovial membrane function.

It would seem that while mechanical and chemical disturbance cause deterioration of synovial cells and articular cartilage chondrocytes, the enzymatic disturbance seems primarily responsible for the degradation of cartilage matrix. Figure 24.1 summarizes a possible pathogenesis of chronic hemophilic arthropathy.

RADIOLOGIC ASSESSMENT OF HEMOPHILIC ARTHROPATHY[20]

The principal value of radiology lies in the assessment of the presence and progression of hemophilic arthropathy. It may be of value in the acute hemarthrosis to know whether such radiologic changes have occurred. Radiographs should be taken when a history of trauma is obtained to exclude bony injury, especially in the less severely affected hemophiliac, in whom hemarthrosis is uncommon.

The radiologic features of hemophilic arthropathy are not diagnostic.[8] A radiologic classification on the basis of changes of surgical significance has been described.[4] However, it is important to correlate the radiologic changes with the patient's age, the number of hemarthroses, periarticular hemorrhages, and the effect of treatment on past hemarthroses. The clinician is then able to evaluate patient management and to determine a more accurate prognosis for each patient.

The radiologic changes in hemophilic arthropathy may be classified in three groups:

1. Those occurring as a direct result of a single or recurrent hemarthrosis.
2. Nonspecific changes, which may result from immobilization of a limb and the reactive hyperemia that accompanies hemorrhage.

3. Specific changes of unknown etiology that occur at certain anatomic sites.

There is generally a gradual increase with age in the percentage of joints showing structural radiologic change. In a radiologic survey of 92 affected knees in 58 patients, 80 percent in the 6- to 10-year-olds had normal or only mildly abnormal radiographs.[20] In 25-year-olds, this figure fell to 38 percent. This progression of radiologic change is a reflection of the repeated hemarthroses of childhood.

Changes associated with hemarthrosis are as follows:

1. Distention of the joint cavity and elevation of the patella, depending on the volume of blood present.
2. Synovial or capsular thickening in the presence of recurrent bleeding or incomplete resolution of a hemarthrosis (Fig. 24.2).

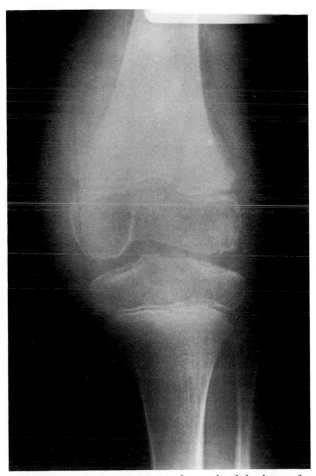

Fig. 24.2. An anteroposterior radiograph of the knee of a 6-year-old boy with a 1-year history of recurrent bleeding and synovial hypertrophy.

3. Osteoporosis and muscle atrophy, a feature of young hemophiliacs, which may account for the relative increase in the synovial density (these features become less apparent as synovial fibrosis and degenerative bony changes supervene with age).
4. Marginal articular erosions.
5. The late changes of secondary degenerative arthritis, namely, loss of joint space, subchondral collapse, cystic changes, and osteophyte formation.
6. Abnormalities of the patellofemoral compartment, which may comprise narrowing of the joint space, loss of congruity of the joint surfaces, and squaring of the inferior pole of the patella.
7. Changes in the tibiofemoral joint may include condylar squaring and enlargement, particularly on the medial side; depression of the tibial table, which is present in 50 percent of cases over the age of 11 years; and may be related to medial condylar enlargement; changes in the late degenerative cases include cyst formation with osteophytosis; all these changes may tend to be more severe in the medial compartment than in the lateral despite the frequent presence of a valgus deformity (Fig. 24.3A,B).

The radiologic changes resulting from immobilization of a joint and secondary hyperemia are not entirely specific to a hemophilic arthropathy, but certain characteristics have been grouped together to form the radiologic appearance most commonly associated with a hemophilic arthropathy:
1. Osteoporosis more marked in the epiphysis than in the shaft of long bones.
2. The preferential resorption of fine bony trabeculae, leading to an open latticework pattern.
3. Transverse growth arrest lines, which become more numerous and prominent.
4. Condylar enlargement, seen in all age groups is more prominent in adult patients (the etiology of condylar enlargement is not yet established). Cartilage overgrowth has been shown to be an important feature of joints of experimental animals subjected to repeated intra-articular injections of blood[24]; calcification of the deeper layers leading to the formation of a ghost head within a head (Fig. 24.4).

Certain radiologic changes have been associated with specific sites in a joint (Fig. 24.5A,B).
1. Squaring of the lower pole of the patella, present

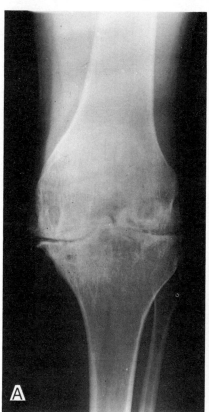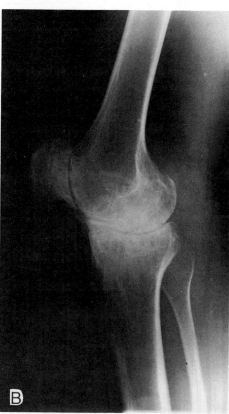

Fig. 24.3. (A,B) Radiographs showing late changes of hemophilic arthropathy in the knee.

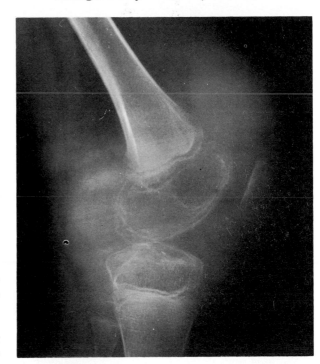

Fig. 24.4. Lateral radiograph of a 6-year-old boy with recurrent bleeding and synovial hypertrophy, showing ghosting of the femoral epiphysis.

Fig. 24.5. (A,B) Radiograph showing squaring of the lower pole of the patella, intercondylar widening, and cyst formation.

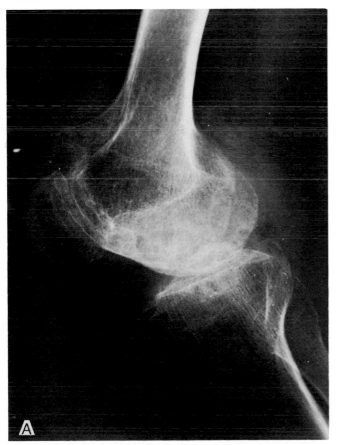

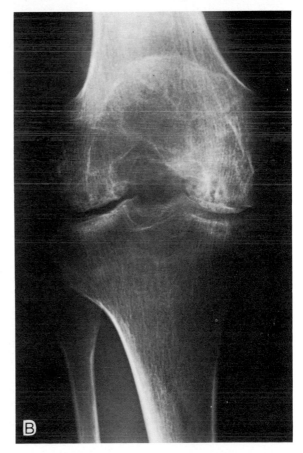

in 20 percent of cases; also found in juvenile rheumatoid arthritis, may be large and wide, long and thin, or even absent.

2. Widening of the intercondylar notch.
3. Cyst formation noted in the tibial intercondylar eminence; both intercondylar widening and cyst formation thought to be associated with bleeding at the site of origin and insertion of the cruciate ligaments.[15]

Changes in the alignment of the femur and tibia, not always clinically apparent owing to soft tissue swelling and hemarthrosis, may be brought to light by radiographs.

The most frequent deformities in the hemophilic knee are flexion, valgus, and external rotation.[12] Posterior and lateral subluxations of the tibia have also been identified as important changes in alignment. Films of the appropriate length and size are necessary to permit accurate assessment of these deformities. A lateral view will only demonstrate posterior subluxation if taken in maximum extension. External rotation of the tibia seen in poliomyelitis and rheumatoid arthritis may play an important part in the progression of deformity. It is thought to result from the imbalance of forces between the relatively strong tensor fascia lata and lateral hamstrings and the weaker medial quadriceps muscles.

ARTICULAR RADIONUCLIDE SCANNING

The skeletal scintigram has become an important clinical tool. Its role and place in the investigation and management of patients with hemophilia have not been fully evaluated.

Technetium-99m has been regarded as the ideal radionuclide. It has a pure γ-ray of appropriate energy (140 keV) with no primary β-radiation and a half-life of 6 hours. The patient therefore receives a low dose of radiation. It is rapidly cleared from the blood with a high target:nontarget ratio when large doses are used. Its advantages include low cost, immediate availability, compatibility with a gamma camera, and the ability to give high doses if required.[53,54]

The mechanism of action of the radiopharmaceuticals has not yet been elucidated. The following types of reaction have been postulated for the ^{99m}Tc-labeled phosphate complexes:

1. The phosphorus groups may become attached onto the calcium of hydroxyapatite in bone.[26]
2. The tracer may be concentrated in the proximity of osteoblastic activity by its affinity for immature collagen.[34]
3. The reduced state of technetium, Tc(IV), may be directly incorporated in bone. The polyphosphates and other agents merely act as chelating agents, preventing colloid formation.

These radiopharmaceutical complexes clear from blood exponentially with a rapid, early phase that distributes through the extracellular space and a slower, later phase that goes intramuscularly and preferentially to bone.

The two features of the radionuclide scan that may be of value to the clinician are (1) an early extracellular flow phase, indicating hyperemic tissue (e.g., synovium), and (2) the later activity in bone, demonstrating osteoblastic activity.

An abnormal scan shows a high radionuclide uptake.[18] It has been shown that isotope is not concentrated by the synovial cells, but that any increased uptake in the early phase is a reflection of the vascularity of the synovium.[60] It has been suggested, but not yet proved, that a radioactive scan may be more sensitive than clinical examination, and an abnormal scan may precede a synovitis.[18] When synovial hypertrophy has become an established clinical entity, the scan may be of value in assessing the effectiveness of adequate nonsurgical therapy and in helping select those patients who would benefit from synovectomy.[17] The completeness of the synovectomy, and further bleeds, and the subsequent regeneration of the synovium may also be assessed in this way.

The place for a radionuclide scintigram in the evaluation of acute hemarthrosis and chronic joint disease still remains to be demonstrated. After acute hemarthroses, bone scintigrams have been shown to correlate well with the clinical signs, but not with the number of bleeding episodes.[18] Bone scintigrams have also been shown to retain a high uptake well after the acute episode has settled, possibly a reflection of synovial hyperemia.[17]

With the use of a large-field-of-view camera and a combined early flow phase and late bone phase scan, it may be possible in the future to establish the pattern of joint disease both in the synovium and in bone. The scan may influence management of the patient.

Scintigraphy has been evaluated in the assessment of chronic joint disease, but no correlation with either the number of bleeding episodes or the clinical grading of the joint disease has been found.[18] Perhaps increased knowledge of the relationship between osteoblastic activity and radionuclide scintigrams will permit a better evaluation of chronic joint disease in the future. Figures 24.6A,B illustrates a bone scintigram and plain films of a 15-year-old boy. Clinically, the disease in the knee was mild in this case. The boy had had one or two small isolated bleeds in the suprapatellar pouch before the scintigram was done. Radiologically, he has moderately advanced changes of a hemophilic arthropathy. An isolated scintigram of the knee is not of any real value, but as part of a serial review of the patient, may prove important in the evaluation of the knee as a whole.

CORRELATION OF RADIOLOGIC CHANGES WITH FREQUENCY OF HEMARTHROSIS

It is now established that the changes of hemophilic arthropathy are clearly related to the frequency of bleeding into a joint. Adults with one radiologically affected knee and one normal knee have a clear history of repeated major hemarthrosis in the affected knee with sparing of the other knee. In children and adolescents, it is possible to watch a steady and progressive deterioration in the radiologic characteristics of the knee in relation to frequent hemarthroses. However, the severe changes of hemophilic arthropathy may be prevented by the prompt administration of the deficient factor. The recognition of this fact and the introduction of home factor treatment must limit the number of severely affected knees seen in the future.

CLINICAL PRESENTATION OF THE HEMOPHILIC KNEE

Acute hemarthrosis is the presenting complaint in the majority of patients with classic hemophilia A and Christmas disease. The fact is confirmed in a summary of the clinical presentation of patients admitted in Oxford (Table 24.4). Intra-articular bleeds of the knee are the single most common cause for admission.

The high incidence and severity of hemarthrosis in any joint is affected by several factors. The following are general factors affecting a hemophiliac patient:

Table 24.4. Clinical Presentation of Patients admitted to the Nuffield Orthopaedic Centre, 1966–1979[a]

Disorder/Site	N	Disorder/Site	N
Hemarthroses		Muscle hematoma	
Knee	363	Ilio psoas	63
Elbow	198	Arm/forearm	35
Ankle	110	Thigh	35
Shoulder	28	Calf	45
Wrist	24	Shoulder	7
Hip	20	Buttock	7
Hand	18	Miscellaneous	4
Foot	12	Total	196
Total	773		
Pseudotumor	7	Peripheral lesions	
Fractures		Femoral	35
Femur	12	Sciatic	3
Tibia	5	Anterior tibial	2
Olecranon	3	Posterior tibial	3
Humerus	1	Median	4
Clavicle	1	Ulnar	5
Radius/ulna	3	Other	3
Axis	1	Total	55
Ankle	1		
Metatarsals	1		
Total	28		
Dislocations	3		

[a]Summary of totals: Hemarthroses, 773; all others, 282.

1. The level of circulating factor (Table 24.3)
2. A traumatic episode
3. The patient's age
   The incidence of hemarthrosis is higher in the teenage years and decreases with age, owing to an overall modified activity, restricted joint activity, and compensatory changes in the hemostatic process that do not affect the clotting defect and which are as yet ill-understood.
4. The presence of antibodies—does not affect the severity or frequency of bleeds[7]
   The knee is particularly at risk, for several specific reasons. It is a hinge joint and subject to angulatory and rotatory strains that it may not be able to withstand. It has a relatively large area of synovium that may be pinched in the articulation. Recurrent bleeding and synovial hypertrophy have a cause-and-effect relationship, one leading to the other and vice versa.

Therefore, a large single bleed or recurrent hemarthrosis, with consequent quadriceps inhibition and wasting, intra-articular fibrosis of clot, and subsynovial and capsular fibrosis, may contribute singly or in

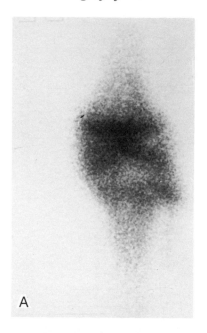
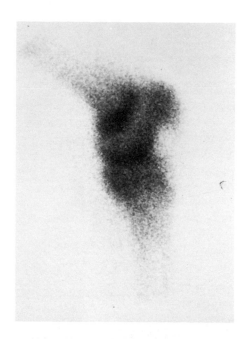

A

Fig. 24.6. (A–C) Anteroposterior and lateral views of a bone scan and plain radiographs of a hemophilic knee. The scan was carried out using a Nuclear Enterprises Mark IV gamma camera, and 12 μCi technetium-99m methylenediphosphonate was injected as a single IV bolus. Scanning was carried out at 5-second intervals after 2 hours.

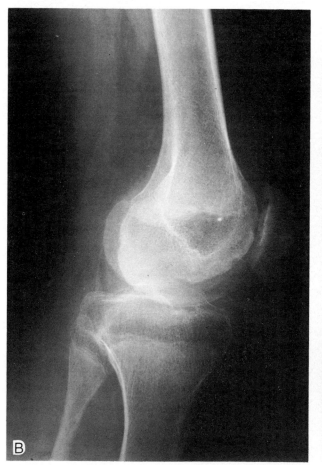

B

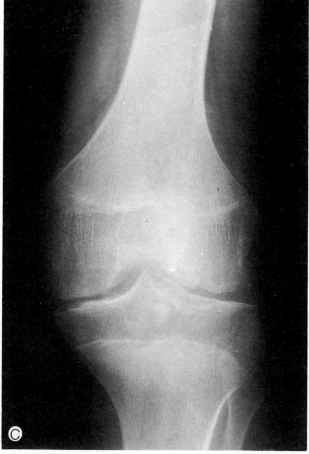

C

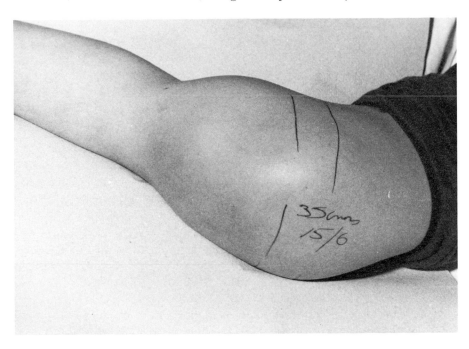

Fig. 24.7. An acute hemarthrosis.

combination with the high incidence of hemarthrosis and later arthropathy of the knee.

The patient presenting with an acute hemarthrosis usually experiences premonitory symptoms, which include a pricking sensation, increased warmth, weakness, and stiffness of the joint. In severe hemophiliacs, a history of trauma is unusual. The pre-

monitory symptoms are followed by pain of variable severity, depending on the size of the hemarthrosis.[11] The joint becomes swollen, tense, and hot; the overlying skin is stretched and red (Fig. 24.7). The knee joint is usually held in flexion of some 75 to 90 degrees, and the range of motion is restricted by flexor spasm (Fig. 24.8). The degree of swelling may not

Fig. 24.8. Flexion deformity after an acute hemarthrosis.

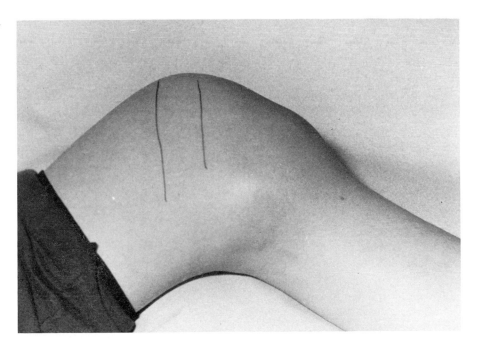

correlate with the severity of pain, especially in the fibrosed joint of an older hemophiliac with reduced joint space. A small bleed into a confined space may produce severe pain with little distention.

The condition of a subacute hemarthrosis often develops after two or more bleeds. It is a relatively painless state associated with a boggy synovial swelling (Fig. 24.9A,B). The etiology of the condition is thought to be related to a late presentation after an acute bleed ineffectively treated, in the presence of antibodies to the specific factor.

The state of chronic hemophilic arthropathy has been recognized since König noted the association of an arthropathy with joint bleeding in 1842. The joints involved are those like the knee, which are subject to repeated hemarthroses with subsequent synovial thickening, intra-articular fibrosis, and cartilage destruction, leading to joint stiffness. Loss of motion, particularly flexion, is the most common finding in this condition and may precede pain and deformity by many years. Fixed flexion contractures occur in 80 percent of knees in which moderate or severe radiologic features are present. Intra-articular adhesions lead to a small stiff joint with a reduced joint cavity. Bleeds into such joints are very painful and tense.

Most patients with chronic hemophilic arthropathy are seen in adult life.[2] The condition presents most commonly in the knee as does osteoarthritis. The two conditions share many symptoms. A persisting ache interspersed with attacks of acute pain and swelling related to an effusion may be the presenting symptom complex. In some cases the progressive loss of motion and fibrosis may terminate in a fibrous ankylosis. If the condition is bilateral, patients may require crutches or a wheelchair to maintain mobility.

Chronic hemophilic arthropathy may be seen in children who have not received adequate treatment for recurrent hemarthroses.

MEDICAL MANAGEMENT

The overall management of hemophilic patients must be supervised by a combined team of hematologists and surgeons familiar with the problems of hemophiliac patients.

The aims of primary medical management of the acute hemarthrosis are to:

1. Secure hemostasis
2. Relieve pain
3. Maintain and restore joint function
4. Prevent chronic hemophilic arthropathy.

Hemostatis is achieved by adequate early infusion of the appropriate factor. The amount of factor required by each patient is calculated according to:
1. Extent of the hemarthrosis
2. Level of circulating factor
3. Presence of antibodies
4. Nature and expected duration of treatment

The half-life of factor VIII in hemophiliacs is approximately 12 hours, and that of factor IX is approximately 18 hours. It is important to assess the level of circulating factor to ensure adequate replacement therapy. Table 24.5 presents the substances available for replacement therapy in hemophilia A and the levels of circulating factor that may be obtained.

A summary of the important points about each source of factor VIII is given in Table 24.6. In practice, lyophilized human AHG or cryoprecipitate is generally used. Plasma, cryoprecipitate, and AHG concentrate contain only small amounts of factor IX and are therefore of little value in the treatment of patients with hemophilia B. Concentrates of factor IX are prepared commercially as a prothrombin complex from human plasma. It contains concentrations of factors II, VII, IX, and X, with the concentration of factors II, VII, and X lower than of factor IX.

The dose factor is calculated using the relationship established between the rise in plasma concentration of clotting factor and the dose in units per kilogram. A rough guide to the dose of factor VIII for patients can be obtained from the average response of the average patient. This has been calculated as about 2 percent U/kg dose. Once the desired rise in concentration of factor VIII has been established by clinical judgment, the dose will be:

Table 24.5. Therapeutic Materials Available for the Treatment of Hemophilia A

Source of Factor VIII	Level of Factor VIII Achievable in Patient's blood (% normal)
Fresh whole blood	4–6
Fresh-frozen plasma	15–20
Cryoprecipitate	60–80
Lyophilized human AHG	60–80
Lyophilized animal AHG	150

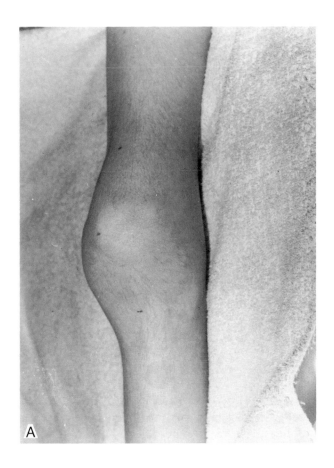

Fig. 24.9. (A,B) Atrophied quadriceps and synovial hypertrophy of a subacute hemarthrosis.

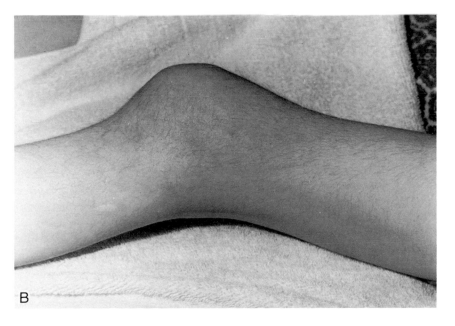

Table 24.6. Important Aspects about the Therapeutic Materials Available for the Treatment of Hemophilia A

Source of Factor VIII	Advantages	Disadvantages
Fresh whole blood	No preparation needed; reserved for whole blood replacement only	Insufficient quantity of factor VIII; factor VIII unstable in stored blood above +4°C
Fresh-frozen plasma	Cheap; can achieve levels of 15 to 20 percent of normal	Circulatory overload; delayed administration of factor: 45 minutes to thaw, 60 minutes to infuse; serum hepatitis in pooled plasma
Cryoprecipitate	Source one donor; little risk of hepatitis or allergic reaction	Cannot be assayed until time of transfusion; variable factor VIII activity; must be stored at −20° to −40°C
Lyophilized human AHG	Standardization of factor VIII content; convenient safe, easy administration; source of choice for elective surgery	Expensive; febrile and allergic reactions; hemolytic anemia in patients with red cell type A, B, or AB; hepatitis risk; protein overload; rapid transfusion; headache, abdominal pain
Lyophilized animal AHG porcine and bovine	Very potent source of factor VIII; useful for life-saving surgery or hemostasis, with high antibody titer	Antigenic

Abbreviation: AHG, Antihemophilic globulin

$$\text{Desired rise in factor VIII percent} = \frac{2 \times \text{units of dose}}{\text{body wt (in kg)}}$$

or

$$\text{Dose units} = \frac{\text{body wt. (in kg)}}{} \times 0.5 \times \text{desired rise in factor VIII percent}$$

Patients with hemophilia B require twice the dose of factor IX expressed as units per kilogram. The concentrates available have given on average a response of 0.6 percent per unit-per kilogram dose. The dose is calculated in exactly the same manner as for factor VIII-deficient patients:

$$\text{Desired rise in factor IX percent} = \frac{0.6 \times \text{units of dose}}{\text{body wt. (in kg)}}$$

or

$$\text{Dose units} = \frac{\text{body wt (in kg)}}{} \times 1.7 \times \text{desired rise in factor IX percent.}$$

Effective hemostatic therapy must be continued until the lesion has completely healed. It must cover subsequent interference with the lesion, such as mobilization of the knee joint after an acute hemarthrosis.

COMPLICATIONS OF TREATMENT WITH SPECIFIC FACTOR REPLACEMENT

Complications may arise as a consequence of the treatment of patients with plasma fractions. They fall into four main groups:

1. The transmission to the patient of an infective organism, which may be contained in the fraction, in particular the agent causing hepatitis.
2. Pyrogenic and other adverse reactions to the infusion factor.
3. Thrombotic episodes.
4. The development of specific antibodies against the coagulation factors, particularly against factor VIII.

Approximately 3 percent of hemophilic patients are Australia antigen positive in the United Kingdom. The incidence is slightly higher in patients with hemophilia A than those with Christmas disease. Screening tests of patients for Australia antigen and antibody show that between 30 and 50 percent of hemophilic patients are Australia antibody positive at any one time. However, illness associated with jaundice occurs in only 4 to 6 percent of hemophilic patients exposed to the virus compared with an infection rate of 50 to 75 percent in the normal population. Presumably hemophilic patients are immunized to viral hepatitis, whereas the normal populations are not. The presence of antibody to the hepatitis B virus may protect the hemophilic patient against infection.[31,32]

As far as treatment is concerned, it is obviously desirable to produce blood products having a low incidence of hepatitis virus contamination. In present circumstances, a balance must be maintained between the risk of transmitting a disease with variable and unpredictable consequences for each individual patient and the hemostatic needs of the patient.

A rational policy might include the selective use of small pool concentrates or cryoprecipitate for patients who have a low incidence of bleeding and therefore receive small infrequent infusions of factor. Patients who have antibody to the hepatitis virus and who are severely affected can receive large pool commercial concentrates. Clearly, treatment should not be withheld from severely affected patients because of the danger of hepatitis. The danger from crippling hemorrhage and death being of more immediate significance.

The infusion of quantities of plasma to achieve safe hemostatic levels of factor VIII has led to hypervolemia even in young patients. In a small number of patients, urticaria to plasma infusion may develop, and bronchospasm, pulmonary congestion, pyrexia, and even death have been reported after plasma infusions. These reactions have been attributed to the presence of white cell antibodies or to anti-Gm(1) precipitins in the donor plasma. Coagulation factor concentrates should always be used in preference to plasma in patients who have had a previous reaction to a plasma infusion.

A hemolytic reaction to infused anti-A or anti-B antibodies may develop in patients of blood groups A, B, or AB who receive a large amount of plasma. Some preparations of factor VIII concentrates contain blood group A and B isoagglutinins. In small doses, such preparations do not cause any problems. However, the large doses required by patients undergoing surgery, or who have antibodies, may cause hemolysis.[55] The development of jaundice in a patient who has no Australia antigen or antibody and who has received large doses of factor VIII may well be caused by the presence of isoagglutinins in the infusion.

Thrombosis of superficial veins was formerly seen when patients received concentrates of animal factor VIII via an indwelling catheter. However, the use of small butterfly needles that are removed and the use of commercial concentrates have eliminated this problem.

Intravascular coagulation as a result of treament with factor IX concentrates has been described.[27–29] Consumption of clotting factors together with evidence of venous thrombosis and pulmonary embolism have been recorded.[16,37,51]

The standardization and safety of commercial factor IX concentrates has not yet been achieved and certain commerical preparations are more liable to cause thrombosis than others. Preparations of concentrates in Oxford and Paris have been used for 15 to 20 years, respectively, with no record of thrombosis or defibrination in any single factor IX-deficient patient. Care must therefore be exercised when considering the long-term use of factor IX concentrates for the day-to-day treatment of patients with a congenital factor IX deficiency.

Patients who have neither factor VIII nor factor IX may have an immune system that may recognize proteins carrying these activities as foreign. Antibodies may then be directed at these foreign proteins. The production of specific antibody occurs in about 6 percent of patients with hemophilia A. It is rare in patients with Christmas disease. The figures have remained constant over the last 10 years despite the increase in the amount of treatment given to patients.

The immunologic processes whereby antibodies may be produced are not fully understood. The presence or absence of abnormal proteins, the type of factor VIII administered and the presence of a familial tendency have been suggested but not proven. It is not possible to identify the patient in whom antibodies to factor VIII will develop and those in whom it will not. The level of antibody usually remains low; this may be attributable to the rapid elimination of factor VIII from the circulation and the normally low plasma concentration being associated with a low potential immunogenic response in terms of the quantity of protein involved. Genetic factors may influence the response of a patient to immunization, which may not be related to the hemophilia gene. Thus one member of a family may be more susceptible to immunization by any foreign protein than a relative.

Antibodies to factor IX are rare. Five patients out of 388 hemophilia B patients treated in the United Kingdom over the 5-year period from 1969 to 1974 have had antibodies to factor IX.[6]

The frequency and severity of bleeding is no greater in the presence of antibodies. The decision to administer factor VIII in the presence of antibody is governed by the severity and site of the bleed. The potency of the antibody and the response of the patients with antibody to previous treatment may also be taken into account. In a review of 38 patients with antibodies in Oxford, 40 percent of the lesions that the patients presented with were treated. Hemarthroses and hematomata formed most of the lesions treated.[45]

Despite adequate measures to relieve pain by rest and careful splinting, bleeding may continue in the patient with antibodies. The continued presence of pain and swelling may be relieved by the use of an appropriate infusion of factor. When the treatment is given, the antibody titer is measured and subsequent dose levels adjusted accordingly. Approximately two to four times the usual dose is given. In the presence of a very severe hemarthrosis, a single large dose of factor VIII will sometimes halt the bleeding, even when no free factor VIII is detectable in the plasma afterward.

Pain of a varying degree is a very common symptom of hemarthrosis of the knee. The speed of onset and the severity of the pain vary from a few hours to several days. The most painful bleeds occur in contracted fibrosed joints accompanying a chronic hemophilic arthropathy. It is the symptom responsible for reflex muscle spasm and the characteristic flexed attitude of the knee.

The pain is relieved by a number of important elements of the treatment of an acute hemarthrosis:

1. Infusion of factor VIII, which has an early, marked, unexplained analgesic effect.
2. Application of a padded wool and domette bandage supported with a plaster-of-Paris backslab with the knee joint in a position of comfort.
3. The careful prescription of analgesics.

Mild to moderate pain may be controlled with oral analgesia. Codeine, paracetamol, and combination preparations including paracetamol are very effective. Aspirin and the nonsteroidal anti-inflammatory drugs are contraindicated owing to their gastric irritant effect and their tendency to reduce platelet adhesion. The nonsteroidal anti-inflammatory agents may also interfere with liver function and the formation of other clotting factors.[1]

Severe pain requires effective intravenous analgesia. The opiates and pethidine (demerol) may be required initially for the relief of pain. These may be administered intravenously for a short period until the pain can be controlled by oral administration of pethidine, pentazocine (Fortral), dextromoramide (Palfium), or dihydrocodeine. On no account should analgesia be administered intramuscularly to a patient with a bleeding diathesis. Drug addiction is not uncommon in patients with chronic hemophilic arthropathy, particularly in those patients with childhood or early adolescent disease. They may be manipulative in seeking analgesia and experience is required to assess the needs of each individual patient; psychiatric advice may be necessary to control an addiction.

The severity of a hemarthrosis in the knee is measured by:

1. Severity of pain
2. Size of a joint as measured by tape measure circumferentially
3. Tension within the joint tissues
4. Presence of a flexion deformity

The response to the initial treatment is measured by the reduction in pain as mirrored by the analgesic requirement, a measured decrease in the joint circumference and decrease in the flexion deformity. Serial plasters in progressive extension may be necessary to support the knee in order to prevent a fixed deformity.

Once the acute phase has settled the knee is progressively mobilised with isometric quadriceps and flexion exercises, supplemented with ice and later hydrotherapy to control the initial weight-bearing phase. Crutches or sticks may be necessary for support on dry land until a satisfactory range of motion is achieved. The speed of a patient's recovery will depend on:

1. Extent of the hemarthrosis
2. Number of previous bleeding episodes
3. Timing and effectiveness of treatment
4. Presence of established hemophilic arthropathy and deformity.

ASPIRATION OF AN ACUTE HEMARTHROSIS

The presence of blood and its effect on the joint are well documented.[24] However, all the conditions required to be fulfilled for joint aspiration are rarely present at one and the same time. The joint should not be affected by degenerative changes, and the hemarthrosis should not be loculated. Aspiration should be carried out within 24 hours of the bleed before clotting occurs. The presence of factor VIII antibodies is a contraindication to aspiration.

Factor VIII infusion should be given simultaneously during aspiration to ensure a seal over the needle hole and to prevent clotting of the hemarthrosis until aspiration is complete. Aspiration should be performed under a general anesthetic with full aseptic precautions. Afterward, the knee should be placed in a wool and domette-padded compression bandage with a plaster-of-Paris backslab support for 48 hours. Factor VIII cover should be continued to cover the period of mobilization. This procedure is now rarely carried out because of the introduction of home factor therapy and the widespread availability of factor VIII and IX concentrates.

HOME THERAPY

Once it was recognized that hemophilia A and B patients should receive prompt treatment for every episode of bleeding and the arrival of cryoprecipitate, the workload of hemophilia centers became impossible. The introduction of the factor replacement administered in the home by the patient, or his relatives, has relieved the pressure and brought benefit to all concerned. The National Hemophilia Foundation in the United States has estimated that 50 percent of hemophiliacs are on home therapy.[4] Home therapy has been in use in Oxford since 1971, where 115 patients with hemophilia A and 10 patients with hemophilia B are currently receiving home therapy. This represents 14 percent of the total number of patients registered in Oxford and approximately 50 percent of those attending the Hemophilia Centre regularly.

The criteria for inclusion in the scheme are (1) frequency of bleeding, and (2) the distance from the patient's home to the center. A patient who bleeds frequently and lives 50 miles from the center will have traveled many thousands of miles per year for treatment.

Other criteria include the willingness and competence of the patient, his or her family, and the general practitioner to administer home therapy and supervise crises. A patient may be excluded for any of the following reasons:
1. The patient may have difficult veins.
2. A difficult child may have a disagreement with his or her parents.
3. The patient may not be able to keep a proper record of therapy.
4. The patient has anti-factor VIII antibodies.

National Health Service freeze-dried factor VIII is used at Oxford.[7] Once the patient, the family, and general practitioner have consented to cooperate with the home therapy program, a course of instruction begins. Only when the patient and relatives are fully conversant with the therapy and its administration are they given a kit containing all that is required.

The period of instruction usually takes about 3 months. The patients are encouraged to maintain close contact with the center, and all attend for a regular 6-month review. It is important to combine all aspects of the program to ensure its maximum efficiency.

Patients are advised to start treatment as soon as possible after the onset of bleeding. For patients with hemophilia A, regular prophylactic doses are only administered for short periods in certain circumstances. The knee may recover a full range of motion faster after a severe bleed if regular treatment is given for a few days or weeks after the bleeding has ceased. Stress may predispose a patient to more frequent bleeding,[7] and patients are advised to have a prophylactic infusion every day during school examinations, before interviews, when starting a new job, or for other special occasions.

Hemophilia B patients are nearly always advised to have a prophylactic dose once every 1 or 2 weeks. This has been found to reduce the frequency of bleeding. The advantages for this form of therapy are as follows:
1. It is much cheaper for the service and the patient.
2. The patient has better medical care.
3. The patient demonstrates overall improvement in physical, mental, and social well-being.

For the future, the amount of factor VIII used will diminish, owing to the preservation of muscle power and tone, which permits patients to take more regular forms of exercise. Exercise is believed to raise patients' level of circulation factor by an as yet unknown mechanism (C.R. Rizza, personal communication, 1980). The earlier that treatment is given, the smaller the dose required to control the bleeding. Chronically inflamed joints will decrease in frequency with the early infusion of factor VIII.

In theory, the complications may include:
1. Hepatitis transmitted to a family member
2. Septicemia
3. Jaundice
4. Lack of controlled therapy and follow-up.

At Oxford, three patients with hemophilia A have developed jaundice and five have had a problem with venipuncture.

Hemophilic arthropathy of the adolescent knee and hence chronic hemophilic arthropathy of the adult knee will decrease in frequency as a result of the increasing speed and efficiency of home therapy.

SUBACUTE HEMARTHROSES

Subacute hemarthrosis is a self-perpetuating pathologic state that results from recurrent hemarthroses. The hypertrophic, hyperemic synovium resulting from a hemarthrosis predisposes to further bleeding in the joint. The knee and elbow are particularly affected by this state, owing to the abundant synovial lining. The vicious circle of events can be broken by effective nonsurgical treatment. Factor VIII replacement and immobilization of the knee joint in a padded plaster splint for a period of 3 or 4 weeks will usually result in a gradual resolution of the swelling. Isometric quadriceps exercises are carried out during this period to prevent muscle atrophy, which may delay the mobilization period and which may be responsible for permitting the condition to recur in some patients.

If after 3 to 4 weeks, the swelling and thickening are resolved the patient is mobilized gradually under factor cover. Hydrotherapy is instituted to give additional support during the initial weight-bearing period, and sticks may be used to aid walking on dry land. Most patients regain a useful range of motion in a further 3 weeks.

If resolution does not take place after 4 weeks, the patient may undergo a further 3-week period of immobilization with factor cover. Most patients will respond to the regime. A program of progressive mobilization under factor cover has been described.[4] The important point about any form of treatment of this condition is that it should be seen to reduce the synovial hypertrophy, reduce the incidence of bleeding, and prevent the progression to a chronic hemophilic arthropathy.

Occasionally the vicious circle cannot be broken and the patient retains a boggy synovial thickening with recurrent hemarthrosis. In these circumstances synovectomy may be necessary as a hemostatic procedure. The value of synovectomy is not yet proved, but its rationale is based on the fact that the synovium is intimately involved in the eventual destruction of the articular surface and the progressive contracture and deformation of the knee joint. The removal of the hypertrophic hyperemic synovium with the elevated levels of cathepsin-D should reduce the risk of further hemorrhage into the joint and halt the destruction of articular cartilage. However, synovectomy may be contraindicated in a patient with high levels of inhibitor or in the very young patient with a chronically swollen knee. In the latter case, the consequences for the nutrition of articular cartilage are unknown. These patients can be immobilized in an ischial bearing caliper with knee support for up to 6 months, with res-

olution of the synovial hypertrophy and recurrent bleeds.

CHRONIC HEMOPHILIC ARTHROPATHY

However, in spite of rigorous attempts to prevent the progression of joint deformity, the radiologic and clinical features of chronic arthropathy may supervene. The knee is the most commonly affected joint. Once this clinical stage is reached, the treatment falls into four categories: physiotherapy, orthotics, corrective devices, and reconstructive surgery.

PHYSIOTHERAPY

The chief aim of physiotherapy to the knee is to maintain good quadriceps muscle power. Bearing in mind that exercise may increase the level of circulating factor VIII, it is a form of prophylactic therapy. Both static and dynamic exercises are carried out to promote mobile and stable joints. However, muscle power alone will not overcome dense intra-articular adhesions. Quadriceps power will be compromised by a fixed flexion deformity owing to mechanical influences. In the presence of these problems other methods have to be employed while physiotherapy continues.

ORTHOTICS

Lightweight plastic splints and calipers are used extensively for the protection and support of joints after repeated hemarthrosis, particularly the knee and ankle. It is important to prevent muscle atrophy while the affected joint is protected by any form of external splintage.

In the presence of a fixed flexion deformity of 20° or less, passive and dynamic quadriceps exercises can be carried out in an open-fronted orthoplast splint (Fig. 24.10A,B). This procedure was first described by Miss D. Boone, Los Angeles, California. Its use is not confined to patients with chronic hemophilic arthropathy but may be used for correcting flexion deformities after acute hemarthrosis or those second-

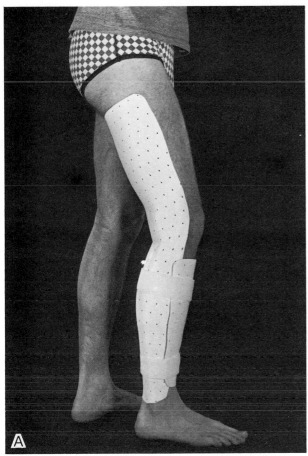 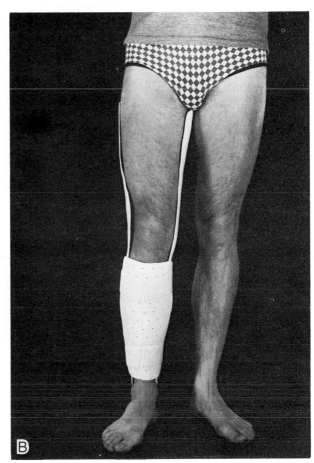

Fig. 24.10. (A,B) Orthoplast open-fronted knee splint. (From Houghton, G.R., Duthie, R.B.: Orthopaedic problems in haemophilia. J.B. Lippincott Co., 1979, pp. 138, 197–216, with permission.)

ary to soft tissue bleeds in the hamstrings and calf muscles.

The final stages of mobilization after the treatment of subacute hemarthrosis and mobilization after surgery to the hemophilic knee may be aided by this splint.

CORRECTIVE APPLIANCES: REVERSED DYNAMIC SLINGS

This technique developed in Oxford over the last 10 years and is now the method of choice for the correction of fixed flexion contracture of the knee. It has the advantage that quadriceps muscle power and tone are improved and enables physiotherapy to be carried out at the same time. Movement of the knee restored by the technique reduces the tendency to intra-articular adhesion formation and aids in the nutrition of the articular cartilage.

METHOD

The patient's leg is supported by balanced traction in a half-ring Thomas splint with a Pearson knee flexion piece attachment (Fig. 24.11 A,B). Longitudinal skin traction is applied to the calf. A padded canvas sling is applied over the distal part of the thigh and is reversed beneath the metal side pieces of the Thomas splint. A traction cord threaded over two pulleys connects the sling to a suitable weight (usual range, 2.7 to 4.1 kg). Therefore, a posterior force is applied to the distal part of the anterior aspect of the thigh against

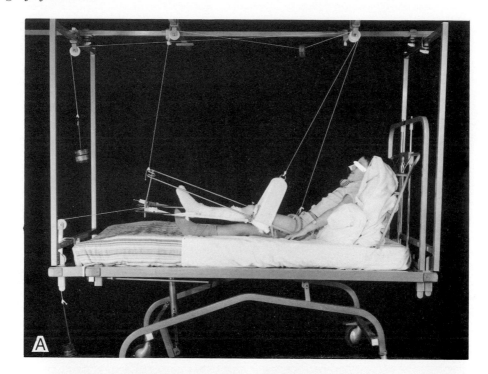

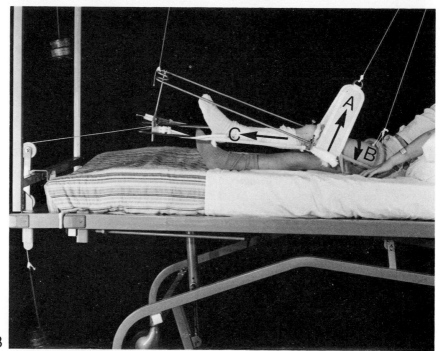

Fig. 24.11. (A) The patient is undergoing correction of a fixed flexion contracture by reversed dynamic slings. (B) Details of the traction. The pressure exerted by the canvas sling A is converted into a downward force B on the knee. The longitudinal force C applied to the tibia allows correction of flexion contractures and posterior subluxation of the tibia.

the counterpressure of the slings on the posterior surface of the calf. Active quadriceps exercises are carried out within the confines of the splint.

The longitudinal traction and thigh weights are increased gradually during the first 48 hours. The combined forces gradually correct the flexion deformity and posterior subluxation of the tibia. The angulation of the Pearson attachment is progressively reduced as the knee straightens. When the knee is straight, or when no further improvement of the deformity in extension has occurred for a week, the patient is mobilized with the knee in an open-fronted molded thermoplastic cylinder (Fig. 24.10A,B).

The further active maximal contraction of unrestricted quadriceps muscle permits further correction of any residual flexion contracture.

A prospective study of this technique comparing the results of reversed dynamic slings with serial plaster casts has shown the slings to be significantly superior.[50] Both groups had severe fixed flexion deformities at the knee for a mean duration of 3 years. The mean age of the cast patients was 19.5 years, and the mean age of the sling patients 17.5 years. In the patients with the reversed dynamic slings, the flexion contracture was reduced by an average of 34.6°, compared with 9.4° in a serial plaster group.

The mean treatment time was significantly reduced in the dynamic sling group (14 days) as compared with the serial cast group (30 days), ($p > 0.01$).

Most patients in each group increased their range of motion. There was no correlation between the duration of fixed flexion contracture and the length of time required to reach the final correction in each group. The method is therefore suitable for the treatment of long-standing deformities. None of the patients treated in this way has had any complications, and factor replacement has not been a routine during the use of reversed dynamic slings.

SURGICAL MANAGEMENT

The ready availability of human factor VIII and IX concentrates has permitted an expansion in the range and severity of surgery, both curative and reconstructive, in hemophilic patients. In particular, joint disease and deformity of the lower limb have come well within the scope of the benefits from surgery. Surgical correction of one severe joint deformity may re-

verse a tendency to further joint involvement, so often the case in the lower limb. The knee in particular has received a lot of attention in recent years and is the crucial joint in many patients with lower limb hemophilic arthropathy

PRINCIPLES OF SURGERY

The surgery of hemophilic patients is governed by certain principles that, if adhered to, limit the margins of error and complications and offer the patient the best possible result.

Standard surgical approaches and techniques are used. A pneumatic tourniquet will ensure a bloodless field. The length of the incision is chosen to give the minimum exposure necessary to carry out the procedure. All dissection is carried out by electrocautery and meticulous hemostasis achieved by diathermy coagulation. Bleeding in patients with von Willebrand's disease may require controlled local pressure. There is minimal dissection of the tissue planes to avoid the pocketing of hematoma in the recovery phase. The wounds are closed by coaptation of tissue planes by continuous hemostatic polyglycolic acid dexon sutures. Wounds are not drained, and the knee joint is compressed with a firm wool and domette compression bandage and immobilized in a plaster-of-Paris back splint. The splintage thereby achieved immobilizes the knee joint after surgery and discourages the formation of hematoma. The use of percutaneous pins and external fixation devices is avoided in order to prevent the inevitable complication of pin tract bleeding with consequent infection. Where indicated internal compression with plates and screws is carried out. In general, definitive operations with predictable and good results are preferred to multiple or staged surgical procedures.

COAGULATION CONTROL DURING AND AFTER SURGERY

Before planning a surgical procedure in a patient with a bleeding disorder, the precise nature of the disorder should be known. The relevant factor deficiency is confirmed and the level of circulating factor should be calculated. Antibodies should be sought for and, if present, are an absolute contraindication to elective surgery. Antibodies are rare in patients with Christmas disease and von Willebrand's disease. The total amount of factor required to cover the procedure and the entire postoperative period and mobilization are calculated and reserved for that particular patient.

The infusion of high levels of factor may lead to the development of antibodies. None of the patients operated on in Oxford has developed antibodies in this situation, but it is a potential hazard. Because of this possibility, however, it is wise to confine surgery to well-tried procedures with a known low complication rate. To conserve factor and to reduce periods of high factor infusion, reconstructive surgery may be combined with minor nonseptic dental or general surgical procedures.

Screening for the presence of hepatitis B antigen must be carried out. Hepatitis occurs in about 3 percent of all hemophiliacs per annum. Jaundice may be attributable to a hemolytic response to the infusion of blood group isoagglutinins or to the transmission of the hepatitis A or B virus in contaminated blood products. Unfortunately a high proportion of hemophilic patients in whom hepatitis develops have no serologic evidence of hepatitis B virus infection. Some may have hepatitis A, which cannot yet be detected serologically, or a long incubation-type of hepatitis the causative agent for which has yet not been identified. Infected patients carry the hepatitis antigen, which is also present in the carrier state when patients are clinically normal. If Australia antigen is detected in a hemophilic before surgery, a scrupulous routine must be instituted in the operating theater:

1. The operating team must be aware of the hazards.
2. The operation must be carried out in an operating theater that will not be required for surgery for at least 24 hours after disinfection.
3. Any cut or accidental prick of the skin from a sharp instrument must be washed immediately with soap and water. Blood stains on the skin must be washed with hypochloride solution followed by immediate liberal washing with soap and water. In the event that the surgeon or surgeon's assistants are cut or blood stained, γ-globulin should be given intramuscularly.
4. Attention to personal hygiene, as well as smoking, eating, and drinking, are prohibited in the theater area. All labels must be self-adhesive and not licked. All specimens should be labeled a hepatitis risk.
5. All the instruments should be placed in a 2 percent

gluteraldehyde solution for 3 hours after use, before autoclaving.
6. The anesthetic room and operating fixtures and fittings should be disinfected with a freshly prepared 10 percent solution of sodium hypochloride.
7. Whenever possible, disposable equipment should be used.
8. Hospital personnel should be made aware of the hepatitis risk of all laundry and laboratory specimens, by appropriate labeling.
9. The surgical team should wear impervious plastic aprons under sterile disposable theater gowns. A face mask and visor should be worn together with two pairs of gloves.

Three patients who have had positive Australia antigen have been operated on under the above conditions in Oxford. A vertical laminar flow operating room was used on each occasion, and this may be a further indication for the provision of this type of theater in specialized centers. In no case did we have an incident of virus hepatitis among any of the hospital staff.

ADDITIONAL SUPPORTIVE MEASURES

The use of an antifibrinolytic agent has been shown to reduce the amount of factor replacement and the amount of bleeding after surgery. This was first demonstrated with ε-aminocaproic acid and factor VIII in the treatment and control of bleeding after dental extraction.[58] ε-aminocaproic acid has produced some undesirable side effects, such as nausea, vomiting, diarrhea, and postural hypotension. These symptoms have seldom been encountered with tranexamic acid (Cyclocapron), which is now preferred in Oxford. It is equally effective in patients with factor VIII or IX deficiency. Although Cyclocapron inhibits plasminogen activation by plasmin, its precise role in the hemostatic process in the hemophiliac is not substantiated. Presumably the clots formed after surgery are stabilized more so than one would expect after the normal healing process. Normal wounds presumably stay dry during the healing phase because clots in the wound area lyse and reform. In the hemophiliac, lysis would normally be accompanied by bleeding, since no new clot would form unless more factor VIII were given.

Cyclocapron is of value in controlling external bleeding from a cut or a wound, especially when surgery has been carried out in a dry field under a tourniquet, hence its value in surgery of the knee. Cyclocapron may also be of value in patients in whom specific antibodies to factor VIII or IX develop during the postoperative phase, as it will enhance the activity of infused factor and stabilize any clot that is formed.

The antifibrinolytic group of drugs are contraindicated in the presence of hematuria or a soft tissue hematoma.

Cyclocapron is administered with the preoperative dose of factor VIII, 1 g being given intravenously; thereafter 1 g is given every six hours orally until the sutures are removed.

Prophylactic antibiotics are also administered to cover any implant surgery. Penicillin and flucloxacillin are administered intravenously with the premedication and at 12 and 24 hours after surgery. Thereafter antibiotics are only used where appropriate to treat specific infections.

POSTOPERATIVE CARE

The postoperative period of wound healing, removal of sutures, mobilization, and additional manipulation of the knee are covered by factor replacement, Cyclocapron, analgesia, and adequate external support. Isometric quadriceps exercises are encouraged by the physiotherapist as soon as the patient is comfortable.

Limb rehabilitation and mobilization are commenced in the hydrotherapy pool and progress to dry land with the appropriate aid of crutches or a stick. The initial postoperative immobilization is always carried out inhospital under the strict control of the surgeon, hematologist, and physiotherapist. Additional factor replacement may be necessary for episodes of spontaneous bleeding, which may occur from time to time. Figure 24.12 illustrates the number of units of factor per dose and the pre- and postinfusion levels of circulatory factor VIII obtained in a patient undergoing synovectomy and patellectomy at the knee.

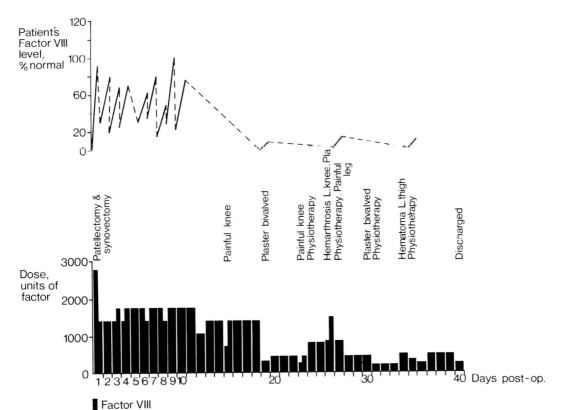

Fig. 24.12. Postoperative requirement of factor VIII in a patient undergoing patellectomy and synovectomy of the knee.

The variable postoperative course which a patient may have and the need for careful assessment of his factor requirement are demonstrated.

SURGERY OF THE HEMOPHILIC PATIENT'S KNEE

Evacuation of hematoma was carried out during the late 1960s on four patients in Oxford (Table 24.7) who fell into the group of patients which we now recognize as having a subacute hemarthrosis. These patients had presented several days or weeks after the initial hemarthrosis with hot, swollen, painful knees. Palpation of the joint contents revealed a doughy semisolid knee, evidence that the hemarthrosis had clotted. The etiology of this state has been discussed. It is now our policy to immobilize these knees in suitably padded compressive splints, to assess their antibody status, and to administer specific factor, if appropriate, as already outlined.

Painful flexion contracture has been treated by manipulation under anesthetic. Both patients who have been treated in this manner in Oxford required further procedures (Table 24.8). One patient had to go into reversed dynamic slings after 6 months because of a recurrence, and the other required a further manipulation for locking associated with a band of medial joint capsule snapping over the medial femoral condyle. On this occasion, the manipulation was successful. The reversed dynamic sling technique would appear superior to a manipulative technique in the management of flexion contractures.

Manipulation is of value in the postoperative phase after patellectomy or synovectomy in order to break down intra-articular adhesions under factor cover.

One patient required the removal of a loose body in his knee, which was giving rise to recurrent hemarthrosis and locking, with complete relief of his symptoms.

The hemophilic patient's knee is subject to internal derangement in the same way as a normal person's would be. Seven medial meniscectomies have been carried out on six patients in the Nuffield Orthopaedic Center in the last 13 years (Table 24.9). Four of the patients had hemophilia A and two had Christmas disease. One of the patients with Christmas disease has undergone bilateral procedures. Three of the patients had a significant rotational injury to the knee, and in four knees the symptoms arose spontaneously. The symptoms have included intermittent pain, swelling, locking, and instability.

Four of the patients had medial joint line tenderness and one had a mechanical block to extension.

Table 24.7. Surgical Procedures Carried out on the Knee, 1966–1979

Procedure	Patients (N)
Evacuation of hematoma	4
Patellectomy	4
Meniscectomy	7
Synovectomy	6
Arthrodesis	11
Removal of exostosis	1
Manipulation under anesthetic	3
Total	36

Table 24.8. Miscellaneous Surgical Procedures Carried out on the Knee

Patient No.	Factor Deficiency	Procedure	Presenting Symptoms	Result
1	VIII	Removal of loose body	Recurrent hemarthrosis and locking	No further bleeding
2	VIII	Manipulation under anesthetic	Painful flexion contracture	Recurrence required; reversed dynamic slings within 6 months
3	VIII	Manipulation under anesthetic	Flexion contracture with fixed flexion deformity	Range of motion restored to 15 to 100°
4	VIII	Further MUA of patient No. 3	Intermittent locking	Range of motion restored; noted to have a subluxing band of medial capsule across the femoral condyle

Abbreviation: MUA, manipulation under anaesthetic

Table 24.9.   Clinical Presentation of Patients Who Required Meniscectomy

Patient No.	Factor Deficiency	Surgical Procedure	Presenting Symptoms	Result
1	VIII	Medial meniscectomy	Clicking, locking, medial joint line tenderness	Full range of motion
2	VIII	Medial meniscectomy	Post-traumatic clicking, instability, locked knee	Good range of motion
3	VIII	Medial meniscectomy	Twisting injury; intermittent locking; swelling, pain, and tenderness on medial joint line	Full range of motion
4	VIII	Medial meniscectomy	Pain, intermittent instability; tender medial joint line	Good result; minimal symptoms
5	IX 5%	Left medial meniscectomy; concomitant vasectomy	Twisting injury with intermittent locking, swelling, instability, quadriceps wasting with a tender medial joint line	Range of motion 1 to 135° after 6 months' small effusion
5b Same patient as 5a	IX 5%	Arthroscopy right knee and medial bucket handle removal only	Spontaneous onset, intermittent painful locking and swelling	Good; full range of motion; no effusion
6	IX	Medial meniscectomy	Recurrent painful swelling and locking	Symptom free

None of the patients had a significant hemophilic arthropathy at surgery, although one patient required a patellectomy and synovectomy 2 years later. This had not been the experience of other centers where the meniscus has not presented as a primary problem in hemophilic arthropathy of the knee.[4] The value of an arthrogram has not been established in the investigation of an internal derangement in a hemophilic knee joint. The presence of an arthropathy, synovial hypertrophy, and concomitant degeneration of the meniscus may make interpretation difficult. The procedure would have to be planned and hemostasis control organized as for a surgical procedure. The arthroscope may permit visualization of the meniscus before an arthrotomy is performed under the same hemostatic cover with the obvious saving in factor and time. One of the patients with Christmas disease (5b) had an arthroscopy before arthrotomy. On this occasion, a bucket-handle lesion could be easily identified and removed. This patient also had a vasectomy carried out under the same anesthetic. In six arthrotomies, a total meniscectomy was carried out, and in one a bucket-handle section was removed. The combined use of the arthroscope and current thoughts on the value of minimal procedures may permit a more selective policy for meniscetomy in the future.[21] Meniscectomy has relieved the patients of their symptoms and permitted full return of existing move-

ment in the knee (Table 24.9). Patients should be mobilized as for a conventional meniscectomy, with the obvious addition of factor cover.

RECONSTRUCTIVE SURGERY: PATELLECTOMY

A patellectomy has been carried out on four patients with hemophilia A at Oxford (Table 24.10). Recurrent pain and swelling have been the presenting symptoms. In one patient the swelling has been proved to be synovial fluid by aspiration. Two patients have had an accompanying synovial hypertrophy, one of whom had also had recurrent hemarthrosis of the knee. All patients had painful retropatellar crepitus and a restricted range of motion. All patients had radiologic evidence of patellofemoral arthritis with variable involvement of the tibiofemoral compartment of the knee joint (Fig. 24.13A–C).

The operation is carried out via a small medial parapatellar incision with careful dissection of the attachments of the quadriceps and patellar tendon fibers from the patella. The defect is closed in layers with opposing dexon sutures, and the leg supported in a padded plaster-of-Paris cylinder for 3 weeks.

Thereafter, the patient is mobilized under factor cover. Figure 24.12 illustrates the hemostatic treat-

Table 24.10. Clinical Presentation of Patients Who Have Had Patellectomy

Patient No.	Factor Deficiency	Surgical Procedure	Presenting Symptoms	Result
1	VIII	Patellectomy	Recurrent pain; instability and swelling requiring frequent bed rest	Symptom free; good range of motion
2	VIII	Patellectomy and synovectomy	Painful retropatellar crepitus; persistent synovial hypertrophy	Simultaneous synovectomy; poor result; persistent pain and recurrent hemarthroses; range of motion 0 to 5 to 68°
3	VIII	Patellectomy	Painful crepitus; recurrent hemarthrosis	Simultaneous synovectomy; one hemarthrosis during mobilization; required a manipulation under anesthesia
4	VIII	Patellectomy	Painful crepitus; recurrent hemarthrosis; range of motion 0 to 90° flexion	Range of motion 0 to 20 to 45° at 4 months; no hemarthroses

ment employed and the relevant milestones in the patient's postoperative mobilization. The results after this procedure have been variable, one patient being rendered symptom free with a range of motion of 5 to 68 degrees. One patient has had persistent pain and hemarthroses with a range of motion of 0 to 5 to 68 degrees. The most recent patient in the series was slow to mobilize and required a manipulation under anesthetic. He had one small bleed after his manipulation. He had concomitant synovectomy, as did the other patient with recurrent hemarthroses. Both patients had a slow postoperative mobilization requiring manipulation. They also had the same small, painful hemarthrosis one associates with chronic hemophilic arthropathy and a fibrosed contracted joint. Patients who have a synovectomy alone are mobilized early, and certainly within 2 weeks of surgery. It would seem that a concomitant synovectomy in a patient having a patellectomy and a longer period of immobilization gives rise to a dry, stiff joint. It is this type of joint that is subject to small, isolated bleeds and postoperative stiffness.

SYNOVECTOMY

Perhaps the most controversial surgical procedure carried out in hemophilic arthropathy of the knee in the last 14 years has been synovectomy. It has been carried out as an isolated procedure and in conjunction with meniscectomy, patellectomy, and total knee arthroplasty.[35,38,40]

The precise role of the physiology of the synovial membrane and synovial fluid and their relationship to normal joint function have not yet been established. After a synovectomy the articular cartilage matrix shows signs of changing from a hyaline to a fibrocartilaginous structure. The biochemical changes precede the morphologic changes by some considerable time. They are caused by alterations in the composition and amount of synovial fluid in the joint. A normal diarthrodial joint is a functional unit of synovial tissue, synovial fluid, and articular cartilage. Normal function must depend on the complex remaining intact. In the hemophilic knee, the complex is not intact, and the synovial lining and fluid are not functioning normally in relationship to the articular cartilage. The increased levels of acid phosphatase, cathepsin-D, prostaglandins, and collagenases all point to the dangerous state of the synovium in the hemophilic knee.

In the initial reports of synectomy, the indications for the necessity to carry out this procedure were not clear.[4,52] However, in recent years the indications for a synovectomy have become clearer and more accepted[4,40,41]:

1. Recurrent frequent hemarthroses
2. Presence of a thickened boggy synovium (Fig. 24.14)
3. Preservation of a good range of motion with minimal radiographic changes of hemophilic arthropathy (Fig. 24.15)
4. Failure to respond to adequate hemostatic and supportive therapy

The hemostatic therapy should consist of adequate factor replacement and firm immobilization in a padded compressive splint for a minimum period of 3 to

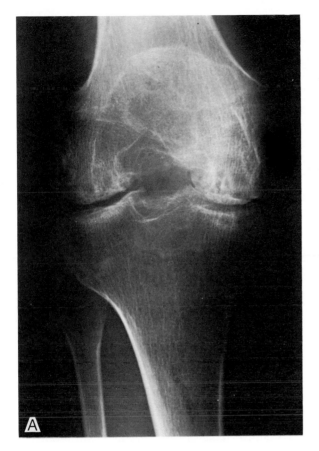

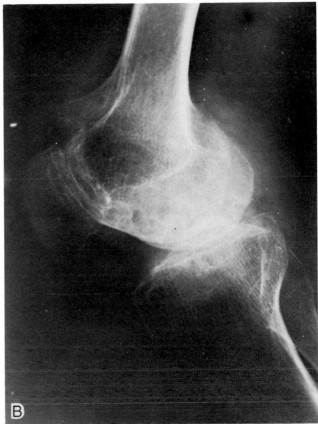

Fig. 24.13. (A–C) Preoperative radiographs of a patient who underwent patellectomy. Note the irregular articular surface of the patella on the skyline view (A).

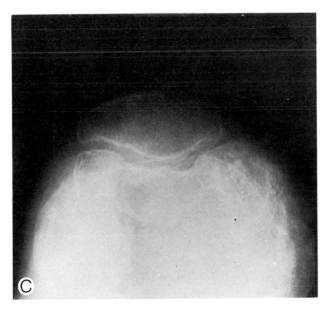

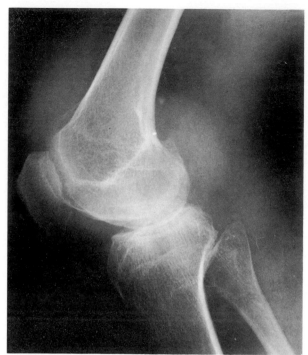

Fig. 24.14. Lateral radiograph showing anterior and posterior soft tissue shadows indicative of thickened synovium.

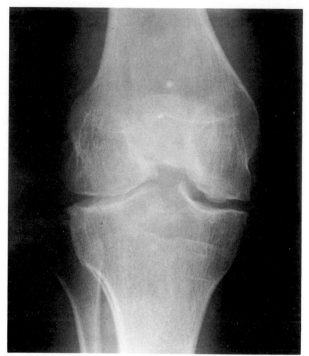

Fig. 24.15. Radiograph showing that the articular cartilage is still preserved.

4 weeks. A short course of steroids has been added to this regime,[40] but they are of no proven value and are not used at Oxford.[5]

The above regime is successful in most patients who present with subacute hemarthrosis. However, should a patient fail to respond, synovectomy is indicated. The continued use of high doses of factor predispose the patient to all the risks of this form of treatment, including the development of antibodies, hepatitis, and hemolytic anemia. Chemical and radioisotopic synovectomy have been described. However, our experience has been confined to six cases of operative synovectomy of the knee. A seventh has been carried out recently, but it is too soon to evaluate the outcome of the procedure.

Under full hemostatic control an anterior two-thirds synovectomy is carried out through a medial parapatellar incision. Hemostatic control is maintained after surgery. The knee is immobilized in a Robert-Jones compression bandage with a plaster-of-Paris backslab until wound healing is complete. Isometric quadriceps exercises are commenced during the initial phase. The optimal time for mobilization of the joint after synovectomy is 2 weeks. Before this time there is a

danger of provoking further bleeding, and prolonged immobilization will favor formation of adhesions and subsequent joint stiffness, as experienced by patients having a concomitant patellectomy. After 2 weeks, active mobilization is commenced in the hydrotherapy pool and on dry land. Once the patient has regained 90 degrees of flexion, full unprotected weight-bearing is allowed.

This procedure would seem to benefit the adolescent patient in the hope of preventing the progression of the hemophilic arthropathy. The advisability of carrying out this procedure on young patients in the first decade is unclear. Some investigators have reported synovectomy in patients 5 years of age.[52] We would not advocate this procedure for an immature joint. The benefits of synovectomy are a reduction in the frequency of bleeding and consequently less factor infusion, preservation of a range of motion, and a more active existence for the patient who becomes less reliant on the hospital services. In carrying out a synovectomy, a boggy swollen knee is converted into a dry somewhat stiffer joint. While there is a marked reduction in the extent, frequency, and severity of bleeding, small punctate and sometimes painful bleeding does occur postoperatively. This has been recorded in two of our series and in other reported series.[4] Complications have been reported after synovectomy and include massive hemarthroses, adherent patellae, reduced range of joint motion, and hemolytic anemia secondary to isoagglutinin infusion.[40] None of these complications has been seen at Oxford.

ARTHRODESIS OF THE KNEE

When a painful fixed-flexion contracture of the knee becomes permanent and functionally disabling, arthrodesis has proved a valuable procedure. Eleven arthrodeses have been carried out over an 11-year period at Oxford.[25] Pain was the main indication in all cases with additional gross deformity, instability, and recurrent hemarthroses, producing disabling symptoms. The average range of motion of the affected joints was 31 degrees compared with 103 degrees in the unaffected knee.

The technique involves full hemostatic control. Approximately 28,000 units of factor VIII is required for each arthrodesis. The following steps are carried out via a median parapatellar incision:

1. Excision of the articular surfaces of the patella, femur, and tibia
2. Internal fixation with compression using cross-threaded cancellous screws (Fig. 24.16A,B)
3. Arthrodesis of the knee between 10 and 30 degrees of flexion, depending on coexistent hip or ankle deformity.

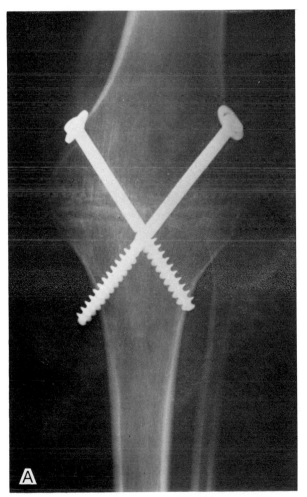
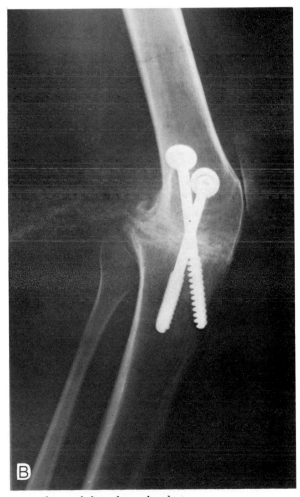

Fig. 24.16. (A,B) Cross-compression screws used to stabilize the arthrodesis.

In the series reported from Oxford, all the arthrodeses united, although there were three cases of delayed union of 7, 11, and 12 months. The mean time taken to accomplish radiologic union was 5.7 months. Complications occurred in two patients. One had a staphylococcal wound infection and the other a wound hematoma. Both settled with conservative therapy and antibiotics appropriate to the organism concerned.

Postoperatively, the leg is protected in a long leg plaster-of-Paris cast, which is changed at 2 weeks when the sutures are removed. The factor VIII levels are raised to 80 to 100 percent during the procedure. Isometric quadriceps exercises are commenced early and maintained until the supportive cast is removed, when there is radiologic union at the site of arthrodesis.

Knee arthrodesis is a successful definitive procedure in the hemophilic patient despite the not uncommon complication of poor wound healing and superficial infection. However, these complications did not require further surgical intervention. The procedure renders the hemophilic knee pain free and thereby avoids the use of further factor and all its attendant dangers.

TOTAL KNEE ARTHROPLASTY

Over the past 5 years, reports of total knee arthroplasty in the hemophilic knee have been appearing in the literature.[4,35,38,40,41] The knee is more frequently affected by hemophilic arthropathy than the hip. Total hip arthroplasty is a predictably successful procedure in the hemophilic patient,[25] whereas total knee arthroplasty is arguably not.

The procedure has been advocated for patients with bilateral disease or in limbs with ipsilateral hip and ankle disease.[40] The main symptom has been pain secondary to destructive disease of the joint. With the exception of one reported case,[35] arthroplasty has not been carried out in order to ease the incidence of bleeding into the joint. It is contraindicated in patients with marked contractural fibrosis and wasting of the quadriceps.[4]

Synovectomy has been carried out simultaneously by most workers.[35,38,40] Most patients have been in their third, fourth, and fifth decades. The operation is definitely contraindicated in the hemophiliac in his first or second decades. The older hemophilic patient seems to require less factor during surgery and in the postoperative phase, as compared with synovectomy in the younger patient. It has been suggested that the older hemophilic patient, like his or her counterpart with rheumatoid arthritis, would not load a knee joint so much.[40]

The main advantage to be gained from total knee arthroplasty would appear to be relief of pain.[23,40,41] The restoration of joint movement would appear to be of secondary consequence and variable in its achievement. The functional gain outweighs any loss of mobility. Any reduction in the incidence of hemarthrosis would have to be evaluated within the context of the individual patient and not advocated as an indication for the technique of total knee arthroplasty. We would not advocate total knee replacement in the adolescent early-onset chronic hemophilic arthropathy. We would also advise caution in using this procedure, even on the older hemophilic patient. Most reports have come from small series of up to eight patients. The only comparable but larger group of patients that have been critically studied after total knee arthroplasty, using both hinged and unconstrained implants, are patients with juvenile chronic polyarthritis (Still's disease).[3]

Among the reported cases of total knee replacement, several investigators have reported minor or no complications.[4,35,38,41] However, McCollough et al.[40] in their comparatively large series of 10 arthroplasties in eight patients, observed several complications, namely, three hemarthroses, two in one patient; one late loosening of the tibial component; and one secondary complication of hemophilia in the form of a large bowel hemorrhage that required subtotal colectomy with a subsequent infection in the prosthetic knee. We reiterate our contention that surgery for hemophilic patients should be definitive with predictably good results. Total knee arthroplasty has not yet come into this category, and the potential complication rate is unacceptable in a group of patients who are already exposed to lethal complications as a result of the natural history and treatment of this disease.(Editor's Note: We do not share this pessimistic and cautious opinion with regard to knee replacement. Since 1973 we have implanted 24 knee prostheses of the total condylar type in hemophilic patients (average age 36 years).[32A] The most common deformity was one of flexion, valgus and external rotation, and the technical difficulties were sometimes formidable due to fibrosis and stiffness. However at follow-up (range 1 to 9 years) 21 knees rated excellent (15 knees) or good (6 knees) and there was improvement in range of motion averaging 23 degrees. There were 2 deep infections (8 percent). We consider hip and knee replacement to be comparable and equally predictable although in both the risk of infection is greater than normal. Both operations should be performed only in properly equipped and experienced centers.—J.N.I.).

CONCLUSION

The management of hemophilic arthropathy makes many demands on the skill and patience of the physicians concerned. It is hoped that the progression toward home therapy and better education of the patient will reduce the problems that must be dealt with in the future.

ACKNOWLEDGMENTS

We should like to acknowledge the skill and dedication of the many members of the medical and nursing staff who are involved with the management of hemophilic patients in Oxford. Dr. Charles Rizza and Dr. James Matthews, consulting physicians at the Oxford Hemophilic Centre, are a constant source of help and advice. Sister Williams of the Hemophilic Centre and Sister Rymill, Sister Wood, and Sister Howard of the Nuffield Orthopaedic Centre have given unstinting support to patients, surgeons, and physicians alike.

REFERENCES

1. Abildgaard, C.F.: Current concepts in the management of hemophilia. Semin. Hematol., *12(3):* 223, 1975.
2. Ahlberg, A.: Hemophilia in Sweden. Acta Orthop. Scand., *77*(suppl.): 1, 1965.
3. Arden, G.P.: Total joint replacement, p. 146. In Arden G.P., and Ansell, B.M. eds.: Surgical Management of Chronic Juvenile Chronic Polyarthritis. London, Academic Press and New York, Grune & Stratton, 1978.
4. Arnold, W.D., and Hilgartner, M.W.: Hemophilic arthropathy. J. Bone Joint Surg. [Am.], *59:* 287, 1977.
5. Bennett, A.E., and Ingram, G.I.: A controlled trial of long-term steroid treatment in hemophilia. Lancet, *1:* 967, 1967.
6. Biggs, R.: Hemophilia treatment in the United Kingdom from 1969 to 1974. Br. J. Hematol., *35:* 487, 1977.
7. Biggs, R.: The treatment of Hemophilia A and B and von Willebrand's disease. Oxford, Blackwell Scientific Publications, 1978.
8. Boldero, J.L., and Kemp, H.S.: The early bone and joint changes in Hemophilia and similar blood dyscrasias. Br. J. Radiol., *39:* 172, 1966.
9. Brighton, C.T., Bigley, E.C., Jr., and Smolenski, B.I.: Iron-induced arthritis in immature rabbits. Arthritis Rheum. *13:* 849, 1970.
10. Davidson, C.S., Epstein, R.D., Miller, G.F., et al: Hemophilia: A clinical study of forty patients. Blood, *4:* 97, 1949.
11. de Andrade, J.R., Grant, C., Dixon, A. St. J.: Joint distension and reflex muscle inhibition in the knee. J. Bone Joint Surg. [Am.], *47:* 313, 1965.
12. DePalma, A.F.: Hemophilic arthropathy. Clin. Orthop., *52:* 145, 1967.
13. DePalma, A.F., and Cotler, J.M.: Hemophilic arthropathy. Arch. Surg., *72:* 247, 1956.
14. Duthie, R.B., and Rizza, C.R.: Rheumatological manifestations of the hemophiliacs. Clin. Rheum. Dis., *1:* 53, 1975.
15. Duthie, R.B., Matthews, J.M., Rizza, C.R., et al.: The management of musculo-skeletal problems in the hemophilias. Oxford, Blackwell Scientific Publications, 1972.
16. Edson, J.R.: Prothrombin—complex concentrates and thromboses. N Engl. J. Med., *290:* 403, 1974.
17. Forbes, C.D., Greig, W.R., Prentice, C.R.M., et al.: Radioisotope knee joint scans in hemophilia and Christmas disease. J. Bone Joint Surg. [Br.], *54:* 468, 1972.
18. Forbes, C.D., James, W., Prentice, C.R.M., et al.: A comparison of thermography, radioisotope scanning and clinical assessment of the knee joints in hemophilia. Clin. Radiol., *26(1):* 41, 1975
19. Ghadially, F.N.: Ultrastructural Pathology of the Cell. London, Butterworth, 1975.
20. Gilbert, M.S., and Cockin, J.: An evaluation of the radiologic changes in hemophilic arthropathy of knee. In Proceedings VII Congress World Federation of hemophilia, Teheran, Iran, 1971. Amsterdam, Excerpta Medica, 1971.
21. Goodfellow, J.: He who hesitates is saved. Editorial. J. Bone Joint Surg. [Br.], *62:* 1, 1980.
22. Hamerman, D.: Synovial joints, aspects of structure and function, p. 1259. In Balazo, E.A., ed.: Chemistry and Molecular Biology of the Intercellular Matrix, Vol. 3. London, Academic Press, 1970.
23. Hilgartner, M.W.: Pathogenesis of joint changes in hemophilia, p. 33. In McCollough, N.C., ed.: Comprehensive Management of Musculo-skeletal Disorders in Hemophilia. Washington, D.C., National Academy of Sciences, 1973.
24. Hoaglund, F.T.: Experimental hemarthrosis. The re-

sponse of canine knees to injections of autologous blood. J. Bone Joint Surg. [Am.], *49:* 285, 1967.

25. Houghton, G.R., and Dickson, R.A.: Lower Limb arthrodesis in hemophilia. J. Bone Joint Surg. [Br.], *60:* 143, 1978.

26. Jones, A.G., Francis, M.D., and Davis, M.A.: Bone scanning: radionuclidic reaction mechanisms. Semin. Nucl. Med., *6*(1): 3, 1976.

27. Kasper, C.K.: Post-operative thromboses in hemophilia B. N. Engl. J. Med., *289:* 160, 1973.

28. Kasper, C.K.: Prothrombin complex concentrates and thromboses. Reply to letter to the editor. N. Engl. J. Med., *290:* 404, 1974.

29. Kasper, C.K.: Thromboembolic complications of Factor IX therapy. Thromb. Haemost. *33:* 642, 1975.

30. Key, J.A.: Hemophilic arthritis. Ann Surg., *95:* 198, 1932.

31. Krugman, S., Giles, J.P., and Hammond, J.: Viral hepatitis type B (MS-2 strain): Prevention with specific hepatitis B immune serum globulin. J.A.M.A., *218:* 1665, 1971.

32. Krugman, S., Giles, J.P., and Hammond, J.: Viral hepatitis (Type B/MS-2 strain): Studies on active immunization. J.A.M.A., *217:* 41, 1971.

32a. Lachiewicz, P.F., Inglis, A.E., Insall, J.N. et al.: Total knee arthroplasty in hemophilia. Presented at the Hemophilia Orthopedic Conference, Los Angeles, California, 1983.

33. Lack, C.H.: Chondrolysis. Ann. Phys. Med., *6:* 93, 1961.

34. Lentle, B.C., Russell, A.S., Percy, J.S., et al.: Bone scintiscanning updated. Ann. Intern. Med., *84*(3): 297, 1976.

35. London, J.T., Kattlove, H., Louie, J.S., et al.: Synovectomy and total joint arthroplasty for recurrent hemarthroses in the arthropathic joint in hemophilia. Arthritis Rheum., *20*(8): 1543, 1977.

36. Luck, J.V.: Articular cartilage. Responses to destructive influences, p. 143. In Bassett, C.A.L., ed.: Cartilage degradation and repair. Washington, D.C., National Academy of Sciences, National Research Council, National Academy of Engineering, 1967.

37. Marchesi, S.L., and Burney, R.: Prothrombin complex concentrates and thromboses. N. Engl. J. Med., *290:* 404, 1974.

38. Marmor, L.: Total knee replacement in hemophilia. Clin. Orthop., *125:* 192, 1977.

39. McCarty, D.J.: Selected aspects of synovial membrane physiology. Arthritis Rheum., *17:* 289, 1974.

40. McCollough, N.C., Enis, J.E., Lovitt, J., et al.: Synovectomy or total replacement of the knee in hemophilia. J. Bone Joint Surg. [Am.], *61:* 69, 1979.

41. Post, M., and Telfer, M.C.: Surgery in hemophilic patients. J. Bone Joint Surg. [Am.], *57:* 1136, 1975.

42. Revel, J.D., and Hay, E.D.: An autoradiographic and electron microscopic study on collagen synthesis in differentiating cartilage. Z. Zellforsch., *61:* 110, 1963.

43. Richter, G.W.: A Study of hemosiderosis with the aid of electron microscopy. J Exp. Med., *106:* 203, 1957.

44. Richter, G.W.: The cellular transformation of injected colloidal iron complexes into ferritin and hemosiderin in experimental animals, J. Exp. Med., *109:* 197, 1959.

45. Rizza, C.R., and Biggs, R.: The treatment of patients who have Factor VIII antibodies. Br. J. Haematol., *24:* 65, 1973.

46. Robinson, H.J., and Granda, J.L.: Prostaglandins in Synovial inflammatory disease. Surg. Forum, *25:* 476, 1974.

47. Roy, S., and Ghadially, F.N.: Synovial membrane in experimentally produced chronic hemarthrosis. Ann. Rheum. Dis., *28:* 402, 1969.

48. Sokoloff, L.: Biochemical and physiological aspects of degenerative joint diseases with special reference to hemophilic arthropathy. Ann. N.Y. Acad. Sci. *240:* 285, 1975.

49. Stein, H.: The interrelationship of synovium and articular cartilage. Ph.D. thesis, University of Oxford, 1975.

50. Stein, H., and Dickson, R.A.: Reversed dynamic slings for knee flexion contractures in the hemophiliac. J. Bone Joint Surg. [Am.], *57:* 282, 1975.

51. Steinberg, M.H., and Breiling, B.J.: Vascular lesions in hemophilia B. N. Engl. J. Med., *289:* 592, 1973.

52. Storti, E., Traldi, A., Tosatti, E., et al.: Synovectomy a new approach to hemophilic arthropathy. Acta Haematol., *41:* 193, 1969.

53. Subramanian, G., and McAfee, J.G.: A new complex of 99mTc for skeletal imaging Radiology, *99:* 192, 1971.

54. Subramanian, G., McAfee, J.G., Bell, E.G., et al.: 99mTc labelled polyphosphate as a skeletal imaging agent. Radiology, *102:* 701, 1972.

55. Tanaginini, G.D., Dormandy, K.M., Ellis, D., et al.: Factor VIII concentrates in hemophilia. Lancet, *2:* 188, 1975.

56. Troyer, H.: The effect of short-term immobilization on the rabbit knee joint cartilage. Clin. Orthop., *107:* 249, 1975.

57. Trueta, J.: Studies on the etiopathology of osteoarthritis of the hip. Clin. Orthop., *31:* 7, 1963.

58. Walsh, P.M., Rissa, C.R.M., Matthews, J.M., et al.: Epsilon amino caproic acid therapy for dental extractions in hemophilia and Christmas disease. A double blind controlled trial. Br. J. Haematol., *20:* 463, 1971.

59. Webb, J.B., and Dixon, A.St.J.: Hemophilia and hemophilic arthropathy. Ann. Rheum. Dis., *19:* 143, 1960.

60. Whaley, K., Pack, A.I., Boyle, J.A., et al.: The articular scan in patients with rheumatoid arthritis: A possible method of quantitating joint inflammation using Radio-technetium. Clin. Sci., *35:* 547, 1968.

25 Congenital and Developmental Abnormalities of the Knee

Robert L. Fisher

ABNORMALITIES OF TIBIOFEMORAL RELATIONSHIP

CONGENITAL HYPEREXTENSION DEFORMITY

Congenital hyperextension of the knee[15] may be classified as simple recurvatum, anterior subluxation, or anterior dislocation, depending on the relationship of the tibiofemoral joint surfaces.[32] Simple recurvatum, the most common type of hyperextension deformity, probably results from intrauterine positioning and usually reponds rapidly to manipulation and splinting or casting in progressive flexion.

Congenital hyperextension knee deformities with subluxation or dislocation are rare—occurring about one-fortieth as frequently as congenital hip dislocation.[9] These deformities are often associated with congenital hip dislocation and arthrogryposis. In contrast to simple recurvatum, congential subluxation or dislocation of the knee frequently do not respond to manipulation or casting and require surgery.

Pathologically, knees with congential subluxation or dislocation of the tibia anterior to the femur show consistent tightness of the extensor mechanism with fibrous replacement of the quadriceps muscle and tightness of the anterior knee capsule.[9] The quadriceps tendon is usually bound down to the femur in the suprapatellar area. The patella may be hypoplastic or absent but is almost always laterally placed. This latter phenomenon may be associated with an external rotation and valgus relationship of the tibia to the femur. When the hyperextension deformity is severe, the collateral ligaments are directed forward, and the hamstring tendons may be displaced anteriorly to the axis of motion such that they perpetuate the hyperextension and subluxation or dislocation. Intra-articular abnormalities, other than bony remodeling, are uncommon except in late cases, in which the absence of cruciate ligaments has been reported.[28]

The diagnosis of congenital hyperextension with subluxation or dislocation may be made on the basis of the clinical appearance of the knee (Fig. 25.1) as well as the resistance to flexion. The axis of joint motion is difficult to determine, and the knees show mediolateral instability in the hyperextended position. Radiologically, there may be delayed ossification of the distal femoral or proximal tibial ossification centers, but the forward luxation of the tibial axis is evident on the lateral projection. Arthrography is technically difficult and not diagnostically useful except to demonstrate obliteration of the suprapatellar pouch.

A trial of manipulation and splinting or casting in progressive flexion is recommended for knees showing hyperextension deformity with subluxation or dislocation. We have had no experience with skeletal

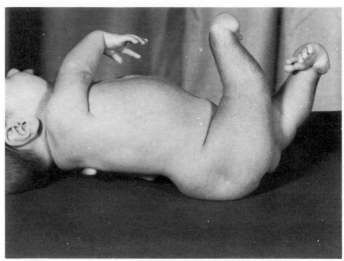

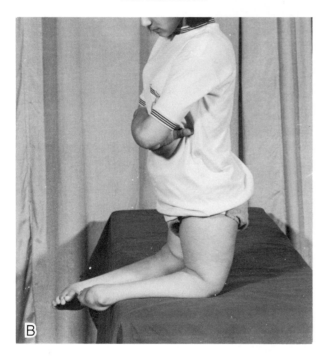

Fig. 25.1. (A,B) Clinical appearance of congenital hyperextension of the knee with subluxation.

of lengthening the quadriceps mechanism at the quadriceps tendon, patellar tendon, or patellar and quadriceps tendons in continuity with the patella. The technique described by Curtis and Fisher will be described in detail.[9] A generous anterior incision extending from the level of the lesser trochanter medially to a point just distal and lateral to the tibial tuberosity is preferred. The quadriceps tendon is divided by an inverted **V** incision superior to the patella (Fig. 25.2). The capsule is divided transversely to the medial and lateral collateral ligaments, which are mobilized by periosteal elevation. The knee should be capable of full flexion at this point. The available quadriceps muscle (in most cases principally vastus medialis) is then sutured to the tongue of quadriceps tendon attached to the patella with the knee in 30 to 40 degrees of flexion. No attempt is made to close the anteromedial or anterolateral capsule.

Postoperatively, the knee is held for 4 to 6 weeks by casting in 30 degrees of flexion. Active and passive exercises are then started. Weight-bearing is commenced about 10 to 12 weeks postoperatively, when optimum motion and strength have been achieved. Older patients are protected by a long leg brace for several additional weeks.

The functional results of surgery have been surprisingly satisfactory, considering the extensive fibrosis of muscle encountered and the coexistence of other musculoskeletal abnormalities. Curtis and Fisher[9] found that seven of 12 knees achieved good to excel-

traction as employed by Griffin.[20] We would recommend surgery for knees failing to respond to manipulation by the age of 6 months, since long-term follow-up of untreated cases would indicate that unstable, even grotesque, deformities may develop.[15]

Many surgical techniques have been described for correcting hyperextension of the knee with subluxation or dislocation.[9,32,39] Almost all involve some method

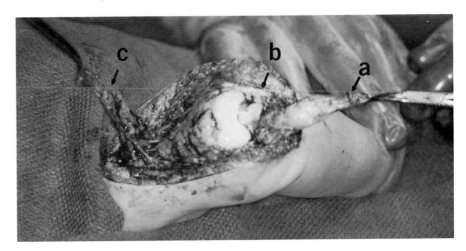

Fig. 25.2. Method of quadriceps lengthening for congenital hyperextension of the knee with subluxation. (a) patella and distal quadriceps tongue (b) medial collateral ligament (c) quadriceps muscles (From Curtis, B.H., and Fisher, R.L.: Congenital hyperextension with anterior subluxation of the knee. Surgical treatment and long-term observations. J. Bone Joint Surg. [Am.], *51*:255, 1969, with permission.)

lent function. Recurrent hyperextension was not observed, and most patients developed at least 90 degrees of flexion and good active extension such that bracing or external support was not required. Residual mediolateral instability and flexion contracture were the most frequent problems. The best results were achieved in younger children. In patients with congenital dislocation of the hip associated with resistant hyperextension of the knee, knee surgery is recommended before reduction of the hip. Otherwise, redislocation of the hip may occur from a tight rectus femoris and an inability to control hip rotation.

HERITABLE CONGENITAL TIBIOFEMORAL SUBLUXATION

Heritable congenital tibiofemoral subluxation is a rare disorder of the knee characterized by anterior tibial subluxation with knee extension and normal tibiofemoral alignment with knee flexion.[10] In contrast to congenital hyperextension with subluxation or dislocation, hyperextension is mild and flexion is unrestricted, and there is no association with congenital hip dislocation or arthrogryposis. The condition has been found in siblings. The major pathology consists of a tight iliotibial band and hypertrophic biceps femoris muscle such that these structures lie anterior to the joint axis and tend to subluxate the tibia forward with extension of the knee. Surgical correction has been described in five cases by sectioning the iliotibial band, excising the distal portion of the intermuscular septum, and transposing the insertion of the

biceps femoris to the vastus lateralis.[10] Postoperatively, the knee should be braced in slight flexion for several weeks with weight-bearing in order to permit remodeling of the joint surfaces and prevent recurrent subluxation. Improvement of gait and prevention of recurrent anterior tibial subluxation have been observed in every instance.

PATELLAR ABNORMALITIES

CONGENITAL DISLOCATION OF THE PATELLA

Although rarely identified at birth, "congenital" dislocation of the patella may be distinguished from habitual or recurrent dislocation by the diagnostic criteria of Conn.[8] These include permanent dislocation, inability to extend the knee actively, unimpaired passive mobility, and absence of the patella from the intertrochlear fossa at birth. Flexion contracture of the knee is another common clinical characteristic.[18] The condition is rare and has been reported in only a few isolated cases or groups of cases.[25,45] Although family history is usually negative, several cases have been associated with Down's syndrome.

The diagnosis can be easily appreciated by careful clinical examination, which indicates a lateral dislocation of the patella. The patella cannot be reduced or, if reducible, promptly dislocates when the knee is flexed. Valgus alignment, flexion contracture, and inability to extend the knee actively should suggest the diagnosis. Radiologic examination in young children before the patellar ossification center has appeared (about age 5 years) may prove unrewarding. In older children, the position and size of the patella and the contour of the patellar surface of the distal femur may be appreciated.

Pathologically, the congenitally dislocated patella is hypoplastic and has underdeveloped or absent facets (Fig. 25.3).[25] Chondromalacia is absent except in late stages. The intercondylar groove of the femur is consistently absent, and the femoral surface may be convex rather than concave. The lateral soft tissues are tight, and the vastus lateralis or iliotibial band may insert abnormally into the patella.

Untreated, congenital dislocation of the patella may be associated with considerable functional disability. In contrast to recurrent dislocation of the patella, which may be treated successfully by quadriceps strengthening or by simple lateral release, congenital dislocation of the patella requires surgical realignment. I have had experience with a procedure that combines an extensive lateral release of capsule, vastus lateralis and synovium combined with medial transposition of the patellar tendon and, when necessary, advancement of the vastus medialis to the upper medial quadrant of the patella (Fig. 25.4)[25] Care must be taken to avoid injury to the proximal tibial epiphysis in young children. By transferring only the patellar tendon to the medial tibia, we have not observed growth disturbance or patella baja. Flexion contracture, if present, must be corrected before patellar realignment by casting or posterior release. Postoperatively, the knee should be protected by cylinder casting for 6 weeks and then rehabilitated by quadriceps strengthening and range of motion exercises.

The results of surgical correction by the above procedure were good, with improvement of knee motion and development of active extension in seven of eight patients in our series.[25] Recurrent dislocation developed in only one patient.

CONGENITAL ABSENCE OF THE PATELLA

Isolated congenital absence of the patella has been reported in rare instances.[1,27] Absence of the patella is usually associated with other anomalies comprising hereditary onycho-osteodysplasia (nail–patella or Fong's syndrome).[12] The characteristics of this syndrome, in addition to absent patellae, include dysplastic nails, dislocation of radial head, and iliac horns (Fig. 25.5). Patients with congenitally absent patellae function sufficiently well without the need for surgery.

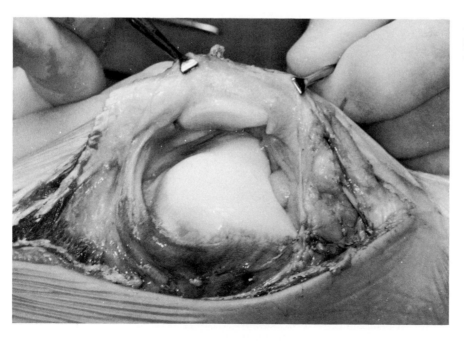

Fig. 25.3. Pathology of congenital dislocation of patella. Note convex femoral sulcus.

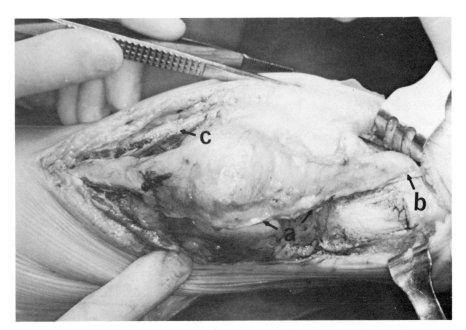

Fig. 25.4. Illustrative drawing of surgery for congenital dislocation of patella. (a) line of lateral release, (b) patellar tendon, (c) vastus medialis.

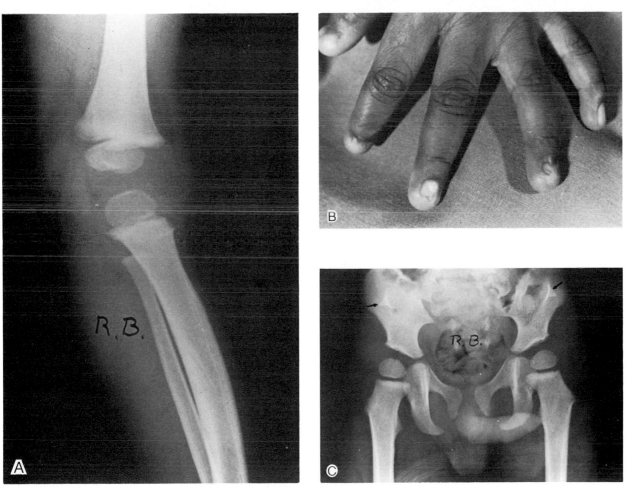

Fig. 25.5. Features of onycho-osteodysplasia (nail–patella syndrome). (a) absent patella, (b) dysplastic nails, (c) disc horns.

BIPARTITE PATELLA

Although there are many forms of patellar fragmentation,[29] all except bipartite patella are extremely uncommon. The vast majority of bipartite fragments occur in the upper outer quadrant of the patella (Fig. 25.6). The etiology of bipartite patella is unclear. Some speculate that the fragment consists of an aberrant ossification center that failed to fuse with the main mass of patella, while others relate it to increased muscle traction on the superolateral portion of the main patellar ossification nucleus at a critical stage of development.[14]

Most bipartite patellae are asymptomatic and are discovered fortuitously. However, pain at the site of bipartite fragment may develop, and the lesion must be distinguished from fracture. Features supporting

a diagnosis of bipartite fragment include bilateral lesions, typical location, and rounded regular margins at the synchondrosis. A painful bipartite patella should be treated initially by analgesics, immobilization by cast or brace, or local steroid injection.[43] Persistent symptoms may be managed successfully by excision of the small bipartite fragment through a short lateral parapatellar incision.[19]

ANGULAR DEFORMITIES

KNOCK-KNEE (GENU VALGUM)

Knock-knee deformity may develop from a number of conditions producing differential growth of the medial and lateral portions of either the distal femoral or proximal tibial epiphyseal plates. These conditions include trauma, infection, nutritional abnormalities (rickets), hereditary conditions (Morquio's disease, metaphyseal dysostosis, familial vitamin D-resistant rickets), muscular imbalance, and endocrinologic abnormality. Developmental (idiopathic) knock-knee is by far the most common etiology.

The development of the knee alignment has been studied clinically in 1,000 examinations of unselected children 1 to 11 years old by Morley.[38] The radiologic measurement of the tibiofemoral angle has been carried out in 979 pediatric patients by Salenius and Vankka.[42] Both investigations indicate that a varus knee alignment at birth rapidly converts to a valgus alignment at about 2 years of age. The valgus alignment increases to an average of about 10 degrees at $3\frac{1}{2}$ years of age. Thereafter, the physiologic tibiofemoral angle decreases to the normal adult measurement of 5 to 9 degrees in females and 4 to 7 degrees in males. After the age of 7 years, only 2 percent of children have significant knock-knees.[38] The bimalleolar distance with the knees together is another clinical estimate of the degree of knock-knee with values greater than 10 cm being abnormal.

Developmental knock-knee deformities may be ignored in younger children in view of the statistical likelihood of spontaneous correction. A medial heel wedge may be employed for more severe deformities if desired. Surgical correction is indicated for cosmetic reasons and theoretically to prevent later lateral compartment arthritis in children with significant deformity after 11 years of age (bimalleolar distances of

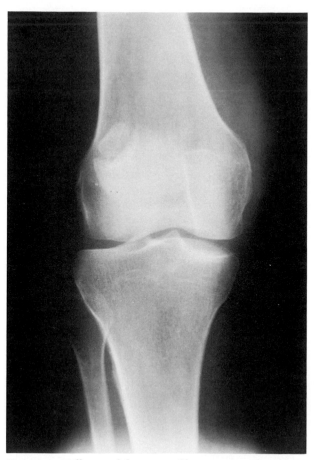

Fig. 25.6. Differential diagnosis of bipartite patella and patellar fracture.

> 10 cm or tibiofemoral angles of > 10 degrees). Epiphyseal stapling has proved a very satisfactory method of correcting developmental knock-knee deformity.[2,3] Zuege et al.[50] reported good results in 41 of 64 valgus knees, while an additional 15 were improved, though not completely corrected. Pistevos and Duckworth[41] found stapling safe and predictable in 49 patients, while Howorth reported good or excellent results in 15 of 16 patients.[24]

Medial stapling of only the distal femoral epiphysis (the site of greatest deformity) is required in most cases. Timing of the operation is critical, with some workers recommending a skeletal age of 11 years in girls and 12 years in boys and others an age of $11\frac{1}{2}$ for both sexes.[41,50] The operation is carried out through a short incision over the medial femoral condyle. Two or three vitallium staples are placed extraperiosteally to straddle the epiphyseal plate (Fig. 25.7).[2,3] The staple shafts should parallel the plate, which is convex distally when viewed from the medial side. The staples should lie flush with the femoral cortex and should be inserted with care to avoid inserting the proximal posterior staple prong into posterior soft tissues. Accurate placement of the staples may be assisted by fluoroscopy or by a small incision through the periosteum, or by both means, to locate the level of the epiphysis. The staples are arranged slightly posterior to the midline when recurvatum deformity coexists and slightly anterior to the midline for flexion deformities. Separate closure of deep fascia and patellar retinaculum is recommended. Postoperatively, the patients may be protected with a cylinder cast for 2 to 3 weeks or managed with soft dressing and crutches.

The staples should be removed when overcorrection has been achieved, recognizing that some re-

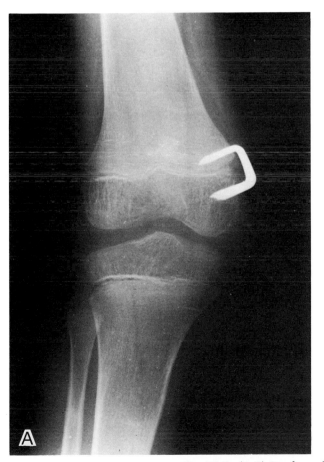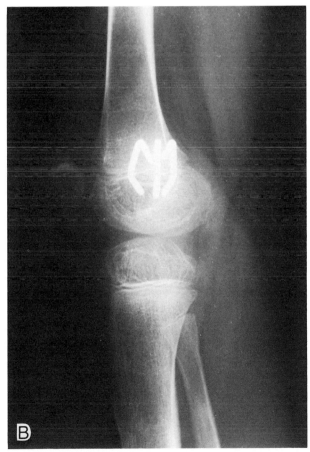

Fig. 25.7. (A,B) Stapling of developmental knock-knee.

bound reversal of about 5 degrees may be expected if growth has not ceased. In older children, or those with severe knock-knee deformity, medial stapling of both distal femoral and proximal tibial epiphyses is required for adequate correction. The technical principles of staple insertion for the tibia are the same as for the femur.

Complications of the stapling procedure have been infrequent. Extrusion of staples, usually from technical errors of insertion, have been seen in a small percentage of cases (5 to 10%).[41,50] These have frequently been salvaged by reinsertion of staples. Closure of the epiphysis with recurvatum or flexion deformity has not been observed. The primary reported complication has been incomplete correction from operating too late or removing the staples too soon.[50]

Tibial osteotomy should be considered for severe knock-knee deformity in older children or those having a short leg or epiphyseal growth abnormality other than developmental knock-knee. The osteotomy must be placed just below the level of the proximal tibial epiphysis and patellar tendon insertion and be combined with a short oblique fibular osteotomy at the junction of proximal and middle thirds. If no tibial torsion requires correction, a dome-shaped tibial osteotomy is preferred. If rotational deformity coexists, a medial based closing wedge osteotomy with appropriate rotation of the distal fragment is accomplished. Internal fixation for additional stability may be provided by crossed K wires or a K wire passing through each fragment and incorporated in plaster. Casting is continued until the osteotomies are well united (8 to 12 weeks). In correcting severe deformities, neurologic compromise from traction on the peroneal nerve or occlusion of the anterior tibial artery at its emergence through the interosseous membrane must be carefully monitored.[46] Less than optimal correction must be accepted to reverse this complication.

BOW LEG DEFORMITY

Bowing of the knees is normal in newborns and involves femur and tibia. This physiologic bowing corrects spontaneously in the first 2 or 3 years of life and usually requires no treatment. Severe cases may be managed with a Denis Browne splint with sufficient length and concavity toward the patient to produce a valgus force on the knees at night and nap time for a few months.

Physiologic bowing must be distinguished from tibia vara (Blount's disease, osteochondrosis deformans tibiae), which represents a failure of growth of the medial part of the upper tibial metaphysis and epiphysis.[4] Tibia vara occurs unilaterally and bilaterally with equal frequency and is seen about twice as often in females as in males. The etiology of tibia vara is unclear, but it is probably related to abnormal stress on physiologically bowed legs during weight-bearing. The infantile form of tibia vara has a particularly high incidence in blacks of the West Indies, who are distinguished by having an early walking age and increased ligamentous laxity.[17] Radiologically, physiologic bowing and tibia vara may be difficult to distinguish in early life. The metaphyseal–diaphyseal angle (Fig. 25.8) is a sensitive measurement that has proved helpful in distinguishing these conditions. Levine and Drennan[33] found that 29 of 30 cases with an initial metaphyseal–diaphyseal angle of >11.0 degrees later developed typical changes of tibia vara, while only three of 58 with a metaphyseal–diaphyseal angle of <11.0 degrees developed any such changes.

Langenskiöld[30] has divided the radiologic course of tibia vara into the following six stages (Fig. 25.9):

Stage I: Irregularity of ossification of metaphysis and beaking of the metaphysis seen in children up to 3 years of age

Stage II: Seen in children between 2½ and 4 years of age, in which there is a sharp depression of the ossification line of the medial one-third of the metaphysis and the medial part of the bony epiphysis becomes more wedge shaped and less developed than the lateral part

Stage III: Seen in the 4- to 6-year age group; shows deepening of the depression of the metaphyseal beak filled by cartilage with a step-shaped appearance to the metaphysis; the medial bony epiphysis is wedge shaped and less distinct, and small areas of calcification may present beneath its medial border

Stage IV: Occurs between 5 and 10 years of age, with the bony epiphysis enlarging and occupying the depression in the medial part of the metaphysis and with irregularity of the medial border of the bony epiphysis

Stage V: Seen in children between 9 and 11 years of age, in which the bony epiphysis is divided by a clear band in its medial portion from the growth

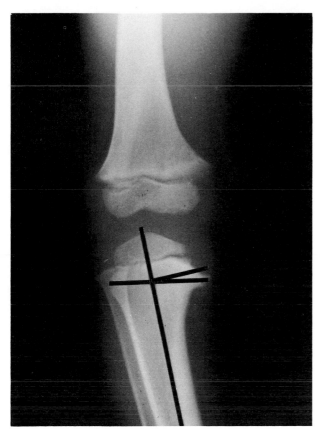

Fig. 25.8. Metaphyseal–diaphyseal angle in Blount's disease. (see text)

plate to articular cartilage; there is a downward slope of the articular surface and irregularity of the medial margin of the epiphysis

Stage VI: Occurs in 10- to 13-year age group, with the growth plate fusing medially and growth proceeding laterally to produce progressive medial sloping deformity

The radiologic progression is accompanied by progressive clinical varus deformity and knee instability. It is agreed that when progressive changes of tibia vara are recognized, prompt corrective valgus osteotomy should be carried out.[17,31] The radiologic deformity is reversible in stages I through IV, while osteotomy alone will not suffice to prevent further deformity in stages V and VI in older children. In Langenskiöld's large series of 61 cases of infantile tibia vara,[31] 47 legs required only one osteotomy. Of these, 25 were operated on before 4 years of age and only three were over 8 years of age. In 21 cases requiring more than one osteotomy, all but five were over 7 years of age. Eleven cases required epiphysiodesis of the lateral tibial epiphyseal and proximal fibular epiphyseal plates. Most of these children did not present for treatment until after 9 years of age.

Treatment for the early case of tibia vara (age 2 to 8 and stages I through IV) should consist of a curved dome-shaped osteotomy of the proximal tibia just distal to the tibial tubercle and a short oblique osteotomy

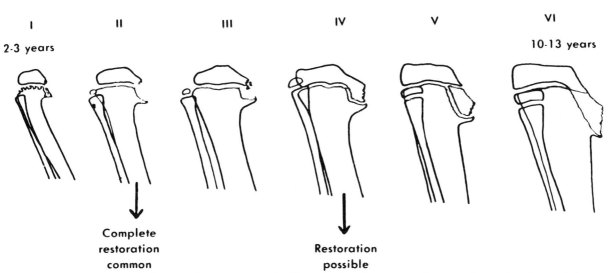

Fig. 25.9. Stages of Blount's disease. (From Langenskiöld, A., and Riska, E.B.: Tibia vara (osteochondrosis deformans tibiae). A survey of 23 cases. Acta Chirurgica Scandinavica, *103*: 1–22, 1952, with permission.)

of the midfibula. Slight valgus overcorrection should be achieved. Postoperative immobilization in a plaster cast for 8 weeks is recommended.

Established deformity in older children with impending or actual arrest of growth of the medial tibial epiphyseal line should have a complete epiphysiodesis of the tibial plate laterally and epiphysiodesis of the proximal fibula. Articular deformity, with downward sloping of the medial tibial condyles (stages V and VI) has been corrected by osteotomy and elevation of the medial condyle combined with epiphysiodesis by Langenskiöld and Riska.[31] This osteotomy extends from the intercondylar eminence to the junction of metaphysis and diaphysis medially. When the medial condyle is elevated, it is secured by placing diaphyseal cortical grafts in the bony defect.

Adolescent tibia vara is uncommon and probably results in most cases from trauma with closure of the medial portion of the epiphyseal plate.[4,31] Spontaneous regression has been described. Corrective surgery prior to completion of growth is recommended in adolescent tibia vara only if progression is observed. A long bridge or partial closure of the epiphyseal line may be ascertained best by tomography in some cases. For progressive deformity and demonstrated bony bridges across the epiphyseal plate, excision of the bony bridge and packing of the resulting defect with subcutaneous fat or corrective osteotomy and completion of the epiphysiodesis as in infantile tibia vara can be considered. If sufficient limb shortening exists (> 2.5 cm) leg lengthening or contralateral proximal tibial and fibular epiphysiodesis should be carried out for equalization of leg length.

In addition to physiologic bowing and tibia vara, bowed deformity of the knee can result from many causes, such as infection, trauma, hereditary conditions, and muscular imbalance. These deformities may be managed surgically by lateral tibial and fibular epiphyseal stapling or tibial osteotomy depending on the severity of deformity and age of the child.

SOFT TISSUE ABNORMALITIES

QUADRICEPS FIBROSIS

Progressive fibrosis of the quadriceps muscle has been reported as a distinct entity in young children to be distinguished from cases of arthrogryposis, congenital dislocation of the knee and congenital dislocation of the patella.[48] This condition typically occurs in children 1 to 7 years of age and is characterized by progressive restriction of knee flexion, a high-riding patella, or laterally dislocating patella or valgus deformity of the knee, depending on the part of muscle predominantly affected. The etiology is obscure,[23] but a high percentage of cases have been reported in children having previous injections of antibiotics and other solutions into the thigh.[22,34]

Pathologically, the vastus lateralis or vastus intermedius or both are involved in almost all cases.[22,48] While scarring of the rectus femoris may also occur, the vastus medialis is rarely affected. Gunn[22] considers the tightness of the iliotibial tract occasionally observed to be secondary to the contracture. The scarring typically occurs in the mid- or distal thigh.

Conservative treatment has been of very little benefit except in mild cases. In children with severe limitation of motion, surgery was successful in restoring a full range of knee motion in all 28 knees reported by Williams[48] and about 90 degrees of flexion in 10 cases reported by Hněvkovský.[23] The surgical release reported by all surgeons has been similar. An incision is made over the lateral border of the rectus femoris in the distal thigh. Any abnormal bands from the iliotibial tract to the patella are released. The usually fibrous vastus lateralis or intermedius tissues, or both, are excised, and the normal muscle tissue is sutured to the rectus femoris with the knee flexed. If the rectus femoris is also involved in scar, a V–Y lengthening of the quadriceps as performed for congenital dislocation of the knee is carried out. Postoperatively, the knee is casted at 90 degrees of flexion for three weeks. An extension lag may be expected for several weeks, particularly if the rectus femoris has been lengthened. The range of motion achieved on the operating table should ultimately be expected.

POPLITEAL CYSTS

Popliteal cysts are swellings in the posterior aspect of the knee which usually occur distal to the skin crease and just medial to the gastrocnemius muscle (Fig. 25.10). They are twice as common in boys as in girls and are almost always unilateral. The presenting complaint is the appearance of a mass in the back of the knee. Significant pain and knee symptoms such as snapping and locking are uncommon. Pathologi-

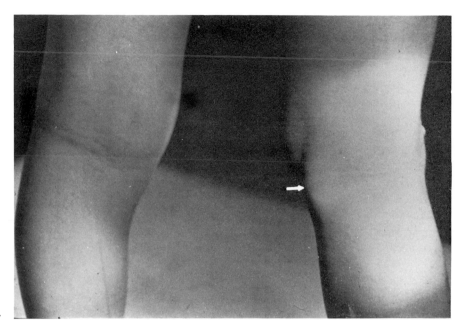

Fig. 25.10. Popliteal cyst.

cally, these lesions have a shiny synovial-like membrane and are generally filled with a thick gelatinous material similar to that found in wrist ganglia.[7] The cysts are associated with the bursa between the gastrocnemius muscle and semimembranosus tendon; in contrast to popliteal cysts of adults, they usually do not communicate with the knee joint or relate to intra-articular pathology.[21] The etiology of childhood popliteal cysts may be direct trauma to the gastrocnemius–semimembranosus bursa.[21]

Popliteal (Baker's) cysts must be distinguished from other rare lesions, such as lipoma, aneurysm, intra-articular pathology, such as rheumatoid arthritis and villonodular synovitis, and soft tissue sarcoma. Popliteal cysts transilluminate and have a higher radiologic density than does a lipoma. When in doubt concerning the diagnosis, aspiration of the typical gelatinous contents through a relatively large bore needle and the use of local anesthesia will confirm the presence of a popliteal cyst. If associated knee pathology is suspected, an arthrogram will demonstrate whether the cyst is communicating with the knee joint.

The evidence now indicates that asymptomatic popliteal cysts of children are best handled by observation and reassurance of the parents. Dinham[11] found that 51 of 70 untreated popliteal cysts disappeared within an average of 1 year, 8 months. MacMahon[35] similarly found a spontaneous disappearance of popliteal cysts in 25 of 42 untreated patients during a period of 6 years. Aspiration and injection of steroids is generally followed by prompt recurrence of the cyst in the hands of the present author and others. This maneuver is primarily of value in confirming the diagnosis and in reassuring the parents that the lesion is not malignant. The results of surgical excision of the cysts has been quite discouraging. Dinham[11] noted a 42 percent recurrence rate within 7 months in 50 excised cysts. Surgery should therefore be reserved for those children with longstanding, painful, or enlarging cysts; patients and their families should be warned of possible recurrence. When surgery is elected, a small transverse skin incision over the lesion is made under general anesthesia and tourniquet control. The cyst is usually readily identified in the subcutaneous tissues. It may be bluntly and sharply dissected from the medial head of the gastrocnemius muscle and semimembranosus tendon with which it is associated. The neurovascular structures lie lateral to the gastrocnemius muscle and should not be encountered. A compression dressing is employed postoperatively.

OSGOOD-SCHLATTER'S DISEASE

Apophysitis of the tibial tuberosity is a common condition in early adolescence. Typically patients present at 12 to 14 years of age with pain and swelling in the region of the tibial tuberosity. The complaints are aggravated by activity and relieved by rest. The etiology is unclear but is probably related to traction of the patellar tendon and microfracture of the developing tibial apophysis.[40] Radiographs show soft tissue swelling in the region of the patellar tendon insertion with or without fragmentation of the tibial apophysis. Treatment for the vast majority of cases should be conservative by restriction of activities and anti-inflammatory agents or a brief period of cast immobilization. Local injection of steroid may be considered but repeated injections should not be carried out because of possible weakening and rupture of the patellar tendon. One hundred and four of 118 patients

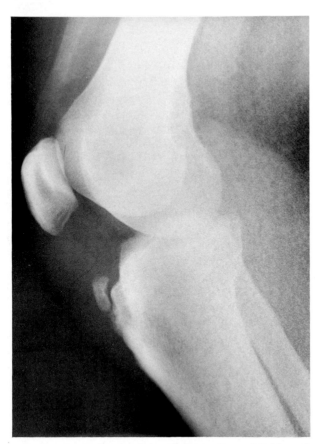

Fig. 25.11. Patellar tendon ossicle in Osgood-Schlatter's disease.

reviewed by Mital and Matzo responded to nonsurgical measures.[37]

Rarely, symptoms related to Osgood-Schlatter's disease persist into adult life. Woolfrey and Chandler[49] have shown that unresolved symptoms are associated with the presence of ossicles in the patellar tendon (Fig. 25.11). In such cases, drilling and bone peg grafting[5] or excision of the tibial tuberosity[13,47] were previously recommended. More recently, simple excision of the patellar tendon ossicles has been shown to relieve symptoms in most cases. In all 13 operated cases reported by Mital and Matzo,[37] patients found complete relief of symptoms and were able to return to work in 6 weeks. In my own experience with 16 patients, 12 were rendered asymptomatic and would repeat the surgery, whereas three who were unchanged and one who was slightly improved would not repeat the surgery.[16]

The operation for unresolved Osgood-Schlatter's disease is carried out under general anesthesia through a small transverse incision over the tibial tuberosity. The patellar tendon is divided in the direction of its fibers to expose the ossicle which is then excised sharply from its attachments to the patellar tendon on its superficial surface. A bursal sac is usually encountered under the cartilaginous deep surface of the ossicle. Postoperatively, patients are managed with a soft dressing and activities as tolerated.

INTRA-ARTICULAR ABNORMALITIES

DISCOID LATERAL MENISCUS

The presence of a discoid rather than semilunar-shaped lateral meniscus is rare. Smillie[44] encountered it in only 2 percent of cases in a large series of arthrotomies for internal derangement. It has been speculated that this meniscal abnormality results from a failure of the embryonal meniscal plate to develop a normal shape,[44] or alternatively from wear of an originally normal-shaped meniscus into a discoid shape resulting from increased mobility from lack of posterior attachments of the meniscus to the tibia.[26] Symptoms of discoid lateral meniscus include snapping or catching of the knee, lateral joint line pain, or the development of a cyst. Diagnosis may be established by arthrogram (Fig. 25.12) or arthroscopy. Tearing or degeneration of the meniscus may be observed in addition to the discoid shape. Traditional treatment for

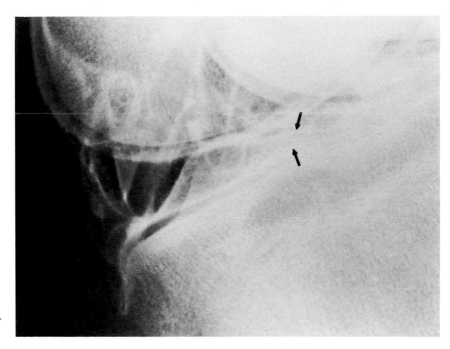

Fig. 25.12. Arthrogram showing discoid lateral meniscus.

symptomatic discoid meniscus has consisted of excision of the meniscus through parapatellar or lateral (Bruser) incision.[6] Recently, arthroscopic surgical reshaping of the meniscus has been carried out with good short term results in a few cases.[36] Figure 25.13A shows the arthroscopic appearance of a discoid meniscus in a 31-year-old soccer referee. His preoperative snapping and pain were eliminated by reshaping the meniscus (Fig. 25.13B) using basket forceps under arthroscopic control.

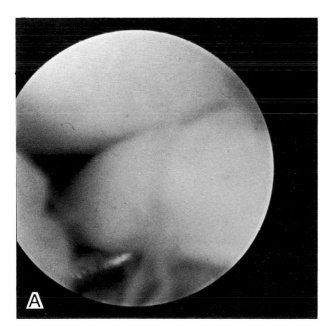

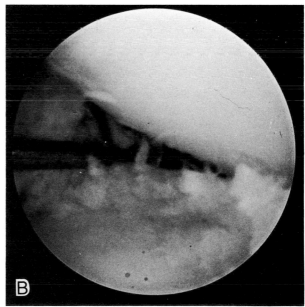

Fig. 25.13. (A,B) Arthroscopic surgery of discoid lateral meniscus.

OSTEOCHONDRITIS DISSECANS

For a discussion of osteochondritis dissecans see Chapter 10.

REFERENCES

1. Bernhang, A.M., and Levine, S.A.: Familial absence of the patella. J. Bone Joint Surg. [Am.], *55:* 1088, 1973.
2. Blount, W.P.: A mature look at epiphyseal stapling. Clin. Orthop., *77:* 158, 1971.
3. Blount, W.P., and Clarke, G.R.: Control of bone growth by epiphyseal stapling—a preliminary report. J. Bone Joint Surg. [Am.], *31:* 464, 1949.
4. Blount, W.P.: Tibia vara. J. Bone Joint Surg., *19:* 1, 1937.
5. Bosworth, D.M.: Autogenous bone pegging for epiphysitis of the tibial tubercle. J. Bone Joint Surg., *16:* 829, 1934.
6. Bruser, D.M.: A direct lateral approach to the lateral compartment of the knee joint. J. Bone Joint Surg. [Br.], *42:* 348, 1960.
7. Burleson, R.J., Bickel, W.H., and Dahlin, D.C.: Popliteal cyst: A clinicopathological survey. J. Bone Joint Surg. [Am.], *38:* 1265, 1956.
8. Conn, H.R.: A new method of operative reduction of congenital luxation of the patella. J. Bone Joint Surg., *7:* 370, 1925.
9. Curtis, B.H., and Fisher, R.L.: Congenital hyperextension with anterior subluxation of the knee. Surgical treatment and long-term observations. J. Bone Joint Surg. [Am.], *51:* 255, 1969.
10. Curtis, B.H., and Fisher, R.L.: Heritable congenital tibiofemoral subluxation. Clinical features and surgical treatment. J. Bone Joint Surg. [Am.], *52:* 1104, 1970.
11. Dinham, J.M.: Popliteal cysts in children. The case against surgery. J. Bone Joint Surg. [Br.], *57:* 69, 1975.
12. Duncan, J.G., and Souter, W.A.: Hereditary onycho-osteodysplasia. The nail-patella syndrome. J. Bone Joint Surg. [Br.], *45:* 242, 1963.
13. Ferciot, C.F.: Surgical management of anterior tibial epiphysis. Clin. Orthop., *5:* 204, 1955.
14. Ficat, R.P., and Hungerford, D.S.: Disorders of the Patello-Femoral Joint. p. 55. Baltimore, Williams & Wilkins, 1977.
15. Finder, J.G.: Congenital hyperextension of the knee. Presented at the Annual Meeting of the American Orthopaedic Association, Vancouver, British Columbia, Canada, June 1964.
16. Fisher, R.L.: Treatment of unresolved Osgood-Schlatter's disease by excision of patellar tendon ossicles. Orthop. Rev., *9(2):* 93, 1980.
17. Golding, J.S.R., and McNeil-Smith, J.D.G.: Observations on the etiology of tibia vara. J. Bone Joint Surg. [Br.], *45:* 320, 1963.
18. Green, J.P., and Waugh, W.: Congenital lateral dislocation of the patella. J. Bone Joint Surg. [Br.], *50:* 285, 1968.
19. Green, W.T., Jr.: Painful bipartite patellae. A report of three cases. Clin. Orthop., *110:* 197, 1975.
20. Griffin, P.P.: The lower limb. p. 881. In Lovell, W.W., Winter, R.B., Ed.: Pediatric Orthopedics. Philadelphia, J.B. Lippincott, 1978.
21. Gristina, A.G., and Wilson, P.D.: Popliteal cysts in adults and children: a review of ninety operative cases. In proceedings J. Bone Joint Surg. [Am.], *45:* 1552, 1963.
22. Gunn, D.R.: Contracture of the quadriceps muscle. A discussion on the etiology and relationship to recurrent dislocation of the patella. J. Bone Joint Surg. [Br.], *46:* 492, 1964.
23. Hněvkovský, O.: Progressive fibrosis of the vastus intermedius muscle in children. A cause of limited knee flexion and elevation of the patella. J. Bone Joint Surg. [Br.], *43:* 318, 1961.
24. Howorth, B.: Knock knees with special reference to the stapling operation. Clin. Orthop., *77:* 233, 1971.
25. Jones, R.D., Fisher, R.L., and Curtis, B.H.: Congenital dislocation of the patella. Clin. Orthop. *119:* 177, 1976.
26. Kaplan, E.B.: Discoid lateral meniscus of the knee joint—nature, mechanism and operative treatment. J. Bone Joint Surg. [Am.], *39:* 77, 1957.
27. Katz, E.R.: Congenital absence of the patellae. J. Pediat., *34:* 760, 1949.
28. Katz, M.P., Grogono, B.J.S., and Soper, K.C.: The etiology and treatment of congenital dislocation of the knee. J. Bone Joint Surg. [Br.], *49:* 112, 1967.
29. Kohler, A., and Zimmer, E.A.: p. 431. In Wilk, S.P., Ed.: Pathologies in Skeletal Roentgenology. 11th Ed. New York, Grune & Stratton, 1968.
30. Langenskiöld, A.: Tibia vara. (Osteochondrosis deformans tibiae.) A survey of 23 cases. Acta Chir. Scand., *103:* 1, 1952.
31. Langenskiöld, A., and Riska, E.B.: Tibia vara (osteochondrosis deformans tibiae). J. Bone Joint Surg. [Am.], *46:* 1405, 1964.
32. Leveuf, J., and Pais, C.: Les dislocations congénitales du genou (genu recurvatum, subluxation, luxation). Rev. Orthop., *32:* 313, 1946.
33. Levine, A.M., and Drennan, J.C.: Physiologic bowing and tibia vara: The metaphyseal-diaphyseal angle in the measurement of bowleg deformities. J. Bone Joint Surg. [Am.], *64:*1158, 1982.

34. Lloyd-Roberts, G.C., and Thomas, T.G.: The etiology of quadriceps contracture in children. J. Bone Joint Surg. [Br.], *46:* 498, 1964.

35. MacMahon, E.B.: Baker's cysts in children—is surgery necessary? In proceedings J. Bone Joint Surg. [Am.], *55:* 1311, 1973.

36. Metcalf, R.W.: Personal communication, 1982.

37. Mital, M.A., Matza, R.A., and Cohen, J.: The so-called unresolved Osgood-Schlatter lesion. J. Bone Joint Surg. [Am.], *62:* 732, 1980.

38. Morley, A.J.M.: Knock knee in children. Br. Med. J., *2:* 976, 1957.

39. Niebauer, J.J., and King, D.E.: Congenital dislocation of the knee. J. Bone Joint Surg. [Am.], *42:* 207, 1960.

40. Ogden, J.A., and Southwick, W.O.: Osgood-Schlatter's disease and tibial tuberosity development. Clin. Orthop., *116:* 180, 1976.

41. Pistevos, G., and Duckworth, T.: The correction of genu valgum by epiphyseal stapling. J. Bone Joint Surg. [Br.], *59:* 72, 1977.

42. Salenius, P., and Vankka, E.: The development of the tibiofemoral angle in children. J. Bone Joint Surg. [Am.], *57:* 259, 1975.

43. Sharrard, W.J.W.: Paediatric Orthopaedics and Fractures. p. 429. 2nd Ed. London, Blackwell Scientific Publications, 1979.

44. Smillie, I.S.: Injuries of the Knee Joint. P. 43 Baltimore, Williams & Wilkins, 1946.

45. Stanisavljevic, S., Zemenick, G., and Miller, D.: Congenital, irreducible, permanent lateral dislocation of the patella. Clin. Orthop., *116:* 190, 1976.

46. Steel, H.H., Sandrow, R.E., and Sullivan, P.D.: Complications of tibial osteotomy in children for genu varum or valgum. Evidence that neurological changes are due to ischemia. J. Bone Joint Surg. [Am.], *53:* 1629, 1971.

47. Thompson, J.E.M.: Operative treatment of osteochondritis of the tibial tubercle. J. Bone Joint Surg. [Am.], *38:* 142, 1956.

48. Williams, P.F.: Quadriceps contracture. J. Bone Joint Surg. [Br.], *50:* 278, 1968.

49. Woolfrey, B.F., and Chandler, E.F.: Manifestations of Osgood-Schlatter's disease in late teen age and early adulthood. J. Bone Joint Surg. [Am.], *42:* 327, 1960.

50. Zuege, R.C., Kempken, T.G., and Blount, W.P.: Epiphyseal stapling for angular deformity at the knee. J. Bone Joint Surg. [Am.], *61:* 320, 1979.

26 Tumors Around the Knee

Brian J. Hurson
and
Joseph M. Lane

INTRODUCTION

Although a large proportion of bone tumors, both benign and malignant, occur in the knee region, it is emphasized that in general orthopaedic practice malignant bone tumors are rare. In the context of this book only those tumors involving the knee joint, the epiphysis, metaphysis and diametaphysis of the distal femur, proximal tibia and fibula are considered. In addition, soft tissue lesions are discussed.

BONE LESIONS

Caffey, in a large survey of "normal children," reported that 43 percent had osseous defects that resolved by adulthood.[2] Fibrous cortical defects occur in 30 to 40 percent of all normal children past 2 years and 90 percent of these are seen in the distal femur.[20] The most common benign tumor of bone is the solitary osteochondroma.[20] It represents 50 percent of benign bone neoplasms and about 12 percent of all neoplasms of bone. Approximately 50 percent of solitary osteochondromas occur around the knee.[5,20] One third of 458 benign chondroblastomas collated in a literature review by Huvos and Marcove occurred about the knee.[21] Over 25 percent of aneurysmal bone cysts in Dahlin's series were in the knee region.[5] Although unicameral bone cysts occur frequently in the growing child they occur uncommonly about the knee. The most common site for giant cell tumors is in and about the knee with about 50 percent of all giant cell tumors occurring in this area evenly distributed between the distal femur and proximal tibia.[16,20,44,56] Almost all of the remaining benign osseous lesions have been reported to occur about the knee including osteoid osteoma, enchondroma, non-ossifying fibroma and chondromyxofibroma.

Excluding multiple myeloma, osteosarcoma is the most common primary malignant tumor of bone.[7,20] The 962 osteosarcomas reviewed by Dahlin comprised 20.2 percent of the total sarcomas of his series.[5] Approximately 50 percent of these occurred about the knee. Although parosteal osteosarcomas are rare, it is noteworthy that 14 of Huvos' series of 24 cases occurred in the posterior aspect of the distal femur.[20] Similarly 26 of the 36 lesions reported by Dahlin were in the same location.[5] A further 4 involved the upper tibia. Approximately 12 percent of the chondrosarcomas seen at Memorial Hospital occurred around the knee.[20] A similar figure was seen in Dahlin's series.[5]

Other malignant spindle cell tumors of bone such as fibrosarcoma, malignant fibrous histiocytoma and haemangiopericytoma present in a similar fashion to osteogenic sarcoma with a similar distribution. Most of these are located in the distal femur followed in frequency by the proximal tibia.[20] They occur in an older age group (i.e., the 3rd, 4th and 5th decades). In addition to the tumors mentioned above, Ewing's sarcoma and reticulum cell sarcoma are rarely seen in the distal femur and proximal tibia. Ewing's sarcoma more frequently occurs in the diametaphysis and is the most common primary bone malignancy of the fibula. Finally, the knee region, although infrequently may be a site for an osteolytic or osteoblastic metastatic deposit from a primary malignancy elsewhere.

CLINICAL

The most common presenting symptoms in patients with bone tumors are those of progressive pain and increasing mass. Classically this pain is unrelieved by position and can occur at night. Occasionally lesions may not be active enough to cause symptoms and will be incidentally diagnosed on a radiograph for an unrelated problem. A small group of patients presents following a pathological fracture. The medical history is usually unhelpful in patients with primary disease, although it may reveal the location of a primary malignancy in metastatic lesions. There is

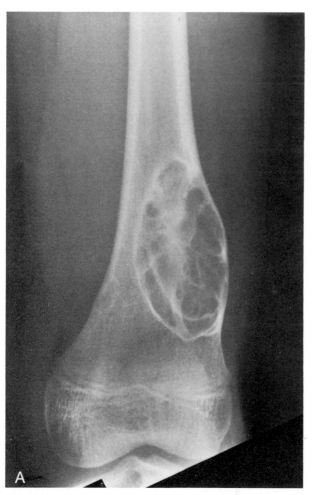 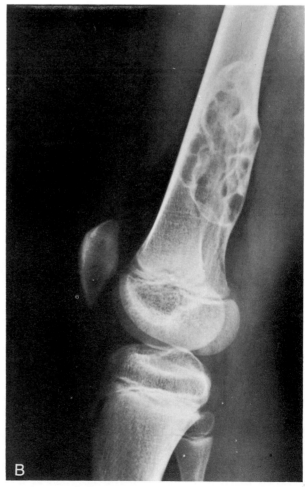

Fig. 26.1 (A and B) Anteroposterior and lateral views of non-ossifying fibroma. Multi-loculated lucent lesion with well-defined margins—classic appearance (see p. 793).

a history of trauma in approximately 30 percent of cases, but evidence suggesting it as an etiologic factor is scant. Physical examination is usually non-specific; a mass, if present, may not be tender. Lymphadenopathy is rare with primary bone tumors. General examination should be directed toward looking for a primary cancer in cases of metastatic disease.

DIAGNOSTIC STUDIES

The single most useful test in the diagnosis of bone lesions is the conventional biplane roentgenograph. It usually suggests the diagnosis of a benign or malignant process and offers a differential diagnosis. Benign lesions most frequently are well marginated and may have cortical expansion. Malignant lesions more commonly are not well marginated, may have a permeative pattern, may evince cortical breakthrough, and may elevate the periosteum (Codman's triangle). The presence or absence of calcification, reactive bone, sarcomatous bone formation, and pure lysis may help in differentiating the specific type of tumor. There are enough exceptions to the rules to force the surgeon to obtain a bone biopsy to provide a definitive diagnosis. Some lesions such as osteochondroma and fibrous cortical defects are about 98 percent diagnostic by radiograph (Figs. 26.1, 2 and 3).

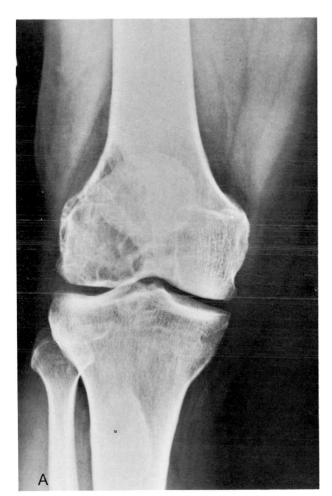
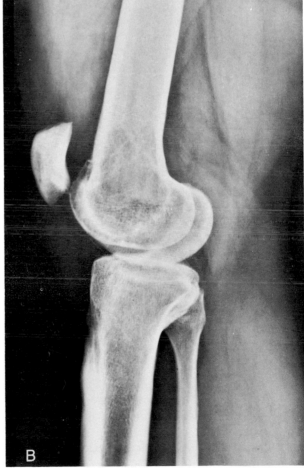

Fig. 26.2 (A and B) Anteroposterior and lateral views of giant cell tumor of distal femur. A typical eccentric lytic lesion extending to the articular surface of the femur. Pseudotrabeculations are well shown.

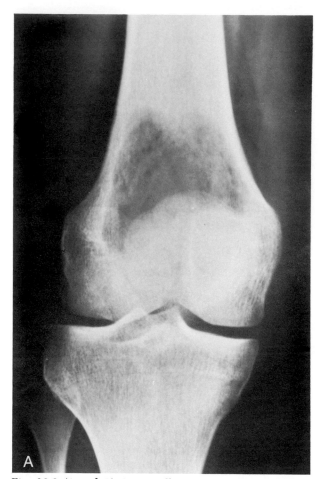
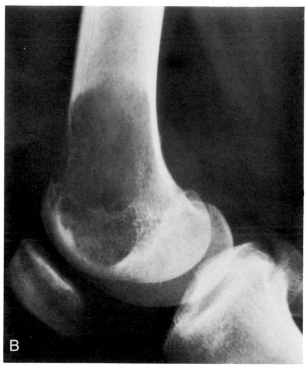

Fig. 26.3 (A and B) Giant cell tumor in a 46-year-old male. Anteroposterior and lateral views. A central lytic lesion extending to articular surface and eroding through cortex anteriorly. No inner texture. Slightly atypical and cannot be differentiated from telangiectatic osteosarcoma, aneurysmal bone cyst or metastasis.

Serological, biochemical and immunological evaluation of these patients has limited value in the diagnosis. The sedimentation rate is non-specific although it may be elevated in round cell tumors such as Ewing's sarcoma and non-Hodgkin's lymphoma of bone. The alkaline phosphatase is commonly elevated in patients with osteogenic sarcoma and, of course, in patients with Paget's disease. Protein immunoelectrophoresis is diagnostic for multiple myeloma. Bone marrow biopsies may assist in the diagnosis of metabolic bone disease, multiple myeloma or leukemia. Patients with chondrosarcoma may have a normal blood glucose level in the face of a diabetic glucose tolerance test.[34]

If at this stage the diagnosis of the lesion may be made with confidence, and particularly if it is benign, then further investigations may not be required. If, however, major surgery is required to remove the lesion, then further radiological and nuclear imaging may be helpful in determining the extent and relationship of the tumor to the neurovascular bundles. Tomography may be used to accurately localize the nidus of an osteoid osteoma or the presence of cortical penetration in a giant cell tumor which may not be detected on plain roentgenograms. Biplane peripheral arteriography will outline the extent of the accompanying soft tissue mass and the relationship of the tumor to the femoral and popliteal vessels and nerves. The soft tissue extent can be distinctly demonstrated by computed axial tomography (with/without contrast), and more importantly the relationship of the tumor to the neurovascular structures can be assessed. Lymphangiography is generally not indicated in primary bone tumors except in the case of lymphoma of bone in order to help in staging.

The search for distant bone disease should include a ^{99}m technetium polyphosphate bone scan. In addition to the detection of distal disease it assists in accurately localizing the primary lesion as well as detecting skip lesions. Gallium scans are helpful in the assessment of the soft tissue component of the tumor and in clarifying the contribution of disuse osteoporosis to a "positive bone scan." Whole lung tomography is helpful in detecting pulmonary metastases so that appropriate staging can be accomplished.

SURGICAL STAGING

With data from investigations made to this point it should be possible to determine a surgical stage for malignant tumors. Enneking, et al, have devised a system for the staging of musculoskeletal sarcomas.[13] In this system neoplasms are histologically graded on their biological aggressiveness, as low grade (G1) or high grade (G2). In general, low grade lesions have a low risk for metastasis (less than 25 percent). They can usually be managed by relatively conservative procedures. High grade lesions (G2) have a significantly higher incidence of metastasis and require more aggressive procedures to achieve local control. In addition to grading the neoplasm an assessment is made as to its anatomical extent. If it is confined to a well-defined anatomical compartment it is designated intracompartmental (T1). A lesion in two or more anatomical compartments is designated (T2). An example of the latter would be a distal femoral tumor extending into the vastus medialis. All lesions in the popliteal fossa are extracompartmental. Staging of the tumor is based upon these two considerations (i.e., grading and anatomical extent). The stages are subdivided into A & B based upon compartmentalization of the lesion Stage IA–(G1, T1), Stage IB (G1, T2), Stage IIA is (G2, T1), Stage IIB (G2, T2) and Stage III is any grade or site with regional or distant metastasis.

Benign tumors can be graded into 3 levels of activity. Grade I tumors, such as fibrous cortical defects, are intracompartmental lesions with little or no chance of expansion. Grade II benign lesions, such as a li-poma or unicameral bone cyst, are intracompartmental lesions with a tendency for slow continuous growth. Grade III lesions are aggressive benign lesions which tend to extend beyond the anatomical compartment and to recur frequently. Occasionally they can transport cells to the lungs as seen in giant cell tumors and chondroblastomas. The treatment in general for Grade I tumors is observation or incisional curettage, for Grade II lesions curettage or marginal excision, and for Grade III lesions excision or curettage beyond the pseudocapsule or reactive bone margin.

THE BIOPSY

In many circumstances the radiological appearances are so characteristic as to be confidently diagnostic (e.g., fibrous cortical defects in the posteromedial cortex of the distal femur or benign osteochondromas).[9] If these lesions are found incidentally and are not the cause of symptoms then surgery is unnecessary. Symptomatic osteochondromas may be treated by excisional biopsy, care being taken to completely excise the perichondrium in order to minimize recurrence. Proximal osteochondromas have a greater tendency to undergo sarcomatous changes than do peripheral ones. Excisional biopsy is also adequate treatment for other lesions which have little or no potential for local recurrence. The diagnosis of osteoid osteoma is usually based on an excisional biopsy.

An incisional biopsy is the most commonly employed type of open biopsy. It is the procedure of choice for open biopsy of most malignant tumors. The placement of the biopsy incision is crucial, as the biopsy scar together with the biopsy tract must be excised en bloc with the malignant tumor at the definitive surgical procedure. The biopsy incision around the knee should be longitudinal and preferably placed either medially or laterally. Posterior knee biopsy scars may jeopardize a further exposure for an en bloc resection, and indeed a large transverse scar may preclude the possibility of performing a limb sparing resection and necessitate an amputation. The smallest incision compatible with obtaining adequate tissue specimen should be employed. The periphery of any tumor offers the best and most representative tissue in malignant tumors. The center may be necrotic. The use of medial and lateral incisions around the knee will minimize unnecessary extracompartmental contamination and avoid contamination of the neurovascular structures. Similarly, a longitudinal incision placed antero-laterally over the fibular head is the incision required for biopsies in this area. The peroneal nerve should not be isolated, otherwise it will need to be resected subsequently if the lesion proves malignant. A small segment of bone may be carefully excised using a sharp osteotome or multiple small drill holes and then an osteotome. The biopsy osteotomy should be round or oval to decrease stress risers. In addition to specimens for permanent sections, frozen sections should be performed to confirm accurate location and adequacy of the biopsy. Special studies such as electron microscopy, lymphoma typing, estrogen binding, etc., may be necessary and can be suggested by the frozen examination. Multiple cultures for fungus aerobic, anaerobic, and acid fast bacilli should be obtained. Antibiotics should not be given prior to biopsy. Tumor blood can also be sent for biochemical analysis (e.g., acid and alkaline phosphatase). Very high values of alkaline phosphatase may be seen in osteosarcomas. Care must be taken to minimize tumor spillage. Meticulous hemostasis during wound closure is of paramount importance because the larger the postoperative hematoma is the greater the contamination of soft tissues with neoplastic cells will be. Gel foam with thrombin and microcrystalline collagen may be necessary. The use of a tourniquet during biopsy is not essential but may be used if preferred. There is no evidence that a tourniquet avoids dissemination of tumor cells into the bloodstream.[50] On no account should an Esmarch bandage be employed to exsanguinate the limb. Suction tubes are not employed to drain the wound. Following biopsy, it is important that the patient be instructed in protective weight bearing to avoid the occurrence of a pathological fracture. In our experience pathological fractures of the distal femur subsequently worsen the prognosis for osteosarcoma.[28]

Percutaneous needle biopsies[45] may be performed in some specialized centers, but again the placement of the needle should be carefully planned so that the needle tract may be excised en bloc. It is just a small open biopsy. It should be remembered that the accuracy with percutaneous needle biopsies is approximately 80 percent compared to a 98 percent accuracy with an open biopsy.[20,37,44] The accuracy and methodology of the biopsy significantly affect the ultimate outcome.[32]

Once the pathological grade of the tumor is determined the tumor may be staged either as IA or IB or IIA or IIB or III. This system of surgical staging assists in the decision of whether a limb sparing procedure is practical or an amputation is required. Stage III lesions with pulmonary metastasis may be considered for limb sparing procedures as in many circumstances the pulmonary metastasis may be amenable to chemotherapy followed by surgical excision.[36]

TREATMENT OF BONE TUMORS

BENIGN LESIONS

Benign lesions showing indisputable diagnostic radiological characteristics (e.g., asymptomatic non-ossifying fibroma and developmental defects in the postero-medial aspect of the distal femur or asymptomatic osteochondromas) do not require surgical treatment or indeed even a biopsy.[9] If, however, any doubt about the benign nature of the lesion exists then a biopsy should be performed. Symptomatic osteochondromas may be treated by excisional biopsy (i.e., marginal excision). Most of the other Grade I or II benign tumors are adequately treated by standard procedures such as curettage and packing with bone chips or by small en bloc excisions. Unicameral bone cysts have been successfully treated by repetitive intra-lesional injection with 40–80 mg of crystalline methyl prednisolone acetate.[4,43] In Campanacci's series, 50 percent disappeared completely, 25 percent had a small residual non-growing cyst and 25 percent persisted.[4] The authors utilize 2 needles to permit through and through irrigation with radiografin to be sure the complete cyst is accessible for injecting the steroid.

MALIGNANT LESIONS

The Surgical Staging System for musculoskeletal sarcomas is linked to a surgical planning system with four surgical procedures for obtaining local control.[13] Each has a well-defined surgical margin based on the relationship of the surgical margin to the neoplasm. An intralesional margin is made when an incision passes through the lesion. Incisional biopsies or curettage of a benign lesion are examples of intralesional procedures which are only adequate for benign lesions. A marginal excision is usually described as an excisional biopsy around the pseudocapsule. It usually leaves microscopic disease at the margin of the wound. In a wide excision the lesion is removed with a surrounding cuff of normal tissue. A wide margin may be achieved when performing a wide local or radical en bloc excision. A radical margin is obtained by removing the tumor en bloc together with all potentially contaminated planes and the entire structures which pass through the involved anatomical compartment or compartments such as in a hip disarticulation for a distal femoral lesion. Amputations need not be more radical however. An amputation plane that enters the tumor is in fact an "intralesional" amputation. Conversely, a total quadriceps resection is a radical procedure for a vastus medialis synovial sarcoma.

Advances in the treatment of malignant lesions around the knee have been made over the past 10–12 years. They include the use of multi-drug chemotherapy and the refinement of the techniques of en bloc or wide resections of distal femoral and proximal tibial lesions.

CHEMOTHERAPY

With modern multi-drug chemotherapy more than three quarters of the patients presenting with malignant bone tumors are now expected to be disease free survivors of their disease following amputation or en bloc resection. In earlier reports, the five year cure rate of patients with osteogenic sarcoma was between 15 20 percent and for Ewing's it was 5–15 percent despite amputation or high dose radiation.[6,15,33] Formerly all patients with malignant lesions around the knee were treated by lower extremity amputation or hip disarticulation. In the past decade, increasing numbers of tumors are being successfully treated with limb preservation. In addition to much improved survival rates the quality of life of many survivors has also improved.

It is assumed that at the time of diagnosis of an osteogenic sarcoma, patients will already have microscopic foci of disease in their lungs. Although surgery can eliminate the primary tumor, chemotherapy is used to destroy these microscopic but undetectable areas of disease. In addition to its use as an adjuvant modality for micrometastases in the treatment of primary bone tumors, chemotherapy employed preoperatively has been shown to be capable of rapidly shrinking bulky primary and metastatic tumors.[53] A particular advantage of this effect in knee lesions is that it allows time for the manufacture of a custom endoprosthesis in cases where en bloc resection of the tumor is feasible rather than performing an amputation (Fig. 26.4).

Many centers now give adjuvant chemotherapy to all patients with high grade spindle cell sarcomas which include osteogenic sarcomas, high grade chondrosarcomas, high grade fibrosarcomas, malignant fibrous histiocytomas and malignant giant cell tumors (Grade III). Small cell sarcomas which include Ewing's sarcoma, non-Hodgkin's lymphoma, angiosarcoma and mesenchymal chondrosarcoma are highly malignant and very sensitive to modern multi-drug chemotherapy. In addition to surgery and chemotherapy, radiation therapy is employed to help obtain local control of primary small cell sarcomas.

The current approach to the treatment of osteogenic sarcoma at Memorial Sloan-Kettering Hospital is to treat all patients preoperatively with multicycle high dose methotrexate with citrovorum factor rescue, bleomycin, cyclophosphamide and dactinomycin (BCD) and adriamycin.[39] This is regardless of whether the patient is to have an amputation or a limb sparing procedure. The effect of 4–12 weeks of pre-operative chemotherapy is assessed by the histological examination of the resected primary tumor. A grading system based on the extent of tumor destruction has been devised.[22] Grade I: little or no effect of chemotherapy noted. Grade II: a partial response with greater than 50 percent tumor necrosis noted and attributable to chemotherapy; Grade III: greater than 90 percent tumor necrosis; Grade IV: no viable-appearing tumor cells noted in any of the histological specimens. In osteogenic sarcoma therapy, patients with Grade III or IV response are continued on the same chemotherapy as preoperatively. Those patients who have a Grade I or II effect of preoperative chemotherapy on the primary tumor have the high dose methotrexate deleted from their postoperative chemotherapy and are placed on a regimen containing cisplatinum with mannitol diuresis combined with adriamycin.[39] Hence the patient's own tumor is evaluated *in vivo* for the efficacy of the chemotherapy protocol.

Combination chemotherapy is also used in the treatment of small cell sarcomas.[41] The patient is given

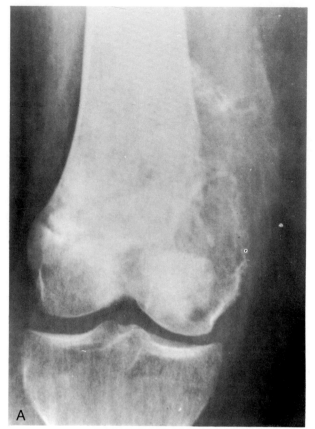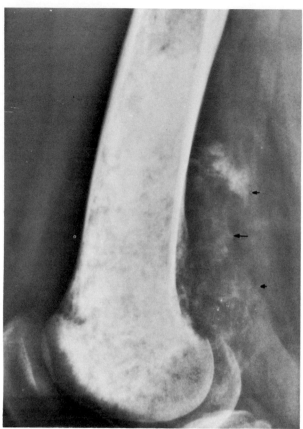

Figure 26.4 (A) An anteroposterior and lateral view of an osteosarcoma of the distal right femur in a 16-year-old female, January 1982. Densely sclerotic lesion with soft tissue mass (arrows) and erosion of medial condyle (figure continues).

early aggressive chemotherapy to eliminate micro-metastasis. Large bulky tumors usually reduce significantly in size. Local therapy is delayed for approximately 3 months, except in cases where there is evidence of a poor response of the tumor as judged by clinical examination, radionuclide imaging or roentgenograms.

Although multi-drug chemotherapy has provided a major advance in the treatment of cancer in general, it is associated with considerable toxicity. High dose methotrexate with citrovorum rescue had a mortality rate of approximately 6 percent in the early days of its use.[24] Although mortality due to chemotherapy has declined with experience, significant temporary morbidity persists. Adriamycin may produce irreversible cardiomyopathy and bleomycin can produce pulmonary fibrosis. Cisplatinum can cause permanent renal toxicity and ototoxicity. Bone healing is delayed so that grafting procedures following resections re-

quire prolonged periods of immobilization. Skin healing is protracted; consequently chemotherapy should not be resumed for 2 weeks following surgery. Skin sutures are usually left in place for approximately 6 weeks.

Although the benefits of chemotherapy are not uniform and several groups do not used adjuvant chemotherapy, the general concensus of orthopaedic oncologists is that adjuvant chemotherapy has a significant role in the treatment of high grade malignant bone tumors particularly osteosarcoma and Ewing's sarcoma.

SURGICAL TREATMENT OF MALIGNANT BONE TUMORS

The choice of surgical procedures for malignant lesions depends on a number of factors. Accurate histological diagnosis and surgical staging are of para-

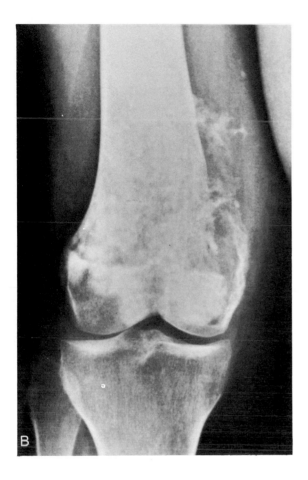

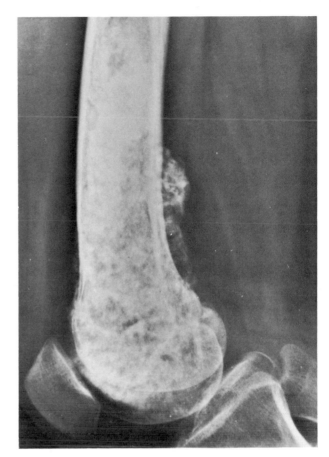

(B) AP and lateral views 3 months following chemotherapy. Good response to chemotherapy with reduction in size of soft tissue mass and well organized spiculation in relation to posterior cortex. (C) CT scan with contrast shows vascular bundle in contrast with tumor at one point but not surrounded or encased by tumor. Vessels thought to be free enough for en bloc resection.

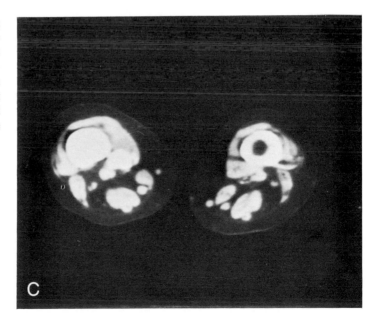

mount importance. The size and extent of both osseous and soft tissue involvement can be determined by biplane roentgenograms, arteriograms, bone and soft tissue imaging procedures together with computerized axial tomography. Perfusion CT scanning is a particularly sensitive method of determining whether or not the major neurovascular structures are involved and will assist in the decision about the resectability of the lesion versus amputation. Preoperative chemotherapy may reduce the size of a tumor rendering it resectable.[22,53] The patient's age plays a major role in determining the type of surgical procedure that should be employed. The projected leg length discrepancy in actively growing young children makes amputation the only realistic choice in proximal tibial lesions. For distal femoral lesions in patients too young for knee replacement, consideration should be given to rotationplasty as developed by Van Nes.[58] Finally, a poorly planned biopsy incision may make a future en bloc resection impossible and necessitate an amputation.

Despite the advances in chemotherapy, amputation remains the most common surgical procedure performed for malignant tumors around the knee.[28,39,48] The level of femoral amputation is selected after careful study of roentgenograms and bone scans. The bone scan is particularly helpful in providing a good approximation of the proximal margin of involved bone. Transmedullary amputation should be approximately 5–7 cm above the proximal margin of increased uptake on the bone scan. The presence of "skip" lesions in the proximal femur should be carefully excluded.

Limb sparing procedures employing en bloc resection is a valid alternative to amputation in carefully selected cases. The ability to restore the integrity of bone or joint function in the resected area is improving, due to the utilization of such procedures as resection arthrodesis, interposition allografts,[27] and custom made total knee replacements.[3,11,23,28,31,38,39,49] Local resectional surgery for malignant lesions is still at the experimental stage and should be done in centers experienced with these techniques. In general limb sparing procedures using en bloc excisional surgery may be considered in fully grown or almost fully grown individuals with a recurrent giant cell tumor, low grade chondrosarcoma, parosteal osteogenic sarcoma, malignant fibrous histiocytoma and carefully selected localized high grade malignancies. These patients must have a potential normal cuff of tissue around

the tumor, no neurovascular involvement, adequate skin coverage, and no pathological fracture.

The first objective in tumor surgery in patients without evidence of skip areas or metastasis is to obtain local control and avoid local recurrence. The second is to preserve as much function as possible without jeopardizing survival. Local recurrence after a high grade sarcoma resection is associated with a poor survival rate. Limb sparing surgery for malignant tumors should be applied with caution and only after careful evaluation of biplane roentgenograms, imaging studies, biplane arteriograms and computerized axial tomography.

En bloc resection of malignant tumors entails the removal of the lesion with an intact cuff of normal tissue that completely surrounds the lesion. Such resections around the knee require the removal of a large segment of bone and muscle tissue. The bony defect requires the insertion of a metal total knee prosthesis, allograft or fusion across the joint using long bony struts with or without intramedullary nails.[3,11,28,31,38,39,49] This can lead to an obvious decrease in function. Careful judgment is required in deciding to proceed with such procedures. The patient and parents should appreciate the realistic functional goals of limb sparing surgery. The patient will have definite weakness and will require bracing, sometimes indefinitely. In some cases an artificial limb will function better, and indeed some patients may prefer amputation. Consent for an alternative procedure such as amputation, if it becomes necessary, should always be obtained preoperatively.

En bloc resection of carefully selected malignant tumors around the knee employs the same principles that are applied to all tumor surgery (i.e., the tumor must never be violated and a surrounding margin of normal soft tissue and bone must be removed en bloc with the lesion). In distal femoral and proximal tibial lesions the resection should include the intact knee joint which must not be entered since in many cases tumor extends into the joint. Special care is taken in the resection of the quadriceps, patella and patellar tendon to avoid entering the joint. The patella is removed en bloc with the joint. In some cases it may be possible to preserve the extensor mechanism by preserving the patellar tendon with the anterior portion of the patella (the patella may be split coronally) together with the anterior portion of the distal rectus femoris. The dictum, "tumor first, function second" should always be kept in mind. If tumor cells spill into the wound, the wound becomes contaminated, and immediate amputation is suggested, following a complete change of gloves and instruments.

A tourniquet is applied to the proximal thigh and is inflated if bleeding becomes troublesome. An Esmarch exsanguination bandage is never used. The incision is carefully planned and should be longitudinal and usually placed either medially or laterally. This is often dictated by the presence of a previous biopsy scar. It should allow excision of the biopsy scar and early estimation of the extent of the tumor and feasibility of local excision. It should not compromise an amputation if such becomes necessary. The saphenous vein should be preserved if possible. The incision is deepened to expose the neurovascular structures. It is only at this stage that one can fully assess whether or not the lesion is resectable. The divisions of the sciatic nerve are mobilized, care being taken to preserve the peroneal nerve (this is nearly always feasible).

The numerous perforating vessels are carefully dissected and ligated. The muscles are incised down to the bone at a predetermined level on the femur (by review of x-rays and bone scans) providing it appears safe to do so. The proximal tibia and distal femur are transected. The remaining muscle and ligamentous attachments are divided, and the tumor with intact cuff of normal tissue is removed. Prior to proceeding with reconstructive procedures confirmation of adequate margins should be made by frozen sections. Frozen section readings of the bone marrow proximally and distally are obtained to ensure that no tumor remains. It is desirable to preserve as much normal muscle as possible (without compromising safety) in order to preserve function and secondly to have muscle between the prosthesis, allograft or arthrodesis and skin. It is critical to be certain that the skin flaps are viable. Intraoperative use of fluorescein may be helpful in this regard.

RECONSTRUCTION

As previously stated, reconstruction of the defect created by en bloc resection of malignant tumors around the knee may be accomplished by (a) arthroplasty using a custom made total knee prosthesis, (b) arthrodesis using large spanning bone grafts, or (c)

the use of osteoarticular allografts. There have been a few reports of the use of autoclaved autografts followed by arthrodesis.[47,54,57]

Currently the preferred method of reconstruction following en bloc resection of the entire knee at the Sloan-Kettering Memorial Hospital is replacement with a custom made total knee prosthesis whenever possible. A selection of modified Guepar prostheses are available for immediate use. A semi-constrained titanium total knee prosthesis can be custom fabricated for each patient following careful study of preoperative lower extremity scanograms and bone scans. Because of the loss of the stabilizing capsule and ligaments these custom made prostheses require the use of constrained or semi-constrained hinges. Since the major extensors of the knee are resected in toto or to such an extent as to severely compromise quadriceps function, the device must be capable of providing stability during weight bearing. Consequently Burstein has designed the axis sufficiently posterior to the center of gravity so as to promote extension during stance.[28] His device requires 8–10° of flexion before it will further flex with weight-bearing. The patient can ambulate by actively plantar-flexing the ankle and extending the hip so as to force the "flail" knee into functional recurvatum and thus stability.

Functionally patients with custom total knee replacements have superior velocity, stride length, endurance, lower oxygen consumption and better utilization of aerobic capacity as compared to patients with amputation. However, en bloc surgery is associated with an 8–9 fold greater complication rate.[28] Fifty percent of these represent small areas of skin necrosis that require minor skin revision. Better experience and use of intraoperative vital dyes can identify potential areas of poor vitality which can be resected before skin closure. Prosthetic failure is decreasing with better metals (titanium). Loosening remains a significant problem but early experience with porous ingrowth suggests that this form of fixation may be superior.

An alternative to the insertion of total knee prostheses following resection of malignant, potentially malignant and recurrent benign tumors is arthrodesis. The defect is spanned with various combinations of autologous grafts and intramedullary rods.[3,11,12] In Campanacci's view attempts to save movement at the knee following the sacrifice of the quadriceps mechanism may be too ambitious. He uses an anterior hemi-cylindrical sliding graft taken from either the tibia or femur and achieves stability by using a long intra-medullary rod which is inserted from the greater trochanter to the distal tibia. In his series, union eventually occurred in 24 (92 percent) of 26 cases (20 primary unions and 4 secondary unions). All patients with union achieved full weight bearing within 2 years of surgery. However, infection occurred in 19 percent of patients. Enneking utilized hemidiaphyseal grafts supplemented by additional autogenous fibular grafts. However, 58 percent of the patients with defects over 12 cm had stress fractures, the majority of which eventually went on to union. When adjunctive chemotherapy is planned, Campanacci delays using these grafts until chemotherapy has been completed. In the interim he uses a polymethylmethacrylate spacer. Recently Gross and McCormack have utilized vascularized autografts with or without allograft supplementation.[17,30]

Massive autoclaved autografts have been used for reconstruction following en bloc resection of the distal femur or proximal tibia for giant cell tumors and chondrosarcomas.[47,54,58] Sijbrandij reported the technique in which the tumor is resected and subsequently autoclaved at 120° for 15 minutes. The soft tissue can then be easily removed from bone. The autoclaved bone is replaced in its original bed and fixed in place. The knee is then arthrodesed and fixed and stabilized with an extended Kuntscher nail. To stimulate union the tumor cavity is filled with autogenous bone graft. Sijbrandij has three cases with a follow-up of 8–11 years, all of which attained solid union. This approach is still experimental.

Allografts as advocated by Mankin and Parrish have mainly been used for aggressive benign tumors, low grade malignancies or chondrosarcomas.[31,38] When used in the face of chemotherapy, Eiler reported an 83 percent complication rate.[10] At this time, allografts should be considered experimental and delegated to those centers with bone banks and broad experience.

OSTEOSARCOMA

Seventy-four consecutive patients at Memorial Hospital with lower extremity osteosarcoma treated by amputation or en bloc resection were recently reviewed.[28] The data showed that limb preserving procedures can achieve comparable survival rates to that of amputation for an equal stage and location of osteogenic sarcoma. Survival rates approaching 80 percent can be expected for the Stage IIA and IIB lower limb lesions (27 months follow-up) treated by amputation or en bloc procedures. Tibial lesions have a significantly better survival rate as compared to distal femoral lesions, and pathological fractures of the distal femur bode poorly. In contradistinction to Stage II lesions only 32 percent of patients presenting with distant metastases can be retrieved, irrespective of whether they are treated with en bloc or amputation for the primary tumor.

Local recurrence did not occur in any of the Stage II lesions following en bloc resection. At Memorial Hospital we perform more amputations than limb preserving procedures. En bloc patients must have free neurovascular bundles, adequate skin, no fractures, achieved full maturity and be fully reliable. Limb preservation must still be considered experimental in light of the continued difficulties of reconstruction. Although function appears superior to similar level amputations, late prosthetic failure and secondary revisional surgery are still frequent.

TREATMENT OF GIANT CELL TUMORS

Forty to 60 percent of giant cell tumors occur at the knee joint.[16,20,44,56] Despite treatment, recurrence rates are high. With simple curettage it can be up to 78 percent and for curettage and bone grafting 24 to 58 percent. The lowest recurrence rate occurs following resection with bone grafting or fusion (7 to 13 percent). Resection, especially of large recurrent lesions, may also be followed by prosthetic knee replacement or allograft replacement. These give early acceptable results in terms of recurrence but may meet with the long term complications of infection, loosening and fatigue failure. Most recurrences occur within 5 years. If there is any evidence of recurrence after this time, one should be highly suspicious of malignant conversion.[20]

Chemical and/or physical modalities have been utilized to extend the margin of tumor necrosis and can improve the results obtained by curettage and bone grafting alone. Cyrosurgery as an adjunct to adequate curettage has been reported to reduce the incidence of local recurrence to about 12 percent in 52 consecutive cases of giant cell tumors.[35] It is achieved by the repetitive exposure of the curetted bony area to liquid nitrogen. Phenol cauterization can extend the necrotic margin by 2–4 mm. In selected cases curettage with acrylic cementation may permit full and early weight-bearing. The thermal necrosis during setting of the methylmethacrylate extends 2–5 mm into the bone margin. Most orthopaedic oncologists advocate thorough curettage with a high speed burr and extension to the cartilage and normal bone. Supplementary use of cryosurgery, phenol or polymethylmethacrylate cement are individual choices. Less than 20 percent recurrence should occur with these techniques.

For large giant cell tumors with knee joint destruction, consideration may be given to en bloc resection with prosthetic or allograft replacement to achieve restoration of knee joint function, or fusion using sliding grafts. Mankin and Parrish have recently reported on their experience with the use of osteochondral allografts as replacements for osteoarticular defects.[31,38] They contend that allografts are relatively easy to obtain and can be stored for long periods of time in the frozen state. The grafts can be matched in size to the segment of bone being replaced. Physiological studies suggest that the foreign bone is slowly revascularized and replaced by normal bone. However, Mankin et al, are careful to point out that the use of osteoarticular allografts should be reserved for young patients with locally aggressive or low grade malignant tumors who will not require adjuvant chemotherapy or radiation as part of the treatment. The procedure should be reserved for the more limited resections. Despite their overall good and excellent results of 74 percent in their entire group of patients, the results in those patients who had osteoarticular replacement about the knee (21 cases) yielded poorer results, 57 percent, excellent and good. Sixteen additional operations were performed on these 21 patients for complications. Four (26.7 percent) of the 15 distal femoral allografts had infections and required amputation.[31]

FIBULAR LESIONS

The proximal fibula may be the site for an aneurysmal bone cyst, unicameral bone cyst, giant cell tumor, malignant fibrous histiocytoma and malignant spindle cell sarcoma. Benign lesions of this area may

be approached through a longitudinal lateral incision, care being taken to isolate the peroneal nerve from proximal to distal. The use of cryotherapy or phenol may be considered in addition to curettage with or without bone grafting. When using cryotherapy great care must be taken to avoid injuring the peroneal nerve and the skin edges. This can be avoided by protecting the nerve with one finger and continuously irrigating the nerve and wound edges. The most common malignant bone tumor of the fibula is Ewing's sarcoma. At Memorial Hospital we advocate the resection of the fibula following a course of multi-drug chemotherapy. Adjunctive perimeter radiotherapy is also employed. En bloc resection of recurrent benign and low grade malignant lesions of the proximal fibula should employ the usual principles of tumor surgery (i.e., never violate the tumor). The proximal tibiofibular joint together with some lateral tibia should be resected with the proximal fibula. On occasion the peroneal nerve may have to be sacrificed if it is incorporated in the lesion. Such procedures are technically very demanding.

METASTATIC KNEE LESIONS

Metastatic lesions in the distal femur or proximal tibia may be the source of pain, swelling or pathological fractures. They may be diagnosed during the workup for metastases during the investigation of a primary lesion. Small isolated lesions that appear unlikely to lead to a pathological fracture may be treated with radiotherapy, protected weight-bearing and careful follow-up. Attention should be directed to the entire femur for evidence of additional areas of metastases. In a patient with a pathological fracture in the supracondylar region who is otherwise in reasonable health, early open reduction and internal fixation using a 95° condylar plate or Zickel supracondylar pins together with methylmethacrylate bone cement can be used. This rigid fixation offers the patients the chance of immediate postoperative ambulation and a better quality of life for the remaining months of their existence. Postoperative radiotherapy may be indicated to gain local control. For isolated lesions in this area cryotherapy following curettage of tumor bone may offer increased local control of the disease.

Localized metastatic disease of either the proximal tibia or distal femur may on occasion be best treated by local resection and total knee replacement. In these lesions, where the aim is palliation rather than cure, the extent of bone excision should be conservative and muscle attachments should be preserved. Rarely palliative amputation may be required for uncontrollable metastatic lesions.

SOFT TISSUE TUMORS

BENIGN LESIONS

Each of the soft tissues of the body can give rise to benign and malignant neoplasms. Most of the benign lesions such as those of fibrous and adipose tissue origin are fully treated by simple excision and do not recur. Lipomas are among the most common of all the benign lesions and may occur in any location where fat is present. They are adequately treated by local enucleation. Atypical lipomas which also occur in subcutaneous tissue and in deep muscle layers can often result in local recurrence.[14] It has no tendency to metastasize and is usually controlled by re-excision. Of the benign fibrous lesions nodular fasciitis can cause difficulty because it can be mistaken for a fibrosarcoma.[1] Extra-abdominal desmoids require aggressive local therapy (wide margins) to prevent local recurrence.

Popliteal cysts are the most common soft tissue masses seen in the posterior aspect of the knee and may be associated with diseases such as rheumatoid arthritis, degenerative arthritis, gout, pigmented villonodular synovitis and rarely with synovial chondromatosis. In the older patient, care must be taken to exclude the presence of a popliteal aneurysm. If an arthrogram does not communicate with the cyst an arteriogram should be performed. Very occasionally a synovioma may present in this manner. Popliteal cysts in children are usually painless and do not require surgery as the majority regress spontaneously.[8]

Synovial chondromatosis is a relatively uncommon monarthropathy which may present with localized or diffuse knee swelling. Foci of cartilage develop in the synovium by metaplasia of the connective tissue membrane. These foci become calcified or ossified, detach, and appear as loose bodies in the joint. It presents with swelling and pain and symptoms of mechanical derangement of the knee in young adults. Radiologically there is evidence of synovial thickening with foci of calcified or ossified areas. Complete removal of the loose bodies together with synovectomy is the treatment indicated.

Pigmented villonodular synovitis although uncommon, occurs as a monarthopathy and is most often seen in the knee. It presents with increasing pain and swelling in young and middle-aged adults. The appearance on roentgenograms is usually that of nonspecific synovitis although erosive and cystic changes may result from pressure and invasion of bone by the hypertrophied synovial tissues. These cysts have been mistaken for giant cell tumors and malignant neoplasms.[25,26] Complete synovectomy with curettage of osseous cysts is indicated if symptoms are disabling. Because of the high recurrence rate perhaps synovectomy should be followed by subsequent radiotherapy either by external beam or with intraarticular radiation with agents such as 90 yttrium or 165 dysprosium.[52]

SOFT TISSUE SARCOMAS

Soft tissue sarcomas comprise 0.7 percent of all cancers including all age groups and 6.5 percent of all cancers in children under the age of 15 years. About 40 percent of these tumors occur in the lower extremity and of these approximately 75 percent occur at or above the knee.[41,42]

The relative incidences of the different sarcomas seen in the lower extremity vary in different studies. This is because there is disagreement among pathologists concerning the exact diagnosis of individual soft tissue sarcomas. Fibrosarcomas, liposarcomas and malignant fibrous histiocytomas accounted for approximately 75 percent of the tumors seen in the Simon and Enneking series.[51] Rhabdomyosarcomas and synoviosarcomas were the next most common. Fibrosarcomas, liposarcomas, rhabdomyosarcomas and synoviosarcomas comprised 79.4 percent of Shui, et al's series of 297 extremity sarcomas.[46] Despite the presence of sarcomas of different histogenetic origins these tumors are grouped together because they have similarities in clinical presentation and biological behavior. They usually present with soft tissue masses with or without pain. There are no reliable physical signs to distinguish between benign and malignant soft tissue lesions. Persistent or growing masses should be biopsied unless they have been present and unchanged for years. Painful masses, regardless of duration also require biopsy. Most soft tissue sarcomas are situated in the deeper planes of the musculo-aponeurotic structures.[19]

The clinical and laboratory investigations are similar to those for bone sarcomas. Physical examination reveals the approximate size of the mass and its attachment to superficial and deep structures. Lymphadenopathy is rare. Evidence of clinical metastases is determined. Full lung tomography should be performed. Biplane roentgenograms, [67]gallium scanning, peripheral arteriography and computerized axial tomography of the knee with contrast will delineate the size of the mass and its relationship to vessels and nerves. If technetium bone scanning shows increased uptake of the isotope in adjacent bones, involvement of the periosteum should be suspected. Soft tissue sarcoma spread is usually hematogenous, and only rarely by the lymphatic system.[59]

Generous quantities of lesional tissue are required for accurate diagnosis of soft tissue sarcomas. For this reason aspiration or needle biopsies are inadequate and an incisional biopsy is necessary. As in biopsies for bone tumors incisions should be longitudinal and carefully placed so as not to compromise subsequent radical excision of the lesion. Meticulous attention should be paid to hemostasis to minimize hematoma formation and avoid subsequent dissection of soft tissue planes with contaminating tumor.

TREATMENT

The most important prognostic factor in patients with soft tissue sarcomas is the histological grading of the tumor (i.e., from Grade I well-differentiated to Grade III poorly differentiated). In addition to the grade, site and size of the lesion are important.[41] Because of the locally invasive nature of these lesions, local recurrence rates of 30 to 50 percent are seen with local excision alone.[14,41] Radical en bloc resections or amputation reduce local recurrences to 7 to 20 percent.[40,51] In both these series amputation was the procedure indicated in approximately 50 percent of a total of 351 lower extremity sarcomas. Amputation achieved local control in 79 percent of 29 patients in Simon and Enneking's series and 93 percent of 139 in Shiu et al's series. Eighty-eight percent of 25 patients in Simon's and Enneking's group and 72 percent of Shiu's et al's group who had en bloc radical

resections were free of local disease. All the patients whose final surgical margins were positive for tumor in Simon's group had local recurrence of their disease. Most of the recurrences in Shiu's et al's group were seen with resections close to the femoral or popliteal neurovascular bundles. Tumors can recur locally even though microscopic examination of the resection margins fail to demonstrate tumor, particularly if the resection is through the reactive pseudocapsule.

Because of the difficulty of obtaining adequate margins during local radical en bloc surgery in the vicinity of the femoral and popliteal neurovascular structures, the use of local excisional surgery to remove gross tumor followed by aggressive radiation therapy to all areas at risk for local tumor spread has been advocated.[29,42,55] This approach leads to a much lower amputation rate, allows for better preservation of limb function, and at the same time obtains acceptable local control of the disease process. However, patients with inadequate margins of resection have a significantly higher incidence of local recurrence compared with those with negative margins even when post-op radiotherapy is used.

The role of adjuvant chemotherapy in the treatment of soft tissue sarcomas is being actively investigated.[18,40,42] Adriamycin containing protocols appear to be the most effective. Although the results using these agents appear promising, experience in controlled trials is awaited. Rosenberg's data suggest that adjuvant chemotherapy using adriamycin with or without external beam radiation can improve survival rates for soft tissue sarcomas of the extremity but not of the body trunk.[42]

Adjunctive postoperative brachytherapy had been used at Memorial Hospital for lower extremity soft tissue sarcomas since 1975.[18] In this treatment schedule, shallow plastic tubes are placed on the operative field at the time of wide excision of the primary tumor. The ends of these geometrically placed catheters come out through normal skin and are "after loaded" with IR-192 seeds. Six-thousand rads can be delivered to a plane of tissue 0.5 cm from the plane of iridium. The catheters are after-loaded as soon as the wound shows evidence of healing. The treatments last 4 to 5 days. This modality delivers a high dose of radiation to a restricted volume of tissue. The preliminary results are being evaluated and are encouraging.

In light of these advances in adjuvant chemotherapy and external and local radiation, there can be guarded optimism for improved survival and an increased opportunity for limb preservation. At Memorial Hospital protocols based on adriamycin, adjuvant chemotherapy, wide en bloc resection, and radiotherapy are providing encouraging survival rates for soft tissue sarcomas about the knee with low rates of local recurrence.

ACKNOWLEDGMENTS

The authors acknowledge the assistance of Dr. Smith from The Department of Radiology, Sloan-Kettering Hospital for help with the radiographs. Our thanks also to Elaine Canzonieri for typing the manuscript.

REFERENCES

1. Allen, P.W.: Nodular fasciitis. Pathology 4:9–26, 1972.
2. Caffey, J.: On fibrous defects in cortical walls of growing tubular bones; their radiological appearance, structure, prevalence, natural course, and diagnostic significance. Adv. Pediatr., 7:13, 1955.
3. Campanacci, M., Costa, P.: Total resection of distal femur or proximal tibia for bone tumors. J. Bone Joint Surg. [Br.], *61*:455, 1979.
4. Campanacci, M.: Personal Communications, 1982.
5. Dahlin, D.C.: Bone Tumors: General Aspects and Data on 6,221 Cases. 3rd Ed., Springfield, Illinois, Charles C Thomas, 1978.
6. Dahlin, D.C., Cupps, R.E., and Johnson, E.W.: Giant cell tumor: a study of 195 cases. Cancer, 25:1061–1070, 1970.
7. Dahlin, D.C., and Coventry, M.B.: Osteogenic sarcoma: a study of 600 cases. J. Bone Joint Surg. [Am.], *49*:101, 1967.
8. Dinham, J.M.: Popliteal cysts in children. J. Bone Joint Surg. [Br.], *57*:69, 1975.
9. Dunham, W.K., Marcus, N.W., Enneking, W.F., and Haun, C.: Developmental defects of the distal femoral metaphysis: J. Bone Joint Surg. [Am.], *62*:801, 1980.
10. Eiler, F.: Personal Communication, 1982.
11. Enneking, W.F., Eady, J.L., and Burchardt, H.: Autogenous cortical bone grafts in the reconstruction of segmental skeletal defects. J. Bone Joint Surg. [Am.], 62:1039, 1980.
12. Enneking, W.F., and Shirley, P.D.: Resection–arthrodesis for malignant and potentially malignant lesions about the knee using an intramedullary rod and local bone grafts. J. Bone Joint Surg. [Am.], 59:223, 1977.
13. Enneking, W.F., Spanier, S.S., and Goodman, M.A.: A system for the surgical staging of musculoskeletal sarcoma. Clinical Orthop., *153*:106, 1980.
14. Evans, H.L., Soule, E.H., and Winkelmann, R.K.: Atypical lipoma: a typical intramuscular lipoma, and well-differentiated retroperitoneal lipsosarcoma: a reappraisal of 30 cases formerly classified as well-differentiated liposarcoma. Cancer, *43*:574, 1979.
15. Falk, S., and Alpert, M.: Five year survival of patients with Ewing's sarcoma. Surg. Gynecol. Obstet., *124*:319, 1967.
16. Goldenberg, R.R., Campbell, C.J., and Bonfiglio, M.: Giant cell tumor of bone: an analysis of two hundred and eighteen cases. J. Bone Joint Surg. [Am.], *52*:619, 1970.
17. Gross, A.E.: Personal Communications, 1982.
18. Hajdu, S.I.: Pathology of Soft Tissue Tumors. Philadelphia, Lee., and Febiger, 1979.
19. Hare, H.F., Cerny, M.J.: Soft tissue sarcoma: a review of 200 cases. Cancer, *16*:1332, 1963.
20. Huvos, A.G.: Bone Tumors: Diagnosis, Treatment and Prognosis. Philadelphia, W.B. Saunders, 1979.
21. Huvos, A.G., and Marcove, R.C.: Chondroblastoma of bone: a critical review. Clin. Orthop., *95*:300, 1973.
22. Huvos, A.G., Rosen, G., and Marcove, R.C.: Primary osteogenic sarcoma: pathologic aspects in 20 patients after treatment with chemotherapy, en bloc resection and prosthetic bone replacement. Arch. Pathol. Lab Med., *101*:14, 1977.
23. Jackson Burrows H., Wilson, J.N., and Scales, J.T.: Excision of tumors of the humerus and femur, with restoration by internal prosthesis. J. Bone Joint Surg. [Br.], *57*:148, 1975.
24. Jaffe, N., and Watts, H.G.: Multidrug chemotherapy in primary treatment of osteosarcoma. J. Bone Joint Surg. [Am.], *58*:634, 1976.
25. Jergensen, H.E., Mankin, H.J., and Schiller, A.L.: Diffuse pigmented villonodular synovitis of the knee mimicking primary bone neoplasm. J. Bone Joint Surg. [Am.], *60*:825, 1978.
26. Kindblom, L.G., and Gunterberg, B.: Pigmented villonodular synovitis involving bone. J. Bone Joint Surg. [Am.], *60*:830, 1978.
27. Koskinen, E.V.S., Salenius, P., and Alho, A.: Allogeneic transplantation in low-grade malignant bone tumors. Acta. Orthop. Scańd., *50*:129, 1979.
28. Lane, J.M., Abou Zahr, K., Boland, P.J., et al.: Surgical management of osteogenic sarcoma of the lower limb. Submitted for Publication, 1983.
29. Lindberg, R.D., Martin, R.G., and Romsdahl, M.M.: Surgery and postoperative radiotherapy in the treat-

ment of soft tissue sarcomas in adults. Am J. Roentgenol. Ther. Nucl. Med., *123*:123, 1975.

30. MacCormack, R.: Personal Communications, 1983.
31. Mankin, H.J., Doppelt, S.H., Sullivan, T., and Tomford, W.W.: Osteoarticular and intercalary allograft transplantation in the management of malignant tumors of bone. Cancer, *50*:613, 1982.
32. Mankin, H.J., Lange, T.A., and Spanier, S.S.: The hazards of biopsy in patients with malignant primary bone and soft tissue tumors. J. Bone Joint Surg. [Am.], *64*:1121, 1982.
33. Marcove, R.C., Mike, V., Hajek, J.V., et al.: Osteogenic sarcoma in childhood. New York State J. Med., *71*:855, 1971.
34. Marcove, R.C., Shoji, H., and Arlen, M.: Altered carbohydrate metabolism in cartilagenous tumors. Contemp. Surg., *5*:53, 1974.
35. Marcove, R.C., Weis, L.D., Vaghaiwalla, M.R., et al.: Cryosurgery in the treatment of giant cell tumors of bone: a report of 52 consecutive cases. Cancer, *41*:957, 1978.
36. Martini, N., Huvos, A.G., Mike, V., et al.: Multiple wedge resections in the treatment of osteogenic sarcoma. Ann. Thorac. Surg., *12*:271, 1971.
37. Moore, T.M., Meyers, M.H., Patzakis, M.J., et al.: Closed biopsy of musculoskeletal lesions. J. Bone Joint Surg. [Am.], *61*:375.
38. Parrish, F.F.: Allograft replacement of all or part of the end of a long bone following excision of a tumor. J. Bone Joint Surg. [Am.], *55*:1, 1973.
39. Rosen, G., Caparros, B., Huvos, A.G., et al.: Preoperative chemotherapy for osteogenic sarcoma. Cancer, *49(6)*:1221, 1982.
40. Rosenberg, S.A., Kent, H., Weber, B.L., et al.: Prospective randomized evaluation of the role of limb sparing surgery: radiation therapy and adjuvant chemo-immunotherapy in the treatment of adult soft tissue sarcomas. Surgery, *84*:62, 1978.
41. Rosenberg, S.A., Suit, H.D., Baker, L.H., and Rosen, G.: Sarcomas of soft tissue and bone. In DeVita, V.T., Hellman, S., Rosenberg, S.A. (eds.): Principles and Practice of Oncology. Philadelphia, J.B. Lippincott, 1037, 1982.
42. Rosenberg, S.A., Tepper, J., Glatstein, E., et al.: Adjuvant chemotherapy for patients with soft tissue sarcomas. Surg. Clin. North Am., *61(6)*:1415, 1981.
43. Scaglietti, O., Marchetti, P.G., and Bartolozzi, P.: The effect of methylprednisolone acetate in the treatment of bone cysts. J. Bone Joint Surg. [Br.], *61*:200, 1979.
44. Schajowicz, F.: Tumors and Tumor-Like Lesions of Bone and Joints. p. 5, New York, Springer-Verlag, 1981.
45. Schajowicz, F., and Derqui, J.C.: Puncture biopsy in lesions of the locomotor system: review of results in 4050 cases including 94 vertebral punctures. Cancer, *21*:531, 1968.
46. Shui, M.H., Castro, E.G., Hajdu, S.I., et al.: Surgical treatment of 297 soft tissue sarcomas of the lower extremity. Ann. Surg., *182*:597, 1975.
47. Sijbrandij, S.: Resection and reconstruction for bone tumors. Acta. Orthop. Scand., *49*:249, 1978.
48. Sim, F.H., Ivins, J.C., and Pritchard, D.J.: The surgical treatment of osteogenic sarcoma at the Mayo Clinic. Cancer Treat. Rep., *62*:205, 1978.
49. Sim, F.H., Pritchard, D.J., Ivins, J.C., et al.: Total joint arthroplasty: applications in the management of bone tumors. Mayo Clinic Proc., *54*:583, 1979.
50. Simon, M.A.: Current concepts review biopsy of musculoskeletal tumors. J. Bone Joint Surg. [Am.], *64*:1253, 1982.
51. Simon, M.A., and Enneking, W.F.: The management of soft tissue sarcomas of the extremities. J. Bone Joint Surg. [Am.], *58*:317, 1976.
52. Sledge, C.B., Atcher, R.W., Lionberger, D.R., Hurson, B.J., et al.: The treatment of knee synovitis with dysprosium: 165 ferric hydroxide macroaggregates. Submitted for Publication in 1983.
53. Smith, J., Hellon, R.T., Huvos, A.G., et al.: Radiographic changes in primary osteogenic sarcoma following intensive chemotherapy, radiological-pathological correlation in 63 patients. Radiology, *143*:355, 1982.
54. Smith, S., and Simon, M.A.: Segmental resection for chondrosarcoma. J. Bone Joint Surg. [Am.], *57*:1097, 1975.
55. Suit, H.D., Russell, W.O., Martin, R.G.: Sarcoma of soft tissue: clinical and histopathologic parameters and response to treatment. Cancer, *35*:1478, 1975.
56. Sung, H.W., Kuo, D.P., Shu, W.P., et al.: Giant cell tumor of bone: analysis of 208 cases in Chinese patients. J. Bone Joint Surg. [Am.], *64*:755, 1982.
57. Thompson, V.P., and Steggall, C.T.: Chondrosarcoma of the proximal portion of the femur treated by resection and bone replacement: a six-year result. J. Bone Joint Surg. [Am.], *38*:357, 1956.
58. Van Nes, C.P.: Rotationplasty for congenital defects of the femur. J. Bone Joint Surg. [Br.], *32*:12, 1950.
59. Weingrad, D.W., and Rosenberg, S.A.: Early lymphatic spread of osteogenic and soft tissue sarcomas. Surgery, *84*:231, 1978.

Index

Illustrations are indicated with an "f" and tables are indicated with a "t" after page numbers.